# Handbuch der experimentellen Pharmakologie
# Handbook of Experimental Pharmacology

Heffter-Heubner New Series

## XXXVIII/1

# Antineoplastic and Immunosuppressive Agents
# Part I

Contributors

R. C. Bagai · M. A. Bagshaw · R. W. Brockman · S. Carter
C. C. Cheng · B. Clarkson · A. L. Cowles · R. L. Dedrick
A. Fefer · J. D. Fenstermacher · E. Frei, III · A. Goldin
J. A. Gottlieb · A. M. Guarino · M. T. Hakala · T. C. Hall · J. E. Harris
J. F. Henderson · E. M. Hersh · L. E. Hopwood · D. G. Johns
L. F. Lamerton · C. L. Litterst · H. Madoc-Jones · N. Mantel · F. Mauro
J. A. R. Mead · L. B. Mellett · M. S. Mitchell · J. A. Montgomery
S. Murphree · V. T. Oliverio · W. C. J. Ross · R. L. Scotte Doggett
E. Stubblefield · P. Todd · L. J. Tolmach · L. B. Townsend
J. M. Venditti · D. S. Zaharko · C. G. Zubrod

Editors

Alan C. Sartorelli and David G. Johns

With 60 Figures

Springer-Verlag Berlin · Heidelberg · New York 1974

Alan C. Sartorelli, Professor, Department of Pharmacology, Yale University School of Medicine, New Haven, Connecticut 06510/USA

David G. Johns, M. D., Laboratory of Chemical Pharmacology, National Cancer Institute, National Institutes of Health, Bethesda, Maryland 20014/USA

This book was co-edited by David G. Johns in his private capacity. No official support or endorsement by the Department of Health, Education and Welfare is intended or should be inferred.

ISBN-13: 978-3-642-65680-4 e-ISBN-13: 978-3-642-65678-1
DOI: 10.1007/978-3-642-65678-1


Softcover reprint of the hardcover 1st edition 1974

# Preface

Over the past two decades a number of attempts have been made, with varying degrees of success, to collect in a single treatise available information on the basic and applied pharmacology and biochemical mechanism of action of antineoplastic and immunosuppressive agents. The logarithmic growth of knowledge in this field has made it progressively more difficult to do justice to all aspects of this topic, and it is possible that the present handbook, more than four years in preparation, may be the last attempt to survey in a single volume the entire field of drugs employed in cancer chemotherapy and immunosuppression. Even in the present instance, it has proved necessary for practical reasons to publish the material in two parts, although the plan of the work constitutes, at least in the editors' view, a single integrated treatment of this research area.

A number of factors have contributed to the continuous expansion of research in the areas of cancer chemotherapy and immunosuppression. Active compounds have been emerging at ever-increasing rates from experimental tumor screening systems maintained by a variety of private and governmental laboratories throughout the world. At the molecular level, knowledge of the modes of action of established agents has continued to expand, and has permitted rational drug design to play a significantly greater role in a process which, in its early years, depended almost completely upon empirical and fortuitous observations. In addition, the rapid expansion in our knowledge of cancer etiology has begun to afford opportunities for the development of new types of agents with the capacity to inhibit the neoplastic process. Recent advances in our knowledge of viral carcinogenesis, and the consequent expansion of the field of cancer chemotherapy to agents which affect the processes of viral replication and virus-induced transformation of mammalian cells, are factors which are already having a profound influence on drug design and development. Modification and enhancement by pharmacological means of immune defenses to neoplastic growth is another area which is only beginning to be exploited by the chemotherapist. Many major advances still remain to be made to take full advantage of potential synergistic interactions between chemotherapy and surgery and/or radiation therapy: these three major modalities have developed almost independently despite the continuing efforts of several outstanding groups of investigators to bridge the gap between them at both the experimental and applied levels.

In addition to the rapid growth of these research areas, a second feature which strikes the editor who attempts to survey cancer chemotherapy and immunotherapy is the frequency with which, as in so many other areas of science, fundamental advances have been made unexpectedly, seemingly almost fortuitously. While such random progress may be expected to be a characteristic of the early development of any new research field, it appears to have played an unusually large role in cancer research, and the recent history of cancer chemotherapy shows that major findings have continued to emerge unpredictably, despite retrospective attempts of scientific historians to detect a previously discernable rationale in such developments. The unusually prominent role of chance in the development of antineoplastic and immunosuppressive agents may be a reflection of the slow and difficult progress in our knowledge of cancer etiology: when the location of a target is still shrouded in darkness, it is probably inevitable that direct hits will continue to be a consequence of accident rather than design. It is to be hoped that current efforts of public and private research funding agencies to superimpose order and modern management techniques on the apparently random development of this and other biomedical sciences will not have the paradoxical effect of slowing the progress they are designed to enhance.

The volume is divided into two parts. The first, has two major sections on general considerations in the areas of antineoplastic and immunosuppressive agents, with chapters included on (a) test systems for both classes of drugs, (b) the clinical utility of both classes of drugs in suppressing the growth of cancer and the immune responses, (c) design of new agents in several major chemical and biochemical classes, (d) the role of cell cycle kinetics in the utility of these therapeutic agents, (e) pharmacologic factors of importance in their optimal utility, (f) selective toxicity, (g) tests predictive of cytotoxic potency, (h) mechanisms of resistance, (i) combination chemotherapy, and (j) among the related modalities, radiation therapy and immunotherapy.

The second part of the volume describes the agents of importance in the treatment of these disease states. It includes major sections on alkylating agents, hormones, antimetabolites and a variety of other cytotoxic compounds, including inhibitors of protein and RNA synthesis, antibiotics and alkaloids, a variety of important synthetic agents and cytotoxic metal-containing compounds.

The Editors wish to express their deepest gratitude to their collaborators who have not only contributed important chapters, but have cooperated fully in the final preparation of this volume. They are also most appreciative of the invaluable editorial assistance provided by Dr. Barbara Renkin and the important secretarial help they have received from Miss Lenora Antinozzi and Miss Lynn A. Bon Tempo. Special thanks go to Dr. William A. Creasey who has compiled the subject index for this volume. It is our deepest hope that research workers in cancer, immunosuppresion and other scientific disciplines will find this volume of use in both their intellectual and laboratory endeavors and that it may aid in the accomplishment of further advances in science for the benefit of man.

New Haven and Bethesda
Summer, 1974

Alan C. Sartorelli
David G. Johns

# Part I Table of Contents

## Section A: General Considerations: Antineoplastic Agents

### Chapter 1

**Agents of Choice in Neoplastic Disease.** C. Gordon Zubrod



### Chapter 2

**Evaluation of Antineoplastic Activity: Requirements of Test Systems.** Abraham Goldin, Stephen Carter, and Nathan Mantel



### Chapter 3

**Rational Design of Alkylating Agents.** W. C. J. Ross

## Chapter 6

**Rational Design of Pyrimidine Nucleoside Analogs.** LEROY B. TOWNSEND and C. C. CHENG



## Chapter 7

**Basic Concepts of Cell Population Kinetics.** L. F. LAMERTON. With 5 Figures



## Chapter 8

**Clinical Applications of Cell Cycle Kinetics.** BAYARD CLARKSON. With 3 Figures

## Chapter 9

**Metabolic Events in the Regulation of Cell Reproduction.** Elton Stubblefield and Sandra Murphree. With 1 Figure



## Chapter 10

**Site of Action of Cytotoxic Agents in the Cell Life Cycle.** H. Madoc-Jones and F. Mauro. With 3 Figures



## Chapter 11

**Pharmacokinetic Models for Antineoplastic Agents.** Daniel S. Zaharko and Robert L. Dedrick. With 4 Figures



## Chapter 12

**Absorption, Distribution, and Excretion of Antineoplastic and Immunosuppressive Agents.** Vincent T. Oliverio. With 3 Figures

## Chapter 13



## Chapter 14

## Chapter 15

**Metabolism of Cancer Chemotherapeutic Agents via Pathways Utilized by Xenobiotics.**
A. M. Guarino and C. L. Litterst. With 3 Figures

## Chapter 16



## Chapter 17



## Chapter 18

## Chapter 19

## Chapter 21

**Combination Chemotherapy: Clinical Considerations.** EMIL FREI, III and JEFFREY A. GOTTLIEB



## Chapter 22

**Tests Predictive of Cytotoxic Activity.** THOMAS C. HALL



## Chapter 23

**Metabolic Changes Induced by Ionizing Radiations.** PAUL TODD. With 2 Figures

## Chapter 26



# Section B: General Considerations: Immunosuppressive Agents

## Chapter 27

## Chapter 28

**Immunosuppressive Agents.** Evan M. Hersh



## Chapter 29

**Clinical Utility of Immunosuppressive Agents.** Jules E. Harris and Ramesh C. Bagai

# Part I Contributors


RAMESH C. BAGAI, Division of Oncology, Department of Medicine, University of Ottawa and Ottawa General Hospital, Ottawa 2/Canada

MALCOLM A. BAGSHAW, Department of Radiology, Stanford University, School of Medicine, Stanford, CA 94305/USA

R. W. BROCKMAN, Kettering-Meyer Laboratories, Southern Research Institute, 2000 Ninth Avenue South, Birmingham, AL 35205/USA

STEPHEN CARTER, Cancer Therapy Evaluation Branch, National Cancer Institute, National Institutes of Health, Bethesda, MD 20014/USA

C. C. CHENG, Cancer Chemotherapy Section, Midwest Research Institute, 425 Volker Building, Kansas City, MO 64110/USA

BAYARD CLARKSON, Hematology Service, Sloan-Kettering Institute for Cancer Research, 444 East 68th Street, New York, NY 10021/USA

ALAN L. COWLES, National Cancer Institute, National Institutes of Health, Bethesda, MD 20014/USA

ROBERT L. DEDRICK, Biomedical Engineering and Instrumentation Branch, Division of Research Services, National Institutes of Health, Bethesda, MD 20014/USA

ALEXANDER FEFER, Division of Oncology, Department of Medicine, University of Washington, School of Medicine, Seattle, WA 98144/USA

JOSEPH D. FENSTERMACHER, National Cancer Institute, National Institutes of Health DCT, Membrane Transport Section, Bethesda, MD 20014/USA

EMIL FREI, III, Children's Cancer Research Foundation, Binney Street, Boston, MS 02115/USA

ABRAHAM GOLDIN, Division of Cancer Treatment, National Cancer Institute, National Institutes of Health, Bethesda, MD 20014/USA

JEFFREY A. GOTTLIEB, Department of Developmental Therapeutics, The University of Texas, M. D. Anderson Hospital and Tumor Institute, Houston, TX 77025/USA

A. M. GUARINO, Laboratory of Toxicology, Division of Cancer Treatment, National Cancer Institute, Bethesda, MD 20014/USA

MAIRE T. HAKALA, Department of Experimental Therapeutics, Roswell Park Memorial Institute, 666 Elm Street, Buffalo, NY 14203/USA

THOMAS C. HALL, Cancer Center and Departments of Medicine and Biochemistry, Los Angeles County-University of Southern California, Medical Center, 1200 North State Street, Los Angeles, CA 90033/USA

JULES E. HARRIS, Division of Oncology, Department of Medicine, University of Ottawa and Ottawa General Hospital, Ottawa 2/Canada

J. FRANK HENDERSON, McEachern Laboratory and Department of Biochemistry, University of Alberta, Cancer Research Unit., Edmonton, Alberta/Canada

EVAN M. HERSH, Department of Developmental Therapeutics, The University of Texas, M. D. Anderson Hospital and Tumor Institute, Houston, TX 77025/USA

L. E. HOPWOOD, Department of Anatomy, Washington University, School of Medicine, 660 S. Euclid, St. Louis, MO 63110/USA

DAVID G. JOHNS, Laboratory of Chemical Pharmacology, National Cancer Institute, National Institutes of Health, Bethesda, MD 20014/USA

L. F. LAMERTON, Institute of Cancer Research, Biophysics Department, Clifton Avenue, Belmont, Sutton, Surrey/Great Britain

C. L. LITTERST, Laboratory of Toxicology, Division of Cancer Treatment, National Cancer Institute, Bethesda, MD 20014/USA

HYWEL MADOC-JONES, Department of Radiology, University of Chicago, Fritzker School of Medicine, 950 East, Fifty-Ninth Street, Chicago, IL 60637/USA

NATHAN MANTEL, Biometry Branch, National Cancer Institute, National Institutes of Health, Bethesda, MD 20014/USA

FRANCESCO MAURO, Laboratorio di Radiobiologia Animale, C.S.N. della Casaccia, Comitato Nazionale Energie Nucleone, 00100 Rome/Italy

JOHN A. R. MEAD, Department of Health, Education and Welfare, National Cancer Institute, National Institutes of Health, Bethesda, MD 20014/USA

L. B. MELLETT, Southern Research Institute, 2000 Ninth Avenue South, Birmingham, AL 35205/USA

MALCOLM S. MITCHELL, Department of Medicine and Pharmacology, Yale University, School of Medicine, 333 Cedar Street, New Haven, CT 06510/USA

JOHN A. MONTGOMERY, Organic Chemistry Research, Southern Research Institute, 2000 Ninth Avenue South, Birmingham, AL 35205/USA

SANDRA MURPHREE, Department of Pharmacology, Yale University, New Haven, CT 06510/USA

VINCENT T. OLIVERIO, Laboratory of Chemical Pharmacology, National Cancer Institute, National Institutes of Health, Bethesda, MD 20014/USA

W. C. J. ROSS, Chester Beatty Research Institute, Institute of Cancer Research, Royal Cancer Hospital, Fulham Road, London SW 3/Great Britain

R. L. SCOTTE DOGGETT, Radiation Therapy Center of Sutter Community Hospitals, 1215 28th Street, Sacramento, CA 95816/USA

ELTON STUBBLEFIELD, Departments of Biology and Biochemistry, The University of Texas at Houston, M. D. Anderson Hospital and Tumor Institute, Houston, TX 77025/USA

PAUL TODD, Department of Biophysics, Pennsylvania State University, College of Science, 618 Life Science Building, University Park, PA 16802/USA

LEONARD J. TOLMACH, Department of Anatomy, Washington University, School of Medicine, 660 S. Euclid, St. Louis, MO 63110/USA

LEROY B. TOWNSEND, Department of Biopharmaceutical Sciences and Department of Chemistry, University of Utah, Salt Lake City, UT 84112/USA

JOHN M. VENDITTI, Drug Evaluation Branch, Division of Cancer Treatment, National Cancer Institute, National Institutes of Health, Bethesda, MD 20014/USA

DANIEL S. ZAHARKO, Laboratory of Chemical Pharmacology, National Cancer Institute, Bethesda, MD 20014/USA

C. GORDON ZUBROD, Division of Cancer Treatment, National Cancer Institute, National Institutes of Health, Bethesda, MD 20014/USA

# Part II Table of Contents

## Section C: Alkylating Agents



## Section D: Hormones



## Section E: Antimetabolites

## Section F: Additional Cytotoxic Agents

Chapter 1

# Agents of Choice in Neoplastic Disease

C. GORDON ZUBROD

## Introduction

A few cancers are highly responsive to drugs and a few are virtually unresponsive. In an intermediate class are a large number of cancers that are partially sensitive to chemotherapy, either in the sense that a sizeable number of patients show some degree of regression of disease, or that a few patients will show a substantial degree of regression. There are now over 30 drugs that are available for the chemotherapy of cancer. Even though some of these are analogs, there are at least 20 different chemical entities capable of causing significant regression of cancer in man. The pathologist recognizes a hundred or more different types of cancer, and chemotherapy is used in about 30 to 40 of these. Finally, intensive research in chemotherapy is continually turning up new drugs and new ways of using old drugs. There is then a vast and heterogeneous body of knowledge governing the choice of drug – a body of knowledge that is evolving rather dynamically. This chapter is written with the objective of providing a general framework for the detailed discussions to follow, so that the reader, should he have the need, may find an orientation to current usage of antitumor drugs. With this in mind, I have not documented the assertions made, nor attempted to provide a text for the treatment of cancer. The references are limited to general reviews.

## General Remarks on Criteria for Drug Choice

The choice of the best drug to use in the treatment of cancer depends upon the demonstration of success; the tables list specific recommendations. There are a few general considerations that sway the physician in his choice and these should be of interest to all who are concerned with the chemical control of cancer since the strategy of control cannot ignore these basic realities. These considerations may be looked at as they relate to the tumor, the patient, the drug, and the physician. Of these, the factors pertaining to the tumor and the patient most often influence drug choice.

## The Tumor

It is clear from much that is written in this book, that the growth fraction of the tumor (i.e. the percentage of cells engaged in DNA synthesis at any one point of time), is probably the most important tumor factor conditioning responsiveness to drugs (SKIPPER, 1971; DEVITA, 1971). Animal tumors with a large growth fraction are most easily cured by means of drugs. In a general way these observations made experimentally have been verified in the clinic. There is only a small amount of data on growth fractions of different tumors of man, and a number of technical advances must be made before these data can be obtained for all cancers. There is a danger at the moment of the circular argument that any highly responsive tumor must have a large growth fraction; in the few instances where valid data exist, the correlation seems to hold true.

The growth fraction is not the only factor controlling susceptibility of tumor cells to drugs, since the cell type or cell of origin is also of importance. In fact, some of the specific usages of several drugs such as the corticosteroids, the vinca alkaloids, streptozotocin, and *o, p'*-DDD were discovered because of their toxicity to specific cell types in normal animals. A more subtle determinant arises from cell type as may be seen in bronchogenic carcinoma, where the oat cell histological type is much more susceptible to drugs than is the adenocarcinoma or epidermoid cell variety. In most cases, the reasons for the susceptibility of a particular cell to a specific drug is unknown, perhaps residing in a metabolic pathway characteristic of that cell or perhaps arising from enhanced transport or binding. At the moment one must be content with the empiric observation that specific drugs do in fact kill particular types of tumor cells and may be ineffective against other cells. The physician must be aware of these in his choice of an agent for a tumor.

The site of tumor growth is important in another respect. Namely, that because of physiologic and pharmacologic reasons, growth within certain areas or organs provides a pharmacologic sanctuary that the drug cannot reach. Thus, a tumor, whether primary or secondary, within the central nervous system cannot be reached by tumoricidal concentrations of drug, and even though the tumor may have a large growth fraction and the cell type be one that is highly susceptible, the drug cannot kill the tumor cells (Rall and Zubrod, 1962). The physician is, therefore, limited to those drugs that will pass the blood brain barrier such as 1,3-*bis*(2-chloroethyl)-1-nitrosourea (BCNU), or can safely be given intrathecally such as methotrexate or cytosine arabinoside. There are presumably other pharmacologic sanctuarics, and there is some evidence that testicular tissue is one of these. Pharmacologists must provide additional data, with respect to each agent, in order that the physician may choose the best drug for these tumor *caches*.

## The Drug

Most of the drug factors concern how the agent is to be given, rather than if it is to be given. Of course, the factors of availability and expense will determine choice, but for the purposes of this chapter we will assume a more ideal circumstance. The specific type of toxicity relating to antitumor drugs is a determinant in its choice, and this will be considered under patient factors. The route of administration may be a consideration in choosing a drug. Some drugs cannot be formulated for parenteral use, and the oral route may be the only one possible. Hence, the physician may, when the patient is unable to take oral medication, choose a drug on the basis of being able to use it parenterally, rather than because it is the ideal drug for this particular tumor.

It is of considerable interest to inquire why it is that some drugs affect relatively few types of tumors while others are effective in a variety of tumors. In Table 1, drugs are categorized as to whether they are effective in less than or more than three different tumors (Livingston and Carter, 1970). While this concept is clearly not so useful as that of the broad spectrum antibiotics in bacterial chemotherapy, it may perhaps be of some help to the physician in the choice of a drug. Even with bacterial chemotherapy the rational approach is to choose the agent known to be effective against a specific microorganism, and it is usually when the

Table 1. *Drugs active in clinical cancer; categorized as to range of usefulness*

| Drugs useful in four or more types of cancer | Drugs useful in three or fewer types of cancer |
|---|---|
| Alkylating agents | |
| Nitrogen mustard (Mechlorethamine) | Busulfan |
| Cyclophosphamide | Pipobroman |
| Melphalan | Dibromomannitol |
| Thiotepa | |
| Chlorambucil | |
| Triethylene melamine | |
| Antimetabolites | |
| Methotrexate | Cytosine arabinoside (Cytarabine) |
| 5-Fluorouracil | Azauridine triacetate |
| Mercaptopurine | Thioguanine |
| Mitotic inhibitors | |
| Vinblastine | TMCA (Trimethyl colchicinic acid) |
| Vincristine | |
| Antibiotics | |
| Dactinomycin | Mithramycin |
| Daunorubicin | Streptozotocin |
| Adriamycin | |
| Random synthetics | |
| BCNU (Carmustine)[a] | Hydroxyurea |
| | Imidazole carboxamide[b] |
| | Procarbazine hydrochloride |
| | Methyl-GAG[c] |
| | *o, p'*-DDD (Mitotane)[c] |
| Hormonal agents | |
| Corticosteroids | ACTH |
| | Androgens |
| | Estrogens |
| | Progesterone |
| Miscellaneous | |
| | L-Asparaginase |

[a] 1,3-*Bis* (2-chloroethyl)-1-nitrosourea.
[b] NSC-45388; 5-(3,3-dimethyl-1-triazeno)-imidazole-4-carboxamide.
[c] Methyl-GAG, methyl glyoxal *bis* (guanylhydrazone); *o, p'*-DDD, 1-(*o*-chlorophenyl)-1-(*p*-chlorophenyl)-2,2-dichloroethane.

sensitivities are unknown, that the physician chooses the drug with the broadest spectrum of coverage. Perhaps in an analogous sense, the "broad spectrum" antitumor agents may have preference to those of narrower range in certain circumstances. The table does not encourage one to think in absolute terms about broad and narrow spectrum drugs, but the trend indicates that alkylating agents and natural products are broader in their effects against cancer than the antimetabolites and hormonal agents. Even here, more clinical data might swell the number of drugs in the broad spectrum column. One may also ask whether a similar analysis would give insights into the types of toxicities produced by the different agents. Inspection of Table 2 leads only to the perhaps trivial observation that most of the alopecia-producing drugs are in the broad spectrum column. Clearly, what is needed to provide the substrate for sharper decisions is a thorough knowledge of the molecular points of action of each compound and the relation of the molecular interference both to site of action within the cell cycle and to the specificity of action for the various tumors.

Table 2. *Comparison of toxicities of antitumor drugs excluding hormones*

| Drug | Bone Marrow | GI Tract | Hair Root | Liver | Others |
|---|---|---|---|---|---|
| Alkylating agents | | | | | |
| Nitrogen mustard | ++++ | + | | | |
| Melphalan | ++++ | + | | | |
| Cyclophosphamide | ++ | + | +++ | | Bladder |
| Myleran | +++ | | | | Endocrinological-Addison-like syndrome<br>Pulmonary fibrosis |
| Chlorambucil | +++ | + | | | |
| Dibromomannitol | +++ | | | | |
| Mitomycin C | ++++ | ++ | | | |
| Antimetabolites | | | | | |
| Methotrexate | ++++ | ++++ | + | +++ | Osteoporosis |
| 6-Mercaptopurine | +++ | + | 0 | ++ | |
| Thioguanine | ++ | | + | | |
| 5-Fluorouracil | ++++ | ++++ | | 0 | Neurological |
| Cytosine arabinoside | +++ | + | 0 | + | |
| Azauridine triacetate | + | | | | |
| Mitotic inhibitors | | | | | |
| Vincristine | + | + | ++++ | | Myoneural junction<br>Dorsal root ganglion |
| Vinblastine | ++ | +++ | + | | |
| TMCA[a] | +++ | | | | |
| Antibiotics | | | | | |
| L-Asparaginase | | + | | +++ | Pancreatitis<br>Diabetes mellitus<br>Anaphylaxis<br>Clotting defects<br>CNS[a] |
| Actinomycin D | +++ | +++ | +++ | | Skin |
| Daunomycin | ++++ | | | | Cardiac failure |
| Adriamycin | +++ | | ++ | | Cardiac failure |
| Mithramycin | ++++ | + | | ++ | Clotting defects |
| Streptozotocin | | | | + | Renal tubular acidosis<br>Diabetes mellitus |
| Miscellaneous synthetics | | | | | |
| BCNU[a] | ++++ | + | | | |
| Procarbazine | +++ | ++ | + | | CNS |
| Imidazole carboxamide | +++ | + | | | |
| Hydroxyurea | +++ | + | | | |
| Methyl-GAG[a] | +++ | ++++ | | | Skin |
| *o, p'*-DDD[a] | | | | | CNS |

[a] Methyl-GAG, methyl glyoxal *bis* (guanylhydrazone); BCNU, 1,3-*bis* (2-chloroethyl)-1-nitrosourea; CNS, central nervous system; *o, p'*-DDD, 1-(*o*-chlorophenyl)-1-(*p*-chlorophenyl)-2,2-dichloroethane; TMCA, Trimethylcolchicinic acid methylether.

## The Patient

The status of the patient is often the controlling determinant in the choice of an antitumor drug. The time is at hand when the physician must consider drugs as primary therapy with curative intent for certain highly responsive tumors. In an older day, when chemotherapy was considered as the last resort for the hopelessly ill cancer patient, antitumor drugs were frequently given too late to do any good. When antitumor drugs are to be used either with the objective of cure or with the intent of effecting marked increase in life expectancy, it makes no sense to wait until the patient is far along in his disease and too ill to permit proper chemotherapy. In analyzing the patient in relation to choice of a particular drug, one factor is the pharmacologic disposition of the drug in relationship to any physiological deficit in the patient. For example, methotrexate is removed from the body largely by renal excretion and even mild renal impairment will result in high plasma concentrations leading to severe toxicity. Hence, it is wiser to choose another drug, unless one is in a position to calculate how small a dose of methotrexate can safely be administered in the presence of renal disease. A more common factor conditioning drug choice has to do with the presence in the patient of organ damage from previous chemotherapy or radiation. Since so many of the drugs are destructive to normal bone marrow, the presence of diminished bone marrow reserve will most often be the conditioning factor. In choosing a drug, a physician should be alert both to a history of previous therapy that might have damaged the bone marrow, and to the present status of the bone marrow. While the peripheral white count is a very rough estimate of degree of bone marrow reserve, it may under or overestimate the patient's resources and hopefully will someday be replaced by more precise methodology. In the presence of uncontrolled active infection, it is sometimes unwise to choose a drug that will depress granulocyte production since this may be followed by uncontrollable extension of the infection (PERRY, 1971). Analogous problems exist with respect to methotrexate in the presence of liver damage, daunomycin in the presence of heart disease, and bleomycin when there is diminished pulmonary function.

The increasing use of combinations of drugs in the treatment of patients with cancer emphasizes the need for the physician to be aware of the organ toxicity of the various agents. It would seem unwise to use a combination of three drugs, all of which result in severe bone marrow damage, when by choosing three drugs whose major toxicities affect different organs, one could obtain three times the antitumor capacity of a single drug without enhancement of toxicity for one particular organ. This has been in part the basis for the success of the combination treatment of acute leukemia and of advanced HODGKIN's disease.

## Physician Factors

The training and attitude of the physician in cancer chemotherapy should be a determinant in the choice of a drug. Clearly, the physician should choose only those drugs with which he has complete familiarity. For example, since there are at least ten different alkylating agents, it would be much better to choose the one that the physician knows best. If the physician's experience is narrow, this imposes certain constraints in the choice of the best possible therapy. As chemotherapy becomes more complex and is given with greater intensity, the physician, in order to have the freedom to choose the best possible therapy, needs to be not only familiar with the various agents, but he should also have available those supportive resources that make intensive chemotherapy feasible and safe (PERRY, 1971). Certainly the availability of dependable laboratory estimations in hematology, bacteriology, and blood chemistry will often be a limiting factor in the choice of drugs and in the intensity with which they can be given. Similarly, easy accessibility to platelet transfusions allows the physician to choose drugs that may cause a fairly severe effect on platelets.

In summary, the choice of those drugs and regimens that will result in prolonged life expectancy or maximum palliation depends upon the familiarity of the physician with the principles of modern curative chemotherapy. These principles, hinted at in this section and fully developed in succeeding chapters, include a knowledge of the available drugs, their toxicity and pharmacology, optimal dosage schedules, cell population kinetics of normal and tumor cells, and the details of laboratory and supportive management of the patient receiving intensive chemotherapy. While deficiencies in our knowledge of cell kinetics and pharmacokinetics will result in compromises, the general principles of potentially curative chemotherapy are well established. A knowledge of these principles will assist the physician in the thicket of 30 drugs and 100 diseases to choose optimal therapy for the individual patient.

## Choice of Drugs for Treatment of Specific Types of Cancer

Recommendations for the choice of drugs are shown in Tables 3 to 5. In selecting a drug to help with the management of a patient with cancer, it is important for the physician to have clearly in mind what he hopes to accomplish by means of the drug. For this purpose it is helpful to classify cancer into three categories: (1) patients with tumors that are highly responsive to drug therapy where one can expect complete remission of the disease and substantial prolongation of life expectancy, (2) patients with tumors sufficiently responsive to chemotherapy that substantial regression of tumor is possible, but increased survival has yet to be demonstrated, and (3) patients with tumors that show little or no response to drugs. In discussing the choice of agents the tables indicate those instances where drugs play a substantial role in the management of cancer when drugs are used as single agents, in combination, or as part of a total effort of eradication of tumor in association with surgery, radiation, or other means of treatment. The tables do not include the details of management or the specific drug schedules, and inclusion of trivial drug effects have been avoided. In the references, only a few general reviews are given (Livingston and Carter, 1970; Holland and Frei, 1973). Finally, I would emphasize once more that the optimal use of a drug depends not only on the choice of the drug, but also upon the manner in which it is given.

## Choice of Drugs for Highly Responsive (Large Growth Fraction) Tumors

A glance at the list of highly responsive tumors in Table 3 reveals that these are tumors sufficiently uncommon that few physicians will see large numbers (Zubrod, 1970; Holland and Frei, 1973). One may also reflect on the fact that all of these tumors are rapidly growing; they have short doubling times, and where measurements have been made, are characterized by a large growth fraction. In spite of the rarity of these tumors, as a group they constitute about 10 to 15% of clinical cancer. It is important for every physician to keep this list in mind since optimal therapy can lead to prolonged survival and, in some instances, cure. If the physician is to treat a patient with one of these diseases, it must be with that intensity and duration of drug therapy, integrated into the total therapy, that will destroy sufficient numbers of tumor cells to achieve complete remission and prolonged survival. When the physician diagnoses one of these diseases and does not wish to undertake treatment himself, he has a clear responsibility to seek early consultation and referral to a center where optimal therapy can be obtained.

In Table 3 an estimate of the optimal drug therapy for these responsive diseases is given. In only two exquisitely drug sensitive tumors, Burkitt's lymphoma and choriocarcinoma, is there an indication for a drug to be used without other drugs or radiation. Even in these two diseases, as it becomes possible to stage the extent

Table 3. *Drugs of choice for tumors that are highly responsive to chemotherapy leading to substantial increases in life expectancy*

| Disease | Best therapy | Drugs recommended | Other drugs that have substantial effect |
|---|---|---|---|
| BURKITT's lymphoma | SD | Cyclophosphamide | Methotrexate<br>Orthomelphalan |
| Choriocarcinoma | SD | Methotrexate<br>Dactinomycin | Mercaptopurine<br>Vinblastine<br>Azauridine |
| Acute lymphocytic leukemia | CD + R | Prednisone<br>Vincristine<br>Methotrexate<br>Mercaptopurine | Cyclophosphamide<br>Daunorubicin<br>L-Asparaginase<br>Cytosine arabinoside |
| Acute myelocytic leukemia | CD | Cytosine arabinoside<br>Thioguanine<br>Daunorubicin | Vincristine<br>Prednisone<br>Mercaptopurine<br>Cyclophosphamide |
| Advanced HODGKIN's disease (stages IIB, IIIB and IVA and B) | CD ("MOPP") | Prednisone<br>Vincristine<br>Nitrogen mustard<br>Procarbazine | BCNU<br>Cyclophosphamide<br>Bleomycin<br>Vinblastine<br>Chlorambucil |
| Lymphosarcoma (Nonlocalized stages) | CD ("COP") | Cyclophosphamide<br>Prednisone<br>Vincristine | Procarbazine<br>Nitrogen mustard<br>Bleomycin |
| Reticulum cell sarcoma (Nonlocalized stages) | CD | Cyclophosphamide<br>Prednisone<br>Vincristine | Procarbazine<br>Nitrogen mustard<br>Bleomycin |
| Mycosis fungoides | SD + EB | Nitrogen mustard (topically) | Azaribine (6-azauridine triacetate) |
| Embryonal testicular cancer | CD | Dactinomycin<br>Methotrexate<br>Chlorambucil | Mithramycin<br>Bleomycin |
| WILMS' tumor | SD + S + R | Dactinomycin<br>Vincristine | |
| EWING's sarcoma | CD + R | Vincristine<br>Cyclophosphamide | Nitrogen mustard<br>5-Fluorouracil<br>BCNU |
| Embryonal rhabdomyosarcoma | CD + R | Vincristine<br>Dactinomycin<br>Cyclophosphamide | Mitomycin C |
| Retinoblastoma | SD + R | Triethylene melamine | Cyclophosphamide<br>Vincristine |

SD = single drug; CD = drugs used in combination; R = x-irradiation; EB = electron beam irradiation; S = surgical excision; MOPP = Mustargen (nitrogen mustard), Oncovin, Procarbazine, prednisone; COP = cyclophosphamide, Oncovin, prednisone.

of disease and relate the amount of disease to prognosis, combination chemotherapy probably should be used at the outset for patients with poorest prognosis. For example, systemic and intrathecal chemotherapy will not cure patients with central nervous system involvement from BURKITT's lymphoma. The value of irradiation of the central nervous system added to chemotherapy, for this situation, is unknown. Such irradiation given prophylactically to patients receiving drug therapy for acute lymphocytic leukemia, has been beneficial in preventing the occurrence of central nervous system leukemia.

The choice of combinations of drugs for the treatment of the acute leukemias and lymphomas is based on the best results published to date (HENDERSON and

SAMAHA, 1969; CARTER, 1971). However, there is intensive investigation going on, with new drugs being added or substituted, and changes in the choice of combinations are to be expected. With respect to the lymphomas, I have completely avoided the issue of combination of drugs with x-irradiation, since this is another rapidly changing area; the degree to which these agents are combined in the treatment of various stages will vary in different institutions until final data are forthcoming.

In mycosis fungoides, the topical administration of nitrogen mustard and the use of electron beam radiation (not x-irradiation), as well as systemic use of azaribine (6-azauridine triacetate), have been used almost always in sequence rather than simultaneously, and no recommendation can be made for concurrent usage. In WILMS' tumor, the drugs have usually been administered as single agents, after surgical removal and x-irradiation of the tumor bed. For metastatic WILMS' tumor, combination chemotherapy is warranted, perhaps with irradiation.

## Drugs of Choice for Patients with Tumors that are Partially Responsive to Chemotherapy (Small Growth Fraction Tumors)

These are seen in Table 4 and require little comment. All of these tumors are slowly growing with doubling times of a week or more. When examined, the growth fraction has been small. Chemotherapy can produce marked tumor regressions, but

Table 4. *Drugs of choice for tumors that are substantially responsive to drugs but where increased survival has not been demonstrated*

| Disease | Best therapy | Drugs recommended | Other drugs that have substantial effect |
|---|---|---|---|
| Chronic myelocytic leukemia | | | |
| Early disease | SD | Busulfan<br>Dibromomannitol | Mercaptopurine<br>Hydroxyurea |
| Blastic crisis | CD | Vincristine<br>Prednisone<br>Arabinosyl cytosine<br>BCNU | Mercaptopurine |
| Chronic lymphocytic leukemia | SD + R | Chlorambucil | Prednisone<br>Other alkylating agents |
| Multiple myeloma | CD | Melphalan<br>Cyclophosphamide<br>Prednisone | BCNU |
| Colo-rectal cancer | SD + R | 5-Fluorouracil | BCNU<br>Mitomycin C |
| Breast cancer | CD | Cyclophosphamide<br>5-Fluorouracil<br>Methotrexate<br>Vincristine<br>Prednisone | BCNU<br>Androgens<br>Estrogens<br>Progestins |
| Ovarian cancer | CD | Melphalan<br>Cyclophosphamide<br>5-Fluorouracil | Hexamethylmelamine |
| Lung cancer | | | |
| Oat cell | CD + R | Cyclophosphamide<br>Methotrexate | CCNU[a]<br>Hexamethylmelamine<br>Procarbazine<br>Nitrogen mustard |

[a] CCNU, 1-(2-chloroethyl)-3-cyclohexyl-1-nitrosourea.

Table 4 (Continued)

| Disease | Best therapy | Drugs recommended | Other drugs that have substantial effect |
|---|---|---|---|
| Squamous cell | CD + R | Nitrogen mustard<br>Methotrexate | CCNU<br>Cyclophosphamide<br>Procarbazine<br>Hexamethylmelamine |
| Adenocarcinoma | CD + R | Nitrogen mustard<br>Methotrexate | CCNU<br>Cyclophosphamide<br>Procarbazine<br>Hexamethylmelamine |
| Undifferentiated | CD + R | Cyclophosphamide<br>Methotrexate | CCNU<br>Nitrogen mustard<br>Procarbazine<br>5-Fluorouracil<br>Hexamethylmelamine |
| Melanoma | CD | Dimethyl triazeno imidazole carboxamide<br>BCNU<br>Vincristine | Melphalan<br>Cyclophosphamide<br>Hydroxyurea<br>Actinomycin D<br>TMCA |
| Skin cancer | | | |
| Multiple basal cell | SD | 5-Fluorouracil | Methotrexate |
| Head and neck cancer | SD + R | Methotrexate | 5-Fluorouracil<br>Bleomycin |
| Brain tumors | | | |
| Glioblastoma | SD | BCNU<br>CCNU | Methotrexate<br>Vincristine<br>Corticosteroids |
| Adrenal cortical carcinoma | SD | o, p′-DDD | |
| Carcinoma of the cervix-endometrium | SD | Methotrexate | Cyclophosphamide<br>5-Fluorouracil<br>Bleomycin<br>Vincristine |
| Pancreatic islet cell carcinoma | SD | Streptozotocin | |
| KAPOSI's sarcoma | CD | Actinomycin D | Chlorambucil |
| Neuroblastoma | CD | Cyclophosphamide<br>Vincristine | Adriamycin<br>5-Fluorouracil |
| Far advanced extremity sarcomas | Hyperthermia + R + SD | Melphalan | Actinomycin D<br>Vincristine<br>Cyclophosphamide<br>Adriamycin |

rarely does complete clinical regression occur. Because of the modest effect of drugs, most physicians have felt that intensive use of drugs is not warranted and drug combinations have usually not been studied. This is particularly true for the chronic leukemias. Recently, more substantial regressions from combinations of drugs have been seen in the accelerated phases of chronic myelocytic leukemia, multiple myeloma, advanced breast and lung cancer, melanoma, KAPOSI's sarcoma, and neuroblastoma. It is in this category, among the surgically resectable tumors, where the best place for drugs used as adjuvants to surgery should be found. The principles of modern chemotherapy are just beginning to be utilized in surgical adjuvant studies and one hopes that ongoing investigations will show the way to reduction in mortality in diseases such as lung and breast cancer.

## Drugs with Some Activity in Patients with Tumors that have Slight or Negligible Drug Responsiveness

These are shown in Table 5. One might rightly ask why bother about the choice of drugs for these patients when there is so little effect. This category was included for several reasons. First, it is mentioned so that the attention of investigators may be focused on these tumors, for perhaps some additional basic biologic difference might be uncovered by intensive study of this adamantine group, as occurred

Table 5. *Drugs with some activity in patients with tumors that have slight or negligible drug responsiveness*

| Disease | Drugs recommended | Other drugs that have some effect |
|---|---|---|
| Pancreatic adenocarcinoma | 5-Fluorouracil | Streptozotocin<br>Tubercidin |
| Hepatoma | 5-Fluorouracil<br>Dichloromethotrexate intra-arterially | |
| Carcinoma of prostate | Estrogens | 5-Fluorouracil |
| Hypernephroma | Progesterone | Hydroxyurea |
| Esophageal carcinoma | Methyl-GAG | 5-Fluorouracil |
| Bladder cancer | | |
| Adenocarcinoma | 5-Fluorouracil | Hydroxyurea |
| Transitional cell | 5-Fluorouracil<br>Adriamycin | |
| Osteogenic sarcoma | Adriamycin | Melphalan<br>Mitomycin C |

following the recognition that the most rapidly growing tumors were the most drug responsive; and second, to emphasize that these are patients usually seen by specialty groups, disinclined to investigate the effects of drugs. Thus, data on drug effects are scanty for many of these tumors. Finally, the wise physician will rarely tell a patient with advanced cancer that there is nothing more to be done, and often a drug with slight effect provides the tenuous thread that keeps the patient free from despair.

## Conclusions

In developing the context for the chapters to follow, I have emphasized the elements involved in selecting a drug for the treatment of cancer. This was done, not as a guideline for physicians, but to illustrate the considerations that make up present day cancer chemotherapy. The design of a successful strategy for chemical control of cancer depends not simply on the discovery of active agents, but also upon their further development with respect to the realities of cell kinetics, toxicity, pharmacokinetics, and the individual patient. Chemotherapy is firmly established along with surgery and radiation as one of the primary modes of treating cancer. It is equally clear, as the biology of tumor growth begins to be understood, that primary modes of therapy by themselves are useful largely only during the earliest portions of the tumor growth curve. When the tumor has grown old, single modalities of therapy are rarely effective and one must call upon all the help available to get rid of the vast number of tumor cells present. In the future, the use of combinations of surgery, radiation, and chemotherapy will expand, and in all likelihood, immunotherapy and hyperthermia will be called upon to help eradicate the last tumor cell. Chemotherapy of cancer should be envisioned not as an isolated method of therapy, but in the context of its maximum contribution in the collaborative effort to eliminate all tumor cells from the patient with minimal side effects.

## References


Carter, S.K.: Clinical trials and combination chemotherapy. Cancer Chemother. Rep. 2, 81—97 (1971).

DeVita, V.: Cell kinetics and the chemotherapy of cancer. Cancer Chemother. Rep. 2, 23—33 (1971).

Henderson, E.S., Samaha, R.J.: Evidence that drugs in multiple combinations have materially advanced the treatment of human malignancies. Symposium: A Critical Evaluation of Cancer Chemotherapy, Cherry Hill, New Jersey, April 9—11, 1969.

Holland, J.F., Frei, E., III. (Eds.): Cancer medicine. Philadelphia, Penn.: Lea & Febiger 1973.

Livingston, R.B., Carter, S.K.: Single agents in cancer chemotherapy. New York: IFI/Plenum 1970.

Perry, S.: Supportive care in cancer therapy. Cancer Chemother. Rep. 2, 99—104 (1971).

Rall, D.P., Zubrod, C.G.: Mechanisms of drug absorption and excretion. Ann. Rev. Pharmacol. 2, 109 (1962).

Skipper, H.E.: Cancer chemotherapy is many things: G. H. A. Clowes Memorial Lecture. Cancer Res. 31, 1173 (1971).

Zubrod, C.G.: Historical perspectives of curative chemotherapy. Proceedings of tenth international cancer congress, Houston, Texas, 1970.

Chapter 2

# Evaluation of Antineoplastic Activity: Requirements of Test Systems

ABRAHAM GOLDIN, STEPHEN CARTER, and NATHAN MANTEL

## Introduction

The primary objectives of test systems for the evaluation of antineoplastic agents include (a) the identification of new agents which may be active against clinical neoplasia, (b) the detailed investigation of the action of drugs on host-tumor parameters and of factors which may influence chemotherapeutic effectiveness, and (c) detailed pharmacologic, toxicologic, biochemical, virologic, immunologic, and other investigations of the basic mechanism of action of antitumor agents.

For these purposes, the primary requirement of any test system is that it have the appropriate design characteristics to meet the level of interest of the investigation being conducted.

For screening, evaluation and fundamental investigation of antitumor agents the test systems should have the requisite quantitative characteristics to provide confidence in the reproducibility of the results. The quantitative aspects of the experimental design must be adjusted and refined in accordance with the demands and complexity of the problems that are posed and the relationship of the studies to potential clinical interest. The test systems should have relevance to the clinic and should be able to predict with some accuracy which drugs will be clinically active. It should be recognized, however, that at the start of any screening program and in the absence of known clinically active drugs, it may only be possible to claim a rational basis for possible predictive properties of a screening test; any actual demonstration of such properties would have to await the identification of clinically effective agents.

The various facets and problems pertaining to screening and evaluation systems, and their relevancy to the clinic may perhaps be best presented in reference to the progression of steps ranging from the initial acquisition of test agents to the clinical usage of active drugs (ZUBROD et al., 1966; GOLDIN, 1968; ROTHENBERG and TERSELIC, 1970; GOLDIN and CARTER, in press; GOLDIN et al., in press).

## Selection and Acquisition of Agents for Screening

The initial step in a screening and evaluation program involves the selection and acquistion of agents for screening. The agents to be tested may fall in various categories:

(1) They may be random synthetic compounds supplied by organic chemists.

(2) They may be natural products including fermentation beers and plant extracts, extracts of marine organisms, etc., also collected on a random basis, or on the basis of previous experience with specific fractions, products, or published information.

(3) They may be compounds for which biological activity has been demonstrated in other systems or programs.

(4) They may be acquired on the basis of specific interest in antitumor structure-activity relationships.

(5) They may be acquired on the basis of the compounds being representative of new structural classes.

(6) They may be new structures or analogs developed through various rationales including chemical, biochemical, pharmacologic, or pharmaceutical, or possess pertinent kinetic characteristics in relation to the cell cycle, etc.

The test agents may have special structural characteristics or elicit interesting biological responses which makes their testing desirable. For example, they may have apparent characteristics for crossing the blood brain barrier with potential for activity against intracranial tumor. They may inhibit specific important enzyme systems such as dihydrofolate reductase (OSBORN et al., 1958), thymidylate synthetase (HARTMANN and HEIDELBERGER, 1961), RNA dependent DNA polymerase (GALLO et al., 1971), etc.

The agents or substances tested, where feasible, should be identified with respect to chemical structure, physical constants, solubility, and stability. Any previously demonstrated biological activity is of interest.

## The Choice of Screening Systems

For the purpose of the examination of a large number of candidate agents it is necessary to select suitable test systems. What systems are worthy of selection for large scale screening? Will the systems employed select compounds of clinical therapeutic value?

Historically there has been a large number of systems employed in cancer chemotherapy in programs designed to identify new antitumor agents for the clinic. The initial report of GELLHORN and HIRSCHBERG (1955), "Investigation of Diverse Systems for Cancer Chemotherapy Screening," served as a basis for the historical development of antitumor systems. In the report there is a detailed analysis of screening methodology involving a broad spectrum of test systems. These included experimental tumor systems, as well as systems utilizing bacteriophage, mouse adapted virus, bacteria, and fungi. Also included were differentiation and development systems, biochemical systems, etc. In all, seventy-four biological test systems were presented. Two important conclusions in this comprehensive review should be noted: (a) there was no evidence for the existence of a nontumor system which could replace tumor systems as a screening tool for carcinostatic agents and (b) there was no single tumor which could be expected to select all useful agents; therefore, the utilization of a spectrum of tumors was suggested. Following this report the Cancer Chemotherapy National Service Center (CCNSC)[1] adopted a three tumor screen in its primary screening program including leukemia L 1210, Sarcoma 180, and adenocarcinoma 755 (LEITER and SCHNEIDERMAN, 1959). After an initial experience with these three tumor systems it was considered desirable to examine a large spectrum of tumor systems in order to determine whether they would provide an advantage for identifying chemotherapeutic agents. In the CCNSC program the total number of tumors examined was over 100 (LEITER et al., 1965; GOLDIN et al., 1966a) and concurrently a spectrum of tumors was utilized in a number of laboratories (HADDOW and SEXTON, 1946; STOCK, 1954; STOCK and SUGIURA, 1958; LOUSTALOT et al., 1958; BURCHENAL and HOLMBERG, 1958;

1 Recently designated: Drug Research and Development, Chemotherapy, National Cancer Institute, U.S. Public Health Service.

YOSHIDA, 1958; HIRSCHBERG, 1963; LARIONOV, 1965; TARNOWSKI et al., 1966; ISSEKUTZ, 1969; SELLEI et al., 1970). Subsequently, following over ten years of experience in the screening program of the CCNSC, a retrospective analysis was conducted to identify those systems which might be most useful for continuation of screening (GOLDIN et al., 1966a). In the retrospective analysis it was determined that only a small number of systems was required in order to identify the established clinically active drugs. It was found that the utilization of leukemia L 1210 plus Walker carcinosarcoma 256 (intramuscular) could have identified almost all of the agents as active for the clinic. The Dunning ascites leukemia and adenocarcinoma 755 would have identified several additional compounds as active. Also, it was determined that the same drugs were selected as active by a number of tumor systems, resulting in duplication of results. Thus, it did not appear desirable or necessary to use a large random body of tumor systems and the screen was revised, with greatest emphasis placed on the utilization of the L 1210 and Walker 256 systems. Subsequently, because of a backlog of compounds that are active in the Walker 256 system which have not as yet received clinical trial, this system has largely been kept in abeyance for generalized screening pending the outcome of clinical testing with the new agents. In the current National Cancer Institute of the U.S.A. program there is continuing judicious entry of tumor systems into the screen based on careful analysis of the characteristics of the screen. An important guide that has been employed in the procedure of introducing new tests, pertains to the ability of the screen to identify drugs that have proven active in the clinic and could not be identified by the L 1210 leukemia system. This includes, for example, the P-388 system. This transplanted neoplasm appears to be somewhat more sensitive than the leukemia L 1210 system and was capable of identifying the clinically active drug mithramycin, which was not identified as active by leukemia L1210. The P-388 system appears particularly useful as a tool for the isolation and purification of natural products, including plant fractions and fermentation products, which are in low concentration and for which a highly sensitive system is required to follow further fractionation and purification (VENDITTI and ABBOTT, 1967). The Lewis lung tumor is of interest since it has the unusual property of differential metastasis to the lung following intramuscular inoculation. With this system it is possible to measure the effects of the drug on the local tumor, on the process of metastasis and on the metastasized cells in the lungs (KARRER et al., 1967). The B16 melanoma has a smaller growth fraction and longer doubling time than leukemia L1210 and may not be as sensitive as the L1210 system to the action of drugs.[2] This system is being investigated to determine whether it will identify compounds which may be active against slower growing solid tumors in man (GOLDIN and CARTER, in press). Leukemia L5178Y may be useful for the selection of drugs such as L-asparaginase. Thus, L-asparaginase is active in the L5178Y system, even though it is not active against leukemia L1210 (VADLAMUDI et al., 1970). The P1798 system which identifies prednisone and vincristine as active may be useful for studies of remission induction and maintenance (VADLAMUDI et al., 1971). The AKR system has also been under intensive investigation for this purpose (SCHABEL et al., 1970). Tumors which are naturally resistant to chemotherapy, and tumor sublines made resistant to various drugs, are useful in the study of cross resistance of drugs and provide leads pertaining to mechanism of action and choise of drugs in chemotherapy. For small quantities of test agent an *in vitro* system, such as the KB system (human epidermoid carcinoma), as employed by the CCNSC, may provide information concerning biological activity.

---

2 I. WODINSKY, unpublished data.

## Determination of Drug Activity

Determination is made of the antitumor activity of candidate agents in appropriate screens, and active compounds are then subjected to a decision network program for the first time (ZUBROD et al., 1966; GOLDIN, 1968; ROTHENBERG and TERSELIC, 1970; GOLDIN and CARTER, in press). At this stage of the decision network, there are a series of questions that may be asked which are pertinent to the further development of a candidate agent.

The primary question is: "Are the criteria for activity met in one of the current screens?" If the new agent is active the question arises: "Is the new agent representative of a new chemical class?" If it is, it is acceptable. If it is not and belongs to some specific chemical class for which there has been demonstrated antitumor activity, then its ranking relative to the parent compound becomes critical. Even if it is not superior to the parent compound this question may still be asked: "Does it have any advantageous biological properties?" For example, it might be more soluble or it might be effective by the oral route which is a more convenient mode of administration, it might have activity against intracranial leukemia, it might not be excreted as rapidly, it might not be as toxic in terms of local application, or it might have diminished undesirable host toxicity not specifically related to antitumor effect. In all such cases a decision could be made to investigate the compound further. For compounds of interest additional basic information may be obtained such as the feasibility of producing radioactive materials, the lipid solubility of the compounds, as well as additional physical constants such as the pKa.

If the criteria for effectiveness are not met in one of the current screens, interest in a potential drug could be maintained if it were active in some other appropriate test system. An agent might also be pursued further if it possessed some special metabolic features, or if it suggested promise of enhanced activity in combination with a second active drug.

## Drug Evaluation and Development

In the next phase of drug progression, information is obtained to guide further preclinical pharmacologic studies. It is important to characterize a drug with respect to its schedule dependency characteristics. Determination of optimal scheduling for maximum therapeutic efficacy may provide a basis for preclinical testing. Information concerning the influence of route of administration on toxicity and antitumor effectiveness may likewise be carried into preclinical pharmacology. Certain practical considerations enter at this point. It is necessary to determine the amount of agent that may be needed for further testing and for formulation, pharmacology, and initial clinical trials. Consideration must be given to feasibility of production of required amounts of the compound and to whether the projected costs are reasonable, taking into account the potential of the agent in terms of chemotherapeutic effectiveness. Additional information on solubility and stability may be necessary and should be acquired. If the agent meets the requirements of solubility and stability for parenteral administration, it is possible to prepare the experimental formulation for evaluation. If not, the question arises as to whether the compound is effective orally. If the test agent meets the requirements for effectiveness on oral administration, a decision may be made to proceed with the oral route. The question also arises as to whether or not the agent is absorbed orally in higher animals. If it is insufficiently absorbed it may be necessary either to obtain some means for increased absorption or to discontinue the compound. It is possible that it may not be active orally in the animal tumor test system, but still be absorbed orally in dogs or monkeys, in which case it might be desirable to continue investigation of the agent. It may be necessary in some cases to actually recycle the drug to obtain additional information. In any event, with the above input a decision can be made at this point as to whether or not a drug is of sufficient interest to introduce it into preclinical pharmacology, and if it is, a priority status is established. High priority would be assigned to a highly active agent representing a new class of compounds, or to an analog of a known clinically important agent if it demonstrates considerably improved effectiveness. The priority status could be influenced by factors such as the extent of cross resistance to known antitumor agents, comparative status in extent and manageability of toxicity, rapidity of origin of resistance, solubility, and stability characteristics, and optimal route of administration.

## Some Principles of Screening and Drug Evaluation

Screening systems, which may be selected for routine use, as indicated by Gellhorn-Hirschberg (1955), may be quite diverse in nature. The simplest type of screening system would be one in which there is an attempt to determine whether or not a test agent exerts biological activity. Various types of *in vitro* tests would fall in this category, including the KB tissue-culture test mentioned above, or other types of tissue-culture screens employing normal or transformed cells. Included could be antiviral or antimicrobial screens, screens involving specific enzymatic inhibition related to growth, differentiation, or embryonic development, or various other types of cytotoxicity testing. In general, in this type of screen, there is no attempt to provide a specificity measure against tumor cells, as compared with any effect against normal cells. Such systems, although not providing any specificity measure, may nevertheless be useful in initial drug characterization, particularly, as mentioned above, in situations where a drug is in short supply.

Screening systems may also involve a single parameter of response, even when the drug is administered *in vivo*. This single parameter may pertain to a measurable characteristic of interest with respect to the host. This may include a measurement of the degree of lethal toxicity for the host, or the extent of damage to a specific organ or tissue. Drugs that are capable of producing leukopenia or bone-marrow depression may be of interest for the treatment of leukemia (Anglesio et al., 1958). Drugs that have selective toxicity for a particular organ or tissue may produce selective toxicity for tumors arising in that organ or tissue. In this category may be mentioned *o, p'*-DDD[3], which on the basis of selective toxicity for the adrenal was tested and appears to have activity against carcinoma of the adrenal cortex (Bergenstal et al., 1960). Streptozotocin, which exerts selective toxicity for the cells of the pancreas (Schein et al., 1967), may have selective action against Islet cell tumors (Livingston and Carter, 1970). The testing can be conducted to determine whether a drug exhibits selective uptake or inhibition of an important cellular component, such as deoxyribonucleic acid.

*In vivo* antitumor testing may also involve the measurement of a single parameter of response. This could include the extent of inhibition of tumor growth, cytotoxic action against the tumor, extent of necrosis, inhibition of metastasis, etc. If the observation is limited to measurement of the effect of the drug on the tumor without regard to any possible concomitant deleterious effect against the host, again, no precise measure is provided of the specificity of action of the drug (Goldin et al., 1961; Goldin, 1968; Goldin and Carter, in press).

---

3 (NSC-38721) ethane, 1,1-dichloro-2-(*o*-chlorophenyl)-2-(*p*-chlorophenyl).

In general, however, the screening and evaluation programs that have been in current use do attempt to provide a measure of drug effectiveness against tumor relative to a limiting effect with respect to the host and, thus, do provide some measure of antitumor specificity (GOLDIN et al., 1961; GOLDIN, 1968; GOLDIN and CARTER, in press).

Where the interest is to compare several drugs, or to compare regimens for the same drug, the problem of drug evaluation is a complex one. It can perhaps be simplified by thinking in terms of the current status of accomplishment and further objectives (MANTEL, 1961, 1962; GOLDIN et al., 1967; GOLDIN, 1968; GOLDIN and CARTER, in press). In some initial stage of attack on a disease situation, the interest may focus on obtaining any moderate prolongation of life. If that goal has been achieved, an attempt may be made to obtain somewhat more extensive prolongation of life, and hopefully some cures. If a therapy has become available which yields some cures, the next step would be to obtain one that yields many if not 100% cures (SKIPPER et al., 1964; GOLDIN, 1969). Yet other successive objectives could include early cure, or curative therapies which minimize certain costs, such as length of hospital stay or requirement of skilled personnel to administer the therapy. An objective of merely reducing drug requirements per se in achieving cure is ordinarily not important, unless it is accompanied by some other important objective, such as reduction of toxicity risk without loss of therapeutic effectiveness. But in instances of limited drug availability, such reduction in drug requirements may become essential.

The processes for identification of useful drugs and determination of optimal modalities undergo progressive development. Where laboratory rather than clinical disease is used for screening and evaluating drugs and drug therapies, research should also be of a progressive nature, with test animals being regarded as representative of patients for whom it is desired to achieve the best possible therapy. This approach has characterized the programs employing primarily leukemia L1210 mice, in seeking effective experimental tumor therapies and has been described in several review articles (GOLDIN et al., 1961; MANTEL, 1961, 1962; GOLDIN et al., 1967; GOLDIN, 1968; GOLDIN and CARTER, in press).

In working with experimental tumor-bearing mice a major obstacle to effective chemotherapy has been the toxicity of the host of the agents employed. But this toxicity provided a means for assessing the value of alternative therapies. The better therapy it was reasoned, was the one yielding the largest antitumor effect for a given amount of damage to the host. Since, in the initial studies, drug administration was on a limited basis, it was possible to assess host toxicity by the frequency of early death, while the amount of antitumor damage could be assessed by the prolongation in life of mice surviving beyond the period of early toxic death (GOLDIN et al., 1953). This approach permitted the identification of a compound such as methotrexate as superior to aminopterin even though the antitumor effects of methotrexate were evidenced only at relatively high dosages (GOLDIN et al., 1955b). Also, the approach was independent of one in which the therapeutic index was used to assess drugs. The therapeutic index is the ratio of drug dosage yielding some defined degree of toxic effect for the host to the dosage yielding some defined antitumor effect (GOLDIN et al., 1961). Where the index is high, protection is provided against inadvertently producing undesired toxicity in the host, but no assurance is provided of a suitably great antitumor effect. Two agents with equal therapeutic indices can differ widely in their therapeutic efficacies, while of two agents, the one with the lower therapeutic index can have the greater therapeutic efficacy (GOLDIN et al., 1961). Nevertheless, for two agents of equal therapeutic efficacy the one with the higher therapeutic index could be employed with the greater margin of safety.

Subsequently, it was necessary to modify the therapeutic efficacy approach, since in using repeated treatment schedules it was not possible to make an effective separation of antitumor and antihost effects. Patterns were observed, however, in which with increasing dosage levels survival time of tumor-bearing mice would initially increase, but beyond the level at which toxicity for the host started to become important, survival times would typically decrease (GOLDIN et al., 1956a; SKIPPER and SCHMIDT, 1962; GOLDIN and VENDITTI, 1962). It was reasoned that the determination of average or median survival time for deaths from any cause, whether from toxicity or due to the malignancy, could provide a means for taking into account both antitumor and antihost effects simultaneously. A summary measure of the efficacy of a drug on a particular regimen was provided by the maximum median survival time which could be elicited with it, irrespective of the dose level at which the maximum occurred (SKIPPER and SCHMIDT, 1962; GOLDIN and VENDITTI, 1962). Because a relatively narrow series of dose levels was used, increasing by factors of only 1.5 or 2, the observed maximum could be considered to be a close approximation of what would have occurred at the unknown true optimum dose. In conducting these studies it is generally advantageous in new situations to use a wide range of dosage levels so as to ensure bracketing the optimum dose. This is particularly important since when drugs are given in repeated doses, some will be much more toxic, others less toxic, than when given as a single dose.

In keeping with the objective of finding effective therapies, comparison is made not only of different drugs (GOLDIN et al., 1960; VENDITTI et al., 1960; SKIPPER and SCHMIDT, 1962; GOLDIN and VENDITTI, 1962), but also a series of studies should be conducted to identify factors which might influence drug effectiveness (GOLDIN, 1968; GOLDIN and CARTER, in press). The same drug administered on different treatment schedules (GOLDIN et al., 1955c, 1956a; VENDITTI et al., 1964; GOLDIN and VENDITTI, 1970; VENDITTI, in press) or by different routes (VENDITTI et al., 1960) could elicit differing therapeutic responses. The time of initiation of therapy could have a marked effect on the therapeutic outcome, with drugs, in general, showing diminished effectiveness against advanced disease (GOLDIN et al., 1954, 1956a; GOLDIN, 1969). One interesting observation was that the antitumor efficacy of a drug could be heightened by appropriate use of an agent antagonistic to its action. Thus, while citrovorum factor reduced the therapeutic efficacy of aminopterin against leukemia L1210 when administered simultaneously or in advance of aminopterin treatment, it could be employed to enhance efficiency by using a 12 to 24 hour delay (GOLDIN et al., 1953). Similar observations have been made with methotrexate (GOLDIN et al., 1966b; SANDBERG and GOLDIN, 1970).

A point was reached in the program where with treatment initiated relatively early it was routinely possible to produce extensive survival times and even some cures of the L1210 leukemia, even though in the interim the challenge had been increased by raising the tumor cell inoculum. The next step then is to duplicate the clinical situation more closely. In treating early experimental leukemia, the "mouse-patients" do not yet display overt neoplasia, as would be true in the clinical situation. The clinical situation could, however, be paralleled by simply delaying initiation until advanced systemic disease was manifest and the mice were within a day or two of dying. Working with so extreme a challenge it was possible initially to produce moderate extensions in survival time. Eventually, however, with advanced leukemia L1210, drugs and regimens were found that elicited progressively better results ranging from rather prolonged survival times to some cures and, finally, to many cures. Noteworthy, were the outstanding successes obtained with two halogenated derivatives of methotrexate, 3′, 5′-dichloroamethopterin and 3′-bromo-5′-chloroamethopterin (GOLDIN et al., 1959). The required dosage levels were considerably greater than with other folic acid antagonists, and it would appear that it was the lesser host toxicity without reduced antitumor effect of these halogenated derivatives that permitted the achievement of greater antitumor effects.

Additional approaches have been taken. In one study (VENDITTI et al., 1957), methotrexate therapy was discontinued at various times as a way of investigating the possibility that cures had been achieved, but that mice were succumbing to chronic toxicity; in that particular study no advantage was found in the discontinuation of therapy. In yet another investigation, the therapy employed was tailored to the individual mouse. Treatment could be delayed for a mouse where there had been body weight loss or overt signs of toxicity (GOLDIN et al., 1955a). In this study management of mouse leukemia L 1210 was accomplished by the employment of a combination of spaced treatment with aminopterin or methotrexate plus delayed administration of citrovorum factor. Other studies were directed to isolating the nonspecific effects of agents. Any agent that was harmful to the host could produce indirect inhibition of tumor growth. Where the antihost effect resulted in weight loss an equivalent weight loss could be obtained through caloric restriction and any resulting antitumor effect could be observed (GOLDIN et al., 1949; SKIPPER et al., 1963). This approach could be particularly relevant in the early stages of an antitumor screen. Other implications of the studies of factors influencing drug effectiveness to antitumor screening methodology have been previously discussed (GOLDIN et al., 1961; MANTEL, 1961, 1962; SKIPPER et al., 1964; GOLDIN, 1968, 1969; GOLDIN and CARTER, in press).

With increasing increments of therapeutic advantage in animal test systems and in the clinic, current emphasis has been on the development and employment of models involving the total eradication of tumor cell populations (GOLDIN et al., 1956b; SKIPPER et al., 1964; SCHABEL et al., 1965; WILCOX et al., 1966; KLINE et al., 1966; BRUCE et al., 1966; GOLDIN, 1969). Drugs may be compared with respect to the degree to which they can eradicate tumor cells. The number of tumor cells destroyed may be estimated by direct count, by transplantation bioassay to recipient animals, by calculation based on the survival time of treated groups and untreated controls, and by measuring the number of tumor-free survivors. The effectiveness of therapy in producing tumor-free survivors may be measured at a series of inoculum concentrations. It has been demonstrated in such studies that the ability of an agent to produce tumor-free survivors may be influenced by a variety of factors including the number of tumor cells present, the schedule of therapy, the degree of metastases and the extent of intracranial disease (GOLDIN, 1969).

An empirical approach is featured in much of the investigations in which each form of therapy is tested to determine whether it is capable of producing a greatly improved result. Kinetic models have been developed and the extent to which experimental data can be usefully interpreted in terms of parameter estimates corresponding to such models is limited only by a knowledge of the precise dynamics of the antitumor and antihost processes. A model, however, can be useful even if not precise, with appropriate recognition of its limitations. For example, drug treatment can produce damage to the tumor with some tumor cells destroyed or made nonviable, while others suffer varying degrees of reversible or irreversible damage. This type of response involving varying degrees of tumor cell injury can be approximated, particularly in the short term, by considering a fixed percentage-kill model in which some percentage of cells is destroyed, the remainder being unaffected. The model directs attention to conducting experiments with a view to rapidly maximizing the cell kill percentage by administration of a large dosage of drug and to the obtaining of the most precise estimates of that percentage. In another approach it may be reasoned that if the damage to the tumor following therapy with relatively small doses of drug is not more than compensated for by cell recovery, then on prolongation of therapy the tumor may at least be kept under control and extended survival times and perhaps even some cures may be achieved. The sequence of experiments which one might perform employing these two approaches could be quite different. The choice of approach including scheduling and dosage may be guided by the cell cycle characteristics of the drug under test, as well as the characteristics of the tumor system. Under any circumstance, total eradication of the tumor is the ultimate objective of both approaches, and these may merge if the results suggested by a cell-kill model are repeatedly checked out by experiments directed at achieving prolonged survival or cures in a high challenge situation.

The overall approaches outlined above have been extended to investigations of viral induced leukemia in which viral induction of tumor and reinduction constitute additional parameters in the study of drug action (CHIRIGOS et al., 1961; GLYNN et al., 1963, 1964; CHIRIGOS, 1964; SCHABEL et al., 1969; SKIPPER et al., 1969).

## Preclinical Toxicology

Following drug evaluation and development, active agents may be entered into preclinical toxicology. At this point two activities are engaged in, somewhat concurrently, including (a) the toxicology in dogs and monkeys, and (b) the production and formulation for clinical trial (ZUBROD et al., 1966; GOLDIN, 1968; ROTHENBERG and TERSELIC, 1970) (the reader is referred to "An Outline of Procedures for Preliminary Toxicologic and Pharmacologic Evaluation of Experimental Cancer Chemotherapeutic Agents," 1964).

The toxicology in dogs and monkeys is conducted taking into account the information pertaining to schedule and route dependency and allied data obtained in the previous studies. With both dogs and monkeys, the primary objectives are to determine the largest nontoxic dose and to identify the nature of the toxicity. Factors taken into account include major organ toxicity, the predictability of the toxicity and the dose-response characteristics of the drug. If the toxicity curve of a drug is steep, more caution must be exercised in dose adjustment upward. Additional queries include: Is the toxicity manageable and reversible? To what extent is there consistency with respect to the quantitative and qualitative nature of the toxicity among species? If the input data are adequate, if there is qualitative and quantitative consistency between species, and if the toxicity of the drug does not mitigate against its use in man, then the drug may be selected for clinical trial. The preclinical toxicology is summarized including a listing of the tolerated doses in mg/kg and also in mg/m$^2$ for each species and the scheduling and route information. Notation is made of potential toxicity for man and this is incorporated with the data pertaining to the therapeutic trials in animals. Specific recommendations are then made for clinical trial.

If there is not internal consistency in the toxicologic findings, consideration may be given to the utilization of other species for further toxicologic study. The question may also arise as to whether the drug should be tested in any special systems and whether additional information should be obtained on other characteristics such as the physiological disposition, in which case the drug may be recycled. On the basis of internal inconsistency or because of undesirable characteristics, forward movement of a drug to the clinic may have to be discontinued.

For active compounds, production and formulation are necessary prior to limited clinical trials. It must be determined that the initial bulk drug is authentic and adequately pure. The formulation must also be determined to be authentic and adequately pure and acceptable for clinical trials. Failure to obtain appropriate formulation of a drug could necessitate deferral of its use.

With favorable input data on toxicity in dogs and monkeys and with appropriate formulation any positive decision to move to the clinic is facilitated. It remains to determine the priority for initial clinical trial, and this is done on the basis of the results of both the chemical and biological characterization of the compound.

## Clinical Evaluation

Chemotherapy programs encompass three phases of clinical evaluation of a new agent, which are specific modifications of the phases required by the United States Food and Drug Administration (GOLDIN and CARTER, in press). These are outlined below:

*Outline of Clinical Evaluation of New Drugs Developed by the National Cancer Institute of the U.S.A.*

Phase I. Clinical pharmacology in advanced cancer patients with or without measurable disease

1. Establish maximally tolerated dose.
2. Establish parameters of toxicity.
3. Pharmacologic evaluation.
4. Antitumor activity not required.

Phase II. Survey for clinical activity in patients with measurable or evaluable disease

1. Nonrandomized studies.
2. 10 to 20 patients in 6 "signal" tumors.
   a) Adenocarcinoma of colon.
   b) Bronchogenic carcinoma.
   c) Adenocarcinoma of breast.
   d) Undifferentiated lymphosarcoma.
   e) Acute myelocytic leukemia.
   f) Acute lymphocytic leukemia.

Phase III. Definitive studies to establish role in cancer therapy armamentarium

1. Controlled clinical trials.
2. Combination studies.

Phase I is limited to clinical pharmacology. The patients who are studied have advanced neoplastic disease and are refractory to standard therapies for their disease. Their estimated survival should be at least two months. It is not required that the disease be measurable or evaluable. The accomplishment of clinical response, although most noteworthy when it occurs, is not essential to evaluation at this stage. The objective is to establish the maximally tolerated dose at the schedule used and to establish the parameters of toxicity. If a tolerated dose can be achieved with toxicity that is predictable, treatable, and reversible, then Phase II trials are begun.

Phase II trial involves a survey for clinical activity against a panel of six signal tumor types. The survey is designed to test for drug activity against tumors which are kinetically described as "fast growing" (leukemia, lymphoma) and "slow growing" (colon, breast, lung). In the studies the patients are ordinarily nonrandomized. Patients are required who are clearly evaluable as to response, having in most

Table 1. *Comparison of experimental and clinical activity of antitumor agents*

| | Rating in two animal tumor test systems[a] | | Pooled data for evaluation of 18 commonly used agents in seven common solid tumor types given in % with numerator and denominator in ( ) | | | | | | |
|---|---|---|---|---|---|---|---|---|---|
| | L1210 leukemia ILS (%) | Walker 256 carcinosarcoma (IM) TWI (%) | Adenocarcinoma of the colon | Adenocarcinoma of the breast | Bronchogenic carcinoma | Malignant melanoma | Ovarian cancer | Head and neck cancer | Cervix and uterine cancer |
| I. Alkylating agents | | | | | | | | | |
| Cyclophosphamide | 80 | 90 | 16 (7/43) | 32 (60/139) | 33 (168/509) | 26 (8/31) | 44 (115/262) | 36 (28/77) | 19 (36/187) |
| Nitrogen mustard | 55 | 62 | 12 (6/50) | 34 (33/98) | 21 (81/391) | 9 (3/34) | 45 (4/9) | 7.5 (5/66) | 0 (0/12) |
| Chlorambucil | 31 | 84 | 9 (5/55) | 20 (11/54) | 8 (2/23) | 9 (2/22) | 52 (222/422) | 15 (5/34) | 25 (11/44) |
| Melphalan (phenylalanine mustard) | 75 | 95 | 15 (12/82) | 23 (20/86) | 10.5 (4/38) | 12 (8/66) | 47 (173/367) | NE | 20 (4/20) |
| Busulfan | 4 | 80 | 10 (1/10) | 0 (0/8) | 32 (6/19) | 10 (1/10) | NE | NE | NE |
| II. Antimetabolites | | | | | | | | | |
| Methotrexate | 100 | 95 | 17 (19/111) | 34 (120/356) | 33 (56/167) | 9 (2/26) | NE | 43.5 (101/232) | 20 (5/25) intra-arterial 46 (33/71) |
| 5-Fluorouracil | 60 | 72 | 24 (305/1270) | 28 (323/1152) | 7.5 (12/158) | 2.5 (1/42) | 32 (32/101) | 15 (18/118) | 25 (48/195) |
| 6-Mercaptopurine | 50 | 86 | 5 (4/75) | 13 (6/45) | 4 (4/95) | 7 (2/30) | 6 (1/17) | 12 (6/45) | NE |

Table 1 (Continued)

| | | | | | | | | | |
|---|---|---|---|---|---|---|---|---|---|
| Arabinosyl cytosine | 94 | 32 | 10<br>(10/103) | 9<br>(6/65) | 0<br>(0/60) | 2<br>(1/51) | NE | NE | NE |
| III. Vinca alkaloids | | | | | | | | | |
| Vincristine | 39 | 80 | 0<br>(0/26) | 21<br>(47/226) | 9<br>(4/43) | 12<br>(6/53) | 0<br>(0/17) | NE | 29<br>(10/34) |
| Vinblastine | 40 | 89 | 7<br>(5/71) | 20<br>(19/95) | 11<br>(12/109) | 15<br>(8/54) | 15<br>(3/20) | 29<br>(10/35) | NE |
| IV. Antibiotics | | | | | | | | | |
| Actinomycin D | 45 | 65 | 15<br>(7/48) | 11<br>(5/45) | 0<br>(0/16) | 33<br>(19/58) | NE | 0<br>(0/11) | NE |
| Mithramycin | 13 | 36 | 16<br>(4/25) | 16<br>(5/32) | 0<br>(0/13) | 15<br>(2/13) | NE | NE | NE |
| Daunorubicin | 58 | 90 | 0<br>(0/2) | 0<br>(0/2) | 0<br>(0/5) | 0<br>(0/6) | NE | NE | NE |
| V. Miscellaneous agents | | | | | | | | | |
| Hydroxyurea | 45 | 47 | 7<br>(4/59) | 19<br>(4/21) | 11<br>(4/36) | 22<br>(47/213) | NE | 39<br>(7/18) | 15<br>(2/13) |
| Procarbazine (Natulan) | 45 | 75 | 20<br>(1/5) | 5<br>(1/21) | 15<br>(26/172) | 18<br>(6/32) | 14<br>(1/7) | NE | NE |
| Imidazole carbox-amide (DTIC) | 55 | 60 | 11<br>(8/71) | 10<br>(4/41) | 10<br>(8/81) | 20<br>(81/419) | 0<br>(0/4) | 0<br>(0/22) | 33<br>(3/9) |
| 1,3-*Bis*(2 chloro-ethyl)-1-nitrosourea (BCNU) | 150 | 98 | 13<br>(17/128) | 35<br>(15/43) | 9<br>(4/46) | 20<br>(17/84) | NE | 16<br>(4/25) | 14<br>(1/7) |

[a] Animal data from Drug Research and Development (see GOLDIN et al., 1966a). For clinical data see LIVINGSTON and CARTER (1970). ILS = % increase in survival time as compared with controls. TWI = Percent inhibition of local tumors; IM = intramuscular inoculation. NE = nonevaluable.

cases measurable indicator lesions. For each signal tumor type the objective response rate is studied in at least 15 to 20 evaluable patients.

Adenocarcinoma of the breast and colon and bronchogenic carcinoma are used to screen against the slow growing tumors which are the most resistant to chemotherapeutic attack. The acute leukemias and lymphoma have been chosen for test against the rapidly growing and more chemotherapeutically sensitive tumor types. It is felt that this kind of disease oriented Phase II trial is superior to the often used general Phase II trial in which a wide range of tumor types are treated, but with numbers for each type usually not large enough to give meaningful results. It is not uncommon in the older literature to see a drug described as inactive based on a low percent of response in 50 or more patients, and to see that only 2 or 3 patients with colon cancer or breast cancer were treated.

In addition, other important parameters of drug action are taken into account. If the agent is a new chemical structure greater interest is shown. Currently, a higher priority is given to agents which are cell-cycle insensitive and have demonstrated the ability to kill nonproliferating cells. Greater emphasis is placed on drugs which can attack cells in pharmacologic sanctuaries such as the central nervous system. Suitability for combination chemotherapy, e.g., lack of bone marrow toxicity, also upgrades interest in moving a drug forward in clinical trial.

If acceptable activity, taking into account the above characteristics, is demonstrated in any of the signal tumors, Phase III trial is begun. This is a definitive study designed to establish the role of the drug in the armamentarium of the clinical oncologist. Discussion of these later trials is outside of the scope of this chapter.

The determination of clinical activity for the six signal tumor types and its correlation with the experimental screen depends significantly on the definition of an adequate trial for a new antitumor agent. As a minimum, an adequate trial requires that a drug be administered in the range of the maximum tolerated dose and on an adequate dosage schedule. Drugs selected by a highly quantitative system such as leukemia L1210 may only tentatively be classified as false positives if, for example, because of poor absorption, systemic inactivation, or limiting toxicity for the modality of therapy employed, they have not received an adequate trial. It would be unfair to label a drug as "inactive" until it has been adequately tested in at least 10 to 15 evaluable patients in the six signal tumor types, and found to have insufficient clinical activity in all of them. In keeping with this reasoning, the Cancer Therapy Evaluation Branch of the National Cancer Institute has instituted an intensive review of all cancer chemotherapeutic agents to see how many have been adequately evaluated by these standards, and to provide a historical background for the data rapidly developing on the new investigational agents. Table 1 is an outline of the data available on the clinical antitumor activity of the commonly used commercially available agents in the seven common solid tumor types. The data are given in percent objective response rate with the actual number of responses per total number of patients in parenthesis. Also included are the ratings for antitumor activity in two experimental test systems, leukemia L1210 and Walker 256 carcinosarcoma (GOLDIN et al., 1966a; GOLDIN and CARTER, in press).

It is clear from this data that most of these drugs have not been fully tested against all seven of these solid tumors. These findings also reveal how tenuous a practice it is to list false positives for any particular preclinical screen for antitumor agents.

Data such as the above do not even begin to take into account the question of whether an adequate dosage schedule was used. In Table 2 are listed the pooled

Table 2. *Pooled clinical data available for cyclophosphamide treatment of solid tumors broken down by dosage schedule given in % with numerator and denominator in parentheses*

| | Intravenous loading dose followed by oral maintenance | Chronic daily to toxicity oral or I.V. | Weekly intravenous | High single dose intermittent (every 2 to 4 wks) intravenous |
|---|---|---|---|---|
| Adenocarcinoma of the colon | 12.5 (2/16) | 0 (0/2) | 0 (0/7) | 100 (3/3) |
| Adenocarcinoma of the breast | 26 (19/73) | 41 (30/74) | 20 (5/25) | NE |
| Bronchogenic carcinoma | 34 (109/317) | 39 (36/93) | 10 (3/30) | 40 (14/35) |
| Malignant melanoma | 25 (4/16) | 30 (3/10) | NE | 8 (1/12) |
| Ovarian cancer | 36 (27/74) | 52 (77/148) | 42 (3/7) | NE |
| Head and neck cancer | Data not sufficiently broken by schedule for analysis | | | |
| Cervix and uterine | 20 (30/147) | 0 (0/2) | 10 (1/10) | NE |

NE = Not evaluable. See LIVINGSTON and CARTER (1970).

clinical data available on cyclophosphamide, grouped in accordance with the schedule used. In the leukemia L1210 system, cyclophosphamide has been shown to be schedule dependent, being most effective in increasing survival time on an intermittent schedule (single dose intermittent with an interval of one week or longer) (LANE, 1959; VENDITTI et al., 1959). On referring to Table 2, it becomes apparent that this highly active drug has had either minimal or no trial in solid tumors on what may be its most active schedule, namely, single large dose intermittent administration. Cyclophosphamide is not considered to be an active agent in the treatment of adenocarcinoma of the colon and in a correlation of activity in an experimental system (such as the L1210 leukemia) and colon cancer, this drug would undoubtedly be listed as a false positive. Yet the data to support this is evidently not available.

Methotrexate is another excellent example of the importance of schedule and the hazards of too simplistic approaches to labeling drugs as inactive. This drug, like cyclophosphamide, is in general not considered to be significantly active against colon carcinoma. The overall response rate from the literature is 15% (19/125) (LIVINGSTON and CARTER, 1970), which is within the range of activity reported for 5-fluorouracil, the standard chemotherapeutic agent for the advanced metastatic stage of this disease. In Table 3 the data for methotrexate in this disease are evaluated in accordance with schedule (CONDIT et al., 1962; WILSON and LOUIS, 1965; ANDREWS and WILSON, 1967; SULLIVAN et al., 1967; MOERTEL et al., 1970), (the reader is referred to "Eastern Cooperative Group in Solid Tumor Chemotherapy. Comparison of Antimetabolites in the Treatment of Breast and Colon Cancer," 1967). When this is done it appears that the most common schedule, a monthly loading dose, has quite a low response rate, but that other schedules, with unfortunately very small numbers, give hints of quite acceptable activity. It is worth noting in this context that trials of the twice weekly or weekly schedule have apparently not been reported in the literature.

Arabinosyl cytosine (Ara-C) is still another good example of the problem. This drug is a relatively new agent in cancer chemotherapy. It is a direct and specific

Table 3. *Methotrexate in colon cancer evaluated by schedule*

| Schedule | No. patients evaluable | No. patients responding | % Responding | Ref. |
|---|---|---|---|---|
| I. Daily single dose | | | | |
| (1) 2 to 5 mg/day P.O. | 6 | 2 | 33 | WILSON and LOUIS (1965) |
| II. Divided daily dose schedule or infusion | | | | |
| (1) 1.25 mg q.i.d. P.O. = 5 mg/day × 5 to 10 days. Repeat when toxicity allows or 5 mg/24 h continuous I.V. Infusion × 5 to 10 days | 17 | 7 | 41 | SULLIVAN et al. (1967) |
| (2) 50 mg/kg Q12h until toxicity or response | 22 | 2 | 9 | MOERTEL et al. (1970) |
| Total | 39 | 9 | 23 | |
| III. High single dose intermittent | | | | |
| (1) 2.5 to 10 mg/kg I.V. Q2 wks. | 12 | 3 | 25 | CONDIT et al. (1962) |
| IV. Monthly leading dose | | | | |
| (1) 0.4 mg/kg/day × 4, then 0.2 mg/kg every other day × 4; repeat in 4 wks. | 40 | 4 | 10 | Eastern Cooperative Group in Solid Tumor Chemotherapy (1967) |
| (2) 0.2 mg/kg/day × 4, then 0.1 mg/kg every other day × 4 P.O.; repeat day 42 | 14 | 1 | 7 | ANDREWS and WILSON (1967) |
| Total | 54 | 5 | 9 | |

inhibitor of DNA synthesis, which may act primarily as an inhibitor of DNA polymerase (FURTH and COHEN, 1968). Ara-C has been shown to have optimal therapeutic effectiveness in the treatment of early leukemia L1210 on an intermittent schedule in which doses are given spaced closely together (every 3 hours, every 4 days) (SKIPPER et al., 1967) (Table 4). In cancer of the colon this drug has only been evaluated on a daily I.V. push for 10 consecutive days schedule. On this schedule a 13% (10/77) response rate has been reported (LIVINGSTON and CARTER, 1970). Based on experimental systems this is a highly inferior schedule and one can only wonder what results exploitation of a possibly more optimal schedule would achieve. The same can be said for hydroxyurea, which is also a specific DNA

Table 4. *Influence of treatment schedule on the antileukemic efficacy of cytosine arabinoside*

| Treatment schedule | Dose range (mg/kg/day) | Optimal dose (mg/kg/day) | % ILS |
|---|---|---|---|
| Daily, days 1—9 | 14— 65 | 39 | 100 |
| Day 1 only, every 3 hours | 500—2313 | 2313 | 33 |
| | 67— 312 | 184 | 78 |
| Days 1, 5, 9, every 3 hours | 500—2313 | 2313 | 128(1) |
| | 40— 184 | 112, 184 | >400(7) |

$1 \times 10^5$ L1210 ascites, i.p.; () = No. of 45-day survivors out of 10 mice.
Data of I. KLINE et al., unpublished observations.
ILS = % increase in life span compared with controls.

synthesis inhibitor and which has identical schedule dependency with Ara-C. This drug has also been reported to have no activity in colon cancer (6/80 = 7.5%) (LIVINGSTON and CARTER, 1970). But again only a few schedules have been used.

The stage of development of the disease may have a profound effect on schedule dependency. Additional studies with Ara-C in the L1210 leukemia system reveal that the schedule dependency involving "around the clock" therapy every 4 days, so marked in the treatment of early leukemia L1210, is less evident for the advanced disease (Table 5). In the treatment of acute myelocytic leukemia with Ara-C, activity has been found on a wide range of schedules, with no clear cut superiority for any of them (Table 6) (HENDERSON and BURKE, 1965; ELLISON et al., 1968; BODEY et al., 1969; CAREY, 1970; GOODELL et al., 1971). The possibility exists that schedule dependency of Ara-C in experimental tumors and in the clinic may be manifest primarily for earlier stages of disease. It is suggested by the observations in the L1210 system that precise correspondence of modalities of therapy in the animal system and the clinic may require detailed analysis of factors, such as stage of disease, in influencing schedule dependency. This in turn, may permit more appropriate assignment of drug scheduling in accordance with patient status.

Table 5. *Comparison of cytosine arabinoside schedule in the treatment of early and advanced leukemia L1210*

| Treatment schedule | Early leukemia IP treatment days 1—9 | | Advanced leukemia IP treatment days 5—13 | |
|---|---|---|---|---|
| | Optimal dose (mg/kg/day) | % ILS | Optimal dose (mg/kg/day) | % ILS |
| *One injection/day* | | | | |
| Daily | 39 | 89 | 23, 39 | 89 |
| Every 2 days | 833 | 178 (1) | 833 | 128 |
| Every 4 days | 2320 | 100 | 2320 | 89 |
| Every 8 days | 2320 | 67 | 2320 | 39 |
| *Eight injections/day* (every 3 hours) | | | | |
| Daily | — | — | — | — |
| Every 2 days | 40 | 222 (3) | 67 | 133 |
| Every 4 days | 184 | >422 (4) | 184 | 122 |
| Every 8 days | 184 | 111 | 184 | 61 |

$1 \times 10^5$ L1210 ascites, i.p.; () = No. of 45-day survivors out of 10 mice.
Data of I. KLINE et al., unpublished observations.
ILS = % increase in life span compared with controls.

Thus, the major point deserving of emphasis is that the labeling of a drug as false positive for a given screening system is not a simple procedure and depends on a rigorous definition of what constitutes an adequate clinical trial. On examining the details of schedule dependency, with its experimental and clinical correlations, it becomes necessary to face the possibility that very few cancer chemotherapeutic agents have been completely characterized. Similarly, correlations of animal and clinical drug action and effectiveness require characterization of other factors influencing drug effectiveness in animal tumor systems and the clinic. Rigorous employment of current and new model test systems is most important to the discovery and optimal application of new antitumor agents with salutary action against clinical neoplasia.

Table 6. *Cytosine arabinoside therapy of acute myelocytic leukemia*

| Group | Regimen | No. Evaluable Cases | No. Cases Responding | % Response |
|---|---|---|---|---|
| Acute leukemia Group B (ELLISON et al., 1968) | 10 $mg/m^2$/day by 12-hour infusion | 12 | 2 | (17) |
| | 10 $mg/m^2$/day by 24-hour infusion | 9 | 2 | (22) |
| | 30 $mg/m^2$/day by 12-hour infusion | 41 | 10 | (23) |
| | 30 $mg/m^2$/day by 24-hour infusion | 36 | 2 | (6) |
| | 30 $mg/m^2$/day by 1-hour infusion | 16 | 3 | (18) |
| | 50 $mg/m^2$/day by 1-hour infusion | 19 | 4 | (21) |
| | 100 $mg/m^2$/day by 1-hour infusion | 20 | 5 | (25) |
| | 30 $mg/m^2$/day by 4-hour infusion | 25 | 3 | (12) |
| (CAREY, 1970) | 100 $mg/m^2$/day by 1-hour infusion | 43 | 6 | (14) |
| Southwest Cancer Chemotherapy Study Group (BODEY et al., 1969)[a] | 800 $mg/m^2$ 48-hour infusion, repeat in 14 days | 55 | 11 | (20) |
| | 1000 $mg/m^2$ 120-hour infusion, repeat in 14 days | 57 | 16 | (28) |
| NCI (HENDERSON, BURKE, 1965; GOODELL et al., 1971) | 75 $mg/m^2$/day given as 15 $mg/m^2$ push and 60 $mg/m^2$ 4-hour infusion × 4 repeated in 4 days | 25 | 11 | (44) |
| Southeastern Cancer Study Group[b] | 100 to 200 $mg/m^2$/wk by 24-hour infusion × 4 to 8 | 5 | 0 | (0) |
| | 100 to 200 $mg/m^2$ twice weekly by 24-hour infusion × 1 to 8 weeks | 9 | 1 | (11) |
| | 20 to 100 mg/day by 120-hour continuous infusion | 13 | 2 | (15) |
| | 50 to 100 mg/day by 72-hour continuous infusion | 3 | 0 | (0) |
| Western Cooperative Cancer Chemotherapy Group[c] | 500 $mg/m^2$ Q2 wks by 2-hour infusion with escalations of 250 $mg/m^2$ at each injection (up to 3000 $mg/m^2$) | 5 | 0 | (0) |
| | 500 $mg/m^2$ Q2 wks by 6-hour infusion with escalation of 250 $mg/m^2$ (up to 1750 $mg/m^2$) | 8 | 2 | (25) |
| Pacific VA[d] | 20 to 35 $mg/m^2$ Q3h × 8 Q4 days × 4 courses | 9 | 0 | (0) |
| | 500 $mg/m^2$/24 h Q3h × 8 on days 1, 3, 6, 8, 11, 13 | 4 | 1 | (25) |

[a] Also FREIREICH, E. Personal Communication.
[b] HUGULEY, C. Personal Communication.
[c] BATEMAN, J. Personal Communication.
[d] BROOKE, J. Personal Communication.

## References


An outline of procedures for preliminary toxicologic and pharmacologic evaluation of experimental cancer chemotherapeutic agents. Cancer Chemother. Rep. 37, 1—34 (1964).

ANDREWS, N. C., WILSON, W. L.: Phase II study of methotrexate (NSC-740) in solid tumors. Cancer Chemother. Rep. 51, 471—474 (1967).

ANGLESIO, E., HIRSCHBERG, E., GELLHORN, A.: Effects of carcinostatic and other biologically active compounds in the normal rat: evaluation as a system for cancer chemotherapy screening. Cancer Res. 18, 113—116 (1958).

BERGENSTAL, D. M., HERTZ, R., LIPSETT, M., MOY, R. H.: Chemotherapy of adrenocortical cancer with *o,p′*-DDD. Ann. int. Med. 53, 672—682 (1960).

BODEY, G., FREIREICH, E., MONTO, R. W., HEWLETT, J. S.: Cytosine arabinoside (NSC-63878) therapy for acute leukemia in adults. Cancer Chemother. Rep. **53**, 59—66 (1969).

BRUCE, W. R., MEEKER, B. E., VALERIOTE, F. A.: Comparison of the sensitivity of normal hematopoietic and transplanted lymphoma colony-forming cells to chemotherapeutic agents administered in vivo. J. nat. Cancer Inst. **37**, 233—245 (1966).

BURCHENAL, J. H., HOLMBERG, E. A. D.: The utility of resistant leukemias in screening for chemotherapeutic activity. Ann. N. Y. Acad. Sci. **76**, 826—837 (1958).

CAREY, R. W.: Comparative study of cytosine arabinoside (CA) therapy alone and combined with thioguanine (TG), mercaptopurine (MP) or daunomycin (DN) in acute myelocytic leukemia (AML). Proc. Amer. Assoc. Cancer Res. **11**, 15 (1970).

CHIRIGOS, M. A.: Studies with the murine leukemogenic Rauscher virus. III. An *in vivo* assay for antiviral agents. Cancer Res. **24**, 1035—1041 (1964).

CHIRIGOS, M. A., MOLONEY, J. B., HUMPHREYS, S. R., MANTEL, N., GOLDIN, A.: Response of a virus-induced murine lymphoid leukemia to drug therapy. Cancer Res. **21**, 803—811 (1961).

CONDIT, P., SHNIDER, B., OWENS, A.: Studies on the folic acid vitamins VII. The effect of large doses of amethopterin in patients with cancer. Cancer Res. **22**, 706—712 (1962).

Eastern Cooperative Group in Solid Tumor Chemotherapy. Comparison of Antimetabolites in the Treatment of Breast and Colon Cancer. J. Amer. med. Assoc. **200**, 770—778 (1967).

ELLISON, R., HOLLAND, J., WEIL, M., JACQUILLAT, C., BOIRON, M., BERNARD, J., SAWITSKY, A., ROSNER, F., GUSSOFF, B., SILVER, R. T., KARANAS, A., CUTTNER, J., SPURR, C. L., HAYES, D. M., BLOM, J., LEONE, L. A., HAURANI, F., KYLE, R., HUTCHISON, J. L., FORCIER, R. J., MOON, J. H.: Arabinosyl cytosine: a useful agent in the treatment of acute leukemia in adults. Blood **32**, 507—523 (1968).

FURTH, J. J., COHEN, S. S.: Inhibition of mammalian DNA polymerase by the 5′-triphosphate of 1-$\beta$-D-arabinofuranosylcytosine and the 5′-triphosphate of 9-$\beta$-D-arabinofuranosyladenine. Cancer Res. **28**, 2061—2067 (1968).

GALLO, R. C., YANG, S. S., SMITH, R. G., HERRERA, F., TING, R. C., BOBROW, S. N., DAVIS, C., FUJIOKA, S.: RNA- and DNA-dependent DNA polymerases of human normal and leukemic cells. In: SILVESTRI, L. G. (Ed.): The biology of oncogenic viruses (Proceedings of the Second Lepetit Colloquium held in Paris, November 1970), pp. 210—220. Amsterdam: North-Holland Publishing Co. 1971.

GELLHORN, A., HIRSCHBERG, E. (Eds.): Investigation of diverse systems for cancer chemotherapy screening. Cancer Res. Supp. **3**, 1—125 (1955).

GLYNN, J. P., BIANCO, A. R., GOLDIN, A.: Variations in drug susceptibility among Moloney virus-induced transplantable leukemias. Cancer Res. **24**, 1303—1307 (1964).

GLYNN, J. P., MOLONEY, J. B., CHIRIGOS, M. A., HUMPHREYS, S. R., GOLDIN, A.: Biological interrelationships in the chemotherapy of Moloney virus leukemia. Cancer Res. **23**, 269—278 (1963).

GOLDIN, A.: Preclinical methodology for the selection of anticancer agents. In: BUSCH, H. (Ed.): Methods in cancer research. IV. pp. 193—254. New York: Academic Press 1968.

GOLDIN, A.: Factors pertaining to complete drug-induced remission of tumor in animals and man. Cancer Res. **29**, 2285—2291 (1969).

GOLDIN, A., CARTER, S. K.: Screening and evaluation of antitumor agents. Cancer Med. pp. 605—628. Philadelphia: Lea & Febiger 1973.

GOLDIN, A., GOLDBERG, B., ORTEGA, L. G., FUGMANN, R., FAIMAN, F., SCHOENBACH, E. B.: Effectiveness of nitrogen mustards in retarding growth of sarcoma 180 with reference to route of administration, age of tumors, food intake and weight loss of the mice. Cancer **2**, 865—876 (1949).

GOLDIN, A., HUMPHREYS, S. R., VENDITTI, J. M., MANTEL, N.: Prolongation of the life span of mice with advanced leukemia L1210 by treatment with halogenated derivatives of amethopterin. J. nat. Cancer Inst. **22**, 811—823 (1959).

GOLDIN, A., MANTEL, N., GREENHOUSE, S. W., VENDITTI, J. M., HUMPHREYS, S. R.: Estimation of the antileukemic potency of the antimetabolite aminopterin, administered alone, and in combination with citrovorum factor or folic acid. Cancer Res. **13**, 843—850 (1953).

GOLDIN, A., MANTEL, N., GREENHOUSE, S. W., VENDITTI, J. M., HUMPHREYS, S. R.: Factors influencing the specificity of action of an acute leukemia agent (aminopterin). Time of treatment and dosage schedule. Cancer Res. **14**, 311—314 (1954).

GOLDIN, A., SANDBERG, J. S., HENDERSON, E. S., NEWMAN, J. W., FREI, E. III., HOLLAND, J. F: The chemotherapy of human and animal acute leukemia. Cancer Chemother. Rep. (in press).

GOLDIN, A., SERPICK, A. A., MANTEL, N.: A commentary — Experimental screening procedures and clinical predictability value. Cancer Chemother. Rep. **50**, 173—218 (1966a).

GOLDIN, A., VADLAMUDI, S., KLINE, I., GANG, M., VENDITTI, J. M.: Test models for evaluating the chemotherapeutic effectiveness of drugs. Proceedings of the Vth International Congress of Chemotherapy, Vienna, Austria, 333—349 (1967).

Goldin, A., Venditti, J. M.: A manual on quantitative drug evaluation in experimental tumor systems. Part II. Quantitative assessment of various classes of agents employing advanced leukemia L1210 in mice. Cancer Chemother. Rep. **17**, 145—178 (1962).

Goldin, A., Venditti, J. M.: *In vivo* testing of antitumor agents. Proceedings of the Sixth International Congress of Chemotherapy, Tokyo, Japan. In: Progress in antimicrobial and anticancer chemotherapy II, pp. 864—877. Tokyo: University of Tokyo Press 1970.

Goldin, A., Venditti, J. M., Humphreys, S. R., Dennis, D., Mantel, N.: Studies on the management of mouse leukemia (L1210) with antagonists of folic acid. Cancer Res. **15**, 742—747 (1955a).

Goldin, A., Venditti, J. M., Humphreys, S. R., Dennis, D., Mantel, N., Greenhouse, S. W.: A quantitative comparison of the antileukemic effectiveness of two folic acid antagonists in mice. J. nat. Cancer Inst. **15**, 1657—1664 (1955b).

Goldin, A., Venditti, J. M., Humphreys, S. R., Dennis, D., Mantel, N., Greenhouse, S. W.: Factors influencing the specificity of action of an antileukemic agent (aminopterin). Multiple treatment schedules plus delayed administration of citrovorum factor. Cancer Res. **15**, 57—61 (1955c).

Goldin, A., Venditti, J. M., Humphreys, S. R., Mantel, N.: Modification of treatment schedules in the management of advanced murine leukemia with amethopterin. J. nat. Cancer Inst. **17**, 203—212 (1956a).

Goldin, A., Venditti, J. M., Humphreys, S. R., Mantel, N.: Influence of the concentration of leukemic inoculum on the effectiveness of treatment. Science **123**, 840 (1956b).

Goldin, A., Venditti, J. M., Kline, I., Mantel, N.: Evaluation of antileukemic agents employing advanced leukemia L1210 in mice. II. Cancer Res. **20**, Cancer Chemotherapy Screening Data VI, 382—448 (1960).

Goldin, A., Venditti, J. M., Kline, I., Mantel, N.: Eradication of leukemic cells (L1210) by methotrexate and methotrexate plus citrovorum factor. Nature (Lond.) **212**, 1548—1550 (1966b).

Goldin, A., Venditti, J. M., Mantel, N.: Preclinical screening and evaluation of agents for the chemotherapy of cancer: a review. Cancer Res. **21**, 1334—1351 (1961).

Goodell, B., Leventhal, B., Henderson, E.: Cytosine arabinoside in acute granulocytic leukemia. Clin. Pharmacol. Ther. **12**, 599—606 (1971).

Haddow, A., Sexton, W. A.: Influence of carbamic esters (urethanes) on experimental animal tumors. Nature (Lond.) **157**, 500—503 (1946).

Hartmann, K. U., Heidelberger, C.: Studies on fluorinated pyrimidines. XIII. Inhibition of thymidylate synthetase. J. biol. Chem. **236**, 3006—3013 (1961).

Henderson, E., Burke, P.: Clinical experience with cytosine arabinoside. Proc. Amer. Ass. Cancer Res. **6**, 26 (1965).

Hirschberg, E.: Patterns of response of animal tumors to anticancer agents. A systematic analysis of the literature in experimental cancer chemotherapy — 1945—1958. Cancer Res. **23**, Cancer Chemotherapy Screening Data XXI, 521—980 (1963).

Issekutz, B.: The chemotherapy of cancer. Budapest: Akademiai Kiado 1969.

Karrer, K., Humphreys, S. R., Goldin, A.: An experimental model for studying factors which influence metastasis of malignant tumors. Int. J. Cancer **2**, 213—223 (1967).

Kline, I., Venditti, J. M., Tyrer, D. D., Mantel, N., Goldin, A.: Chemotherapy of leukemia L1210 in mice with 1-$\beta$-D-arabinofuranosylcytosine hydrochloride II. Effectiveness against intracerebrally and subcutaneously inoculated leukemic cells. Cancer Res. **26**, 1930—1937 (1966).

Lane, M.: Some effects of cyclophosphamide (cytoxan) on normal mice and mice with L1210 leukemia. J. nat. Cancer Inst. **23**, 1347—1357 (1959).

Larionov, L. F.: Cancer chemotherapy. London: Macmillan (Pergamon) 1965.

Leiter, J., Abbott, B. J., Schepartz, S. A.: Screening data from the Cancer Chemotherapy National Service Center Screening Laboratories. XXVIII. Cancer Res. Supp. **25**, 1626—1769 (1965).

Leiter, J., Schneiderman, M. A.: Screening data from the Cancer Chemotherapy National Service Center Screening Laboratories. Cancer Res. **19**, 31—193 (1959).

Livingston, R. B., Carter, S. K.: Single agents in cancer chemotherapy. New York: Plenum Press 1970.

Loustalot, D., Desaulles, P. A., Meier, R.: Characterization of the specificity of action of tumor-inhibiting compounds. Ann. N. Y. Acad. Sci. **76**, 838—849 (1958).

Mantel, N.: Principles of chemotherapeutic screening. Proc. Berkley Symp. math. Statist. Probabil. Biol. Probl. Health **4**, 293—306 (1961).

Mantel, N.: Preclinical cancer chemotherapy. Biometrie-Praximetrie **3**, 17—30 (1962).

Moertel, C., Reitemeier, R. J., Hahn, R.: Oral methotrexate therapy of gastrointestinal cancer. Surg. Gyn. Obstet. **130**, 292—294 (1970).

OSBORN, M. J., FREEMAN, M., HUENNEKENS, F. M.: Inhibition of dihydrofolic reductase by aminopterin and amethopterin. Proc. Soc. exp. Biol., N. Y. **97**, 429—431 (1958).

ROTHENBERG, L., TERSELIC, R. A.: Commentary: management of the National Cancer Institute's drug research program through application of the linear array concept. Cancer Chemother. Rep. **54**, 303—310 (1970).

SANDBERG, J. S., GOLDIN, A.: The use of leucovorin orally in normal and leukemic L1210 mice to prevent the toxicity and gastrointestinal lesions caused by high doses of methotrexate. Cancer Res. **30**, 1276—1280 (1970).

SCHABEL, F. M., JR., SKIPPER, H. E., LASTER, W. R., JR., TRADER, M. W., WELLS, J. R.: Remission induction of spontaneous lymphoma in AKR mice with prednisone + vincristine. Proc. Amer. Ass. Cancer Res. **11**, 69 (1970).

SCHABEL, F. M., JR., SKIPPER, H. E., TRADER, M. W., LASTER, W. R., JR., SIMPSON-HERREN, L.: Spontaneous AK leukemia (lymphoma) as a model system. Cancer Chemother. Rep. **53**, 329—344 (1969).

SCHABEL, F. M., JR., SKIPPER, H. E., TRADER, M. W., WILCOX, W. S.: Experimental evaluation of potential anticancer agents. XIX. Sensitivity of nondividing leukemic cell populations to certain classes of drugs *in vivo*. Cancer Chemother. Rep. **48**, 17—30 (1965).

SCHEIN, P. S., COONEY, D. A., VERNON, M. L.: The use of nicotinamide to modify the toxicity of streptozotocin diabetes without loss of antitumor activity. Cancer Res. **27**, 2324—2331 (1967).

SELLEI, C., ECKHARDT, S., NEMETH, L.: Chemotherapy of neoplastic diseases. Budapest: Akademiai Kiado 1970.

SKIPPER, H. E., SCHABEL, F. M., JR., TRADER, M. W., LASTER, W. R., JR.: Response to therapy of spontaneous, first passage, and long passage lines of AK leukemia. Cancer Chemother. Rep. **53**, 345—366 (1969).

SKIPPER, H. E., SCHABEL, F. M., JR., WILCOX, W. S.: Experimental evaluation of potential anticancer agents. XIII. On the criteria and kinetics associated with "curability" of experimental leukemia. Cancer Chemother. Rep. **35**, 1—111 (1964).

SKIPPER, H. E., SCHABEL, F. M., JR., WILCOX, W. S.: Experimental evaluation of potential anticancer agents. XXI. Scheduling of arabinosylcytosine to take advantage of its *S*-phase specificity against leukemia cells. Cancer Chemother. Rep. **51**, 125—165 (1967).

SKIPPER, H. E., SCHMIDT, L. H.: A manual on quantitative drug evaluation in experimental tumor systems. Part I. Background, description of criteria, and presentation of quantitative therapeutic data on various classes of drugs obtained in diverse experimental tumor systems. Cancer Chemother. Rep. **17**, 1—143 (1962).

SKIPPER, H. E., WILCOX, W. S., SCHABEL, F. M., JR., LASTER, W. R., JR., MATTIL, L.: Experimental evaluation of potential anticancer agents. X. A specificity test for distinguishing false positives. Cancer Chemother. Rep. **29**, 1—62 (1963).

STOCK, C. C.: Experimental cancer chemotherapy. In: GREENSTEIN, J., HADDOW, A. (Eds.): Advances in cancer research 2, pp. 425—492. New York: Academic Press 1954.

STOCK, C. C., SUGIURA, K.: Screening steroids against a spectrum of tumors. Ann. N. Y. Acad. Sci. **76**, 720—728 (1958).

SULLIVAN, R., MILLER, E., ZUREK, W., OBERFIELD, R., OJIMA, Y.: Re-evaluation of methotrexate as an antitumor drug. Surg. Gynec. Obstet. **125**, 819—824 (1967).

TARNOWSKI, G. S., SCHMID, F. A., CAPPUCCINO, J. G., STOCK, C. C.: Chemotherapy studies in an animal tumor spectrum. II. Sensitivity of tumors to fourteen antitumor chemicals. Cancer Res. **26**, Cancer Chemotherapy Screening Data XLIII, 181—206 (1966).

VADLAMUDI, S., PADARATHSINGH, M., WARAVDEKAR, V. S., and GOLDIN, A.: Factors influencing the therapeutic activity of L-asparaginase (NSC-109229) in leukemic (L5178Y) mice. Cancer Res. **30**, 1467—1472 (1970).

VADLAMUDI, S., PADARATHSINGH, M., WARAVDEKAR, V. S., GOLDIN, A.: Leukemia P1798 as a possible experimental model for remission induction and remission maintenance for acute leukemia. Proc. Amer. Assoc. Cancer Res. **12**, 16 (1971).

VENDITTI, J. M.: A commentary. Treatment schedule dependency of experimentally active antileukemic (L1210) drugs. Cancer Chemother. Rep. (in press).

VENDITTI, J. M., ABBOTT, B. J.: Studies on oncolytic agents from natural sources. Correlations of activity against animal tumors and clinical effectiveness. Lloydia **30**, 332—348 (1967).

VENDITTI, J. M., HUMPHREYS, S. R., GOLDIN, A.: The effectiveness of cytoxan against mouse leukemia L1210 and resistant sublines. Cancer Chemother. Rep. **3**, 6—8 (1959).

VENDITTI, J. M., HUMPHREYS, S. R., MANTEL, N., GOLDIN, A.: Influence of the duration of treatment with A-methopterin on the survival time of mice with advanced leukemia (L1210). Cancer Res. **17**, 917—922 (1957).

VENDITTI, J. M., HUMPHREYS, S. R., MANTEL, N., KLINE, I., GOLDIN, A.: Evaluation of antileukemic agents employing advanced leukemia L1210 in mice. III. Congeners of folic acid. Cancer Res. **20**, Cancer Chemotherapy Screening Data VIII, 698—733 (1960).

VENDITTI, J. M., KLINE, I., GOLDIN, A.: Evaluation of antileukemic agents employing advanced leukemia L1210 in mice. VIII. Cancer Res. **24**, Cancer Chemotherapy Screening Data XXXI, 827—879 (1964).
VENDITTI, J. M., SCHRECKER, A. W., MEAD, J. A. R., KLINE, I., GOLDIN, A.: Influence of the route of administration on the relative effectiveness of 3′, 5′-dichloroamethopterin and amethopterin against advanced leukemia (L1210) in mice. Cancer Res. **20**, 1451—1456 (1960).
WILCOX, W. S., SCHABEL, F. M., JR., SKIPPER, H. E.: Experimental evaluation of potential anticancer agents XV. On the relative rates of growth and host kill of "single" leukemia cells that survive *in vivo* cytoxan therapy. Cancer Res. **26**, 1009—1014 (1966).
WILSON, H., LOUIS, J.: The use of low dosage regimens in the treatment of neoplastic disease. Ann. intern. Med. **63**, 918 (1965).
YOSHIDA, T.: Screening with ascites hepatoma. Ann. N. Y. Acad. Sci. **76**, 610—618 (1958).
ZUBROD, C. G., SCHEPARTZ, S., LEITER, J., ENDICOTT, K. M., CARRESE, L. M., BAKER, C. G.: The chemotherapy program of the National Cancer Institute: history, analysis and plans. Cancer Chemother. Rep. **50**, 349—540 (1966).

Chapter 3

# Rational Design of Alkylating Agents

W. C. J. Ross

## Introduction

The cytotoxic effects of agents that are able to alkylate biological material under physiological conditions were first reported by Meyer (1887) and Ehrlich (1898), and the application of this class of compounds to the treatment of human cancers was introduced by Gilman and Philips (1946). This followed the observation that derivatives of mustard gas such as HN2 (nitrogen mustard, I) were particularly toxic towards lymphoid tissue

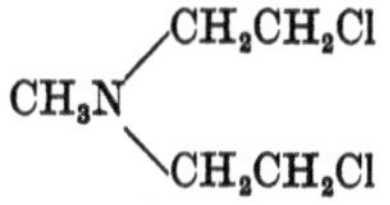

(I)

and led to the use of such agents in the treatment of lymphatic leukemia. It was later established that other classes of compounds which had comparable alkylating ability, for example, aziridines, epoxides, and alkanesulfonates, also exerted a cytotoxic action on a variety of rapidly dividing cell types (Ross, 1953, 1962). This action is not, however, specific for neoplastic tissue, for all rapidly proliferating cells are affected: normal bone marrow, intestinal mucosa, hair forming cells, and testicular and ovarian tissues are also damaged. The cancer chemotherapist has the problem of modifying the structure of the so-called biological alkylating agents in such a way as to render them specifically cytotoxic towards neoplastic tissue.

By 1957 several thousand derivatives of alkylating drugs had been prepared and an impression was developing that no significant advance in the development of truly specific agents was being made; therefore, Schmidt et al. (1965) began their impressive study of 114 representative compounds. They concluded that though there were demonstrable differences in the activities of the various alkylating agents against the more susceptible tumors, these were of a quantitative nature. Generally the agents showed a broad spectrum of activity and two types of compounds were outstanding in this respect: these were cyclophosphamide (LXIV) and the isomeric phenylalanine mustards (IX, X, XI). The view is now being expressed that agents with a wide cytotoxic spectrum are unlikely to be of lasting value since they must inevitably affect many normal proliferating tissues with attendant unwanted side effects.

The future advancement would seem to lie in the discovery of compounds that are toxic towards a limited range of neoplasms. It is of interest to recall that though Schmidt et al. (1965) expressed the view that their survey offered little hope that any agent of the alkylating type would be found which would affect some neoplasm in a unique way, they did draw attention to the specific antitumor activity of methyl methanesulfonate (II) and 2-chloroethyl methanesulfonate (III) against lymphoma 8 and of another methanesulfonate (IV) towards the Yoshida ascites hepatoma.

$CH_3OO_2SCH_3$ (II) $ClCH_2CH_2OO_2SCH_3$ (III)

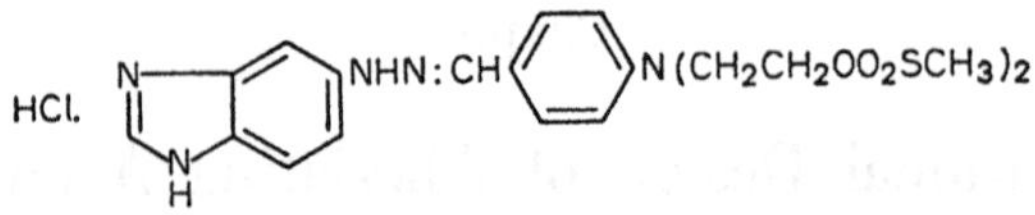

(IV)

The present author agrees with Heidelberger (1969) that much of the work done on alkylating derivatives has involved the random attachment of alkylating moieties to a "fanciful collection of carriers dreamed up *ad hoc*". Nevertheless, this criticism cannot be justifiably leveled at those groups of workers who have attempted to synthesize new compounds based on reasonably exploitable differences between cell types. This approach, largely initiated since the above mentioned survey, forms the subject of this chapter.

## General Principles of Rational Design of Agents

Danielli (1954, 1961) pointed out that the selectivity of action of a drug can be enhanced by the number of variables on which the drug depends for its activity. Some of the parameters that can be considered individually or in combination are: 1. physical characteristics (water and/or lipid solubility, water/lipid partition coefficients, affinity for macromolecules) which will affect the transport characteristics and pharmacological disposition of the drug, 2. chemical reactivity (absolute velocity of reaction, mechanism of reaction, influence of pH and redox potential on reactivity) which will determine the persistence of the drug after administration, and influence the site of maximum action, and 3. potentiation by enzymic modification (e.g. hydrolysis, reduction, and oxidation) that will influence the tissue specificity of action. These factors will now be considered in detail:

### A. Exploitation of Physico-Chemical Characteristics

#### I. Solubility and Partition Coefficients

Since alkylating drugs almost certainly produce their cytotoxic effects by reacting chemically with some cell component, an adequate concentration of the agent must reach the target site. The disposition of the drug will be related to its solubility in aqueous and lipid media (Ross, 1962, p. 121). Water solubility is advantageous for agents that are to be administered by intravenous injection and an example of a compound designed for this purpose is chlorambucil (V).

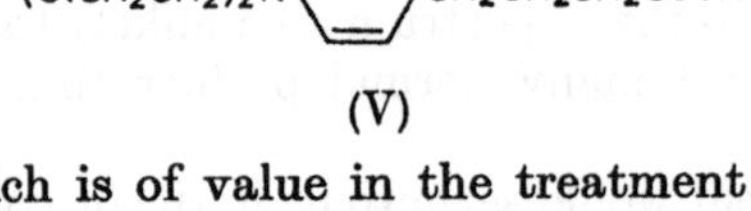

(V)

This compound, which is of value in the treatment of chronic lymphocytic leukemia and adenocarcinoma of the ovary, is particularly well suited for regional perfusion techniques (Ross, 1962, p. 193). Localization of drug action, with sparing of distal sites, is achieved by introducing the agent into the blood supply of a specific region which is maintained in closed circulation by the use of a pump-oxygenator. Chlorambucil and other water soluble drugs (e.g., cyclophosphamide and triethylenemelamine) have been used for treating neoplasms in the following regions: brain, lung, head and neck, liver, abdomen, and the extremities.

Lipid solubility is desirable in compounds that are required to penetrate the blood-brain barrier and this property probably accounts for the efficacy of the potential alkylating agent, 1,3-*bis*-2-chloroethyl-1-nitrosourea (BCNU, VI) against

$$CO\begin{cases} N(NO)CH_2CH_2Cl \\ NHCH_2CH_2Cl \end{cases} \qquad \text{(VI)}$$

intracerebral L1210 mouse leukemia (SCHABEL et al., 1963) and human meningeal leukemia (RALL et al., 1963).

The nature of the partition of a drug between aqueous and lipid phases will also influence the manner in which the agent is distributed throughout an organism and the eventual diffusion through cellular membranes. Two studies have shown that maximum biological activity is associated with a lipid-water partition coefficient that is close to unity. HUDSON et al. (1958) showed that, in a series of $\alpha$, $\omega$-dimethanesulfonoxyalkanes (VII), maximum cytotoxic effects on neutrophils was exhibited by derivatives with distribution coefficients near unity. A similar result was obtained by KHAN and ROSS (1969, 1970) in their study of derivatives of the highly specific carcinostatic 5-aziridino-2,4-dinitrobenzamide (VIII, CB 1954).

$$CH_3SO_2O(CH_2)_nOO_2SCH_3 \qquad \text{(VII)}$$

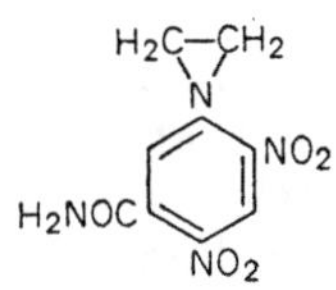


(VIII)

It would appear that compounds with this distribution characteristic are able to pass with equal ease throughout aqueous and lipid media and thus achieve universal disposition. This factor is worth consideration in the future design of cytotoxic drugs of all types.

## II. Derivatives with Active Transport Potentialities

As alkylating agents need to penetrate cellular and nuclear membranes to reach the presumed target sites it seemed logical to attach the cytotoxic group to carrying structures that are related to substances normally involved in cell growth. For such structures mechanisms of activated or facilitated transport have been evolved. This approach has led to the synthesis of some of the most potent carcinostatic derivatives, although, on the whole, the improvement in the selectivity of action has been disappointing. Structures investigated have included naturally occurring amino acids, carbohydrates, nucleic acid bases, and steroids.

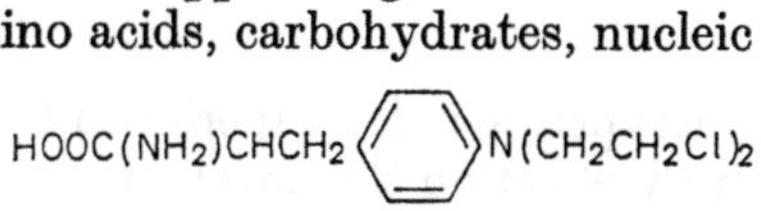


(IX)

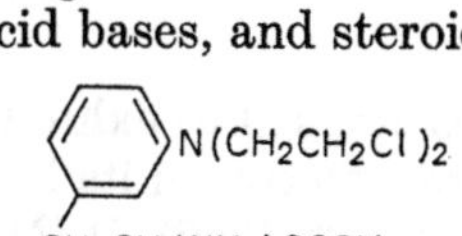


(X)

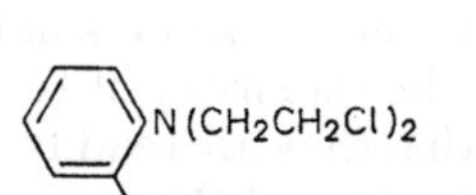


(XI)

Derivatives of phenylalanine, in which the di-2-choroethylamino group is attached to the three available positions on the aromatic ring, are sarcolysin (IX, DL-form) (LARIONOV et al., 1955), melphalan (IX, L-form) (BERGEL and STOCK, 1954), *m*-sarcolysin (X, DL-form) (GRAM et al., 1959; OSDENE et al., 1959) and *o*-sarcolysin (XI, DL-form, merophan) (CONNORS and ROSS, 1960).

Reference has already been made to the wide spectrum of activity exhibited by these derivatives against a range of animal tumors, and they have proved equally versatile in the treatment of human neoplasms. The *p*-substituted derivative (IX) has been extensively used in the clinic (WHITE, 1960; LARIONOV, 1965) especially in the treatment of seminoma of the testis, EWING's bone tumor, and reticulum cell sarcoma. CLIFFORD (1970) regards the ortho analog (XI) as the agent of choice for the treatment of BURKITT's lymphoma, and some success has attended the use of this compound in the treatment of solid tumors (SALMON et al., 1966; YOUNT et al., 1967).

The tryptophan derivative (XII) proved effective against the mouse plasma cell tumor YPC1 and the mast cell tumor P815 (FISHBEIN et al., 1964) and also in the treatment of human plasmacytic melanoma (KYLE et al., 1967).

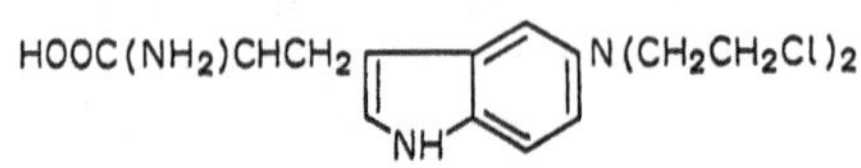


(XII)

The use of carrying structures related to carbohydrates has led to the preparation of a number of derivatives that have merited clinical application. The mannitol derivatives, Degranol (XIII, mannomustine, BCM), 1,6-dibromo- (XIV, X = Br, DBM) and 1,6-dimethanesulfonoxy- (XIV, X = $CH_3SO_2O$, mannitol myleran) 1,6-dideoxy-D-mannitol and 1,6-dibromo-1,6-dideoxygalactitol (XV, dibromodulcitol) are representative.

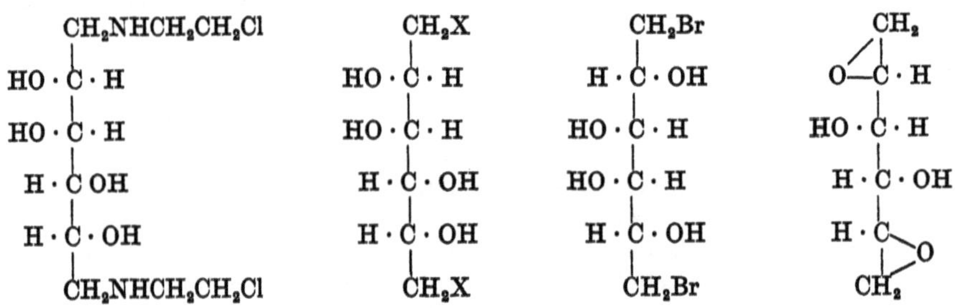


(XIII) (XIV) (XV) (XVI)

Degranol is claimed to exhibit a therapeutic index superior to that of HN2 (I) and to be more effective in its inhibitory effect on the development of metastases (LAPIS and HEMETH, 1956). DBM (XIV, X = Br) has given encouraging results in the treatment of myeloid leukemia (ECKHARDT et al., 1963; CASSAZZA et al., 1967). A phase I study of dibromodulcitol (XV) has indicated that this agent may be useful in the palliative treatment of some solid tumors (ANDREWS et al., 1971).

A recent development in the chemistry of 1,6-disubstituted 1,6-dideoxyhexitols has been the demonstration that they are readily converted into dianhydrides under physiological conditions (JARMAN and ROSS, 1967). The mannitol derivative (XVI) is some 50 times as potent as a carcinostatic agent compared with the parent compounds (XIV, X = Br or $CH_3SO_2O$) and its use in the treatment of human my elogenous leukemia has been advocated (ELSON et al., 1968).

The use of nucleic acid bases as carriers of cytotoxic groups is exemplified by three uracil derivatives, 5-(di-2-chloroethyl)aminouracil (XVII, uracil mustard), its 6-methyl derivative (XVIII, Dopan) and the riboside (XIX, BELIKOVA et al., 1967).

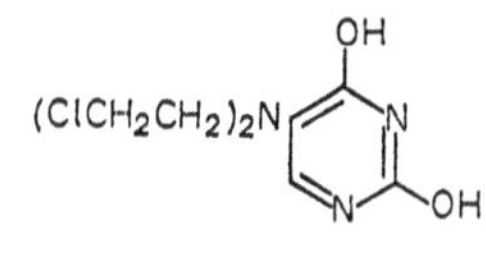

(XVII)

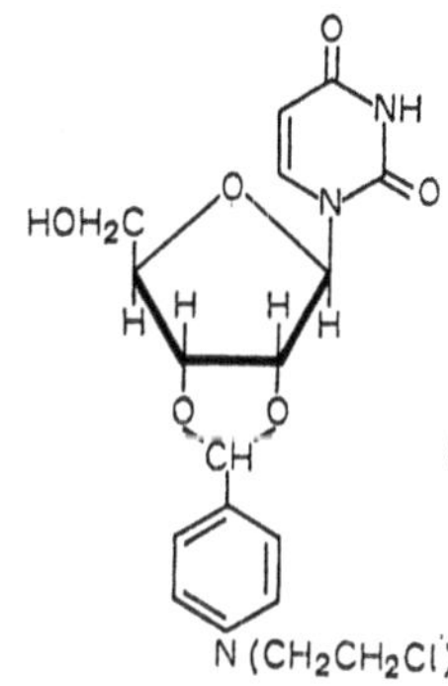

(XIX)

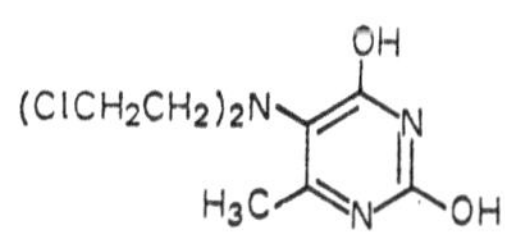

(XVIII)

Clinical evaluation of uracil mustard (WILLIAMS, 1963) and Dopan (WHITE, 1961) has indicated that these agents are effective against tumors of the hematopoietic system and occasionally against solid tumors.

Alkylating steroid derivatives that have been examined as antitumor agents include the cholesterol derivative (XX, phenestrin) which is claimed to be particularly effective against brain tumors (DEGTEVA and LARIONOV, 1966) and the hormonal derivatives (XXI, R = estrone, estradiol, testosterone and deoxycorticosterone) which produced excellent inhibition of DMBA induced and transplantable mammary adenocarcinoma (WALL et al., 1969).

Certain aziridine derivatives (e.g., XXII) have also shown activity against an implanted mammary carcinoma ($C_3H$/An) in mice (BUKVA and GASS, 1967).

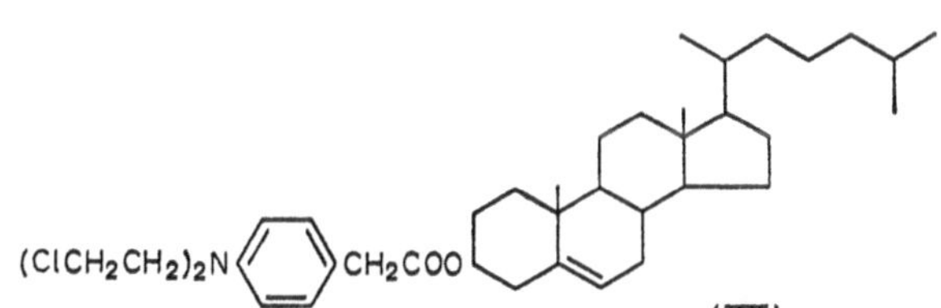

(XX)

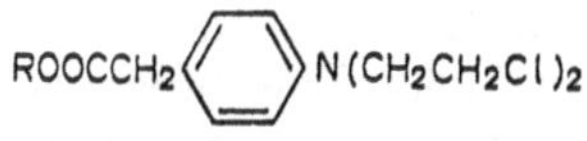

(XXI)

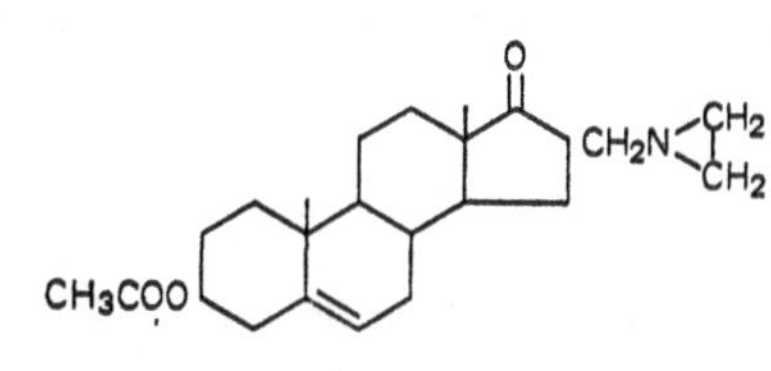

(XXII)

## III. Derivatives with Tissue Specific Affinity

COBB (1970) has suggested an approach to cancer chemotherapy which is based on the preferential uptake of chemicals by particular tissues. He argues that, in certain cases, it would be acceptable to destroy practically all the normal tissue as well as the neoplastic tissue at a given site (e.g., in cancer of the breast, ovary, and prostate, and possibly in some melanomas). If this compromise is feasible, then there are a number of carrying structures for cytotoxic groups that have been proposed for this type of tissue specificity.

Compounds with structures related to the antimalarial drugs, chloroquine and quinacrine, will localize in the cell nucleus and also have affinity for melanomatous tissue (Counsell et al., 1967; Blois, 1968). The chloroquine (XXIII) and quinacrine (XXIV) mustards prepared by Jones et al. (1958) would seem to merit further assessment in the treatment of melanomas.

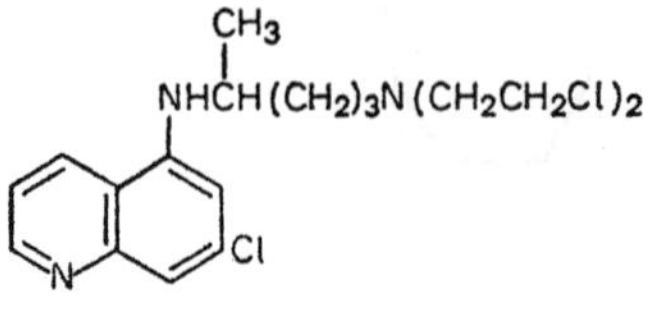


(XXIII)

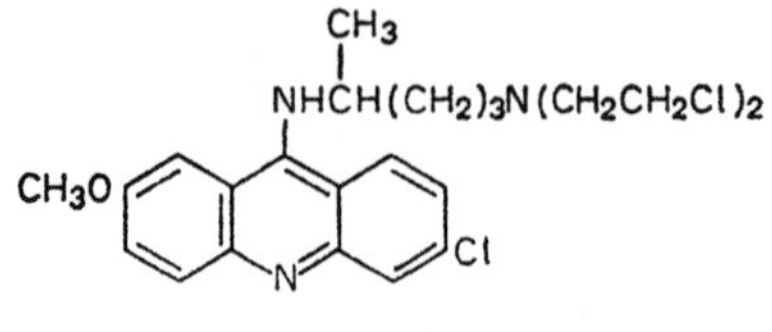


(XXIV)

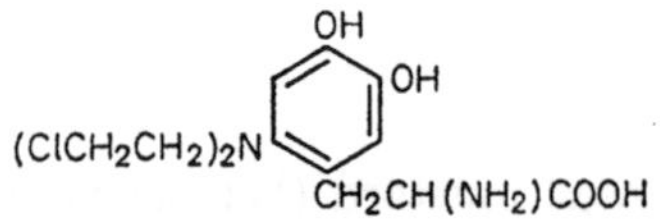


(XXV)

Melanin precursors (e.g., 3,4-dihydroxyphenylalanine, Dopa) are incorporated into the insoluble melanin which deposits in melanotic melanomas (Blois and Kallman, 1964) and this has prompted the synthesis of a dopa-mustard (XXV) (Vasil'Eva et al., 1970).

Csaba and Korosi (1968) synthesized the phenazathionium mustard chloride (XXVI) and later showed that this substance exhibited the expected affinity for neoplastic cells (Csaba et al., 1969).

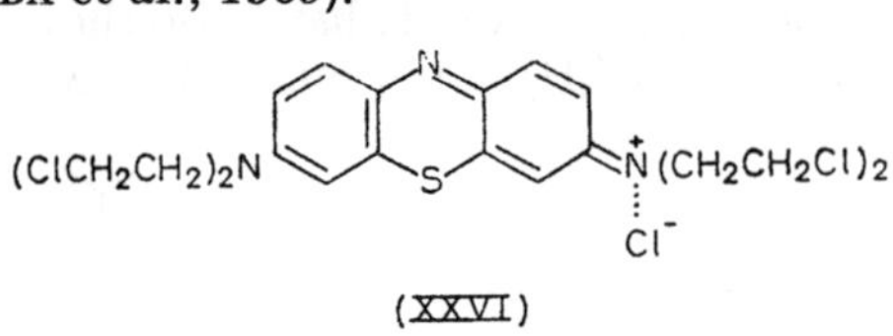


(XXVI)

Unexpected indications of binding to specific cell types has arisen in the study of agents designed to exploit other characteristics. For example, the urethane mustards (L and LI), although having the potential for enzymic activation, may owe their specific cytotoxic activity towards Walker tumor cells to the selective uptake by receptors unique to this tumor (Bardos et al., 1969; Hebborn et al., 1970).

Cancer tissue often has a higher hydrogen ion concentration than most normal tissue: this has been demonstrated both in animal (Kahler and Robertson, 1943; Eden et al., 1955) and in human tumors (Ashby, 1966). This difference, which can be accentuated by glucose administration, is even more pronounced in the micrometastases (von Ardenne et al., 1969) for which chemotherapy appears to be the only reasonable method of attack.

It is known that basic drugs with the appropriate dissociation constant will concentrate in cells with lower internal pH as a consequence of the lower permeability of the cellular membrane to charged molecules. This led to the preparation of some aromatic nitrogen mustards containing basic side chains with the desired characteristic, and to the demonstration that their activity against tumors was enhanced by prior glucose administration. *NN*-Dimethyl-*p*-(di-2-chloroethylamino)phenylethylamine (XXVII) is representative of this class of agent (Ross, 1961).

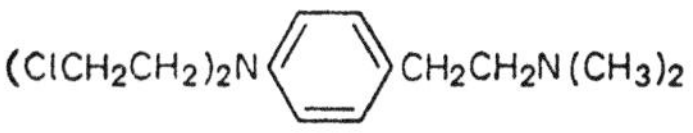

(XXVII)

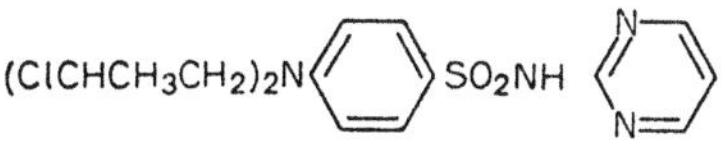

(XXVIII)

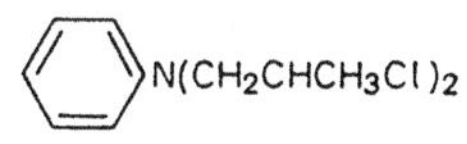

(XXIX)

Certain sulfonamides will deposit in the more acidic cell, on account of the insolubility of the undissociated form that predominates at lower pH, and this property has been exploited by the synthesis of alkylating derivatives of such sulfonamides. The sulfadiazine mustard (XXVIII) was shown to exhibit a chemotherapeutic index (median lethal dose/dose to produce 90% inhibition of tumor growth) of 24.5 in the Walker tumor assay as compared with an index of 10.8 for the parent aniline derivative (XXIX) (Calvert et al., 1968).

## B. Exploitation of Differences in Chemical Reactivity

### I. Highly Reactive Agents for Intra-Arterial Infusion

Systemic administration of alkylating drugs usually suffers from the disadvantage that unacceptable damage to the bone marrow and the gastrointestinal tract ensues. In order to overcome this handicap, regional intra-arterial therapy using agents with short half-lives has been developed. It was hoped that the drugs, on being introduced directly into the blood supply to the tumor, would exert a carcinostatic effect therein and minimal toxicity would occur on escape into the general circulation because of chemical lability. The pioneering work in this area was carried out by Seligman and his colleagues (1962) in the course of which they developed a series of sulfur mustard gas derivatives with very short half-lives (e.g. XXX, half-life 1.3 min, and XXXI, half-life 0.6 sec at pH 7.4, 37°). Compound (XXX) was administered by the intracarotid, lower aortic and intracoeliac routes and palliation in cases of head and pelvic cancers was reported.

$[ClCH_2CH_2S(CH_2)_3CONHCH_2\cdot]_2$ (XXX)

$[ICH_2CH_2S(CH_2)_4CONHCH_2\cdot]_2$ (XXXI)

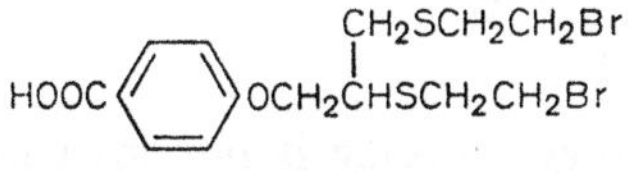

(XXXII)

Another sulfur mustard gas derivative designed for use in this manner was *p*-(2,3-di-(2-bromoethylthio)-*n*-propyloxy) benzoic acid (XXXII) which has a half-life of 4 to 5 seconds under physiological conditions (Davis and Ross, 1965). Clinical trials (Meyza and Cobb, 1971) against a variety of carcinomas, melanomas, and sarcomas indicated that the drug showed significant antitumor activity; in particular, the sarcomas, which are normally resistant to therapy, showed marked responses. The drug produced alleviation of pain, whereas other agents failed to produce this effect. Furthermore, there was no toxicity towards the sensitive elements in bone marrow and intestine.

## II. Mechanistic Differences

Alkylation of biological receptors can occur by two mechanisms, the unimolecular ($S_N1$) and the bimolecular ($S_N2$) processes (Ross, 1962). Compounds reacting by an $S_N1$ mechanism should distribute throughout an organism and react at a rate determined by the dielectric constant of the medium, whereas the rate of reaction of compounds reacting by an $S_N2$ mechanism will be dependent on the concentration of alkylatable centres. Although it was hoped that this mechanistic difference would result in different spectra of cytotoxicity this has generally not been borne out. For example, aromatic nitrogen mustards, which react for all practical purposes by a unimolecular mechanism, do not differ significantly in their effects from those of the epoxides and C-unsubstituted aziridines, which react essentially by a bimolecular mechanism.

One instance where the biological effect is probably determined by the mechanism of reaction is the relative action of two methanesulfonates on the hematopoietic system. Busulfan (XXXIII), which reacts by an $S_N2$ mechanism, produces a greater depressant action on circulating neutrophils, whereas the azo-compound (XXXIV), which reacts by an $S_N1$ mechanism, produces a greater effect on lymphocytes (Elson, 1963).

$$CH_3SO_2O(CH_2)_4OO_2SCH_3$$

(XXXIII)

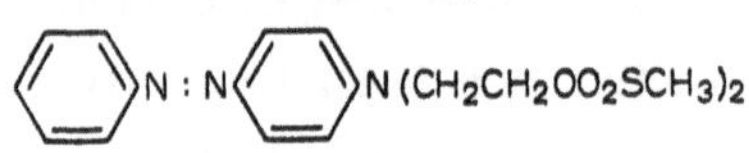


(XXXIV)

Another recent example was reported by Bardos et al. (1969). Although triethylenephosphoramide (XXXV, TEPA) had little or no activity against the mouse leukemia, L1210, the C-dimethyl analog (XXXVI) produced a significant number of cures in this tumor system. It was suggested that this interesting difference in antitumor activity may be related to the fact that (XXXV) reacts by an $S_N2$ mechanism, whereas the compound (XXXVI) has an ability to undergo $S_N2$ reaction with the unsubstituted ring carbon atoms and also $S_N1$ reactions through the formation of a tertiary carbonium ion, i.e. with the charge centered on the substituted carbon atoms of the opened aziridine ring.

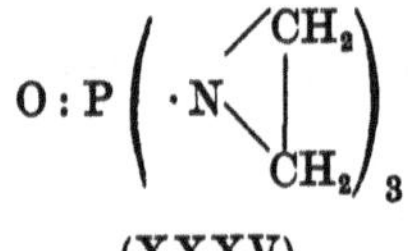


(XXXV)

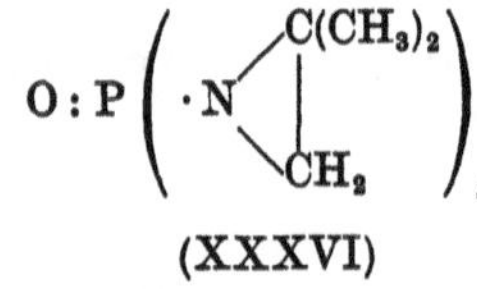


(XXXVI)

Nevertheless, tumor inhibitory activity is not invariably potentiated by *C*-substitution in the aziridine ring, for, whereas 5-aziridinyl-2,4-dinitrobenzamide (VIII) is highly effective in the Walker tumor assay, the 2,2-dimethyl analog (XXXVII) is without activity in this system or against the L1210 leukemia (Khan and Ross, 1969 and 1970).

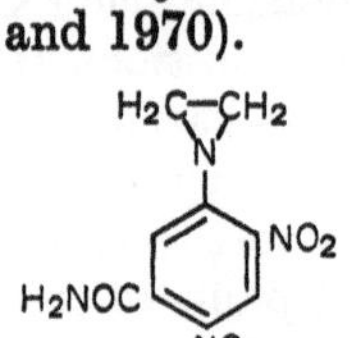


(VIII)

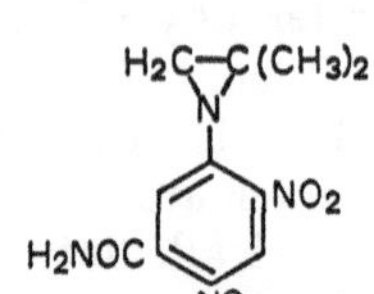


(XXXVII)

## III. Chemical Reactivity Influenced by Tissue pH

Correlations between the chemical reactivity of alkylating agents and their carcinostatic activity have been established. Two classes of these agents become more reactive at lower pH, namely the aziridines and the epoxides. As the hydrogen ion concentration in cancer tissue is often higher than that in most normal tissues (see above), these agents should be selectively toxic to malignant tissue, especially if the pH differential is accentuated by glucose administration to the host. This predicted enhancement of activity has been demonstrated for the aziridine derivative, triethylenemelamine (XXXVIII, TEM) in assays against the Walker rat tumor (CONNORS et al., 1964). The chemotherapeutic index (defined above) for this compound is raised from 9 to 28 by glucose pretreatment of the host rat.

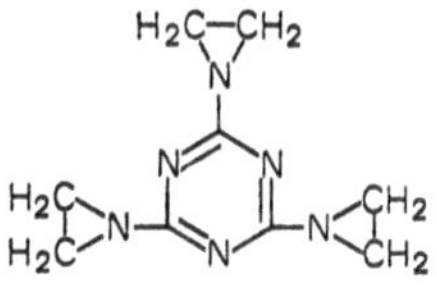


(XXXVIII)

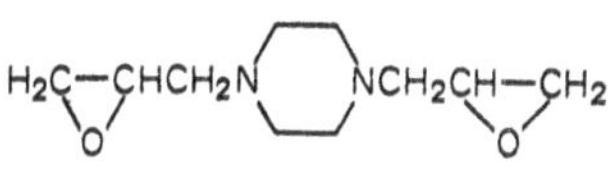


(XXXIX)

The attachment of cytotoxic aziridine groups to new carrying structures designed to produce the maximum difference in reactivity between the pH of normal tissue (pH 7.4) and that achieveable in cancer tissue (about pH 6.5) would seem to be a profitable venture for the future.

The basic epoxide derivatives (e. g. XXXIX, prepared by GERZON et al., 1959) are also well suited to exploit any pH difference since the activating effect of the protonation of the nitrogen atoms reinforces the acid-catalyzed reaction of the epoxide groups.

## IV. Chemical Reactivity Influenced by Tissue Redox Potential

CATER and PHILLIPS (1954) established the lower oxidation-reduction potential of tumor tissue relative to that of most normal tissues. This feature has been exploited in the design of potentially more selective agents by the synthesis of derivatives that are more reactive at the lower redox potential of neoplastic tissue. Two types of compound satisfying this requirement are quinone derivatives (e.g. XL) and indophenol derivatives (e.g. XLI). The expected higher chemical reactivity of the reduced forms (XLII and XLIII, respectively) has been confirmed and their carcinostatic activity has been demonstrated (ROSS, 1964).

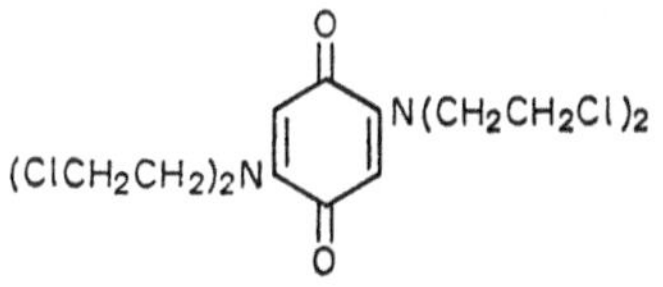


(XL)

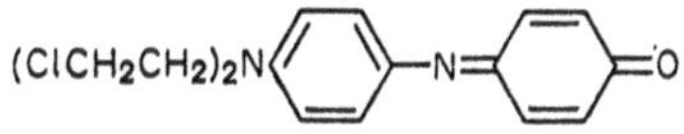


(XLI)

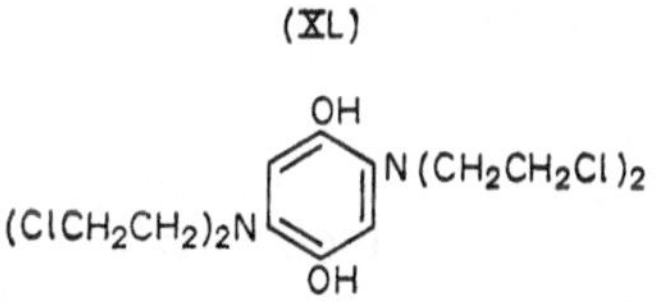


(XLII)

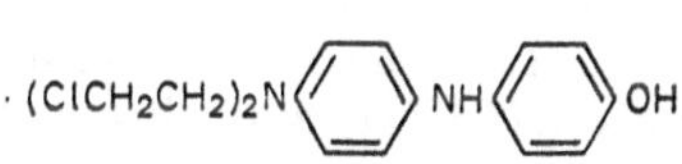


(XLIII)

## C. Exploitation of Differences in Enzyme Constitution of Tissues

Rapidly dividing cells of all kinds are especially sensitive towards alkylating agents. Each cellular species possesses a characteristic enzymic constitution (GREENSTEIN, 1947). If one could design agents that are biologically inactive by virtue of low chemical reactivity, but which could become activated by an increase in reactivity following enzymic modification, then there is a hope of obtaining cytotoxic specificity. Such agents could be regarded as having latent activity. The earlier work in this field has already been reviewed (ROSS, 1962) and only some of the more recent work will be dealt with in this section.

### I. Agents Modified by Hydrolytic Enzymes

Esters of *p*-(di-2-chloroethylamino)phenol (XLIV, $R =$ methyl or phenyl) (ROSS et al., 1955) were shown to have antitumor activity superior to that of the parent phenolic mustard and this activity could be correlated with the presence of the appropriate esterase (HEBBORN and DANIELLI, 1958).

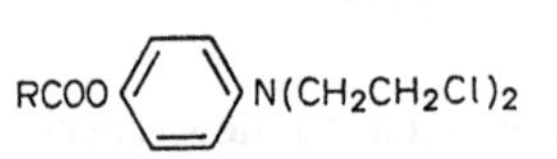

(XLIV)

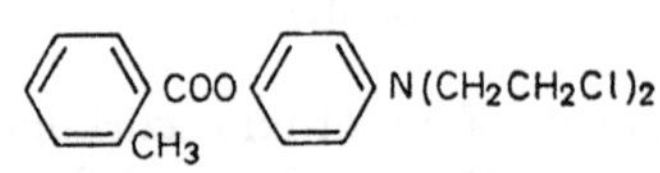

(XLV)

Compounds of this type are still being investigated. VICKERS et al. (1969) and BARDOS et al. (1969) consider that the optimum rate of hydrolytic activation is that shown by the *o*-methylbenzoate (XLV) which exhibits the highest chemotherapeutic index in their Walker tumor assays.

CONNORS and WHISSON (1965) showed that the PC5 mouse plasma cell tumor, was highly sensitive towards *N*,*N*-di-2-chloroethylaniline (XLVI, R = H). It was considered that this specificity of action was due to the initial conversion of the aniline mustard into the less toxic *O*-glucuronide (XLVII) of its *p*-hydroxylated derivative (XLVI, R = OH) (CONNORS and WHISSON, 1966; WHISSON et al., 1966). Owing to the high *β*-glucuronidase activity of the plasma cell tumor, it was suggested that this conjugate would be selectively transformed into the much more toxic *p*-di-2-chloroethylaminophenol (XLVI, R = OH) within the tissues of this neoplasm.

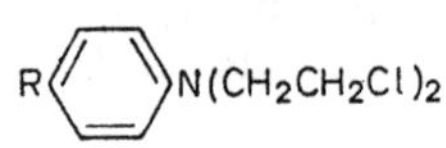

(XLVI)

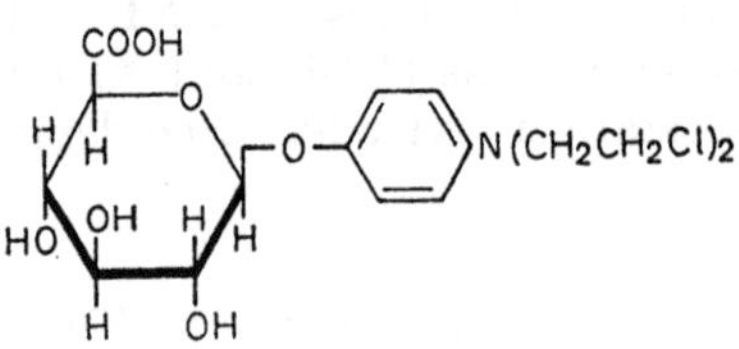

(XLVII)

An approach to the chemotherapy of malignancies could be based on their ability to potentiate the cytotoxic effect of conjugates of the *p*-hydroxy derivative. BUKHARI et al. (1971) have synthesized the glucuronide (XLVII) and also the ethereal sulfate (XLVIII) and phosphate (XLIX). These conjugates should be applicable to the treatment of tumors which possess high activity of the appropriate esterases, e.g., those malignancies reported to have higher sulfatase activity than corresponding normal tissue (DZIALOSZYNSKI et al., 1966; ZBYTNIEWSKI,

1969), and prostatic carcinomas that have high phosphatase activity (GREENSTEIN, 1947).

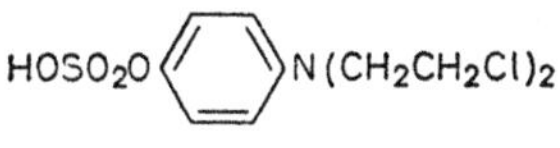


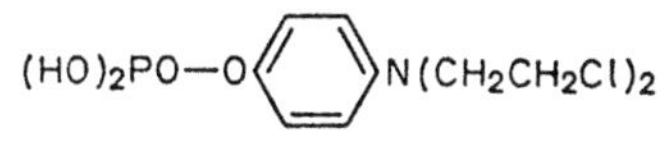


(XLVIII) (XLIX)

High chemotherapeutic indices have been exhibited by two types of agent which were designed to be potentiated by hydrolysis of a urethane linkage. These are *p*-di-2-chloroethylaminophenyl *p*-carboxycarbanilate (L, IC 140) and the reverse carbamates (LI, R = 3 or 4-COOH and R = 2 or 4-COOMe).

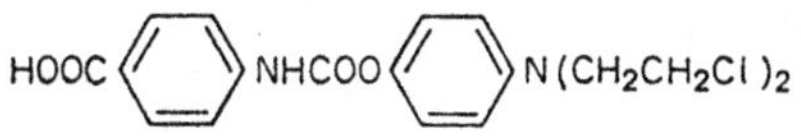


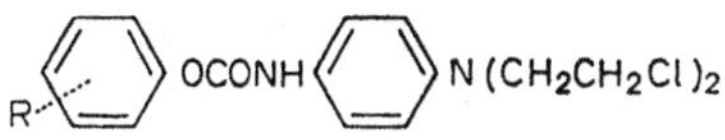


(L) (LI)

Outstanding in this group of compounds were the two esters (LI, R = 2 or 4-COOMe) which showed indices of 126 and 137, respectively, in the Walker tumor assay system (BARDOS et al., 1969). Although designed for activation by hydrolysis of the carbamate linkage there are indications that selective uptake by specific receptors and site directed catalysis also play a part in determining the high activity of these derivatives.

The widely used cyclophosphamide (LXIV) was originally designed to be activated by phosphoesterases and/or phosphoramidases, and though these enzymes may have a role to play in the potentiation of activity, it would now appear that an essential stage in the activation process is a prior oxidative modification (see below).

The design of compounds with latent activity that can be potentiated by enzymic modification relies on the greater ability of neoplastic tissue to effect the required transformation. While this may be true for some tumors, the general picture is that the enzymic activity of the tumor is lower than that of most normal tissue. To meet such a situation one would need to design an agent that was active but which could be more readily deactivated in normal tissues.

A brief account of this approach has already been given (ROSS, 1962) and its application has been extended by SELIGMAN and his coworkers in an impressive series of papers (SELIGMAN et al., 1962; WITTEN et al., 1962a, b; GOODMAN et al., 1962, 1965; SCHILLING et al., 1963; WILLIAMSON et al., 1963; KRAMER et al., 1963; SASS et al., 1965). For example, amides of the general formula (LII, X = Cl, Br, or I) were prepared, and it was demonstrated that, as expected, these bifunctional alkylating agents were more toxic than the monofunctional hydrolysis products (LIII).

$$XCH_2CH_2S(CH_2)_nCONH(CH_2)_xNHCO(CH_2)_nSCH_2CH_2X \qquad \text{(LII)}$$

$$XCH_2CH_2S(CH_2)_nCOOH\,. \qquad \text{(LIII)}$$

Impetus was given to this work by the fact that many of the compounds had short half-lives rendering them especially suited for intra-arterial infusion techniques (see above). The compound (LII, X = Cl, $n = 1, x = 2$; S 46) had a half-life of 26 minutes at 37°, pH 7.4 and in clinical trials on 43 patients with advanced cancers of various types, improvement was reported in 18% of the cases (GOODMAN et al., 1962).

Bifunctional aziridine derivatives (e.g., LIV) were also synthesized as agents that should be more readily converted into the less toxic $\beta$-(aziridinyl)alanine (LV) in normal tissues with higher esterase activity than most cancer tissues (Tsou et al., 1963). The compound (LIV) inhibits the growth of four experimental tumors (sarcoma 180, carcinoma 755, L1210 lymphoma, and the Walker 256 tumor) at well tolerated doses.

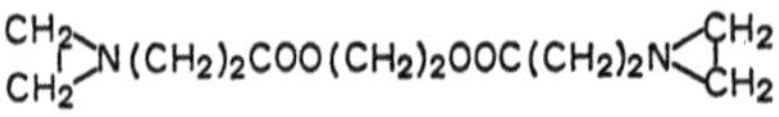

(LIV)

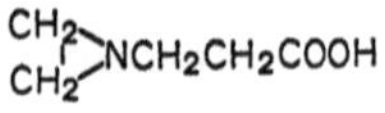

(LV)

## II. Agents Activated by Reducing Enzymes

It has been shown that di-2-chloroethylamino derivatives of various substituted azobenzenes are effective antitumor agents and that this activity can be correlated with the reducibility of the azo-linkage by an enzyme system (Ross and Warwick, 1955; Ross, 1962). Substitution in the aromatic rings at positions ortho to the azo-linkage promotes reduction to derivatives of the very reactive *p*-phenylenediamine derivative (LVII) and one of the most effective compounds of this type is 4-(di-2-chloroethylamino)-2-methylazobenzene-2′-carboxylic acid (LVI, CB 1414). Clinical responses in cases of chronic lymphocytic leukemia and in one case of astrocytoma were reported following the administration of this agent (Israels and Ritzmann, 1960; Duvall, 1961). CB 1414 (LVI) was one of the few alkylating agents to exhibit significant activity against established lymphoma 8 (Schmidt, 1960).

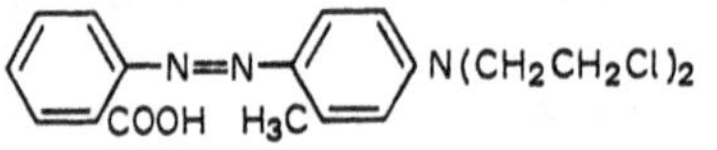

(LVI)

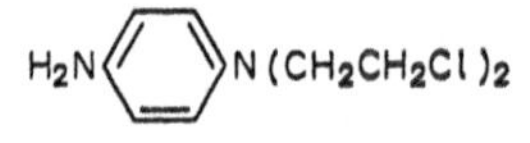

(LVII)

Liver is particularly rich in azo-reductases and so hepatic tissues should be a major site of activation of this type of agent. It would, therefore, appear that azo-derivatives are suitable for the treatment of primary hepatomas, for even if a considerable amount of normal liver tissue is damaged, this organ has considerable capacity for regeneration. Ideally the reactive reduction product should have a very short half-life so that distant tissues are spared, and the synthesis of suitable precursors is now being pursued in the author's laboratories. This work involves the replacement of the 2-chloroethyl groups by the more reactive 2-bromoethyl and 2-iodoethyl groups, as well as by 2-methanesulfonoxyethyl and 2-halogeno-*n*-propyl groups.

The antitumor activity of the tetrazolium (LVIII) and formazan (LIX) derivatives prepared by Tsou and Su (1963) would also be potentiated by reduction *in vivo* to the *p*-phenylenediamine derivative (LVII). (LVIII) and (LIX) were tested

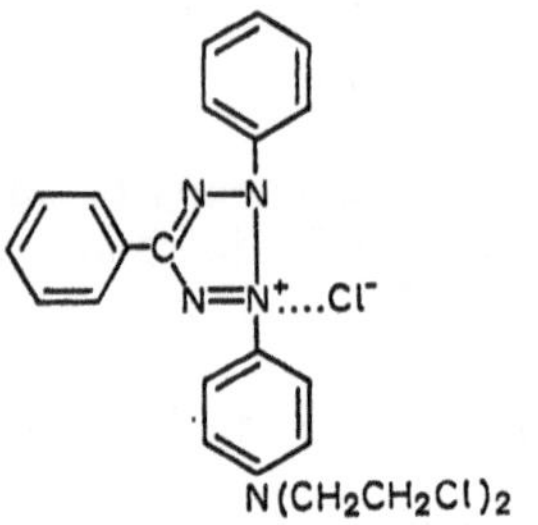

(LVIII)

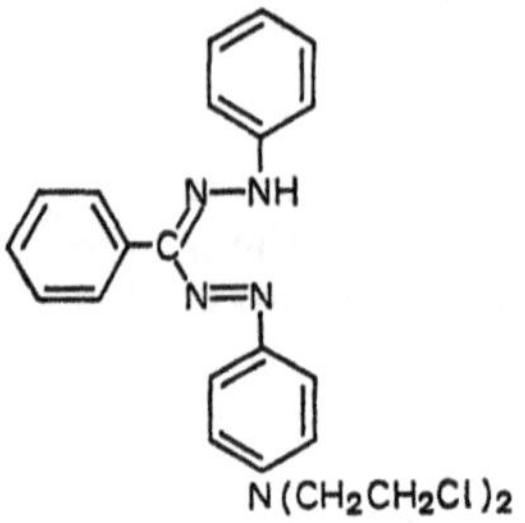

(LIX)

in the Walker tumor assay and the formazan derivative showed the higher activity; this could be accounted for by the relative inability of the cationic tetrazolium compound to diffuse through cellular membranes.

*p*-Nitroso-*N*, *N*-(di-2-methanesulfonoxyethyl)aniline (LX), which exhibits a wide spectrum of antitumor activity (28 out of 37 animal tumors being sensitive to the agent) (Papanastassiou et al., 1966), almost certainly owes its high carcinostatic activity to a similar reduction of the nitroso group giving the diamine derivative. The exceptional activity of the nitroso compound against the intracerebral form of the Dunning leukemia indicates that this lipid soluble derivative is able to penetrate the blood-brain barrier.

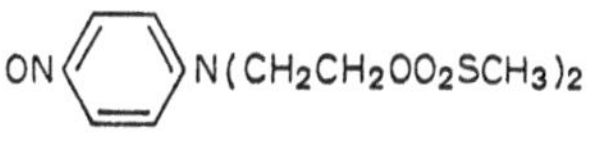


(LX)

The carcinostatic activity of the antibiotic mitomycin C (LXI) evidently depends on potentiation by conversion *in vivo* into the reduced form (LXII) which, after loss of methyl alcohol giving (LXIII), is able to cross-link DNA molecules by the reaction of two alkylating sites (the aziridine ring and the marked * methylene group) (Iyer and Szybalski, 1964).

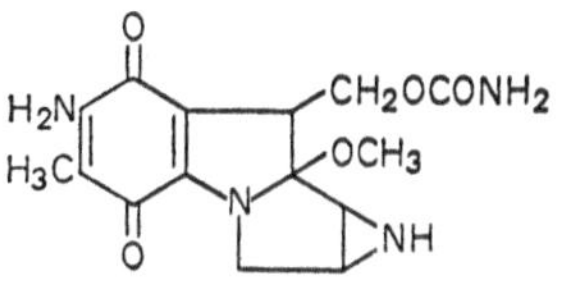


(LXI)

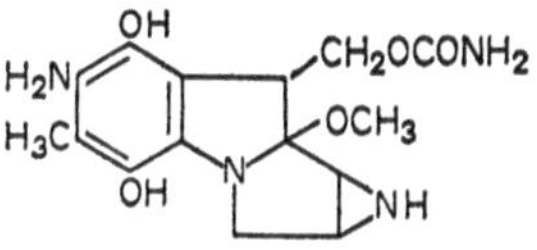


(LXII)

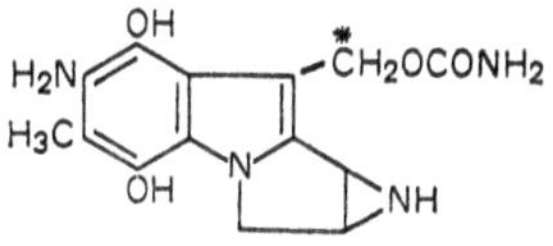


(LXIII)

## III. Agents Activated by Oxidative Enzymes

In view of the lower redox potential of tumor cells (Cater and Phillips, 1954), which can be associated with a lower level of cofactors concerned with electron transport (Weinhouse, 1955), it has generally not been considered profitable to design agents that would be activated by oxidative enzymes. However, two instances where oxidative transformation plays an important initial role have emerged from metabolic studies.

The potentiation of the activity of aniline mustard (XLVI) involves a preliminary attachment of a *p*-hydroxy group, clearly an oxidative process. A second example is the potentiation of the activity of cyclophosphamide (LXIV) which was originally designed to be activated by hydrolysis of ester and/or amide bonds. According to Brock (1967) "in contrast to our initial hypothesis, the mechanism of activation is based not on hydrolysis catalyzed by phosphatases and phosphamidases, but on oxidation (or on a multistage reaction sequence induced by the oxidative process) which occurs in liver microsomes." The mechanism of the activation of cyclophosphamide is still under investigation and a recent significant development is the isolation of 4-ketocyclophosphamide (LXV) from the urine of dogs treated with this drug (Hill et al., 1970). This metabolite is about fifty times as toxic towards cultured human epidermal cancer cells as is the parent compound (LXIV). It still remains to be determined whether (LXV) is the active form or a precursor which undergoes hydrolysis, possibly yielding N-2-chloroethylaziridine (LXVI) by way of nor-HN2 (LXVII)) Ochoa and Hirschberg, 1967).

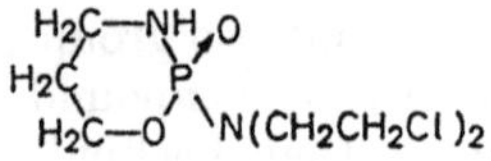

(LXIV)

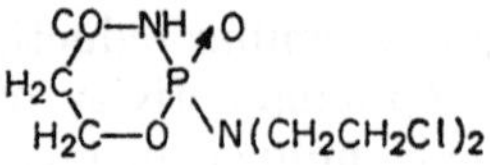

(LXV)

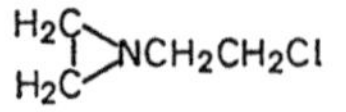

(LXVI)

$HN(CH_2CH_2Cl)_2$

(LXVII)

## Conclusions

Since the statement of Schmidt et al. (1965) that their survey offered little hope that any alkylating agent would affect some neoplasm in a unique way, with its implication that all such agents would ultimately be found to possess similar spectra of activity, there have been significant developments that should make one reconsider this somewhat pessimistic view.

Cyclophosphamide (LXIV) and merophan (XI) are greatly superior to other alkylating drugs [e.g., HN2 (I) and chlorambucil (V)] in the treatment of Burkitt's lymphoma. The aziridine (VIII, CB 1954) exerts a highly specific carcinostatic effect on Walker tumor cells, but has little or no effect on other experimental tumors that are normally very sensitive towards alkylating agents (Cobb et al., 1969). A mouse plasma cell tumor (PC5) responds to aniline mustard (XLVI, R = H) but not to most alkylating drugs. The

$$HN(CH_2CH_2CH_2OO_2SCH_3)_2 \qquad \text{(LXVIII)}$$

dimethanesulfonoxy derivative (LXVIII) inhibits the growth of AH 7974 and AH 66 tumors which are refractory to 250 other alkylating agents and yet does not affect the normally alkylating agent sensitive Yoshida sarcoma (Mandel, 1969). These findings make it apparent that it is possible to design an agent that will affect some neoplasm in a unique way.

The development of more specific agents will require a new approach to the application of such drugs. Henderson (1969) suggests that a drug used for a particular patient should be chosen on the basis of the biochemical characterization of the individual tumor. The assessment of the response of cultured biopsy specimens to a range of drugs would be invaluable in making the selection. More needs to be known about the pharmacodynamic characteristics of carcinostatic drugs, e.g. their persistence in tumors and in normal tissues, and the newer techniques of mass spectrometry coupled with gas-liquid chromatography will have an important role to play in such studies (Nichol, 1969). Advances are being made in the use of combinations of drugs. Dose regimens should be based on a knowledge of tumor growth kinetics and a rational approach to the treatment of malignant disease based on sequential therapy with highly reactive and cell cycle nonspecific agents (e.g., alkylating agents) followed by cell cycle specific agents (e.g., antimetabolites) has been suggested by Schabel (1969).

Potential antineoplastic drugs are still being evaluated in assays using experimental animal tumors and the relevance of these systems continues to be a subject for discussion (LARIONOV, 1970; SCHNEIDERMAN et al., 1970). Only a handful of new agents that show activity in these systems ever proceed to clinical trial. This probably follows from the former obsession with obtaining agents with a wide spectrum of activity; the clinician is at a loss to decide which malignancy to treat with any novel drug. The situation could be changed if the organic chemist set out to design a drug for the treatment of a particular type of tumor, an example being the development of azo mustards for the treatment of liver cancers.

This approach will be dependent on a greater knowledge of the biochemical characteristics of tumors at different sites and the acquiring of such information must go hand in hand with any future attempts to design specific antitumor agents. Since the screening of all tumors for all possible biochemical differences is an impossible pursuit, clues from the study of existing agents must be actively followed up. In this way the asparagine dependence of certain lymphomas and the high glucuronidase activity of some plasma cell tumors was highlighted. The discovery of the biochemical peculiarity of Walker tumor cells that makes them uniquely susceptible to the aziridine CB 1954 should point the way to the design of more specific agents. CONNORS and MELZACK (1971) have suggested that the purine synthetic pathway may be selectively blocked by CB 1954. Screening of human tumors for a similar peculiarity would indicate the type of malignancy likely to respond to this drug.

As HARPER (1959) has stated "the development of comparative biochemistry of various tissues and cells has lagged behind the ingenuity of the synthetic chemist, so that although in many cases the gun could be loaded with suitable ammunition we lack information about the target."

## References


ANDREWS, N. C., WEISS, A. J., ANSFIELD, F. J., ROCHLIN, D. B., MASON, J. H.: Phase 1 study of dibromodulcitol (NSC 104800). Cancer Chemother. Rep. **55**, 61—65 (1971).

ARDENNE, VON, M., REITNAUER, P. G., ROHDE, K., WESTMEYER, H.: *In vivo*-pH-Messung in Krebs-Micrometastasen bei optimierter Übersauerung. Z. Naturforschung. **24**, 1610—1619 (1969).

ASHBY, B. S.: pH studies in human malignant tumors. Lancet II, 312—315 (1966).

BARDOS, T. J., CHMIELEWICZ, Z. F., HEBBORN, P.: Structure-activity relationships of alkylating agents in cancer chemotherapy. Ann. N. Y. Acad. Sci. **163**, 1006—1025 (1969).

BELIKOVA, A. M., ZARYTOVA, V. F., GRINEVA, N. I.: Synthesis of ribonucleosides and diribonucleoside phosphates containing 2-chloroethylamine and nitrogen mustard residues. Tet. Letters 3357—3562 (1967).

BERGEL, F., STOCK, J. A.: Cytoactive amino acid and peptide derivatives. Part I. Substituted phenylalanines. J. chem. Soc. 2409—2417 (1954).

BLOIS, M. S.: Melanoma detection with radioiodoquinoline. J. nuclear Med. **9**, 492—493 (1968).

BLOIS, M. S., KALLMAN, K. F.: The incorporation of $C^{14}$ from 3,4-dihydroxyphenylalanine-2-$C^{14}$ into the melanin of mouse melanoma. Cancer Res. **24**, 863—868 (1964).

BROCK, N.: Pharmacological characterization of cyclophosphamide (NSC 26271) and cyclophosphamide metabolites. Cancer Chemother. Rep. **51**, 315—325 (1967).

BUKHARI, M. A., EVERETT, J. L., ROSS, W. C. J.: Aryl-2-halogenoalkylamines. Part XXVI. Glucuronic, sulphuric and phosphoric esters of *p*-di-2-chloroethylaminophenol. Biochem. Pharmacol. **21**, 963—967 (1972).

BUKVA, N. F., GASS, G. H.: Oncolytic effect of four C-16 aziridine steroidal alkylating agents. Cancer Chemother. Rep. **51**, 431—433 (1967).

CALVERT, N., CONNORS, T. A., ROSS, W. C. J.: Aryl-2-halogenoalkylamines. XXV. Derivatives of sulphanilamide designed for selective deposition in neoplastic tissue. Europ. J. Cancer **4**, 627—636 (1968).

CASSAZZA, A. R., CAHN, E. L., CARBONE, P. P.: Preliminary studies with dibromomannitol in patients with chronic myelogenous leukaemia. Cancer Chemother. Rep. **51**, 91—97 (1967).

Cater, D. B., Phillips, A. F.: Measurement of electrode potentials in living and dead tissues. Nature (Lond.) **174**, 121—123 (1954).

Clifford, P.: Response to particular chemotherapeutic and other agents and treatment of CNS involvement. In: Burkitt, D. P., Wright, D. H. (Eds.): Burkitt's lymphoma, pp. 52—63. Edinburgh-London: Livingstone 1970.

Cobb, L. M.: Tissue specific chemotherapy. Cancer Chemother. Rep. **54**, 375—378 (1970).

Cobb, L. M., Connors, T. A., Elson, L. A., Khan, A. H., Mitchley, B. C. V., Ross, W. C. J., Whisson, M. E.: 2,4-Dinitro-5-ethyleneimino-benzamide (CB 1954): a potent and selective inhibitor of the growth of the Walker carcinoma 256. Biochem. Pharmacol. **18**, 1519—1527 (1969).

Connors, T. A., Melzack, D. H.: Studies on the mechanism of action of 5-aziridinyl-2,4-dinitrobenzamide (CB 1954), a selective inhibitor of the Walker tumour. Int. J. Cancer **7**, 86—92 (1971).

Connors, T. A., Mitchley, B. C. V., Rosenoer, V. M., Ross, W. C. J.: The effect of glucose pretreatment on the carcinostatic and toxic activities of some alkylating agents. Biochem. Pharmacol. **13**, 395—400 (1964).

Connors, T. A., Ross, W. C. J.: New chloroethylaminoaryl substituted amino acids. Chem. and Ind. 492—493 (1960).

Connors, T. A., Whisson, M. E.: Cure of mice bearing advanced plasma cell tumours with aniline mustard. Nature (Lond.) **206**, 689—691 (1965).

Connors, T. A., Whisson, M. E.: Cure of mice bearing advanced plasma cell tumours with aniline mustard: the relationship between glucuronidase activity and tumour sensitivity. Nature (Lond.) **210**, 866—867 (1966).

Counsell, R. E., Pocha, P., Morales, J. O., Beierwaltes, W. H.: Tumour localising agents. III. Radioiodinated quinoline derivatives. J. pharm. Sci. **56**, 1042—1044 (1967).

Csaba, G., Kiss, J., Korosi, J.: Intratumoral localisation of phenazathionium mustard chloride: a new anti-tumour agent. Neoplasma **16**, 145—149 (1969).

Csaba, G., Korosi, J.: A new anti-tumour agent: phenazathionium mustard salt. Neoplasma **15**, 443—445 (1968).

Danielli, J. F.: The designing of selective drugs. Ciba Found. Symp. Leukaemia Res. 263—273 (1954).

Danielli, J. F.: General cell theory and drug design. In: Biological approaches to cancer chemotherapy. (Harris, R. J. C., Ed.) London and New York: Academic Press 1961, pp. 1—9.

Davis, W., Ross, W. C. J.: A highly reactive sulphur mustard gas derivative for localised infusion studies. J. med. Chem. **8**, 757—759 (1965).

Degteva, S. A., Larionov, L. F.: Toxicity and anti-tumor effect of $\beta$-sitosterol and cholesterol esters of *p*-di(2-chloroethyl)aminophenylacetic acid. Vopr. Onkl. **12**, 51—53 (1966).

Duvall, L. R.: Ross' azo mustard. Cancer Chemother. Rep. **14**, 174—179 (1961).

Dzialoszynski, L. M., Kroll, J. L., Frömlich, A.: Arylsulphatase activity of some malignant tumours. Clin. chim. Acta **14**, 450—453 (1966).

Eckhardt, S., Sellei, C., Horvath, P., Institoris, L.: Effect of 1,6-dibromo-1,6-dideoxy-D-mannitol on chronic granulocytic leukaemia. Cancer Chemother. Rep. **33**, 57—61 (1963).

Eden, M., Haines, B., Kahler, H.: The pH of rat tumors measured *in vivo*. J. nat. Cancer Inst. **16**, 541—556 (1955).

Ehrlich, P.: Über die Beziehungen von chemischer Constitution, Verteilung und pharmakologischer Wirkung (1898). In: Himmelweit, F. (Ed.): The collected papers of Paul Ehrlich, vol. I., pp. 570—595. New York: MacMillan (Pergamon) 1965.

Elson, L. A.: Radiation and radiomimetic chemicals. London: Butterworths 1963.

Elson, L. A., Jarman, M., Ross, W. C. J.: Toxicity, haematological effects and anti-tumor activity of epoxides derived from disubstituted hexitols. Mode of action of mannitol myleran Europ. J. Cancer **4**, 617—625 (1968).

Fishbein, W. N., Carbone, P. P., Owens, A. H., Jr., Kelly, M. G., Rall, D. P., Tarr, N.: Preliminary studies with 5-[*bis*(2-chloroethyl)amino]-DL-tryptophan. Cancer Chemother. Rep. **42**, 19—24 (1964).

Gerzon, K., Cochran, J. E., White, A. L., Monahan, R., Krumkalns, E. V., Scroggs, R. E., Mills, J.: Structure activity relationships of some diamine *bis*-epoxides in mouse leukaemia. J. med. pharm. Chem. **1**, 223—243 (1959).

Gilman, A., Philips, F. S.: The biological actions and therapeutic applications of the $\beta$-chloroethyl amines and sulphides. Science **103**, 409—415 (1946).

Goodman, L. E., Kramer, S. P., Gaby, S. D., Bakal, D., Solomon, R. D., Williamson, C. E., Miller, J. I., Sass, S., Witten, B., Seligman, A. M.: Enzyme-alterable alkylating agents. II. Clinical evaluation of N,N'-*bis*[(2-chloroethylthio)acetyl]-1,2-ethylenediamine (S-46). Cancer **15**, 1056—1061 (1962).

GOODMAN, L. E., ULFOHN, A., KRAMER, S. P., CENDANA, E. H., FLORES, A. B., BAKAL, D., ABRAMS, S. J., HIRSCHFIELD, R. L., CALLE, S., WILLIAMSON, C. E., SASS, S., WITTEN, B., SELIGMAN, A. M.: Enzyme alterable alkylating agents. VIII. Clinical trials with intra-arterial infusion of an alkylating agent with a half life of 0.2 second. Ann. Surg. **162**, 663—688 (1965).

GRAM, H. F., MOSHER, C. W., BAKER, B. R.: Potential anticancer agents. XVII. Alkylating agents to phenylalanine mustard. J. Amer. chem. Soc. **81**, 3103—3108 (1959).

GREENSTEIN, J. P.: Biochemistry of cancer. New York: Academic Press 1947.

HARPER, N. J.: Drug latentiation. J. med. pharm. Chem. **1**, 467—500 (1959).

HEBBORN, P., DANIELLI, J. F.: The increased tumour inhibitory effect of enzyme-activated nitrogen mustards. Biochem. Pharmacol. **1**, 19—24 (1958).

HEBBORN, P., SIMPSON, C. L., MIHICH, E.: Anti-tumour and toxicological effects of *p*-carboxy-carbanilic acid, N-[*p*-*bis*((2-chloroethyl)amino]phenyl ester (NSC 130998, IC 140). Cancer Chemother. Rep. **54**, 23—31 (1970).

HEIDELBERGER, C.: The need for additional alkylating agents and antimetabolites. Cancer Res. **29**, 2435—2442 (1969).

HENDERSON, J. F.: Variation in selective toxicity: causes and consequences. Cancer Res. **29**, 2404—2406 (1969).

HILL, D. L., KIRK, M. C., STRUCK, R. F.: Isolation and identification of 4-ketocyclophosphamide, a possible active form of the anti-tumour agent, cyclophosphamide. J. Amer. chem. Soc. **92**, 3207—3208 (1970).

HUDSON, R. F., TIMMIS, G. M., MARSHALL, R. D.: A physicochemical investigation into the biological action of myleran and related sulphonic esters. Biochem. Pharmacol. **1**, 48—59 (1958).

ISRAELS, L. G., RITZMANN, S. E.: Laboratory and clinical studies on a new azo-mustard, 4-di-2″-chloroethylamino-2-methylazobenzene-2′-carboxylic acid (CB 1414). Acta Unio intern. contra cancrum. **16**, 665—671 (1960).

IYER, V. N., SZYBALSKI, W.: Chemical basis of the activation of mitomycin C and its ability to cross link DNA molecules. Bact. Proc. 40—41 (1964).

JARMAN, M., ROSS, W. C. J.: Formation of 1,2 : 5,6-dianhydro-D-mannitol from 1,6-dibromo- and 1,6-dimethanesulphonoxy-1,6-dideoxy-D-mannitol. Chem. and Ind. 1789—1790 (1967).

JONES, R., JR., JONSSON, U., BROWNING, M., LESSNER, H., PRICE, C. C., SEN, A. K.: Initial clinical trial of the nitrogen mustard analogues of chloroquine and quinacrine: a preliminary report. Ann. N. Y. Acad. Sci. **68**, 1133—1150 (1968).

KAHLER, H., ROBERTSON, W. B.: pH of normal liver and hepatic tumours. J. nat. Cancer Inst. **3**, 495—501 (1943).

KHAN, A. H., ROSS, W. C. J.: Tumour-growth inhibitory nitrophenylaziridines and related compounds: structure-activity relationships. Chem. biol. Interact. **1**, 27—47 (1969/70).

KRAMER, S. P., GOODMAN, L. E., DORFMAN, H., SOLOMON, R., RUTENBERG, A. M., PINEDA, E., NASON, L. L., ULFOHN, A., GABY, S. D., BAKAL, D., WILLIAMSON, C. E., MILLER, J. I., SASS, S., WITTEN, B., SELIGMAN, A. M.: Enzyme alterable alkylating agents. VI. Synthesis, chemical properties, toxicities, and clinical trial of haloacetates and haloacetamides containing enzyme-susceptible bonds. J. nat. Cancer Inst. **31**, 297—327 (1963).

KYLE, R. A., CARBONE, P. P., LYNCH, J. J., OWENS, A. H., JR., COSTA, G., SILVER, R. T., CUTTNER, J., HARLEY, J. B., LEONE, L. A., SHNIDER, B. I., HOLLAND, J. F.: Evaluation of tryptophan mustard (NSC 62403) in patients with plasmacytic myeloma. Cancer Res. **27**, 510—515 (1967).

LAPIS, K., NEMETH, L.: Die Wirkung des BCM auf die Metastasenbildung transplantierter Tiergeschwulste. Klin. Wochschr. **34**, 864—867 (1956).

LARIONOV, L. F.: Cancer chemotherapy. Oxford: Pergamon Press 1965.

LARIONOV, L. F.: Methods of screening anticancer drugs in the Soviet Union. Cancer Chemother. Rep. **54**, 71—77 (1970).

LARIONOV, L. F., KHOKHLOV, A. S., SHKODINSKAJA, E. N., VASINA, O. S., TROOSHEIKINA, V. I., NOVIKOVA, M. A.: Studies on the antitumor activity of *p*-di-(2-chloroethyl)aminophenylalanine (sarcolysine). Lancet **269**, 169—171 (1955).

MANDEL, H. G.: Summary of informal discussion on the basis for future approaches to cancer chemotherapy. Cancer Res. **29**, 2475—2477 (1969).

MEYER, V.: Medicinisch-chemische Notizen. II. Physiologische Wirkung der gechlorten Schwefelaethyle. Ber. **20**, 1729—1731 (1887).

MEYZA, J., COBB, L. M.: The clinical trial of an alkylating agent with a short half-life designed for intra-arterial chemotherapy. Cancer **27**, 369—373 (1971).

NICHOL, C. A.: The application of new knowledge to the effective administration of anticancer agents. Cancer Res. **29**, 2469—2470 (1969).

OCHOA, M., JR., HIRSCHBERG, E.: Alkylating agents. Exp. Chemother. **5**, 1—132 (1967).

Osdene, T. S., Ward, D. N., Chapman, W. H., Rakoff, H.: The synthesis of *m*-(di-(2-chloroethyl)amino]-DL-phenylalanine. J. Amer. chem. Soc. **81**, 3100—3102 (1959).
Papanastassiou, Z. B., Bruni, R. J., White, E., Levins, P. L.: Potential carcinolytic agents. IV. Diazoamino mustards. J. med. Chem. **9**, 725—729 (1966).
Rall, D. P., Ben, M., McCarthy, D. M.: 1,3-*Bis*-β-chloroethyl-1-nitrosourea (BCNU). Toxicity and initial clinical trial. Proc. Amer. Assoc. Cancer Res. **4**, 55 (1963).
Ross, W. C. J.: The chemistry of cytotoxic alkylating agents. Advanc. Cancer Res. **1**, 397—449 (1953).
Ross, W. C. J.: Increased sensitivity of the Walker tumour towards aromatic nitrogen mustards carrying basic side chains following glucose pretreatment. Biochem. Pharmacol. **8**, 235—240 (1961).
Ross, W. C. J.: Biological alkylating agents. London and Washington (D.C.): Butterworths 1962.
Ross, W. C. J.: Aryl-2-halogenoalkylarylamines. XXI. The design of agents to exploit differences in cellular oxidation-reduction potentials. Biochem. Pharmacol. **13**, 969—982 (1964).
Ross, W. C. J., Warwick, G. P.: Reduction of cytotoxic azo compounds by hydrazine and by the xanthine oxidase-xanthine system. Nature (Lond.) **176**, 298—299 (1955).
Ross, W. C. J., Warwick, G. P., Roberts, J. J.: Aryl-2-halogenoalkylamines. Part XIV. Some compounds possessing latent cytotoxic activity. J. chem. Soc. 3110—3116 (1955).
Salmon, S. E., Yount, W. J., Shadduck, R. K., Hall, T. C., Shilling, A.: *o*-DL-Sarcolysin (NSC 57199) in solid tumours. Cancer Chemother. Rep. **50**, 685—692 (1966).
Sass, S., Williamson, C. E., Kramer, S. P., Goodman, L. E., Ulfohn, A., Seligman, A. M., Witten, B.: Enzyme-alterable alkylating agents. VII. The design of short lived mustards. J. med. Chem. **8**, 14—17 (1965).
Schabel, F. M., Jr.: The use of tumour growth kinetics in planing "curative" chemotherapy of advanced solid tumours. Cancer Res. **29**, 2384—2389 (1969).
Schabel, F. M., Jr., Johnston, T. P., McCaleb, G. S., Montgomery, J. A., Laster, W. R., Skipper, H. E.: Experimental evaluation of potential anti-cancer agents. VIII. Effects of certain nitrosoureas on intracerebral L1210 leukaemia. Cancer Res. **23**, 725—733 (1963).
Schilling, A., Ulfohn, A., Aybar, O., Miller, S., Kravitz, S., Goodman, L. E., Gaby, S. D., Bakal, D., Kramer, S. P., Williamson, C. E., Sass, S., Miller, J. I., Witten, B., Seligman, A. M.: Enzyme-alterable alkylating agents. IV. Treatment of cancer in children with repetitive massive doses of S-46, protecting the extremity marrow by tourniquets. Cancer **16**, 727 (1963).
Schmidt, L. H.: Observations on the therapeutic activity and toxicity of 2-chloroethyl methanesulphonate — CB 1506 (NSC 18016). Cancer Chemother. Rep. **9**, 56—68 (1960).
Schmidt, L. H., Fradkin, R., Sullivan, R., Flowers, A.: Comparative pharmacology of alkylating agents. Cancer Chemother. Rep. suppl. 2, 1—1528 (1965).
Schneiderman, M. A., Goldin, A., Carter, S. K., Mantel, N., Stock, C. C.: On screening procedures. Cancer Chemother. Rep. **54**, 294—301 (1970).
Seligman, A. M., Ulfohn, A., Gaby, S. D., Goodman, L. E., Aybar, O., Kramer, S. P., Bakal, D., Haber, S., Williamson, C. E., Miller, J. I., Sass, S., Witten, B.: Enzyme alterable alkylating agents: a new approach to regional chemotherapy by intra-arterial infusion of new short-lived alkylating agents. Ann. Surg. **156**, 429—441 (1962).
Tsou, K. C., Hoegerle, K., Su, H. C. F.: Synthesis of possible cancer chemotherapeutic compounds based on enzyme approach. IV. Aziridine derivatives. J. med. Chem. **6**, 435—439 (1963).
Tsou, K. C., Su, H. C. F.: Synthesis of possible cancer chemotherapeutic compounds based on enzyme approach. V. Tetrazolium nitrogen mustards. J. med. Chem. **6**, 693—696 (1963).
Vasil'eva, M. N., Martynov, V. S., Berlin, A. Y.: Synthesis of bis(2-chloroethyl)amino derivatives of pyrocatechol. III. Derivatives of 3-(3,4-dihydroxyphenyl)alanine (dopa). Zh. org. Khim. **6**, 1677—1682 (1970).
Vicker, S., Hebborn, P., Moran, J. F., Triggle, D. J.: Synthesis and evaluation of esters of *N,N-bis*(2-chloroethyl)-*p*-aminophenol and *N,N-bis*(2-bromoethyl)-*p*-aminophenol as potential antitumour agents. J. med. Chem. **12**, 491—494 (1969).
Wall, M. E., Abernethy, S., Jr., Carol, F. I., Taylor, D. J.: The effects of some steroidal alkylating agents on experimental animal mammary tumour and leukaemia systems. J. med. Chem. **12**, 810—818 (1969).
Weinhouse, S.: Oxidative metabolism of neoplastic tissue. Advanc. Cancer Res. **3**, 270—325 (1955).
Whisson, M. E., Connors, T. A., Jeney, A.: A mechanism of cure of large plasma cell tumours. Arch. Immunologia Therapiae Exp. **14**, 825—831 (1966).
White, F. R.: Sarcolysin and related compounds. Cancer Chemother. Rept. **6**, 61—93 (1960).
White, F. R.: Agent data summaries. Dopan. Cancer Chemother. Rep. **14**, 169—173 (1961).

WILLIAMS, H. M.: Clinical evaluation of uracil mustard. Cancer Chemother. Rep. **32**, 73—75 (1963).

WILLIAMSON, C. E., MILLER, J. I., SASS, S., CASANOVA, J., KRAMER, S. P., SELIGMAN, A. M., WITTEN, B.: Enzyme alterable alkylating agents. V. Design of sulphur mustards with varying degrees of hydrolytic stability in a search for short biological half-life agents. J. nat. Cancer Inst. **31**, 273—296 (1963).

WITTEN, B., SASS, S., MILLER, J. I., WILLIAMSON, C. E., GUERRERO, H. G., KRAMER, S. P., SOLOMON, R. D., GOODMAN, M. D., SELIGMAN, A. M.: Enzyme-alterable alkylating agents. III. Synthesis, chemical properties, and toxicities of mustards containing enzyme-susceptible ester bonds. Cancer **15**, 1062—1072 (1962a).

WITTEN, B., WILLIAMSON, C. E., SASS, S., MILLER, J. I., BEST, R., WICKS, G. E., JR., KRAMER, S. P., WEINBURG, T., SOLOMON, R. D., GOODMAN, L. E., SELIGMAN, A. M.: Enzyme-alterable alkylating agents. I. Synthesis, chemical properties, and toxicities of sulphur mustards containing enzyme-susceptible amide bonds. Cancer **15**, 1041—1055 (1962b).

YOUNT, W. J., HALL, T. C., SCHILLING, A., SHADDUCK, R. K.: DL-ortho-Sarcolysin (NSC 57199) in treatment of multiple myeloma. Cancer Chemother. Rep. **51**, 517—523 (1967).

ZBYTNIEWSKI, Z.: Activity of arylsulphatase in transplantable melanotic and amelanotic melanoma in golden hamster (Mesocricetus auratus Waterhouse). Nowotwory **19**, 165—172 (1969).

Chapter 4

# Rational Design of Folic Acid Antagonists

J. A. R. MEAD

With 2 Figures

## Introduction

Although the title of this chapter implies that there has been a successful rational approach to the design of folic acid antagonists, a review of the history of these agents suggests quite the opposite. In more recent years the light of rationalism has begun to gleam more strongly and there promises to be an "age of reason" in the design of antifolates. The objectives of this chapter are two-fold. First, by reviewing the properties of existing agents it is hoped to demonstrate that perhaps a retrospective approach to old agents might be extremely productive in light of our current knowledge of folate biochemistry, and second, by consideration of new areas of considerable promise, more truly rational approaches will be discussed which could greatly enhance the therapeutic utility of these agents.

While it is recognized that folic acid antagonists are extremely useful in the chemotherapy of bacterial diseases, as well as in the treatment of malaria and certain other conditions, it is in cancer chemotherapy that their greatest potential lies. For this reason this chapter will be confined to this aspect of antifolate therapy, and the reader is referred to the excellent book by BLAKLEY (1969) and the recently published New York Academy of Sciences Symposium entitled, "Folate Antagonists as Chemotherapeutic Agents" edited by BERTINO (1971) for comprehensive accounts of the extent of current knowledge across the length and breadth of the folate-antifolate fields.

## Historical Aspects

When ANGIER et al. (1946) elucidated the structure of folate (pteroylglutamic acid) it is doubtful whether the authors could have envisioned the enormous volume of papers, articles and reviews which were to follow their discovery. Much attention is still being focused on the biochemical functions of folate derivatives. The high citation frequency of articles in this field is certainly an accurate measure of the importance of these compounds in the biochemical economy of most higher animals. Although delayed by two years, accompanying the literature explosion which ensued after the discovery of folate, was a parallel increase in the literature citations of aminopterin and methotrexate, two of the earliest folate antagonists to be synthesized. Aminopterin was synthesized by SEEGER et al. (1947) and methotrexate by SEEGER et al. (1949). These two synthetic folate analogs were immediately recognized as potent antagonists of the bacterial growth-promoting action of folate, but it remained for FARBER et al. (1948) to demonstrate that aminopterin was able to produce temporary remissions in acute leukemia in children. This observation not only established aminopterin, and subsequently methotrexate, as valuable drugs, it also showed that cancer chemotherapy, until then a stepchild of pharmacology, had come of age. After this auspicious beginning to the antifolate era it was to be expected that more and better antifolates would soon be available. This was not to be, and twenty-five years after the synthesis of aminopterin, the folic acid antagonist of choice in the treatment of human malignant disease remains the closely related compound methotrexate (amethopterin). Since this chapter is concerned with the rational design of folic acid antagonists, it will therefore be instructive to explore what has happened to attempts to produce "rational" antifolates in the period since the advent of the two trail-blazing agents. Consideration will also be given to the thesis that it is not possible to improve significantly on the biological effects of methotrexate and that it will remain the pre-eminent 4-aminopteroylglutamate antagonist in clinical use for the foreseeable future. This is not to suggest, however, that other folate antagonists will not be discovered, but rather a recognition of the fact that all approaches employed so far have failed to yield an agent with clinical activity superior to methotrexate.

There are many ways in which a drug may be selected as an agent of potential clinical interest. Random empirical screening in all available biological systems has sometimes uncovered useful agents. Molecular manipulation of a prototype active drug has in some instances been a very useful method of improving activity and at the same time can contribute to an understanding of its mechanism of action. Structural modification of important metabolites to give an antimetabolite has been a most profitable approach in cancer chemotherapy where the majority of active drugs seem to influence the synthesis of DNA and/or RNA. When an enzyme is known to be important in biochemical processes involved in cell replication, inhibitors of the step which it catalyzes can result in pharmacologically active compounds (e.g. at the present time a considerable effort is being concentrated on a search for inhibitors of reverse transcriptase in the hope of obtaining a selective inhibitor of viral carcinogenesis). More commonly, however, after the pharmacological activity of an agent is detected by empirical approaches, the biochemical lesion it induces is discovered, and its activity can then be related to inhibition of a specific enzyme. Finally, serendipity or, "the chance which favors the prepared mind," has made spectacular contributions to chemotherapy and pharmacology and is perhaps best exemplified by the discovery of penicillin. Unfortunately, this latter approach is notoriously unpredictable and therefore unreliable as a systematic source of new drugs.

Historically the folate antagonists have followed the developmental course illustrated in Table 1. The discovery of folate and the elucidation of its structure and synthesis made possible the synthesis of a large group of antimetabolites very soon afterwards. These antimetabolites were in large part produced before the biochemistry of folate was understood even slightly. Because of this, the activity of these antagonists can only be assessed in relation to the knowledge existing at the time of their initial synthesis. Most of them have not been examined in the light of current knowledge of folate metabolism. The pre-eminence of methotrexate in clinical medicine today is perhaps all the more remarkable since its development was purely empirical and not guided by any knowledge of biochemical mechanisms other than the clear understanding that folate was an essential growth factor for microbe and mammal. Parenthetically, it might be added that among a very large number of purine antagonists which have been synthesized in the last two decades, one of the first, 6-mercaptopurine, remains the major drug of choice when an antipurine-sensitive condition requires treatment (GOLDIN et al., 1971). After the conversion of folate to citrovorum factor was shown to be an important 4-amino-

Table 1. *A chronology of events in the development of antifolates structurally related to folates*

| Year | Event | Reference |
|---|---|---|
| 1940 | Identification of norite eluate factor in yeast extract | SNELL and PETERSON |
| 1941 | Identification of "folic acid" in autolysed spinach leaves as growth factor for *S. faecalis R* | MITCHELL et al. |
| 1946 | Elucidation of the structure and synthesis of folate | ANGIER et al. |
| 1947 | Synthesis of aminopterin | SEEGER et al. |
| 1948 | Identification of "citrovorum factor", a growth factor for *Leuconostoc citrovorum (Pediococcus cerevisiae)* | SAUBERLICH and BAUMAN |
| | First clinical use of aminopterin | FARBER et al. |
| 1949 | Synthesis of amethopterin (methotrexate) | SEEGER et al. |
| 1950 | Demonstration of the conversion of folic acid to citrovorum factor in rats and its inhibition by aminopterin. Protection of rats from aminopterin-induced toxicity by citrovorum factor | NICHOL and WELCH |
| 1952 | Elucidation of the structure and synthesis of citrovorum factor | COSULICH et al., and ROTH et al. |
| 1957 | Aminopterin inhibition of inactivation of folic acid by liver | FUTTERMAN and SILVERMAN |
| | Inhibition of the enzymatic reduction of folic acid and dihydrofolic acid to tetrahydrofolic acid by aminopterin | FUTTERMAN |
| 1958 | Noncompetitive inhibition of dihydrofolate reductase by aminopterin and methotrexate | OSBORN et al. |
| 1959 | Synthesis of dichloroamethopterin (dichloromethotrexate) | ANGIER and CURRAN, |
| | Indefinite survivors in L1210 leukemic mice produced by treatment of advanced disease with dichloroamethopterin | GOLDIN et al. |
| 1960 | Synthesis and antimicrobial activity of tetrahydroaminopterin and tetrahydroamethopterin | KISLIUK |
| 1961 | Increased levels of dihydrofolate reductase associated with resistance to methotrexate in murine leukemia L1210 | MISRA et al. |
| | Activity of tetrahydromethotrexate against leukemia L1210 | MEAD et al. |
| | Recognition of 5-methyltetrahydrofolate as a source of the methyl group of methionine | LARRABEE et al. |
| 1964 | Synthesis of tetrahydrohomofolate, a potent inhibitor of thymidylate synthetase | GOODMAN et al. |
| 1965 | Clinical trial of dichloromethotrexate showing it to be not greatly superior to methotrexate in treatment of human lymphoma and leukemia | FREI et al. |
| | Identification of the 7-hydroxy derivative as a metabolite of dichloromethotrexate in man | LOO and ADAMSON |
| | Identification of rabbit liver methotrexate oxidase as aldehyde oxidase | JOHNS et al. |
| 1966 | Demonstration of the antileukemic activity of tetrahydrohomofolate in a methotrexate-resistant variant of leukemia L1210 | MEAD et al. |
| 1970 | Potent inhibition of thymidylate synthetase by a 2-amino-4-hydroxyquinazoline antifolate | BIRD et al. |
| 1971 | Synthesis of 5-methyltetrahydrohomofolate — a stable derivative of tetrahydrohomofolate | KNOTT et al. |
| 1972 | Demonstration of activity of 5-methyltetrahydrohomofolate against leukemia L1210 and its methotrexate-resistant variant | MISHRA et al. |
| | Preliminary clinical trial of methasquin | ETCUBANAS et al. |

pteroylglutamate-sensitive step, eight years passed before the potent "irreversible" inhibition of dihydrofolate reductase by aminopterin and methotrexate was first observed. The term irreversible is in quotes because, while there is no doubt that the binding to the enzyme is very strong, it is not by a covalent link; in fact, recent work suggests that appreciable enzymic activity may be restored *in vivo* relatively soon after administration of methotrexate (MISHRA et al., 1972). This important demonstration of a potent biochemical property of aminopterin and methotrexate resulted in a concentrated effort to understand this relationship in more detail. The studies of BERTINO (1964) and WERKHEISER (1964) are particularly noteworthy. However, apart from the fact that these and later studies confirmed the extreme sensitivity of dihydrofolate reductase to inhibition by 2,4-diaminopteroylglutamate derivatives, as well as other compounds, the discovery of this inhibitory effect did not readily explain other results. Among these were the finding that methotrexate exerted a greater antileukemic effect against leukemia L1210 in mice when given in larger doses on an intermittent schedule than on a daily schedule. Presumably, inhibition of dihydrofolate reductase was similar in extent and duration on both schedules according to the thinking at the time. Another finding (GOLDIN et al., 1959) showed that a derivative of methotrexate, 3′,5′-dichloromethotrexate, was much less toxic to mice and had a remarkable effect on the survival time of mice with advanced leukemia L1210. Animals treated with the drug for prolonged periods not only were cured of the disease, but were resistant to reimplantation of the parent tumor. Since methotrexate and dichloromethotrexate do not differ much in their ability to inhibit dihydrofolate reductase from leukemia L1210, the differences in the biological effects of the two drugs must have their origins in other systems. The differences in toxicity to the mouse can most probably be explained by the ability of the host to metabolize dichloromethotrexate more rapidly than methotrexate (JOHNS and VALERINO, 1971), but this does not explain, for example, the greater persistence of the inhibitory effect of dichloromethotrexate on the incorporation of formate into acid-soluble adenine in leukemic mouse spleen reported by SCHRECKER et al. (1960). It was, therefore, something of a disappointment when dichloromethotrexate was subjected to a limited clinical trial only to be found not greatly superior to methotrexate (FREI et al., 1965). Even the dose levels were not too different in spite of the demonstration of the metabolism of dichloromethotrexate in man (OLIVERIO and DAVIDSON, 1962). So it remains to the present that methotrexate is the clinical antifolate of choice, but perhaps even more significantly the evaluation of new antifolates tends to be based on their biological effect (usually antitumor activity) and the potency of their inhibition of dihydrofolate reductase. In other words, the selection mechanisms are geared to identifying more of the same general type of drug when what appears to be needed is another system by which to make the selection.

There have been two fairly extensive reviews of the relationship of structure to antitumor activity in structural analogs of pteroylglutamate (VENDITTI et al., 1960; MEAD et al., 1968). The major determinant of antitumor activity in these studies was the presence of a free 4-amino group in the pteridine ring. Since this was also necessary for strong inhibition of dihydrofolate reductase (ZAKRZEWSKI, 1963), the correlation of antitumor activity and enzyme inhibition was reinforced. An additional conclusion drawn from the later study by MEAD et al. (1968), was that antitumor activity in a series of compounds which were structurally derived from at least part of the folate molecule was confined to two arbitrarily defined classes of compound. These were the compounds derived from folate itself which contained all three moieties (i.e. pteridine, *p*-aminobenzoic acid, and an amino acid) and the 2,4-diaminopyrimidine and 4,6-diaminodihydrotriazine related compounds which were considered as one class. Both classes of active compounds contained the diamino configuration with one exception and that was tetrahydrohomofolate (MEAD et al., 1966) which had borderline activity against leukemia L1210. This latter compound will be discussed in detail later in this chapter. Compounds with the diamino function which did not demonstrate important antitumor activity included those related to pteroic acid and a large group of simple pteridines. These very general conclusions do not make it possible to design a rational approach to the synthesis of new antifolates, but they at least focus on some general requirements for this type of agent.

Perhaps the most rational approach to the search for antifolates with specific enzyme binding properties was employed by BAKER who developed the concept of active-site-directed irreversible inhibitors of pharmacologically important enzymes. This concept formed the basis of a book by BAKER (1967) in which an extensive discussion is presented relating the concept to inhibition of dihydrofolate reductase. A more recent review by BAKER (1970) discusses some of his later findings related to the enzyme and also to the antitumor activity of some enzyme inhibitors made in accordance with the concept. Essentially this approach requires that there be a difference in the susceptibility of the enzyme in tumor tissue and in normal tissue leading to the ultimate disadvantage of the tumor cell. This can readily be shown to be the case for mammalian cell dihydrofolate reductase, relative to bacterial reductase as this forms the basis for the potent inhibitory effect of trimethoprim on bacterial growth, with relatively no toxicity for the host (HITCHINGS and BURCHALL, 1965). Similarly, malarial dihydrofolate reductase is far more sensitive to pyrimethamine than is the mammalian enzyme (FERONE et al., 1969). Thus, BAKER'S approach was an attempt to find an exploitable biochemical difference between the tumor and host cell based on the difference in properties of dihydrofolate reductase in the two cell species. This approach is in contrast to the extensive but unsuccessful efforts to find a therapeutically exploitable biochemical difference, of any kind, between tumor and host which was carried out in the early 1960's (ZUBROD et al., 1966). Several compounds which were synthesized by BAKER had significant activity *in vivo* against both leukemia L 1210 in mice and the Walker 256 tumor in rats. It is not clear at present whether the antitumor activity seen *in vivo* represents a positive correlation with BAKER'S concept or whether the possession of the 4,6-diaminodihydro-*s*-triazine moiety is sufficient to account for the activity by whatever mechanism is involved in their antitumor action.

When one considers the many enzyme systems involved in folate metabolism as depicted in Fig. 1 and also how little is known about the effect of methotrexate and other 4-amino antifolates on these individual reactions, there must be some doubt as to whether the correlation between the inhibition of dihydrofolate reductase and antitumor effect is complete. In view of the relatively high selectivity shown by methotrexate when it is used as a therapeutic agent, the statement by GEILS et al. (1971) should be borne in mind. These authors stated, "The extreme degree of dihydrofolate reductase binding by methotrexate, inhibiting formation of all folate coenzymes, must diminish the specificity of methotrexate for neoplastic cells, and probably accounts for the prolonged severe toxicity of methotrexate." Since it now appears that this inhibition may not be as prolonged *in vivo* as previously supposed (MISHRA et al., 1972), a detailed assessment of the effects of methotrexate on other folate-dependent systems is urgently required to guide more rationally the synthesis of other types of antifolates which do not have as their dominant property the ability to inhibit dihydrofolate reductase stoichiometrically.

In 1961 there was a development which may yet lead to a rational approach to chemotherapy with antifolates. This was the discovery by MISRA et al. (1961) that when successive resistance to methotrexate and dichloromethotrexate was accomplished in murine leukemia L1210, there was an associated progressive and dramatic increase in the dihydrofolate reductase content of the tumor. This phenomenon once again focused attention on the methotrexate-dihydrofolate reductase interaction. However, it also marked the beginning of a new era because subsequently it led to the proposal that it might be possible to take advantage of

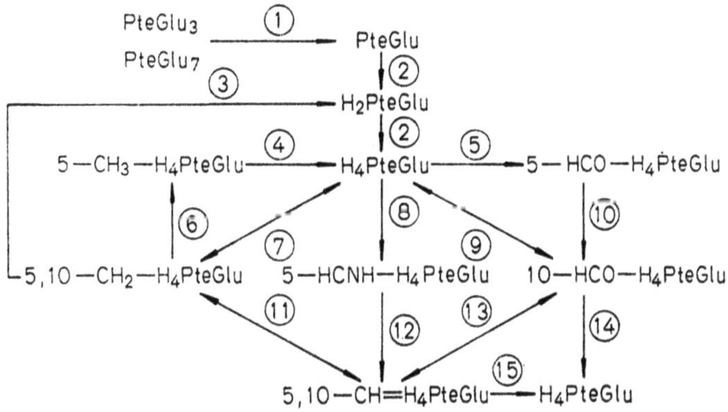


Fig. 1. Enzymic reactions of folates, *1* conjugase, *2* dihydrofolate reductase, *3* thymidylate synthetase, *4* methionine synthetase, *5* formylglutamate formyl transferase, *6* $N^5$, $N^{10}$-methylenetetrahydrofolate reductase, *7* L-serine hydroxymethyl transferase, *8* formiminoglutamate formimino transferase, *9* $N^{10}$-formyltetrahydrofolate synthetase, *10* $N^5$-formyltetrahydrofolate isomerase, *11* $N^5$, $N^{10}$-methylenetetrahydrofolate dehydrogenase, *12* $N^5$-formiminotetrahydrofolate cyclodeaminase, *13* $N^5$, $N^{10}$-methenyltetrahydrofolate cyclohydrolase, *14* 5-amino-4-imidazole carboxamide ribonucleotide transformylase, *15* glycinamide ribonucleotide transformylase. Abbreviations: $PteGlu_3$ = pteroyltriglutamate; $PteGlu_7$ = pteroylheptaglutamate; PteGlu = pteroylglutamate (folate); $H_2PteGlu$ = dihydropteroylglutamate; $H_4PteGlu$ = tetrahydropteroylglutamate; 5-$CH_3$—$H_4PteGlu$ = 5-methyl-tetrahydropteroylglutamate; 5-HCO—$H_4PteGlu$ = 5-formyltetrahydropteroylglutamate (citrovorum factor); 5,10-$CH_2$—$H_4$-PteGlu = 5,10-methylene-tetrahydropteroylglutamate; 5-HCNH—$H_4PteGlu$ = 5-formimino-tetrahydropteroylglutamate; 10-HCO—$H_4PteGlu$ = 10-formyl-tetrahydropteroylglutamate; 5,10-CH=$H_4PteGlu$ = 5,10-methenyl-tetrahydropteroylglutamate

this biochemical change to accomplish a lethal synthesis within the resistant tumor cells. These authors suggested that a fraudulent substrate for dihydrofolate reductase might be able to produce an inhibitor of enzymes, such as thymidylate synthetase, which require reduced folate cofactors to function, and a search commenced for such a compound. The major advantages of this approach was that it had the potential of taking advantage of a biochemically unique property of the resistant tumor cell and thus would result in what all cancer chemotherapists are searching for (i.e., a high degree of specificity for the tumor relative to the host).

From the perspective of the last twenty-five years it would appear that there are some important considerations to be taken into account by any program involved in the synthesis of new antifolates. For instance, a 4-aminopteroylglutamate derivative which inhibited the growth of L1210 leukemia *in vivo* and dihydrofolate reductase *in vitro* could hardly expect to be given a high priority for clinical trial in the absence of some property which distinguished it from methotrexate. Thus, if a congener of methotrexate were made, which in contrast to methotrexate was rapidly metabolized by human liver, this property would certainly influence its pharmacology and could possibly change the antitumor potential of the compound. Another type of agent might be a pteroylglutamate without a 4-amino group. If this compound had a minimal inhibitory effect on dihydrofolate reductase, but a potent inhibitory effect on another folate-dependent enzyme, as well as good *in vivo* antitumor activity, it should be of compelling interest to cancer chemotherapists because of its differences from, rather than similarities to, methotrexate. Thus, although knowledge of the effect of a new antifolate's inhibitory effect on dihydrofolate reductase may be of some value, it probably should not be regarded as the dominant method of selection of antifolates for the clinic. Biological activities, such as inhibition of tumor cells in culture or the demonstration of antitumor activity *in vivo*, should almost certainly be considered as equally important selection methods.

It has become fairly obvious in the last few years that many classes of antitumor agents, including the antifolates, lack good secondary evaluation systems. Thus, when significant numbers of experimentally active antitumor agents are accumulated in a certain category (e.g. alkylating agents), it is very difficult to select candidates for clinical trial other than on a purely random basis. There is then a most urgent need to develop secondary selection mechanisms to permit a more rational identification of potentially useful clinical agents.

Rational design of antitumor agents would necessarily imply a more or less complete understanding of the biochemical effects of existing agents. In the case of the antifolates, while it is true that the influence of structural change on the interaction of compounds of this class with dihydrofolate reductase is fairly well understood, there are many other enzyme systems which are involved in folate biochemistry. Rational design of antifolates has therefore been built on the assumption that inhibition of dihydrofolate reductase is the property necessary to achieve the desired biological activity. This chapter will attempt to demonstrate that this approach may have prevented a truly rational design of new antifolates by literally "pitting all the structures against one enzyme" thus preventing the maximum exploitation of the tumor cell's very real dependence on many different folate derivatives.

## Structural Analogs of Pteroylglutamate

Although this chapter is concerned with the rational design of folic acid antagonists, a review of the agents which have been made to the present time suggests quite strongly that, rather than a rational approach, the synthetic programs in this area have represented a "state of the art" approach on the part of medicinal and organic chemists. In a molecule such as folate the opportunities for structural modification are numerous.

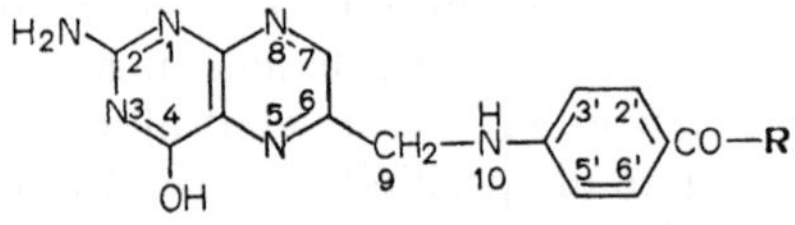


Folate R = L - Glutamate

However, once it was established that the substitution of an amino group for the 4-hydroxyl resulted in an effective antitumor agent, virtually all compounds in this category contained this 2,4-diamino configuration. It is not too surprising, therefore, that the biological activities which resulted from the changes tended to differ quantitatively rather than qualitatively. Thus, the successive structural change from aminopterin, to methotrexate, to dichloromethotrexate resulted in major quantitative differences in activity in the L1210-bearing mouse even though these agents are probably acting via a similar mechanism. The differences in toxicity, however, are not so readily explained, and a more detailed understanding of this aspect of their pharmacology would be most valuable.

Since methotrexate was among the first group of antagonists synthesized, all subsequent analogs have had to stand comparison with it. The passage of time has tended to reinforce its pre-eminent position because increased therapeutic activity has accompanied its employment in new modalities of treatment. One of the most recent of the latter has been the successful use of large doses of methotrexate, with the delayed administration of citrovorum factor, to treat human osteogenic sarcoma (JAFFE et al., 1972). Against this background it is easy to see why there have been so very few clinical trials of this type of compound since the advent of methotrexate. The two notable entries that have had a modest trial were dichloromethotrexate (FREI et al., 1965) and methasquin (ETCUBANAS et al., 1972). In a very limited trial the first showed no advantage over methotrexate in spite of the dramatic therapeutic difference in activity in mice and the second showed activity comparable to aminopterin, to which it is structurally analogous, although there were sufficient differences from methotrexate in its experimentally determined biological properties to hope for a potent tumor-inhibitory effect in man (HUTCHISON, 1968).

Although several structural analogs of folate were considered in the two reviews of structure-antitumor activity relationships by VENDITTI et al. (1960) and MEAD et al. (1968), the listing of analogs was by no means a complete one. Only those agents were included which had been examined in the standardized animal tumor systems of the Cancer Chemotherapy National Service Center, United States National Cancer Institute. There are, therefore, many compounds which have not been tested under standardized conditions and in light of present day knowledge it could be profitable to reexamine some of these compounds. It should also be noted that until the synthesis of tetrahydroaminopterin and tetrahydromethotrexate by KISLIUK (1960), virtually all the folate analogs contained an oxidized pyrazine ring, so that the likelihood of interaction with enzymes distal to dihydrofolate reductase was probably not great.

To illustrate the problems encountered in undertaking the synthesis of new antitumor antifolates it is useful to consider the compounds synthesized around 1950 and listed in the paper by WILLIAMS (1952). Some of these are presented in Table 2, together with an indication of their activity against leukemia L1210. As can readily be seen with those agents in which the activity is known, there is a difference in antitumor activity between those compounds containing the pteroylglutamate configuration and those containing the 4-aminopteroylglutamate configuration. It is therefore quite apparent why the emphasis, since this time, has been placed on 4-aminopteroylglutamate derivatives. It is not apparent, however, why methotrexate was selected to become the primary antifolate. The report by VENDITTI et al. (1960) shows quite clearly that three 4-aminopteroylglutamates had more or less equivalent activity against advanced leukemia L1210 in mice. These were amethopterin ($N^{10}$-methylaminopterin), adenopterin (9,$N^{10}$-dimethylaminopterin) and 3′,5′,-dichloroaminopterin. Aninopterin (9-methylaminopterin) could possibly have been included, but was not examined in the study. It seems that the historical sequence of clinical trials determined the fate of the three drugs more than any other single factor. Their inhibitory effect on dihydrofolate reductase was not even a factor in the decision. Certainly no comparative clinical trial was conducted among them and yet methotrexate became the drug of choice. This example from the early days of the antifolate period demonstrates the problems of rational design of new drugs of this kind. Pharmacological investigations using modern techniques might well indicate some significant differences in their

Table 2. *Pteroylglutamate analogs*

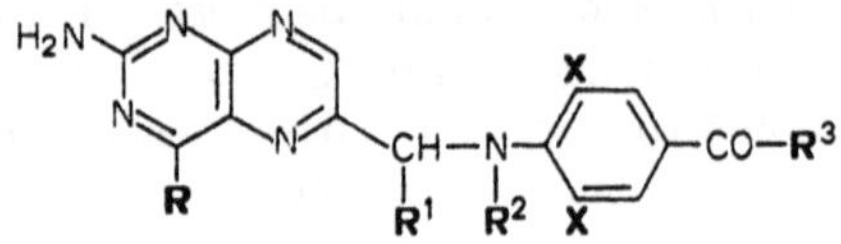

| Name | R | $R^1$ | $R^2$ | X | $R^3$ | Leukemia L1210 activity |
|---|---|---|---|---|---|---|
| Anfol-A | OH | H | H | H | L-aspartate | ? |
| Anfol-R | OH | H | H | H | DL-aspartate | ? |
| Metfol-B | OH | H | $CH_3$ | H | OH | — |
| Bremfol | OH | $CH_3$ | H | H | L-glutamate | — |
| Teropterin | OH | H | H | H | γ-glutamyl-γ-glutamyl-glutamate | ? |
| Teralpherin | OH | H | H | H | α-glutamyl-α-glutamyl-glutamate | ? |
| $N^{10}$methylfolate | OH | H | $CH_3$ | H | L-glutamate | — |
| Dimetfol | OH | $CH_3$ | $CH_3$ | H | L-glutamate | ? |
| Dichlorofolate | OH | H | H | Cl | L-glutamate | — |
| Aminopterin | $NH_2$ | H | H | H | L-glutamate | + |
| Amino-anfol | $NH_2$ | H | H | H | L-aspartate | + |
| A-methopterin | $NH_2$ | H | $CH_3$ | H | L-glutamate | + |
| A-ninopterin | $NH_2$ | $CH_3$ | H | H | L-glutamate | ? |
| A-denopterin | $NH_2$ | $CH_3$ | $CH_3$ | H | L-glutamate | + |
| Aminoteropterin | $NH_2$ | H | H | H | γ-glutamyl-γ-glutamyl-glutamate | + |
| Aminoalanfol | $NH_2$ | H | H | H | L-alanine | + |
| Aminotreofol | $NH_2$ | H | H | H | DL-threonine | ? |
| Dichloroaminopterin | $NH_2$ | H | H | Cl | L-glutamate | + |

(After: WILLIAMS, 1952)

behavior *in vitro* and *in vivo* such as metabolism, transport, protein binding, biliary secretion, or excretion pattern. If differences were found, then a more rational base for future synthesis would have been attained because the analysis of structure-activity relationship would then depend on a multifactorial approach rather than one or two properties. To give an indication of the number of compounds prepared over the last 25 years as pteroylglutamate analogs, Table 3 lists the type of compound with the appropriate reference.

As was the case with the listing in Table 2, the compounds have been divided into those derived from folate and those from aminopterin. There is virtually no part of the pteroylglutamate structure which has not been modified in some way. In spite of these changes, no compounds other than aminopterin and methotrexate have emerged from either series with biological activity of sufficient interest to warrant development to the clinical level, with the exception of 3′,5′-dichloromethotrexate and methasquin which demonstrated no clinical advantages over methotrexate. Mention has already been made in Table 1 of the potent inhibition of thymidylate synthetase by the 2-amino-4-hydroxyquinazoline derivative (BIRD et al., 1970). Unfortunately, the antitumor activity of this compound has not been reported, but if it turns out to have significant activity, this agent might well be the first antitumor pteroylglutamate analog which does not have dihydrofolate reductase as its primary target enzyme. If compounds such as this do have useful antitumor effects, then the progressive modification to the $N^{10}$-methyl and 3′,5′-dichloro-$N^{10}$-methyl derivatives would certainly be justified. It might also be

Table 3. *An historical survey of some pteroylglutamate analogs*

| Year | Structural change | Reference |
|---|---|---|
| | *4-hydroxypteroylglutamates* | |
| 1947 | aspartate for glutamate | HUTCHINGS et al. |
| 1948 | $N^{10}$-alkylpteroic acid | COSULICH and SMITH |
| 1949 | 9-methyl substitution | HULTQUIST et al. |
| | poly-$\alpha$-glutamates | BOOTHE et al. |
| | $\gamma$-$\alpha$ diglutamate | MOWAT et al. |
| | $\gamma$-$\gamma$, $\gamma$-$\alpha$ and $\alpha$-$\gamma$ triglutamates | SEMB et al. |
| | amino acids for glutamate | WRIGHT et al. |
| 1951 | 3′, 5′ halogen substitution of benzene ring | COSULICH et al. |
| | 4-alkoxy derivatives | ROTH et al. |
| | 2′, 3′ monosubstitution of benzene ring | BACKER and HOUTMAN |
| | 2-alkylamino derivatives | ROTH et al. |
| 1952 | 7-isomer | WALLER et al. |
| | 7-methyl substitution | BOOTHE et al. |
| 1953 | 3′- and 3′,5′-substitution of benzene ring | COSULICH et al. |
| 1954 | sulfanilamide analogs | FAHRENBACH et al. |
| 1959 | 3′- and 3′5′-halogenation of benzene ring | ANGIER and CURRAN |
| 1965 | homofolic acid | DEGRAW et al. |
| | 2′- and 3′-azafolate | ROBERTS and SHEALY |
| | $N^{10}$-deazapteroate, deazafolate, and 9,10-dehydroderivatives | STRUCK et al. |
| | 5,8-dideazafolate | DAVOLL and JOHNSON |
| 1971 | polyglutamates, mixed dipeptides and homofolate di- and tri-glutamates | BAUGH and KRUMDIECK |
| | *4-aminopteroylglutamates* | |
| 1947 | aminopterin | SEEGER et al. |
| 1949 | methotrexate | SEEGER et al. |
| | aspartate for glutamate in aminopterin | HUTCHINGS et al. |
| 1950 | 4-alkylamino derivatives | ROTH et al. |
| 1951 | 3′,5′-dihalogenation of benzene ring | COSULICH et al. |
| 1959 | 3′-and 3′,5′-halogenation of methotrexate | ANGIER and CURRAN |
| 1961 | 3′-and 3′,5′-fluoromethotrexate | TOMCUFCIK and SEEGER |
| 1965 | aspartate for glutamate in methotrexate | MEAD et al. |
| | 3′-iodoaminopterin | LOO et al. |
| 1968 | 11-azahomoaminopterin | SLAVIK et al. |
| 1970 | 2,6-diaminopurine congeners of aminopterin and methotrexate | WEINSTOCK et al. |
| | 5,8,-dideazaaminopterin derivatives | DAVOLL and JOHNSON |
| 1971 | 1- and 3-deazamethotrexate | ELLIOTT et al. |
| 1972 | 7-hydroxy, 7-methylmethotrexate, 7-methylaminopterin | FARQUHAR et al. |

anticipated that compounds such as these would exhibit a different antitumor spectrum than the 4-amino derivatives. The quinazoline antifolates remain a very interesting group of agents and are worthy of continued attention in spite of the modest results observed with methasquin in the clinic. For example, methasquin strictly speaking is an analog of aminopterin, whereas its $N^{10}$-methyl derivative would be analogous to methotrexate. Thus, a comparison of methotrexate with its quinazoline analog might reveal subtle differences between them which could be exploited therapeutically. Regretably, the synthesis of this latter analog has not been reported.

As was pointed out earlier in the historical section, many of the pteroylglutamate derivatives were synthesized before much was known about the biochemistry of folate derivatives. The emphasis was, therefore, placed on those analogs which contained a fully oxidized pyrazine ring. With recent developments in the reduced pteroylglutamate field, the question arises as to whether any of the reduced derivatives of some of the older analogs might have useful therapeutic activity. It would seem that the best hope for new agents in the pteroylglutamate category might well lie in the reduced derivatives of existing agents, unless it becomes possible to enhance the selective permeability, or some other property of the 4-amino analogs, for tumor and not for sensitive host tissues. Recognizing that any compound in this category will be compared to methotrexate, the probabilities would certainly favor increased attention to those areas where new leads with new types of antifolate are presently being developed.

## Folate Antagonists which are not Structural Analogs of Reduced Pteroylglutamate

In the limited structure-antitumor activity studies reported by MEAD et al. (1968), significant antitumor activity was observed in two related classes of compounds that were not structurally analogous to pteroylglutamate. These were the 2,4-diaminopyrimidine derivatives and the 4,6-diamino-1-substituted-1,2-dihydro-*s*-triazines. To date these compounds have exhibited their most useful clinical activity in the antibacterial and antimalarial fields and for this reason do not fall within the necessarily limited scope of this chapter. For a detailed and extended discussion of this type of agent the review by HITCHINGS and BURCHALL (1965) is highly recommended. These authors point out that the small molecular inhibitors of dihydrofolate reductase, with the basic structure shown in Fig. 2, are far more likely to detect differences in the enzyme from different species than are the structural analogs of folate such as methotrexate. It is of course this very difference between the inhibitory effects that permits the selective inhibition of dihydrofolate reductase in bacteria and protozoal parasites such as malaria with relatively little effect on the host enzyme.

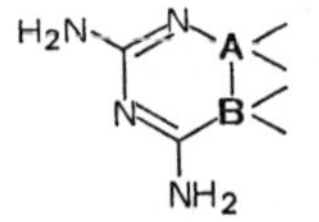


Fig. 2. Basic structural features of inhibitors of dihydrofolate reductase not analogous to folate. A—B = C=C, N=C, C=N. (After HITCHINGS and BURCHALL, 1965)

Thus, the successful employment of trimethoprim as an antibacterial agent in man in conjunction with sulfamethoxazole (DREW et al., 1967a, 1967b) relied, among other things, on the fact that the human enzyme can be up to 10000 times less sensitive to inhibition by trimethoprim than is the bacterial enzyme (HITCHINGS and BURCHALL, 1965). There is no doubt that a range of susceptibilities between species exists to a given inhibitor in this category. It was also found, however, in the study of MCCORMACK and JAFFE (1969) that a group of 2,4-diaminopyrimidines exhibited a wide range of inhibitory effects against dihydrofolate reductases from three different sources, *Trypanosoma equiperdum*, chicken liver, and rat liver. This variation between species almost certainly accounts for the usefulness of these compounds in the chemotherapy of infectious diseases. In addition, it has made possible a far more rational approach to the design of this type of agent because the influence of chemical change on biological and biochemical activity has been very extensively investigated.

It is appropriate to consider in this group of materials two of the compounds recently synthesized by BAKER (1971). Compound I was shown to have a fair

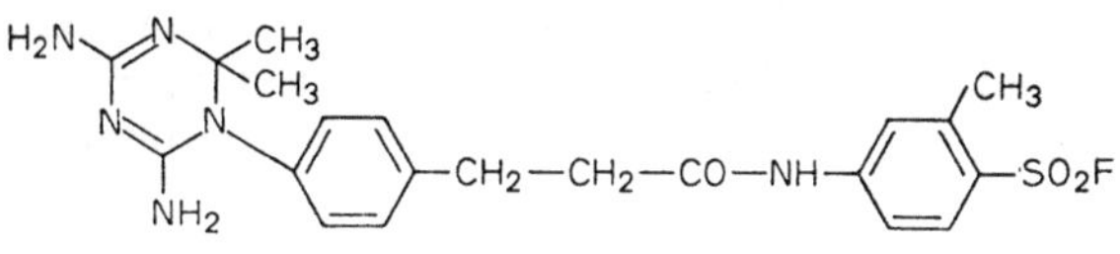

I

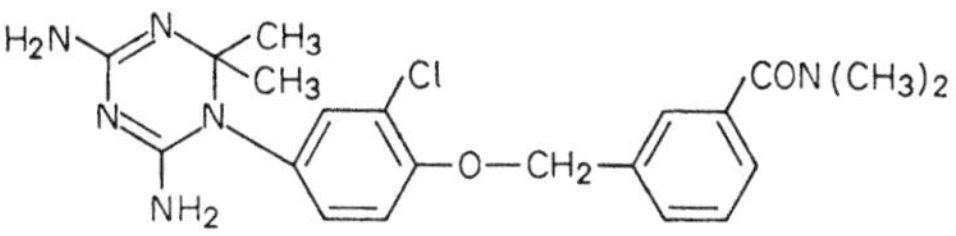

II

degree of specificity for inactivation of the dihydrofolate reductase of the Walker 256 tumor relative to normal rat tissues and was able to "cure" animals with Walker 256 ascites tumor. It was not as effective against leukemia L1210 because the drug was strongly bound to serum proteins in the mouse, much less so in the rat, and not at all in man (FÖLSCH and BERTINO, 1970). Also there was observed a disconcerting lack of correlation between *in vitro* and *in vivo* test systems in the rat. This had its basis in the metabolism of the sulfonyl fluoride group to sulfonic acid which, although a good inhibitor of dihydrofolate reductase, was unable to penetrate cell membranes efficiently. To these complicating factors in the rational design of this antitumor agent was added the extra one of insolubility, so the compound was not pursued further. Compound II was synthesized and met the basic requirements of solubility, inhibitory action on dihydrofolate reductase, and antitumor activity against the Walker 256 tumor, and is currently under development by the United States National Cancer Institute as a potential clinical agent. If this compound, a dihydrotriazine derivative, should turn out to have good activity in the clinic, then the question must be raised as to whether there are other useful structures with clinical potential as antitumor agents among the literally hundreds of compounds of this type that have been synthesized over the past few years. The problem will be to select those agents with the greatest potential; it is doubtful whether inhibition of dihydrofolate reductase will permit the necessary level of discrimination unless there is a dramatic difference in the susceptibility to inhibition of the enzyme of human tumors relative to the enzyme of corresponding normal tissues.

There are some important pharmacological differences between the compounds in this group and those in the pteroylglutamate category. Thus, a differential ability to cross bacterial cell membranes was clearly demonstrated by WOOD et al. (1961) for methotrexate and pyrimethamine. This differential permeability is apparently the basis for the successful treatment of human meningeal leukemia with pyrimethamine by GEILS et al. (1971). Methotrexate is unable to traverse the blood-brain barrier in therapeutic amounts when administered systemically and has to be given intrathecally for the treatment of meningeal leukemia. Pyrimethamine, being uncharged at body pH, is readily lipid soluble and enters the cerebrospinal fluid easily. This lack of a permeability barrier by at least some of the "small molecule" compounds suggests that these agents may find an important application in the treatment of tumors which are pharmacologically inaccessible to compounds such as methotrexate. Since meningeal leukemia is a problem of considerable magnitude in the chemotherapy of leukemia, the possibility might well be entertained of treating patients with a combination of pyrimethamine and methotrexate. Thus, the leukemic cells which become sequestered in sites inaccessible to methotrexate might still be exposed to effective levels of a less potent, but better distributed agent.

Metabolism may also be a factor in the activity of small molecule drugs. Trimethoprim can be metabolized in man and animals to four metabolites (BROSSI et al., 1971) and thus the possibility of species variation in pharmacology is greatly increased.

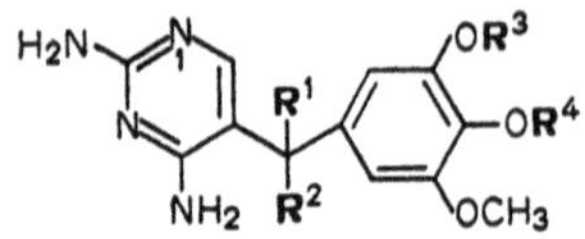


Trimethoprim $R_1, R_2 = H; R_3, R_4 = CH_3$.
Metabolite I $R_1, R_2 = H; R_3 = CH_3; R_4 = H$.
Metabolite II $R_1 = H; R_2 = OH; R_3, R_4 = CH_3$.
Metabolite III $N_1 = \rightarrow O; R_1, R_2 = H; R_3, R_4 = CH_3$.
Metabolite IV $R_1, R_2 = H; R_3 = H; R_4 = CH_3$.

In contrast, methotrexate is metabolized to a very small extent by the mouse, although metabolism by intestinal bacteria of the rat and mouse has been described (VALERINO et al., 1971). The extent to which other "small molecule" dihydrofolate reductase inhibitors are subject to pharmacological variation has not been intensively studied, but it is worthwhile recalling that one of the first antimalarial dihydrotriazines (cycloguanil) to be described was formed *in vivo* by the transformation of proguanil (Paludrine) (CARRINGTON et al., 1951, 1954).

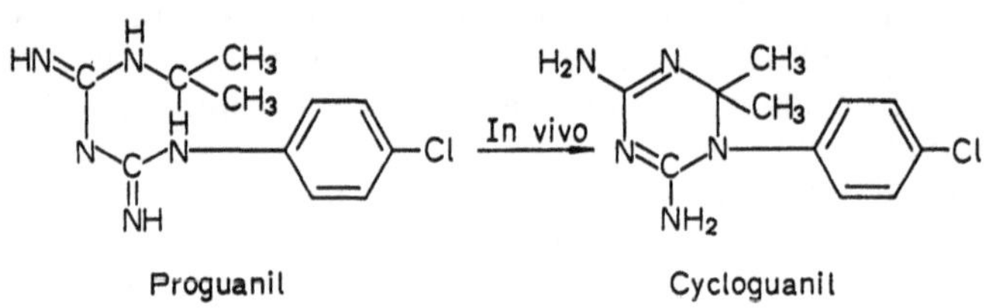


In summary, the rational design of agents in this category of antifolate has proceeded much further than the pteroylglutamate analogs as HITCHINGS and BURCHALL (1965) have documented. However, most of the agents are used for the treatment of protozoal or bacterial infections, with some application of pyrimethamine to the treatment of polycythemia vera (JONES and JELLIFFE, 1963). The rational approach has therefore tended to optimize the development of agents with good antiprotozoal or antibacterial properties, but with unknown qualities as clinical antitumor agents, although many of them have demonstrated significant antitumor activity in experimental tumor systems. From the historical perspective it may well be that the synthesis of dihydrotriazines by MODEST et al. (1951) came so soon after the development of methotrexate that their potential as clinical antitumor agents was not fully explored, and as methotrexate became more firmly established, the incentive to use other dihydrofolate reductase inhibitors greatly diminished. It remains to be seen whether future investigations will uncover useful clinical antitumor activity among these compounds. It should, however, be pointed out that, as with the pteroylglutamate analogs, a primary selection tool for these agents has been the inhibition of dihydrofolate reductase with relatively little attention being given to the effects on the 14 other enzyme systems depicted in Fig. 1. In his book BAKER (1967) discussed the inhibition of *E. coli B* thymidylate synthetase by several different pyrimidine derivatives; it is worth noting that while the inhibitions observed were considerably less potent than those with the dihydrofolate reductase inhibitors, there was inhibition which varied according to structure.

By analogy with dihydrofolate reductase inhibitors, it might also be anticipated that there would be some difference in the inhibition of thymidylate synthetase from other species. It remains to be determined whether there is a difference between the inhibition of thymidylate synthetase in tumor relative to normal host tissue.

## Structural Analogs of Reduced Pteroylglutamates

The emphasis which has been placed on the inhibition of dihydrofolate reductase as a prerequisite for antifolate activity has necessarily diverted some attention from the effects of the drugs on those enzyme systems which utilize tetrahydrofolate cofactors directly (i.e. steps 3 to 15 in Fig. 1). The conclusion has generally been drawn that after the inhibition of dihydrofolate reductase there will be a decline in the intracellular levels of tetrahydrofolate derivatives. When the depletion of the cofactors is accomplished, the biosynthetic steps and metabolic interconversions which depend on them will necessarily be inhibited. There has, however, been only one preliminary report of possible tissue depletion of tetrahydrofolate compounds. This was the report by WERKHEISER (1969), on the effect of methotrexate on tetrahydrofolate levels in mouse intestinal mucosa. A massive dose of methotrexate (400 mg/kg) was employed in this study, and it could be argued that the apparent reduction in the levels of tetrahydrofolate reported could have been due to displacement by methotrexate or perhaps to massive cell death and breakdown. This author made a statement which is generally accepted, namely: "The major requirement for this enzyme (dihydrofolate reductase) in growing tissues is to regenerate tetrahydrofolate from the dihydrofolate formed by the action of thymidylate synthetase" (WERKHEISER, 1969). Although there is no doubt that this is a very important function for dihydrofolate reductase, it is probably a little too narrow as a definition. With the exception of 5-formyltetrahydrofolate (citrovorum factor), none of the tetrahydrofolate cofactors is particularly stable to oxidative degradation in the absence of reducing agents (CHIPPEL and SCRIMGEOUR, 1970). In the case of tetrahydrofolate, the primary product seems to be dihydrofolate and it is perhaps this intrinsic property of the tetrahydro derivative which gives dihydrofolate reductase its *raison d'être*. Thus, in any environment *in vivo* where dihydrofolate could be formed nonenzymically from tetrahydrofolate it would be of prime importance to the organism to be able to convert spontaneous oxidation products back to the fully reduced state whenever needed. As far as is known, the only tetrahydrofolate-dependent enzyme system which produces dihydrofolate is thymidylate synthetase. If thymineless death is solely responsible for the toxicity and antitumor effects of agents like methotrexate, then the inhibition of thymidylate synthetase would seem to be the major objective of antifolate therapy. It is, however, questionable as to whether this is so and although identification of tetrahydrofolate has not always been confirmed as a product, it has been tacitly assumed that when a one-carbon unit is transferred enzymically from a tetrahydrofolate cofactor, tetrahydrofolate remains and could be utilized again for biosynthetic purposes, unless it is not recycled because of oxidative breakdown. If tetrahydrofolate can act catalytically, similarly to NAD and NADP, then inhibition of dihydrofolate reductase should not, by itself, seriously impair steps such as 14 or 15 in Fig. 1, which are involved in purine nucleotide biosynthesis *de novo*. This is not the case, however, and there is a rapid and almost complete inhibition of the incorporation of $^{14}C$-formate into acid-soluble purines by methotrexate. It was also shown that there was a good correlation between the inhibition of formate incorporation into the acid-soluble adenine of leukemic spleen and the relative antitumor effectiveness of methotrexate and 3′,5′-dichloromethotrexate (SCHRECKER et al., 1960). More recently HRYNIUK (1972) has suggested that purineless death may be a link between growth rate and the cytotoxicity of methotrexate. The importance of purine nucleotide biosynthesis to cell growth was also emphasized by HAKALA (1971) who showed that homofolate and tetrahydrohomofolate were able to inhibit the growth of Sarcoma 180 cells *in vitro* and that the analog's primary effect was on step 14 of Fig. 1. It would appear, therefore, that antifolates may also act to reduce the level of purine nucleotides, as well as thymine nucleotides, so that inhibition of purine nucleotide biosynthesis may be just as important an objective as inhibition of thymidylate synthesis.

The preceding discussion was included as a necessary introduction to an account of the currently available analogs of reduced pteroylglutamate. Numerically these do not amount to anything like the number of pteroylglutamate analogs, but from the limited experience available with these compounds they may have an even greater selectivity of action than provided by methotrexate. It should also be remembered that methotrexate may act as a tetrahydrofolate antagonist under circumstances similar to the inhibition of thymidylate synthetase by quinazoline antifolates (BIRD et al., 1970); however, there is no evidence at present that this occurs directly.

The first analogs of reduced pteroylglutamate to be synthesized were 5,8-dideaza-5,6,7,8-tetrahydrofolate and the corresponding 4-amino derivative (KOEHLER et al., 1958; DEGRAW et al., 1959, 1961, 1962). When the 5,8-dideazatetra-

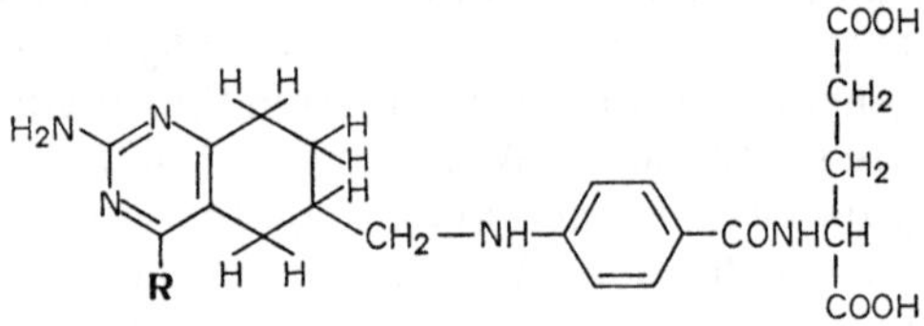

R = OH, 5,8 - Dideaza - 5,6,7,8, - Tetrahydrofolate
R = $NH_2$, 5,8 - Dideaza - 5,6,7,8, - Tetrahydroaminopterin

hydrofolate was examined as a bacterial growth inhibitor it gave 50% inhibition at a concentration of 50 ng/ml in the presence of 3 ng folate. This was not a particularly potent effect, and interest in the compound was dropped, apparently without determination of the antitumor activity. The 5,8-dideazatetrahydroaminopterin was examined in the L1210 system (MEAD et al., 1968) and found to be toxic at dose levels in the µg/kg range. It did not prolong the lifespan of the mice and was also dropped from further consideration as an antitumor agent. The metabolic basis for its toxicity was not ascertained and neither was its ability to inhibit dihydrofolate reductase. These two early reduced pteroylglutamate derivatives did not raise any hope for antitumor activity. From the rational design standpoint the synthesis of other analogs in the series, for example, the $N^{10}$-methyl derivative or the 5-methyl derivative would appear justifiable. Also, a complete examination of their biochemical effects, especially those of the aminopterin analog, would indicate whether this synthetic approach might have any therapeutic application, even if only in combination with other drugs. Both compounds did not seem to present any problems with regard to their chemical stability which, as will be seen later, is of some consequence for other reduced pteroylglutamates.

The next compounds to be made in this class were the fully reduced derivatives of aminopterin (KISLIUK, 1960) and methotrexate (MEAD et al., 1961). The latter compound was an L1210-active antitumor agent, although its activity was less than that of methotrexate. In addition, it was inactive against a methotrexate-resistant variant of the L1210 leukemia and was considerably more toxic than the parent compound. The activity of tetrahydroaminopterin was attributed by ZAKRZEWSKI et al. (1962) to the presence of dihydroaminopterin as a degradation product. This claim was disputed by KISLIUK and LEVINE (1964) who argued for a sequential effect of dihydro and tetrahydroaminopterin. Both authors recognized the need for protective measures against oxidative breakdown. Further chromatographic studies with tetrahydromethotrexate revealed that it contained several components (MEAD, 1962). These compounds were not identified, but it was clear from these initial experiences that the reduced pteroylglutamate analogs would pose stabilization problems if used in chemotherapy. The synthesis of 5-alkyl derivatives of tetrahydromethotrexate has recently been described by BLAIR and SAUNDERS (1971), but no biological activity was reported. By analogy with tetrahydrofolate, 5-substitution might increase the stability of these compounds considerably, but an answer to this question is needed before the merit of this approach can be determined.

The reduced pteroylglutamate analogs described above were probably synthesized originally on structural grounds coupled with a desire to attack those enzymic reactions dependent on reduced folates. Probably the first direct evidence that reduced analogs could inhibit such a reaction was provided by WAHBA and FRIEDKIN (1961) who demonstrated that tetrahydroaminopterin and tetrahydromethotrexate were potent inhibitors of *Escherichia coli* thymidylate synthetase, compared to the parent compounds. More recently, SLAVIK and ZAKRZEWSKI (1967) have shown that a series of dihydro and tetrahydro analogs of pteroylglutamate derivatives were able to inhibit *E. coli* thymidylate synthetase quite well.

The final class of compounds to be considered in this group resulted from the highly imaginative reasoning of FRIEDKIN and his colleagues (MISRA et al., 1961; FRIEDKIN et al., 1962) who were studying the development of resistance to methotrexate in leukemia L1210. Their observation that the development of resistance to methotrexate was accompanied by a considerable increase in tumor dihydrofolate reductase led them to propose a novel approach to antifolate chemotherapy. Rather than attempting to inhibit dihydrofolate reductase, the objective would be to take advantage of the elevated enzyme levels by providing an analog of the substrate which after reduction would produce *in situ* a tetrahydro analog capable of inhibiting enzymes such as thymidylate synthetase. The attractive aspect of this approach was the potential for a highly selective attack on the tumor cells with a minimum effect on normal cells, since they would not contain elevated enzyme levels. The search for a suitable compound began and shortly thereafter the synthesis of homofolate was accomplished (DEGRAW et al., 1965). This compound,

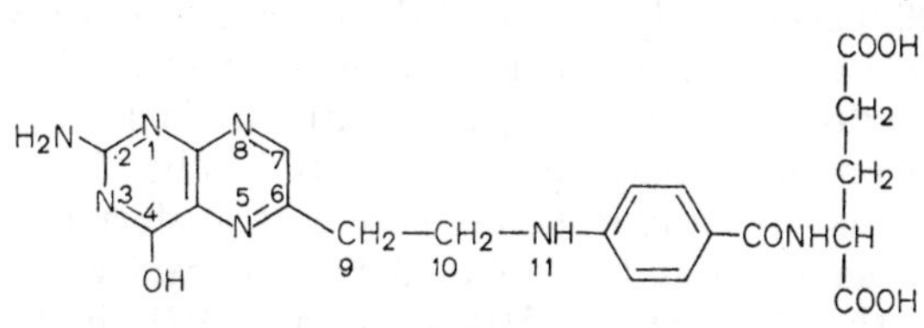


Homofolate

after conversion to its dihydroderivative, was a good substrate for dihydrofolate reductase and the product, tetrahydrohomofolate, proved to be a specific inhibitor of thymidylate synthetase (GOODMAN et al., 1964). The basic requirements suggested by MISRA et al. (1961) were fulfilled and it remained to test this compound in an experimental tumor system. Because the supply of compound was limited, a complete test for antitumor activity was performed with tetrahydrohomofolate instead of the dihydro derivative (MEAD et al., 1966). Significant antitumor activity was seen against an antifolate-resistant variant of leukemia L1210 with greatly elevated levels of dihydrofolate reductase, but the compound had only a borderline effect on the parent, antifolate-sensitive L1210. A selectivity of action was thus realized, although the antitumor activity of the dihydrohomofolate remained in question until recently when MISHRA and MEAD (1972) demonstrated that it had antitumor activity comparable to that of tetrahydrohomofolate. Based on the initial observations of antitumor activity, attempts were made to prepare a clinically acceptable formulation of tetrahydrohomofolate as a prelude to a clinical trial. It soon became apparent, however, that the instability of the compound would constitute a major barrier to this objective. In addition, synthetic problems during this early period contributed to some confusion as to the active principle. Thus, it was reported by KISLIUK et al. (1967) that impure tetrahydrohomofolate exhibited antimalarial activity in monkeys, whereas the purified material did not. The active antimalarial impurity proved to be tetrahydrohomopteroate. Tetrahydrohomofolate itself was devoid of antimalarial activity, although it was found to have full antileukemic potency.

There have been two studies of the distribution of tetrahydrohomofolate in mice (NAHAS and FRIEDKIN, 1969; MISHRA et al., 1970). The former studied the distribution of the drug using a measurement of radioactivity coupled with a microbiological assay, and the good agreement observed between the two, prompted the authors to conclude that the bulk of this inherently unstable drug was excreted intact. The later studies of MISHRA et al. (1970) used the Bratton-Marshall reaction as a colorimetric assay for unchanged tetrahydrohomofolate and could only account for 26% of the dose. The low urinary recovery with the Bratton-Marshall assay could be attributed to breakdown *in vivo* to compounds which do not give a color. Since the radioactive measurements could have included more than one compound under the chromatographic peak, a concomitant Bratton-Marshall assay would have been most useful. The microbiological assay seemed at the time to have a high degree of specificity. This is now known not to be the case. KISLIUK and GAUMONT (1970) showed that only the unnatural diastereoisomer of *dl*,L-tetrahydrohomofolate was inhibitory to the assay organism *Streptococcus faecium* (ATCC 8043), whereas only the natural isomer was inhibitory to *E. coli* thymidylate synthetase (PLANTE et al., 1967). Thus, if tetrahydrohomofolate showed any instability *in vivo* and broke down nonenzymically to dihydrohomofolate which was then converted stereospecifically back to the tetrahydro level by dihydrofolate reductase (e.g. in the liver) it would not be measured by the microbiological assay, but would presumably retain its antileukemic properties. NAHAS and FRIEDKIN (1969) specifically excluded the formation of dihydrohomofolate *in vivo* based on the close agreement of the microbiological assay and isotopic determination of tetrahydrohomofolate together with the lack of a separate peak of dihydrohomofolate on chromatography. Later studies by MISHRA et al. (1971) do suggest, however, that tetrahydrohomofolate is transformed *in vivo* and that dihydrohomofolate should not be excluded from consideration. There are two reasons to suspect that this occurs. MISHRA et al. (1971) have shown that after administration of either dihydrohomofolate or tetrahydrohomofolate to mice the sole material present in liver up to 4 hours later is tetrahydrohomofolate. However, if the animals are pretreated with methotrexate before administration of either agent, it is possible to detect sizeable amounts of both di- and tetrahydrohomofolate in the liver. If tetrahydrohomofolate was as stable *in vivo* as suggested, the inhibition of dihydrofolate reductase with methotrexate should not have resulted in the appearance of dihydrohomofolate after administration of tetrahydrohomofolate. Similarly, MISHRA and MEAD (1972) have shown that when mice bearing an antifolate-resistant tumor are treated with di- or tetrahydrohomofolate their antileukemic effect can be greatly diminished by pretreatment with methotrexate. Taken together with the effect of methotrexate on the tetrahydrohomofolate levels in the liver these observations provide very strong evidence that tetrahydrohomofolate can be transformed *in vivo* to dihydrohomofolate. Depending on the availability of adequate levels of dihydrofolate reductase this will be converted to tetrahydrohomofolate which is presumably the active form of the drug.

The major question to be resolved concerning the reduced homofolates is whether the original hypothesis of MISRA et al. (1961) is still tenable. The answer would seem to be a qualified "yes", although there is evidence to suggest that in some tumors reduction of the substrate dihydrohomofolate does not occur (NAHAS and FRIEDKIN, 1972). Overall, however, the evidence favors the formation of tetrahydrohomofolate *in vivo* from dihydrohomofolate, and dihydrofolate reductase levels in the tumor seem to be an important determinant of antitumor activity (MISHRA and MEAD, 1972).

Before the decision was made to stop the further development of tetrahydrohomofolate the synthesis of 5-methyltetrahydrohomofolate was reported (KNOTT et al., 1971).

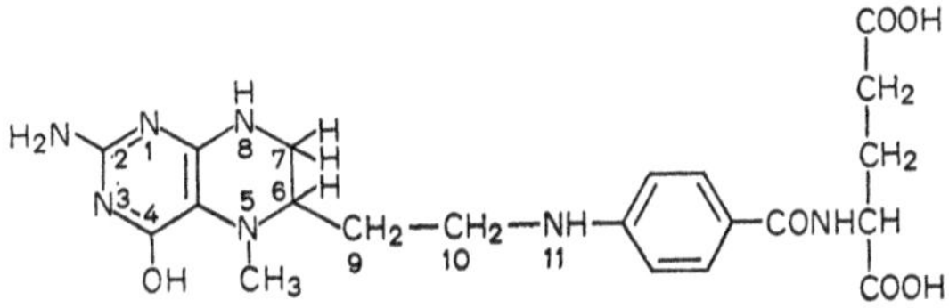

5-Methyl-D,L,-Tetrahydrohomofolate

This compound was found to be quite stable relative to tetrahydrohomofolate and showed improved antileukemic activity (MISHRA et al., 1972). Not only was it more active than tetrahydrohomofolate against the antifolate-resistant variant of L1210, but it was also significantly more active against the parent L1210 leukemia. 5-Methyltetrahydrohomofolate is presently undergoing further development and it promises to have much better prospects of reaching clinical trial because of its stability. It has also shown some interesting differences from tetrahydrohomofolate. Thus KISLIUK (personal communication) has shown that the 5-methyl analog is a relatively poor inhibitor of thymidylate synthetase compared to tetrahydrohomofolate. The two compounds may well have different loci of action, and a logical site for the 5-methyl derivative would seem to be step 4 in Fig. 1.

The exploration of the potential of reduced pteroylglutamates as antitumor agents is in a very early stage and would seem to hold great promise. There are, however, certain factors to be taken into consideration. The intrinsic instability of these compounds will, as discussed above, be a major drawback to their use in chemotherapy. For those derivatives which break down to form substrates for dihydrofolate reductase, biological activity related to the enzyme levels may be seen. On the other hand, tetrahydro derivatives of 4-aminopteroylglutamates would presumably break down to form inhibitors of dihydrofolate reductase and might be expected to have a chemotherapeutic spectrum similar to methotrexate. The best strategy for future developments in this area would seem to be the preparation of stable analogs such as the 5-methyl or 5-formyl derivatives. This chapter contains references to many pteroylglutamate analogs which have been described in the literature. Plante et al. (1967) reported the synthesis and properties of several folate and homofolate derivatives. Kisliuk et al. (1971) have described the effects of polygammaglutamyl derivatives of homofolate on thymidylate synthetase. All of these agents are potential antileukemic agents in a reduced and stabilized form. The opportunities for a greater biochemical selectivity appear to be more promising with this class of compound and offer great hope for fruitful investigations.

The antileukemic properties of the reduced homofolates may have actually revealed a strategy for increasing the productivity of a preclinical screening program. Tetrahydrohomofolate did not prolong the survival of L1210 leukemic mice sufficiently to be selected for future study; however, in a tumor which had been made refractory to methotrexate it had significant activity. The basis for this collateral sensitivity may be related to the elevated dihydrofolate reductase levels, but regardless of the mechanism a specific change has occurred which renders the tumor cell much more sensitive to the agent than both the non-resistant tumor and the host tissues. This would mean that a prime objective of chemotherapy has been achieved, namely, there has been a therapeutically exploitable biochemical change induced selectively in the tumor. Since new agents are usually introduced into clinical trial after established agents cease to be effective, it would seem logical to test new compounds against experimental tumors resistant to the commonly used clinical agents. In this way heightened sensitivity in resistant tumors would not be overlooked and might well enrich the output of a primary screening system for antitumor agents.

## Conclusions

The first twenty-five years of the antifolate chemotherapy of tumors have been dominated by the dihydrofolate reductase inhibitor methotrexate. This drug has probably been studied as intensively as any drug employed in clinical medicine. Although many derivatives and analogs of folate have been synthesized during the above period, only two agents, 3′,5′-dichloromethotrexate and methasquin, demonstrated preclinical attributes sufficiently different from methotrexate to warrant a clinical trial. Neither of these compounds proved to be better than methotrexate. It must however be emphasized that the clinical trial of dichloromethotrexate in particular was not an extensive one and for this reason serious consideration should certainly be given to further comparisons with methotrexate. The main objective would be to look for significant differences in activity relating to the treatment schedule employed or the nature of the tumor treated. The real question then is whether it will be possible to develop 4-aminopteroylglutamate analogs with clinical properties superior to methotrexate. At the present time the answer to this question is probably "no", albeit a qualified one. Derivatives of methotrexate with improved lipid solubility might be of use for special applications, such as the treatment of meningeal leukemia. If biotransformability is an important factor in the reduction of toxicity of methotrexate derivatives then a systematic study of the effects of molecular changes on this property would be highly desirable. Many of the antifolates which have already been described have only been studied superficially. More detailed examination of their pharmacology and biochemical effects could be extremely useful for the development of a rational 4-aminopteroylglutamate superior to methotrexate. As Friedkin et al. (1971) have said "... a reasonable strategy involves looking for differences between normal and neoplastic cells, taking advantage of these differences in designing new compounds and then systematically modifying the drugs, as the feedback of pharmacologic information on efficacy, selectivity and toxicity becomes available." Unfortunately the feedback has not been too informative and many of the recent synthesis programs have not had much guidance along the lines suggested. Also, a major problem continues to be the lack of information on exploitable differences between normal and neoplastic cells. If these differences could be induced in some way before chemotherapy with a given agent starts, then the prospects for selective chemotherapy would be much brighter.

The experience with the small molecule dihydrofolate reductase inhibitors as effective antimalarial and antibacterial agents shows quite clearly that when a selective action against dihydrofolate reductase can be achieved chemotherapy is highly effective. Whether dihydrofolate reductase of human tumors will ever reveal a sufficient difference in its properties from normal tissue to yield a therapeutic advantage by its selective inhibition is problematic. In the event that such a difference was uncovered then a major attempt should be made to take advantage of this potential for selective tumor cell destruction.

The reduced pteroylglutamate analogs probably deserve a major emphasis in the future, especially those compounds which do not inhibit dihydrofolate reductase, because these agents are most likely to be clearly distinct from methotrexate in their mechanism of action. The possibility of a selective approach would also appear to be much greater because exploitable differences in enzyme properties or levels would be much more likely when several enzymes are involved.

As methotrexate has become more deeply enmeshed in the fabric of modern cancer chemotherapy it represents one of the signal successes of the equation of antimetabolites with chemotherapeutic agents. Although the synthesis of a better agent has not been demonstrated, at least new directions have opened up for investigation and further development. To quote HITCHINGS and BURCHALL (1965), ". . . if (antifolate) chemotherapy is not presently 'rational' it is at least much less irrational than it once was", or as FRIEDKIN et al. (1971) have described it "semirational chemotherapy." Regardless of their philosophical origin the fact remains that antifolates have been, are, and will continue to be the basis of much activity in cancer chemotherapy.

*Acknowledgment.* The author is particularly indebted to Dr. ABRAHAM GOLDIN for introducing him to the antifolates and for participating in many stimulating discussions. Many thanks are also due Mrs. JO CLEM, Mrs. ZELDA MONTGOMERY and Miss LAVERNE SPATES for their invaluable help in the preparation of this article.

## References


ANGIER, R. B., BOOTHE, J. H., CURRAN, W. V.: The halogenation of 4-amino-4-deoxy-$N^{10}$-methylpteroylglutamic acid (methotrexate) and other pteroylglutamic acid derivatives. J. Amer. chem. Soc. **81**, 2814—2818 (1959).

ANGIER, R. B., BOOTHE, J. H., HUTCHINGS, B. L., MOWAT, J. H., SEMB, J., STOKSTAD, E. L. R., SUBBAROW, Y., WALLER, C. W., COSULICH, D. B., FAHRENBACH, M. J., HULTQUIST, M. E., KUH, E., NORTHEY, E. H., SEEGER, D. R., STICKELS, J. P., SMITH, J. M.: The structure and synthesis of the liver *L. casei* factor. Science **103**, 667—669 (1946).

BACKER, H. J., HOUTMAN, A. C.: Quelques acides ptéroylglutamiques (foliques) substitués dans le noyau benzénique. Rec. Trav. chim. Pays-Bas **70**, 738—746 (1951).

BAKER, B. R.: Design of active-site-directed irreversible enzyme inhibitors. New York: John Wiley and Sons 1967.

BAKER, B. R.: Specific irreversible enzyme inhibitors. Ann. Rev. Pharmacol. **10**, 35—50 (1970).

BAKER, B. R.: Active-site directed irreversible inhibitors of dihydrofolate reductase. Ann. N. Y. Acad. Sci. **186**, 214—226 (1971).

BAUGH, C. M., KRUMDIECK, C. L.: Naturally occurring folates. Ann. N. Y. Acad. Sci. **186**, 7—28 (1971).

BERTINO, J. R.: The mechanism of action of the folate antagonists in man. Cancer Res. **23**, 1286—1306 (1963).

BIRD, O.D., VAITKUS, J.W., CLARKE, J.: 2-Amino-4-hydroxyquinazolines as inhibitors of thymidylate synthetase. Molec. Pharmacol. **6**, 573—575 (1970).

BLAIR, J.A., SAUNDERS, K.J.: Preparation of analogs of *dl*-tetrahydromethotrexate (4-amino-4-deoxy-N[10]-methyl-*dl*-5,6,7,8-tetrahydropteroyl-*l*-monoglutamic acid). Anal. Biochem. **41**, 482—486 (1971).

BLAKLEY, R.L.: The biochemistry of folic acid and related pteridines, Amsterdam: North Holland Publishing Co. 1969.

BOOTHE, J.H., SEMB, J., WALLER, C.W., ANGIER, R.B., MOWAT, J.H., HUTCHINGS, B.L., STOKSTAD, E.L.R., SUBBAROW, Y.: Pteroic acid derivatives. III. Pteroyl-γ-glutamylglutamic acid and pteroyl-γ-glutamyl-γ-glutamylglutamic acid. J. Amer. chem. Soc. **71**, 2304—2308 (1949).

BOOTHE, J.H., MOWAT, J.H., WALLER, C.W., ANGIER, R.B., SEMB, J., GAZZOLA, A.L.: 7-Methylpteroylglutamic acid and some related compounds. J. Amer. chem. Soc. **74**, 5407—5409 (1952).

BROSSI, A., GRUNBERG, E., HOFFER, M., TEITEL, S.: Synthesis and chemotherapeutic activity of two metabolites of trimethoprim. J. med. Chem. **14**, 58—59 (1971).

CARRINGTON, H.C., CROWTHER, A.F., DAVEY, D.G., LEVI, A.A., ROSE, F.L.: A metabolite of "paludrine" with high antimalarial activity. Nature (Lond.) **168**, 1080 (1951).

CARRINGTON, H.C., STACEY, G.J.: Synthetic antimalarials. XLIX. The structure and synthesis of the dihydrotriazine metabolite of proguanil. J. chem. Soc. 1017—1031 (1954).

CHIPPEL, D., SCRIMGEOUR, K.G.: Oxidative degradation of dihydrofolate and tetrahydrofolate. Canad. J. Biochem. **48**, 999—1009 (1970).

COSULICH, D.B., SMITH, J.M.: Analogs of pteroylglutamic acid. I. N[10]-alkylpteroic acid and derivatives. J. Amer. chem. Soc. **70**, 1922—1926 (1948).

COSULICH, D.B., SEEGER, D.R., FAHRENBACH, M.J., ROTH, B., MOWAT, J.H., SMITH, J.M., HULTQUIST, M.E.: Analogs of pteroylglutamic acid. VI. 3′,5′-Dihalopteroyl derivatives. J. Amer. chem. Soc. **73**, 2554—2557 (1951).

COSULICH, D.B., ROTH, B., SMITH, J.M., HULTQUIST, M.E., PARKER, R.P.: Chemistry of leucovorin. J. Amer. chem. Soc. **74**, 3252—3263 (1952).

COSULICH, D.B., SEEGER, D.R., FAHRENBACH, M.J., COLLINS, K.H., ROTH, B., HULTQUIST, M.E., SMITH, J.M.: Analogs of pteroylglutamic acid. IX. Derivatives with substituents on the benzene ring. J. Amer. chem. Soc. **75**, 4675—4680 (1953).

DAVOLL, J., JOHNSON, A.M.: Quinazoline analogues of folic acid. J. chem. Soc. C8, 997—1002 (1970).

DEGRAW, J., GOODMAN, L., KOEHLER, R., BAKER, B.R.: Potential anticancer agents. XXIV. Tetrahydroquinazoline analogs of tetrahydrofolic acid. II. J. org. Chem. **24**, 1632—1640 (1959).

DEGRAW, J., GOODMAN, L., BAKER, B.R.: Potential anticancer agents. XLII. Tetrahydroquinazoline analogs of tetrahydrofolic acid. III. An improved synthesis of 5,8-dideaza-5,6,7,8-tetrahydrofolic acid. J. org. Chem. **26**, 1156—1161 (1961).

DEGRAW, J., GOODMAN, L., WEINSTEIN, B., BAKER, B.R.: Potential anticancer agents. LXIX. Tetrahydroquinazoline analogs of tetrahydrofolic acid. IV. The synthesis of 5,8-dideaza-5,6,7,8-tetrahydroaminopterin. J. org. Chem. **27**, 576—580 (1962).

DEGRAW, J., MARSH, J.P., ACTON, E.M., CREWS, O.P., MOSHER, C.W., FUJIWARA, A.N., GOODMAN, L.: The synthesis of homofolic acid. J. org. Chem. **30**, 3404—3409 (1965).

DREW, C.D.M., HUGHES, D.T.D., FOWLE, A.S.E., CASSELL, M.A.: Effective treatment of chronic bronchitis with short term trimethoprim and sulphamethoxazole. Proc. 5th int. Congr. Chemoth. **1**, 293—296 (1967).

DREW, C.D.M., HUGHES, D.T.O., JENKINS, G.C.: Long term treatment of chest infections with a combination of trimethoprim and sulphonamide, the clinical, bacteriological and haematological effects. Proc. 5th int. Congr. Chemother. **5**, 107—109 (1967).

ELLIOTT, R.D., TEMPLE, C., FRYE, J.L., MONTGOMERY, J.A.: Potential folic acid antagonists. VI. The syntheses of 1- and 3-deazamethotrexate. J. org. Chem. **36**, 2818—2823 (1971).

ETCUBANAS, E., TAN, C., GO, S.C., KRAKOFF, I.H.: Preliminary clinical trials of the quinazoline antifolate methasquin. Proc. Amer. Ass. Cancer Res. **13**, 48 (1972).

FAHRENBACH, M.J., COLLINS, K.H., HULTQUIST, M.E., SMITH, J.M.: Analogs of pteroylglutamic acid. X. N[1]-(pteridyl-2)-sulfanilamides. J. Amer. chem. Soc. **76**, 4006—4010 (1954).

FARBER, S., DIAMOND, L.K., MERCER, R.D., SYLVESTER, R.F., WOLFF, J.A.: Temporary remissions in acute leukemia in children produced by folic acid antagonist, 4-aminopteroylglutamic acid (aminopterin). New Engl. J. Med. **238**, 787—793 (1948).

FARQUHAR, D., LOO, T.L.: Synthesis and biologic evaluation of 7-hydroxymethotrexate, 7-methylaminopterin, and 7-methylmethotrexate. J. med. Chem. **15**, 567—569 (1972).

FERONE, R., BURCHALL, J.J., HITCHINGS, G.H.: *Plasmodium berghei* dihydrofolate reductase isolation, properties, and inhibition by antifolates. Molec. Pharmacol. **5**, 49—59 (1969).

FÖLSCH, E., BERTINO, J.R.: Inactivation by mouse serum of a tightly bound inhibitor of dihydrofolate reductase. Molec. Pharmacol. **6**, 93—96 (1970).

FREI, E., SPURR, C. L., BRINDLEY, C. O., SELAWRY, O., HOLLAND, J. F., RALL, D. P., WASSERMAN, L. R., HOOGSTRATEN, B., SHNIDER, B. I., McINTYRE, O. R., MATTHEWS, L. B., MILLER, S. P.: Clinical studies of dichloromethotrexate (NSC 29630). Clin. Pharmacol. Ther. **6**, 160—171 (1965).

FRIEDKIN, M., CRAWFORD, E., HUMPHREYS, S. R., GOLDIN, A.: The association of increased dihydrofolate reductase with amethopterin resistance in mouse leukemia. Cancer Res. **22**, 600—606 (1962).

FRIEDKIN, M., CRAWFORD, E., PLANTE, L. T.: Empirical *vs* rational approaches in cancer chemotherapy. Ann. N. Y. Acad. Sci. **186**, 209—213 (1971).

FUTTERMAN, S., SILVERMAN, M.: The "inactivation" of folic acid by liver. J. biol. Chem. **224**, 31—40 (1957a).

FUTTERMAN, S.: Enzymatic reduction of folic acid and dihydrofolic acid to tetrahydrofolic acid. J. biol. Chem. **228**, 1031—1038 (1957b).

GEILS, G. F., SCOTT, C. W., BAUGH, C. M., BUTTERWORTH, C. E.: Treatment of meningeal leukemia with pyrimethamine. Blood **38**, 131—137 (1971).

GOLDIN, A., HUMPHREYS, S. R., VENDITTI, J. M., MANTEL, N.: Prolongation of the lifespan of mice with advanced leukemia (L1210) by treatment with halogenated derivatives of amethopterin. J. nat. Cancer Inst. **22**, 811—823 (1959).

GOLDIN, A., SANDBERG, J. S., HENDERSON, E. S., NEWMAN, J. W., FREI, E., HOLLAND, J. F.: The chemotherapy of human and animal acute leukemia. Cancer Chemother. Rep. **55**, 309—507 (1971).

GOODMAN, L., DEGRAW, J., KISLIUK, R. L., FRIEDKIN, M., PASTORE, E. J., CRAWFORD, E. J., PLANTE, L. T., AL-NAHAS, A., MORNINGSTAR, J. F., KWOK, G., WILSON, L., DONOVAN, F., RATZAN, J.: Tetrahydrohomofolate, a specific inhibitor of thymidylate synthetase. J. Amer. chem. Soc. **86**, 308—309 (1964).

HAKALA, M. T.: Homofolate and tetrahydrohomofolate, inhibitors of purine synthesis. Cancer Res. **31**, 813—816 (1971).

HITCHINGS, G. H., BURCHALL, J. J.: Inhibition of folate biosynthesis and function as a basis for chemotherapy. Adv. Enzymol. **27**, 417—468 (1965).

HRYNIUK, W. M.: Purineless death as a link between growth rate and cytotoxicity by methotrexate. Cancer Res. **32**, 1506—1511 (1972).

HULTQUIST, M. E., SMITH, J. M., SEEGER, D. R., COSULICH, D. B., KUH, E.: Analogs of pteroylglutamic acid. II. 9-Methylpteroylglutamic acid and derivatives. J. Amer. chem. Soc. **71**, 619—622 (1949).

HUTCHINGS, B. L., MOWAT, J. H., OLESON, J. J., STOKSTAD, E. L. R., BOOTHE, J. H., WALLER, C. W., ANGIER, R. B., SEMB, J., SUBBAROW, Y.: Pteroylaspartic acid, an antagonist for pteroylglutamic acid. J. biol. Chem. **170**, 323—328 (1947).

HUTCHINGS, B. L., MOWAT, J. H., OLESON, J. J., GAZZOLA, A. L., BOGGIANO, E. M., SEEGER, D. R., BOOTHE, J. H., WALLER, C. W., ANGIER, R. B., SEMB, J., SUBBAROW, Y.: Synthesis and some biological properties of 4-aminopteroylaspartic acid. J. biol. Chem. **180**, 857—863 (1949).

HUTCHISON, D. J.: Quinazoline antifolates: Biologic activities. Cancer Chemother. Rep. **52**, 697—705 (1968).

JAFFE, N., FARBER, S., TRAGGIS, D., GEISER, C., DAS, L., KIM, B., FRAUENBERGER, G., DJERRASSI, I.: Favorable response of metastatic osteogenic sarcoma to pulse high dose methotrexate . . . citrovorum administration (HDMC). Proc. Amer. Ass. Cancer Res. **13**, 27 (1972).

JENKINS, G. C., HUGHES, D. T. D., HALL, P. C.: A haematological study of patients receiving long term treatment with trimethoprim and sulphonamide. J. clin. Path. **23**, 392—396 (1970).

JOHNS, D. G., IANNOTTI, A. T., SARTORELLI, A. C., BOOTH, B. A., BERTINO, J. R.: The identity of rabbit-liver methotrexate oxidase. Biochim. biophys. Acta (Amst.) **105**, 380—382 (1965).

JOHNS, D. G., VALERINO, A. M.: Metabolism of folate antagonists. Ann. N. Y. Acad. Sci. **186**, 378—386 (1971).

JONES, J. S. P., JELLIFFE, A. M.: Pyrimethamine: An alternative to radiophosphorus in the treatment of polycythemia rubra vera. Clin. Radiol. **14**, 424 (1963).

KISLIUK, R. L.: Reduced folic acid analogues as antimetabolites. Nature (Lond.) **188**, 584—585 (1960).

KISLIUK, R. L., LEVINE, M. D.: Properties of reduced derivatives of aminopterin. J. Biol. Chem. **239**, 1900—1904 (1964).

KISLIUK, R. L., FRIEDKIN, M., SCHMIDT, L. H., ROSSAN, R. N.: Antimalarial activity of tetrahydrohomopteroic acid. Science **156**, 1616—1617 (1967).

KISLIUK, R. L., GAUMONT, Y.: *d*,L-Tetrahydrohomofolate: A growth inhibitor. Fed. Proc. **29**, 807 (1970).

KISLIUK, R. L., GAUMONT, Y., KRUMDIECK, C., BAUGH, C. M.: Effect of polygammaglutamyl derivatives of homofolate (homopteroylmonoglutamate) on thymidylate synthetase. Pharmacologist **13**, 208 (1971).

KISLIUK, R. L.: Personal communication (1972).
KNOTT, R., TAUNTON-RIGBY, A.: The synthesis of $N^5$-methyltetrahydrohomofolic acid and related reduced derivatives of homofolic acid. Abstract, 162nd national meeting, Medicinal Chemistry 27. Washington, D.C.: Amer. Chem. Soc. 1971.
KOEHLER, R., GOODMAN, L., DEGRAW, J., BAKER, B. R.: Potential anticancer agents. IX. Tetrahydroquinazoline analogs of tetrahydrofolic acid. I. J. Amer. chem. Soc. **80**, 5779—5786 (1958).
LARRABEE, A. R., ROSENTHAL, S., CATHOU, R. E., BUCHANAN, J. M.: Enzymatic synthesis of the methyl group of methionine. IV. Isolation, characterization, and role of 5-methyl tetrahydrofolate. J. biol. Chem. **238**, 1025—1031 (1963).
LOO, T. L., ADAMSON, R. H.: The metabolite of 3′,5′-dichloro-4-amino-4-deoxy-$N^{10}$-methylpteroylglutamic acid (dichloromethotrexate). J. med. Chem. **8**, 513—515 (1965).
LOO, T. L., DION, R. L., ADAMSON, R. H., CHIRIGOS, M. A., KISLIUK, R. L.: 3′-Iodo-4-amino-4-deoxypteroylglutamic acid (3′-iodoaminopterin). J. med. Chem. **8**, 713—715 (1965).
LOO, T. L., DION, R. L., FU, S. C. J.: 3′-Iodopteroylglutamic acid (iodofolic acid). J. org. Chem. **30**, 2837 (1965).
MCCORMACK, J. J., JAFFE, J. J.: Dihydrofolate reductase from *Trypanosoma equiperdum*. II. Inhibition by 2,4-diaminopyrimidines and related heterocycles. J. med. Chem. **12**, 662—668 (1969).
MEAD, J. A. R., VENDITTI, J. M., SCHRECKER, A. W., GOLDIN, A., KISLIUK, R. L.: Toxicity and anti-leukaemic effectiveness, in mice, of 4-amino-4-deoxy-$N^{10}$-methyl-5,6,7,8-tetrahydropteroylglutamic acid (tetrahydroamethopterin). Nature (Lond.) **189**, 937—939 (1961).
MEAD, J. A. R.: Unpublished observations (1962).
MEAD, J. A. R., GREENBERG, N. H., SCHRECKER, A. W., SEEGER, D. R., TOMCUFCIK, A. S.: The pharmacological and biochemical activity of 4-amino-4-deoxy-10-methylpteroylaspartic acid. Biochem. Pharmacol. **14**, 105—114 (1965).
MEAD, J. A. R., GOLDIN, A., KISLIUK, R. L., FRIEDKIN, M., PLANTE, L., CRAWFORD, E. J., KWOK, G.: Pharmacologic aspects of homofolate derivatives in relation to amethopterin-resistant murine leukemia. Cancer Res. **26**, 2374—2379 (1966).
MEAD, J. A. R., WOOD, H. B., GOLDIN, A.: Relationship of structure to antitumor activity in compounds related to folic acid. Cancer Chemother. Rep. **1**, 273—361 (1968).
MISHRA, L. C., PARMAR, A. S., MEAD, J. A. R.: Distribution studies of tetrahydrohomofolic acid (NSC 89473) in mice. Cancer Res. **30**, 642—649 (1970).
MISHRA, L. C., PARMAR, A. S., MEAD, J. A. R.: Effect of pretreatment with methotrexate on the reduction of dihydrohomofolic acid in mice. Biochem. Pharmacol. **20**, 2871—2878 (1971).
MISHRA, L. C., PARMAR, A. S., MEAD, J. A. R., KNOTT, R., TAUNTON-RIGBY, A., FRIEDMAN, O. M.: Comparative antitumor activity of 5-methyltetrahydrohomofolate ($CH_3$—$H_4HF$) and tetrahydrohomofolate ($H_4HF$) in mice. Proc. Amer. Ass. Cancer Res. **13**, 76 (1972).
MISHRA, L. C., PARMAR, A. S., MEAD, J. A. R.: A method for assessing dihydrofolate reductase inhibition *in vivo*. Anal. Biochem. **48**, 515—523 (1972).
MISHRA, L. C., MEAD, J. A. R.: Further evaluation of the antitumor activity of homofolate and its reduced derivatives against methotrexate-insensitive tumors. Chemother. **17**, 283—292 (1972).
MISRA, D. K., HUMPHREYS, S. R., FRIEDKIN, M., GOLDIN, A., CRAWFORD, E. J.: Increased dihydrofolate reductase activity as a possible basis of drug resistance in leukaemia. Nature (Lond.) **189**, 39—42 (1961).
MODEST, E. J., FOLEY, G. E., PERCHET, M. M., FARBER, S.: A series of new, biologically significant dihydrotriazines. J. Amer. chem. Soc. **74**, 855—856 (1952).
MONTGOMERY, J. A., HEWSON, K., PIPER, J. R.: 3′-Fluorofolic acid. J. med. Chem. **8**, 727 (1965).
MOWAT, J. H., GAZZOLA, A. L., HUTCHINGS, B. L., BOOTHE, J. H., WALLER, C. W., ANGIER, R. B., SEMB, J., SUBBAROW, Y.: Pteroic acid derivatives. IV. Pteroyl-$\alpha$, $\gamma$-glutamyldiglutamic acid. J. Amer. chem. Soc. **71**, 2308—2310 (1949).
NAHAS, A., FRIEDKIN, M.: Fate of tetrahydrohomofolate in mice. Cancer Res. **29**, 1937—1943 (1969).
NAHAS, A., FRIEDKIN, M.: Lack of intracellular conversion of dihydrohomofolate to tetrahydrohomofolate in leukemia cells with high levels of dihydrofolate reductase. Molec. Pharmacol. **8**, 353—361 (1972).
OLIVERIO, V. T., DAVIDSON, J. D.: The physiological disposition of dichloromethotrexate-$Cl^{36}$ in animals. J. Pharmacol. exp. Ther. **137**, 76—83 (1962).
OSBORN, M. J., FREEMAN, M., HUENNEKENS, F. M.: Inhibition of dihydrofolic reductase by aminopterin and amethopterin. Proc. Soc. exp. Biol. (N. Y.) **97**, 429—431 (1958).
PLANTE, L. T., CRAWFORD, E. J., FRIEDKIN, M.: Enzyme studies with new analogues of folic acid and homofolic acid. J. biol. Chem. **242**, 1466—1476 (1967).
ROBERTS, E. C., SHEALY, Y. F.: Folic acid analogs. Modifications in the benzene-ring region. 1. 2′- and 3′-azafolic acids. J. med. Chem. **14**, 125—130 (1971).

ROTH, B., SMITH, J. M., HULTQUIST, M. E.: Analogs of pteroylglutamic acid. V. 4-Alkylamino derivatives. J. Amer. chem. Soc. 72, 1914—1918 (1950).
ROTH, B., SMITH, J. M., HULTQUIST, M. E.: Analogs of pteroylglutamic acid. VII. 2-Alkylamino derivatives. J. Amer. chem. Soc. 73, 2864—2868 (1951 a).
ROTH, B., SMITH, J. M., HULTQUIST, M. E.: Analogs of pteroylglutamic acid. VIII. 4-Alkoxy derivatives. J. Amer. chem. Soc. 73, 2869—2871 (1951 b).
ROTH, B., HULTQUIST, M. E., FAHRENBACH, M. J., COSULICH, D. B., BROQUIST, H. P., BROCKMAN, J. A., SMITH, J. M., PARKER, R. P., STOKSTAD, E. L. R., JUKES, J. H.: Synthesis of leucovorin. J. Amer. chem. Soc. 74, 3247—3252 (1952).
SCHRECKER, A. W., MEAD, J. A. R., LYNCH, M. R., GOLDIN, A.: Comparative effect of amethopterin and its 3′,5′-dichloro derivative on purine biosynthesis in leukemic mice. Cancer Res. 20, 876—886 (1960).
SEEGER, D. R., COSULICH, D. B., SMITH, J. M., HULTQUIST, M. E.: Analogs of pteroylglutamic acid. III. 4-Amino derivatives. J. Amer. chem. Soc. 71, 1753—1758 (1949).
SEEGER, D. R., SMITH, J. M., HULTQUIST, M. E.: Antagonist for pteroylglutamic acid. J. Amer. chem. Soc. 69, 2567 (1947).
SEMB, J., BOOTHE, J. H., ANGIER, R. B., WALLER, C. W., MOWAT, J. H., HUTCHINGS, B. L., SUBBAROW, Y.: Pteroic acid derivatives. V. Pteroyl-α glutamyl-α-glutamylglutamic acid, pteroyl-γ-glutamyl-α-glutamylglutamic acid, pteroyl-α-glutamyl-γ-glutamylglutamic acid. J. Amer. chem. Soc. 71, 2310—2315 (1949).
SLAVIK, K., ZAKRZEWSKI, S. F.: Inhibition of thymidylate synthetase by some analogs of tetrahydrofolic acid. Molec. Pharmacol. 3, 370—377 (1967).
SLAVIK, K., SLAVÍKOVÁ, V., MOTYČKA, K., HERMANOVÁ, E., SOUČEK, J., TOMSOVÁ, Z., ŠPUNDOVÁ, M., NOVÁKOVÁ, E.: Azahomoaminopterin, a new type of folic acid antimetabolite. Molec. Pharmacol. 5, 137—147 (1969).
STRUCK, R. F., SHEALY, Y. F., MONTGOMERY, J. A.: Potential folic acid antagonists. 5. Synthesis and biologic evaluation of $N^{10}$-deazapteroic acid and $N^{10}$-deazafolic acid and their 9,10-dehydro derivatives. J. med. Chem. 14, 693—698 (1971).
TOMCUFCIK, A. S., SEEGER, D. R.: The synthesis of the 3′-fluoro and 3′,5′-difluoro derivatives of 4-amino-4-deoxy-$N^{10}$-methylpteroylglutamic acid (methotrexate). J. org. Chem. 26, 3351—3356 (1961).
VALERINO, D. M., ZAHARKO, D. S., JOHNS, D. G., OLIVERIO, V. T.: Studies of the metabolism of methotrexate by the intestinal flora of the mouse. Fed. Proc. 30, 388 (1971).
VENDITTI, J. M., HUMPHREYS, S. R., MANTEL, N., KLINE, I., GOLDIN, A.: Evaluation of antileukemic agents employing advanced leukemia L1210 in mice. III. Congeners of folic acid. Cancer Res. 20, 698—733 (1960).
WAHBA, A. J., FRIEDKIN, M. E.: Direct spectrophotometric evidence for the oxidation of tetrahydrofolate during the enzymatic synthesis of thymidylate. J. biol. Chem. 237, PC11—PC12 (1961).
WALLER, C. W., FAHRENBACH, M. J., BOOTHE, J. H., ANGIER, R. B., HUTCHINGS, B. L., MOWAT, J. H., POLETTO, J. F., SEMB, J.: 7-Isomer of pteroylglutamic acid. J. Amer. chem. Soc. 74, 5405—5407 (1952).
WEINSTOCK, L. T., GRABOWSKI, B. F., CHENG, C. C.: Folic acid analogs. II. p-{[(2,6-diamino-8-purinyl)methyl]amino}-benzoyl-L-glutamic acid and related compounds. J. med. Chem. 13, 995—997 (1970).
WERKHEISER, W. C.: The biochemical, cellular and pharmacological action and effects of the folic acid antagonists. Cancer Res. 23, 1277—1285 (1963).
WERKHEISER, W. C.: Influence of methotrexate on the level of tetrahydrofolate ($FH_4$) compounds in mouse intestinal mucosa. Fed. Proc. 28, 362 (1969).
WILLIAMS, J. H.: Proceedings of second conference on folic acid antagonists in leukemia treatment. Blood 7, 100—107 (1952).
WOOD, R. C., FERONE, R., HITCHINGS, G. H.: The relationships of cellular permeability to the degree of inhibition by amethopterin and pyrimethamine in several species of bacteria. Biochem. Pharmacol. 6, 113—124 (1961).
WRIGHT, W. B., COSULICH, D. B., FAHRENBACH, M. J., WALLER, C. W., SMITH, J. M., HULTQUIST, M. E.: Analogs of pteroylglutamic acid. IV. Replacement of glutamic acid by other amino acids. J. Amer. chem. Soc. 71, 3014—3017 (1949).
ZAKRZEWSKI, S. F., HAKALA, M. T., NICHOL, C. A.: Preparation and biological activity of dihydroaminopterin. Biochem. 1, 842—846 (1962).
ZAKRZEWSKI, S. F.: The mechanism of binding of folate analogues by folate reductase. J. biol. Chem. 238, 1485—1490 (1963).
ZUBROD, C. G., SCHEPARTZ, S. A., LEITER, J., ENDICOTT, K. M., CARRESE, L. M., BAKER, C. G.: The chemotherapy program of the National Cancer Institute: History, analysis and plans. Cancer Chemother. Rep. 50, 378 (1966).

Chapter 5

# Rational Design of Purine Nucleoside Analogs

John A. Montgomery

## Introduction

The rational design of cancer chemotherapeutic agents must ultimately be based on an exploitable biochemical difference between normal host cells and the invading cancer cells. Although much is known about the biologic activity of certain agents, such as 6-mercaptopurine and 6-thioguanine, the basis of their selective action on cancer cells is still not fully understood. This selectivity could result from greater catabolism of the drug by normal cells, since it is known that the xanthine oxidase level of cancer cells is generally lower than that of normal cells (Bergel et al., 1957). The metabolic state of treated cells must also be important, since established solid tumors with a low growth fraction do not normally respond well to antimetabolites, purines or otherwise (Laster et al., 1969). Because of our limited knowledge about the basis of selective toxicity of purine antagonists, we must base the design of new agents on what is known about the metabolism and the mechanisms of action of purine analogs and the effects of structural changes on both of these. Although some of these topics will be discussed in more detail later in this volume, our knowledge of the biologically active purine analogs will be summarized briefly here.

An analog of a naturally occurring purine, purine nucleoside, or a metabolic product of either, is potentially a substrate for and/or an inhibitor of the enzymes involved in the cellular metabolism of the naturally occurring purines, their nucleosides, and their nucleotides (Bennett and Montgomery, 1967; Montgomery, 1970). In addition, certain analog nucleotides can, by negative pseudo-feedback, inhibit the *de novo* synthesis of inosinic acid, and others can be incorporated into nucleic acids (Henderson, 1965; Bennett and Montgomery, 1967; Montgomery, 1970).

Biologically active purines can be divided into two major classes: (1) those that are active per se and (2) those that are metabolized to active forms. Only puromycin and its relatives (Guarino et al., 1963; Nathans, 1967), nucleocidin (Florini, 1967), psicofuranine (Hanka, 1967), and decoyinine (Guarino, 1967), and certain 9-alkylpurines (Montgomery, 1970) belong to the first class. Puromycin and its relatives, because of their resemblance to aminoacyl tRNA, interfere with protein synthesis by causing the premature release of growing polypeptide chains from ribosomes (Guarino et al., 1963; Nathans, 1967). Nucleocidin, which is perhaps an even more potent inhibitor of protein synthesis, forms a complex with ribosomes which is inactive in peptide bond formation (Florini, 1967). The anticancer activity of these inhibitors of protein synthesis is at best marginal.

The second step in the conversion of inosinic acid to guanylic acid is the aminolysis of xanthylic acid with glutamine by xanthosine 5′-phosphate aminase. This aminase is inhibited allosterically by adenosine and adenylic acid (Fukuyama and Moyed, 1964; Kuramitsu and Moyed, 1966), noncompetitively by psicofuranine (HANKA, 1967), and less effectively by decoyinine (Chart I), which appears to be interconvertible with psicofuranine in cells (GUARINO, 1967). This inhibition is thought to be allosteric also at a site normally occupied by a metabolic

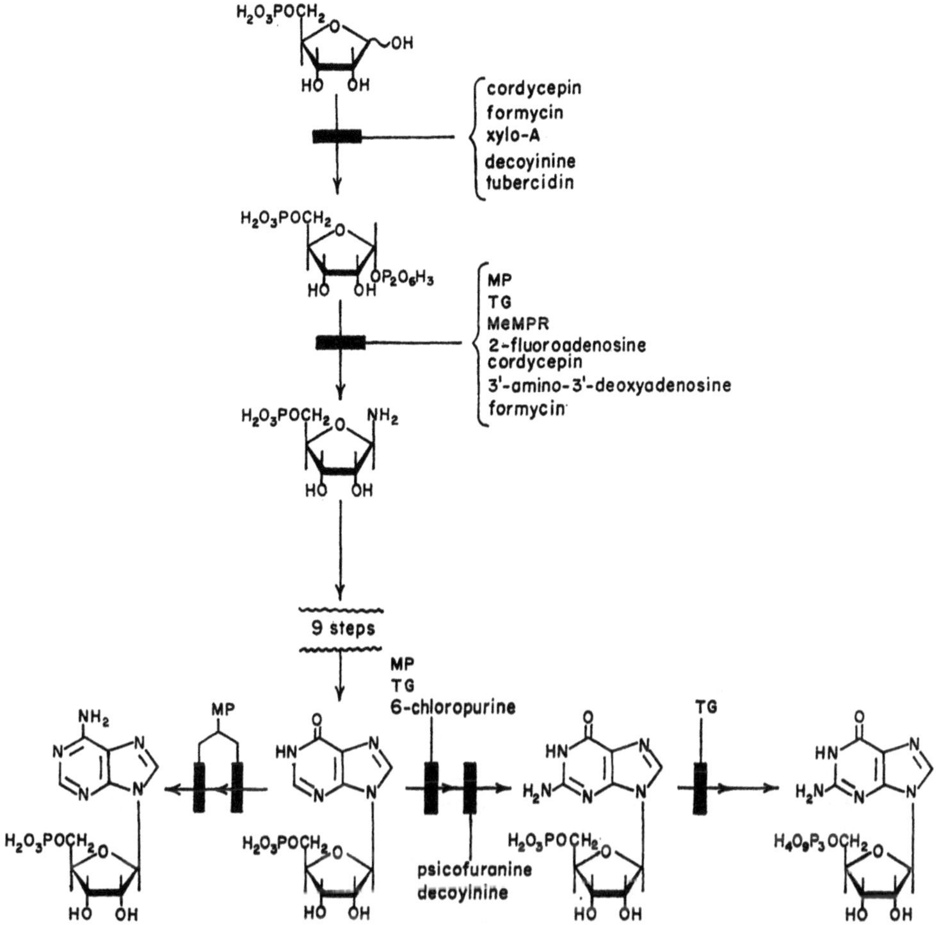


Chart I. Inhibition of the *de novo* synthesis of inosinic acid and purine nucleotide interconversions.

regulator. Psicofuranine and decoyinine have shown anticancer activity in a variety of experimental animal systems (SCHROEDER and HOEKSEMA, 1959; TANAKA et al., 1961).

The vast majority of biologically active purines and their nucleosides, however, are anabolized to active forms, some of which are among the best anticancer agents known. These agents can be grouped according to structure as analogs of adenine or its nucleosides on the one hand or as analogs of the 6-oxopurines – hypoxanthine, xanthine, guanine – or their nucleosides on the other (Chart II). In some cases, such as 2-fluoroadenosine (MONTGOMERY and HEWSON, 1957), the classification of an analog is obvious and predictable, but in others, such as the adenosine analog 6-(methylthio)purine ribonucleoside, the classification is deceptive and was correctly made in retrospect (BENNETT et al., 1965).

Certain purine analogs are anabolized to their ribonucleotides by purine phosphoribosyltransferases. Two such enzymes are known to function in mammalian cells: (1) adenine phosphoribosyltransferase and (2) hypoxanthine-guanine

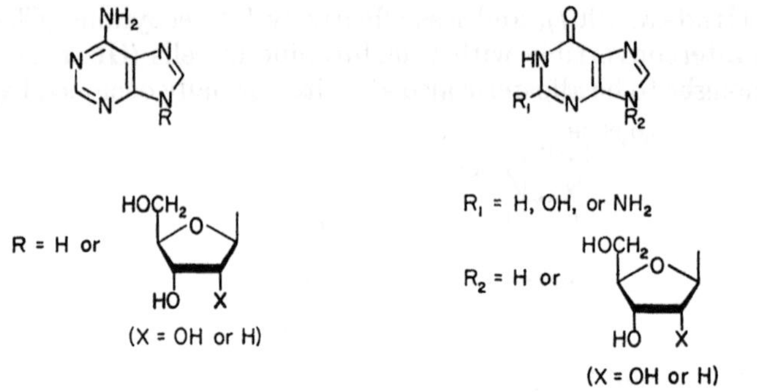


Adenine and nucleosides 6-Oxypurines and nucleosides

Chart II

phosphoribosyltransferase (Kornberg et al., 1955; Flaks, 1957). Substrates for the adenine enzyme include certain 2- and *N*-substituted adenines, other 6-substituted purines, and ring analogs of adenine (Way and Parks, 1958; Roy et al., 1960; Bennett et al., 1966a). Substrates for the hypoxanthine-guanine enzyme include 6-mercaptopurine, thioguanine, and ring analogs of hypoxanthine and guanine (Brockman and Anderson, 1963; Brockman, 1963; Krenitsky et al., 1969).

A large number of adenosine analogs are phosphorylated by adenosine kinase, an enzyme of relatively low substrate specificity (Schnebli et al., 1967; Lindberg et al., 1967). The sugar moiety of the substrate is the most restrictive part of the molecule, but even here certain changes can be made without serious loss of substrate activity. Adenosine can be substituted at *N*-1 and *C*-2 to give active substrates. A number of groups can be substituted for the amino group of adenosine; a variety of changes in the imidazole ring can be made, but changes in the pyrimidine ring of adenosine appear to be less favorable (Schnebli et al., 1967). Kinase activity for inosine or its analogs in most mammalian cells is either absent or very weak under normal *in vivo* conditions, but 6-mercaptopurine ribonucleoside, in certain cell lines (Pierre et al., 1967; Pierre and LePage, 1968), and 8-azainosine (Allan and Bennett, 1970) are converted to their nucleotides to a small extent.

There is evidence that the nucleotides of a number of adenine and adenosine analogs are phosphorylated by nucleoside phosphokinases (Montgomery, 1970). Substitution on the amino group of adenylic acid, however, prevents phosphorylation (Shigeura et al., 1966; Coddington, 1962), indicating that adenylate kinase has little bulk tolerance at the point where the amino group fits. There is no evidence for the formation of di- and triphosphates of inosinic acid analogs such as 6-thioinosinic acid. 8-Azaguanylic acid is a good substrate for GMP-ATP phosphotransferase (Roy et al., 1961), whereas 6-thioguanylic acid is a poor substrate and a good inhibitor of the enzyme (Miech et al., 1967, 1969).

Other anabolic enzymes such as aminases, methylases, and reductases may be important to the action of certain purine analogs. For example, 7-deazainosine (Bloch et al., 1969), formycin B (Sawa et al., 1968), and 8-azainosine (Allan and Bennett, 1970) are all converted to adenine analog nucleotides. 6-Thioinosinic acid and 6-thioguanylic acid are both *S*-methylated (Allan et al., 1966; Allan and Bennett, 1971), and the incorporation of 6-mercaptopurine (Scannell and Hitchings, 1966) and thioguanine (LePage, 1960) into DNA may depend on the ribonucleoside diphosphate reductase (Montgomery, 1970).

The catabolism of purine analogs must also be considered. The cleavage of nucleotides to nucleosides by phosphatases may be of some consequence (Heppel,

1961; WHEELER and ALEXANDER, 1961; MONTGOMERY et al., 1963; BENNETT et al., 1965). The cleavage of inosine analogs by nucleoside phosphorylase is certainly important (PATERSON and SUTHERLAND, 1964; KRENITSKY et al., 1968). Although there is evidence for the cleavage by mammalian cells of certain adenosine analogs (BENNETT et al., 1966b; MONTGOMERY and HEWSON, 1968b), they are much less susceptible to this catabolic process. The relatively high inosine phosphorylase activity coupled with the low inosine kinase activity of cells precludes much direct conversion of inosine analogs to the nucleotides. The reverse obtains with the adenosine metabolizing enzymes, but, with certain exceptions, adenosine analogs are catabolized by adenosine deaminase to the corresponding inosine analogs even though the rate of catabolism varies greatly (MONTGOMERY, 1970). Thioguanine (CURRIE, 1967) and 8-azaguanine (KREAM and CHARGAFF, 1952) are deaminated by guanase to the less active or inactive xanthine analogs. Many purine analogs unsubstituted at *N*-9 are oxidized by xanthine oxidase (BRAY, 1963) to 2-oxo-, 2,8-dioxopurines, or uric acid, and thus detoxified.

6-Chloropurine is converted to its ribonucleoside monophosphate (HAMPTON and PATERSON, 1966), which is degraded eventually to uric acid (DUGGAN and TITUS, 1959). Its ribonucleoside is rapidly converted to inosine by adenosine deaminase (CORY and SUHADOLNIK, 1965; WOLFENDEN, 1966) and, therefore, is less toxic than 6-chloropurine (MONTGOMERY, 1970). 2-Fluoroadenine is not readily degraded, but is anabolized to the triphosphate and incorporated into RNA (SHIGEURA et al., 1965). 2-Fluoroadenosine appears to be cleaved to 2-fluoroadenine (BENNETT et al., 1966a), but is not detoxified. Tubercidin and 6-methylpurine are metabolized in a similar, but not identical, fashion (MONTGOMERY, 1970). 9-$\beta$-D-Arabinofuranosyladenine is poorly converted to the monophosphate (SCHNEBLI et al., 1967), which is readily phosphorylated to the triphosphate (BRINK and LEPAGE, 1964), but is not incorporated into RNA. It is rapidly deaminated to 9-$\beta$-D-arabinofuranosylhypoxanthine (YORK and LEPAGE, 1966), a catabolite inactive against cancer. 9-$\beta$-D-Xylofuranosyladenine (YORK and LEPAGE, 1966) and formycin (SAWA et al., 1968; CALDWELL et al., 1969) are similarly metabolized. The metabolism of the thiopurines is more complicated than that of the analogs discussed above (ELION and HITCHINGS, 1967; ELION, 1967; MONTGOMERY, 1970). They are readily catabolized and are anabolized primarily to the ribonucleoside monophosphates (BENNETT and MONTGOMERY, 1967; MONTGOMERY, 1970), which are *S*-methylated to varying extents (ALLAN et al., 1966; ALLAN and BENNETT, 1971).

To determine the ultimate fate and mechanism of action of a purine analog, one must determine not only what enzymes can metabolize it but the relative rates of these enzymic transformations and the $K_i$ values for the enzymes that the purine analog or its anabolites inhibit. A number of adenosine analogs as their triphosphates are known or thought to inhibit PRPP synthetase, thus blocking the first step of the *de novo* synthesis of inosinic acid (Chart I) (OVERGAARD-HANSEN, 1964; BLOCH and NICHOL, 1964; HENDERSON et al., 1967; ELLIS and LEPAGE, 1965). The second step of this pathway, the conversion of PRPP to phosphoribosylamine, is under allosteric control and is inhibited by negative pseudofeedback by adenosine analogs and the 6-thiopurines as their nucleotides (CASKEY et al., 1964; ROTTMAN and GUARINO, 1964; NIERLICH and MAGASANIK, 1965; MCCOLLISTER et al., 1964; BROCKMAN and CHUMLEY, 1965; BENNETT and SMITHERS, 1964; HILL and BENNETT, 1969). 6-Mercaptopurine ribonucleotide also inhibits both steps in the conversion of inosinic to adenylic acid (DAVIDSON, 1960; SALSER et al., 1960; HAMPTON, 1962) and inosinic dehydrogenase (HAMPTON, 1963), the enzyme that catalyzes the first step of the conversion of inosinic to guanylic acid. Thioguanine ribonucleotide, in addition to its allosteric inhibition of PRPP-amidotransferase, inhibits inosinic dehydrogenase (HAMPTON, 1963) and GMP-ATP phosphotransferase (MIECH et al., 1967, 1969).

In addition to the enzyme inhibitions mentioned above, the 6-thiopurines are incorporated into DNA as 2′-deoxythioguanylic acid (LEPAGE, 1960; SCANNELL and HITCHINGS, 1966), which may affect RNA synthesis. 8-Azaguanine is incorporated into RNA (MITCHELL et al., 1950), and this incorporation is known to affect protein synthesis (MANDEL, 1967).

Thus, the metabolism and the effects of the anabolites of many purine analogs, particularly the important 6-thiopurines, is complex, and it would appear likely that many, if not most, of these analogs owe their biologic activity to multiple sites of action. Recent investigations of drug combinations such as arabinosylcytosine and thioguanine, which show not only therapeutic synergism but subadditive toxicity in the L1210 leukemia system in mice (SCHMIDT et al., 1970), indicate that it may be possible to manipulate these multiple sites advantageously by the use of drug combinations, and similar results may be attainable by the proper structural modification of known agents.

## Chemistry

### A. Ring Analogs of Purines

#### I. Azapurines

Among the earliest biologically active purine analogs were the 8-azapurines (*v*-triazolo[4,5-*d*]pyrimidines) prepared by ROBLIN et al. (1945) in which the carbon in the eight position of the purine ring is replaced by nitrogen. These compounds were made by the action of nitrous acid on variously substituted 4,5-diaminopyrimidines [synthesized by ring closure reactions followed by the introduction of the amino function at *C*-5 (BROWN, 1962)]. Among the more active structures are 8-azaadenine (1), 8-azahypoxanthine (6) and 8-azaguanine (7). The ribonucleosides of 8-azaadenine and 8-azaguanine were first prepared (DAVOLL, 1958) by the chloromercuri procedure of DAVOLL and LOWY (1951) from the suitably protected bases and 2,3,5-tri-*O*-benzoyl-D-ribofuranosyl chloride (KISSMAN et al., 1955). Methanolic sodium methoxide was then used to remove the acyl groups from the intermediate nucleosides to give 8-azaadenosine (2) and 8-azaguanosine (9). 8-Azaguanosine was also prepared by a more involved route *via* 2-(methylthio)-8-azaadenine, and 8-azaadenosine was deaminated to give 8-azainosine (8). A detailed discussion of the *trans* rule (BAKER, 1957) is beyond the scope of this section, but it is sufficient to say the benzoyloxy group at *C*-2 of the sugar exerts steric control over its reactions with chloromercuri purines so that the desired *trans* (or in the case of ribose the $\beta$) anomers (2 and 9) are formed almost exclusively. Although substitution could theoretically take place at any of the five ring nitrogens, it occurs primarily at *N*-9 (purine numbering system) with a small amount of an isomer being formed (DAVOLL, 1958). Reaction of 2,3,5-tri-*O*-acetyl-D-ribofuranosyl chloride with the chloromercuri derivative of *N*-nonanoyl-8-azaadenine, however, gave only the isomer that was identified as the 8-isomer (MONTGOMERY et al., 1970). 8-Azaadenosine has also been prepared by the fusion reaction (SATO et al., 1960) of *N*-octanoyl-8-azaadenine and tetra-*O*-acetyl-$\beta$-D-ribofuranose (LEE et al., 1963). The fusion reaction is acid catalyzed and undoubtedly proceeds through a carbonium ion mechanism, and although it usually gives predominantly the *trans* anomer (MONTGOMERY and HEWSON, 1968b), it does not always do so (LEE et al., 1963). 8-Azainosine (8) has also been prepared from a derivative of 6-chloro-9-$\beta$-D-ribofuranosylpurine by ring opening and reclosure, with nitrous acid, of the imidazole ring (MONTGOMERY and THOMAS, 1971), but the best method for the synthesis of 8-azaadenosine now appears to be by the reaction of *N*-nonanoyl-8-azaadenine with 2,3,5-tri-*O*-acetyl-D-ribofuranosyl chloride in the presence of a molecular sieve (MONTGOMERY et al., 1970b). This procedure has also been used for the preparation of 2′-deoxy-8-azaadenosine and its $\alpha$-anomer ($\beta$- and $\alpha$-3), 9-$\alpha$- and $\beta$-D-arabinofuranosyl-8-azaadenine ($\alpha$- and $\beta$-4), and 9-$\beta$-D-xylofuranosyl-8-azaadenine (5) (MONTGOMERY and THOMAS, 1972a). The 2′-deoxyribose nucleosides were also prepared by the chloromercuri procedure (TONG et al., 1965).

9- and *O*-Substituted derivatives (10 and 11) of 8-azaguanine have been prepared from the appropriately substituted 4,5-diamino-6-chloropyrimidines

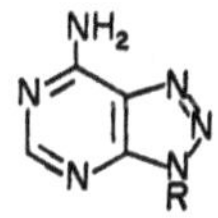

1: R = H

2: R = 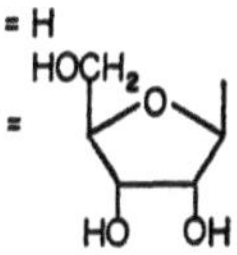

3: R = 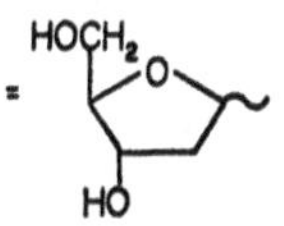

4: R = 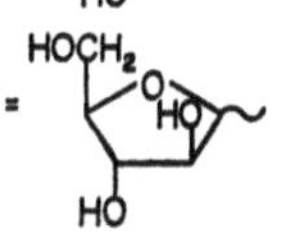

5: R = 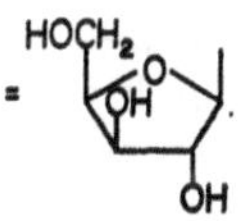

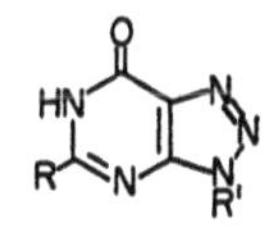

6: R = R′ = H

7: R = $NH_2$, R = H

8: R = H, R′ = 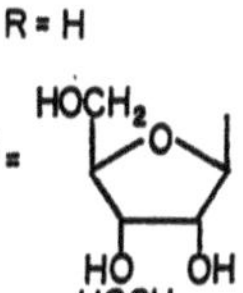

9: R = $NH_2$, R′ = 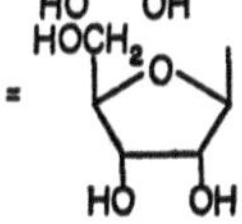

10: R = $NH_2$, R′ = alkyl

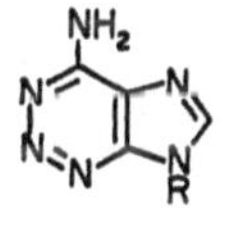

12: R = H

13: R = 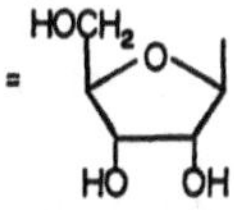

14: R = 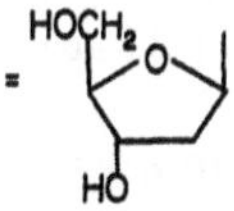

15: R = 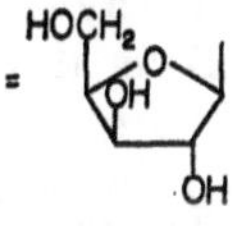

16: R = 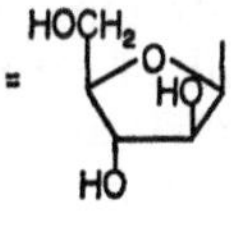

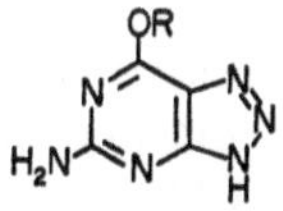

11: R = alkyl

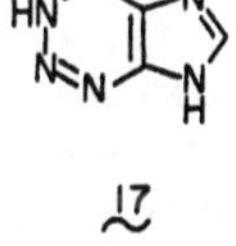

17

by ring closure with nitrous acid followed by displacement of the chloro group (SHEALY et al., 1961, 1962).

SHAW and WOOLLEY (1949) synthesized 5-aminoimidazole-4-carboxamide hydrochloride from ethyl cyanoacetate, and SHAW (1950) prepared the corresponding carboxamidine hydrochloride in a similar manner from malononitrile. Treatment of these imidazoles with sodium nitrite in aqueous media gave 2-azahypoxanthine (imidazo[4,5-*d*]-*v*-triazin-4(3*H*)-one (17) and 2-azaadenine (4-aminoimidazo[4,5-*d*]-*v*-triazine (12) (WOOLLEY and SHAW, 1951). The ribonucleoside (13) of 2-azaadenine has been prepared from adenosine-1-oxide by *O*-benzylation, treatment with methanolic ammonia, catalytic hydrogenolysis of the benzyloxy group, and reclosure of the resultant carboxamidine with nitrous acid (MONTGOMERY and THOMAS, 1969). This procedure has been applied to the preparation of other nucleosides of 2-azaadenine (14–16) (MONTGOMERY and THOMAS, 1972b). The 2-azapurines are highly cytotoxic but have shown less anticancer activity than the 8-azapurines (MONTGOMERY et al., 1970a).

## II. Pyrazolopyrimidines

4-Aminopyrazolo[3,4-*d*]pyrimidine (18), an adenine analog in which the carbon at position 8 has been interchanged with the nitrogen at position 7, was prepared by ROBINS (1956) in two steps from ethoxymethylenemalononitrile. The intermediate aminonitrile was hydrolyzed to the amide, which was converted to a number of other pyrazolo[3,4-*d*]pyrimidines (19–21, 24). 4-Aminopyrazolo[3,4-*d*]pyrimidine, prepared almost simultaneously by FALCO and HITCHINGS (1956) by a much more involved route, is active in a number of experimental animal tumor systems, but because of hepatotoxicity had to be abandoned as a clinical agent. Using substituted hydrazines in the reaction with ethoxymethylenemalononitrile, 1-alkylpyrazoles were prepared and converted into 1-alkyl derivatives (18–21, 24) (CHENG and ROBINS, 1956; SUTCLIFFE et al., 1962), which are also active against experimental animal neoplasms. 4-Chloropyrazolo[3,4-*d*]pyrimidine (19) and its methyl analog (22) react readily with amines to produce *N*-alkyl derivatives (21 and 23) of 18, which are also active (NOELL and ROBINS, 1958). DAVOLL and KERRIDGE (1961) used the chloromercuri procedure to convert 18 to its ribonucleoside 25, but the fusion procedure using the *N*-benzoyl derivative of 18 and tetra-*O*-acetyl-*β*-D-ribofuranose appears to be superior in this case (MONTGOMERY et al., 1964). Compound 25 has also been prepared (REVANKAR and TOWNSEND, 1971) by the trimethylsilyl procedure first used by BIRKOFER et al. (1963) for the synthesis of 3-*β*-D-ribofuranosyluric acid and later applied to the synthesis of pyrimidine nucleosides (NISHIMURA and IWAI, 1964). In this procedure, the trimethylsilylheterocycle, prepared by the action of trimethylsilyl chloride, is fused with an acylglycosyl halide followed by removal of the protecting groups. Deamination of 25 gave the ribonucleoside of allopurinol (26) (KRENITSKY et al., 1967).

The isomeric 7-aminopyrazolo[4,3-*d*]pyrimidine (27) was prepared by ROBINS et al. (1956) from 5-methyl-4-nitropyrazole-3-carboxylic acid by a seven-step sequence. Although 27 is devoid of biologic activity, presumably because it cannot be converted *in vivo* to a ribonucleotide (MONTGOMERY et al., 1970a), its 3-ribonucleoside, formycin (28) – a *C*-nucleoside antibiotic isolated by HORI et al. (1964) – is readily phosphorylated *in vivo* and is a highly active structure. Although the synthesis of formycin itself has not yet been accomplished, oxyformycin B (29, R = OH) and formycin B (29, R = H) have been prepared from 2,3,5-tri-*O*-benzoyl-D-ribofuranosyl bromide by eleven- (BOBEK et al., 1970a) and fourteen-step (ACTON et al., 1971) sequences. The key to this sequence is the preparation of 2,3,5-tri-*O*-benzyl-1-deoxy-1-diazomethyl-$\beta$-D-ribofuranose and its reaction with the methyl ester of acetylenedicarboxylic acid to form the pyrazole ring. Formycin B has been converted to a number of other 7-substituted 3-$\beta$-D-ribofuranosylpyrazolo[4,3-*d*]pyrimidines (LONG et al., 1971).

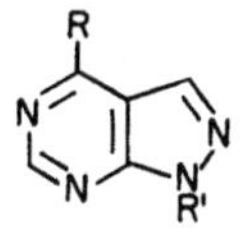

R' = H

**18**: R = $NH_2$
**19**: R = Cl
**20**: R = SR''
**21**: R = NR''R'''

R' = $CH_3$

**22**: R = Cl
**23**: R = NR''R'''

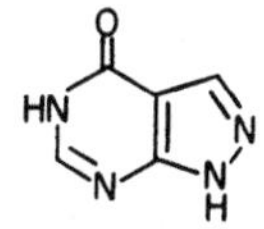

**24**

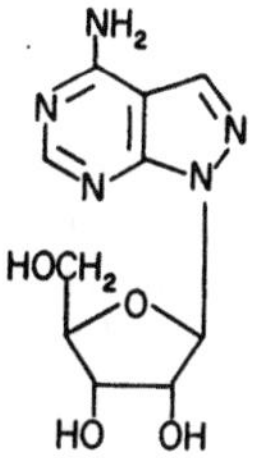

**25**

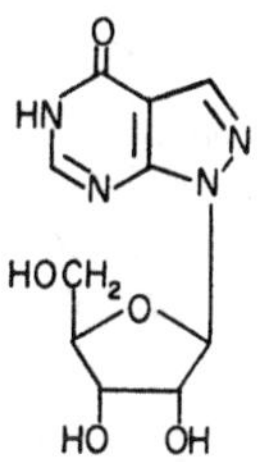

**26**

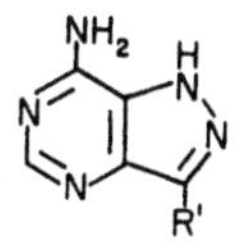

**27**: R' = H
**28**: R' = 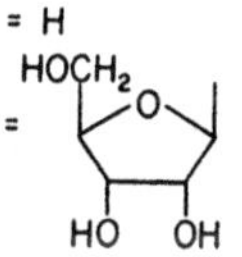

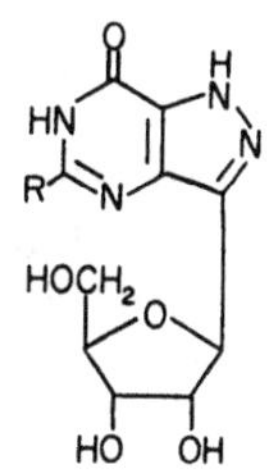

**29**

## III. Deazapurines

The pyrrolo[2,3-*d*]pyrimidine (7-deazapurine) ring system was first prepared by DAVOLL (1960) by constructing the appropriately substituted pyrimidine and then effecting ring closure of the pyrrole ring to give 6-oxopurine analogs (30–33). The adenine (34) and 2,6-diaminopurine (35) analogs were prepared in a similar manner from malononitrile. Although it is possible for these 7-deazapurines to be phosphoribosidated *in vivo* by cellular phosphoribosyltransferases, they apparently are not and they are biologically inactive. Tubercidin (7-deazaadenosine, 37) (ANZAI et al., 1957) and its relatives toyocamycin (38) (NISHIMURA et al., 1956) and sangivamycin (39) (RAO and RENN, 1963), all nucleoside antibiotics that are highly active biologically, are phosphorylated *in vivo* and have demonstrated anticancer activity in experimental animal systems. Although tubercidin was converted to a number of analogs by replacement of its 4-amino group (PIKE et al., 1964; GERSTER et al., 1967) and by electrophilic substitution at the five position (HINSHAW et al., 1969), it resisted synthesis and has still not been prepared directly from 7-deazaadenine. In the first approach to its synthesis, MIZUNO et al. (1963) used Todd's purine nucleoside synthesis involving the reaction of 4-aminopyrimidines with sugars followed by cyclization of the sugar and closure of the heterocyclic ring (KENNER et al., 1948). This approach allowed the preparation of 7-deazainosine (43) and its conversion to 7-deaza-6-thioinosine (44), which was *S*-methylated, but conversion of the methylthio compound to tubercidin itself was not successful.

TOLMAN et al. (1967) prepared the 7-*β*-D-ribofuranosylpyrrolo[2,3-*d*]pyrimidine (40) *via* fusion of 4-chloro-5-cyano-6-(methylthio)pyrrolo[2,3-*d*]pyrimidine with tetra-*O*-acetyl-*β*-D-ribofuranose followed by deblocking and displacement of the 4-chloro group of the resultant nucleoside. Compound 40 was also prepared by the fusion reaction from 4-acetamido-7-acetyl-5-cyano-6-(methylthio)pyrrolo-[2,3-*d*]pyrimidine (IWAMURA and HASHIZUME, 1968a). Application of this procedure (TOLMAN et al., 1969) to 4-acetamido-5-cyano-6-bromopyrrolo[2,3-*d*]pyrimidine gave 6-bromotoyocamycin (41) which was converted to 6-bromosangivamycin (42). Catalytic hydrodebromination gave toyocamycin (38) and sangivamycin (39) themselves. Toyocamycin was hydrolyzed to the corresponding acid, which was decarboxylated to tubercidin (37).

Better yields of 7-*β*-D-ribofuranosylpyrrolo[2,3-*d*]pyrimidines have been obtained by the reaction of 2,3,5-tri-*O*-benzoyl-D-ribofuranosyl bromide with silylated pyrrolo[2,3-*d*]pyrimidines in the presence of mercuric cyanide (TOLMAN et al., 1970). Several tubercidin analogs (36) have been prepared from 4,6-dichloro-5-pyrimidineacetaldehyde (MONTGOMERY and HEWSON, 1967).

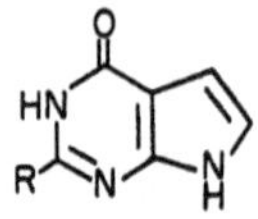

30: R = H
31: R = $NH_2$
32: R = OH
33: R = SH

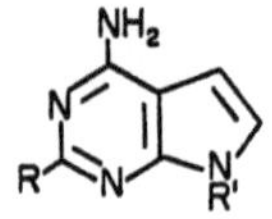

R' = H
34: R = H
35: R = $NH_2$
R' = alkyl
36: R = H

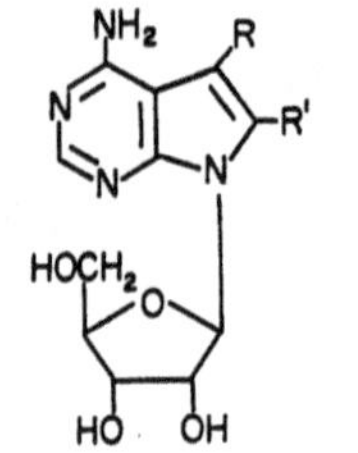

37: R = R' = H
38: R = CN, R' = H
39: R = $CONH_2$, R' = H
40: R = CN, R' = $SCH_3$
41: R = CN, R' = Br
42: R = $CONH_2$, R' = Br

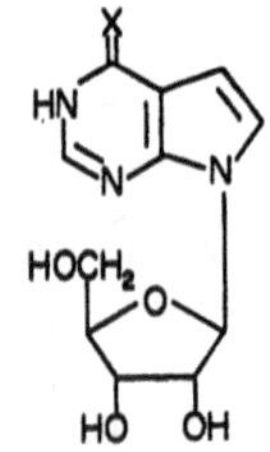

43: X = O
44: X = S

Although a number of 1-deazapurines (imidazo[4,5-*b*]pyridines) (KÖGL et al., 1948; MONTGOMERY and HEWSON, 1965a), 3-deazapurines (imidazo[4,5-*c*]-pyridines) (SALEMINK and VAN DER WANT, 1949; MONTGOMERY and HEWSON, 1965a), 9-deazapurines (pyrrolo[3,2-*d*]pyrimidines) (ROSE, 1954; PFLEIDERER and MOSTHAF, 1957; IMAI, 1964; TANAKA et al., 1964; MONTGOMERY and HEWSON, 1965b), and nucleosides of the first two ring systems (MIZUNO et al., 1964; MONTGOMERY and HEWSON, 1966a, b; ROUSSEAU et al., 1966; JAIN et al., 1966) have been prepared, none of these compounds have shown significant cytotoxicity or anticancer activity.

## B. Unnatural Purines and Their Nucleosides

### I. Adenine Analogs

#### 1. 2-Substituted Adenines

The first adenine analog, 2-aminoadenine (2,6-diaminopurine, 45), was synthesized by TRAUBE in 1904 from tetraaminopyrimidine, which in turn was prepared from guanidine and malononitrile by a three-step sequence. Formylation of tetraaminopyrimidine was carried out with sodium formate in acetic acid, and ring closure was effected by fusion of the dry formamide. The ring closure is better carried out by heating tetraaminopyrimidine in formamide with (BENDICH et al., 1948) or without (ROBINS et al., 1959) formic acid. TAYLOR et al. (1959) have synthesized 2,6-diaminopurine (45) in 89% yield by a two-step sequence starting with guanidine carbonate and the potassium salt of isonitrosomalononitrile. 2,6-Diaminopurine was the first purine to exhibit anticancer activity in experimental systems. The ribonucleoside (48) of 2,6-diaminopurine was first prepared by DAVOLL and LOWY (1951) from 2,3,5-tri-*O*-acetyl-D-ribofuranosyl chloride by the chloromercuri procedure that they developed for a highly successful synthesis of adenosine. The intermediate 9-(2,3,5-tri-*O*-acetyl-$\beta$-D-ribofuranosyl)-2,6-diacetamidopurine ribonucleoside was also converted to crotonoside (57) by deacylation followed by deamination of the 2-amino group. SHIMIZU and MIYAKI (1966) have more recently shown that the chloromercuri procedure initially gives 3- as well as 9-glycosylpurines and that the 3-isomer rearranges on continued heating to the more thermodynamically stable 9-isomer. The xylonucleoside (53) of 2,6-diaminopurine was also prepared by DAVOLL and LOWY (1951) in low yield by the chloromercuri procedure. Diazotization of 2,6-diaminopurine ribonucleoside (48) in 48% fluoroboric acid gave the highly biologically active 2-fluoroadenosine (49) (MONTGOMERY and HEWSON, 1957). 2-Fluoroadenine (46) and other 2-fluoropurines were prepared in a similar manner (MONTGOMERY and HEWSON, 1960). More satisfactory procedures for the synthesis of 2-fluoroadenine (EATON and DENNY, 1969) and 2-fluoroadenosine were developed later. The latter procedure consists of conversion of 2,6-dichloro-9-(2,3,5-tri-*O*-acetyl-$\beta$-D-ribofuranosyl)purine, prepared by MONTGOMERY and HEWSON (1964) by the fusion reaction of SATO et al. (1960), to 2,6-diazido-9-(2,3,5-tri-*O*-acetyl-$\beta$-D-ribofuranosyl)purine, which was reduced catalytically to 2,6-diamino-9-(2,3,5-tri-*O*-acetyl-$\beta$-D-ribofuranosyl) purine. Application of the modified Schiemann reaction to this acetylated nucleoside followed by deacetylation with ammonia gave much better yields of 2-fluoroadenosine (MONTGOMERY and HEWSON, 1968a) because of the increased stability of the glycosyl linkage and more desirable solubility characteristics of the acetylated nucleosides. This procedure has also been used to prepare the 9-$\beta$-D-xylofuranosyl- (54), 9-$\alpha$- and $\beta$-D-arabinofuranosyl- (55), and 2′-deoxy-$\alpha$- and $\beta$-ribofuranosyl- (56) 2-fluoroadenines (MONTGOMERY and HEWSON, 1969). This work also resulted in the preparation of 2,6-difluoro-9-(2,3,5-tri-*O*-acetyl-$\beta$-D-ribofuranosyl) purine (58), which was converted to a number of new 2-fluoropurine ribonucleosides (59) by selective nucleophilic displacement of the 6-fluoro group (MONTGOMERY and HEWSON, 1970). Although 2-chloroadenosine (50) can also be prepared in low yields by the diazotization of 2,6-diaminopurine ribonucleoside (MONTGOMERY and HEWSON, 1960) or from 2-chloroadenine (47) by the chloromercuri procedure (DAVOLL and LOWY, 1952; BROWN and WELIKY, 1958) (prior acylation of the 6-amino group is not necessary in this case), it is better prepared from 2,6-dichloro-9-(2,3,5-tri-*O*-acyl-$\beta$-D-ribofuranosyl)purine by treatment with methanolic ammonia (SCHAEFFER and THOMAS, 1958; MONTGOMERY and HEWSON, 1964). 2-Bromoadenosine (51) has been prepared in the same way from 2,6-dibromo-9-(2,3,5-tri-*O*-acetyl-$\beta$-D-ribofuranosyl)purine (MONTGOMERY and HEWSON, 1964).

2-Methoxyadenosine (spongosine, 52) was originally isolated from the Caribbean sponge and then synthesized from 2-methoxyadenine (BERGMANN and STEMPIEN, 1957). It has also been prepared from 2,6-dichloro-9-(2,3,5-tri-*O*-benzoyl-$\beta$-D-ribofuranosyl)purine *via* 2-chloroadenosine (50) (SCHAEFFER and THOMAS, 1958).

The 2-substituted adenine nucleosides have shown a high degree of biologic activity, but unfortunately only modest and, so far, unexploitable anticancer activity.

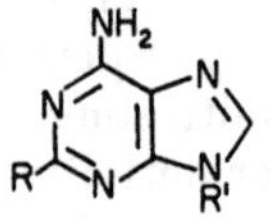

R' = H
45: R = $NH_2$
46: R = F
47: R = Cl

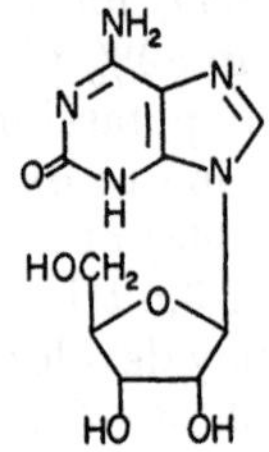

57

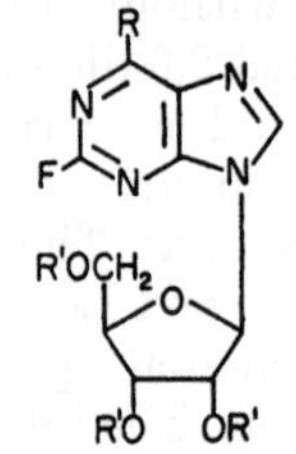

58: R = F, R' = Ac
59: R' = H

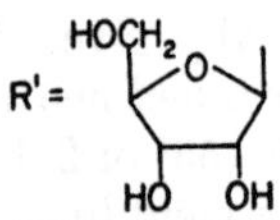

48: R = $NH_2$
49: R = F
50: R = Cl
51: R = Br
52: R = $OCH_3$

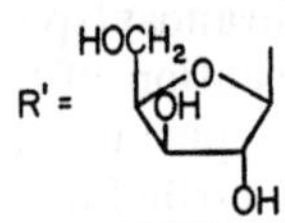

53: R = $NH_2$
54: R = F

55: R = F, R' =
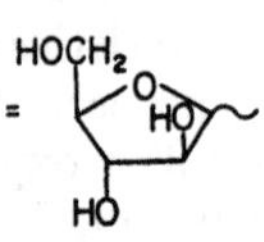

56: R = F, R' =
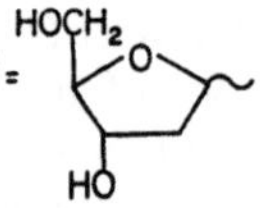

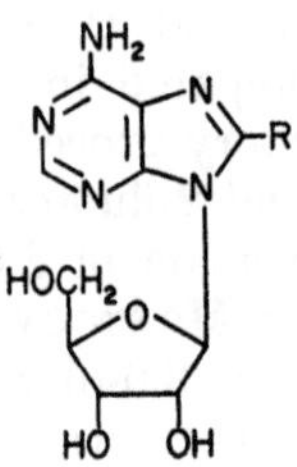

60: R = Br
61: R = I
62: R = F

## 2. 8-Substituted Adenosines

8-Bromoadenosine (60), which has shown some activity in experimental animal tumor systems, was prepared by the bromination of adenosine (IKEHARA et al., 1967) or its triacetate (HOLMES and ROBINS, 1964). The intermediate 8-bromo-adenosine triacetate was deacetylated with methanolic ammonia. The direct iodination of adenosine failed (LIPKIN et al., 1963; YOSHIDA et al., 1968), but 8-iodoadenosine (61) has been prepared from the bromo compound *via* 8-mercaptoadenosine (HOLMES and ROBINS, 1964). 8-Fluoroadenosine (62) was prepared in very low yield (IKEHARA and YAMADA, 1971) by the diazotization of 8-amino-adenosine triacetate in fluoroboric acid by the procedure of MONTGOMERY and HEWSON (1968) followed by deacetylation.

### 3. 9-D-Furanosyladenines

Originally 9-$\beta$-D-xylofuranosyladenine (63), a congener of adenosine in which the hydroxyl group of $C$-3 of the sugar moiety is epimerized, was prepared by the reaction of the silver salt of 2,8-dichloroadenine with 2,3,5-tri-$O$-acetyl-D-xylofuranosyl chloride followed by deacylation and catalytic hydrodechlorination (CHANG and LYTHGOE, 1950). It was later prepared from $N$-benzoyladenine by the chloromercuri procedure (BAKER and HEWSON, 1957).

9-$\beta$-Arabinofuranosyladenine (64) was prepared from 9-$\beta$-xylofuranosyladenine (63) by a five-step sequence (REIST et al., 1962a). Reaction of 2,3,5-tri-$O$-acetyl-D-arabinofuranosyl bromide with $N$-benzoyladenine chloromercuri (DAVOLL and LOWY, 1952) gave $\alpha$-, not $\beta$-, D-arabinofuranosyladenine because of intervention of the orthoester ion as explained by the *trans* rule. But GLAUDEMANS and FLETCHER (1963) were able to prepare the $\beta$-anomer directly from $N$-benzoyladenine by using 2,3,5-tri-$O$-benzyl-$\alpha$-D-arabinofuranosyl chloride, which reacts by an $S_N2$ mechanism with inversion at $C$-1 of the sugar (molecular sieve was the acid acceptor). The $O$-benzyl protecting groups were removed catalytically to give 64, but more effective procedures for debenzylation have been developed (REIST et al., 1964; FLETCHER and DIEHL, 1971).

These adenine nucleosides, which are epimeric with adenosine, and their 1-$N$-oxides (REIST et al., 1967a) have shown modest activity in experimental animal test systems. 2-Substituted derivatives of these nucleosides were discussed above.

Cordycepin (3′-deoxyadenosine, 65), the first nucleoside antibiotic, was isolated from the culture filtrates of *C. militaris* by CUNNINGHAM et al. (1951). Cordycepin was correctly identified by KACZKA et al. (1964) as 3′-deoxyadenosine, rather than the branched-chain pentofuranosyladenine originally proposed by BENTLEY et al. (1951). Cordycepin was first synthesized from adenosine by TODD and ULBRICHT (1960). It was also synthesized by LEE et al. (1961) in low yield by a complex route, which also gave 2′-deoxyadenosine. Both of these syntheses appeared before the correct identity of cordycepin was established. Since then, two procedures have been described for its preparation by the condensation of chloromercuri $N$-benzoyladenine with appropriately blocked 3′-deoxyribofuranosyl chlorides (WALTON et al., 1064; MURRAY and PROKOP, 1965). More recently it has been prepared *via* the cyclonucleoside 66 (IKEHARA and TADA, 1966). Other 3′-deoxy-$\beta$-D-ribonucleosides have been synthesized (WALTON et al., 1965; DICKINSON et al., 1967).

Although puromycin (67), which was isolated from the culture filtrates of *S. alboniga* by PORTER et al. (1952), did not show significant anticancer activity in experimental animal systems, the aminonucleoside (68) did. The total chemical synthesis of 3-amino-3-deoxy-D-ribose (BAKER et al., 1955b; SOWA, 1968) permitted BAKER et al. (1955c) to synthesize the aminonucleoside (68) (which was converted to puromycin) by a variation of the chloromercuri procedure employing the titanium chloride complex of the amino sugar and the chloromercuri derivative of 2-(methylthio)-6-dimethylaminopurine. Dethiolation followed by stepwise deacylation gave 68. Reaction of the amino sugar titanium chloride complex with the chloromercuri derivative of $N$-benzoyladenine, followed by stepwise deacylation, gave 3′-amino-3′-deoxyadenosine (69) (BAKER et al., 1955a), a nucleoside with anticancer activity that was later isolated from the culture filtrates of *Helminthosporium* sp. No. 215 by AMMANN and SAFFERMAN (1958).

Psicofuranine (angustmycin C) and decoyinine (angustmycin A) were both isolated from *Streptomyces* sp. 6A-704 by YÜNTSEN et al. (1954, 1956). As a result of degradation studies, YÜNTSEN (1958a, b) proposed the structure of angustmycin C to be 9-β-D-psicofuranosyladenine (70) and that of angustmycin A to be 9-(L-1,2-fucopyranoseenyl)adenine. The former structure proved to be correct, but the latter structure had to be revised. HOEKSEMA et al. (1964) correctly identified

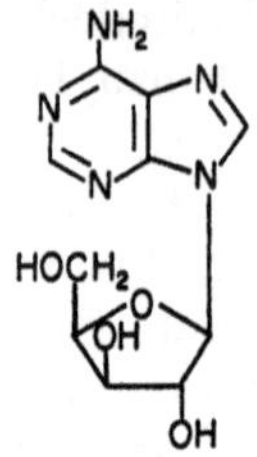

63

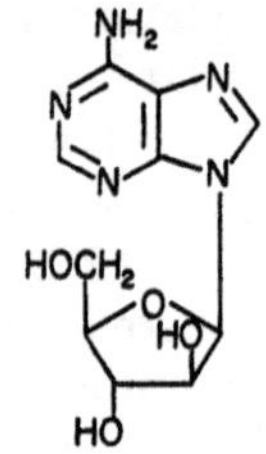

64

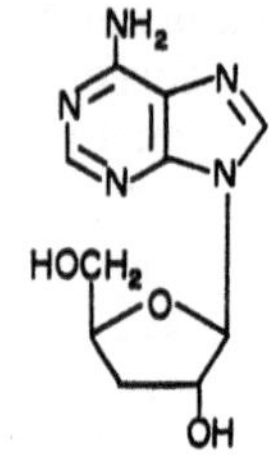

65

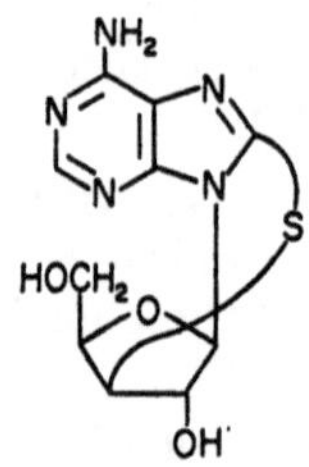

66

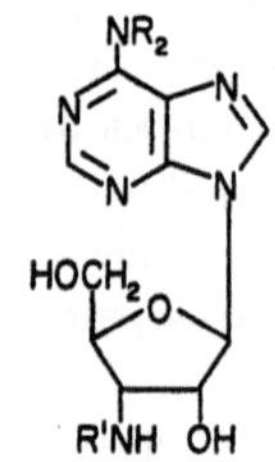

67: R = Me,
R' = MeO-$C_6H_4$-$CH_2CHCO$-($NH_2$)

68: R = Me, R' = H
69: R = R' = H

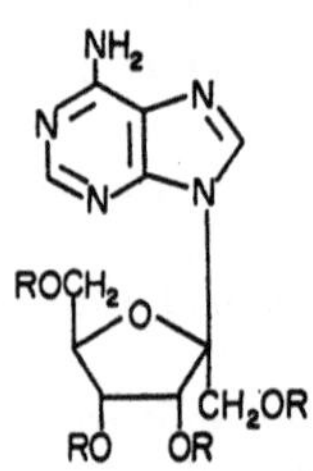

70: R = H
71: R = Ac

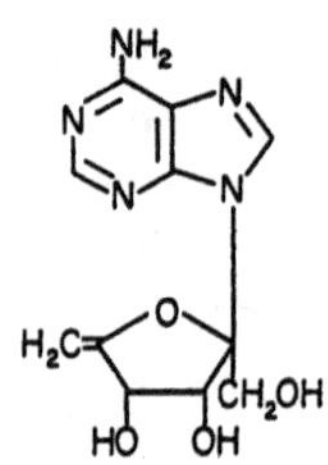

72

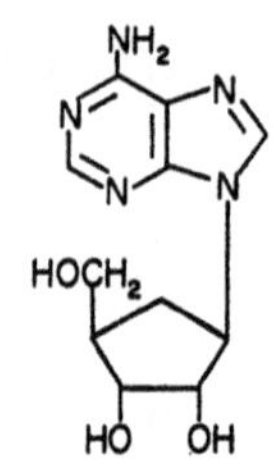

73

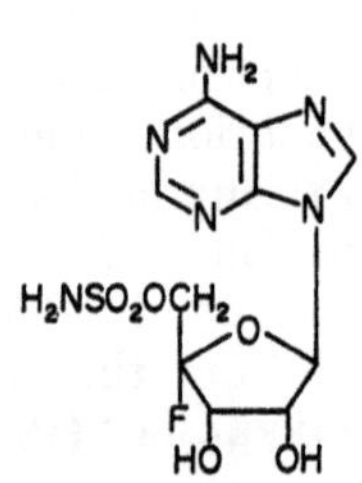

74

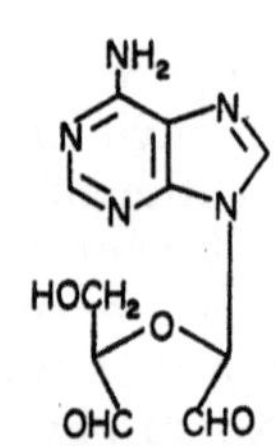

75: R = $NH_2$

the structure of angustmycin A as 9-(β-D-5,6-psicofuranoseenyl)adenine (72). D-Psicose (WOLFROM et al., 1945) was converted to 1,3,4,5-tetra-*O*-acetylpsicofuranosyl chloride, which on reaction with chloromercuri *N*-acetyladenine followed by deacetylation of the resulting nucleoside, gave psicofuranine (SCHROEDER and HOEKSEMA, 1957). FARKAŠ and ŠORM (1963) synthesized psicofuranine in a similar manner. MCCARTHY et al. (1968) synthesized decoyinine from psicofuranine and proved unequivocally the β configuration of these nucleosides. HOEKSEMA et al. (1961) improved the oral absorption of psicofuranine by the selective acetylation of the hydroxyls of the sugar moiety to give 71.

Other nucleoside antibiotics such as aristeromycin – the carbocyclic analog of adenosine (73) (SHEALY and CLAYTON, 1966; KUSAKA et al., 1968) – and nucleocidin (74) (THOMAS et al., 1957; MORTON et al., 1969; JENKINS et al., 1971) have not shown significant anticancer activity.

Treatment of nucleosides such as adenosine with metaperiodate results in oxidation of the *cis* hydroxyls to aldehyde functions. The oxidation product from adenosine, represented by the dialdehyde structure 75, which is in equilibrium with other forms, is active against leukemia L1210 (DVONCH et al., 1966), as is the oxidation product from 6-(methylthio)purine ribonucleoside (BELL et al., 1968).

## 4. Other 6-Substituted Purines

6-Chloropurine (76) and its ribonucleoside (77) not only are among the most active purine analogs against cancer, but they are key intermediates in the synthesis of a number of other active compounds. 6-Chloropurine (76) was first prepared by the phosphorus oxychloride chlorodehydroxylation of hypoxanthine (79) (BENDICH et al., 1954; ELION and HITCHINGS, 1956), later by the ring closure of

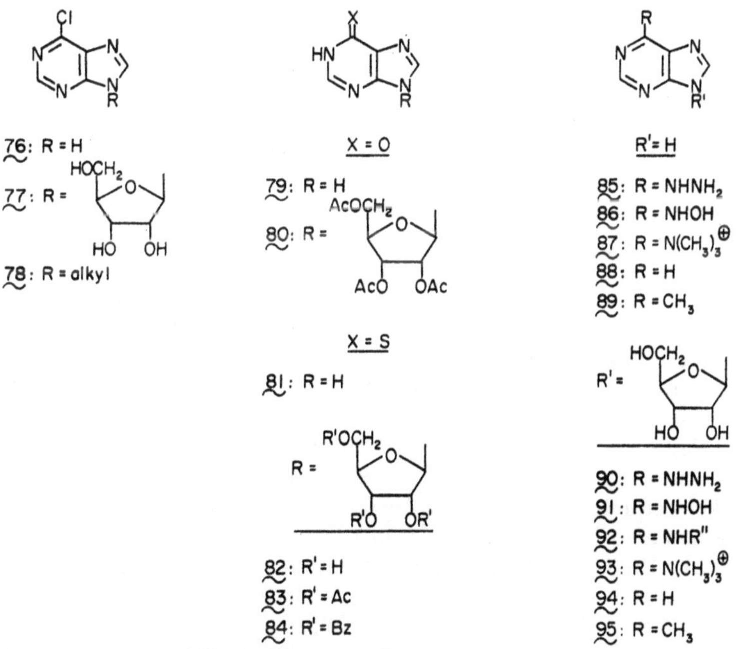


4,5-diamino-6-chloropyrimidine with ethyl orthoformate and acetic anhydride (MONTGOMERY, 1956), and also by the chlorodethiolation of 6-mercaptopurine (81) with chlorine in methanol (HITCHINGS and ELION, 1957; BEAMAN and ROBINS,

1962). Similar procedures have been used to prepare other halopurines (ELION and HITCHINGS, 1956; BEAMAN et al., 1962). 6-Chloropurine ribonucleoside (77) has been prepared from both 2,3,5-tri-*O*-acetyl- and benzoyl-D-ribofuranosyl chloride by the chloromercuri procedure (BROWN and WELIKY, 1953; BAKER et al., 1957). It has also been prepared from tetraacetyl-D-ribofuranose by the fusion reaction (ISHIDO et al., 1967), by chlorodethiolation of 6-mercaptopurine ribonucleoside (82) (ROBINS, 1960), or its triacyl derivatives 83 and 84 (LETTRÉ and BOLLWEG, 1962; GERSTER et al., 1963), and by the chlorodehydroxylation of inosine triacetate (80) (GERSTER et al., 1963). The intermediate nucleosides were deacylated with methanolic ammonia. Alkylation of 6-chloropurine gave 9-alkyl-6-chloropurines (78) along with small amounts of the 7-isomers (MONTGOMERY and TEMPLE, 1961). 9-Alkyl-6-chloropurines have also been prepared by the ring closure of 4-alkylamino-5-amino-6-chloropyrimidine with diethoxymethyl acetate (MONTGOMERY and TEMPLE, 1957, 1958) and ethyl orthoformate and hydrochloric acid (TEMPLE et al., 1962).

The nucleophilic displacement of the chloro group of 6-chloropurine (BENDICH et al., 1954) and its ribonucleoside (JOHNSON et al., 1958), or its ribonucleoside tribenzoate (KISSMAN and WEISS, 1956), takes place readily giving rise to a variety of *N*-substituted adenines and adenosines, a number of which are active against cancer. Thus, 6-hydrazinopurine (85) (MONTGOMERY and HOLUM, 1957) and its ribonucleoside (90) (JOHNSON et al., 1958) both demonstrated modest activity against Adenocarcinoma 755, while *N*-hydroxyadenosine (91), prepared by the reaction of 6-chloropurine ribonucleoside with hydroxylamine (CHANG, 1965; GINER-SOROLLA et al., 1966a), is highly active against leukemia L1210 in mice [in contrast to the inactivity of *N*-hydroxyadenine (86)], although its toxicity appears likely to prevent its use in man. A number of other hydroxylaminopurines and their nucleosides have been prepared (GINER-SOROLLA et al., 1966b, 1968a, b; GINER-SOROLLA, 1969; MONTGOMERY and HEWSON, 1970), but none of these compounds are as active as *N*-hydroxyadenosine. Several *N*-alkyl- and *N*-aralkyladenosines (92), synthesized from 6-chloropurine ribonucleoside (FLEYSHER et al., 1968, 1969), have demonstrated activity against leukemia L1210. Compounds of this type have also been prepared by the Dimroth rearrangement of 1-substituted adenines or adenosines (LEONARD et al., 1966). Also of interest are trimethylpurin-6-ylammonium chloride (87) (HORWITZ and VAITKEVICIUS, 1961) and its ribonucleoside (93) (GERSTER et al., 1963), prepared by the reaction of trimethylamine with 6-chloropurines 76 and 77. Purine 88, first prepared from 2,6,8-trichloropurine by iododechlorination followed by chemical reduction (FISCHER, 1898), is better prepared by catalytic reduction of 6-chloropurine (BENDICH et al., 1954), the ribonucleoside (77) of which can also be reduced to nebularine (purine ribonucleoside, 94) (BROWN and WELIKY, 1953). Purine has also been prepared by the cyclization with formic acid of 4,5-diaminopyrimidine (ISAY, 1906; BENDICH et al., 1954) and by the Raney nickel reduction of 6-mercaptopurine (BENDICH et al., 1954), and purine ribonucleoside by the Raney nickel reduction of 6-mercaptopurine ribonucleoside (FOX et al., 1958). Nebularine has also been prepared from purine by the chloromercuri procedure (MIZUNO et al., 1965) and by the fusion reaction, which also gave a 20% yield of 7-isomer and was used to prepare other nucleosides of purine (IWAMURA and HASHIZUME, 1968b). BREDERECK et al. (1956) reported a remarkable synthesis of purine by heating formamide saturated with dry ammonia. Although the yield was low, it could be markedly improved by the addition of aminoacetonitrile in place of ammonia (BREDERICK et al., 1962). 6-Methylpurine (89), prepared from 4,5-diamino-6-methylpyrimidine (GABRIEL and COLMAN, 1901), has been converted to its ribonucleoside (95) by the chloromercuri procedure (GORDON et al., 1957; VINCZE and COHEN, 1966) and by the fusion procedure, which was also used to prepare a number of other 6-methylpurine nucleosides (MONTGOMERY and HEWSON, 1968).

## II. 6-Thiopurines

### 1. 6-Mercaptopurine and Thioguanine

Of all the purines synthesized and evaluated as anticancer agents, 6-mercaptopurine [purin-6(1*H*)-thione, 96 (R = H)] and thioguanine [2-aminopurin-6(1*H*)-thione, 96 (R = $NH_2$)] are by far the most effective thus far produced, particularly against human cancer, although many promising compounds have had little or no clinical study. Despite this relatively high level of activity, the 6-thiopurines only affect a small percentage of human cancers, and many chemical modifications of them have been made in an effort to improve their efficacy.

6-Mercaptopurine was originally prepared by ELION et al. (1952) by the thiation of hypoxanthine (79) with phosphorus pentasulfide in tetralin. Treatment of 6-mercaptopurine with either dimethylsulfate or methyl iodide in aqueous base gave the *S*-methylated derivative 6-(methylthio)purine (110, R = R″ = H, R′ = $CH_3$), which on treatment with amines gave a series of *N*-alkyladenines. Thiation of guanine to give thioguanine could not be carried out in tetralin but was successful in pyridine (ELION and HITCHINGS, 1955), which is also a better solvent for the thiation of hypoxanthine (79) (ČERNÝ and SEMONSKÝ, 1958). These 6-thiopurines (96) have also been prepared by fusion of the sodium salts of the 4-amino-5-formylaminopyrimidin-6(1*H*)-thiones (114 and 115) (ELION et al., 1956). Refluxing formic acid converts the corresponding diaminopyrimidines

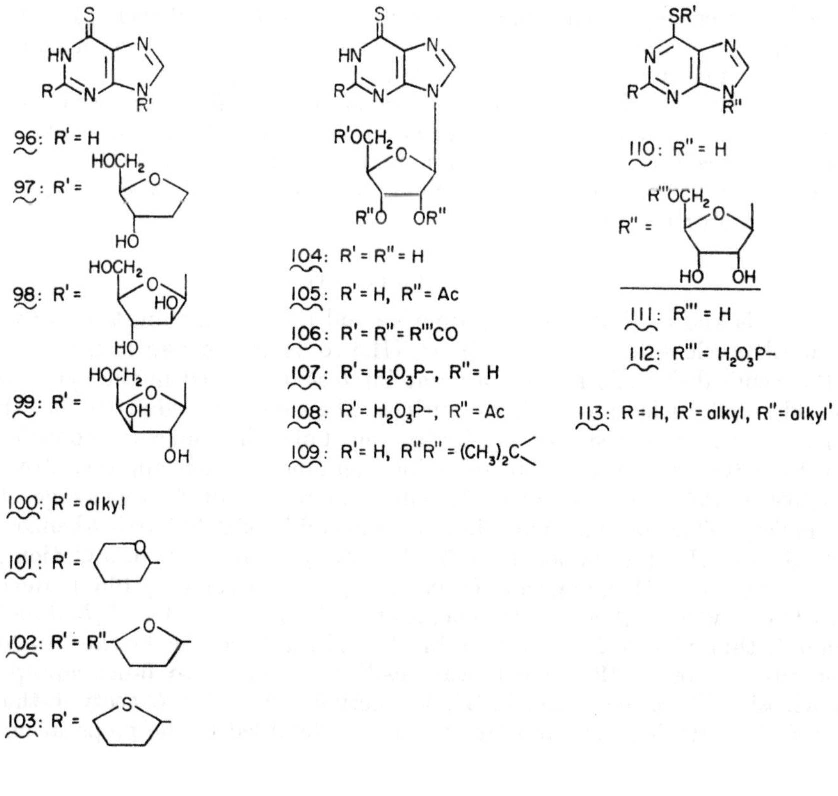

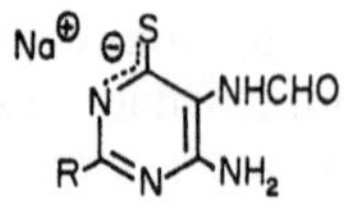

114: R = H

115: R = $NH_2$

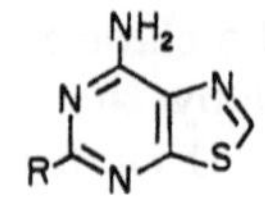

116: R = H

117: R = $NH_2$

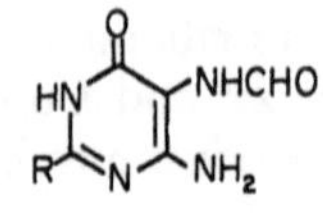

118: R = H

119: R = $NH_2$

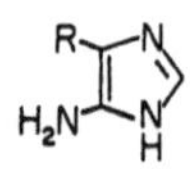

120: R = $CONH_2$

121: R = $CSNH_2$

122: R = CN

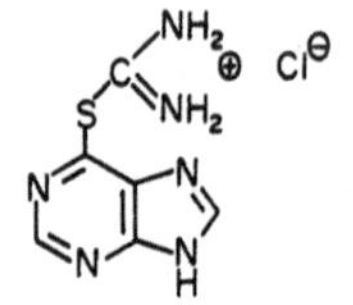

123

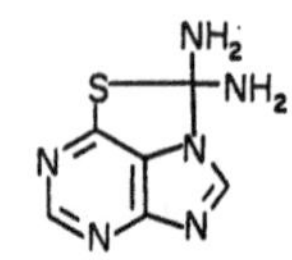

124

to the aminothiazolo[5,4-*d*]pyrimidines (116 and 117) rather than to the desired purines (96). Treatment of the 4-amino-5-formamidopyrimidin-6(1*H*)-ones (118 and 119) with phosphorus pentasulfide in pyridine results in thiation followed by ring closure to the 6-thiopurines (HITCHINGS and ELION, 1954; DAVES et al., 1960).

Another route to 6-mercaptopurine involves the phosphorus pentasulfide thiation of 5-aminoimidazole-4-carboxamide (120) (SHAW and WOOLLEY, 1949) followed by closure of the pyrimidine ring with formamide (HITCHINGS and ELION, 1956). The intermediate 5-aminoimidazole-4-thiocarboxamide (121) can also be prepared in three steps from cyanothioacetamide (SHAW and BUTLER, 1959) or by the reaction of 5-aminoimidazole-4-carbonitrile (122) with hydrogen sulfide in methanolic potassium hydroxide (YAMAZAKI et al., 1968).

Displacement of the chloro group of 6-chloropurine (76) with sodium hydrosulfide or thiourea gave 6-mercaptopurine in good yield (BENDICH et al., 1954). The thiourea reaction proceeds through the isothiouronium salt 123, which also cyclizes to give a 10% yield of 2,2-diamino-2*H*-thiazolo[3,4,5-*gh*]purine (124) (TEMPLE and MONTGOMERY, 1966).

## 2. Nucleosides and Derivatives

Since it is known that 6-mercaptopurine and thioguanine must be converted to their ribonucleotides (107, R = H or $NH_2$) to exert their anticancer activity (see Biochemical Considerations), a great interest developed in the synthesis of nucleosides and nucleotides of these purines. The ribonucleoside (104, R = H) of 6-mercaptopurine was first prepared by treatment of 6-chloropurine ribonucleoside (77) with sodium hydrosulfide in refluxing methanol for ten minutes (JOHNSON and THOMAS, 1956). Treatment of 77 with thiourea resulted in cleavage of the sugar moiety. Thiation with phosphorus pentasulfide of 2′,3′,5′-tri-*O*-benzoylinosine (125, R = H) and guanosine (125, R = $NH_2$) followed by deacylation gave 6-thioinosine and 6-thioguanosine (FOX et al., 1958; IKEHARA, 1960). Reaction of 5′-*O*-benzoyl-2′,3′-*O*-isopropylideneinosine (126) with the *N*,*N*-dimethylformamide-thionyl chloride complex in chloroform gave the blocked 6-chloropurine ribonucleoside 127, which was readily converted to 6-mercaptopurine ribonucleoside (IKEHARA et al., 1964). The activity of 2′,3′-di-*O*-acetyl-6-thioinosine (105, R = H) (THOMAS and MONTGOMERY, 1962) led to the preparation of a number of *O*-acyl derivatives of 6-thioinosine (106, R = H) (LEWIS et al., 1964). The ribonucleotides of 6-mercaptopurine (107, R = H) and thioguanine (107, R = $NH_2$) (as well as that of 8-azaguanine) were prepared for biologic study by the reaction of the 2′,3′-*O*-isopropylidene nucleosides (109, R = H, $NH_2$) with a phosphorylating agent, preferably cyanoethyl phosphate, followed by removal of the blocking groups (MONTGOMERY and THOMAS, 1961; HAMPTON and MAGUIRE, 1961; ROY et al., 1961). The 6-thiopurine ribonucleotides have also been prepared by the thiation of 2′,3′-di-*O*-acetyl-6-thioinosinic acid (108, R = H) and 2′,3′-di-*O*-acetylguanylic acid (108, R = $NH_2$) (SANEYOSHI, 1971), followed by deacetylation. Phosphorylation of the 6-thiopurine ribonucleosides (104, R = H, $NH_2$) with phosphorus oxychloride in trimethyl phosphate by the procedure of YOSHIKAWA et al. (1967) gave the expected nucleotides (107, R = H, $NH_2$) and also their *S*-methyl derivatives (112, R′ = $CH_3$, R = H, $NH_2$) (PERINI and HAMPTON, 1970). Although those nucleotides are important in the study of enzyme inhibitions, they are of no special value as chemotherapeutic agents because they fail to gain entry into cells and are cleaved by extracellular phosphatases (see Biochemical Considerations). For this reason a number of esters of 6-thioinosinic acid were prepared (MONTGOMERY et al., 1961a; THOMAS and MONTGOMERY, 1962, 1968), and one of these, *bis*(thioinosine)-5′,5‴-phosphate (128), proved to be of particular interest because of its activity against cell lines resistant to 6-mercaptopurine (MONTGOMERY et al., 1963).

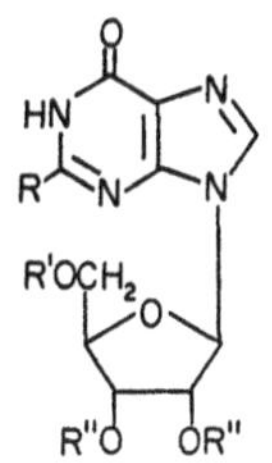

125: R′ = R″ = Bz

126: R = H, R′ = Bz, R″R″ = $(CH_3)_2C<$

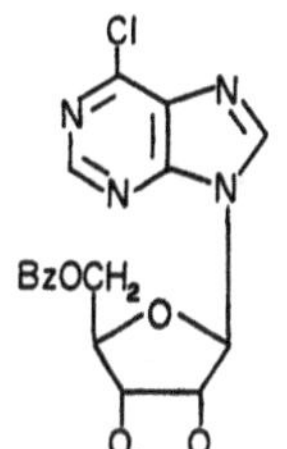

127

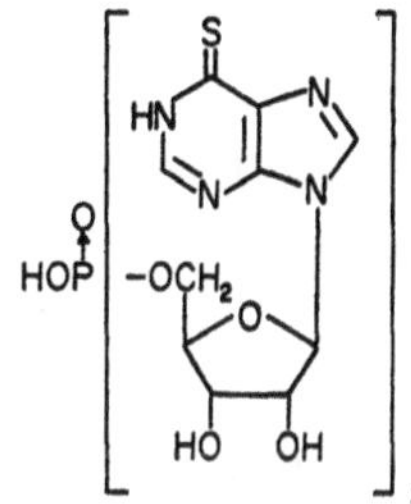

128

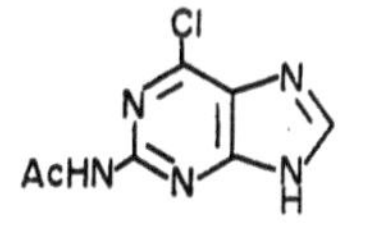

129

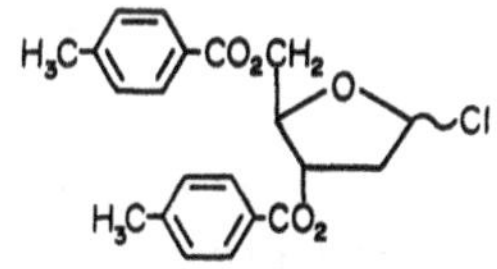

130

A number of other nucleosides of 6-mercaptopurine and thioguanine have been prepared (REIST et al., 1961, 1962b, 1967b; TONG et al., 1967a, b; MARTINEZ and LEE, 1969; BOBEK et al., 1970b; LEE et al., 1970), but the most interesting compounds from the point of view of anticancer activity are the 2′-deoxy-D-ribofuranosyl-6-mercaptopurines (IWAMOTO et al., 1962) and thioguanines (ACTON et al., 1963) and the 9-β-D-arabinofuranosyl- (98, R = H) (REIST et al., 1962a) and 9-β-D-xylofuranosyl-6-mercaptopurines (99, R = H) (SATO et al., 1966). The anomeric 2′-deoxy-D-ribofuranosylpurin-6(1*H*)-thiones (97, R = H, $NH_2$) were prepared by the chloromercuri coupling of 6-chloropurine and 2-acetamido-6-chloropurine (129) with 2-deoxy-3,5-di-*O*-(*p*-toluoyl)-D-ribofuranosyl chloride (130), followed by thiation and deacylation. Since there is no acyloxy group at *C*-2 of this sugar, both the α- and the β-anomers are formed in approximately equal amounts.

The arabino- and xylonucleosides (98 and 99, R = H) were both derived from the corresponding nucleosides of adenine by deamination followed by acylation of the sugar hydroxyls, thiation of the 6-oxy function with phosphorus pentasulfide in pyridine, and finally deacylation of the protected 6-thiopurine nucleosides.

9-β-D-Arabinofuranosylpurin-6(1*H*)-thione and 9-β-D-xylofuranosylpurin-6-(1*H*)-thione do not appear to be metabolized to their nucleotides but are active per se, although their mechanism of action has not been fully elucidated. Both 2′-deoxy-6-thioguanosine and its α-anomer are phosphorylated and then incorporated into DNA. It is claimed that the α-anomer is preferentially incorporated into the DNA of cancer cells because it is phosphorylated by responsive tumor cells but not by bone marrow cells (LEPAGE, 1968).

### 3. *S*-Substituted Derivatives

As mentioned above, ELION et al. (1952) found that 6-mercaptopurine is subject to *S*-methylation in aqueous base, and this reaction led to the preparation of a large number of active *S*-substituted derivatives of both 6-mercaptopurine (110, R = H) (SKINNER et al., 1956a, b, 1958; JOHNSTON et al., 1958; ELION et al., 1959; KOPPEL et al., 1959a; SEMONSKÝ et al., 1960) and thioguanine (110, R = $NH_2$) (ELION et al., 1959). 4-(Purin-6-ylthio)butyric acid [110, R = H, R′ = $(CH_2)_3CO_2H$] and its derivatives and analogs have received considerable attention (ČERNÝ et al., 1962, 1966, 1967; SEMONSKÝ et al., 1968, 1970; KOTVA et al., 1969, 1970). A superior procedure for the preparation of these *S*-substituted derivatives resulted from the use of *N*,*N*-dimethylformamide as a solvent and potassium carbonate as the proton acceptor for the reaction, although the use of excess halides under these conditions leads to *N*-alkylation also (JOHNSTON et al., 1958). *S*-Substituted derivatives of the 6-thiopurines (110, R = H, $NH_2$) are less conveniently prepared by the reaction of the alkali metal salts of thiols with 6-chloropurine (JOHNSTON et al., 1958; KOPPEL et al., 1959a) (although for most aryl derivatives this procedure must be used) and by the ring closure of 4,5-diamino-6-(*S*-substituted thio)pyrimidines (131 and 132) (ELION et al., 1956; DAVES et al., 1960; ČERNÝ and SEMONSKÝ, 1967). *S*-Glycosyl derivatives of 6-mercaptopurine, such as 133, were prepared by the reaction of acylglycosyl halides with the sodium salt of 6-mercaptopurine followed by deacylation or by the reaction of salts of the thio sugars with 6-chloropurine (GOODMAN et al., 1968), and heterocyclic derivatives of thioguanine (134) by the reaction of thioguanine with a number of 4-chloropyrimidines in aqueous ammonia (KOPPEL et al., 1962a), but the most promising *S*-substituted derivatives of the 6-thiopurines, Imuran (135) and Guaneran (136), prepared by the reaction of their salts with 1-methyl-5-chloro-4-nitroimidazole (HITCHINGS and ELION, 1962), are protected from catabolism by the covering group but are converted *in vivo* back to the 6-thiopurines (96, R = H, $NH_2$), which are then metabolized to active forms – a very practical example of latentiation. 6-(Methylthio)purine ribonucleoside (111, R = H, R′ = $CH_3$), prepared from 6-(methylthio)purine (110, R = H, R′ = $CH_3$) by the chloromercuri coupling reaction (HAMPTON et al., 1956) and by the alkylation of 6-mercaptopurine ribonucleoside (MONTGOMERY et al., 1961b), is phosphorylated by adenosine kinase and, therefore, is active against certain 6-mercaptopurine-resistant cancers and therapeutically synergistic with 6-mercaptopurine. Other

*S*-substituted derivatives of 6-thioinosine (111, R = H) have been prepared by the chloromercuri coupling (ČERNÝ et al., 1968) and by *S*-alkylation (MONTGOMERY et al., 1961b), and of thioguanosine (111, R = $NH_2$) by *S*-alkylation (IKEHARA et al., 1962; NOELL and ROBINS, 1962b).

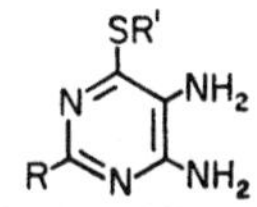

131: R = H

132: R = $NH_2$

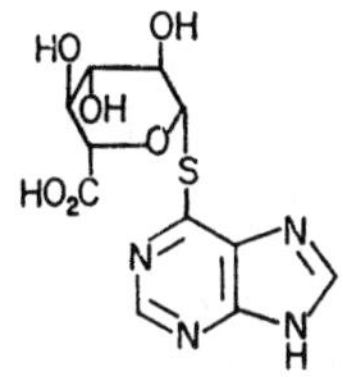

133

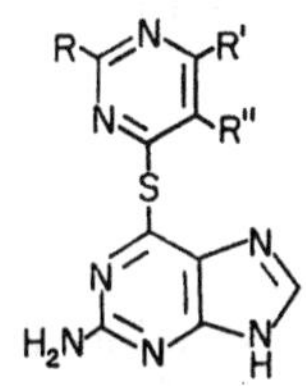

134

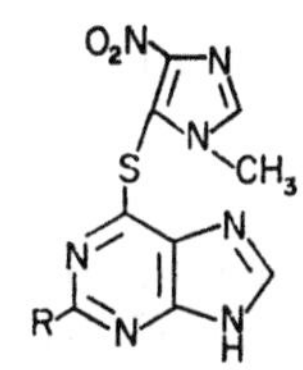

135: R = H

136: R = $NH_2$

## 4. Other *C*- and *N*-Substituted Derivatives

6-Thiopurines substituted at position 2 (96) (HITCHINGS and ELION, 1954; TEMPLE and MONTGOMERY, 1966) and position 8 (137) (MONTGOMERY and TEMPLE, 1960; KOPPEL and ROBINS, 1958) have been prepared by procedures similar to those already described but, save for thioguanine and its nucleosides, have all been essentially inactive.

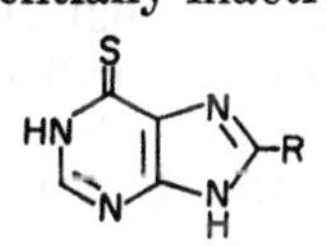

137

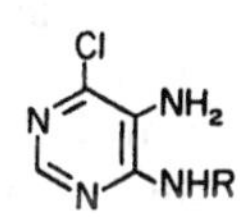

138

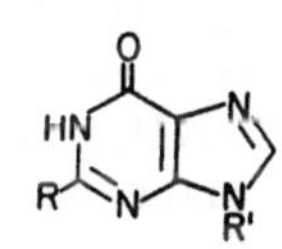

139: R = H, R' = $CH_3$

140: R = $NH_2$, R' = alkyl

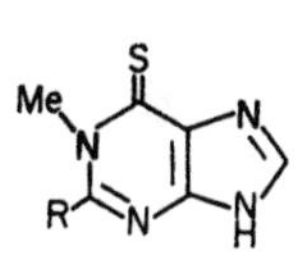

141: R = H

142: R = $NH_2$

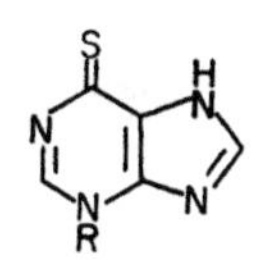

143: R = $CH_3$

144: R = $C_6H_5CH_2$

145: R = O

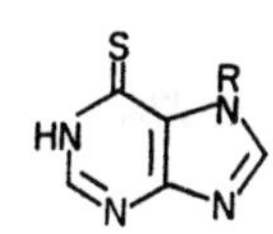

146: R = alkyl

9-Alkyl derivatives of 6-mercaptopurine (100, R = H) have been prepared by the reaction of thiourea with the corresponding 6-chloropurines (78) – which in turn were prepared by the diethoxymethyl acetate or ethyl orthoformate ring closure of the 4-alkylamino-5-amino-6-chloropyrimidines (138) (MONTGOMERY and TEMPLE, 1957, 1958; TEMPLE et al., 1962) or by the alkylation of 6-chloropurine (76) (MONTGOMERY and TEMPLE, 1961) – or by the thiation of 9-methylhypoxanthine (139) (ELION, 1962), a reaction which has also been applied to 9-alkylguanines (140) (KOPPEL et al., 1959b; NOELL and ROBINS, 1962a). The acid catalyzed addition of 6-chloropurine to 2,3-dihydropyran (ROBINS et al., 1961) and to 2,3-dihydrofuran and 2,3-dihydrothiophen (LEWIS et al., 1961; BOWLES et al., 1963) gave the corresponding 9-substituted 6-chloropurines, which on reaction with sodium hydrosulfide gave the 6-thiopurines (101–103). A series of lipid-soluble 9,*S*-disubstituted derivatives of 6-mercaptopurine (113) have shown activity against intracerebrally implanted tumors (TEMPLE et al., 1968) demonstrating their ability to cross the blood-brain barrier.

6-Thiopurines with alkyl groups at the 1-, 3-, or 7-nitrogens of the purine ring (141–144, 146) (HITCHINGS and ELION, 1958; MONTGOMERY and HEWSON, 1961; NOELL et al., 1962; ELION, 1962; MONTGOMERY and THOMAS, 1963, 1965) are, in general, less active than the parent compounds or are inactive.

## 5. Oxidation Products

6-Mercaptopurine-3-*N*-oxide (145), prepared from 7-aminothiazolo[5,4-*d*]-pyrimidine (116) by *N*-oxidation with hydrogen peroxide to *N*-oxide (147) followed by opening of the thiazole ring and reclosure to form the imidazole ring (BROWN et al., 1965), has shown good anticancer activity, perhaps as a result of *in vivo* reduction to 6-mercaptopurine. The reaction sequence outlined above for the preparation of 145 was necessary to prevent preferential oxidation at sulfur. Iodine oxidation of the 6-thiopurines and their nucleosides gave the corresponding disulfides (148, R = H, $NH_2$) (HITCHINGS and ELION, 1954; DOERR et al., 1961; KELLER and BUNKER, 1969), which have also shown good activity. Reduction *in vivo* by disulfide interchange is probably responsible for this activity, and, if so, these compounds represent another example of latentiation. Oxidation of 6-(alkylthio)purines with chlorine or *N*-chlorosuccinimide gave the 6-(alkylsulfonyl)purines (149) (NOELL and ROBINS, 1959; IKEHARA et al., 1962). Oxidation of the 6-thiopurines with iodine under basic conditions gave the purine-6-sulfinates (150, R = H, $NH_2$), an oxidation that probably proceeds through the disulfides. Alkaline permanganate oxidation of the 6-thiopurines (96, R = H, $NH_2$) or the sulfinates (150, R = H, $NH_2$) gave the purine-6-sulfonates (151, R = H, $NH_2$)

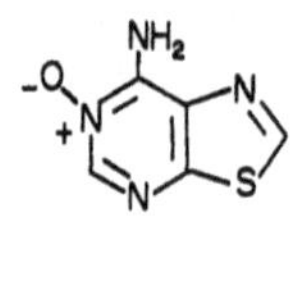

147

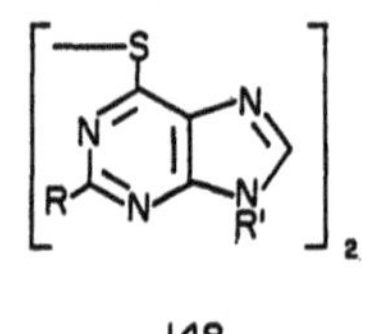

148

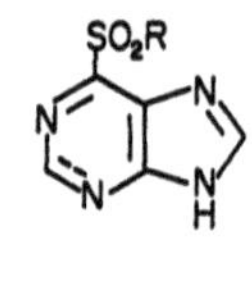

149

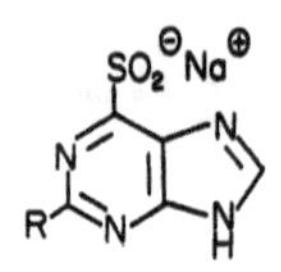

150

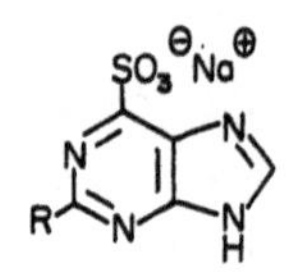

151

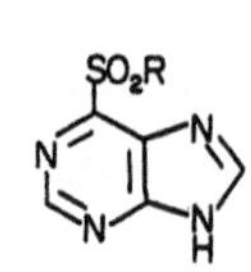

152: R = F

153: R = NHR'

(DOERR et al., 1961). Although these oxidation products (150 and 151) are inactive, probably due to their instability *in vivo*, 6-mercaptopurine can be oxidized by chlorine in the presence of potassium fluoride and hydrofluoric acid in methanol to give the stable purine-6-sulfonyl fluoride (152), which was converted to a series of purine-6-sulfonamides (153) (BEAMAN and ROBINS, 1961; LEWIS et al., 1962). These compounds (149, 152, and 153) have also shown anticancer activity, and, although nothing is known about the mechanism of action of these derivatives containing sulfur in its higher oxidation states, they do not appear to offer any therapeutic advantage over the 6-thiopurines.

### 6. Selenium Analogs

The selenium analogs of the 6-thiopurines (154, R = H, $NH_2$) and their ribonucleosides (155, R = H, $NH_2$), prepared by the appropriate modification of procedures described above (MAUTNER, 1956; MAUTNER et al., 1963; CHU, 1971; MILNE and TOWNSEND, 1971), differ somewhat in their physical and chemical properties but again do not appear to offer any advantage over the 6-thiopurines from a therapeutic point of view.

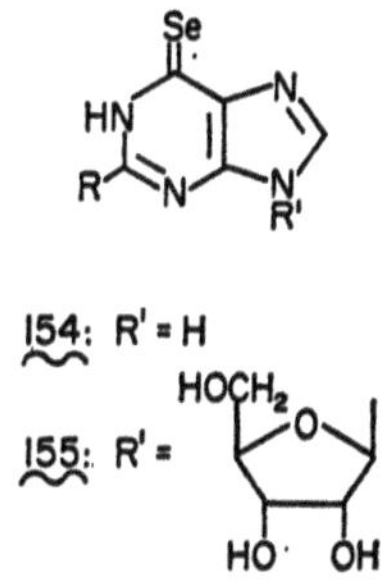


## III. Purines Containing Chemically Reactive Groups

The first attempt at combining an alkylating agent with the purine nucleus resulted in failure: treatment of 2,2′-(purin-6-ylimino)diethanol (156), prepared by the reaction of 2,2′-iminodiethanol with 6-chloropurine, with thionyl chloride (HÜBER, 1956) gave, instead of the desired *N*,*N*-*bis*(2-chloroethyl)adenine (157), the tricyclic derivative 9-(2-chloroethyl)-7,8-dihydro-9*H*-imidazo[2,1-*i*]purine hydrochloride (158), resulting from intramolecular alkylation (JOHNSTON et al., 1962). This compound was biologically inactive. More success was encountered in attempts to prepare sulfur mustard analogs. Alkylation of 6-mercaptopurine with bromochloroethane gave the active anticancer agent 6-(2-chloroethylthio)purine (160) (JOHNSTON et al., 1958), which, although easily cyclized to the inactive 7,8-dihydrothiazolo[2,3-*i*]purine (159) (BALSIGER et al., 1961), could be isolated as such in pure form. 2-(2-Chloroethylthio)purine (161) was similarly prepared from 2-mercaptopurine, but 8-mercaptopurine gave only a mixture of the two possible tricyclic purines (162 and 163). Whether or not the several reported 8-*bis*(2-chloroethylamino)-substituted purines (164) (CHU et al., 1960) cyclize as readily as the thio compound has apparently not been established, except in a case in which one of the imidazole nitrogens is blocked (165) (KOPPEL et al., 1962b). Adenine mustards (166) in which the *bis*(2-chloroethyl)amino group is not attached directly to the heterocyclic ring, prepared from 6-chloropurine by a sequence similar to that described for 158 (LIN and PRICE, 1961), are not subject to intramolecular cyclization and are active. The nitrogen mustard group has been similarly attached to *N*-9 of some 6-(alkylthio)purines to give active agents (170) (O'BRIEN et al.,

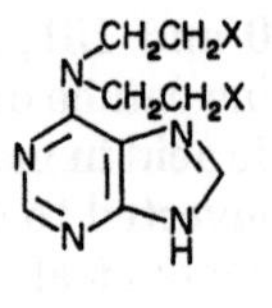

156: X = OH

157: X = Cl

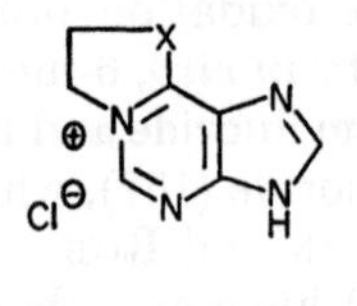

158: X = $NCH_2CH_2Cl$

159: X = S

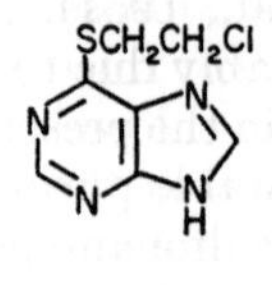

160

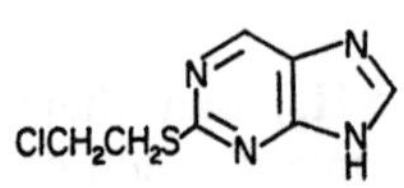

161

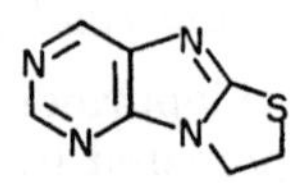

162

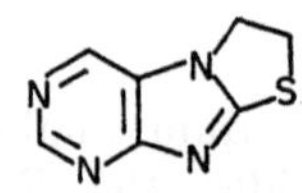

163

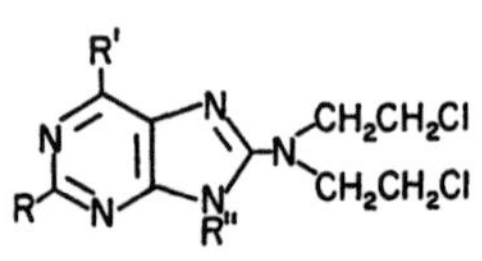

164: R'' = H

165: R'' = $CH_3$

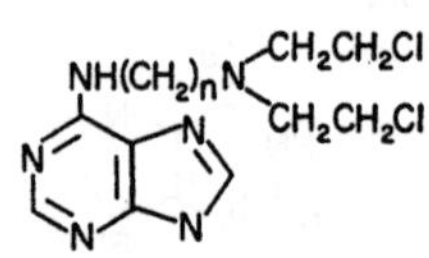

166: n = 2,3

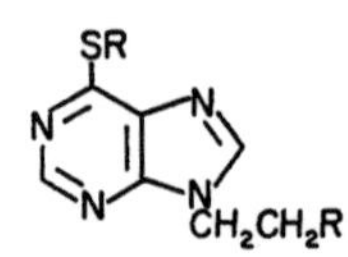

167: R = OH

168: R = Cl

169: R = $N(CH_2CH_2OH)_2$

170: R = $N(CH_2CH_2Cl)_2$

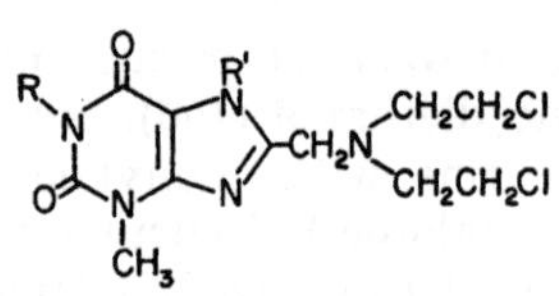

171

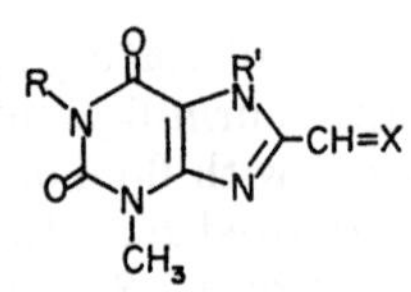

172: X = O

173: X = $NN(CH_2CH_2OH)_2$

174: X = $NN(CH_2CH_2Cl)$

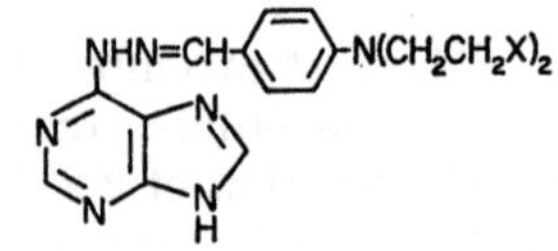

175: X = Cl

176: X = $OSO_2CH_3$

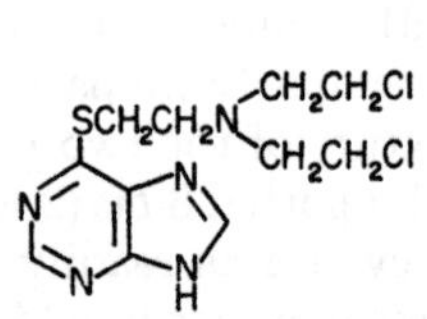

177

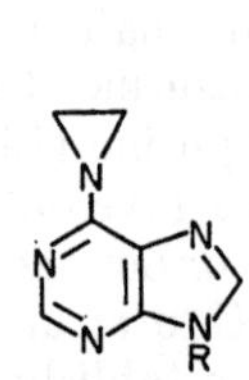

178: R = Et

179: R = $C_6H_5CH_2$

180: R = 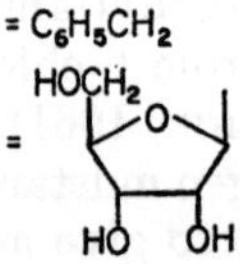

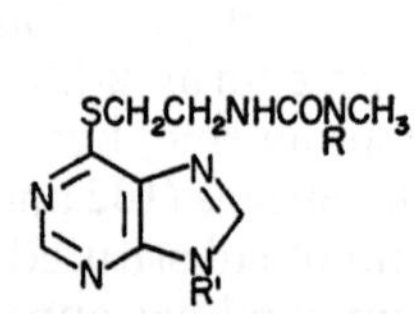

181: R = R' = H

182: R = H, R' = Bu

183: R = NO, R' = H

184: R = NO, R' = Bu

1965). The reaction sequence leading to these compounds involved alkylation of 6-chloropurine or the 6-(alkylthio)purines with ethylene bromohydrin, followed in the case of 6-chloropurine by conversion to 9-(2-hydroxyethyl)purin-6(1*H*)-thione, which was then alkylated to the 6-(alkylthio)purines (167). These compounds (167) were chlorinated to the 9-(2-chloroethyl)purines (168), which in turn were allowed to react with 2,2′-iminodiethanol. The 2,2′-(purin-9-ylethylimino)-diethanols (169) were then chlorinated to give the nitrogen mustards (170). A similar sequence gave nitrogen mustard linked through a methylene group to the 8-carbon of the methylated xanthines (171) (KOPPEL et al., 1962b). Reaction of the purine-8-carboxaldehydes (172) with 1,1-*bis*(2-hydroxyethyl)hydrazine followed by thionyl chloride chlorination of 173 gave a different type of purine mustard (174) (KOPPEL et al., 1962b). Condensation of 6-hydrazinopurine with *p*-[*N*,*N*-*bis*(2-chloroethyl)amino]benzaldehyde gave *p*-[*bis*(2-chloroethyl)-amino]-benzaldehyde purin-6-ylhydrazone (175) as the hydrochloride. Similarly, *p*-[*N*,*N*-*bis*(2-methanesulfonoxyethyl)amino]benzaldehyde and 6-hydrazinopurine gave the corresponding methanesulfonate derivative (176) (ELDERFIELD et al., 1962). Reaction of *tris*(2-chloroethyl)amine (HN3) with the salt of 6-mercaptopurine gave a structure (177) with broad-spectrum antitumor activity (LEVIN et al., 1964). Most of these purines containing an alkylating function have shown anticancer activity, particularly against tumors known to be sensitive to alkylating agents. Whether the purine nucleus contributes significantly to this activity has not really been established.

The activity of the monofunctional alkylating agent *N*-(2,4-dinitrophenyl)-aziridine provided the basis for the synthesis of some 6-(1-aziridinyl)purines (178–180), which showed activity against Adenocarcinoma 755, a tumor not normally sensitive to alkylating agents (MONTGOMERY et al., 1962). These compounds were prepared by the reaction of aziridine with the corresponding 6-chloropurines.

The activity of 1-methyl-1-nitrosourea suggested the incorporation of this moiety into a purine structure. Reaction of 6-chloropurine with 1-(2-mercaptoethyl-3-methylurea or 6-mercaptopurine with 1-(2-chloroethyl)-3-methylurea gave 1-methyl-3-[2-(purin-6-ylthio)ethyl]urea (181), which on nitrosation gave 183, a compound more active against leukemia L1210 than simple 6-(alkylthio)purines. The 9-butyl derivative (184) was prepared similarly *via* 182 (JOHNSTON et al., 1963). Again, the contribution of the purine nucleus to the activity of these compounds is not known.

## References


ACTON, E. M., GOODMAN, L., IWAMOTO, R. H.: 2′-Deoxythioguanosine and related nucleosides. J. med. Chem. **6**, 684—688 (1963).

ACTON, E. M., RYAN, K. J., HENRY, D. W., GOODMAN, L.: Synthesis of the nucleoside antibiotic formycin B. Chem. Commun. 986—988 (1971).

ALLAN, P. W., BENNETT, L. L., JR.: Metabolism of 8-azainosine. Proc. Amer. Assoc. Cancer Res. **11**, 2 (1970).

ALLAN, P. W., BENNETT, L. L., JR.: 6-Methylthioguanylic acid, a metabolite of 6-thioguanine. Biochem. Pharmacol. **20**, 847—852 (1971).

ALLAN, P. W., SCHNEBLI, H. P., BENNETT, L. L., JR.: Conversion of 6-mercaptopurine and 6-mercaptopurine ribonucleoside to 6-methylmercaptopurine ribonucleotide in human epidermoid carcinoma No. 2 cells in culture. Biochim. biophys. Acta (Amst.) **114**, 647—650 (1966).

AMMANN, C. A., SAFFERMAN, R. S.: The onion test as a possible screening method for anti-tumor agents. Antibiot. Chemother. **8**, 1 (1958).

ANZAI, K., NAKAMURA, G., SUZUKI, S.: A new antibiotic, tubercidin. J. Antibiot. (Tokyo) **10**, 201—204 (1957).

Baker, B. R.: Stereochemistry of nucleoside synthesis. In: Ciba foundation symposium on chemistry and biology of purines. London: J. and A. Churchill, Ltd. 1957.
Baker, B. R., Hewson, K.: Synthesis of potential anticancer agents. VIII. Nucleosides derived from L-rhamnofuranose. J. org. Chem. **22**, 966—971 (1957).
Baker, B. R., Schaub, R. E., Kissman, H. M.: Puromycin. Synthetic studies. XV. 3′-Amino-3′-deoxyadenosine. J. Amer. chem. Soc. **77**, 5911—5915 (1955a).
Baker, B. R., Schaub, R. E., Williams, J. H.: Puromycin. Synthetic studies. VIII. Synthesis of 3-amino-3-deoxy-D-ribofuranoside derivative. A second synthesis of 3-amino-3-deoxy-D-ribose. J. Amer. chem. Soc. **77**, 7—12 (1955b).
Baker, B. R., Schaub, R. E., Joseph, J. P., Williams, J. H.: Puromycin. Synthetic studies. IX. Total synthesis. J. Amer. chem. Soc. **77**, 12—15 (1955c).
Baker, B. R., Hewson, K., Thomas, H. J., Johnson, J. A., Jr.: Synthesis of potential anticancer agents. VI. Use of O-benzoyl blocking group for synthesis of 6-chloropurine nucleosides. J. org. Chem. **22**, 954—959 (1957).
Balsiger, R. W., Fikes, A. L., Johnston, T. P., Montgomery, J. A.: (2-Chloroethyl)thiopurines and the corresponding dihydrothiazolopurines. J. org. Chem. **26**, 3446—3451 (1961).
Beaman, A. G., Robins, R. K.: Potential purine antagonists. XXVII. Synthesis and reactions of some purinesulfonyl fluorides. J. Amer. chem. Soc. **83**, 4038—4044 (1961).
Beaman, A. G., Robins, R. K.: Potential purine antagonists. XXXIII. Synthesis of chloropurines. J. appl. Chem. **12**, 432—437 (1962).
Beaman, A. G., Gusta, J. F., Robins, R. K.: Potential purine antagonists. XXVIII. The preparation of various bromopurines. J. org. Chem. **27**, 986—990 (1962).
Bell, J. P., Faures, M. L., LePage, G. A., Kimball, A. P.: Immunosuppressive and antitumor activity of the periodate oxidation product of β-D-ribosyl-6-methylthiopurine. Cancer Res. **28**, 782—787 (1968).
Bendich, A., Russell, P. J., Jr., Fox, J. J.: The synthesis and properties of 6-chloropurine and purine. J. Amer. chem. Soc. **76**, 6073—6077 (1954).
Bendich, A., Tinker, J. F., Brown, G. B.: A synthesis of isoguanine labeled with isotopic nitrogen. J. Amer. chem. Soc. **70**, 3109—3113 (1948).
Bennett, L. L., Jr., Montgomery, J. A.: Design of anticancer agents, problems and approaches. In: Methods in cancer research, vol. 3. New York: Academic Press 1967.
Bennett, L. L., Jr., Smithers, D.: Feedback inhibition of purine biosynthesis in H.Ep. No. 2 cells by adenine analogs. Biochem. Pharmacol. **13**, 1331—1339 (1964).
Bennett, L. L., Jr., Vail, M. H., Chumley, S., Montgomery, J. A.: Activity of adenosine analogs against a cell culture line resistant to 2-fluoroadenine. Biochem. Pharmacol. **15**, 1719—1728 (1966a).
Bennett, L. L., Jr., Schnebli, H. P., Vail, M. H., Allan, P. W., Montgomery, J. A.: Purine ribonucleoside kinase activity and resistance to some analogs of adenosine. Molec. Pharmacol. **2**, 432—443 (1966b).
Bennett, L. L., Jr., Brockman, R. W., Schnebli, H. P., Chumley, S., Dixon, G. J., Schabel, F. M., Jr., Dulmadge, E. A., Skipper, H. E., Montgomery, J. A., Thomas, H. J.: Activity and mechanism of action of 6-methylthiopurine ribonucleoside in cancer cells resistant to 6-mercaptopurine. Nature (Lond.) **205**, 1276—1279 (1965).
Bentley, H. R., Cunningham, K. G., Spring, F. S.: Cordycepin, a metabolic product from cultures of *Cordyceps militaris* (Linn.) link. Part II. The structure of cordycepin. J. chem. Soc., 2301—2305 (1951).
Bergel, F., Bray, R. C., Haddow, A., Lewin, I.: Enzyme control of purines by xanthine oxidase. In: Ciba foundation symposium on chemistry and biology of purines. London: J. and A. Churchill, Ltd. 1957.
Bergmann, W., Stempien, M. F.: Contributions to the study of marine products. XLIII. The nucleosides of sponges. V. The synthesis of spongosine. J. org. Chem. **22**, 1575—1577 (1957).
Birkofer, L., Ritter, A., Kuhlthau, H. P.: Harnsäure-3-ribofuranosid und harnsäure-3-glucopyranosid. Angew. Chem. **75**, 209—210 (1963).
Bloch, A., Nichol, C. A.: Inhibition of ribosephosphate pyrophosphokinase activity by decoyinine, an adenine nucleoside. Biochem. biophys. Res. Commun. **16**, 400—403 (1964).
Bloch, A., Mihich, E., Leonard, R. J., Nichol, C. A.: Studies on the biologic activity and mode of action of 7-deazainosine. Cancer Res. **29**, 110—115 (1969).
Bobek, M., Farkaš, J., Šorm, F.: Synthesis of 3-(β-D-ribofuranosyl)-5,7-dihydroxy-1H-pyrazolo[4,3-*d*]pyrimidine. Tetrahedron Let., 4611—4614 (1970a).
Bobek, M., Whistler, R. L., Bloch, A.: Preparation and activity of the 4′-thio derivatives of some 6-substituted purine nucleosides. J. med. Chem. **13**, 411—413 (1970b).
Bowles, W. A., Schneider, F. H., Lewis, L. R., Robins, R. K.: Synthesis and antitumor activity of 9-(tetrahydro-2-furyl)purine analogs of biologically important deoxynucleosides. J. med. Chem. **6**, 471—480 (1963).

BRAY, R. C.: Xanthine oxidase. In: The enzymes, 2nd ed., vol. 7, New York and London: Academic Press 1963.
BREDERECK, H., ULMER, H., WALDMANN, H.: Purin aus Formamid. Methylierung und Bromierung des Purins (Synthesenin der Purinreihe VII. Mitteil). Chem. Ber. **89**, 12—18 (1956).
BREDERECK, H., EFFENBERGER, F., RAINER, G., SCHOSSER, H. P.: Saureamid-reactionen, XXXI. Eine einfache Synthese des Purins. Ann. Chem. Liebigs. **659**, 133—138 (1962).
BRINK, J. J., LEPAGE, G. A.: Metabolism and distribution of 9-β-D-arabinofuranosyladenine in mouse tissues. Cancer Res. **24**, 1042—1049 (1964).
BROCKMAN, R. W.: Mechanism of resistance to anticancer agents. Adv. Cancer Res. **7**, 129—234 (1963).
BROCKMAN, R. W., ANDERSON, E. P.: Biochemistry of cancer (metabolic aspects). Ann. Rev. Biochem. **32**, 463—512 (1963).
BROCKMAN, R. W., CHUMLEY, S.: Inhibition of formylglycinamide ribonucleotide synthesis in neoplastic cells by purines and analogs. Biochim. biophys. Acta (Amst.) **95**, 365—379 (1965).
BROWN, D. J.: The pyrimidines: The chemistry of heterocyclic compounds. (A. Weissberger, Ed.) New York: Wiley and Sons 1962.
BROWN, G. B., WELIKY, V. S.: The synthesis of 9 β-D-ribofuranosylpurine and the identity of nebularine. J. biol. Chem. **204**, 1019—1024 (1953).
BROWN, G. B., WELIKY, V. S.: 2-Chloroadenine and 2-chloroadenosine. J. org. Chem. **23**, 125—126 (1958).
BROWN, G. B., LEVIN, G., MURPHY, S., SELE, A., REILLY, H. C., TARNOWSKI, G. S., SCHMID, F. A., TELLER, M. N., STOCK, C. C.: Purine N-oxides. XV. The synthesis of 6-mercaptopurine 3-N-oxide. Its chemotherapeutic possibilities. J. med. Chem. **8**, 190—195 (1965).
CALDWELL, I. C., HENDERSON, J. F., PATERSON, A. R. P.: The metabolism of formycin, an adenosine analog. Can. J. Chem. **47**, 901—908 (1969).
CASKEY, C. T., ASHTON, D. M., WYNGAARDEN, J. B.: The enzymology of feedback inhibition of glutamine phosphoribosylpyrophosphate amidotransferase by purine ribonucleotides. J. biol. Chem. **239**, 2570—2579 (1964).
ČERNÝ, A., SEMONSKÝ, M.: Contribution to the synthesis of 6-mercaptopurine. Cs. Farm. **7**, 402—403 (1958).
ČERNÝ, A., SEMONSKÝ, M.: Substances with antineoplastic activity XVII. Preparation of 6-(4-carboxybutyl)thiopurine. Arzneim.-Forsch. **17**, 1034—1036 (1967).
ČERNÝ, A., SEMONSKÝ, M., JELÍNEK, V.: Substances with antineoplastic activity. III. Some derivatives and analogs of 6-(1-carboxy-4-butyl)thiopurine. Coll. Czech. Chem. Comm. **27**, 57—63 (1962).
ČERNÝ, A., KOTVA, R., VESELA, H., JELÍNEK, V., SEMONSKÝ, M.: Substances with antineoplastic activity. XXIII. Synthesis of 6-(4-carboxybutyl)thionebularin and its effect on some transplantable animal tumors. Coll. Czech. Chem. Comm. **33**, 1474—1479 (1968).
ČERNÝ, A., KOTVA, R., FRANCOVA, V., FRANC, Z., RAZ, K., SEMONSKÝ, M.: Substances with antineoplastic activity. XIV. Some nuclear hydroxylated 6-(4-carboxybutyl)- and 6-(2-carboxyethyl)thiopurines. Coll. Czech. Chem. Comm. **31**, 1824—1830 (1966).
ČERNÝ, A., SEMONSKÝ, M., JELÍNEK, V., FRANCOVA, V., RAZ, K., FRANC, Z.: Substances with antineoplastic activity. XV. Some esters of 6-(4-carboxybutyl)thiopurine. Coll. Czech. Chem. Comm. **32**, 1035—1044 (1967).
CHANG, P. K.: Synthesis of some hydroxylamine derivatives of pyrimidines and purines. J. med. Chem. 8, 884 (1965).
CHANG, P., LYTHGOE, B.: Experiments on the synthesis of purine nucleosides. Part XXVII. 1:2:3:5-Tetra-acetyl-D-oxylofuranose and the D-xylofuranosides of theophylline and adenine. J. chem. Soc. 1992—1993 (1950).
CHENG, C. C., ROBINS, R. K.: Potential purine antagonists. VI. Synthesis of 1-alkyl- and 1-aryl-4-substituted pyrazolo[3,4-*d*]pyrimidines. J. org. Chem. **21**, 1240—1256 (1956).
CHU, S. H.: Potential antitumor agents. Selenoguanosine and related compounds. J. med. Chem. **14**, 254—255 (1971).
CHU, S., HARRIS, I. S., MAUTNER, H. G.: Synthesis of some 8-purinyl nitrogen mustards. J. org. Chem. **25**, 1759—1761 (1960).
CODDINGTON, A.: The preparation of 6-*N*-methyldeoxyadenosine. Biochim. biophys. Acta (Amst.) **59**, 472—474 (1962).
CORY, J. G., SUHADOLNIK, R. J.: Dechloronase activity of adenosine deaminase. Biochemistry **4**, 1733—1734 (1965).
CUNNINGHAM, K. G., HUTCHINSON, S. A., MANSON, W., SPRING, F. S.: Cordycepin, a metabolic product from cultures of *Cordyceps militaris* (Linn) link. Part I. Isolation and characterization. J. chem. Soc. 2299—2300 (1951).
CURRIE, R., BERGEL, F., BRAY, R. C.: Enzymes and cancer, preparation and some properties of guanase from rabbit liver. Biochem. J. **104**, 634—638 (1967).

Daves, G.D., Jr., Noell, C.W., Robins, R.K., Koppel, H.C., Beaman, A.G.: Potential purine antagonists. XXII. The preparation and reactions of certain derivatives of 2-amino-6-purinethiol. J. Amer. chem. Soc. **82**, 2633—2640 (1960).

Davidson, J.D.: Studies on the mechanism of action of 6-mercaptopurine in sensitive and resistant L1210 leukemia *in vitro*. Cancer Res. **20**, 225—232 (1960).

Davoll, J.: The synthesis of the *v*-triazolo[*d*]pyrimidine analogues of adenosine, inosine, guanosine, and xanthosine, and a new synthesis of guanosine. J. chem. Soc. 1593—1599 (1958).

Davoll, J.: Pyrrolo[2,3-*d*]pyrimidines. J. chem. Soc. 131—138 (1960).

Davoll, J., Kerridge, K.A.: The preparation of some 1- and 2-β-D-ribofuranosylpyrazolo-[3,4-*d*]pyrimidines. J. chem. Soc. 2589—2591 (1961).

Davoll, J., Lowy, B.A.: A new synthesis of purine nucleosides. The synthesis of adenosine, guanosine, and 2,6-diamino-9-β-D-ribofuranosylpurine. J. Amer. chem. Soc. **73**, 1650—1655 (1951).

Davoll, J., Lowy, B.A.: Some synthetic analogs of the natural purine nucleosides. J. Amer. chem. Soc. **74**, 1563—1566 (1952).

Dickinson, M.J., Holly, F.W., Walton, E., Zimmerman, M.: 3′-Deoxynucleosides. V. 3′-Deoxy-2-fluoroadenosine. J. med. Chem. **10**, 1165—1166 (1967).

Doerr, I.L., Wempen, I., Clarke, D.A., Fox, J.J.: Thiation of nucleosides. III. Oxidation of 6-mercaptopurines. J. org. Chem. **26**, 3401—3409 (1961).

Duggan, D.E., Titus, E.: 6-Chloropurine and 6-chlorouric acid as substrates and inhibitors of purine-oxidizing enzymes. J. biol. Chem. **234**, 2100—2104 (1959).

Dvonch, W., Fletcher, H., III., Gregory, F.J., Healy, E.-M., Warren, G.H., Alburn, H. E.: Antitumor activity of periodate oxidation products of carbohydrates and their derivatives. Cancer Res. **26**, 2386—2389 (1966).

Eaton, C.N., Denny, G.H., Jr.: Convenient synthesis of 2-fluoroadenine. J. org. Chem. **34**, 747—748 (1969).

Elderfield, R.C., Prasad, R.N., Liao, T.-K.: Synthesis of potential anticancer compounds. XIV. Methanesulfonic acid ester analogs of nitrogen mustards. J. org. Chem. **27**, 573—575 (1962).

Elion, G.B.: Condensed pyrimidine systems. XXII. *N*-methylpurines. J. org. Chem. **27**, 2478—2491 (1962).

Elion, G.B.: Biochemistry and pharmacology of purine analogues. Fed. Proc. **26**, 898—904 (1967).

Elion, G.B., Hitchings, G.H.: The synthesis of 6-thioguanine. J. Amer. chem. Soc. **77**, 1676 (1955).

Elion, G.B., Hitchings, G.H.: Studies on condensed pyrimidine systems. XVII. Some halogenopurines. J. Amer. chem. Soc. **78**, 3508—3510 (1956).

Elion, G.B., Hitchings, G.H.: Metabolic basis for the actions of analogs of purines and pyrimidines. Advanc. Chemother. **2**, 91—177 (1967).

Elion, G.B., Burgi, E., Hitchings, G.H.: Studies on condensed pyrimidine systems. IX. The synthesis of some 6-substituted purines. J. Amer. chem. Soc. **74**, 411—414 (1952).

Elion, G.B., Lange, W.H., Hitchings, G.H.: Studies on condensed pyrimidine systems. XVI. Purines and thiazolo[5,4-*d*]pyrimidines from 4-amino-5-formamido-6-mercaptopyrimidines. J. Amer. chem. Soc. **78**, 2858—2863 (1956).

Elion, G.B., Goodman, I., Lange, W., Hitchings, G.H.: Condensed pyrimidine systems. XX. Purines related to 6-mercaptopurine and thioguanine. J. Amer. chem. Soc. **81**, 1898—1902 (1959).

Ellis, D.B., LePage, G.A.: Some inhibitory effects of 9-β-D-xylofuranosyladenine, an adenosine analog, on nucleotide metabolism in ascites tumor cells. Molec. Pharmacol. **1**, 231—238 (1965).

Falco, E.A., Hitchings, G.H.: Studies on condensed pyrimidine systems. XV. Some pyrazolo-[3,4-*d*]pyrimidines. J. Amer. chem. Soc. **78**, 3143—1345 (1956).

Farkaš, J., Šorm, F.: Nucleic acid components and their analogues. XXX. The synthesis of psicofuranine. Coll. Czech. Chem. Comm. **28**, 882—886 (1963).

Fischer, E.: Über das Purin und seine methyl-derivate. Ber. **31**, 2550—2574 (1898).

Flaks, J.G., Erwin, M.J., Buchanan, J.M.: Biosynthesis of purines. XVI. The synthesis of adenosine 5′-phosphate and 5-amino-4-imidazolecarboxamide ribotide by a nucleotide pyrophosphorylase. J. biol. Chem. **228**, 201—213 (1957).

Fletcher, H.G., Jr., Diehl, H.W.: De-*O*-benzylation of benzyl ethers of carbohydrate derivatives by thiols in the presence of boron trifluoride. Carbohyd. Res. **17**, 383—391 (1971).

Fleysher, M.H., Bloch, A., Hakala, M.T., Nichol, C.A.: Synthesis and biological activity of some new *N*(6)-substituted purine nucleosides. J. med. Chem. **12**, 1056—1061 (1969).

FLEYSHER, M. H., HAKALA, M. T., BLOCH, A., HALL, R. H.: Synthesis and biological activity of some $N(6)$-alkyladenosines. J. med. Chem. 11, 717—720 (1968).
FLORINI, J. R.: Nucleocidin. In: Antibiotics, Vol. 1. Berlin-Heidelberg-New York: Springer 1967.
FOX, J. J., WEMPEN, I., HAMPTON, A., DOERR, I. L.: Thiation of nucleosides. I. Synthesis of 2-amino-6-mercapto-9-β-D-ribofuranosylpurine ("Thioguanosine") and related purine nucleosides. J. Amer. chem. Soc. 80, 1669—1675 (1958).
FUKUYAMA, T. T., MOYED, H. S.: A separate antibiotic-binding site in xanthosine-5'-phosphate aminase: Inhibitor- and substrate-binding studies. Biochemistry 3, 1488—1492 (1964).
GABRIEL, S., COLMAN, J.: Synthesen in der purinreihe. Ber. 34, 1234—1257 (1901).
GERSTER, J. F., JONES, J. W., ROBINS, R. K.: Purine nucleosides. IV. The synthesis of 6-halogenated 9-β-D-ribofuranosylpurines from inosine and guanosine. J. org. Chem. 28, 945—948 (1963).
GERSTER, J. F., CARPENTER, B., ROBINS, R. K., TOWNSEND, L. B.: Pyrrolopyrimidine nucleosides. I. The synthesis of 4-substituted 7-(β-D-ribofuranosyl) pyrrolo(2,3-*d*)pyrimidines from tubercidin. J. med. Chem. 10, 326—331 (1967).
GINER-SOROLLA, A.: The synthesis and properties of 9-β-D-arabinofuranosyl-6-hydroxylaminopurine. J. Heterocycl. Chem. 6, 405—406 (1969).
GINER-SOROLLA, A., MEDREK, L., BENDICH, A.: Synthesis and biological activity of 9-β-D-ribofuranosyl-6-hydroxylaminopurine. J. med. Chem. 9, 143—144 (1966a).
GINER-SOROLLA, A., O'BRYANT, S., BURCHENAL, J. H., BENDICH, A.: The synthesis and properties of substituted 6-hydroxylaminopurines. Biochemistry 5, 3057—3061 (1966b).
GINER-SOROLLA, A., NANOS, C., BURCHENAL, J. H., DOLLINGER, M., BENDICH, A.: The synthesis and properties of 2,6-dihydroxylaminopurine and its 9-β-D-ribofuranosyl derivative. J. med. Chem. 11, 52—54 (1968a).
GINER-SOROLLA, A., O'BRYANT, S. A., NANOS, C., DOLLINGER, M. R., BENDICH, A., BURCHENAL, J. H.: The synthesis and biological properties of hydroxylaminopurines and related derivatives. J. med. Chem. 11, 521—523 (1968b).
GLAUDEMANS, C. P. J., FLETCHER, H. G.: Syntheses with partially benzylated sugars. III. A simple pathway to a "*cis*-nucleoside" 9-β-D-arabinofuranosyladenine (spongoadenosine). J. org. Chem. 28, 3004—3006 (1963).
GOODMAN, I., SALCE, L., HITCHINGS, G. H.: Purine thioglycosides. I. *S*-Glycosides of 6-mercaptopurine. J. med. Chem. 11, 516—521 (1968).
GORDON, M. P., WELIKY, V. S., BROWN, G. B.: A study of the action of acid and alkali on certain purines and purine nucleosides. J. Amer. chem. Soc. 79, 3245—3250 (1957).
GUARINO, A. J.: Angustmycin A. In: Antibiotics, Vol. 1. Berlin-Heidelberg-New York: Springer 1967.
GUARINO, A. J., IBERSHOF, M. L., SWAIN, R.: Inhibition of protein synthesis in cell-free systems by homocitrullylamino adenosine. Biochim. biophys. Acta (Amst.) 72, 62—68 (1963).
HAMPTON, A.: Studies of the action of adenylosuccinase with 6-thio analogues of adenylosuccinic acid. J. biol. Chem. 237, 529—535 (1962).
HAMPTON, A.: Reactions of ribonucleotide derivatives of purine analogues at the catalytic site of inosine 5'-phosphate dehydrogenase. J. biol. Chem. 238, 3068—3074 (1963).
HAMPTON, A., MAGUIRE, M. H.: Nucleotides. I. Syntheses of 6-chloro-, 6-mercapto-, and 2-amino-6-mercapto-9-β-D-ribofuranosylpurine 5'-phosphates. J. Amer. chem. Soc. 83, 150—157 (1961).
HAMPTON, A., PATERSON, A. R. P.: Conversion of 6-chloropurine to its ribonucleotide by ascites tumor cells. Biochim. biophys. Acta (Amst.) 114, 185—187 (1966).
HAMPTON, A., BIESELE, J. J., MOORE, A. E., BROWN, G. B.: 6-Furfurylamino-9-β-D-ribofuranosylpurine: Synthesis and differential toxicity to mammalian cells *in vitro*. J. Amer. chem. Soc. 78, 5695 (1956).
HANKA, L. J.: Psicofuranine. In: Antibiotics, Vol. 1. Berlin-Heidelberg-New York: Springer 1967.
HENDERSON, J. F.: Effects of anticancer drugs on biochemical control mechanisms. Progr. exp. Tumor Res. 6, 84—126 (1965).
HENDERSON, J. F., PATERSON, A. R. P., CALDWELL, I. C., HORI, M.: Biochemical effects of formycin, an adenosine analog. Cancer Res. 27, 715—719 (1967).
HEPPEL, L. A.: 5'-Nucleotidase. In: The enzymes, 2nd ed., Vol. 5. New York and London: Academic Press 1961.
HILL, D. L., BENNETT, L. L., JR.: Purification and properties of 5-phosphoribosyl pyrophosphate amidotransferase from adenocarcinoma 755 cells. Biochemistry 8, 122—130 (1969).
HINSHAW, B. C., GERSTER, J. F., ROBINS, R. K., TOWNSEND, L. B.: Pyrrolopyrimidine nucleosides. IV. The synthesis of certain 4,5-disubstituted-7-(β-D-ribofuranosyl) pyrrolo-(2,3-*d*) pyrimidines related to the pyrrolo(2,3-*d*)pyrimidine nucleoside antibiotics. J. Heterocycl. Chem. 6, 215—221 (1969).

HITCHINGS, G. H., ELION, G. B.: Mercapto heterocycles. U.S. Patent 2,697,709 (1954).
HITCHINGS, G. H., ELION, G. B.: 6-Mercaptopurine from aminoglyoxaline-5-thiocarboxamide. U.S. Patent 2,756,228 (1956).
HITCHINGS, G. H., ELION, G. B.: Novel 6-chloropurine compounds. U.S. Patent 2,815,346 (1957).
HITCHINGS, G. H., ELION, G. B.: 1-Methylthioguanine. Brit. Patent 798,165 (1958).
HITCHINGS, G. H., ELION, G. B.: Purine derivatives. U.S. Patent 3,056,785 (1962).
HOEKSEMA, H., SLOMP, G., VAN TAMELEN, E. E.: Angustmycin A and decoyinine. Tetrahedron Let. 1787—1795 (1964).
HOEKSEMA, H., WHITFIELD, G. B., RHULAND, L. E.: Effect of selective acylation on the oral absorption of a nucleoside by humans. Biochem. biophys. Res. Comm. 6, 213—216 (1961).
HOLMES, R. E., ROBINS, R. K.: Purine nucleosides. VII. Direct bromination of adenosine, deoxyadenosine, guanosine, and related purine nucleosides. J. Amer. chem. Soc. 86, 1242—1245 (1965).
HORI, M., ITO, E., TAKITA, T., KOYAMA, G., TAKEUCHI, T., UMEZAWA, H.: A new antibiotic, formycin. J. Antibiot. (Tokyo) 17 A, 96—99 (1964).
HORWITZ, J. P., VAITKEVICIUS, V. K.: Purin-6-yltrimethylammonium chloride: A new purine antimetabolite. Experientia (Basel) 17, 552—553 (1961).
HUBER, G.: Stickstofflost-analoge der purin-reihe. Angew. Chem. 68, 706 (1956).
IKEHARA, M.: Studies on coenzyme analogs. II. A convenient synthesis of "Thioinosine". Chem. pharm. Bull. (Tokyo) 8, 367—368 (1960).
IKEHARA, M., TADA, H.: Studies on nucleosides and nucleotides. XXXII. Purine cyclonucleosides. 3. Synthesis of 2′-deoxy- and 3′-deoxyadenosine from adenosine. Chem. pharm. Bull. 15, 94—100 (1966).
IKEHARA, M., YAMADA, S.: Studies of nucleosides and nucleotides. 49. Synthesis of 8-fluoroadenosine. Chem. pharm. Bull. 19, 104—109 (1971).
IKEHARA, M., UESUGI, S., KANEKO, M.: Bromination of adenine nucleoside and nucleotide. Chem. Commun. 17—18 (1967).
IKEHARA, M., UNO, H., ISHIKAWA, F.: Studies of nucleosides and nucleotides. XXIII. A versatile method for replacement of 6-hydroxyl group of purine nucleoside. Chem. pharm. Bull. 12, 267—271 (1964).
IKEHARA, M., YAMAZAKI, A., FUJIEDA, T.: Studies on coenzyme analogs. XIII. Oxidation of methylmercaptopurine and its nucleoside by means of $N$-chloro- and $N$-bromosuccinimide. Chem. pharm. Bull. 10, 1075—1080 (1962).
IMAI, K.-I.: Studies on nucleic acid antagonists. VII. Synthesis and characterization of 1,4,6-triazaindenes (5$H$-pyrrolo[3,2-$d$]pyrimidines). Chem. pharm. Bull. 12, 1030—1042 (1964).
ISAY, O.: Eine synthese des purins. Ber. 39, 259—265 (1906).
ISHIDO, Y., MATSUBA, T., HOSONO, A., FUJII, K., SATO, T., ISOME, S., MARUYAMA, A., KIKUCHI, Y.: Non-catalytic fusion reaction of 1,2,3,5-tetra-$O$-acetyl-$\beta$-D-ribofuranose with purine derivatives. Bull. chem. Soc. Jap. 40, 1007—1009 (1967).
IWAMOTO, R. H., ACTON, E. M., GOODMAN, L.: Potential anticancer agents. LXXXI. 2′-Deoxyribofuranosides of 6-mercaptopurine and related purines. J. org. Chem. 27, 3949—3953 (1962).
IWAMURA, H., HASHIZUME, T.: Synthesis in nucleoside antibiotics. III. Synthesis of 4-amino-5-cyano-6-methylmercaptopyrrolo(2,3-$d$)pyrimidine-7-$\beta$-D-ribosides (toyocamycin analogs). Agr. biol. Chem. 32, 1010—1015 (1968a).
IWAMURA, H., HASHIZUME, T.: Synthesis in nucleoside antibiotics. II. Facile synthesis of nebularine and its analogs by a modified fusion procedure. J. org. Chem. 33, 1796—1799 (1968b).
JAIN, P. C., CHATTERJEE, S. K., ANAND, N.: Potential purine antagonists: Part VII—Synthesis of 3-$\beta$-D-ribofuranosyl-7-aminoimidazo(4,5-$b$)pyridine (1-deazaadenosine). Ind. J. Chem. 4, 403—405 (1966).
JENKINS, I. D., VERHEYDEN, J. P. H., MOFFATT, J. G.: Synthesis of the nucleoside antibiotic nucleocidin. J. Amer. chem. Soc. 93, 4323—4324 (1971).
JOHNSON, J. A., JR., THOMAS, H. J.: Synthesis of potential anticancer agents. II. 6-Mercapto-9-$\beta$-D-ribofuranosylpurine. J. Amer. chem. Soc. 78, 3863 (1956).
JOHNSON, J. A., JR., SCHAEFFER, H. J., THOMAS, H. J.: Synthesis of potential anticancer agents. XIII. Ribosides of 6-substituted purines. J. Amer. chem. Soc. 80, 699—702 (1958).
JOHNSTON, T. P., FIKES, A. L., MONTGOMERY, J. A.: The structure of the tricyclic purine derived from the purin-6-yl analog of nitrogen mustard. J. org. Chem. 27, 973—976 (1962).
JOHNSTON, T. P., HOLUM, L. B., MONTGOMERY, J. A.: Synthesis of potential anticancer agents. XVI. $S$-Substituted derivatives of 6-mercaptopurine. J. Amer. chem. Soc. 80, 6265—6271 (1958).
JOHNSTON, T. P., MCCALEB, G. S., MONTGOMERY, J. A.: The synthesis of antineoplastic agents. XXXII. $N$-Nitrosoureas. I. J. med. Chem. 6, 669—681 (1963).

KACZKA, E. A., TRENNER, N. R., ARISON, B., WALKER, R. W., FOLKERS, K.: Identification of cordycepin, a metabolite of *Cordyceps militaris* as 3′-deoxyadenosine. Biochem. biophys. Res. Commun. **14**, 456 (1964).
KELLER, F., BUNKER, J. E.: 6,6′-Dithiobispurinyl nucleosides. J. med. Chem. **12**, 1117—1118 (1969).
KENNER, G. W., LYTHGOE, B., TODD, A. R.: Experiments on the synthesis of purine nucleosides. Part XVII. The preparation of 4-glycofuranosidaminopyrimidines, and a synthesis of 9-L-arabofuranosido-2-methylthioadenine. J. chem. Soc. 957—964 (1948).
KISSMAN, H. M., WEISS, M. J.: Kinetin riboside and related nucleosides. J. org. Chem. **21**, 1053—1055 (1956).
KISSMAN, H. M., DACKS, C. P., BAKER, B. R.: Puromycin synthetic studies. XI. D-Ribofuranosyl derivatives of 6-methylaminopurine. J. Amer. chem. Soc. **77**, 18—24 (1955).
KÖGL, F., VAN DER WANT, G. M., SALEMINK, C. A.: Über 1-des-aza-adenin (7-amino-1-imidazo (b) pyridin). 1. Mitteilung über des-aza-purin derivate. Rec. trav. chim. **67**, 29—44 (1948).
KOPPEL, H. C., ROBINS, R. K.: Potential purine antagonists. XIII. Synthesis of some 8-methylpurines. J. org. Chem. **23**, 1457—1460 (1958).
KOPPEL, H. C., O'BRIEN, D. E., ROBINS, R. K.: Potential purine antagonists. XVIII. Preparation of some 6-alkylthiopurines and 4-alkylthiopyrazolo [3,4-*d*] pyrimidines. J. org. Chem. **24**, 259—261 (1959a).
KOPPEL, H. C., O'BRIEN, D. E., ROBINS, R. K.: Potential purine antagonists. XIX. Synthesis of some 9-alkyl (aryl)-2-amino-6-substituted purines and related v-triazolo[*d*]pyrimidines. J. Amer. chem. Soc. **81**, 3046—3051 (1959b).
KOPPEL, H. C., SPRINGER, R. H., ROBINS, R. K., CHENG, C. C.: Pyrimidines. VIII. Pyrimidine derivatives of thioguanine. J. med. pharm. Chem. **5**, 639—641 (1962a).
KOPPEL, H. C., SPRINGER, R. H., ROBINS, R. K., SCHNEIDER, F. H., CHENG, C. C.: Synthesis of some 8-substituted *bis*($\beta$-chloroethyl) amino derivatives of naturally occurring *N*-methylated purines. J. org. Chem. **27**, 2173—2177 (1962b).
KORNBERG, A., LIEBERMAN, I., SIMMS, E. S.: Enzymatic synthesis of purine nucleotides. J. biol. Chem. **215**, 417—427 (1955).
KOTVA, R., SEMONSKÝ, M., VACHEK, J., JELÍNEK, V.: Substances with antineoplastic activity. 41. $\delta$-(8-Aza-6-purinylthio) valeric acid and some of its 9-alkyl and 9-cycloalkyl derivatives. Coll. Czech. Chem. Commun. **35**, 1610—1613 (1970).
KOTVA, R., ČERNÝ, A., SEMONSKÝ, M., VACHEK, J., JELÍNEK, V.: Substances with antineoplastic activity. XXXII. Some 9-alkyl and 9-cycloalkyl-6-(4-carboxybutylthio) purines. Coll. Czech. Chem. Commun. **34**, 2114—2121 (1969).
KREAM, J., CHARGAFF, E.: Procedures for the study of purine and pyrimidine deaminases in small amounts. J. Amer. chem. Soc. **74**, 4274—4277 (1952).
KRENITSKY, T. A., PAPAIOANNOU, R., ELION, G. B.: Human hypoxanthine phosphoribosyltransferase. I. Purification, properties, and specificity. J. biol. Chem. **244**, 1263—1270 (1969).
KRENITSKY, T. A., ELION, G. B., HENDERSON, A. M., HITCHINGS, G. H.: Inhibition of human purine nucleoside phosphorylase, studies with intact erythrocytes and the purified enzyme. J. biol. Chem. **243**, 2876—2881 (1968).
KRENITSKY, T. A., ELION, G. B., STRELITZ, R. A., HITCHINGS, G. H.: Ribonucleosides of allopurinol and oxoallopurinol. J. biol. Chem. **242**, 2675—2682 (1967).
KURAMITSU, H., MOYED, H. S.: A separate antibiotic binding site in xanthosine 5′-phosphate aminase. J. biol. Chem. **241**, 1596—1601 (1966).
KUSAKA, T., YAMAMOTO, H., SHIBATA, M., MUROI, M., KISHI, T., MIZUNO, K.: *Streptomyces citricolor* nov. sp. and a new antibiotic, aristeromycin. J. Antibiot. (Tokyo) 255—263 (1968).
LASTER, W. R., JR., MAYO, J. G., SIMPSON-HERREN, L., GRISWOLD, D. P., JR., LLOYD, H. H., SCHABEL, F. M., JR., SKIPPER, H. E.: Success and failure in the treatment of solid tumors. II. Kinetic parameters and "cell cure" of moderately advanced carcinoma 755. Cancer Chemother. Rep. **53**, 169—188 (1969).
LEE, W. W., MARTINEZ, A. P., TONG, G. L., GOODMAN, L.: Simultaneous formation of both $\alpha$- and $\beta$-nucleosides by the fusion method. Chem. Ind. (Lond.) 2007—2008 (1963).
LEE, W. W., TONG, G. L., BLACKFORD, R. W., GOODMAN, L.: Nucleosides from 3-deoxy-3-methylamino-D-ribofuranose. J. org. Chem. **35**, 3808—3814 (1970).
LEE, W. W., BENITEZ, A., ANDERSON, C. D., GOODMAN, L., BAKER, B. R.: Potential anticancer agents. LV. Synthesis of 3′-amino-2′,3′-dideoxyadenosine and related analogs. J. Amer. chem. Soc. **83**, 1906—1911 (1961).
LEONARD, N. J., ACHMATOWICZ, S., LOEPPKY, R. N., CARRAWAY, K. L., GRIMM, W. A. H., SZWEYKOWSKA, A., HAMZI, H. Q., SKOOG, F.: Development of cytokinin activity by rearrangement of 1-substituted adenines to 6-substituted aminopurines. Inactivation by N6,1-cyclization. Proc. nat. Acad. Sci. (Wash.) **56**, 709—716 (1966).

LEPAGE, G. A.: Incorporation of 6-thioguanine into nucleic acids. Cancer Res. **20**, 403—408 (1960).
LEPAGE, G. A.: The metabolism of α-2′-deoxythioguanosine in murine tumor cells. Can. J. Biochem. **46**, 655—661 (1968).
LETTRÉ, H., BALLWEG, H.: Ribosides of some cytotoxic purine derivatives. Ann. Chem., Liebigs. **656**, 158—162 (1962).
LEVIN, G., SUGIURA, K., BROWN, G. B.: A nitrogen mustard derivative of 6-mercaptopurine. J. med. Chem. **7**, 357—358 (1964).
LEWIS, L. R., ROBINS, R. K., CHENG, C. C.: The preparation and antitumor properties of acylated derivatives of 6-thiopurine ribosides. J. med. Chem. **7**, 200—204 (1964).
LEWIS, L. R., SCHNEIDER, F. H., ROBINS, R. K.: Purine nucleosides. II. The preparation of 6-substituted 9-(tetrahydro-2-furyl) purines and 6-substituted 9-(tetrahydro-2-thienyl)-purines as models of purine deoxynucleosides. J. org. Chem. **26**, 3837—3842 (1961).
LEWIS, L. R., NOELL, C. W., BEAMAN, A. G., ROBINS, R. K.: The preparation and antitumor activity of certain derivatives of 6-mercaptopurine. J. med. pharm. Chem. **5**, 607—617 (1962).
LIN, H. H., PRICE, C. C.: Some 6-*bis*(2-chloroethyl) aminoalkyladenines. J. org. Chem. **26**, 264—265 (1961).
LINDBERG, B., KLENOW, H., HANSEN, K.: Some properties of partially purified mammalian adenosine kinase. J. biol. Chem. **242**, 350—356 (1967).
LIPKIN, D., HOWARD, F. B., NOWOTNY, D., SANO, M.: The iodination of nucleosides and nucleotides. J. biol. Chem. **238**, 2249—2250 (1963).
LONG, R. A., LEWIS, A. F., ROBINS, R. K., TOWNSEND, L. B.: Pyrazolopyrimidine nucleosides. Part II. 7-Substituted 3-β-D-ribofuranosylpyrazolo [4,3-*d*] pyrimidines related to and derived from the nucleoside antibiotics formycin and formycin B. J. chem. Soc. 2443—2446 (1971).
MANDEL, H. G.: Comparative actions of some purine analogues on growing *Bacillus cereus*. Fed. Proc. **26**, 905—906 (1967).
MARTINEZ, A. P., LEE, W. W.: Pentopyranosyl nucleosides. II. 6-Mercapto and other substituted derivatives of 9-D-arabino- and 9-D-xylopyranosylpurine. Synthesis and spectral properties. J. org. Chem. **34**, 416—421 (1969).
MAUTNER, H. G.: The synthesis and properties of some selenopurines and selenopyrimidines. J. Amer. chem. Soc. **78**, 5292—5294 (1956).
MAUTNER, H. G., CHU, S.-H., JAFFE, J. J., SARTORELLI, A. C.: The synthesis and antineoplastic properties of selenoguanine, selenocytosine and related compounds. J. med. Chem. **6**, 36—39 (1963).
McCARTHY, J. R., ROBINS, R. K., ROBINS, M. J.: Purine nucleosides. XXII. The synthesis of angustmycin A (decoyinine) and related unsaturated nucleosides. J. Amer. chem. Soc. **90**, 4993—4999 (1968).
McCOLLISTER, R. J., GILBERT, W. R., ASHTON, D. M., WYNGAARDEN, J. B.: Pseudofeedback inhibition of purine synthesis by 6-mercaptopurine ribonucleotide and other purine analogues. J. biol. Chem. **239**, 1560—1563 (1964).
MIECH, R. P., YORK, R., PARKS, R. E., JR.: Adenosine triphosphate-guanosine 5′-phosphate phosphotransferase. II. Inhibition by 6-thioguanosine 5′-phosphate of the enzyme isolated from hog brain and sarcoma 180 ascites cells. Molec. Pharmacol. **5**, 30—37 (1969).
MIECH, R. P., PARKS, R. E., JR., ANDERSON, J. H., SARTORELLI, A. C.: An hypothesis on the mechanism of action of 6-thioguanine. Biochem. Pharmacol. **16**, 2222—2227 (1967).
MILNE, G. H., TOWNSEND, L. B.: The synthesis and chemical reactivity of 6-selenoguanosine and certain related derivatives. J. Heterocycl. Chem. **8**, 379—382 (1971).
MITCHELL, J. H., JR., SKIPPER, H. E., BENNETT, L. L., JR.: Investigation of the nucleic acids of viscera and tumor tissue from animals injected with radioactive 8-azaguanine. Cancer Res. **10**, 647—649 (1950).
MIZUNO, Y., ITOH, T., SAITO, K.: Studies on condensed systems of aromatic nitrogenous series. XXIII. Synthesis of 1-(β-D-ribofuranosyl)-1 *H*-imidazo[4,5-*c*]pyridines. J. org. Chem. **29**, 2611—2615 (1964).
MIZUNO, Y., IKEKAWA, N., ITOH, T., SAITO, K.: Studies on condensed aromatic nitrogenous compounds. XXV. Product distribution in ribosylation of purines and deazapurines by the mercuri method. J. org. Chem. **30**, 4066—4071 (1965).
MIZUNO, Y., IKEHARA, M., WATANABE, K. A., SUZAKI, S.: Synthetic studies of potential antimetabolites. X. Synthesis of 4-hydroxy-7-β-D-ribofuranosyl-7*H*-pyrrolo [2,3-*d*] pyrimidine, a tubercidin analog. J. org. Chem. **28**, 3331—3336 (1963).
MONTGOMERY, J. A.: Synthesis of potential anticancer agents. I. Chloropurines. J. Amer. chem. Soc. **78**, 1928—1930 (1956).
MONTGOMERY, J. A.: The biochemical basis for the drug actions of purines. Progr. med. Chem. **7**, 69—122 (1970).

MONTGOMERY, J. A., HEWSON, K.: Synthesis of potential anticancer agents. X. 2-Fluoroadenosine. J. Amer. chem. Soc. 79, 4559 (1957).
MONTGOMERY, J. A., HEWSON, K.: Synthesis of potential anticancer agents. XX. 2-Fluoropurines. J. Amer. chem. Soc. 82, 463—468 (1960).
MONTGOMERY, J. A., HEWSON, K.: 7-Substituted-7*H*-purines. J. org. Chem. 26, 4469—4472 (1961).
MONTGOMERY, J. A., HEWSON, K.: The synthesis of 2-bromoadenosine. J. Heterocycl. Chem. 1, 213—214 (1964).
MONTGOMERY, J. A., HEWSON, K.: Deaza analogs of 6-mercaptopurine. J. med. Chem. 8, 708—710 (1965a).
MONTGOMERY, J. A., HEWSON, K.: New approaches to the synthesis of 5 *H*-pyrrolo[3,2-*d*]-pyrimidines. J. org. Chem. 30, 1528—1532 (1965b).
MONTGOMERY, J. A., HEWSON, K.: 1-Deaza-6-methylthiopurine ribonucleoside. J. med. Chem. 9, 354—357 (1966a).
MONTGOMERY, J. A., HEWSON, K.: 2-Deaza-6-methylthiopurine ribonucleoside. J. med. Chem. 9, 105—107 (1966b).
MONTGOMERY, J. A., HEWSON, K.: Analogs of tubercidin. J. med. Chem. 10, 665—667 (1967).
MONTGOMERY, J. A., HEWSON, K.: A convenient method for the synthesis of 2-fluoroadenosine. J. org. Chem. 33, 432—434 (1968a).
MONTGOMERY, J. A., HEWSON, K.: Analogs of 6-methyl-9-β-D-ribofuranosylpurine. J. med. Chem. 11, 48—52 (1968b).
MONTGOMERY, J. A., HEWSON, K.: Nucleosides of 2-fluoroadenine. J. med. Chem. 12, 498—504 (1969).
MONTGOMERY, J. A., HEWSON, K.: 2-Fluoropurine ribonucleosides. J. med. Chem. 13, 427—430 (1970).
MONTGOMERY, J. A., HOLUM, L. B.: Synthesis of potential anticancer agents. III. Hydrazino analogs of biologically active purines. J. Amer. chem. Soc. 79, 2185—2188 (1957).
MONTGOMERY, J. A., TEMPLE, C., JR.: Synthesis of potential anticancer agents. IX. 9-Ethyl-6-substituted purines. J. Amer. chem. Soc. 79, 5238—5242 (1957).
MONTGOMERY, J. A., TEMPLE, C., JR.: Synthesis of potential anticancer agents. XII. 9-Alkyl-6-substituted-purines. J. Amer. chem. Soc. 80, 409—411 (1958).
MONTGOMERY, J. A., TEMPLE, C., JR.: Synthesis of potential anticancer agents. XXII. Reactions of orthoesters with 4,5-diaminopyrimidines. J. org. Chem. 25, 395—399 (1960).
MONTGOMERY, J. A., TEMPLE, C., JR.: Synthesis of potential anticancer agents. XXVI. The alkylation of 6-chloropurine. J. Amer. chem. Soc. 83, 630—635 (1961).
MONTGOMERY, J. A., THOMAS, H. J.: Synthesis of potential anticancer agents. XXVII. The ribonucleotides of 6-mercaptopurine and 8-azaguanine. J. org. Chem. 26, 1926—1929 (1961).
MONTGOMERY, J. A., THOMAS, H. J.: Directive influences in the preparation of purine nucleosides. J. org. Chem. 28, 2304—2310 (1963).
MONTGOMERY, J. A., THOMAS, H. J.: The use of the allyl group as a blocking group for the synthesis of *N*-substituted purines. J. org. Chem. 30, 3235—3236 (1965).
MONTGOMERY, J. A., THOMAS, H. J.: 2-Azaadenosine (4-amino-7-β-D-ribofuranosyl-7 *H*-imidazo-[4,5-*d*]-*v*-triazine). Chem. Commun. 458 (1969).
MONTGOMERY, J. A., THOMAS, H. J.: A new approach to the synthesis of nucleosides of 8-azapurines (1-glycosyl-*v*-triazolo[4,5-*d*]pyrimidines). J. org. Chem. 36, 1962—1967 (1971).
MONTGOMERY, J. A., THOMAS, H. J.: Nucleosides of 8-azapurines (*v*-triazolo[4,5-*d*]pyrimidines). J. med. Chem. 15, 305—307 (1972a).
MONTGOMERY, J. A., THOMAS, H. J.: Nucleosides of 2-azapurines and certain ring analogs. J. med. Chem. 15, 182—187 (1972b).
MONTGOMERY, J. A., CLAYTON, S. J., FITZGIBBON, W. E., JR.: The ribonucleosides of 4-aminopyrazolo[3,4-*d*]pyrimidines. J. Heterocycl. Chem. 1, 215—216 (1964).
MONTGOMERY, J. A., HEWSON, K., TEMPLE, C., JR.: Synthesis of potential anticancer agents. XXX. (1-aziridinyl)purines. J. med. Pharm. Chem. 5, 15—24 (1962).
MONTGOMERY, J. A., JOHNSTON, T. P., SHEALY, Y. F.: Drugs for neoplastic diseases. In: Medicinal chemistry, 3rd. ed. New York: Wiley Interscience 1970a.
MONTGOMERY, J. A., THOMAS, H. J., CLAYTON, S. J.: A convenient synthesis of 8-azaadenosine. J. Heterocycl. Chem. 7, 215—217 (1970b).
MONTGOMERY, J. A., THOMAS, H. J., SCHAEFFER, H. J.: Synthesis of potential anticancer agents. XXVIII. Simple esters of 6-mercaptopurine ribonucleotide. J. org. Chem. 26, 1929—1933 (1961a).
MONTGOMERY, J. A., JOHNSTON, T. P., GALLAGHER, A., STRINGFELLOW, C. R., SCHABEL, F. M., JR.: A comparative study of the anticancer activity of some *S*-substituted derivatives of 6-mercaptopurine and their ribonucleosides. J. med. pharm. Chem. 3, 265—288 (1961b).

MONTGOMERY, J. A., DIXON, G. J., DULMADGE, E. A., THOMAS, H. J., BROCKMAN, R. W., SKIPPER, H. E.: Inhibition of 6-mercaptopurine-resistant cancer cells in culture by *bis*(thioinosine)-5'-5'''-phosphate. Nature (Lond.) **199**, 769—772 (1963).

MORTON, G. O., LANCASTER, J. E., VAN LEAR, G. E., FULMOR, W., MEYER, W. E.: The structure of nucleocidin. III. (A new structure). J. Amer. chem. Soc. **91**, 1535—1537 (1969).

MURRAY, D. H., PROKOP, J.: Synthesis of 3'-deoxynucleosides. II. Synthesis of 9-(3-deoxyaldofuranosyl) adenines derived from 3-deoxy-D-glucose. J. pharm. Sci. **54**, 1468—1473 (1965).

NATHANS, D.: Puromycin. In: Antibiotics, vol. 1. Berlin-Heidelberg-New York: Springer-Verlag, 1967.

NIERLICH, D. P., MAGASANIK, B.: Regulation of purine ribonucleotide synthesis by end product inhibition. The effect of adenine and guanine ribonucleotides on the 5'-phosphoribosylpyrophosphate amidotransferase of *Aerobacter aerogenes*. J. biol. Chem. **240**, 358—365 (1965).

NISHIMURA, T., IWAI, I.: Studies on synthetic nucleosides. II. Novel synthesis of pyrimidine glucosides. Chem. pharm. Bull. **12**, 357—361 (1964).

NISHIMURA, H., KATAGIRI, K., SATO, K., MAYAMA, M., SHIMAOKA, N.: Toyocamycin, a new antibiotic. J. Antibiot. (Tokyo) **9**, 60—62 (1956).

NOELL, C. W., ROBINS, R. K.: Potential purine antagonists. XIV. Synthesis of some 4-(substituted amino)pyrazolo[3,4-*d*]pyrimidines. J. org. Chem. **23**, 1547—1550 (1958).

NOELL, C. W., ROBINS, R. K.: Potential purine antagonists. XX. The preparation and reactions of some methylthiopurines. J. Amer. chem. Soc. **81**, 5997—6001 (1959).

NOELL, C. W., ROBINS, R. K.: Potential purine antagonists. XXXI. The preparation of certain 9-alkyl-2-amino-6-purinethiols and related derivatives as antitumor agents. J. med. pharm. Chem. **5**, 558—588 (1962a).

NOELL, C. W., ROBINS, R. K.: The antitumor activity of 2-amino-6-alkylthio-9-β-D-ribofuranosylpurines and related derivatives of 2-amino-6-purinethiol (thioguanine). J. med. pharm. Chem. **5**, 1074—1085 (1962b).

NOELL, C. W., SMITH, D. W., ROBINS, R. K.: Synthesis and antitumor activity of 2-amino-1-methylpurine-6-thione. J. med. pharm. Chem. **5**, 996—999 (1962).

O'BRIEN, D. E., WESTOVER, J. D., ROBINS, R. K., CHENG, C. C.: Synthesis and antitumor activity of 9-substituted nitrogen mustard derivatives of 6-alkylthiopurines. J. med. Chem. **8**, 182—187 (1965).

OVERGAARD-HANSEN, K.: The inhibition of 5-phosphoribosyl-1-pyrophosphate formation by cordycepin triphosphate in extracts of Ehrlich ascites tumor cells. Biochim. biophys. Acta (Amst.) **80**, 504—507 (1964).

PATERSON, A. R. P., SUTHERLAND, A.: Metabolism of 6-mercaptopurine ribonucleoside by Ehrlich ascites carcinoma cells. Can. J. Biochem. **42**, 1415—1423 (1964).

PERINI, F., HAMPTON, A.: A simplified procedure for the synthesis of 6-methylthiopurine ribonucleoside 5'-phosphates. J. Heterocycl. Chem. **7**, 969—971 (1970).

PFLEIDERER, W., MOSTHAF, H.: Untersuchungen in der pyrimidinreihe, II. Über die Darstellung von Pyrido-[3.2-*d*]- und pyrrolo-[3.2-*d*]-pyrimidinen. Chem. Ber. **90**, 738—745 (1957).

PIERRE, K. J., LEPAGE, G. A.: Formation of inosine-5'-monophosphate by a kinase in cell-free extracts of Ehrlich ascites cells *in vitro*. Proc. Soc. exp. Biol. N. Y. **127**, 432—440 (1968).

PIERRE, K. J., KIMBALL, A. P., LEPAGE, G. A.: The effect of structure on nucleoside kinase activity. Can. J. Biochem. **45**, 1619—1632 (1967).

PIKE, J. E., SLECHTA, L., WILEY, P. F.: Tubercidin and related compounds. J. Heterocycl. Chem. **1**, 159—161 (1964).

PORTER, J. N., HEWITT, R. I., HESSELTINE, C. W., KRUPKA, G., LOWERY, J. A., WALLACE, W. S., BOHONOS, N., WILLIAMS, J. H.: Achromycin: A new antibiotic having trypanocidal properties. Antibiot. Chemother. **2**, 409—410 (1952).

RAO, K. V., RENN, D. W.: BA-90912: An antibiotic substance. Antimicrob. Agents Chemother. 77—79 (1963).

REIST, E. J., BARTUSKA, V. J., GOODMAN, L.: Sodium-liquid ammonia debenzylation in nucleoside synthesis. J. org. Chem. **29**, 3725—3726 (1964).

REIST, E. J., CALKINS, D. F., GOODMAN, L.: *N*-Oxides of 9-(β-D-xylofuranosyl) adenine and 9-(β-D-arabinofuranosyl) adenine. J. med. Chem. **10**, 130 (1967a).

REIST, E. J., CALKINS, D. F., GOODMAN, L.: Purine nucleosides of β-D-lyxofuranose. J. org. Chem. **32**, 169—173 (1967b).

REIST, E. J., HART, P. A., GOODMAN, L., BAKER, B. R.: Potential anticancer agents. LI. Synthesis of 2-amino-9-(5'-deoxy-β-D-ribofuranosyl)-9-*H*-purine-6-thiol. J. org. Chem. **26**, 1557—1562 (1961).

REIST, E. J., BENITEZ, A., GOODMAN, L., BAKER, B. R., LEE, W. W.: Potential anticancer agents. LXXVI. Synthesis of purine nucleosides of β-D-arabinofuranose. J. org. Chem. **27**, 3774—3779 (1962a).

REIST, E. J., BENITEZ, A., LEE, W. W., BAKER, B. R., GOODMAN, L.: Potential anticancer agents. LXXVII. Synthesis of nucleosides of purine-6-thiol (6-mercaptopurine) containing "fraudulent" sugars. J. org. Chem. **27**, 3279—3283 (1962b).

REVANKAR, G. R., TOWNSEND, L. B.: Pyrazolopyrimidine nucleosides. Part. I. Synthesis of pyrazolopyrimidine nucleosides related to the nucleoside antibiotic tubercidin. J. chem. Soc. 2440—2442 (1971).

ROBINS, R. K.: Potential purine antagonists. I. Synthesis of some 4,6-substituted pyrazolo-[3,4-*d*]pyrimidines. J. Amer. chem. Soc. **78**, 784—790 (1956).

ROBINS, R. K.: A new synthesis of chloropurine ribonucleosides. J. Amer. chem. Soc. **82**, 2654—2655 (1960).

ROBINS, R. K., DILLE, K. J., WILLITS, C. H., CHRISTENSEN, B. E.: Purines. II. The synthesis of certain purines and the cyclization of several substituted 4,5-diaminopyrimidines. J. Amer. chem. Soc. **75**, 263—266, 6359 (1959).

ROBINS, R. K., FURCHT, F. W., GRAUER, A. D., JONES, J. W.: Potential purine antagonists. II. Synthesis of some 7- and 5,7-substituted pyrazolo[4,3-*d*]pyrimidines. J. Amer. chem. Soc. **78**, 2418—2422 (1956).

ROBINS, R. K., GODEFROI, E. F., TAYLOR, E. C., LEWIS, L. R., JACKSON, A.: Purine nucleosides. I. The synthesis of certain 6-substituted-9-(tetrahydro-2-pyranyl) purines as models of purine deoxynucleosides. J. Amer. chem. Soc. **83**, 2574—2579 (1961).

ROBLIN, R. O., JR., LAMPEN, J. O., ENGLISH, J. P., COLE, Q. P., VAUGHN, J. R., JR.: Studies in chemotherapy. VIII. Methionine and purine antagonists and their relation to the sulfonamides. J. Amer. chem. Soc. **67**, 290—294 (1945).

ROSE, F. L.: 1:2:4:6-Tetraazaindenes and 1:4:6-triazaindan-2-ones from 5-aminopyrimidines. J. chem. Soc. 4116—4126 (1954).

ROTTMAN, F., GUARINO, A. J.: The inhibition of phosphoribosylpyrophosphate amidotransferase activity by cordycepin monophosphate. Biochim. biophys. Acta (Amst.) **89**, 465—472 (1964).

ROUSSEAU, R. J., TOWNSEND, L. B., ROBINS, R. K.: The synthesis of 4-amino-$\beta$-D-ribofuranosyl-imidazo[4,5-*c*]pyridine (3-deazaadenosine) and related nucleotides. Biochemistry **5**, 756—760 (1966).

ROY, J. K., HAAVIK, A. G., PARKS, R. E., JR: Nucleotides of adenine analogs. Proc. Amer. Assoc. Cancer Res. **3**, 146 (1960).

ROY, J. K., KVAM, D. C., DAHL, J. L., PARKS, R. E., JR.: Effect of triphosphate nucleosides of 8-azaguanine, 6-thioguanine, and 6-mercaptopurine on amino acid incorporation *in vitro* into microsomal protein. J. biol. Chem. **236**, 1158—1162 (1961).

SALEMINK, C. A., VAN DER WANT, G. M.: Über 3-desaza-adenin (4-amino-1-imidazo-(*c*)-pyridin) und verwandte basen. 3. Mitteilung über desazapurin-derivate. Rec. trav. chim. **68**, 1013—1029 (1949).

SALSER, J., HUTCHISON, D. J., BALIS, M. E.: Studies on the mechanism of action of 6-mercaptopurine in cell-free preparations. J. biol. Chem. **235**, 429—432 (1960).

SANEYOSHI, M.: Synthetic nucleosides and nucleotides. 8. Direct synthesis of the 5′-phosphate of 4-thiouridine, 6-thioinosine and 6-thioguanosine from the corresponding oxy nucleotide via Lathiation procedure. Chem. pharm. Bull. **19**, 493—498 (1971).

SATO, K., LEPAGE, G. A., KIMBALL, A. P.: The metabolism of 9-$\beta$-D-xylofuranosyl-6-mercaptopurine. Cancer Res. **26**, 741—747 (1966).

SATO, T., SHIMADATE, T., ISHIDO, Y.: A new method for syntheses of purine nucleosides. Parts 1 and 2. Nippon Kagaku Zasshi **81**, 1440—1444 (1960).

SAWA, T., FUKAGAWA, Y., HOMMA, I., WAKASHIRO, T., TAKEUCHI, T., HORI, M., and KOMAI, T.: Metabolic conversion of formycin B to formycin A and to oxoformycin B in *Nocardia interforma*. J. Antibiot. **21**, 334—339 (1968).

SCANNELL, J. P., HITCHINGS, G. H.: Thioguanine in deoxyribonucleic acid from tumors of 6-mercaptopurine-treated mice. Proc. Soc. exp. Biol. N. Y. **122**, 627—629 (1966).

SCHAEFFER, H. J., THOMAS, H. J.: Synthesis of potential anticancer agents. XIV. Ribosides of 2,6-disubstituted purines. J. Amer. chem. Soc. **80**, 3738—3742 (1958).

SCHMIDT, L. H., MONTGOMERY, J. A., LASTER, W. R., JR., SCHABEL, F. M., JR.: Combination therapy with arabinosyl cytosine and thioguanine. Proc. Amer. Assoc. Cancer Res. **11**, 70 (1970).

SCHNEBLI, H. P., HILL, D. L., BENNETT, L. L., JR.: Purification and properties of adenosine kinase from human tumor cells of type H.Ep. No. 2. J. biol. Chem. **242**, 1997—2004 (1967).

SCHROEDER, W., HOEKSEMA, H.: A new antibiotic, 6-amino-9-D-psicofuranosylpurines. J. Amer. chem. Soc. 81, 1767—1768 (1959).

SEMONSKÝ, M., ČERNÝ, A., JELÍNEK, V.: Substanzen mit antineoplastischer wirksamkeit. II. Einige 6-carboxylalkylthiopurine. Coll. Czech. Chem. Commun. **25**, 1091—1099 (1960).

Semonský, M., Černý, A., Jelínek, V.: Substances with antineoplastic activity. 29. N-(δ-(6-purinylthio) valeryl) amino acids and analogous dipeptide and trigflycine derivatives. Arzneim.-Forsch. **20**, 316—323 (1970).

Semonský, M., Kotva, R., Vachek, J., Jelínek, V.: Substances with antineoplastic activity. XXVII. Some α-substitution derivatives of δ-(6-purinylthio) valeric and ε-(6-purinylthio)-caproic acids. Coll. Czech. Chem. Commun. **33**, 3823—3832 (1968).

Shaw, E.: A new synthesis of the purines adenine, hypoxanthine, xanthine, and isoguanine. J. biol. Chem. **185**, 439—447 (1950).

Shaw, E., Woolley, D. W.: A new and convenient synthesis of 4-amino-5-imidazolecarboxamide. J. biol. Chem. **181**, 89—93 (1949).

Shaw, G., Butler, D. N.: Purines, pyrimidines, and glyoxalines. Part XIV. The preparation and some reactions of α-amino-α-cyanothioacetamide, leading to 6-mercaptopurines and adenines. J. chem. Soc. 4040—4045 (1959).

Shealy, Y. F., Clayton, J. D.: 9-[β-DL-2α,3α-Dihydroxy-4β-(hydroxymethyl)cyclopentyl]-adenine, the carbocyclic analog of adenosine. J. Amer. chem. Soc. **88**, 3885—3887 (1966).

Shealy, Y. F., Clayton, J. D., O'Dell, C. A., Montgomery, J. A.: *v*-Triazolo[4,5-*d*] pyrimidines II. *O*-Substituted derivatives of 8-azaguanine and 8-azahypoxanthine. J. org. Chem. **27**, 4518—4523 (1962).

Shealy, Y. F., Struck, R. F., Clayton, J. D., Montgomery, J. A.: *v*-Triazolo[4,5-*d*]pyrimidines. I. Synthesis and nucleophilic substitution of 7-chloro derivatives of 3-substituted *v*-triazolo[4,5-*d*]pyrimidines. J. org. Chem. **26**, 4433—4440 (1961).

Shigeura, H. T., Sampson, S. D., Melon, M. L.: Limited phosphorylation of some 6-methylaminopurine nucleosides. Arch. Biochem. Biophys. **115**, 462—467 (1967).

Shigeura, H. T., Boxer, G. E., Sampson, S. D., Meloni, M. L.: Metabolism of 2-fluoroadenosine by Ehrlich ascites cells. Arch. Biochem. Biophys. **111**, 713—719 (1965).

Shimizu, B., Miyaki, M.: Glycosyl migration of derivatives of 3-isoadenosine and its 5'-phosphate. Chem. Ind. 664—665 (1966).

Skinner, C. G., Claybrook, J. R., Ross, D. L., Shive, W.: Synthesis of some α- and β-(6-purinylthio) carboxylic acids. J. org. Chem. **23**, 1223—1224 (1958).

Skinner, C. G., Ham, R. G., Fitzgerald, D. C., Jr., Eakin, R. E., Shive, W.: Synthesis and biological activity of some 6-(substituted) thiopurines. J. org. Chem. **21**, 1330—1332 (1956a).

Skinner, C. G., Shive, W., Ham, R. G., Fitzgerald, D. C., Jr., Eakin, R. E.: Effects of some 6-(substituted)-purines on regeneration of hydra. J. Amer. chem. Soc. **78**, 5097—5100 (1956b).

Sowa, W.: Convenient synthesis of 3-amino-3-deoxy-D-ribose. Can. J. Chem. **46**, 1586—1589 (1968).

Sutcliffe, E. Y., Zee-Cheng, K. Y., Cheng, C. C., Robins, R. K.: Potential purine antagonists. XXXII. The synthesis and antitumor activity of certain compounds related to 4-amino-pyrazolo[3,4-*d*]pyrimidine. J. med. pharm. Chem. **5**, 588—607 (1962).

Tanaka, K., Sugawa, T., Nakamori, R., Sanno, Y., Ando, Y., Imai, K.-I.: Studies on nucleic acid antagonists. VI. Synthesis of 1,4,6-triazaindenes (5*H*-pyrrolo[3,2-*d*]pyrimidines). Chem. pharm. Bull. **12**, 1024—1030 (1964).

Tanaka, N., Nishimura, T., Yamaguchi, H., Umezawa, H.: Activity of angustmycins against experimental infections and transplantable tumors. J. Antibiot. (Tokyo) **14**, 98—102 (1961).

Taylor, E. C., Vogl, O., Cheng, C. C.: Studies in purine chemistry. II. A facile synthesis of 2-substituted adenines. J. Amer. chem. Soc. **81**, 2442—2448 (1959).

Temple, C., Jr., Montgomery, J. A.: Some unusual reactions of 6-chloropurines with thioureas. 6-Alkylthiopurines and 2,2-diamino-2*H*-thiazolo[3,4,5-*gh*]purines from 2-(purin-6-yl)-2-thiopseudoureas. J. org. Chem. **31**, 1417—1422 (1966).

Temple, C., Jr., Kussner, C. L., Montgomery, J. A.: Synthesis of potential anticancer agents. XXXI. 9-Alkyl-9*H*-purines. J. med. pharm. Chem. **5**, 866—870 (1962).

Temple, C., Jr., Kussner, C. L., Montgomery, J. A.: Lipid-soluble derivatives of 6-mercaptopurine. J. med. Chem. **11**, 41—44 (1968).

Thomas, H. J., Montgomery, J. A.: Complex esters of thioinosinic-(5') acid. J. med. pharm. Chem. **5**, 24—32 (1962).

Thomas, H. J., Montgomery, J. A.: Derivatives and analogs of 6-mercaptopurine ribonucleotide. J. med. Chem. **11**, 44—48 (1968).

Thomas, S. O., Singleton, V. L., Lowery, J. A., Sharpe, R. W., Preuss, L. M., Porter, J. N., Mowat, J. H., Bohonos, N.: Nucleocidin, a new antibiotic with activity against trypanosomes. Antibiot. Ann. 716—721 (1956—1957).

Todd, A., Ulbricht, T. L. V.: Deoxynucleosides and related compounds. Part IX. A synthesis of 3'-deoxyadenosine. J. chem. Soc. 3275—3277 (1960).

TOLMAN, R. L., ROBINS, R. K., TOWNSEND, L. B.: Pyrrolopyrimidine nucleosides. II. The total synthesis of 7-β-D-ribofuranosylpyrrolo(2,3-*d*)pyrimidines related to toyocamycin. J. Heterocycl. Chem. **4**, 230—238 (1967).
TOLMAN, R. L., TOWNSEND, L. B., ROBINS, R. K.: Pyrrolopyrimidine nucleosides. III. The total synthesis of toyocamycin, sangivamycin, tubercidin, and related derivatives. J. Amer. Chem. Soc. **91**, 2102—2108 (1969).
TOLMAN, R. L., TOLMAN, G. L., ROBINS, R. K., TOWNSEND, L. B.: Pyrrolopyrimidine nucleosides. 6. Synthesis of 1,3 and 7-β-D-ribofuranosylpyrrolo(2,3-*d*)pyrimidines via silylated intermediates. J. Heterocycl. Chem. **7**, 799—806 (1970).
TONG, G. L., LEE, W. W., GOODMAN, L.: Synthesis of some 3-*O*-methyl purine ribonucleosides. J. org. Chem. **32**, 1984—1985 (1967a).
TONG, G. L., RYAN, K. J., LEE, W. W., ACTON, E. M., GOODMAN, L.: Nucleosides of thioguanine and other 2-amino-6-substituted purines from 2-acetamido-6-chloropurine. J. org. Chem. **32**, 859—862 (1967b).
TONG, G. L., LEE, W. W., GOODMAN, L., FREDERIKSEN, S.: Synthesis of some 2′-deoxyribosides of 8-azaadenine. Arch. Biochem. Biophys. **112**, 76—81 (1965).
TRAUBE, W.: Über 2-amino-adenin (2,6-diaminopurin). Ber. **37**, 4544—4547 (1904).
VINCZE, A., COHEN, S.: Some *N*-substituted 6-methylpurines. Israel J. Chem. **4**, 23—30 (1966).
WALTON, E., NUTT, R. F., JENKINS, S. R., HOLLY, F. W.: 3′-Deoxynucleosides. I. A synthesis of 3′-deoxyadenosine. J. Amer. chem. Soc. **86**, 2952 (1964).
WALTON, E., HOLLY, F. W., BOXER, G. E., NUTT, R. F., JENKINS, S. R.: 3′-Deoxynucleosides. II. Purine 3′-deoxynucleosides. J. med. Chem. **8**, 659—663 (1965).
WAY, J. L., PARKS, R. E.: Enzymatic synthesis of 5′-phosphate nucleotides of purine analogues. J. biol. Chem. **231**, 467—480 (1958).
WHEELER, G. P., ALEXANDER, J. A.: Searches for exploitable biochemical differences between normal and cancer cells. VIII. Catabolism of purines and purine nucleotides by sonicates. Cancer Res. **21**, 407—421 (1961).
WOLFENDEN, R.: Enzymatic hydrolysis of 6-substituents on purine ribosides. J. Amer. chem. Soc. **88**, 3157—3158 (1966).
WOLFROM, M. L., THOMPSON, A., EVANS, E. F.: The action of diazomethane upon acyclic sugar derivatives. VII. D-Psicose. J. Amer. chem. Soc. **67**, 1793—1797 (1945).
WOOLLEY, D. W., SHAW, E.: Some imidazo-1,2,3-triazines and their biological relationship to the purines. J. biol. Chem. **189**, 401—410 (1951).
YAMAZAKI, A., KUMASHIRO, I., TAKENISHI, T., IKEHARA, M.: Synthesis of thio-AICA, 6-thioxanthine, isoguanine analogs, and their ribosides. Chem. pharm. Bull. **16**, 2172—2181 (1968).
YORK, J. L., LEPAGE, G. A.: A kinetic study of the deamination of some adenosine analogues, substrate specificity of adenosine deaminase. Can. J. Biochem. **44**, 331—337 (1966).
YOSHIDA, H., DUVAL, J., EBEL, J. P.: Halogenation of nucleic acids. VI. Iodination of nucleosides in dimethylformamide. Biochim. biophys. Acta (Amst.) **161**, 13—22 (1968).
YOSHIKAWA, M., KATO, T., TAKENISHI, T.: A novel method for phosphorylation of nucleosides to 5′-nucleotides. Tetrahedron Let. 5065 (1967).
YÜNTSEN, H.: Chemical structure of angustmycin A. J. Antibiot. (Tokyo) **11**, 233—243 (1958a).
YÜNTSEN, H.: Structure of angustmycin C. J. Antibiot. (Tokyo) **11**, 244—249 (1958b).
YÜNTSEN, H., YONEHARA, H., UI, H.: A new antibiotic, angustmycin. I. J. Antibiot. (Japan) **7**, 113—115 (1954).
YÜNTSEN, H., OHKUMA, K., ISHII, Y.: A new antibiotic, angustmycin. III. J. Antibiot. (Japan) **9**, 195—201 (1956).

Chapter 6

# Rational Design of Pyrimidine Nucleoside Analogs

LEROY B. TOWNSEND and C. C. CHENG

## Introduction

The uncontrolled growth of cells is characteristic of a group of diseases known as cancer. The major difficulty in coping with this problem is that there is, as yet, little information of particular significance on the biochemical differences between normal and malignant tissues. Out of necessity, the chemotherapeutic approach to oncology has been rather empirical with the major successes being noted with drugs which are generally more toxic to rapidly proliferating cells. Most of these cytotoxic anticancer agents act primarily as inhibitors of nucleic acid synthesis at various sites and by different mechanisms.

A number of pyrimidine nucleosides have been reported to be cytotoxic agents. Among these, some were obtained as a consequence of rational design, whereas

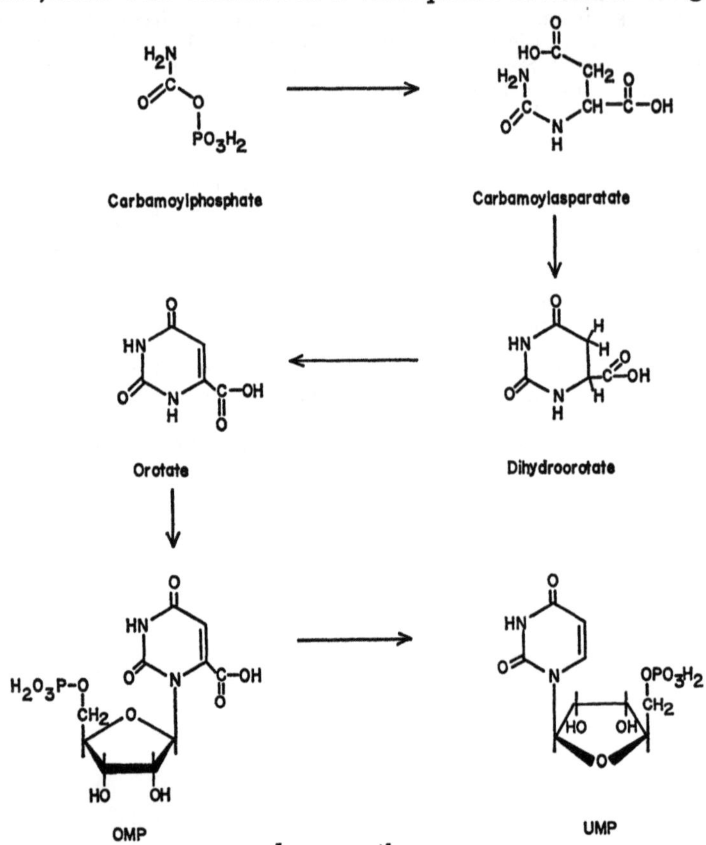


*de novo* pathway

others were recognized through random screening. The present chapter will encompass compounds in both areas and, in addition, will include those which might be involved in future synthetic approaches with a rationale based on existing information. Comprehensive reviews of the pyrimidines per se, with a

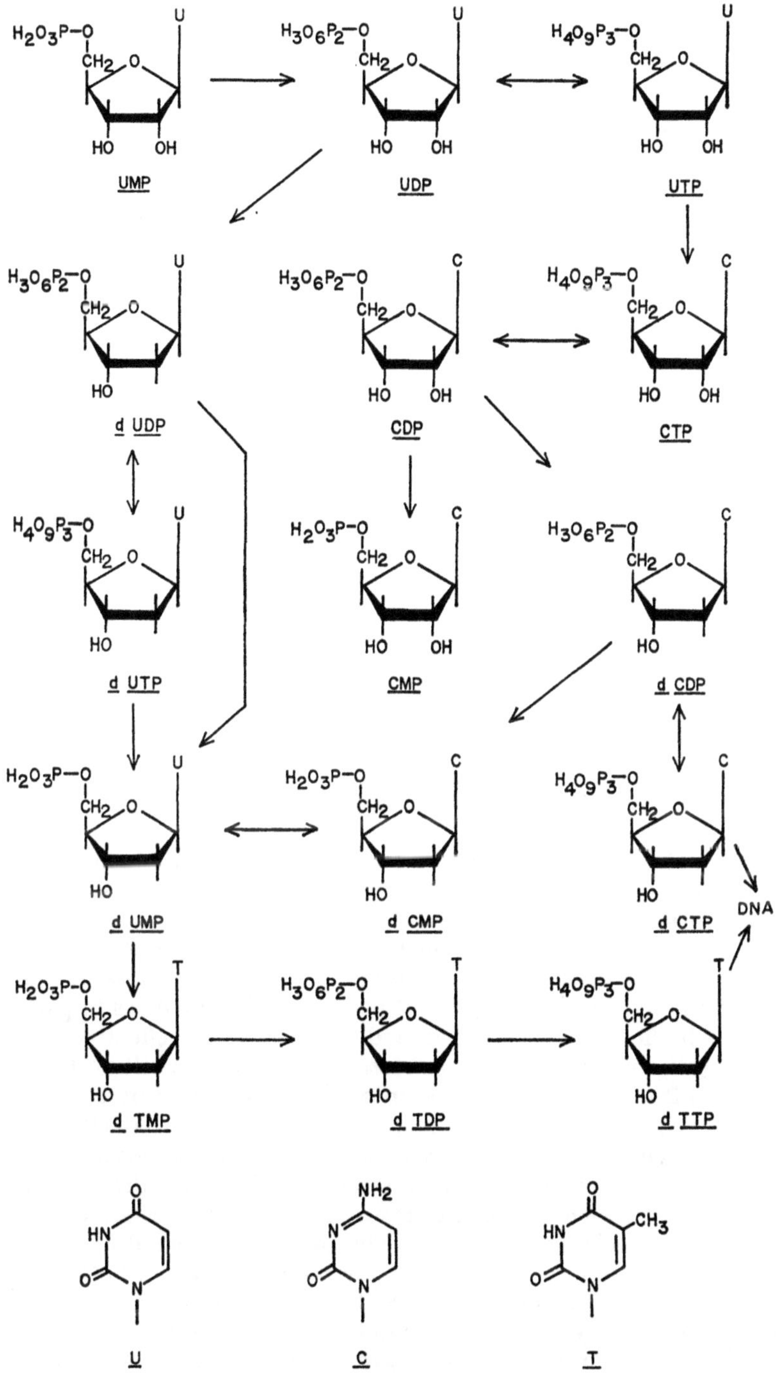


*de novo* pathway

brief mention of pyrimidine nucleosides included, have been published (CHENG, 1969; CHENG and ROTH, 1970, 1971). The pyrimidines, as well as the corresponding nucleosides, may interfere with nucleic acid synthesis in several ways, e. g., the inhibition of a specific enzyme essential for the normal biosynthesis of pyrimidine nucleotides via the *de novo* pathway or in the polymerization to RNA or DNA by competing with the normal substrate. In general, the synthetic compounds function as antimetabolites and are converted into the corresponding analog nucleotides which may then be incorporated into nucleic acids to form fraudulent, but not necessarily defective, polymers, or they may exert a regulatory influence by acting in place of a natural feedback inhibitor either at an allosteric site or in enzyme synthesis. Another area of importance is the "salvage" pathway which uses the products from nucleic acid degradation for the resynthesis of pyrimidine nucleotides. This pathway, shown to be operative in various mammalian tumors

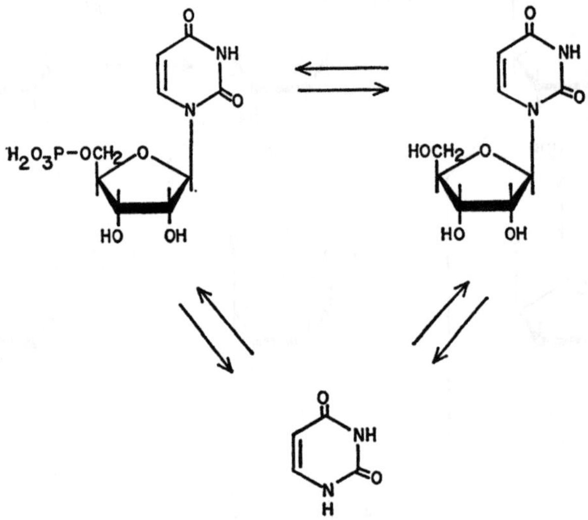


Salvage pathway

(MATSUSHITA and FANBURG, 1970), plays a major role in pyrimide nucleotide synthesis with the two most active enzymes (uridine phosphorylase and uridine kinase) using uracil and uridine as substrates.

The main problem in the development of an effective chemotherapeutic agent is that of selective cytotoxicity, the killing or producing a loss of viability of cancer cells without harming the normal host cells. This involves in part a determination of whether an agent exerts a differential lethal effect on cells at all stages of the cell cycle or acts only in certain phases of the cell cycle.

The entry or transport of nucleosides into cells is also of considerable importance (OLIVER and PATERSON, 1970). In fact, it has been reported (PATERSON and OLIVER, 1971) that the transport of nucleosides does not occur via a simple diffusion process but rather by the interaction of nucleosides with a carrier mechanism in the cell membrane, since it was observed that certain purine nucleosides could inhibit nucleoside transport. This system was found to possess broad specificity in that ribonucleosides and deoxyribonucleosides of both purines and pyrimidines may act as substrates. A recent report (LIEU et al., 1971) suggests that the transport of pyrimidine nucleosides in human erythrocytes occurs by a facilitated diffusion mechanism, although the possibility of a complex carrier mechanism was not ruled out. Phosphorylation may also act as a regulating factor for pyrimidine nucleoside uptake across the cell membrane (SCHUSTER and HARE, 1971), since uptake appears to be directly correlated with the level of the specific kinase which is available in the cell.

The rate at which deoxyribonucleoside triphosphates are formed is believed to be a major control point in regulating the synthesis of DNA, and the inhibition of ribonucleotide reductase appears to be an important site for inhibiting the synthesis of DNA. The conversion of pyrimidine nucleosides into the corresponding deoxyribonucleotides by rat thymus cells can be inhibited *in vitro* by the addition of certain purine deoxyribonucleosides. These deoxyribonucleosides seem to affect not only the reductase system, but also cellular uptake and initial phosphorylation (THOMSON et al., 1971).

An in depth discussion (JONES, 1971) of the regulation of pyrimidine nucleotide biosynthesis in mammals has emphasized that future studies on the regulation of the pyrimidine nucleotide biosynthetic pathways requires a more detailed knowledge of the enzymes in these pathways. These studies are essential for rational design and synthesis of cytotoxic agents (e.g. pyrimidine nucleosides) designed to inhibit pyrimidine nucleotide biosynthesis. Complicating factors exist, however, as shown by a recent report which indicates that the first three enzymes [carbamyl phosphate synthetase (CPSase), aspartate transcarbamylase (ATCase) and dihydroorotase (DHOase)] of the *de novo* pyrimidine nucleotide biosynthetic pathway in Ehrlich ascites tumor cells may exist as a complex, rather than as separate entities. A further complication is provided by the finding (SHOAF and JONES, 1971) that the enzyme pyrimidine nucleoside phosphorylase, possesses both uridine phosphorylase and thymidine phosphorylase activities and cleaves both ribonucleosides and deoxyribonucleosides. The relative $\Delta_{max}$ values were noteworthy, since for several common substrates, uridine was the best substrate, followed by 5-bromodeoxyuridine, 5-bromouridine, 5-methyluridine, thymidine, and deoxyuridine. The rate for 5-bromodeoxyuridine was approximately 5 times that of the other deoxynucleosides used and would indicate that this enzyme may possess greatest affinity for pyrimidine deoxynucleosides halogenated at position 5. Uracil arabinoside was cleaved at about 10% the rate of uridine, while cytidine was not cleaved. Thus, the source as well as the purity of specific enzymes remains a critical factor in the design of pyrimidine nucleosides as potential antineoplastic agents with selective toxicity. The isolation and characterization of enzymes previously undetected will also have a major effect on the design of cytotoxic agents, e.g., the isolation of a reverse-transcriptase (RNA-dependent DNA-polymerase) associated with RNA oncogenic viruses has revived considerable interest in the synthesis of deoxyribonucleosides (TEMIN and MITZUTANI, 1970; BALTIMORE, 1970). This interest has been further stimulated by a report (REID and ALBERT, 1972) of RNA dependent DNA polymerase activity in human tumors with no observed activity in the corresponding normal tissues. The space provided is insufficient for a comprehensive treatment of the area described by the title of this section. Therefore, we shall illustrate by the use of specific examples, e.g. the epimerization of a hydroxyl group on a carbohydrate, the change in lipophilic and hydrophobic character, the conversion of functional groups on the heterocycle, the effect of introducing halogens on both the carbohydrate and heterocycle, the exchange of an original atom in the heterocycle for another atom, the extrusion of an atom from the heterocycle, how conformation may be a factor, and how certain changes may be used in a general fashion for the rational design of cytotoxic agents. We should like to emphasize that these examples are used only to illustrate the principles of rational design for the synthesis of pyrimidine nucleoside derivatives exhibiting cytotoxicity.

## Design of Pyrimidine Nucleosides as Cytotoxic Agents

We shall start our discussion on the actual rational design of pyrimidine nucleosides as cytotoxic agents by illustrating how a minor structural change in the naturally occurring pyrimidine nucleosides can affect their cytotoxicity and chemotherapeutic activity. The classic example in this area is the simple epimerization of the 2'-hydroxyl group of the carbohydrate moiety of cytidine to afford 4-amino-1-(β-D-arabinofuranosyl)pyrimidin-2-one (I, ara-C) (WALWICH et al., 1959). Ara-C has been found to inhibit human leukemia (HOWARD et al., 1966) and

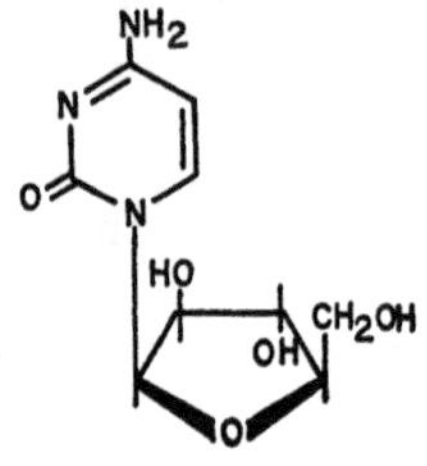

I

various other tumors both *in vivo* and *in vitro*. It has been established (NODINSKI and KENSLER, 1965) that 2'-deoxycytidine can partially reverse the cytostatic activity of ara-C in certain instances. Ara-C has also been found (CHU and FISCHER, 1968a, b) to inhibit the incorporation of radioactive precursors into DNA via the *de novo* synthetic pathway but not into RNA. Furthermore, it has been shown that ara-C as the 5'-triphosphate acts as a potent inhibitor of DNA polymerase (FURTH and COHEN, 1968) and possibly of the reduction of CDP to dCDP. This has been supported by the finding (SCHRECKER and URSHEL, 1968) that ara-C enhances the incorporation of deoxycytidine into DNA through a stimulation of deoxycytidine kinase which favors the phosphorylation of deoxycytidine over ara-C. Ara-C has been found (KARON and SHIRAKAWA, 1969) to be most effective in the *S*-phase of the mitotic cycle and also to be an inhibitor at sites other than those described above. The above reports afford only a brief and incomplete insight into the chemotherapeutic and biological activity of ara-C; however, this subject is covered in detail in another chapter.

There has been found an increase in dCTP in cells resistant to ara-C, a finding consistent with increased activity of CDP reductase (CAMIENER and SMITH, 1965). A large increase in dCMP deaminase activity, which can convert ara-C monophosphate into the inactive uridine analog spongouridine *(vide infra)* via the corresponding nucleotide, has also been observed and was followed by other studies on the physiological distribution of ara-C in tumor-bearing mice (UCHIDA and KREIS, 1969). Inhibition of this enzymatic deamination should enhance the cyototoxicity and presumably the chemotherapeutic and biological activity of ara-C.

1-(β-D-Ribofuranosyl)-4-hydroxytetrahydropyrimidin-2-one (HANZE, 1967) (II, $H_4U$), also termed tetrahydrouridine, is a potent and specific inhibitor of the enzymatic deamination of ara-C by a preparation from human liver, mouse kidney, rhesus monkey liver (CAMIENER, 1968) and a purified cytidine deaminase from *E. coli* (COHEN and WOLFENDEN, 1971). $H_4U$ requires preincubation with the enzyme for optimum effectiveness and this results in a noncompetitive inhibition of enzyme action. This action is in direct contrast to that of hydroxylamino-5-methyl-1-(2-deoxy-β-D-ribofuranosyl)pyrimidin-2-one (III) (FOX et al., 1959), which was reported (CAMIENER, 1967) to be in direct competition with ara-C for the active site. These results are of interest since 4-hydroxylamino-1-(β-D-ribofuranosyl) pyrimidin-2-one will substitute for uridine as a pyrimidine supplement for the growth of *E. coli*, but only after it is converted to cytidine or

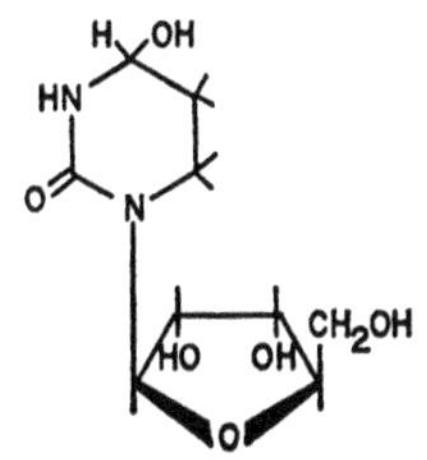

II

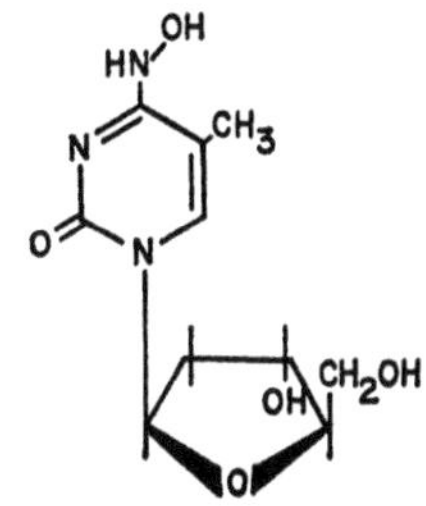

III

uridine. Further study (Trimble and Maley, 1971) suggested that a direct dehydroxylamination occurred rather than a reduction to cytidine with a subsequent deamination.

A new approach to preventing the inactivation of ara-C involves a modification of ara-C per se, which would (a) inhibit deamination and (b) subsequently furnish ara-C by an *in vivo* conversion of this derivative to ara-C. This prompted the synthesis of ara-C-3-*N*-oxide (IV) which furnished (Panzica et al., 1971) a nucleoside designed to be resistant toward cytidine deaminase and yet be slowly released *in vivo* to ara-C by a reduction of the *N*-oxide function. Another nucleoside in this same category is 2,2′-*O*-cyclocytidine (V) (Kanai et al., 1970; Kigukawa and Ichino, 1972), which is effective against L1210 leukemia (Hoshi et al., 1971). This activity is most likely due to the resistance of V toward deamination by cytidine deaminase (cytidine aminohydrolase) (Hoshi et al., 1972).

L-Adenosine is deaminated by adenosine deaminase (Shimizu et al., 1965) only 50% as fast as D-adenosine. By analogy, it could be assumed that 1-(β-L-arabinofuranosyl)cytosine (VI, L-ara-C) should undergo deamination by cytidine deamin-

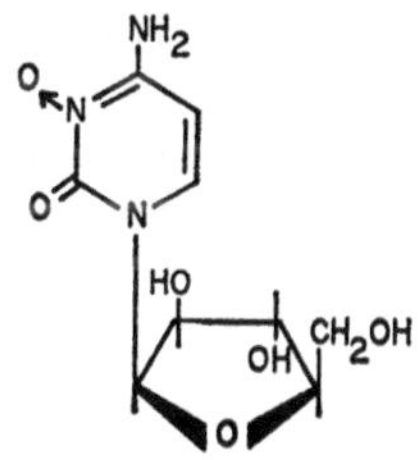

IV

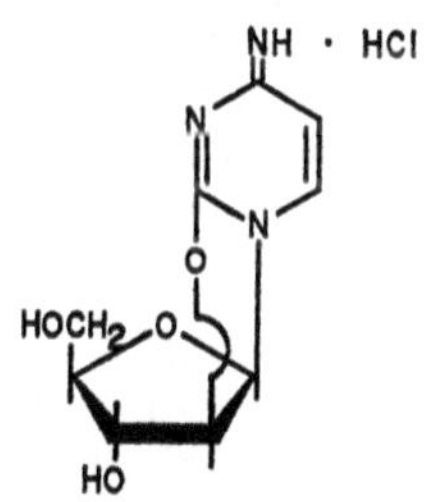

V

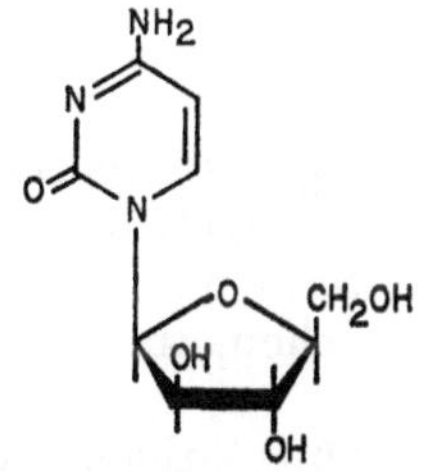

VI

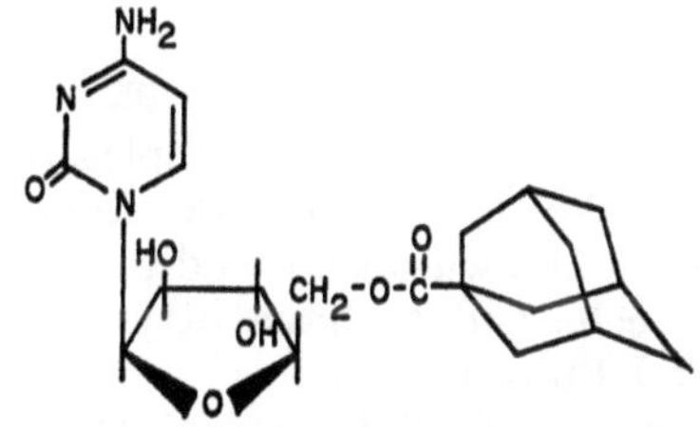

VII

ase much more slowly than ara-C. Such a decrease in the rate of deamination was indeed observed in *E. coli* (Tolman and Robins, 1971; Gish et al., 1971) presumably due to the fact that (VI) did not function as a substrate for cytidine deaminase in this system. However, (VI) was found (Tolman and Robins, 1971; Gish et al., 1971) to be devoid of any significant antitumor activity against leukemia L1210 and Ridgeway osteogenic sarcoma. These results are similar to those reported (Yamaoka et al., 1968) for several α-L-arabino-, α-L-xylo- and α-L-lyxo derivatives of thymine, uracil and cytosine, and would seem to indicate that both the α and β anomers of L-glycosyl pyrimidines may be one of the less rewarding areas for future anticancer research.

When uridine was administered in conjunction with a suboptimal dose of ara-C to BDF1 mice bearing leukemia L1210, a very significant increase in life span was observed (Saslaw et al., 1968); there was essentially no effect produced by thymidine and several other uracil derivatives. However, the use of uridine with an optimal dose of ara-C caused toxicity which was apparently due to increased localization of ara-C in the spleen.

Synthesis of an ara-C derivative [Adamantoyl Cytarabine, 1-(5′-1-adamantanecarboxylate)-β-D-arabinofuranosylcytosine (AdOCA) (VII)], was followed by a report (Neil et al., 1970) on its efficacy as a significant inhibitor of growth in a mouse leukemia system (L1210). Compound VII exhibits an increase in duration of antileukemic and immunosuppressive activity in comparison with ara-C per se. Subsequent studies (Gish et al., 1971; Gray et al., 1972) have used a series (19) of 5′-esters of ara-C to establish that the properties of VII were due not only to the adamantane moiety, but would probably be exhibited by any group that would appropriately affect the rate of dissolution, lipophilicity, rate of hydrolysis, resistance to cytidine deaminase and other essential properties of these nucleoside derivatives (Howard et al., 1966). It may well be that the efficacy of these 5′-esters is dependent on their ability to act as substrates for specific *in vivo* esterases and this selectivity or specificity may be the predominant factor in the distribution and ultimate availability of ara-C at the active site.

Derivatives of uridine might be expected to exhibit some properties similar to those discussed above for cytidine. A simple epimerization of the hydroxyl group at *C*-2 of the carbohydrate moiety of uridine has furnished 1-(β-D-arabinofuranosyl)pyrimidin-2,4(3H)-dione (VIII, ara-U) which is the uridine analog of ara-C. Although one might expect antitumor activity on the basis of the reported activity

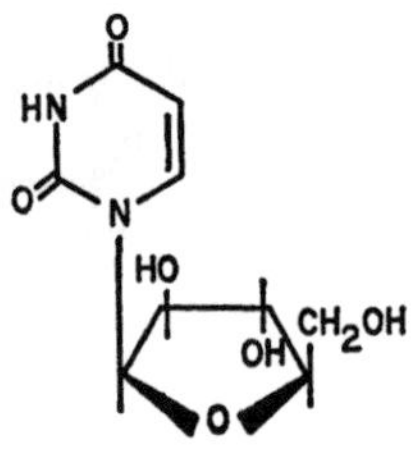


VIII

of ara-C, VIII was found to be completely inactive against several tumor lines (Goldin et al., 1968). A nucleoside, isolated from *C. crypta* and subsequently characterized as VIII, was also found to possess essentially no toxicity or activity against tumor cells and to have little biological or chemotherapeutic activity (Bergmann and Burke, 1955).

The thio analogs of uridine are of some interest since 2-thiouridine (Carbon et al., 1965) and 4-thiouridine (Lipsett, 1965) have both been isolated as minor nucleosides from tRNA, as well as chemically synthesized (Fox et al., 1959; UEDA et al., 1968). Several thiopyrimidine nucleosides which have been isolated from yeast and *E. coli* tRNA were postulated to be in the first position of the anticodon with a possible specific role in codon recognition. The first thiopyrimidine nucleoside isolated from a mammalian tRNA was characterized (KUMURA-HARADA et al., 1971) as 5-methyl-2-thiouridine (IX). This minor nucleoside was also postulated to reside in the first position of the anticodon of rat liver $tRNA^{glu}$

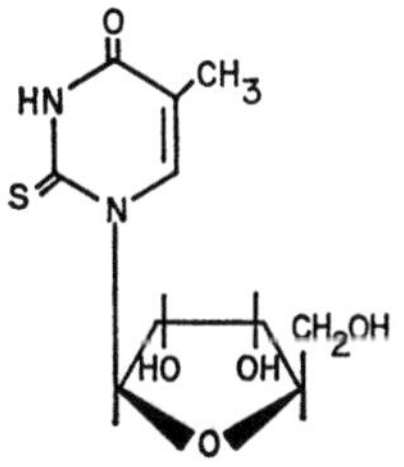

IX

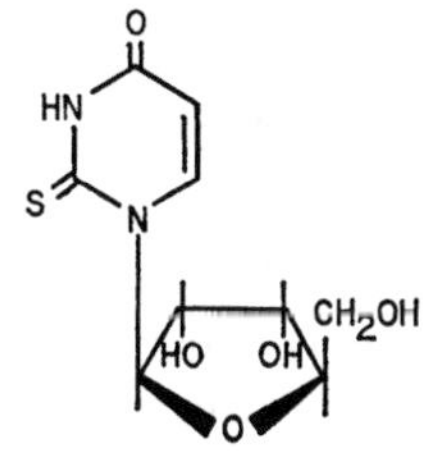

X

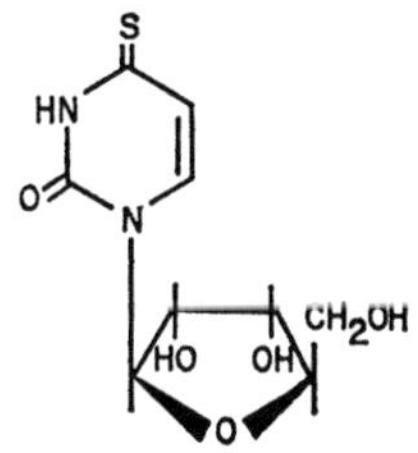

XI

and $tRNA^{Lys}$. A study (LOZZIO and WIGLER, 1971) on the cytotoxicity of 2-thiouridine and 4-thiouridine (X and XI, respectively) in cultures of Chinese hamster cells revealed maximum sensitivity at the late $G_1$ and $G_2$ phases of the cell cycle. It was postulated on this basis that inhibition was possibly due to interference with the synthesis of some species of RNA. In fact, it was postulated that inhibition of the formation of cytoplasmic RNA was due to interruption of the synthesis of ribosomal RNA which in turn would also interfere with protein synthesis. It was also established that DNA synthesis was not affected by the same concentrations of cytotoxic thiopyrimidine nucleosides. Of considerable interest, is the recent report (PLEISS and CERUTTI, 1971) on the selective transformation of 4-thiouridine in *E. coli* $tRNA^{Val}$ to uridine upon irradiation in t-butanol. This resulted in only a 19% reduction in the capacity of the tRNA to accept valine, suggesting that 4-thiouridine in tRNA, at least from this source, was not required as a specific recognition site for valyl-tRNA synthetase. This indicates that the activity of 4-thiouridine is most probably related to conformation rather than to the recognition site. The initial product formed during irradiation of $tRNA^{Val}$ is covalently linked between 4-thiouridine in the 8th position, and cytidine in the 13th position (FAVRE et al., 1971). There did not appear to be any change in the size and shape of the molecule and it was postulated that this modification exerts only a small local change in the tertiary structure of the tRNA. The change in biological properties of this irradiated tRNA also seems to be very minor in nature (YANIV et al., 1971) and has been corroborated by a study which demonstrated that the chemical modification of 4-thiouridine does not result in a loss of aminoacyl-$tRNA^{Phe}$ formation (SHUGART, 1972). This latter finding has led to the proposal that the cognate ligase recognition site for this specific $tRNA^{Phe}$ is located in the non-hydrogen bonded dihydrouridine loop area of the molecule and supports the proposal that 4-thiouridine is not in this area, but resides in a region adjacent to this loop. The facile conversion of 4-thiouridine to other products, e.g. treatment with nitrous acid to furnish uridine via *bis*-4-thiouridine (IIDA and HAYATSU, 1971), photoreduction to afford the product, 1-(β-D-ribofuranosyl)hexahydropyrimidin-2-one (XII) (SATO and KANAOKA, 1969), which was also obtained by sodium borohydride reduction of 4-thiouridine in the dark (CERUTTI et al., 1965), etc., would suggest that this is indeed a fertile area for the synthesis of cytotoxic pyrimidine nucleosides. The incorporation of thiopyrimidine nucleosides into RNA and DNA could provide an excellent method for the introduction of controlled cytotoxicity due to a selective modification of the macromolecule at a specific site, i.e., the specific thiopyrimidine nucleoside. In this respect, a recent

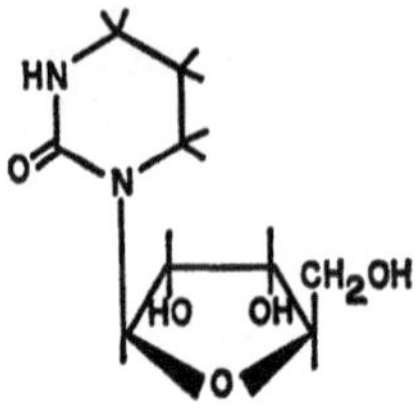


XII

study of some interest is the report that 2-thiouracil can be converted to 2-thiouridylic acid by the salvage pathway enzyme UMP pyrophosphorylase isolated from *Lactobacillus leichmannii* (LINDSAY et al., 1972). 2-Thiouridylic acid was also found to function as a substrate for a 5′-nucleotidase to afford 2-thiouridine.

A closely related area with considerable potential involves the synthesis of corresponding selenopyrimidine nucleosides, particularly since the seleno analogs of the naturally occurring sulfur containing amino acids have been isolated and found to function as substrates for certain enzymatic reactions as effectively as the naturally occurring sulfur-containing amino acids., e.g. the use of selenomethionine in place of methionine during aminoacyl-tRNA synthesis in *E. coli* (HOFFMANN et al., 1970). These nucleosides, have not (at the present time) been isolated from naturally occurring sources; however, this may only be due to hydrolysis during isolation and a specific modification of isolation procedures in the future may well provide several selenopyrimidine nucleosides as minor components of certain RNA species. In fact, the synthesis of 2-selenouridine and 4-selenouridine (WISE and TOWNSEND, 1972) has established that the lability of the exocyclic seleno group of these selenopyrimidine nucleosides is very similar to that reported for selenopurine nucleosides (TOWNSEND and MILNE, 1970; MILNE and TOWNSEND, 1972; MILNE and TOWNSEND, 1973) and tends to support the assumption that selenonucleosides will be isolated in the very near future from RNA species. The introduction of a mercapto or thio group at the 5-position of 2′-deoxyuridine furnished 5-mercapto-2′-deoxyuridine (XIII) (KOTICK et al., 1969) which has demonstrated cytotoxicity and some *in vivo* and *in vitro* antitumor activity against

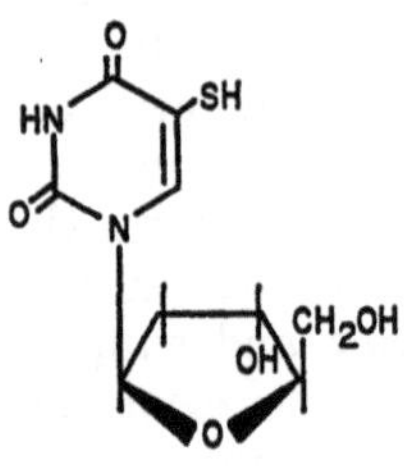


XIII

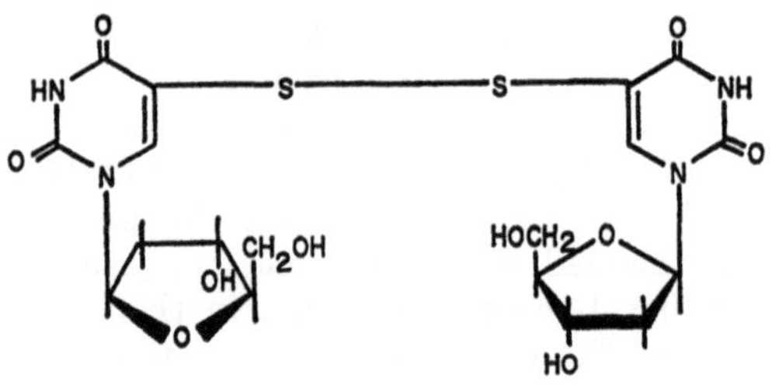


XIV

leukemia L1210 in mice, and the complete eradication of multiple superfical basal cell carcinomas in man (SCHWARTZ et al., 1970). A recent study on the mode of action of XIII has established that it is converted to the 5′-phosphate derivative by thymidine kinase and the 5′-phosphate derivative then inhibits thymidylate synthetase (Kalman and Bardos, 1970). The same study indicated that the *S*-methyl derivative of XIII was also phosphorylated by thymidine kinase, while the disulfide nucleoside (XIV) was apparently not a substrate. It is tempting to assume that the reason XIV is not a substrate, may be a conformational problem, since XIV most likely exists in the anti conformation, and if this nucleoside should assume the anti-anti conformation, there would be a considerable amount of steric inhibition in approaching the active or binding site of thymidine kinase. The seleno derivatives of these nucleosides should also be of considerable interest, since the seleno group would most likely be in anionic form, whereas the thio group would be predominately in the nonionized form.

The introduction of other groups at the 5-position of uridine has induced a significant change in cytotoxicity and other biological activity. 5-Aminouridine (XV) (Roberts and Visser, 1952) possesses a wide range of biological activity including some antitumor activity (Visser, 1955). This compound has also been shown to be incorporated into the RNA of Ehrlich ascites cells and metabolized to 5′-mono-, di-, and triphosphate derivatives, with the 5′-monophosphate derivative being a potent inhibitor of orotidylic (OMP) decarboxylase (Smith et al., 1966). It has been reported (Eidinoff et al., 1959) that XV can also inhibit the incorporation of carbamylaspartate into pyrimidine nucleotides of RNA and DNA in rat liver. The closely related compound, 5-methylamino-2-deoxyuridine, was found to be a potent antiherpes agent (Shen et al., 1966). Several derivatives related to XV, 5-*N*-peptidyl derivatives of 5-aminouridine, have been recently prepared (Ivanovics et al., 1971) because of the isolation of 5-alanyluracil from

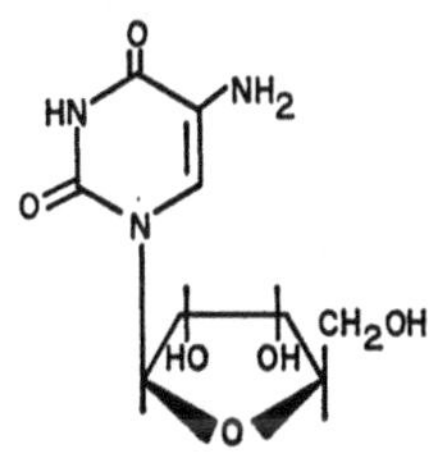

XV

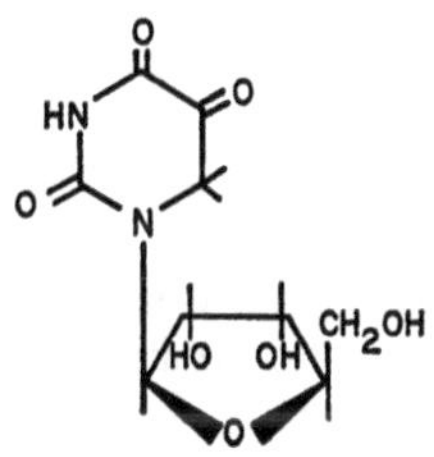

XVI

germinating pea seeds (Brown and Silver, 1966). This nucleoside possesses essentially no activity against L1210 leukemia, Walker carcinosarcoma 256, or adenocarcinoma 755 (Goldin et al., 1968). A conversion of XV into 1-(β-D-ribofuranosyl)isobarbituric acid (XVI) was found to provide a small increase, albeit not of a significant magnitude, in activity against leukemia L1210 (Goldin et al., 1968). However, a conversion of the 5-amino group of XV to a 5-diazo group by treatment with nitrous acid has furnished the only uracil riboside derivative (5-diazouridine) with antitumor activity of significant magnitude to be included in a comprehensive study (Goldin et al., 1968). The structure reported in the study has been revised to 1-(β-D-ribofuranosyl)-$O^5$-6(*S*)-cyclo-5-diazo-1,6-dihydropyrimidin-2,4-(3H, 6H)-dione (XVIII, 5-diazouridine) (Thurber and Townsend, 1971; Abraham et al., 1971). However, a more recent evaluation of antitumor potency has revealed only marginal activity against leukemia L1210 for both XVII and the corresponding 2-deoxy derivative, 1-(2-deoxy-β-D-ribofuranosyl)-$O^5$-6(*S*)-cyclo-5-diazo-1,6-dihydropyrimidin-2,4-(3H,6H)-dione (XVIII, 5-diazo-2-deoxyuridine) (Townsend, 1972a). A visual inspection of structures XVII and XVIII reveals that there may be some conjecture as to whether these compounds should even be classified as uracil ribofuranosides. This diazotization is of interest since it has been shown that Newcastle disease and Western equine encephalomyelitis viruses, which were grown in the presence of XV, were hypersensitized toward the action of nitrous acid (Thiry, 1966). There was observed a

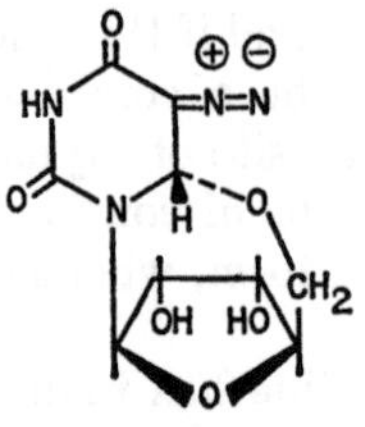

XVII

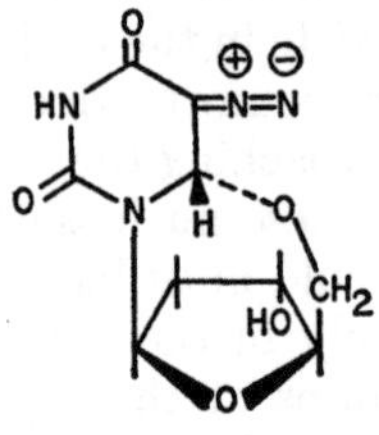

XVIII

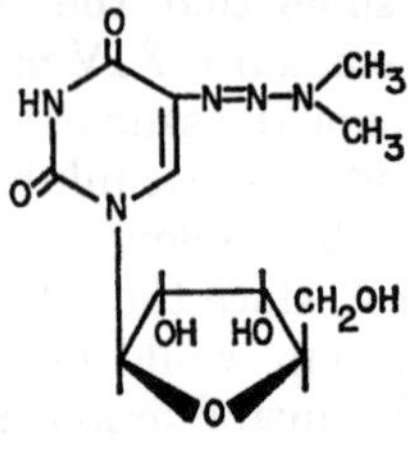

XIX

7-fold increase in susceptibility toward nitrous acid, presumed to be substitution of XV for uridine during biosynthesis. The obvious effect of simple deamination would be the conversion of XV to XVI, while diazotization would convert XV to XVII, and if prior incorporation of XV into nucleic acids had occurred, there would be observed either a cleavage of the glycosidic bond or a cleavage of a phosphodiester bond. Treatment of XVII with dimethylamine has furnished 5-(3,3-dimethyl-1-triazenol)-1-(β-D-ribofuranosyl)pyrimidin-2,4-(3H)dione (XIX) and the antitumor activity against leukemia L1210 of XIX is far superior to that reported for XVII (Goldin et al., 1968; Townsend, 1972a). In fact, it has been recently reported that XIX exhibited a $T/C$ (ratio of the survival time of treated to untreated tumor-bearing animals) of 300 at 200 mg/kg, 100 mg/kg, and 50 mg/kg with 6 of 6 cures at the 2 lower dose levels, against P-388 lymphocytic leukemia (Townsend, 1971). There is no data available at the present time for the corresponding 2-deoxy derivative of XIX.

The 5-halo uracil ribosides have shown some very interesting activity and will be discussed very briefly since this area will be covered in detail in other chapters of this book. The antitumor activity of 5-fluorouracil has prompted the synthesis and evaluation of numerous derivatives. 5-Fluorouridine (XX) has

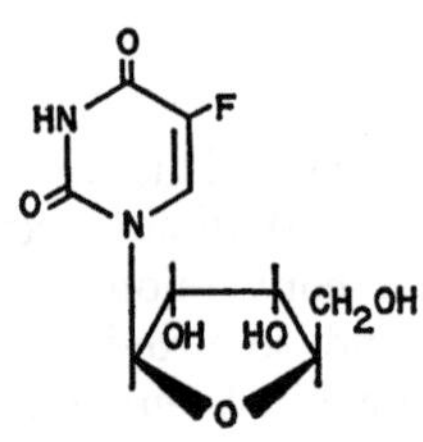

XX

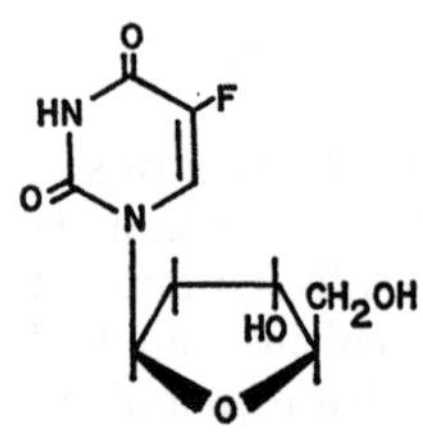

XXI

demonstrated some antitumor activity, although 5-fluoro-2′-deoxyuridine (XXI) has shown greater activity than XX against leukemia L1210, Walker carcinosarcoma 256, adenocarcinoma 755, sarcoma 180, and Lewis lung carcinoma (Goldin et al., 1968). The α-anomer of XXI and the arabinosyl derivative [1-(β-D-arabinofuranosyl)-5-fluorouracil] demonstrated essentially no activity against leukemia L1210 (Goldin et al., 1968). This finding is of interest, since 5-fluoro-1-(tetrahydrofuran-2-yl)pyrimidin-2,4(3H)-dione (XXII, fluorafur or ftorafur) (Hiller et al., 1967) possesses essentially the same antitumor activity against certain tumors of the gastro-intestinal tract as 5-FU, but with a 5- to

6-fold decrease in toxicity, thereby increasing the chemotherapeutic index (KRAVCHENKO and ZIDERMANE, 1968; HILLER et al., 1968). An alternate route has been reported for the preparation of XXII and involves a direct fluorination of 1-(tetrahydrofuran-2-yl)uracil (EARL and TOWNSEND, 1972). A number of closely related tetrahydrofuran-2-yl 5-substituted pyrimidines and the correspond-

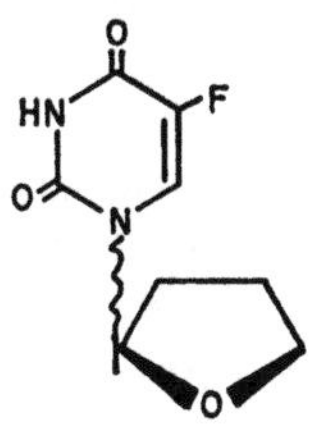


XXII

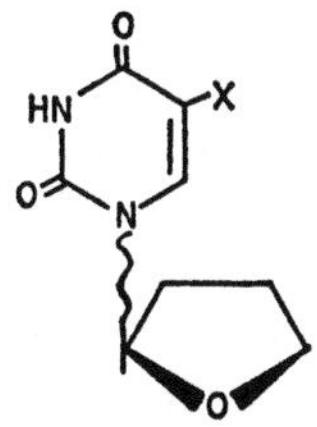


XXIII

X = $CH_3$, Br, I

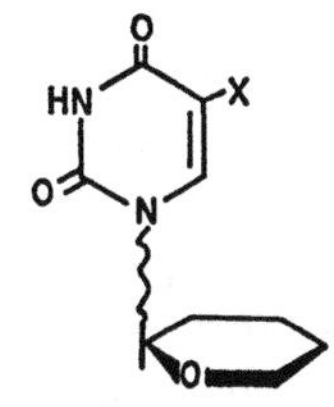


XXIV

ing tetrahydropyran-2-yl analogs of the general formulas XXIII and XXIV, as well as the cytidine analogs, had been synthesized earlier (NOELL and CHENG, 1966, 1968), but have shown very little antitumor activity. This would suggest that a study on ftorafur should be initiated to determine if this modification has merely provided an increase in mobility *in vivo* and possibly acts as a depot form of 5-FU. However, in general it appears that the other 5-halo (bromo, iodo, chloro) uracil furanosides possess very little antitumor activity, although the 5-halo-2′-deoxyribofuranosyluracils have shown some biological and chemotherapeutic activity, e. g., XXV. In this same general area, 5-trifluoro-

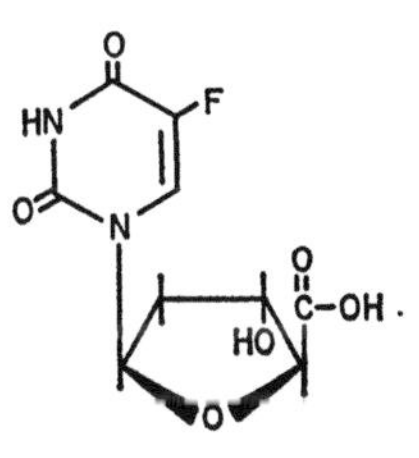


XXV

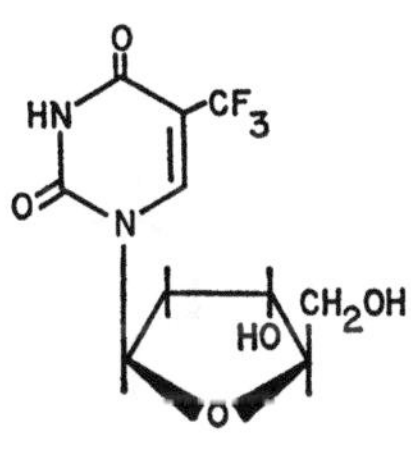


XXVI

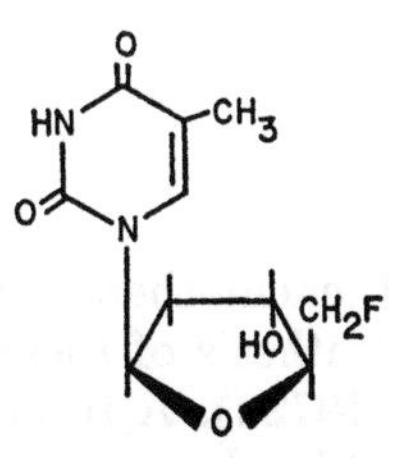


XXVII

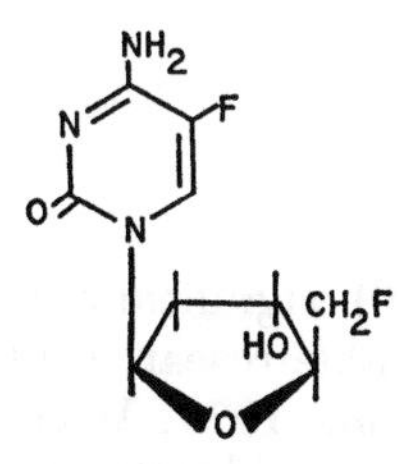


XXVIII

methyl-2′-deoxyuridine (XXVI, $F_3$TDR) (HEIDELBERGER et al., 1964) is presently being studied in the clinic (ANSFIELD and RAMIREZ, 1971), and has been reported to be less toxic than 5-FU and 5-FUDR in the monkey, but more toxic in the dog. A recent study has established that no correlation exists between the extent of catabolism of XXVI and its clinical efficacy (DEXTER et al., 1972).

5′-Fluoro-5′-deoxythymidine (XXVII) and several related derivatives were tested as inhibitors of thymidylate kinase in cells obtained from the Ehrlich ascites carcinoma and XXVII was found to be the most effective. Synthesis of the corresponding cytidine derivative has also been accomplished, as well as several additional 5-substituted derivatives, e. g. XXVIII (LANGEN et al., 1969, KOWOLLIK et al., 1970a, b). 1-β-D-Arabinofuranosyl-5-fluorocytosine (ara-FC) was found to be a somewhat more active derivative than ara-C (BURCHENAL et al., 1966). The 2,2′-anhydro derivative of ara-FC has been prepared (FOX et al., 1972) and exhibited an increase in antitumor activity, apparently due to its ability to act as a slow-release form of ara-FC. Several other pyrimidine nucleosides with halogen groups residing on the carbohydrate moiety have been synthesized, although none of them has displayed outstanding anticancer activity.

The isolation and characterization of blasticidin S (TAKEUCHI et al., 1958; YONEHARA and OTAKE, 1966) and gougerotin (KANZAKI et al., 1962; FOX et al., 1968) as cytosine nucleosides which exhibited (TOWNSEND and ROBINS, 1970;

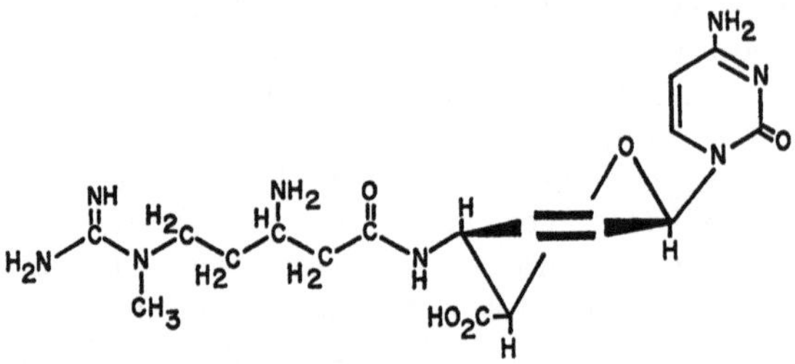

Gougerotin

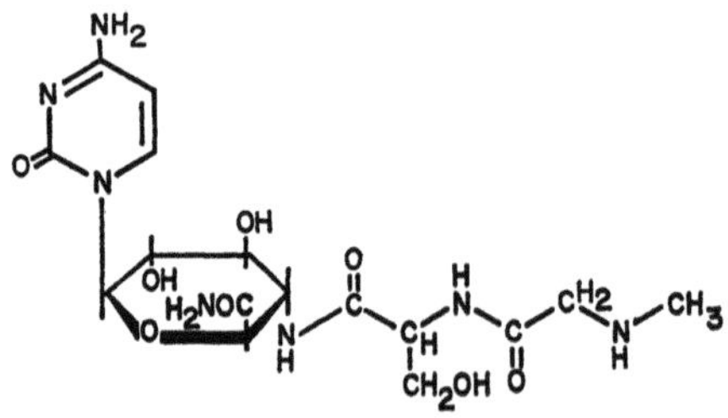

Blasticidin S

SUHADOLNIK, 1970) significant biological and chemotherapeutic activity has prompted considerable research into the total synthesis of these nucleoside antibiotics (GOODY et al., 1970; WATANABE et al., 1972a). A total synthesis of the nucleoside component of blasticidin S (cytosinine) has been accomplished (KONDO et al., 1972), and should stimulate additional interest in this area which will lead to a total synthesis of blasticidin S. In the case of gougerotin, this has stimulated research in the area of 4-amino-4-deoxy-hexo-pyranose derivatives. This has prompted research in the total synthesis of "C-substance" (WATANABE et al., 1970, 1972b), a degradation product of gougerotin which was required as a precursor for the total chemical synthesis of gougerotin. The synthesis of a nucleoside, 1-(4-amino-4-deoxy-β-D-glucopyranosyl)uracil, which is very closely related to "C-substance" and its immediate precursors, has been reported (KONDO and GOTO, 1971); however, since it is a uridine analog, there is some doubt as to its potential as an antineoplastic agent.

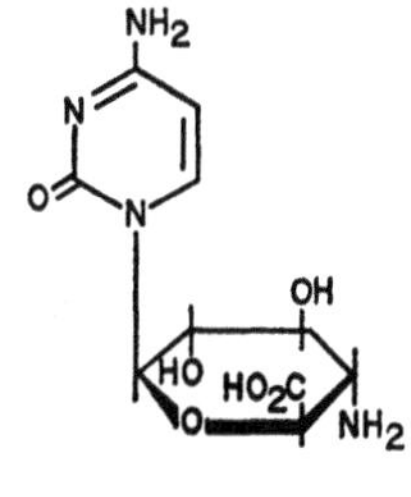


C-SUBSTANCE

A number of antibiotics have been isolated from a broth produced by *Streptomyces cocaoi var. asoensis* (HORI et al., 1971), characterized as uridine derivatives (ISONO et al., 1969), and given the names polyoxins A–M. These antibiotics have demonstrated the ability to inhibit cell wall chitin synthesis of some phytopatho-

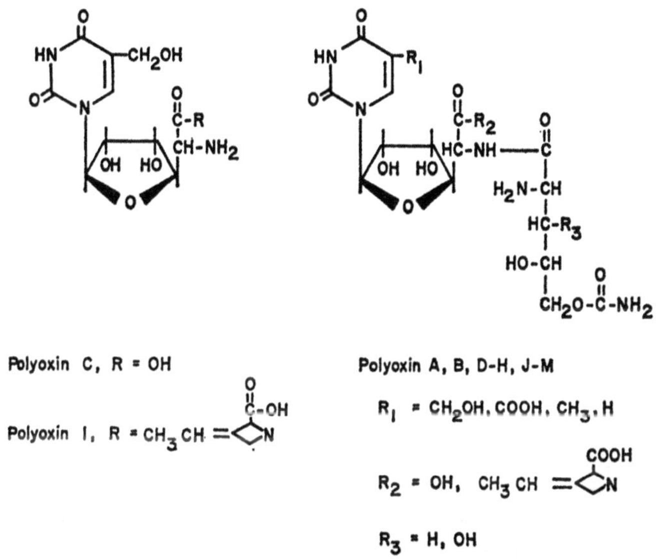


genic fungi. The polyoxins can be classified as aminoacyl nucleosides and may therefore be considered in the same general category as the nucleoside antibiotics gougerotin and blasticidin S, which have been established as inhibitors of protein synthesis. The one feature of especial interest in this area is the fact that most of the effective pyrimidine nucleoside antibiotics have been cytosine nucleosides, whereas the polyoxins are uracil nucleosides. The basic nucleoside structure of the polyoxins (XXVIII a) has been recently synthesized chemically from uridine (DAMODARAN et al., 1971) and a route for the synthesis of 1-(5-amino-5-deoxy-$\beta$-D-allofuranuronosyl)thymine (thymine polyoxin C) has been reported (OHRUI et al., 1971) from a condensation of silylated thymine and the appropriate carbohydrate precursor followed by functional group modifications. This would appear to provide alternate routes for the synthesis of polyoxin analogs in several diverse areas. These reports should prompt a significant increase in synthetic activity in this area which will involve not only the direct glycosylation route and chemical transformations of preformed pyrimidine nucleosides, but also modifications of the preformed polyoxins (Isono et al., 1971) and may provide derivatives with

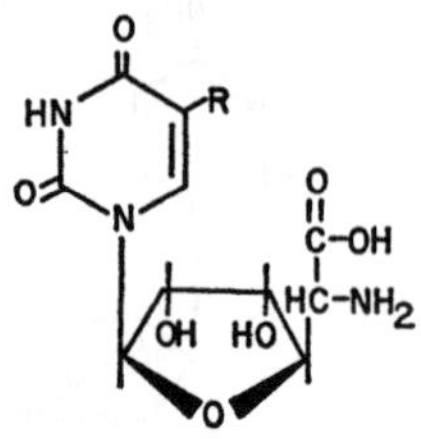

XXVIIIa, R = $-CH_2OH$

Thymine Polyoxin C, R = $-CH_3$

potential antitumor activity. In fact, several 5-fluoropolyoxins have been prepared by a fermentation process (Isono et al., 1973) and were found to inhibit not only fungi, but also *Streptococcus faecalis* and *Escherichia coli*.

5-Allyl-2-deoxyuridine (XXIX) exhibited the capacity to inhibit nucleoside phosphorylase activity associated with mycoplasma contaminated HeLa cells (Holland et al., 1967) and possessed only slight activity against leukemia L1210,

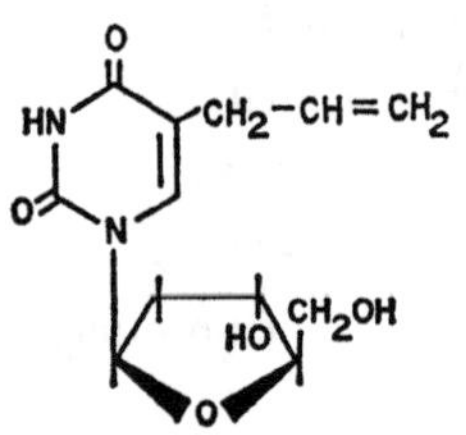

XXIX

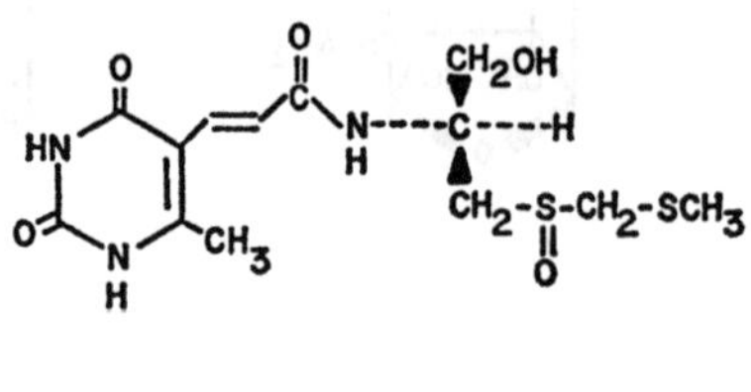

SPARSOMYCIN

but better activity against Walker 256 carcinosarcoma (Goldin et al., 1968). A visual comparison of XXIX and the antibiotic sparsomycin (Wiley and Mackeller, 1970) is of some interest and the synthesis and antitumor evaluation of sparsomycin deoxyriboside should be investigated rather than the riboside derivative, since 5-allyluridine has shown no antitumor activity (Minnemeyer et al., 1963).

Due to the tremendous amount of research which has been accomplished in these areas, which involve cytosine, uracil, cytidine, and uridine derivatives, this discussion could continue almost indefinitely. However, we feel that the above examples, although very brief, should be sufficient to illustrate the primary purpose of this chapter. We should now like to discuss some ancillary aspects of this subject which, although they are not as obvious, are just as interesting and perhaps more important from the standpoint of future research in this area.

The aza and deazapyrimidine nucleosides will be discussed only briefly, since this type of nucleoside will be presented at length in another chapter. 5-Azacytidine (XXX) is the most interesting and important nucleoside of this class and, as the name implies, can be viewed as a simple insertion of a ring nitrogen for the methine group at position five of cytidine. The initial chemical synthesis of XXX

(PÍSKALLA and ŠORM, 1964; WINKLEY and ROBINS, 1970) was followed by the isolation of XXX from *Streptoverticillium ladakanus* (HAŇKA et al., 1966). This latter report (HAŇKA et al., 1966) was of some interest since the usual sequence was reversed with the isolation of XXX being preceded by a chemical synthesis (PÍSKALLA and ŠORM, 1964). 5-Azacytidine is presently in the clinic and shows considerable promise (HRODEK and VESELÝ, 1971). 5-Azacytidine is a substrate for cytidine deaminase which results in the formation of the inactive nucleoside 5-azauridine (ČIHÁK and ŠORM, 1965). This is of interest since 6-azauridine (XXXI) which is structurally almost identical to 5-azauridine, has demonstrated sufficient

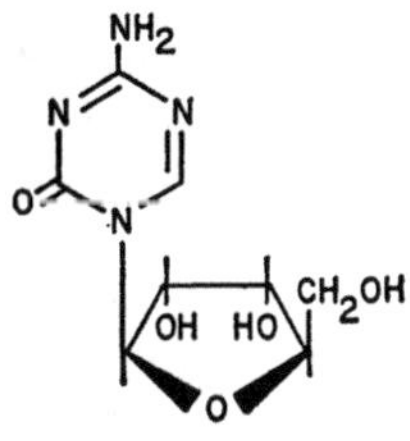


XXX

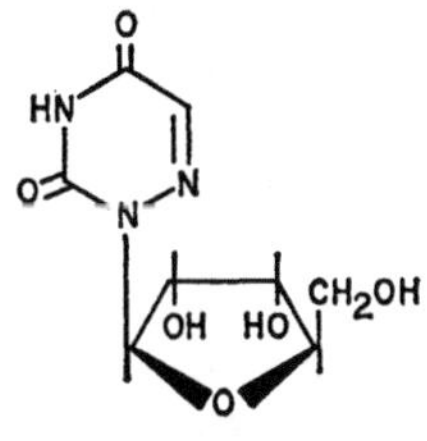


XXXI

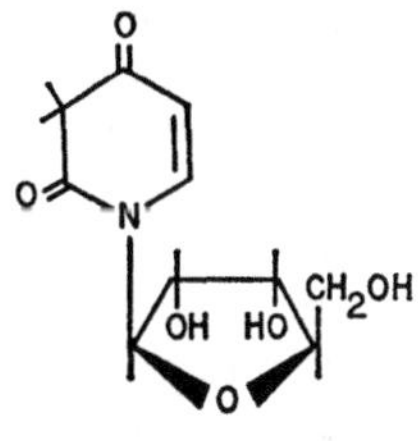


XXXII

activity to be recommended at one time for clinical trial against leukemia (HERNANDEZ et al., 1969). The nucleoside XXXI has shown resistance toward uridine phosphorylase (PONTIS et al., 1961), acts as a substrate for uridine kinase (SKÖLD, 1960) and, as the 5′-nucleotide, has been found to interfere with the *de novo* synthesis of uridine nucleotides by inhibiting orotidylic acid decarboxylase (BRUEMMER et al., 1962). 6-Azauridine has been prepared chemically (HANDSCHUMACHER, 1960; PRYSTAŠ and ŠORM, 1962) and by fermentation procedures (MORAVEK and ŠKODA, 1969). The tri-*O*-acetyl derivative of XXXI has also been used as an antitumor agent; it has been found to produce a high level of certain abnormal amino acids in the serum and would appear to require further study in animals (SLAVÍK et al., 1971). The deaza analogs, 3-deazauridine (XXXII) and 3-deazacytidine, have been synthesized (CURRIE et al., 1970) and on the basis of preliminary studies, the uridine analog appears to be the more active antitumor agent (ROBINS et al., 1969; BLOCH et al., 1972; WANG and BLOCH, 1972).

The minor nucleoside pseudouridine has been isolated (COHN, 1957; DAVIS and ALLEN, 1957; COMB and KATZ, 1964; LANE, 1965), from a variety of tRNA's; in fact, from all tRNA species which have been sequenced (PHILLIPS, 1969). The structure of pseudouridine (XXXIII) was initially established as being 5-D-ribosyluracil (COHN, 1960), with the remaining structural features (anomeric configuration and ring size of the carbohydrate moiety) being subsequently established as beta and furanose (MICHELSON and COHN, 1962). A visual inspection reveals a very close structural similarity between pseudouridine and uridine; there is some evidence for the existence of a pseudouridine kinase since labeled pseudouridine was isolated as mono-, di- and triphosphates from the metabolic pool of a pyrimidine requiring mutant of *E. coli* (GINSBERG and DAVIS, 1968). However, it is not too surprising to find that pseudouridine (like uridine) possesses essentially no antineoplastic activity and that several pyrimidine C-nucleosides derived from pseudouridine are also devoid of antitumor activity (CHAMBERS, 1966; HO and GILHAM, 1971). The chemical synthesis of XXXIII and related derivatives have involved the condensation of a preformed pyrimidine derivative with the appropriate carbohydrate derivative (SHAPIRO and CHAMBERS,

1961; Asbun and Binkley, 1966, 1968; Brown et al., 1968; Leich et al., 1971). The 2′-deoxy derivative of pseudouridylic acid has been prepared enzymatically and was found to be an effective inhibitor of thymidylate synthetase (Kalman, 1972). It is of interest that the 5′-triphosphate derivative of XXXIII can be incorporated into RNA *in vitro* (Zachau, 1969) which would indicate that this derivative can function as a substrate for RNA polymerase and would suggest that appropriate chemical modification of pseudouridine could lead to a pseudouridine derivative with significant antitumor activity. In this respect, another antibiotic has been isolated from the culture filtrate of *Streptomyces tanesashiensis* and assigned the C-nucleoside structure XXXIV and the name oxazinomycin (Haneishi et al., 1972). Oxazinomycin is identical to another C-nucleoside antibiotic (minimycin) which was subsequently isolated from a *Streptomyces* strain sp. 80432 (Kusakabe et al., 1972). These C-nucleosides possess a very close structural similarity to pseudouridine and on the basis of this similarity it is tempting to assume that oxazinomycin and minimycin would possess essentially no chemotherapeutic or biological activity. However, XXXIV has not only been reported to possess activity against gram positive and gram negative bacteria, but also to have significant antitumor activity against the Ehrlich ascites carcinoma and both the ascites and solid forms of Sarcoma 180 (Haneishi et al., 1972; Kusakabe et al., 1972; Sasaki et al., 1972).

Another closely related C-nucleoside antibiotic is showdomycin which was isolated from *Streptomyces showdoensis* (Nishimura and Mayama, 1964) and assigned the structure 3-($\beta$-D-ribofuranosyl) maleimide (XXXV) on the basis of chemical and pmr studies (Darnall et al., 1967). The initial structural assignment was subsequently corroborated by an x-ray study (Nakagawa et al., 1967). The close structural similarity between showdomycin and pseudouridine would suggest that they might have similar properties, e.g. substrate affinity for certain enzymes, chemotherapeutic and biological activity, conformation, etc.; however, a recent x-ray study has established that showdomycin definitely exists in the syn conformation in the solid state, although in solution there is probably a considerable amount of the anti conformation (Tsukuda and Koyama, 1970). The chemical synthesis of XXXV has been accomplished via a long but elegant route (Kal-

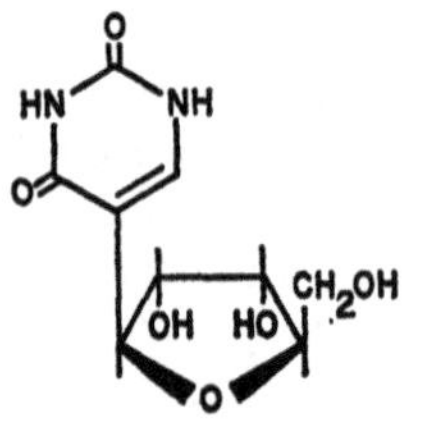


XXXIII

Pseudouridine

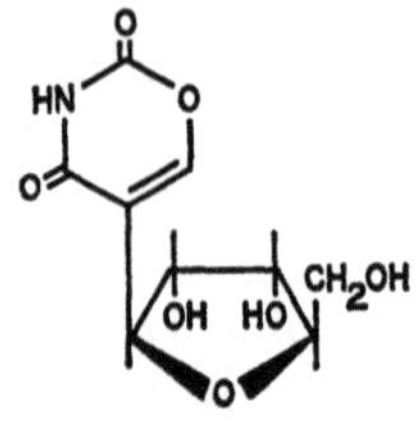


XXXIV

Oxazinomycin

or

Minimycin

voda et al., 1970) and a recent study on the biosynthesis of XXXV has established that the Krebs cycle is involved rather than the *de novo* pyrimidine nucleotide biosynthetic pathway (Elstner and Suhadolnik, 1971). Showdomycin has been found to inhibit RNA and DNA polymerases isolated from

*E. coli* (Maryanka and Johnston, 1970) and also inhibits the incorporation of amino acids and heterocyclic bases (pyrimidine and purine) into *E. coli* K-12 cells (Komatsu and Tanaka, 1970). However, on the basis of current information, the biological and chemotherapeutic activity of XXXV appears to be a function of the chemical reactivity of the heterocyclic moiety (maleimide) with sulfhydryl

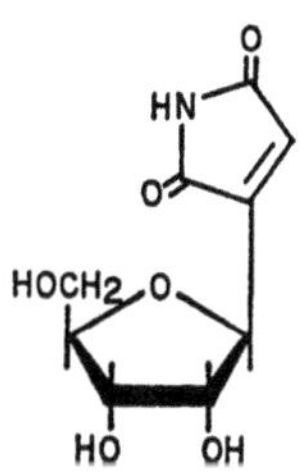


XXXV

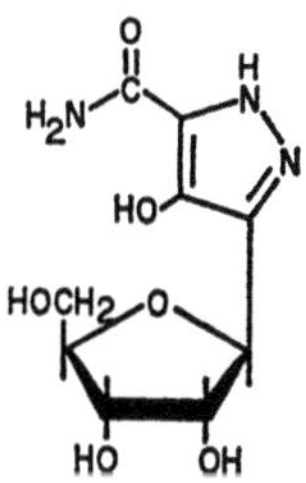


XXXVI

groups, including sulfhydryl groups of proteins, rather than as a pyrimidine nucleoside analog (Hadler et al., 1968; Watanabe, 1970). Yet there is a definite difference in the mode of action of showdomycin and *N*-ethylmaleimide, which has been rationalized by the assumption that showdomycin has a dual role and acts as a nucleoside for entry into the cell, but as a maleimide derivative once inside the cell (Komatsu, 1971).

Showdomycin has been found to inhibit certain nucleotide interconversions, presumably due to blockage of UMP kinase, and to cause a drastic reduction in the utilization of orotic acid (Roy-Burman et al., 1968). This inhibition does not appear to be due to interference with orotidylic acid decarboxylase, although this is one of the major sites of inhibition for the 5′-phosphate derivative of the C-nucleoside pyrazomycin (XXXVI) (Gerzon et al., 1969). Pyrazomycin was initially reported to possess only antiviral activity (Williams et al., 1969) but has now demonstrated significant antitumor activity against several tumor lines (Walker carcinosarcoma 256, adenocarcinoma 755, CA-115 mammary carcinoma and Gardner lymphosarcoma) (Sweeney et al., 1972). Therefore, it would appear that although pseudouridine possesses essentially no antitumor activity, the area encompassed by pseudouridine derivatives and C-nucleosides which are closely related to pyrimidine analogs, is indeed a fertile area for anticancer research.

Pyrazolo[3,4-*d*]pyrimidin-4-one (allopurinol) was synthesized as a purine antagonist (Robins, 1956) and has been proposed to inhibit purine nucleotide biosynthesis *de novo* by acting as either a feedback inhibitor at the ribonucleotide level or by depleting the supply of phosphoribosyl pyrophosphate (PRPP) (Kelley et al., 1971). It was established that allopurinol and oxipurinol, presumably as the ribonucleotide derivatives XXXVII and XXXVIII, respectively, were also potent inhibitors of pyrimidine nucleotide biosynthesis *de novo*, by interfering with the activity of orotidylic decarboxylase. This activity by allopurinol and oxipurinol was observed in cells with normal hypoxanthine-guanine phosphoribosyltransferase activity, as well as in cell strains deficient in such activity and would indicate that there may be other mechanisms or sites of action involved, in addition to those described above. The ribonucleoside derivatives of XXXVII and XXXVIII have been isolated from the urine of patients on allopurinol therapy (Beardmore and Kelley, 1971). On the basis of further study it would appear that the 7-oxipurinol nucleotide is primarily responsible for the inhibition of pyrimidine nucleotide biosynthesis *in vivo*. The formation of 7-oxipurinol ribonucleoside and ribonucleotide was not completely unexpected since it had been previously reported that certain purine derivatives with a diketo type of pyrimidine moiety could serve as substrates for hypoxanthine-guanine phosphoribosyltransferase (HGPRT) and orotate phosphoribosyltransferase (OPRT) and

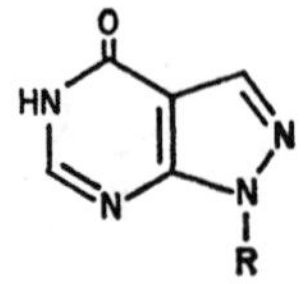


XXXVII

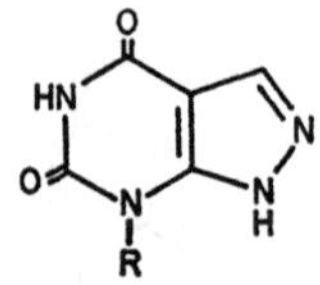


XXXVIII

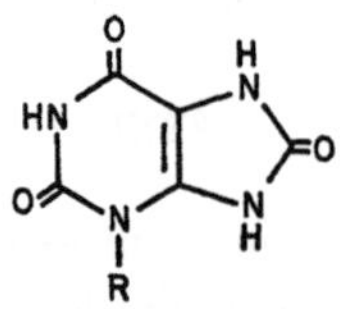


XXXIX

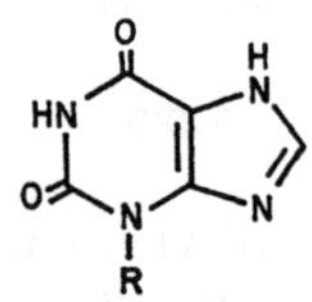


XL

R = D-ribosyl or D-glucosyl

with OPRT, nucleotides very similar to the 5′-phosphate derivative of 7-oxipurinol ribonucleoside were obtained (Hatfield and Wyngaarden, 1964a, b). The first example of this type of nucleoside was a uric acid ribonucleoside which was isolated from ox blood and subsequently characterized as 3-D-ribosyluric acid (XXXIX) (Falconner and Gulland, 1939; Lohrmann et al., 1964). This was of some interest, since at that time, there was no reason to suspect that a purine would be capable of functioning as a substrate for an enzyme in the pyrimidine nucleotide biosynthetic pathway. A close structural analog (3-D-glucosylxanthine, XL) was prepared chemically by utilization of the silylation procedure (Birkofer et al., 1964). Several purines were subsequently found to function as substrates for uridine and thymidine phosphorylase which furnished a number of 3-D-2′-deoxyribosylpurines (Zimmerman, 1966), and pyrimidine deoxynucleoside phosphorylase

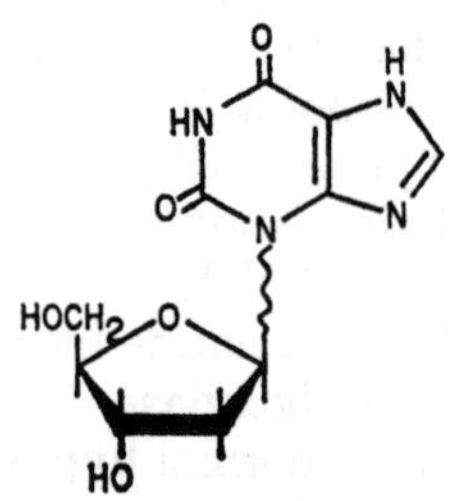


XLI

has also produced 3-D-2′-deoxyribosylxanthine (XLI) from xanthine and deoxyribose 1-phosphate (Tarr et al., 1968). These examples have created some interest in the synthesis of other bicyclic nucleosides which are closely related to uridine and cytidine. The synthesis of 4-(β-D-ribofuranosyl)thiazolo[5,4-d]pyrimidin-5,7-

dione (XLII) via the silylation procedure is an example in this area (SCHMIDT et al., 1971). A visual inspection of XLII reveals that a close structural resemblance between XLII and uridine exists. The ara-U analog [4-(β-D-arabinofuranosyl)-thiazolo[5,4-d]pyrimidin-5,7-dione (XLIII)] has also been prepared from XLII

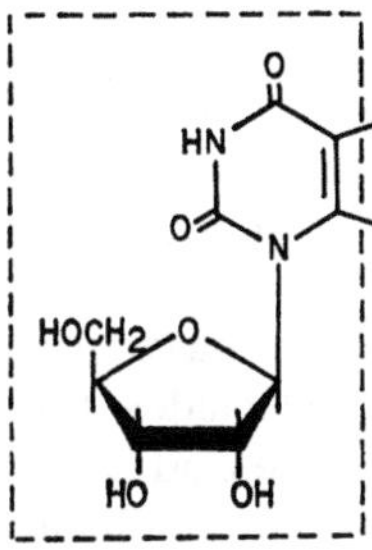

XLII

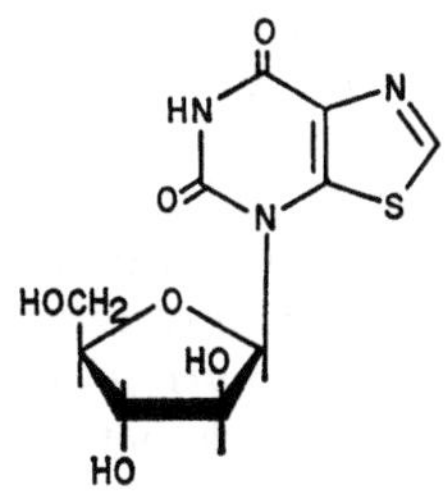

XLIII

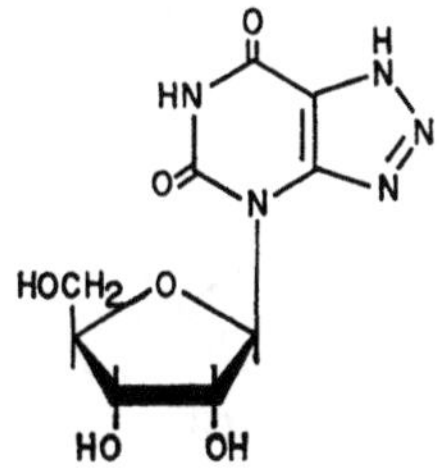

XLIV

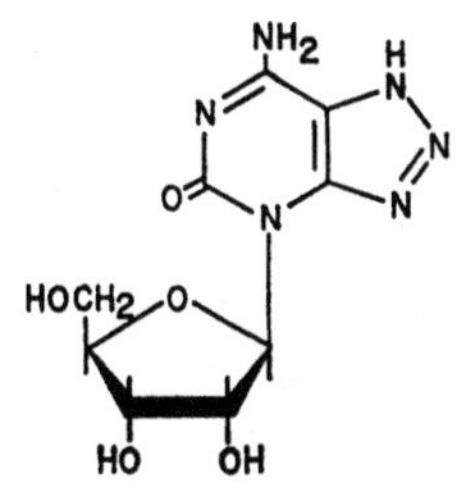

XLV

via the anhydronucleoside with subsequent opening of the anhydro linkage. The synthesis of 3-(β-D-ribofuranosyl)-8-azaxanthine (XLIV) and 3-(β-D-ribofuranosyl)-8-aza-*iso*-guanine (XLV) was accomplished by treatment of the 5-nitro derivatives of uridine and cytidine with sodium azide in dimethylformamide (BLANK and FOX, 1968) which provided additional examples in this area. The cytidine analog in the purine series, 3-(β-D-ribofuranosyl)purin-2-one [3-β-D-ribofuranosylisoguanine (*iso*-isoguanine)], has been synthesized (SCHMIDT and TOWNSEND, 1973) and as the 2-keto derivative of 3-isoadenosine it should function much more effectively as a cytidine derivative than as an adenosine analog.

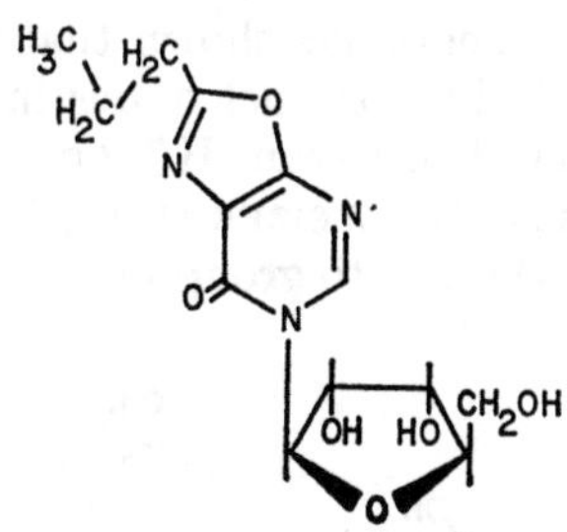

XLVI

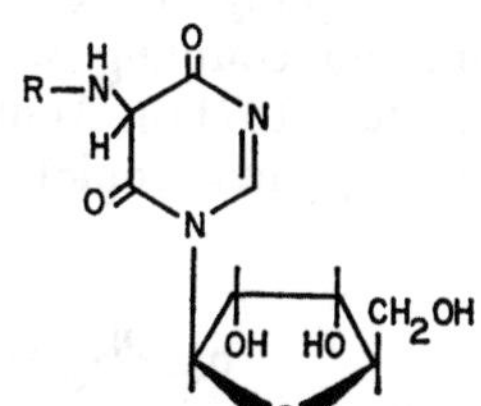

XLVII

Another bicyclic (5,6) nucleoside with the carbohydrate moiety in the six membered ring is 2-ethyl-6-(β-D-ribofuranosyl)oxazolo[5,4-*d*]-pyrimidin-7-one (XLVI) which was prepared via the silylation procedure and reported to possess significant activity against L1210 leukemia (Townsend et al., 1971). It was postulated that this nucleoside may actually be a latent form, and opening of the oxazole ring to yield a pyrimidine nucleoside of the general structure XLVII may be necessary for activity. This is a relatively new area and should provide some interesting pyrimidine nucleoside type compounds in the near future. The approximate conformation (syn, anti, or a conformation somewhere between) of these bicyclic nucleosides is still undetermined and may play an important role in their ability to function as substrates for specific enzymes.

In fact, this area which involves the orientation of the heterocyclic base (pyrimidine) relative to the carbohydrate (primarily ribose and 2-deoxyribose) moiety is of considerable interest and will undoubtedly have increased importance in future research. In pyrimidine and purine nucleosides (and in nucleosides generally) the torsion angle between the carbohydrate and heterocycle about the glycosyl bond ($\Phi$) has been designated as syn and anti depending on the angle (Donohue and Trueblood, 1960). It has been established that the majority (there are exceptions) of the naturally occurring pyrimidine nucleosides (tRNA, etc.) exist preferentially in the anti conformation in the crystalline state, as well as in solution, e.g. uridine (XLVIII). However, as would be expected, orotidine

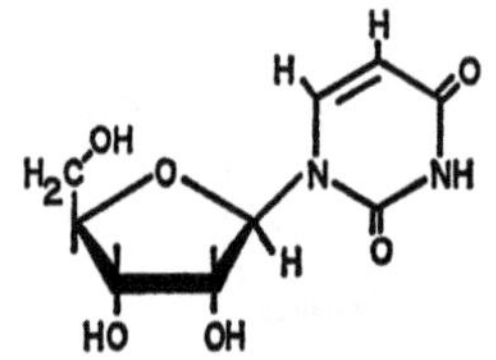

XLVIII

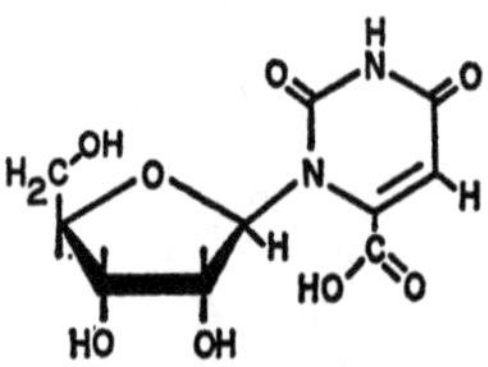

XLIX

has been shown to exist predominantly in the syn conformation (XLIX) in aqueous solution, presumably due to the steric effect of the 6-carboxyl group (Hruska, 1971a). This is of some interest, since if the 5′-phosphate derivatives of these two nucleosides possess the same conformation as the nucleosides, then in the biosynthetic pathway, orotidylic acid, which is in the more restricted and crowded conformation (*syn*), is converted to uridylic acid in the anti conformation. This has been a very active area and there have been numerous reports and techniques described for ascertaining the correct conformation of pyrimidine nucleosides. Proton magnetic resonance spectroscopy has been found to be very informative in this area (Townsend, 1972b). A recent report has shown that there exists a small long range coupling between H5 and H1′ for nucleosides in the anti conformation, while no coupling was observed between H5 and H1′ for orotidine (syn) (Hruska, 1971b). Another study (Schweizer et al., 1971) has correlated the deshielding (anisotropic) effect of the 2-keto group primarily on the H2′

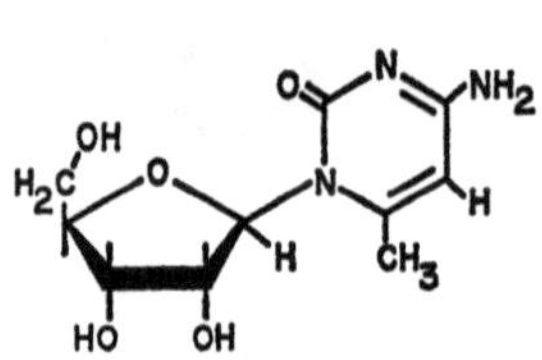

L

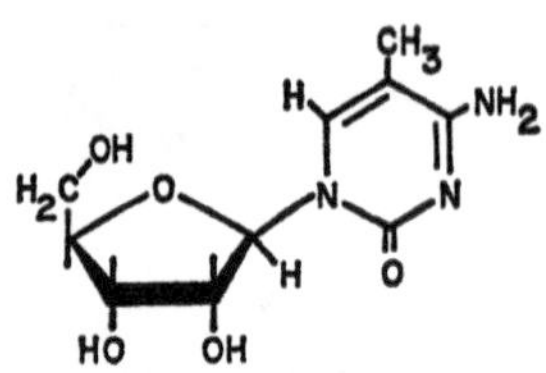

LI

proton. The difference between the chemical shift for the H2′ proton of 6-methylcytidine (L) and 5-methylcytidine (LI) (WINKLEY and ROBINS, 1968; PRYSTAŠ and ŠORM, 1968, 1969) was found to be (5.30−4.71 = Δδ0.59) and the downfield shift to δ5.30 for L was attributed to the proximity of the 2-keto group in the syn conformation. These same assignments were also made on the basis of spectral studies (MILES et al., 1969; ROGERS and ULBRICHT, 1971), where L displayed a negative CD curve, while LI displayed the usual positive cotton effects observed for pyrimidine nucleosides in the anti conformation. 6-Methyluridine (LII) has been the subject of a recent x-ray study which established

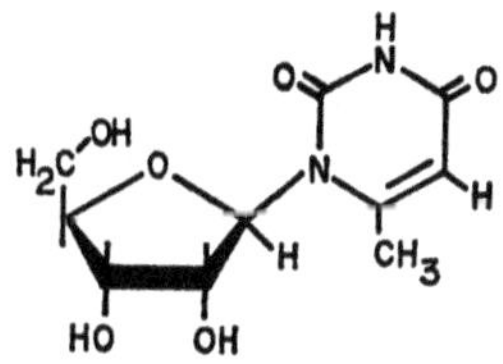

LII

that LII exists in the syn conformation in the solid state with the normal *C*(2′)-endo puckering for the ribofuranosyl moiety (SUCK et al., 1972). This is in direct contrast to 4-thiouridine which also exists in the syn conformation, but exhibits an unusual *C*(3′)-endo-*C*(4′)-exo conformation for the ribofuranosyl moiety (SAENGER and SCHEIT, 1970). 6-Methyluridine and 4-thiouridine exist in the syn conformation (solid state) and appear to exhibit a stacking pattern for the heterocyclic moieties with the same general features, alternating hydrophobic and hydrophilic bands. However, considerable caution should be used in applying the results obtained for a nucleoside by x-ray to the results obtained for the same nucleoside under biological or physiological conditions, e.g. although 4-thiouridine has been definitely shown to exist in the syn conformation by x-ray (SAENGER and SCHEIT, 1970), a recent study (SCHWEIZER et al., 1971) of 4-thiouridine has indicated that in solution it probably prefers the anti conformation. Some synthetic pyrimidine and pyrimidine type nucleosides, *e.g.* barbituric acid riboside, XLII, etc., probably exist predominantly in a conformation somewhere between (*amphi*) the classical *syn* and *anti* conformation (CHENON et al., 1973). The full impact of the significance that conformation will play in the chemotherapeutic and biological activity of pyrimidine nucleosides will require additional research similar to a recent study on 6-methylcytidine triphosphate (6-MeCTP) (KAPULER and REICH, 1971). It was found (KAPULER and REICH, 1971) that 6-MeCTP is not a substrate for RNA polymerase and may, in fact, be a competitive inhibitor of CTP. It was proposed that this finding may be due to the fact that the initial binding of the substrate to the enzyme may be independent of the conformation, with conformation only becoming important at a subsequent step. Therefore, in this instance, although the initial binding may be independent of conformation, a subsequent step (e.g. the formation of the phosphodiester bond) may require the *anti* conformation for incorporation. This a priori explanation could presumably be extended to include several other analogous situations in the pyrimidine nucleoside area and will obviously be one of the fertile areas of research in the near future.

## References

ABRAHAM, D. J., COCHRAN, T. C., ROSENSTEIN, R. D.: Single-crystal X-ray structures of chemotherapeutic agents. V. The structures of 5-diazo-6-methoxy-6-hydrouracil and 2'-deoxy-5-diazo-6-hydro-$O^6$, 5'-cyclouridine hemihydrate. J. Amer. chem. Soc. **93**, 6279—6281 (1971).

ANSFIELD, F. J., RAMIREZ, G.: Phase I and II studies of 2'-deoxy-5-(trifluoromethyl)uridine (NSC-75520). Cancer Chemother. Rep. **55**, 205—208 (1971) and references cited therein.

ASBUN, W., BINKLEY, S. B.: Synthesis of 5-substituted pyrimidines. J. org. Chem. **31**, 2215—2219 (1966).

ASBUN, W., BINKLEY, S. B.: Synthesis of 5-substituted pyrimidines. II. J. org. Chem. **33**, 140—142 (1968).

BALTIMORE, D.: RNA-dependent DNA-polymerase in virions of RNA tumour viruses. Nature (Lond.) **226**, 1209—1211 (1970).

BEARDMORE, T. D., KELLEY, W. N.: Mechanism of allopurinol-mediated inhibition of pyrimidine biosynthesis. J. Lab. clin. Med. **78**, 696—704 (1971).

BERGMANN, W., BURKE, D. C.: Contributions to the study of marine products. XXXIX. The nucleosides of sponges. III. Spongothymidine and spongouridine. J. org. Chem. **20**, 1501—1507 (1955).

BIRKOFER, L., RITTER, A., KUHLTHAU, H. P.: Alkylierungen und Glykosidierungen über Silyl-Derivate. Chem. Ber. **97**, 934—945 (1964).

BLANK, H. U., FOX, J. J.: Pyrimidines VII. A simple conversion of 2-oxo-5-nitro heterocycles to *v*-triazolo derivatives by sodium azide. J. Amer. chem. Soc. **90**, 7175—7176 (1968).

BLOCH, A., DUTSCHMAN, G., GRINDEY, G.: Nucleoside hormone interaction: toxicity of 3-deazauridine in male vs. female mice, as affected by androgens and estrogens. Proc. Amer. Ass. Cancer Res. **13**, 19 (1972).

BROWN, D. M., BURDON, M. G., SLATCHER, R. P.: A synthesis of pseudouridine and of 5-β-D-ribofuranosyluridine. J. chem. Soc. *C*, 1051—1053 (1968).

BROWN, E. G., SILVER, A. V.: The natural occurrence of a uracil 5-peptide and its metabolite relationship to guanosine 5'-monophosphate. Biochim. biophys. Acta (Amst.) **119**, 1—10 (1966).

BRUEMMER, N. C., HOLLAND, J. F., SHEEHE, P. R.: Drug effects on a target metabolic pathway and on mouse tumor growth: azauridine and decarboxylation of orotic acid-7-$C^{14}$. Cancer Res. **22**, 113—119 (1962).

BURCHENAL, J. H., ADAMS, H. H., NEWELL, N. S., FOX, J. J.: Comparative activity of 1-β-D-arabinofuranosyl-5-fluorocytosine and related compounds against transplanted mouse leukemias *in vitro* and *in vivo*. Cancer Res. **26**, 370—373 (1966).

CAMIENER, G. W.: Studies of the enzymatic deamination of cytosine arabinoside-III. Substrate requirements and inhibitors of the deaminase of human liver. Biochem. Pharmacol. **16**, 1691—1702 (1967).

CAMIENER, G. W.: Studies on the enzymatic deamination of ara-cytidine-V. Inhibition *in vitro* and *in vivo* by tetrahydrouridine and other reduced pyrimidine nucleosides. Biochem. Pharmacol. **17**, 1981—1991 (1968).

CAMIENER, G. W., SMITH, C. G.: Studies of the enzymatic deamination of cytosine arabinoside I. Enzyme distribution and species specificity. Biochem. Pharmacol. **14**, 1405—1416 (1965).

CARBON, J. A., HUNG, L., JONES, D. S.: A reversible oxidative inactivation of specific transfer RNA species. Proc. nat. Acad. Sci. (Wash.) **53**, 979—986 (1965).

CERUTTI, P., IKEDA, K., WITKOP, B.: The selective photoreduction of uridine in polynucleotides. J. Amer. chem. Soc. **87**, 2505—2507 (1965).

CHAMBERS, R. W.: The chemistry of pseudouridine. Progr. nucl. Acid. molec. Biol. **5**, 349—398 (1966) and references cited therein.

CHENG, C. C.: Some pyrimidines of biological and medicinal interest, Part I. Progr. med. Chem. **6**, 67—134 (1969).

CHENG, C. C., ROTH, B.: Some pyrimidines of biological and medicinal interest, Part II. Progr. med. Chem. **7**, 285—341 (1970).

CHENG, C. C., ROTH, B.: Some pyrimidines of biological and medicinal interest, Part III. Progr. med. Chem. **8**, 61—117 (1971).

CHENON, M.-T., PUGMIRE, R. J., GRANT, D. M., PANZICA, R. P., TOWNSEND, L. B.: Carbon-13 NMR Spectra of C-nucleosides showdomycin and β-pseudouridine. J. Heterocyclic Chem., **10**, 427—429 (1973).

CHU, M. Y., FISCHER, G. A.: Effects of cytosine arabinoside on the cell viability and uptake of deoxypyrimidine nucleosides in L5178Y cells. Biochem. Pharmacol. **17**, 741—751 (1968a).

CHU, M. Y., FISCHER, G. A.: The incorporation of $^3$H-cytosine arabinoside and its effect on murine leukemic cells (L5178Y). Biochem. Pharmacol. **17**, 753—767 (1968b).

Čihák, A., Šorm, F.: Biochemical effects and metabolic transformations of 5-azacytidine in *Escherichia coli*. Coll. Czech. Chem. Commun. **30**, 2091—2102 (1965).

Cohen, R. M., Wolfenden, R.: Cytidine deaminase from *Escherichia coli*. Purification, properties and inhibition by the potential transition state analog 3,4,5,6-tetrahydrouridine. J. biol. Chem. **246**, 7561—7565 (1971).

Cohn, W. E.: Minor constituents of ribonucleic acids. Fed. Proc. **16**, 166 (1957).

Cohn, W. E.: Pseudouridine, a carbon-carbon linked ribonucleoside in ribonucleic acids: isolation, structure, and chemical characteristics. J. biol. Chem. **235**, 1488—1489 (1960).

Comb, D. G., Katz, S.: Studies on the biosynthesis and methylation of transfer RNA. J. molec. Biol. **8**, 790—800 (1964) and references cited therein.

Currie, B. L., Robins, R. K., Robins, M. J.: The synthesis of 3-deazapyrimidine nucleosides related to uridine and cytidine and their derivatives. J. heterocyclic Chem. **7**, 323—329 (1970).

Damodaran, N. P., Jones, G. H., Moffat, J. G.: Synthesis of the basic nucleoside skeleton of the polyoxin complex. J. Amer. chem. Soc. **93**, 3812—3813 (1971).

Darnall, K. R., Townsend, L. B., Robins, R. K.: The structure of showdomycin, a novel carbon-linked nucleoside antibiotic related to uridine. Proc. nat. Acad. Sci. (Wash.) **57**, 548—553 (1967).

Davis, F. F., Allen, F. W.: Ribonucleic acids from yeast which contain a fifth nucleotide. J. biol. Chem. **227**, 907—915 (1957).

Dexter, D. L., Wolberg, W. H., Ansfield, F. J., Helson, L., Heidelberger, C.: The clinical pharmacology of 5-trifluoromethyl-2′-deoxyuridine. Cancer Res. **32**, 247—253 (1972).

Donohue, J., Trueblood, K. N.: Base pairing in DNA. J. molec. Biol. **2**, 363—371 (1960).

Earl, R. A., Townsend, L. B.: The synthesis of 1-(tetrahydro-2-furanyl)-5-fluorouracil (ftorafur) via direct fluorination. J. heterocyclic Chem. **9**, 1141—1143 (1972).

Eidinoff, M. L., Knoll, J. E., Marano, B. J., Klein, D.: Pyrimidine studies II. Effect of 5-bromodeoxyuridine and related nucleosides on incorporation of precursors into nucleic acid pyrimidines. Cancer Res. **19**, 738—745 (1959).

Elstner, E. F., Suhadolnik, R. J.: Nucleoside antibiotics. Biosynthesis of the maleimide nucleoside antibiotic, showdomycin, by *Streptomyces showdoensis*. Biochemistry **10**, 3608—3614 (1971).

Falconner, R., Gulland, J. M.: The constitution of the purine nucleosides. Part VIII. Uric acid riboside. J. chem. Soc. 1369—1371 (1939).

Favre, A., Michelson, A. M., Yaniv, M.: Photochemistry of 4-thiouridine in *Escherichia coli* transfer $RNA^{Val}$. J. molec. Biol. **58**, 367—379 (1971).

Fox, J. J., Falco, E. A., Wempen, I., Pomeroy, D., Dowling, M. D., Suichenal, J. H.: Oral and parenteral activity of 2,2′-anhydro-1-β-D-arabinofuranosyl-5-fluorocytosine against both intraperitoneally and intracerebrally inoculated mouse leukemia. Cancer Res. **32**, 2269—2272 (1972).

Fox, J. J., Kuwada, Y., Watanabe, K. A.: Nucleoside LVI. On the structure of the nucleoside antibiotic gougerotin. Tetrahedron Let. 6029—6032 (1968).

Fox, J. J., van Praag, D., Wempen, I., Doerr, I. L., Cheong, L., Knace, J. E., Edinoff, M. L., Bendich, A., Brown, G. B.: Thiation of nucleosides. II. Synthesis of 5-methyl-2′-deoxycytidine and related pyrimidine nucleosides. J. Amer. chem. Soc. **81**, 178—187 (1959).

Furth, J. J., Cohen, S. S.: Inhibition of mammalian DNA polymerase by the 5′-triphosphate of 1-β-D-arabinofuranosylcytosine and the 5′-triphosphate of 9-β-D-arabinofuranosyladenine. Cancer Res. **28**, 2061—2067 (1968).

Gerzon, K., Williams, R. H., Hoehn, M., Gorman, M., DeLong, D. C.: Pyrazomycin, a *C*-nucleoside with antiviral activity. 2nd int. Congr. heterocyclic Chem., Montpellier, France (July 1969), p. 131, Abst. C-30.

Ginsberg, T., Davis, F. F.: The biosynthesis of pseudouridine in ribonucleic acids of *Escherichia coli*. J. biol. Chem. **243**, 6300—6305 (1968).

Gish, D. T., Kelley, R. C., Camiener, G. W., Wechter, W. J.: Nucleic acids. 11. Synthesis of 5′-esters of 1-β-D-arabinofuranosylcytosine possessing antileukemic and immunosuppressive activity. J. med. Chem. **14**, 1159—1162 (1971).

Gish, D. T., Neil, G. L., Wechter, W. J.: Nucleic acids. 12. Synthesis of the L-enantiomer of 1-β-D-arabinofuranosylcytosine and of $O^2$, $O^{2'}$-anhydro-1-β-D-ribofuranosylcytosine. J. med. Chem. **14**, 882—883 (1971).

Goldin, A., Wood, H. B., Jr., Engle, R. R.: Relation of structure of purine and pyrimidine nucleosides to antitumor activity. Cancer Chemother. Rep. Part 2, **1**, 1—269 (1968).

Goody, R. S., Watanabe, K. A., Fox, J. J.: Nucleoside LXVI. Synthetic studies on nucleoside antibiotics. 4. Synthesis of methyl 4-amino-2,3,4-trideoxy-α-D-*erythro*-hex-2-enopyranosiduronic acid, the carbohydrate moiety of blasticidin S. Tetrahedron Let. 293—296 (1970).

Gray, G. D., Nichol, F. R., Camiener, M. M., Gish, D. T., Kelly, R. C., Wechter, W. J., Moxley, T. E., Neil, G. L.: Immunosuppressive, antiviral and antitumor activities of cytarabine derivatives. Biochem. Pharmacol. **21**, 465—475 (1972).
Hadler, H. I., Claybourn, E. B., Tschang, T. P.: Mitochondrial volume changes induced by the antibiotic showdomycin. Biochem. biophys. Res. Commun. **31**, 25—31 (1968).
Handschumacher, R. E.: Azauracil ribonucleoside and ribonucleotides: isolation and chemical synthesis. J. biol. Chem. **235**, 764—768 (1960).
Haneishi, T., Okazaki, T., Hata, T., Tamura, C., Nomura, M., Naito, A., Seki, I., Arai, M.: Oxazinomycin, a new carbon-linked nucleoside antibiotic. J. Antibiot. (Tokyo) **24** A, 797—799 (1972).
Hanka, L. J., Evans, J. S., Mason, D. J., Dietz, A.: A microbiological production of 5-azacytidine I. Production and biological activity. Antimicrob. Agents Chemother. 619—630 (1966).
Hanze, A. R.: Nucleic acids. IV. The catalytic reduction of pyrimidine nucleosides (human liver deaminase inhibitors). J. Amer. chem. Soc. **89**, 6720—6725 (1967).
Hatfield, D., Wyngaarden, J. B.: 3-Ribosylpurines I. Synthesis of (3-ribosyluric acid) 5′-phosphate and (3-ribosylxanthine) 5′-phosphate by a pyrimidine ribonucleotide pyrophosphorylase of beef erythrocytes. J. biol. Chem. **239**, 2580—2586 (1964a).
Hatfield, D., Wyngaarden, J. B.: 3-Ribosylpurines II. Studies on 3-ribosylxanthine-5′-phosphate and on ribonucleotide derivatives of certain uracil analogues. J. biol. Chem. **239**, 2587—2592 (1964b).
Heidelberger, C., Parsons, D. G., Remy, D. C.: Synthesis of 5-trifluoromethyl-2′-deoxyuridine. J. med. Chem. **7**, 1—5 (1964).
Hernandez, K., Pinkel, D., Lee, S., Leone, L.: Chemotherapy with 6-azauridine (NSC-32074) for patients with leukemia. Cancer Chemother. Rep. **53**, 203—207 (1969).
Hiller, S. A., Zhuk, R. A., Lidaks, M. Y.: Analogs of pyrimidine nucleosides I. $N_1$($\alpha$-furanyl) derivatives of pyrimidine bases as antimetabolites. Dokil. Akad. Nauk. (USSR) **176**, 332—335 (1967).
Hiller, S. A., Lidaks, M. Y., Zhuk, R. A., Pets, K. I., Getsova, I. N., Berzinya, A. E.: Analogues of pyrimidine nucleosides in chemotherapy of cancer. First All-Union Conference on Chemotherapy of Malignant Tumors, Riga, USSR, 7—11 October **1968**, p. 111.
Ho, N. W. H., Gilham, P. T.: Reaction of pseudouridine and inosine with *N*-cyclohexyl-*N*-$\beta$-(4-methylmorpholinium) ethylcarbodiimide. Biochemistry **10**, 3651—3657 (1971), and references cited therein.
Hoffman, J. L., McConnell, K. P., Carpenter, D. R.: Aminoacylation of *Escherichia coli* methionine t-RNA by selenomethionine. Biochim. biophys. Acta (Amst.) **199**, 531—534 (1970).
Holland, J. F., Korn, R., O'Malley, J., Minnemeyer, H. J., and Tieckelmann, H.: 5-Allyl-2′-deoxyuridine, inhibition of nucleoside phosphorylase in HeLa cells containing mycoplasma. Cancer Res. **27**, 1867 (1967).
Hori, M., Kakiki, K., Suzuki, S., Misato, T.: Studies on the mode of action of polyoxins, Part III. Relation of polyoxin structure to chitin synthetase inhibition. Agr. biol. Chem. (Tokyo) **35**, 1280—1291 (1971).
Hoshi, A., Kanzawa, F., Kuretani, K., Saneyoshi, M., Arai, Y.: 2,2′-*O*-Cyclocytidine, an antitumor cytidine analog resistant to cytidine deaminase. Gann **62**, 145—146 (1971).
Hoshi, A., Kanazawa, F., Kuretani: Antitumor activity of cyclocytidine in a variety of tumors. Gann. **63**, 353—360 (1972).
Howard, J. P., Cevik, N., Murphy, M. L.: Cytosine arabinoside (NSC-63878) in acute leukemia in children. Cancer Chemother. Rep. **50**, 287—291 (1966).
Hrodek, O., Veselý, J.: 5-Azacytidine in childhood leukemia. Neoplasma (Bratisl.) **18**, 493—503 (1971), and references cited therein.
Hruska, F. E.: Molecular conformation of orotidine, a naturally occurring nucleoside, in the *syn* conformation in aqueous solution. J. Amer. chem. Soc. **93**, 1795—1797 (1971).
Hruska, F. E.: Long-range spin-spin coupling in pyrimidine nucleosides. Canad. J. Chem. **49**, 2111—2118 (1971).
Iida, S., Hayatsu, H.: Chemical transformation of 4-thiouridine with nitrous acid. Biochem. biophys. Res. Commun. **43**, 163—167 (1971).
Isono, K., Asaki, K., Suzuki, S.: Studies on polyoxins, antifungal antibiotics. XIII. The structure of polyoxins. J. Amer. chem. Soc. **91**, 7490—7505 (1969), and references cited therein.
Isono, K., Crain, P. F., Odiorne, T. J., McCloskey, J. A., Suhadolnik, R. J.: Biosynthesis of the 5-fluoropolyoxins, aberrant nucleoside antibiotics. J. Amer. Chem. Soc. **95**, 5788—5789 (1973).
Isono, K., Suzuki, S., Azumo, T.: Semisynthetic polyoxins; aminoacyl derivatives of polyoxin C and their *in vitro* activity. Agr. biol. Chem. (Tokyo) **35**, 1986—1989 (1971).

IVANOVICS, G. A., ROUSSEAU, R. J., ROBINS, R. K.: Nucleoside peptides. 2. Synthesis of certain 5-*N*-aminoacyl and 5-*N*-peptidyl derivatives of 5-aminouridine. J. med. Chem. **14**, 1155—1158 (1971).

JONES, M. E.: Regulation of pyrimidine and arginine biosynthesis in mammals, in Advances in Enzyme Regulation. Vol. 9. pp. 19—49. George Weber, (Ed)., New York: Pergamon Press 1971.

KALMAN, T. I.: Enzymatic synthesis of 2′-deoxy-pseudouridylic acid. Biochem. biophys. Res. Commun. **46**, 1194—1200 (1972).

KALMAN, T. I., BARDOS, T. J.: Enzymatic studies relating to the mode of action of 5-mercapto-2′-deoxyuridine. Molec. Pharmacol. **6**, 621—630 (1970).

KALVODA, L., FARKAŠ, J., ŠORM, F.: Synthesis of showdomycin. Tetrahedron Let. 2297—2300 (1970).

KANAI, T., KOJIMA, T., MARUYAMA, O., ICHINO, M.: Pyrimidine nucleosides III. Reaction of cytidine or $N^4$-acetylcytidine with partially hydrolyzed phosphorus oxychloride. Chem. pharm. Bull. (Tokyo) **18**, 2569—2571 (1970).

KANZAKI, T., HIGASHIDE, E., YAMAMOTO, H., SHIBATA, M., NAKAZAWA, K., IWASAKI, H., TAKEWAKA, T., MIYAKE, A.: Gougerotin, a new antibacterial antibiotic. J. Antibiot. (Tokyo) **15 A**, 93—97 (1962).

KAPULER, A. M., REICH, E.: Some stereochemical requirements of *Escherichia coli* ribonucleic acid polymerase interaction with conformationally restricted ribonucleoside 5′-triphosphates: 8-bromoguanosine, 8-ketoguanosine, and 6-methylcytidine triphosphates. Biochemistry **10**, 4050—4061 (1971).

KARON, M., SHIRAKAWA, S.: The locus of action of 1-$\beta$-D-arabinofuranosylcytosine in cell cycle. Cancer Res. **29**, 687—696 (1969).

KELLEY, W. N., FOX, I. H., BEARDMORE, T. D., MEADE, J. C.: Allopurinol and oxipurinol: alteration of purine and pyrimidine metabolism in cell culture. Ann. N. Y. Acad. Sci. **179**, 588—595 (1971).

KIKUGAWA, K., ICHINO, M.: Studies on the VILSMEIR-HAACK reaction. IV. Convenient synthesis of 2,2′-anhydro-1-$\beta$-D-arabinofuranosylcytosine (2,2′-cyclocytidine) and its derivatives. J. org. Chem. **37**, 284—288 (1972).

KOMATSU, Y.: Mechanism of action of showdomycin, Part IV. Interactions between the mechanisms for transport of showdomycin and of various nucleosides. Agr. biol. Chem. (Tokyo) **35**, 1328—1339 (1971).

KOMATSU, Y., TANAKA, K.: Mechanism of action of showdomycin, Part II. Effect of showdomycin on the synthesis of deoxyribonucleic acid in *Escherichia coli*. Agr. biol. Chem. (Tokyo) **34**, 891—899 (1970).

KONDO, T., GOTO, T.: Synthesis of 1-(4-amino-4-deoxy-$\beta$-D-glucopyranosyl)uracil. Agr. biol. Chem. (Tokyo) **35**, 625—628 (1971).

KONDO, T., NAKI, H., GOTO, T.: Synthesis of cytosine, the nucleoside component of the antibiotic blasticidin S. Tetrahedron Let. 1881—1884 (1972).

KOTICK, M., SZANTAY, C., BARDOS, T. J.: Synthesis of 5-*S*-substituted 2′-deoxyuridines. Study of the factors influencing the stereo-selectivity of the silyl modification of the Hilbert-Johnson reaction. J. org. Chem. **34**, 3806—3822 (1969).

KOWOLLIK, G., GAERTNER, K., ETZOLD, G., LANGEN, P.: Nucleoside von Fluor-Zuckern, Teil III. Synthese 5′-fluorsubstituierter Desoxyribonucleoside. Carbohydrate Res. **12**, 301—311 (1970a).

KOWOLLIK, G., GAERTNER, K., LANGEN, P.: Nucleoside von Fluor-Zuckern; Synthese neuer potentieller DNS-Hemmstoffe. Z. Chem. **10**, 141—142 (1970b).

KRAVCHENKO, I. M., ZIDERMANE, A. A.: Antineoplastic activity of fluorafur [$N_3$-(2′-furanidyl)-5-fluorouracil] in experiment. First All-Union Conference on Chemotherapy of Malignant Tumors, Riga, USSR, 7—11 October 1968 p. 214—215.

KUMURA-HARADA, F., SANEYOSHI, M., NISHIMURA, S.: 5-Methyl-2-thiouridine: a new sulfur-containing minor constituent from rat liver glutamic acid and lysine t-*RNAs*. Febs Letters, **13**, 335—338 (1971).

KUSAKABE, Y., NOGATSU, J., SHIBUYA, M., KAWAGUCHI, O., HIROSE, C., SHIRATO, S.: Minimycin, a new antibiotic. J. Antibiot. (Tokyo) **25 A**, 44—47 (1972).

LANE, B. G.: The alkali-stable trinucleotide sequences and the chain termini in 18S and 28S ribonucleates from wheat germ. Biochemistry **4**, 212—219 (1965).

LANGEN, P., KOWOLLIK, G., SCHUTT, M., ETZOLD, G.: Thymidylate kinase as target enzyme for 5′-deoxythymidine and various 5′-deoxy-5′-halogeno pyrimidine nucleosides. Acta biol. Med. germ. **23**, K 19—22 (1969).

LEICH, U., BURDON, M. G., MOFFAT, J. G.: *C*-Glycosyl nucleosides. I. Studies on the synthesis of pseudouridine and related compounds. J. org. Chem. **36**, 1507—1513 (1971).

LIEU, T. S., HUDSON, R. A., BROWN, R. K., WHITE, B. C.: Transport of pyrimidine nucleosides across human erythrocyte membranes. Biochim. biophys. Acta (Amst.) **241**, 884—893 (1971).

Lindsay, R. H., Tillery, C. R., Wong Yu, M. Y.: Conversion of the antithyroid drug 2-thiouracil to 2-thio-5'-UMP by UMP pyrophosphorylase. Arch. Biochem. Biophys. **148**, 466—474 (1972).
Lipsett, M. N.: The isolation of 4-thiouridylic acid from the soluble ribonucleic acid of *Escherichia coli*. J. biol. Chem. **240**, 3975—3978 (1965).
Lohrmann, R., Lagowski, J. M., Forrest, H. S.: 3-Ribosyluric acid. Part III. Unambiguous syntheses of 3-ribosyluric acid and related compounds. J. Chem. Soc. 451—459 (1964).
Lozzio, C. B., Wigler, P. W.: Cytotoxic effects of thiopyrimidines. J. cell. Physiol. **78**, 25—32 (1971).
Maryanka, D., Johnston, I. R.: The inhibition of *DNA*-dependent *RNA* polymerase of *E. coli* by showdomycin. Febs Let. **7**, 125—128 (1970).
Matsushita, S., Fanburg, B. L.: Pyrimidine nucleotide synthesis in the normal and hypertrophying rat heart, relative importance of the *de novo* and salvage pathways. Circulation Res. **27**, 415—428 (1970).
Michelson, A. M., Cohn, W. E.: Cyclo-pseudouridine and the configuration of pseudouridine. Biochemistry **1**, 490—495 (1962).
Miles, D. W., Robins, M. J., Robins, R. K., Winkley, M. W., Eyring, H.: Circular dichroism of nucleoside derivatives IV. Uracil derivatives. J. Amer. chem. Soc. **91**, 824—831 (1969).
Milne, G. H., Townsend, L. B.: The synthesis of $\alpha$- and $\beta$-2'-deoxyselenoguanosine. Biochim. Biophys. Acta **269**, 344—346 (1972).
Milne, G. H., Townsend, L. B.: Purine nucleosides XXXII, synthesis and reactivity of 6-alkylseleno-9-($\beta$-D-ribofuranosyl)purines. J. Chem. Soc. Perk. Trans I, 313—315 (1973).
Minnemeyer, H. J., Tieckelman, H., Holland, J. F.: 5-Allyluridine. J. med. Chem. **6**, 602 (1963).
Moravek, J., Škoda, J.: Biochemically important labelled compounds. IV. Biosynthetic preparation of 6-azauridine [4,5-$^{14}$C] and its isolation by gel filtration. Coll. Czech. Chem. Commun. **34**, 1837—1840 (1969).
Nakagawa, Y., Kano, H., Tsukuda, Y., Koyama, H.: Structure of a new class of *C*-nucleoside antibiotic, showdomycin. Tetrahedron Let. 4105—4109 (1967).
Neil, G. L., Wiley, P. F., Manak, R. C., Moxley, T. E.: Antitumor effect of 1-$\beta$-D-arabinofuranosylcytosine 5'-adamantoate (NSC 117614) in L1210 leukemic mice. Cancer Res. **30**, 1047—1054 (1970).
Nishimura, H., Mayama, M., Komatsu, Y., Kato, H., Shimaoka, N., Tanaka, T.: Showdomycin, a new antibiotic from a *Streptomyces* sp. J. Antibiot. (Tokyo) **17 A**, 148—155 (1964).
Nodinski, L., Kensler, C. J.: Activity of cytosine arabinoside (NSC 117614) in L1210 leukemic mice. Cancer Chemother. Rep. **47**, 65—68 (1965).
Noell, C. W., Cheng, C. C.: Pyrimidines XVII. 1-(Tetrahydro-2-pyranyl) cytosine, -uracil, -thymine. J. heterocyclic Chem., **3**, 5—8 (1966).
Noell, C. W., Cheng, C. C.: Pyrimidines XXI. 1-(Tetrahydro-2-furyl)-pyrimidines. J. heterocyclic Chem. **5**, 25—28 (1968).
Ohrui, H., Kuzuhara, H., Emato, S.: Synthesis of deoxypolyoxin C, thymine polyoxin C. Tetrahedron Let. 4267—4270 (1971).
Oliver, J. M., Paterson, A. R. P.: Nucleoside transport I. A mediated process in human erythrocytes. Canad. J. Biochem. **49**, 262—270 (1970).
Panzica, R. P., Robins, R. K., Townsend, L. B.: Synthesis and anticancer activity of cytosine arabinoside 3-*N*-oxide (ara-C 3-*N*-oxide). J. med. Chem. **14**, 259 (1971).
Paterson, A. R. P., Oliver, J. M.: Nucleoside transport II. Inhibition of *p*-nitrobenzylthioguanosine and related compounds. Canad. J. Biochem. **49**, 271—274 (1971).
Phillips, G. R.: Primary structure of transfer *RNA*. Nature (Lond.) **223**, 374—377 (1969).
Pískala, A., Šorm, F.: Nucleic acid components and their analogues. LI. Synthesis of 1-glycosyl derivatives of 5-azauracil and 5-azacytosine. Coll. Czech. Chem. Commun. **29**, 2060—2076 (1964).
Pleiss, M. G., Cerutti, P. A.: Phototransformation of 4-thiouridine in *Escherichia coli* valine transfer ribonucleic acid to uridine, cytidine and $N^4$-methylcytidine. Biochemistry **10**, 3093—3099 (1971).
Pontis, H., Degerstedt, G., Reichard, P.: Uridine and deoxyuridine phosphorylases from Ehrlich ascites tumor. Biochim. biophys. Acta (Amst.) **51**, 138—147 (1961).
Prystaš, M., Šorm, F.: Nucleic acid components and their analogues. XXII. Synthesis of 6-azauridine and 5-methyl-6-azauridine. Coll. Czech. Chem. Commun. **27**, 1578—1584 (1962).
Prystaš, M., Šorm, F.: Synthesis of 6-methyl- and 5,6-dimethyluridines and cytidines. Coll. Czech. Chem. Commun. **33**, 331—335 (1968).
Prystaš, M., Šorm, F.: Nucleic acid components and their analogues. CXXVII. Synthesis of uridine and cytidine 6-methyl and 5,6-dimethyl derivatives. Coll. Czech. Chem. Commun. **34**, 2316—2347 (1969).

REID, T. W., ALBERT, D. M.: RNA-dependent DNA-polymerase activity in human tumors. Biochem. biophys. Res. Commun. **46**, 383—389 (1972).

ROBERTS, M., VISSER, D. W.: Antimetabolite activity of uridine and cytidine derivatives. J. biol. Chem. **194**, 695—701 (1952).

ROBINS, M. J., CURRIE, B. L., ROBINS, R. K., BLOCH, A.: The biological activity of 3-deazapyrimidine nucleosides. Proc. Amer. Ass. Cancer Res. **10**, 73 (1969).

ROBINS, R. K.: Synthesis of some 4,6-substituted pyrazolo[3,4-*d*]pyrimidines. J. Amer. chem. Soc. **78**, 784—790 (1956).

ROGERS, G. T., ULBRICHT, T. L. V.: Optical rotatory studies on nucleic acid derivatives, *n*-transitions and the relation of the $B_{2u}$ cotton effect of conformation in pyrimidine and azapyrimidine nucleosides. Europ. J. Biochem. **22**, 457—466 (1971), and references cited therein.

ROY-BURMAN, S., ROY-BURMAN, P., VISSER, D. W.: Showdomycin, a new nucleoside antibiotic. Cancer Res. **28**, 1605—1610 (1968).

SAENGER, W., SCHEIT, K. H.: A pyrimidine nucleoside in the *syn* conformation: molecular and crystal structure of 4-thiouridine hydrate. J. molec. Biol. **50**, 153—169 (1970).

SASAKI, K., KUSAKABE, Y., ESUMI, S.: The structure of minimycin, a novel carbon-linked nucleoside antibiotic related to β-pseudouridine. J. Antibiot. (Tokyo) **25** A, 152—154 (1972).

SASLAW, L. D., GRINDEY, G. B., KLINE, I., WARAVDEKAR, V. S.: Sparing action of uridine on the activity of arabinosylcytosine with normal and leukemic mice. Cancer Res. **28**, 11—20 (1968).

SATO, E., KANAOKA, Y.: Photoreduction of 4- and 2-thiouracil and 4-thiouridine. Tetrahedron Let. 3547—3548 (1969).

SCHMIDT, C. L., RUSHO, W. J., TOWNSEND, L. B.: The synthesis of bicyclic nucleosides related to uridine, 4-(β-D-ribofuranosyl)thiazolo[5,4-*d*]pyrimidines. Chem. Commun. 1515—1516 (1971).

SCHMIDT, C. L., TOWNSEND, L. B.: The synthesis of bicyclic nucleosides related to cytidine; 3-(β-D-ribofuranosyl)isoguanine. J. Heterocyclic Chem. **10**, 687—688 (1973).

SCHRECKER, A. W., URSHEL, M. J.: Metabolism of 1-β-D-arabinofuranosylcytosine in leukemia L1210: studies with intact cells. Cancer Res. **28**, 793—801 (1968).

SCHUSTER, G. S., HARE, J. D.: The role of phosphorylation in the uptake of thymidine in mammalian cells. In Vitro **6**, 427—436 (1971).

SCHWARTZ, S. H., BARDOS, T. J., BURGESS, G. H., KLEIN, E.: Cytostatic and immunologic activity of 5-mercaptouracil deoxyriboside in the management of multiple superficial basal cell epitheliomas. J. Med. **1**, 174—179 (1970).

SCHWEIZER, M. P., WITOWSKI, J. T., ROBINS, R. K.: Nuclear magnetic resonance determination of syn and anti conformations in pyrimidine nucleosides. J. Amer. chem. Soc. **93**, 277—279 (1971).

SHAPIRO, R., CHAMBERS, R. W.: Synthesis of Pseudouridine. J. Amer. chem. Soc. **83**, 3920—3921 (1961).

SHEN, T. Y., MCPHERSON, J. F., LINN, B. O.: Nucleosides III. Studies on 5-methylamino-2'-deoxyuridine as a specific antiherpes agent. J. med. Chem. **9**, 366—369 (1966).

SHIMUZU, B., ASAI, M., HIEDER, H., MIYAKI, M., OKAZAKI, H.: Preparation of L-β-ribonucleotides. Chem. pharm. Bull. (Tokyo) **13**, 616—618 (1965).

SHOAF, W. T., JONES, M. E.: Initial steps in pyrimidine synthesis in Ehrlich ascites carcinoma. Biochem. biophys. Res. Commun. **45**, 796—802 (1971).

SHUGART, L.: Effect of selective chemical modification of 4-thiouridine of phenylalanine transfer ribonucleic acid on enzyme recognition. Arch. Biochem. Biophys. **148**, 488—495 (1972).

SKÖLD, O.: Uridine kinase from Ehrlich ascites tumor: purification and properties. J. biol. Chem. **235**, 3273—3279 (1960).

SLAVÍK, M., KEISER, H. R., LOVENBERG, W., SJÖERDSMA, A.: Hyperaminoacidemia in rabbits treated with 6-azauridine triacetate. Life Sci. **10**, 1293—1295 (1971).

SMITH, D. A., ROY-BURMAN, P., VISSER, D. W.: Studies of 5-aminouridine. Biochim. biophys. Acta (Amst.) **119**, 221—228 (1966).

SUCK, D., SAENGER, W., VORBRUGGEN, H.: Conformation of 6-methyl-uridine — a pyrimidine nucleoside in the syn conformation. Nature (Lond.) **235**, 333—334 (1972).

SUHADOLNIK, R. J.: Nucleoside antibiotics. pp. 172—202. New York: Wiley-Interscience 1970.

SWEENY, M. J., GUTOWSKI, G. E., POORE, G. A., HAMILL, R. L.: Pyrazomycin: a new antitumor antibiotic. Proc. Amer. Ass. Cancer Res. **13**, 108 (1972).

TAKEUCHI, S., HIRAYAMA, K., UEDA, K., SAKAI, H., YONEHARA, H.: Blasticidin S, a new antibiotic. J. Antibiot. (Tokyo) **11** A, 1—5 (1958).

TARR, H. L. A., ROY, J. E., YAMAMOTO, M.: Fish liver pyrimidine deoxynucleoside phosphorylase and deoxyribosyltransferase. Canad. J. Biochem. **46**, 407—415 (1968).

Temin, H. M., Mitzutani, S.: *RNA*-dependent *DNA* polymerase in virions of Rous sarcoma virus. Nature (Lond.) **226**, 1211—1213 (1970).

Thiry, L.: Viruses grown in the presence of base analogs. Specific alteration of susceptibility to inactivation by radiation, mutagens, and protodyes. Virology **28**, 543—554 (1966).

Thomson, M. J., Garland, M. R., Richards, J. F.: Metabolic effects of nucleosides in rat thymus cells *in vitro*. J. cell. Physiol. **77**, 17—30 (1971).

Thurber, T. C., Townsend, L. B.: A structural study of 5-diazouracil, 5-diazouridine, and 5-diazo-2′-deoxyuridine by *PMR* spectroscopy and a discussion of certain reactions in view of the revised structures. 3rd Intern. Cong. Heterocyclic Chem., Sendai, Japan, August 1971.

Tolman, R. L., Robins, R. K.: Synthesis of 1-β-L-arabinofuranosylcytosine the enantiomer of cytosine arabinoside. J. med. Chem. **14**, 1112 (1972).

Townsend, L. B.: Selection of specific compounds with potential antitumor activity for synthesis on the basis of screening data. 2nd Annual NCI Contractors meeting, Annapolis, Maryland, 3—5 November, 1971.

Townsend, L. B.: Unpublished testing data received from NCI for XVII and XVIII against leukemia L 1210, 1972a.

Townsend, L. B.: Synthetic procedures in nucleic acid chemistry, vol. II, Chapt. 7. W. W. Zorbach and R. S. Tipson (Eds.) New York: Intersience 1972b.

Townsend, L. B., Milne, G. H.: Synthesis of the selenium congener of the naturally occurring guanosine nucleoside, 6-selenoguanosine. J. Heterocyclic Chem. **7**, 753—754 (1970).

Townsend, L. B., Robins, R. K.: Nucleoside antibiotics. Physicochemical constants, spectral, chemotherapeutic and biological properties. In: Sober (Ed.): Handbook of Biochemistry and Molecular Biology pp. G 115—G 213. 2 ed. Cleveland, Ohio: The Chemical Rubber Co. 1970.

Townsend, L. B., Patil, V. D., Bloch, A.: Synthesis and biological activity of ribofuranosyl derivatives of oxazolo[5,4-*d*]pyrimidines. Proc. Amer. Ass. Cancer Res. **12**, 74 (1971).

Trimble, R. B., Maley, F.: Metabolism of 4-N-hydroxycytidine in *Escherichia coli*. J. Bact. 145—153 (1971).

Tsukuda, Y., Koyama, H.: Crystal and Molecular Structure of Showdomycin. J. chem. Soc. 1709—1712 (1970).

Uchida, K., Kreis, W.: Studies on drug resistance — I. Distribution of 1-β-D-arabinofuranosylcytosine, cytidine and deoxycytidine in mice bearing ara-C sensitive and resistant P815 neoplasms. Biochem. Pharmacol. **18**, 1115—1127 (1969).

Ueda, T., Iida, Y., Ikeda, K., Mizuno, Y.: Synthesis of 2,4-dithiouridine and 2-thiocytidines. Chem. pharm. Bull. (Tokyo) **16**, 1788—1794 (1968), and references cited therein.

Visser, D. W.: Antimetabolites and cancer, p. 47. C. P. Rhoads (Ed.). Washington, D. C.: Amer. Assoc. for the Adv. of Sci. 1955.

Walwich, E. R., Dekker, C. A., Roberts, W. K.: Cyclisation during the phosphorylation of uridine and cytidine by polyphosphoric acid: a new route to the $O^2$, 2′-cyclonucleosides. Proc. chem. Soc. **84** (1959).

Wang, M. C., Bloch, A.: Studies on the mode of action of 3-deazapyrimidines. Biochem. Pharmacol. **21**, 1063—1073 (1972).

Watanabe, K. A., Kotick, M. P., Fox, J. J.: Nucleosides LXIII. Synthetic studies on nucleoside antibiotics. 3. Total synthesis of 1-(4-amino-4-deoxy-β-D-glucopyranosyluronic acid)-cytosine, the nucleoside moiety of gougerotin. J. org. Chem. **35**, 231—236 (1970).

Watanabe, K. A., Falco, E. A., Fox, J. J.: Total synthesis of gougerotin. J. Amer. chem. Soc. **94**, 3272—3274 (1972a).

Watanabe, K. A., Wempen, I. M., Fox, J. J.: Nucleosides Part LXXII. Synthetic studies on nucleoside antibiotics. 7. An improved synthesis of C-substance. Carbohydrate Res. **21**, 148—153 (1972b), and references cited therein.

Watanabe, S.: Equimolecular reaction of showdomycin with thiols. J. Antibiot. **23** A, 313—314 (1970).

Wiley, P. F., Mackellar, F. A.: The structure of sparsomycin. J. Amer. chem. Soc. **92** 417—418 (1970).

Williams, R. H., Gerzon, K., Hoehn, M., Gorman, M., Delong, D. C.: Pyrazomycin — a novel carbon-linked nucleoside. 158th Nat. Amer. Chem. Soc. Meeting, September 1969, New York: MICR 038.

Winkley, M. W., Robins, R. K.: Pyrimidine nucleosides I. The synthesis of 6-methylcytidine, 6-methyluridine, and related 6-methylpyrimidine nucleosides. J. org. Chem. **33**, 2822—2827 (1968).

Winkley, M. W., Robins, R. K.: Direct glycosylation of 1,3,5-triazinones. A new approach to the synthesis of the nucleoside antibiotic 5-azacytidine (4-amino-1-β-D-ribofuranosyl-1,3,5-triazin-2-one) and related derivatives. J. org. Chem. **35**, 491—495 (1970).

WISE, D. S., TOWNSEND, L. B.: Synthesis of the selenopyrimidine nucleosides 2-seleno and 4-selenouridine. J. Heterocyclic Chem. **10**, 1461—1462 (1972).

YAMAOKA, N., OTTER, B. A., FOX, J. J.: Nucleosides. XLV. 1-α-L-aldopentofuranosylpyrimidines. J. med. Chem. **11**, 55—59 (1968).

YANIV, M., CHESTIER, A., GROS, A., FAVRE, A.: Biological activity of irradiated $tRNA^{Val}$ containing a 4-thiouridine-cytosine dimer. J. molec. Biol. **58**, 381—388 (1971).

YONEHARA, H., OTAKE, N.: Absolute configuration of Blasticidin S. Tetrahedron Let. 3785—3791 (1966).

ZACHAU, H. G.: Transfer ribonucleic acids. Angew. Chem. 8, Int. Ed. 711—727 (1969).

ZIMMERMAN, M.: Deoxyribosyl transfer, III. Catalysis of 3-pentosylpurine formation by pyrimidine nucleoside phosphorylases. J. biol. Chem. **241**, 4914—4916 (1966).

Chapter 7

# Basic Concepts of Cell Population Kinetics

L. F. LAMERTON

With 5 Figures

## Introduction

The subject of cell population kinetics covers two related fields of study. One is concerned with the various stages or phases of the cell cycle. The other relates to the dynamic characteristics of cell populations, including rates of cell proliferation, of cell migration, and of cell death, and the changes in these parameters involved in tissue response to injury.

The importance of this subject in cancer therapy and in immunosuppression, which are the subjects of this book, is that the response of tissues to cytotoxic agents, both in initial damage and in repair, will often depend on the cell population kinetics of the tissues concerned. This will be particularly so when recognized proliferation-dependent drugs are used, although cell population kinetic factors must be involved to some extent in the response to any form of cytotoxic treatment.

The subject has developed rapidly over the last 15 to 20 years, following the recognition that the period of DNA synthesis is of limited duration and so allows the intermitotic time to be divided up into discrete phases. As a basis of techniques for studying cell population kinetics, four phases may be distinguished (Fig. 1) –

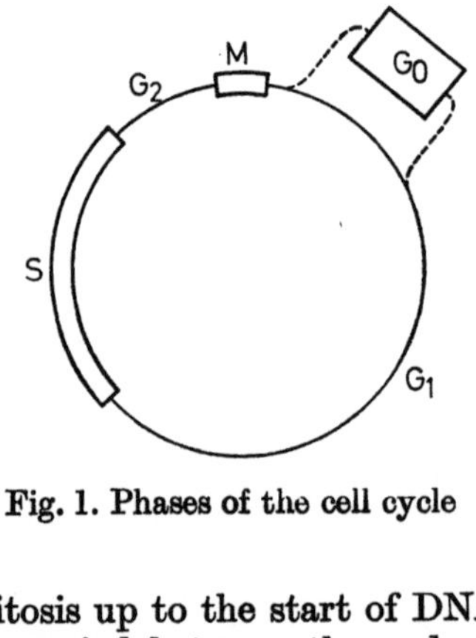


Fig. 1. Phases of the cell cycle

$G_1$, the period following mitosis up to the start of DNA synthesis; $S$, the period of DNA synthesis; $G_2$, the period between the end of DNA synthesis and the start of the next mitosis; $M$, the period of cell mitosis. These various phases must not be regarded as representing biochemically homogeneous states of the cells, and advances now being made in the characterization of the fine structure of these states, and the nature and timing of the various trigger points, will greatly extend the present range of techniques for studying the proliferation characteristics of cells. For reviews of the present state of knowledge in the biochemistry of the cell cycle, the reader is referred to BASERGA (1968) and LALA (1971).

In certain tissues it appears that cells can enter a "resting" or "$G_0$" stage in which they retain proliferative capacity, but will not actively prepare for division unless appropriately stimulated. In the "conditional renewal" tissues of the body, such as the liver, it appears that most cells are in the $G_0$ state and enter it immediately after mitosis, that is, within the $G_1$ period. However, in certain other tissues, for instance in the skin, there is evidence that cells may also rest in the $G_2$ stage. Thus $G_0$ cells may represent cells in various biochemical states, all characterized by being stopped in the cell cycle at some critical point. Such arrest of cells at points in the cycle may be part of a normal tissue control system; on the other hand, it may also arise as the result of some nutritional deficiency, and this effect may sometimes be of importance in tumors. For further discussion of the "$G_0$" state the reader is referred to the review of the subject by EPIFANOVA and TERSKIKH (1969).

Various terms are used to describe the interval between successive mitoses. The term "cell cycle" suggests a well-defined periodic event, which is not very appropriate when the interval varies considerably in length and especially if it includes a $G_0$ period. The term "generation time" also has limitations and as a general term "intermitotic time" seems to be the most satisfactory.

## The Identification of the Proliferative State of Cells

The study of the dynamic characteristics of cell populations depends on the ability to recognize cells in the various stages of the division process. Until fairly recently the only generally available marker of the proliferative state of a cell was mitosis itself. However, with the availability of radioactively-labeled DNA precursors, particularly tritiated-thymidine, and the development of autoradiographic techniques, the opportunity was provided to identify cells in the $S$ period. The label is effectively nonexchangeable and reduced only by dilution at cell division, so that a cohort of cells within the cell cycle could be labeled and their subsequent behaviour investigated, greatly extending the type of investigation that could be made. A third means of identification of the proliferative state of a cell is provided by measurement of DNA content, using microspectrometry, since cells in $G_2$ will have twice the amount of DNA as those in $G_1$. The lack of a distinct boundary, because of the varying amounts of DNA in cells in process of synthesis, can be largely overcome by combination of microspectrometry and autoradiography (HALE et al., 1965).

The above techniques may be considered as "physiological" in that the cell marker studied does not itself affect the behavior of the cell; in the case of labeled DNA this requires, of course, that the intensity of labeling is kept sufficiently low. However, these markers provide direct recognition of the proliferative state of a cell only when in the DNA synthetic, mitotic, or $G_2$ stages. There is as yet no morphological marker which will distinguish $G_1$ cells from $G_0$ cells, or from cells that have lost capacity for division. This is a major limitation, particularly in the study of human tissues, where the more elaborate transplantation and other techniques used in experimental animals may not be possible.

Another class of techniques is provided by phase-specific cytotoxic drugs. When a proliferating cell population is exposed to a sufficient concentration of such a drug, all cells in the sensitive phase of the cycle will be killed, and an assay for cell survival will indicate the proportion of cells in the given phase. Also, if the concentration of the drug is maintained over an extended period of time, a determination can be made of the rate at which cells move into the sensitive phase, and a value can be found for the "Turnover Time" (see below) of the cell population concerned. This technique can only be used when a quantitative assay for cell survival is available, and is therefore restricted mainly to "stem" cells, but it does not require the particular cell population to be identified morphologically. However, in the interpretation of results, it has to be recognized that the cell death produced may affect the proliferative characteristics of the population.

## The Kinetic Parameters of Cell Populations

For a cell population in which at a given time some cells are in the division cycle and some not, there are two classes of kinetic parameters. There are those which are concerned with the "instantaneous" state of the population, for instance, the classification of cells into the various phases of the cycle; these are capable of clear definition and, at least in theory, of precise measurement. One such parameter of considerable importance is the specific birth rate, that is, the mean rate of cell division per cell present, appropriate to the time of measurement. This will be given by the mitotic index of the population divided by the duration of mitosis.

The second class of kinetic parameter involves, however, a prospective element, which introduces certain difficulties both in concept and in measurement. Important examples of this class are distribution of intermitotic time, and the related concept of "Growth Fraction". In principle, the distribution of intermitotic time in a proliferating cell population will normally be defined as the distribution of time intervals, for each cell present, between its last division and its next division. However, experiments can only continue for a limited time and unless it is known, or can be shown, that there is a maximum intermitotic time, there will always be uncertainty about the intermitotic times of the more slowly dividing cells. The presence of "resting" cells within the population will introduce additional problems of measurement unless and until morphological markers are available to distinguish $G_0$ cells from cells in extended $G_1$, and from sterile cells. With regard to the definition of a "sterile" cell, advances in knowledge of the internal control system in cells make it increasingly difficult to be certain that any given cell has lost all capacity for division. In some cases there can be no doubt, i.e., when a cell has lost its nucleus, but the apparent sterility of other classes of cells may be due to the fact that the appropriate stimulus has been lacking. Additional problems, both in concept and in measurement, arise when the distribution of intermitotic times is itself changing with time.

These considerations demonstrate that great care must be taken in stating what is meant by the "Growth Fraction" of a population. The term was introduced by Mendelsohn (1962) to denote the fraction of proliferating cells in the population. But clearly it is an ill-defined concept unless it can be shown that there is a defined maximum intermitotic time for the cells present. An assumption about the time that must elapse since the last division before a cell is defined as "nonproliferating" is, in fact, implicit in the methods available for measurement of the Growth Fraction. These problems concerning the distribution of intermitotic time and Growth Fraction imply that, in practice, operational definitions have to be employed, particularly concerning the distinction between proliferating and nonproliferating cells. This is quite justifiable, so long as proper account is taken of the assumptions made in any practical use to which the data are put.

Another "prospective" and important characteristic of cell populations is the extent to which the proliferating cells present at any given time can continue to produce fertile daughters. At one extreme there will be cells that will continue to produce fertile daughters indefinitely or, at least, for a large number of generations. Such cells will make up the "stem cells" of normal tissues, where they have the dual property of self-maintenance and of providing cells for the maturation pathways. At the other extreme some cells may produce daughters at the first division that will play no further part in proliferation, and there can be intermediate groups with the capacity for limited numbers of divisions. These distinctions are of importance in the understanding of tissue control mechanisms.

Bearing in mind the qualifications that have been discussed above, short accounts will now be given of methods for measuring the main kinetic parameters, introduced by a discussion of the cell "age distribution".

## "Age Distribution" of Cells

A knowledge of the apportionment of cells to the various phases of the cell cycle is a necessary preliminary to the interpretation of labeling indices and of a number of other kinetic measures of cell populations. In a proliferating cell population in steady state, that is, when the rates of cell birth and of cell loss are equal, the proportion of cells in the various phases of the cycle will, in general, be proportional to the duration of the phases. This is expressed by saying that the cells have a "rectangular age distribution" since, if the time since the last division is considered to be the "age" of the cell, the curve of cell number against age will have a rectangular form (Fig. 2a). In point of fact, a steady state renewal popula-

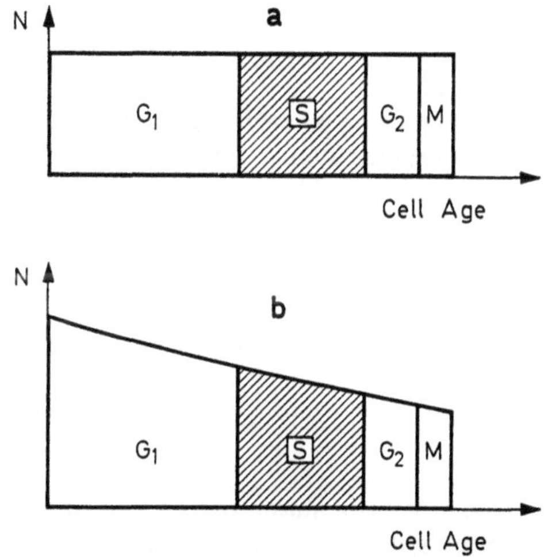


Fig. 2. Age distribution diagrams for two model cell populations; (a) an ideal steady state population, and (b) a no-loss exponentially growing population with two proliferative cells produced at each division

tion will only have a true rectangular age distribution when the loss of cells from the system occurs immediately following mitosis. If loss occurs later, the curve will fall at the cell age where loss occurs. A rectangular age distribution will not hold for growing populations. For a population of proliferating cells with no cell loss, and therefore exponential growth, the age distribution of the cells will be as in Fig. 2b, with the cell number rising to twice the number at the start of $G_1$, since twice as many cells leave $M$ as enter it. For growing cell populations with some cell loss the age distribution will be intermediate between that for a steady-state and a no-loss population.

It should be noted that while a steady-state population will, overall, have a rectangular age-distribution, it may include a subpopulation in which all cell divisions produce proliferative daughters. This subpopulation will have the characteristics of exponential growth and will have a nonrectangular age-distribution. An example of this is found in the small intestine (CAIRNIE et al., 1965). When there is substantial spread in the duration of the phases, the presentation of age distribution curves has to be modified. For a fuller treatment of the subject, the reader is referred to various reviews (STEEL, 1968; LALA, 1971).

## Measurement of "Turnover Time" and "Potential Doubling Time"

The simplest index of the proliferative state of a cell population is the birth rate, that is, the rate of cell production per cell present. It is often conceptually easier, however, to think in terms of "Turnover Time" or "Potential Doubling Time". The term "Turnover Time" is normally applied to steady-state populations and is the time required to produce a number of cells equal to that of the population. It is given by the reciprocal of the birth rate:

$$\text{Turnover Time} = \frac{T_m}{M.\,I.} = \frac{T_s}{L.\,I.}$$

where $M.I.$ is the mitotic index, $L.I.$ is the labeling index, $T_m$ the duration of mitosis, and $T_s$ that of synthesis.

Under conditions of cell population growth, as in tumors, it is more convenient to use the term "Potential Doubling Time" (STEEL, 1968), which represents the time within which the population would double if the same specific birth rate persisted, in the absence of cell loss, and thus represents the doubling time for exponential growth.

It is given by:

$$\text{Potential Doubling Time} = \log_e 2 \times \frac{T_m}{M.\,I.}$$

$$= \log_e 2 \times K \times \frac{T_s}{L.\,I.}$$

where $K$ is a correction factor for the shape of the age distribution of the cells. The error involved in assuming that $K$ has a value of unity will normally be relatively small.

Both Turnover Time and Potential Doubling Time are measures of cell production rate, as opposed to actual growth rate. The application of Potential Doubling Time in considerations of tumor growth is discussed below.

There are a number of different ways in which $T_s$ may be measured to allow the calculation of turnover time from the labeling index. An accurate direct measurement of $T_m$ presents more problems, because there are fewer methods available and because it is much shorter than $T_s$. However, the difficulty can be circumvented to some extent by the use of metaphase arrest agents. The ideal agent will arrest all metaphases, at least over several hours, and will not affect the behavior of cells in other parts of the cycle. Under these conditions, the initial slope of the curve of metaphase index against time will give the turnover time of the population and will also allow a value for $T_m$ to be determined (STEVENS-HOOPER, 1961). However, much care must be taken with this technique since it is unlikely that any of the available metaphase agents, either colchicine derivatives or the vinca alkaloids, are ideal. The work of TANNOCK (1967) shows that there can be considerable departure from ideal behaviour, depending both on the agent used and the type of tissue studied. In all cases, a test must be made to ensure that the metaphase collection increases linearly with time over the period of observation.

## Measurement of the Intermitotic Time and Duration of the Constituent Phases

The most widely used, and most informative, technique for studying intermitotic time and the duration of the various phases is that of "labeled mitoses" (QUASTLER and SHERMAN, 1959), in which the passage of a cohort of cells labeled in *S* is followed through successive mitotic divisions. The method depends on the use of a labeled DNA precursor whose availability time is short compared with the duration of the phases measured, and this will normally be the case with *in vivo* administration of labeled thymidine. For an asynchronous cell population in which there is not spread in the duration of the different phases, a determination of the fraction of mitotic figures labeled at various times after a single administration of the labeled DNA precursor will show a periodic variation, as shown in Fig. 3a, from which the phase durations can be read off.

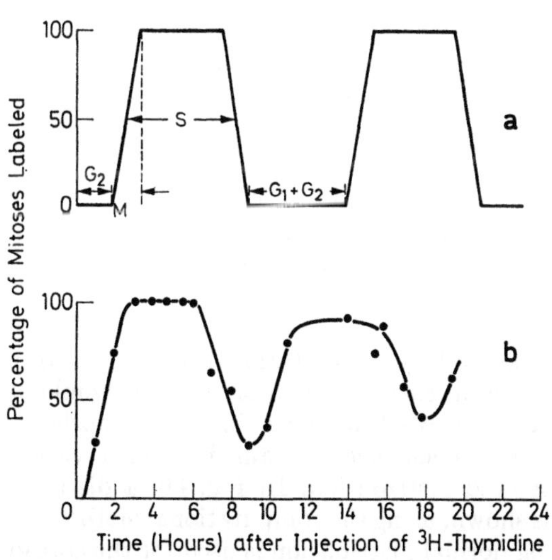


**Fig. 3. Labeled mitoses curves; (a) "Ideal" curve, and (b) experimental curve for tail bud of embryo mouse (12th to 13th day of gestation)**

Some tissues will show labeled mitoses curves corresponding quite closely to the theoretical curve. An example is shown in Fig. 3b. One can deduce from this result that the great majority of cells have a narrow spread of phase durations and intermitotic times, and reasonably precise values can be obtained. However, such a curve does not rule out the existence of a small subpopulation of slowly dividing cells, since this will have very little effect on the shape of the labeled mitoses curve.

In many tissues, and this applies particularly to most primary tumors, there is a considerable spread in intermitotic time and in the duration of the individual phases. This leads to a damping-out of the curve, as seen in Fig. 4a, which is a curve obtained from human epithelial tumor data of FRINDEL et al. (1968). The interpretation of such curves has been the subject of a great deal of published work. One approach is to assume a particular mathematical form for the spread of

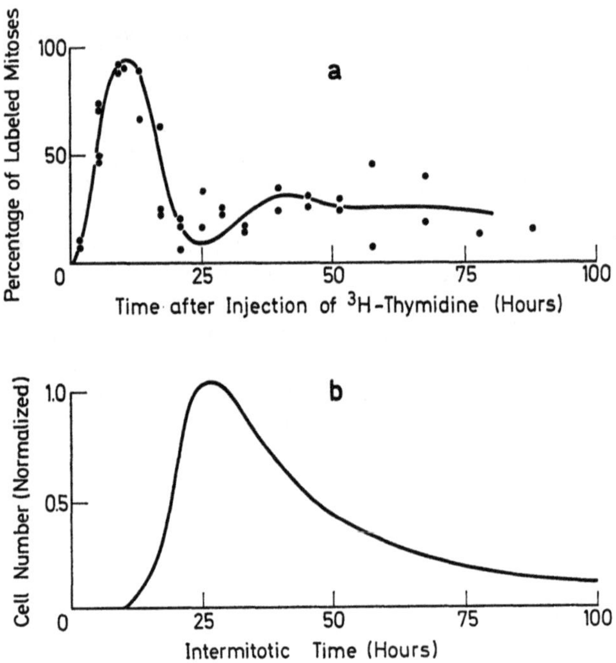


Fig. 4. (a) Labeled mitoses curve for human epithelial tumor cells. (b) Computed distribution of intermitotic times

duration of the phases and by computational or analytical methods to attempt to match the experimental curve. For most tissues it would appear that a distribution of phase duration skewed to longer time is appropriate, and good matching with experimental curves has been obtained using a variety of mathematical expressions for a skewed distribution. In Fig. 4b, a distribution obtained from the data of Fig. 4a is shown, using the computational method described by BARRETT (1966), in which a log normal distribution is used for the spread of phase duration.

Distributions of intermitotic time obtained in this way can only be taken as giving a general guide to the true situation in the cell population concerned, particularly when the spread is considerable. Depending on the period over which experimental observations were made, and the assumptions in the analysis, the distribution represented by the "tail" of the curve can be highly inaccurate, and the contribution from the more slowly dividing cells can be seriously underestimated.

A simulation approach, as described above, will frequently not be available, or even justified, for the interpretation of labeled mitoses curves. When the curve is well-defined, average values may be read off directly from the curve. One of the most commonly applied methods is to take the intervals at which the curve crosses the 50% level as the appropriate phase durations. This will sometimes give a poor estimate of the mean duration, but in most cases a rather better estimate of the median values. The value of such an estimate depends, of course, on the practical use to which the data is being put. The general problems of extraction of information from labeled mitoses curves have been reviewed in two recent papers (MENDELSOHN and TAKAHASHI, 1971; STEEL, 1972).

Under certain circumstances, information on the spread of intermitotic time and, in particular, of the more slowly dividing members of the population can be obtained from continuous or frequently repeated administration of a labeled DNA precursor. If the population is known to have a Growth Fraction of unity, that is, all cells are proliferating, the maximum intermitotic time will be given by the time taken for the whole population to become fully labeled, added to the duration of synthesis. However, if the population contains a nonproliferative fraction, derived from the proliferating cells, which is so in many types of normal and malignant tissues, the interpretation of the data becomes uncertain. The interpretation of continous labeling data in tumors has been discussed by LALA (1971) and by STEEL et al. (1966).

In principle, measurement of the rate of decrease of the mean grain count of labeled cells should give information on intermitotic time. When there is a narrow spread of intermitotic time, and little or no movement of cells from proliferating to nonproliferating compartments (or vice versa) the technique is reasonably straightforward. However, a spread of intermitotic time and a low Growth Fraction can make interpretation of data difficult, quite apart from problems arising due to reutilization of label. Nevertheless, this may be one of the few techniques applicable under certain circumstances, for instance with some human studies. Reports of its application in cases of human leukemia are discussed in a series of papers by CLARKSON and his colleagues (FRIED, 1968; CLARKSON, 1969).

Perhaps the most reliable method for obtaining information on the slowly dividing cells in a population was referred to earlier: the survival of the cells is determined after various periods of administration of a phase-specific cytotoxic agent. This requires a quantitative assay for cell survival and thus has limited application. Examples of its use in studies of stem cells of normal tissues and of tumors are mentioned below.

Apart from the labeled mitoses method, there are additional techniques available for the measurement of $T_s$ and, to a lesser extent, for other phases of the cell cycle. The double labeling technique is one that has been used extensively to measure $T_s$. This requires the use of two differently labeled DNA precursors, usually $^3$H-labeled thymidine and $^{14}$C-labeled thymidine, and an autoradiographic technique capable of distinguishing between the two labels. The method is to inject the tritiated precursor and, after an interval $t$ (which must be less than $G_2$ and is normally about 1 hour), to inject the $^{14}$C-labeled precursor. Cells leaving $S$ during the period $t$ will carry only the $^3$H label, so that if the population is examined autoradiographically soon after the second injection $T_s$ can be determined from the expression:

$$T_s = t \times \frac{\text{proportion of cells labeled with } ^{14}\text{C (and } ^{14}\text{C} + {}^3\text{H)}}{\text{proportion of cells labeled with } ^3\text{H only}}$$

For details of the technique the general review of LALA (1971) can be consulted.

## Measurement of Growth Fraction

Most of the methods for measuring the Growth Fraction of a population are based on an assessment of the labeling index of the proliferating fraction, since the Growth Fraction, defined as the ratio of proliferating cells to total cells, will be equal to the ratio of the labeling index of the proliferating cells to that of the whole population. The usual approach is to use the labeled mitoses curve to estimate the durations of $S$ and of the intermitotic time $T$ and from the ratio to derive labeling index of the proliferating fraction. This can be considerably in error if the labeled mitosis curve is very damped, because of the problems of analyzing a highly damped curve and because the slowly dividing component of the population may be underestimated.

Another method, originally proposed by Mendelsohn (1962), is to continue the labeled mitoses curve until it levels out, due to asynchrony of the originally labeled cohort of cells. With corrections, the final level will give the labeling index of the proliferative fraction. The problem here is to ensure that the true final level is measured; the label may be diluted below a measurable value before the level is reached and also reutilization of label may distort the curve at later intervals.

A third method is to assess the Growth Fraction from the shape of the continuous or repeated labeling curve of the population. It is sometimes assumed that the Growth Fraction is equal to the value at which the labeling index of the population levels off. The difficulty here is that the nonproliferating cells which have been derived from the proliferating cells will at later time intervals themselves be labeled. Frequently the curve will not level off, and when it does the interpretation may not be straightforward. Steel et al. (1966) and Lala (1971) have, as already mentioned, considered the problem of interpretation of continuous labeling curves in some detail.

Growth Fraction is a clear concept and measurable with precision when the intermitotic time of the proliferating cells is short and covers only a narrow range of values. When substantial numbers of slowly dividing cells are present, the quantitative assessment of the Growth Fraction may have little significance.

## Measurement of Cell Loss

The Potential Doubling Time ($T_{pot}$), measured as described above, will give for a growing population, the time taken for the cell population to double in size, assuming that the specific birth rate remains constant, and in the absence of any form of cell loss. A comparison of $T_{pot}$ with the observed doubling time of the cell population can therefore give a measure of the extent of cell loss, which may include ineffective division, cell death within the tissue and cell escape from the tissue. Application of this procedure to tumors indicates that cell loss is a major factor in the relatively slow growth rate of many primary tumors. Results and further discussion will be found in papers by Iversen (1967) and Steel (1968).

## Cell Population Kinetics of Normal Tissues

A brief summary of the cell population kinetics of the normal proliferating tissues of the body can usefully be based on the compartmental diagram shown below (Fig. 5), though not all compartments will be found in each tissue.

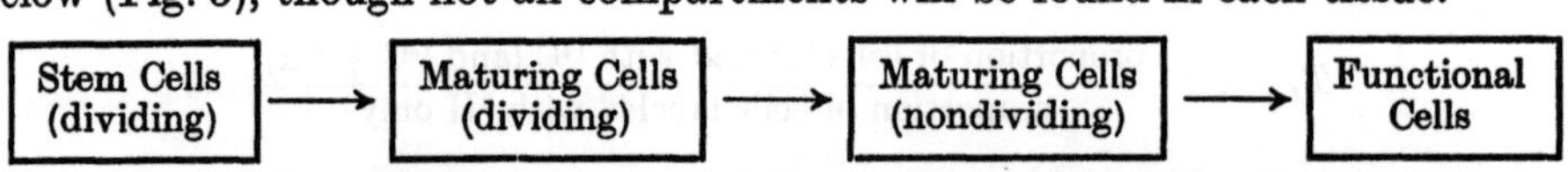


Fig. 5. Generalized compartmental diagram of normal proliferating tissues

In the blood forming tissues of the bone marrow all four compartments are found, and investigations by a number of workers have provided a considerable amount of data on the cell population kinetics of the system. The stem cells represent only a small subpopulation of the nucleated cells present and cannot yet be recognized morphologically. Consequently, functional techniques based on stem cell assay procedures have to be used to study their properties. Such investigations, carried out mainly in rodents (LAHIRI and VAN PUTTEN, 1969) have demonstrated that the stem cell content of the bone marrow is small, 1% or possibly considerably less, and that, in the unstimulated marrow, the stem cells are relatively slowly dividing. Precise intermitotic times are not known, but present data, obtained by the technique involving selective killing of cells using phase-specific cytotoxic drugs, suggest that in the rat the intermitotic time may be of the order of two days (BLACKETT, 1968). In the mouse, the mean intermitotic time may be considerably longer than this (BECKER et al., 1965) and some workers have concluded that the stem cell compartment will include a population of resting cells. This slow rate of proliferation is in contrast to that found in the recognizable dividing precursors of the erythropoietic and granulocytic series, that is, in Compartment II of Fig. 5. Here, labeled mitoses and other direct techniques may be used, and the mean intermitotic times in the rat and mouse are found to be of the order of 10 hours (FRINDEL et al., 1967; HANNA et al., 1969). Studies on the red cell system suggest that the change from proliferating to nonproliferating cells in the maturation sequence is not accompanied by any substantial lengthening of this short intermitotic time.

The compartmental scheme given above is highly simplified as far as the bone marrow is concerned. There are extra compartments between the progenitor cells and recognizable precursors, whose characteristics and interrelationships are not fully understood, but this uncertainty does not affect the general concept, in unstimulated tissue, of slowly dividing stem cells and rapidly dividing later precursors.

The small intestine is another tissue in which the cell population kinetics have been extensively studied (FRY et al., 1963; CAIRNIE et al., 1965). The proliferating cells are found in the lower part of the crypts of Lieberkuhn, and labeled mitosis studies carried out in rats, mice and in some other species show that at least the great majority of these cells are dividing rapidly, with intermitotic times of the order of ten hours. However, it now appears that this fast rate of cell division does not hold throughout the proliferative zone. Both labeling index, and mitotic index, are lower in cells at the base of the crypts (CAIRNIE, 1967; WRIGHT, personal communication). Making the reasonable assumption that the growth fraction in these lower cell positions is unity, the mitotic index data of WRIGHT indicates that the cell at the base of the mouse crypt has an intermitotic time of at least 40 hours. Recent unpublished work by WRIGHT on human intestinal material obtained by biopsy, indicates that the slower turnover of cells at the base of the crypt is more marked in man than in rodents. Thus, the small intestine appears to resemble the bone marrow in having a slower rate of proliferation among the earliest precursors of the series. The small intestine does not, however, lend itself so easily to stem cell assay, and it is not yet clear whether stem cell capacity in the crypt is confined to the lowest cells or also includes the remaining more rapidly dividing cells in the proliferative zone. In other words, it is not yet known whether Compartment II, containing dividing nonstem cells, exists in this tissue. As in the case of bone marrow, the change from dividing to nondividing cells is not accompanied by any marked lengthening of intermitotic time.

The skin is another normal renewal tissue which has been the subject of considerable cell kinetic study. Here the stem cells, which are a recognizable population comprising the basal layer adjacent to the basement membrane, also have a slow rate of division in unstimulated tissue, the mean intermitotic time being of several days in rodents. The extent to which these cells contain a $G_0$ population has been studied (Burns and Tannock, 1970). It is possible that all the basal cells enter a $G_0$ state after mitosis, but proof is difficult. In normal mouse skin, cells leaving the basal layer appear to lose their capacity for division immediately, or at least very quickly, so that effectively there is no Compartment II.

Response to injury and a demand for new cells call into play homeostatic mechanisms which affect the cell population kinetics of these tissues in various ways. One is by a shortening of the intermitotic time of the stem cells, and this is shown clearly in skin in response to loss of the overlying keratinized cells (Hennings and Elgjo, 1970). This effect is also demonstrated in the bone marrow, where the stem cells are speeded up considerably following treatment with radiation or other agents causing depletion of proliferating cells. However, it should be noted that removal of mature red cells from the animal does not necessarily cause a speeding up of stem cells. Here the recovery mechanism appears to act, at least to a large extent, by stimulation of the erythropoietin-sensitive cells, which are a cell population subsequent to the progenitor cells of the system.

Some shortening of intermitotic time also occurs in the small intestine after cell depletion by radiation (and this may be very substantial in the cells in the lowest cell positions, though this has not yet been confirmed), but another, and very important, effect is the temporary extension of the zone of proliferation up the crypt (Lesher et al., 1967), which greatly increases the output of mature cells. A similar effect has been observed in the bone marrow under continuous irradiation, where there is some shortening of intermitotic time in the dividing and recognizable precursors, but also a marked lengthening of time spent in the various morphological stages, allowing more divisions to occur and the amplification factor of the compartment to be increased.

Further work is required on the cell population kinetics of tissue response in these and other proliferating tissues of the body if proper therapeutic use is to be made of the proliferation-dependent cytotoxic agents now available. Of special importance is new information on the timing of the proliferative changes in the stem cell populations and the nature and extent of feed-back between the later precursors and mature cells and the stem cell compartments.

## Cell Population Kinetics of Tumors

The nature of tumors, their diversity of types, and the range in degree of histological disorganization do not allow the same type of broad generalizations to be made as with normal tissues. The main compartmental distinction will be between cells having stem cell capacity, that is, the capacity for indefinitely continued proliferation, and those that have not. The kinetics of the nonstem cell population will be of less concern than in normal tissues, particularly in regrowth. The usefulness of cell kinetic studies on tumors will depend largely on how far the stem cells can be studied independently of the other cells present.

In certain normal tissues the presumptive stem cells can be identified on architectural grounds, but this is generally not the case with tumors. In some of the more highly differentiated tumors there may be opportunities for architectural identification of stem cells, though this is a field which has so far been little explored, but in most tumors the disorganization of structure is likely to make their direct identification impossible and knowledge of kinetic characteristics must be based on indirect methods.

With some of the rapidly growing transplantable tumors used in experimental work, the situation is relatively straightforward, since the observed rate of tumor doubling is found to be only slightly less than the mean intermitotic time determined by the method of labeled mitoses, indicating a low rate of cell loss, a high growth fraction, and showing that the majority of cells present are behaving as stem cells. Nevertheless, it is difficult to be certain that there is not a small subpopulation of slowly dividing stem cells, which could be of considerable practical significance.

However, with some transplantable tumors and with most primary tumors, the situation is different, and the estimation of numbers and proliferative characteristics of the stem cell population presents several problems. These neoplasms often grow very slowly, which can be shown to be due to a combination of high cell loss, low Growth Fraction, and a relatively long intermitotic time for the dividing cells, with considerable spread (STEEL, 1972). The proportion of stem cells may in some cases be quite low, due to differentiation or to the presence of many cells destined to death or loss from the tissue. Under these conditions the distribution of intermitotic times derived from the labeled mitoses curve (of which an example is given in Fig. 4a)] may not be representative of the stem cells. In the first place, the shape of the labeled mitoses curve may be strongly influenced by the presence of cells on their way to death or differentiation, but which still retain a limited capacity for division. Secondly, stem cells might be found in a "resting" state, or in the population of very slowly dividing cells which is not estimated by the labeled mitoses method.

Only a few studies have so far been made of the proliferative characteristics of the stem cell population using the technique of phase specific cytotoxic agents combined with a tumor stem cell assay. Using spontaneous leukemia in AKR mice, SKIPPER (personal communication) demonstrated a difference between distribution of intermitotic times for the stem cells and for the tumor cell population taken as a whole. In this case the stem cells were the more rapidly dividing.

Tumor repopulation after damage by cytotoxic agents will originate from the surviving stem cells, though not necessarily all surviving stem cells will take part in repopulation. The particular environment of a surviving stem cell, for instance, its distance from a blood vessel, may well determine whether or not it can express its proliferative potential, though this is an area in which at the moment there is very little information. With regard to possible change in the proliferation rate of tumor cells during repopulation, HERMENS and BARENDSEN (1969) have reported a shortening in intermitotic time following irradiation of an experimental tumor. The measurements could not distinguish the stem cells from "doomed" cells which were damaged but still able to divide several times. However, it is likely that the surviving stem cells were speeded up. It is very important to know how far this is a general characteristic of repopulating tumors, and, in particular, how far very slowly dividing cells can be speeded up and "resting" cells triggered into preparation for cell division. Some information on these matters comes from studies on human acute leukemia (SAUNDERS and MAUER, 1969) but, as with normal tissues, one of the challenges to the subject of cell population kinetics at the present time is a better understanding of the nature and timing of the various processes of tumor repopulation.

## References


Barrett, J.C.: A mathematical model of the mitotic cycle and its application to interpretation of percentage labeled mitoses data. J. nat. Cancer Inst. **37**, 443—450 (1966).

Baserga, R.: Biochemistry of the cell cycle: a review. Cell and Tissue Kinet. **1**, 167—191 (1968).

Becker, A.J., McCulloch, E.A., Siminovitch, L., Till, J.E.: The effect of differing demands for blood cell production on DNA synthesis by hemopoietic colony forming cells of mice. Blood **26**, 296—308 (1965).

Blackett, N.M.: Investigation of bone-marrow stem cell proliferation in normal, anaemic and irradiated rats, using methotrexate and tritiated thymidine. J. nat. Cancer Inst. **41**, 909—918 (1968).

Burns, F.J., Tannock, I.F.: On the existence of a $G_0$ phase in the cell cycle. Cell and Tissue Kinet. **3**, 321—334 (1970).

Cairnie, A.B.: Cell proliferation studies in the intestinal epithelium of the rat: response to continuous irradiation. Radiat. Res. **32**, 240—264 (1967).

Cairnie, A.B., Lamerton, L.F., Steel, G.G.: Cell proliferation studies in the intestinal epithelium of the rat. Exp. cell Res. **39**, 528—538, 539—553 (1965).

Clarkson, B.D.: Review of recent studies of cellular proliferation in acute leukemia. In: Human tumour cell kinetics. National Cancer Institute Monograph 30, (1969), pp. 81—119.

Epifanova, O.I., Terskikh, V.V.: On the resting periods in the cell life cycle. Cell and Tissue Kinet. **2**, 75—93 (1969).

Fried, J.: Estimating the median generation time of proliferating cell systems in steady state. Biophys. J. 8, 710—729 (1968).

Frindel, E., Malaise, E.P., Tubiana, M.: Cell proliferation kinetics in five human solid tumours. Cancer **22**, 611—620 (1968).

Frindel, E., Tubiana, M., Vassort, F.: Generation cycle of mouse bone marrow. Nature (Lond.) **214**, 1017—1018 (1967).

Fry, R.J.M., Lesher, S., Kisieleski, W.E., Sacher, G.: Cell proliferation in the small intestine. In: Cell proliferation — a Guiness symposium. Oxford: Blackwell Scientific Publications (1963).

Hale, A.J., Cooper, E.H., Milton, J.D.: Studies of the incorporation of pyrimidines into DNA in single leukaemic and other proliferating leucocytes. Brit. J. Haematol. **11**, 144—161 (1965).

Hanna, I.R.A., Tarbutt, R.G., Lamerton, L.F.: Shortening of cell-cycle time of erythroid precursors in response to anaemia. Brit. J. Haematol. **16**, 381—387 (1969).

Hennings, H., Elgjo, K.: Epidermal regeneration after cellophane tape stripping of hairless mouse skin. Cell and Tissue Kinet. **3**, 243—252 (1970).

Hermens, A.F., Barendsen, G.W.: Changes of cell proliferation characteristics in a rat rhabdomyosarcoma before and after x-irradiation. Europ. J. Cancer **5**, 173—189 (1969).

Iversen, O.H.: Kinetics of cellular proliferation and cell loss in human carcinoma: a discussion of methods available for *in vivo* studies. Europ. J. Cancer **3**, 389—394 (1967).

Lahiri, S.K., Van Putten, L.M.: Distribution and multiplication of colony forming units from bone marrow and spleen after injection in irradiated mice. Cell and Tissue Kinet. **2**, 21—28 (1969).

Lala, P.K.: Studies on tumor cell population kinetics. In: Methods in Cancer Research, Vol. 6, pp. 3—95. New York: Academic Press 1971.

Lesher, S., Sallese, A., Jones, M.: Effects of 1000 R whole-body x-irradiation on DNA and mitosis in the duodenal crypts of the BCF-1 mouse. Z. Zellforsch. mikrosk. Anat. **77**, 144—146 (1967).

Mendelsohn, M.L.: Autoradiographic analysis of cell proliferation in spontaneous breast cancer of C3H mouse. III. The growth fraction. J. nat. Cancer Inst. **28**, 1015—1029 (1962).

Mendelsohn, M.L., Takahashi, M.: A critical evaluation of the fraction of labelled mitoses method as applied to the analysis of tumor and other cell cycles. In: The cell cycle and cancer. New York: Marcel Dekker 1971.

Quastler, H., Sherman, F.G.: Cell population kinetics in the intestinal epithelium of the mouse. Exp. cell Res. **17**, 420—438 (1959).

Saunders, E.F., Mauer, A.M.: Re-entry of nondividing leukemic cells into a proliferative phase in acute childhood leukaemia. J. clin. Invest. **48**, 1299—1305 (1969).

STEEL, G. G.: Cell loss from experimental tumors. Cell and Tissue Kinet. **1**, 193—207 (1968).

STEEL, G. G.: The cell cycle in tumours: an examination of data gained by the technique of labelled mitoses. Cell and Tissue Kinet. **5**, 87—100 (1972).

STEEL, G. G., ADAMS, K., BARRETT, J. C.: Analysis of the cell population kinetics of transplanted tumours of widely differing growth rate. Brit. J. Cancer **20**, 784—800 (1966).

STEVENS-HOOPER, C.E.: Use of colchicine for the measurement of mitotic rate in the intestinal epithelium. Amer. J. Anat. **108**, 231—244 (1961).

TANNOCK, I.F.: A comparison of the relative efficiencies of various metaphase arrest agents. Exp. cell Res. **47**, 345—356 (1967).

Chapter 8

# Clinical Applications of Cell Cycle Kinetics

BAYARD CLARKSON

With 3 Figures

## Introduction

Clinicians experienced in treating cancer have long been aware of the great variability in growth rates among different types of cancer and even within the same type, but until recently estimates of growth rates were largely limited to measurements of volume doubling times of solid tumors visible externally or roentgenographically (COLLINS et al., 1956; COLLINS, 1962; GARLAND et al., 1963; SPRATT and SPRATT, 1964; CHARBIT et al., 1971). These estimates were necessarily rough and gave little insight into the many factors which can influence the doubling time, such as the tumor cells' intermitotic time and its variability, the relative proportions of actively proliferating and resting tumor cells, changes in the tumor's proliferative behavior during different stages of growth, rate of cell loss, influence of vascular supply, contribution of stromal tissues, hemorrhage or necrosis to the tumor mass, and perturbations caused by therapy. Information about the comparative proliferative rates of normal tissues was also largely lacking.

These crude estimates of tumor growth were of limited value in guiding treatment, and therapeutic programs to date have been almost entirely empirical. Radiation therapy and cytotoxic drugs which showed therapeutic promise in subclinical tumor screening systems were tested for their activity against different types of human tumors; dosage schedules for both chemotherapy and radiotherapy were arrived at largely by trial and error. Sometimes two or more agents, each with demonstrable activity against a given neoplastic disease, were combined, and the combination often produced better therapeutic results than any single agent (HENDERSON and SAMAHA, 1969). However, little thought was given to cytokinetic considerations in designing treatment schedules.

During the last decade, a great deal has been learned about the proliferative behavior of tumors in both experimental animals and man. In some experimental tumors, intelligent application of chemotherapeutic tactics, based at least in part on kinetic principles, have succeeded in curing a high proportion of animals (BRUCE et al., 1966, 1969; BRUCE and BERGSAGEL, 1967; BRUCE and VALERIOTE, 1968; SCHABEL, 1968; SKIPPER, 1968, 1971a; SCHABEL et al., 1969; SKIPPER et al., 1969; VENDITTI, 1971). However, for the most part, the human cytokinetic studies have succeeded only in demonstrating the complexities of the tumors' proliferative behavior and have given few clues as to how to use this knowledge for therapeutic advantage. Moreover, the initial studies have posed many new problems which had previously not been appreciated.

It has become apparent that in spontaneous human neoplasms there is often no sharp distinction between the proliferative behavior of the neoplastic cells and that of the normal cells from which they arose, and that there is generally an intimate relationship between the normal and neoplastic populations. In some tumors the proliferative rate of the tumor cells far outstrips that of their normal ancestors, and the host is quickly overwhelmed by massive tumor. In other cases the normal and neoplastic populations may coexist in a fine state of balance, at least for a time, so that there is little net gain in the size of the tumor (e.g. *in situ* tumors and indolent forms of leukemia or other tumors). In still other instances, a tumor may start to develop and then disappear due to degeneration or maturation. The possibility that spontaneous regression may sometimes occur has been well-documented in the case of neuroblastoma and to a lesser extent in nephroblastoma in infants (Farber, 1940; Koop et al., 1955; Everson and Cole, 1966). It has been estimated that the incidence of neuroblastoma *in situ* in fetuses and newborns dying of other causes may be as high as 67 times that of clinically apparent neuroblastoma of childhood (Shanklin and Sotelo-Avila, 1969). It is not known how frequently a similar phenomenon might occur in adults without being recognized, but spontaneous regression of established tumors is extremely rare. In a recent review only 176 adequately documented cases were collected from the world medical literature in which temporary or permanent spontaneous regression occurred (Everson and Cole, 1966). Once a tumor has become large enough to give rise to symptoms and be diagnosed, it almost invariably grows progressively, although the rate of growth may vary enormously.

## Classification of Tumors Based on Response to Treatment

In terms of response to treatment, it is useful to separate human tumors into five broad categories; examples of each will be given, but a comprehensive listing is not intended.

1. Tumors, usually localized, which are frequently amenable to cure, either by surgical resection, radiotherapy, chemotherapy, or by combined forms of these treatments: carcinoma of the cervix, Wilms' tumor, endometrial cancer, carcinoma of the larynx, astrocytoma, some cases of breast or colon cancer, epidermoid cancers of the head and neck, retinoblastoma, some thyroid cancers; some lymphomas, and some testicular cancers.

2. Disseminated tumors which are frequently curable by chemotherapy alone. There are presently only two such examples: (a) metastatic uterine choriocarcinoma, and (b) Burkitt's lymphoma.

3. Disseminated tumors which are usually highly responsive to chemotherapy and probably sometimes curable (in some cases only after the primary tumor has been surgically resected or irradiated): acute lymphoblastic leukemia, Wilm's tumor, Ewing's sarcoma, childhood embryonal rhabdomyosarcoma, some testicular cancers, and some lymphomas.

4. Disseminated tumors usually moderately responsive to chemotherapy (and/or radiotherapy), but rarely if ever curable, and in which therapy generally causes no increase or only a slight increase in survival time: acute myeloblastic and other nonlymphoblastic forms of acute leukemia, chronic myelogenous leukemia, chronic lymphocytic leukemia, polycythemia vera, neuroblastoma, multiple myeloma, some ovarian cancers, and often many of the tumors listed in categories 1 and 3.

5. Locally invasive or disseminated tumors rarely curable with surgery and/or radiation, and so poorly responsive to any form of treatment that there is usually no significant increase in survival time: glioblastoma multiforme, esophageal cancer, lung cancer, stomach cancer, pancreatic cancer, hepatoma, and metastatic melanoma.

This section will deal mainly with tumors in categories 3 and 4. Treatment is as yet so poorly developed for most category 5 tumors that cytokinetic information, even if it were available, would probably be of little value at the present time. With regard to category 2, these tumors are often so exquisitely sensitive to chemotherapy that cytokinetic considerations are probably less important in designing treatment regimes than in the case of tumors in categories 3 and 4. The reason why uterine choriocarcinoma is so responsive to chemotherapy is unknown. It is widely assumed that host defense mechanisms may play a role in the tumor's regression, in view of this tumor's unique characteristic of metastasizing from the fetal portion of the placenta to the mother, but there is as yet no proof of this. It was discovered empirically that it was possible to cure a high proportion of women with metastatic choriocarcinoma with several different cytotoxic drugs long before any thought was given to possible peculiarities in the tumor's kinetic behavior (Li et al., 1956; Bagshawe, 1969). There is still only limited information about the proliferative characteristics of choriocarcinoma; available data are based either on volume doubling times of pulmonary metastases or on estimations of growth rate as related to chorionic gonadotrophin excretion (Bagshawe, 1969).

Similarly, many patients with Burkitt's lymphoma were shown to be curable with cyclophosphamide (and sometimes by other drugs) before any information about the tumor's kinetic behavior was available (Carbone et al., 1969). It has subsequently been shown that this tumor's rapid clinical growth is a consequence of a short cell cycle time and a high growth fraction; there is also indirect evidence that the spontaneous death rate of the tumor cells is high (Cooper et al., 1966; Iverson et al., 1972). Stage I or II Burkitt's lymphoma can sometimes be cured with a single dose of cyclophosphamide, but the reason for this extraordinary sensitivity is not known (Ziegler et al., 1970; Carbone et al., 1971). There are other types of lymphomas that grow just as rapidly, but that are not nearly as amenable to cure with chemotherapy. Host immunity has also been assumed to be important in contributing to the regression of Burkitt's lymphoma following treatment, but here too definitive evidence is still lacking.

Cytokinetic information might be expected to be most helpful in formulating more effective treatment protocols for tumors in categories 3 and 4, which are partially responsive to treatment but which are presently rarely or never curable. No easy kinetic solution has been discovered which can be used to selectively destroy neoplastic cells without damaging normal ones. If, for example, there were a clear difference between the cell cycles of neoplastic and normal cells, it might be possible to capitalize on this difference and to design a therapeutic strategem to selectively kill the former. However, since no major differences have been found between the cell cycle or other kinetic parameters of neoplastic and normal cells, and since no highly selective antitumor drugs have been found, the approach to treatment must be more subtle and comprehensive. One must take advantage of minor kinetic, biochemical, or other differences between neoplastic and normal cells which may make the former more vulnerable to available methods of treatment.

## Integration of Cytokinetic Strategems with other Therapeutic Considerations

If it is assumed that the eventual goal is to eradicate the entire neoplastic population without causing irreversible toxicity, it is of course desirable to have as precise an understanding as possible of the proliferative behavior of not only the neoplastic population but also of any normal cell populations which may be susceptible to injury by the therapy employed. Unfortunately, detailed cytokinetic information is available for only a few human tumors. Moreover, the measurements which have been made are generally semiquantitative at best, and data about several crucial parameters are almost entirely lacking (e.g. size of clonogenic fraction of tumor cells, rate of cell loss, etc.). It must also be realized that cytokinetic considerations are only one facet in the design of a rational clinical treatment protocol, and it is necessary to integrate kinetic strategems with any other pertinent information about using available therapeutic modalities most effectively. The most important other considerations are:

1. Appreciation of the clinical patterns and natural courses of evolution and spread of different neoplasms in order to be able to judge intelligently when and how aggressively to treat them.

2. Knowledge about the biochemical mechanisms of action of different drugs and of their physiological distributions and metabolic fates when administered by different routes and dosage schedules.

3. Correlation of extracellular and (when possible) intracellular drug concentrations in tumors with levels known to be cytocidal for specific types of tumor cells.

4. Appreciation of how a given agent exerts its lethal effect in relation to the cell cycle (i.e. does it kill cells in all phases of the cycle or is its lethal action restricted to one or more phases of the cycle ?)

5. Choice of therapeutic agents which have been demonstrated empirically in clinical trials to be at least partially effective in treating specific neoplastic diseases.

6. Awareness of the injurious effects of cytotoxic agents on the hematopoietic and other sensitive normal tissues and of their expected rates of recovery.

7. Estimation on the basis of past experience of the maximum amount of therapy it is possible to deliver consistent with tolerable toxicity. Intelligent use of combinations of agents with proven effectiveness based on their different mechanisms of action in order to try to (a) circumvent development of resistance to any one, and (b) obtain synergistic or additive therapeutic activity while at the same time minimizing damage to any single critical normal organ system by taking advantage of the different agents' differing patterns of toxicity.

One must learn to manipulate the different agents in complex treatment schedules in a manner most consistent with maximum therapeutic effect and minimal toxicity.

Because there are important differences in their proliferative behavior and response to treatment, tumors which become widely disseminated early in their course, such as those of the hematopoietic system, will be considered separately from "solid" tumors which arise locally at one or more sites and which become inoperable by direct extension or metastatic spread. Attention will be focused mainly on the few tumors about which kinetic information is most complete and where initial attempts have already been made to use this information to improve treatment. Different modes of treatment will also be considered separately, concentrating on chemotherapy for widely disseminated tumors and radiotherapy for localized tumors. We will then consider combined conventional methods of treatment, and finally other possible but as yet unproved approaches to therapy.

# Hematopoietic Tumors

## A. Acute Leukemia

### I. General Characteristics and Potential Curability

More is known about the proliferative behavior of cells in acute leukemia than any other human tumor (KILLMANN, 1968; CLARKSON et al., 1969, 1971b; GAVOSTO and PILERI, 1971). Acute leukemia has been postulated to originate from (neoplastic) transformation of a single hematopoietic (stem) cell (CLARKSON and FRIED, 1971a). The transformed cell and its descendents have unlimited proliferative potential coupled with relative unresponsiveness to normal regulatory mechanisms. Whatever surveillance mechanisms might normally operate to dispose of such cells are presumably defective, at least temporarily, in patients who develop leukemia. To maintain a constant number of cells, a normal hematopoietic stem cell on the average generates one daughter committed to differentiation (which may then undergo a limited number of maturation divisions), and one daughter which remains as a stem cell in order to carry on the line (CLARKSON and FRIED, 1971a). The transformed (leukemic) cell and its progeny instead produce a greater than 1:1 ratio of stem: committed cells and therefore the leukemic population becomes progressively larger.

No specific chromosomal abnormality has been found in acute leukemia; approximately half of the patients have microscopically normal diploid karyotypes in their leukemic marrow cells, while the rest have one or more chromosomal deviations. The latter are not specific or consistent and have no apparent therapeutic or prognostic significance (FITZGERALD et al., 1964; KIOSSOGLOU et al., 1965; SANDBERG, 1966). The lack of detectable abnormalities in some patients and the diversity and variability of changes in others suggest that the abnormalities are either due to multiple causative factors or, more likely, that they represent secondary changes as a consequence of greater fragility of leukemic metaphases, disorder of the DNA replicative process, or other metabolic alterations.

In patients who have recognizable karyotypic abnormalities prior to treatment and in whom serial cytogenetic studies have been performed, the abnormal metaphases disappear from the marrow or are greatly reduced in number, and normal diploid modes are present during drug-induced remissions (JENSEN, 1967; ZUELZER and COX, 1969; HART et al., 1971). When relapse occurs, the original abnormal leukemic line reappears; in some cases, one or more secondary abnormal lines may appear, probably most often as a result of clonal evolution. These observations provide fairly compelling evidence that acute leukemia (both myeloblastic and lymphoblastic) usually has a unicentric origin, and that the leukemic population is separate and distinct from the normal hematopoietic stem line[1]. Thus, relapse is ordinarily caused by regrowth of residual cells from the

1 A contrary alternative concept has been expressed with varying emphasis by several investigators who have suggested that at least sometimes in acute myeloblastic leukemia there may be only one population of hematopoietic cells which are defective in their maturation, but which might be forced to differentiate under appropriate circumstances (PARAN et al., 1970; ROBINSON and PIKE, 1970; METCALF et al., 1971b, 1972; ICHIKAWA, 1972; KILLMANN, 1972; MCCULLOCH and TILL, 1972). In some patients with acute leukemia, especially those in whom the disease becomes manifest after a prolonged period of marrow hypoplasia, it may well be true that the normal stem cells are defective, and there is no doubt that acute leukemic cells often undergo partial maturation (CLARKSON et al., 1968, 1969, 1970b). However, the aforementioned cytogenetic evidence and the demonstration that the proliferative kinetics of leukemic cells are quite different than those of residual normal hematopoietic cells in the same marrow environment (CLARKSON et al., 1967, 1970c, 1971b; CLARKSON and FRIED, 1971a) lend strong support to the view that in the majority of cases there are in fact two competing populations of cells, one leukemic and one normal.

original leukemic population rather than as a result of reinduction of a new leukemia.

Since the normal and leukemic stem cells generally coexist as two separate populations, it should be possible to achieve a cure with chemotherapy by killing all of the leukemic cells, if enough normal stem cells can be spared to permit the host's survival. It is recognized that some conditions, both congenital and acquired, are associated with an increased risk of developing leukemia, and that curing the original disease might not necessarily eliminate the risk that such patients could develop a new leukemia (MACMAHON and LEVY, 1964; FRAUMENI, 1968; MILLER, 1968; CLARKSON, 1970a). There is in fact one reported instance in which a girl with acute leukemia was heavily irradiated to destroy most of her marrow and then given a marrow transplant from her normal brother (FIALKOW, 1971). When the disease recurred, the leukemic cells were found to have a male karyotype and it was therefore presumed that leukemic transformation had occurred in the grafted cells.

There are already a substantial number of patients with well-documented evidence of acute leukemia who have survived over 5 years even with the use heretofore of fairly conservative chemotherapy, and it has been estimated that at least half of these patients should have normal life spans (BURCHENAL, 1970a). During the last 5 years there have been significant advances in the treatment of lymphoblastic leukemia, and it seems reasonable to predict that within the next several years the number of long survivors will greatly increase.

## II. Cytokinetic Considerations

Acute leukemia is ordinarily already in an advanced stage when diagnosed, and there are usually around one to several trillion ($10^{12}$) leukemic cells present (CLARKSON, 1969; HART et al., 1969). A 13 decade ($\log_{10}$) reduction is therefore necessary to eliminate all of them, but, depending on the extent of disease, only a 1 to 3 decade reduction is necessary to bring about a "complete remission" according to conventional criteria. Thus a billion or more leukemic cells can still be present during remission and not be detected. Following a 2 decade reduction only 7 doublings are required for the population to return to its original number. It has not been possible to determine the doubling time of leukemic populations *in vivo* with any precision, but the doubling time is undoubtedly always significantly greater than the cells' mean cell cycle time because of (spontaneous) cell death and entry of cells into a prolonged $G_1$ phase (CLARKSON and FRIED, 1971a).

Reported estimates of cell cycle parameters in acute leukemic cells have varied widely (LALA et al., 1965; MAUER and FISHER, 1966; CLARKSON et al., 1967, 1969, 1970b, 1971b; SAUNDERS et al., 1967; KEISER et al., 1968; GOODELL et al., 1970; GAVOSTO and PILERI, 1971; STEEL, 1972; WAGNER et al., 1972). However, some of the extreme values reported are based on methods of questionable validity and require confirmation. In the best documented studies, the mean duration of DNA synthesis ($S$ phase) has usually been found to be around 20 hours or longer (16 to 47 hours). The mean intermitotic or generation time of the leukemic cells varies greatly in different patients (2 to $>10$ days), and there is also considerable variability within any one population of cells and probably also according to the stage of disease. Most of the variability is in the length of $G_1$. The 20-hour or greater values for $S$ are based on percent labeled mitoses experiments performed during advanced disease, and it is possible that when they are less crowded, the cells have a shorter synthetic period, possibly close to the 13 to 16 hour estimates found for the $S$ phase of normal granulocyte precursors (STRYCKmans et al., 1966; Todo, 1968). Because of technical considerations, it has not been possible to perform labeled mitoses experiments of leukemic blasts during minimal disease (i.e., not enough mitoses are present and one usually cannot distinguish leukemic blasts from normal ones). Drugs which exert their lethal effect by blocking DNA synthesis (Mauro and Madoc-Jones, 1970; Skipper, 1971 a) should be cytocidal during the greater part of the $S$ period, although there is as yet no precise information as to the exact drug concentration and duration of exposure needed to kill human leukemic cells during any portion of the $S$ phase *in vivo*.

Administration of an $S$ phase active drug in adequate dosage and with sufficient frequency to provide a cytocidal blood concentration every 12 hours should therefore kill all leukemic cells passing through $S$. However, if 20 hours or more are allowed to elapse between effective blood levels, some cells may be able to complete $S$ and thereby escape being killed. The rate of progression of leukemic cells from $G_1$ into $S$ varies greatly among different patients and probably also with the stage of disease (i.e. the fraction in $S$ may increase as the population is reduced by treatment) (Clarkson et al., 1969, 1971 b, 1972 b). The rate of cell kill with $S$ phase active drugs thus varies considerably, but the extent of variability under different conditions is still uncertain.

Since many leukemic cells may die spontaneously and only some of them are clonogenic (i.e. here defined as having the capacity to proliferate to a lethal number of cells), a greater reduction in cell number may occur than can be accounted for by drug kill. The fraction of leukemic cells which are clonogenic is unknown, and undoubtedly varies in different populations. In most patients, the leukemic cells have a substantial spontaneous death rate, and in many cases a sizeable fraction of the cells mature to the extent of losing their ability to divide (Clarkson et al., 1968, 1969, 1970 b, 1971 b).

By means of continuous infusions of $^3$H-thymidine, it has been shown that a significant number of leukemic cells remain in a prolonged $G_1$ phase or possibly in $G_0$ for at least 20 days and probably much longer (Clarkson et al., 1969, 1970 b, 1971 b; Ohara et al., 1971). Such "dormant" cells appear morphologically to be viable, and they are still metabolically active in terms of continuing RNA and protein synthesis. The fraction of cells in an extended $G_1$ phase is generally small; this may vary in different patients and in any one patient in relation to the stage of disease. The great majority of cells in prolonged $G_1$ are very small cells; apparently they must attain a sufficient critical mass before they are able to begin DNA synthesis. It has been reported that a correlation between the mass of a cell after mitosis and the duration of its $G_1$ phase also exists for bacteria (Kubitschek et al., 1967) and for both normal and neoplastic mammalian cells (Killander, 1965, 1967). On the other hand, Fox and Pardee (1970), studying Chinese hamster cells, recently reported there was no correlation between the length of $G_1$ and cell size. However, the latter experiments were short-term ones, and there seems to be little doubt from the long-term *in vivo* $^3$H-thymidine continuous infusion studies in patients with leukemia that the great majority of leukemic cells in a prolonged resting phase are very small cells, although, as with the Chinese hamster cells, there is considerable size variability at the time of initiation of DNA synthesis (Clarkson et al., 1968, 1969, 1970 b, 1971 b; Ohara et al., 1971).

The small dormant cells almost certainly have the potential to later resume proliferation at about the same rate as the original whole population and to reproduce the disease; although the evidence for this in human leukemia is only indirect (Clarkson et al., 1967, 1969; Gabutti and Pileri, 1969; Saunders and Mauer, 1969; Stryckmans et al., 1970; Clarkson and Fried, 1971 a); the leukemogenic potential of the small resting cells has been well demonstrated in spontaneous AKR leukemia in mice (ROSEN et al., 1970).

The normal hematopoietic precursors are generally greatly reduced in advanced leukemia, probably due to inhibition at the stem cell level by the mass of leukemic cells (CLARKSON et al., 1967, 1970c, 1971a, 1971b; LAJTHA, 1971). The mechanism of inhibition is unknown. However, virtually all the remaining erythrocyte and megakaryocyte precursors are proliferating faster than, and the normal granulocyte precursors at least as fast as, the great majority of leukemic cells. On the other hand, it appears that plasma cells, lymphocytes, and histiocytes generally proliferate more slowly in the marrow than do the leukemic cells. Because of their rapid rate of division, the residual normal erythrocyte, granulocyte, and megakaryocyte precursors are rapidly killed by $S$ phase active drugs, leaving only the slowly dividing lymphocytes, plasma cells, histiocytes, and the inactive leukemic and normal stem cells. If chemotherapy reduces the leukemic population sufficiently, the normal stem cells are released from inhibition, and because of their faster proliferative rate, the normal precursors may repopulate the marrow faster than can the leukemic cells. If enough leukemic cells have been destroyed, this will result in a remission.

Once a remission has been accomplished the most important obstacles to eliminating all of the remaining leukemic cells appear to be:

1. Development of drug resistance. To try to circumvent resistance, most current intensive treatment regimens employ combinations of drugs with different mechanisms of action, either concurrently or sequentially, in as high dosage as tolerated. Because of the probability of emergence of a drug-resistant population of cells, it seems obvious that the best chance to eliminate all the cells is when the disease is first diagnosed (rather than after the disease has relapsed following inadequate therapy).

2. In some patients, leukemic cells may become sequestered in the central nervous system (and possibly other physiological sanctuaries, although this is less clear), into which most drugs fail to penetrate in effective lethal concentrations. Since previous attempts at treating symptomatic central nervous system disease have generally had only limited and temporary success, the best procedure is to include prophylactic intrathecal chemotherapy (and/or x-irradiation to the neuro-axis) during the initial course of remission induction. It is not yet known how vigorous or protracted such therapy must be in order to destroy all leukemic cells.

3. The third major obstacle is the persistence of a small but significant fraction of leukemic cells in an extended $G_1$ phase, where they are relatively insensitive to the cytotoxic agents. No reliable way has yet been found to eliminate these long-term dormant cells. Reducing the population pressure by therapy probably induces more of them to enter $S$, but it appears that some still persist in $G_1$ (CLARKSON and FRIED, 1971a).

## III. Application of Cytokinetic Principles to Treatment

If one accepts the general concepts outlined above regarding the kinetic behavior of leukemic and normal cells, what therapeutic strategy is most appropriate to destroy the entire leukemic population without causing irreversible damage to the normal hematopoietic system? Several intensive treatment regimens for lymphoblastic leukemia are undergoing clinical trials (HENDERSON, 1969; HOLLAND and GLIDEWELL, 1970, 1972; MATHÉ et al., 1970; PINKEL, 1971; VIETTI et al., 1971), and it is not yet certain which will prove to be most effective.

The "L-2" protocol, which was designed in accordance with the principles outlined above and which is currently in use at Memorial Hospital in New York, is shown in Fig. 1 and 2 (CLARKSON and FRIED, 1971a). This protocol was designed for previously untreated patients in whom the leukemic cells could be expected to have some sensitivity to each component of the regimen.

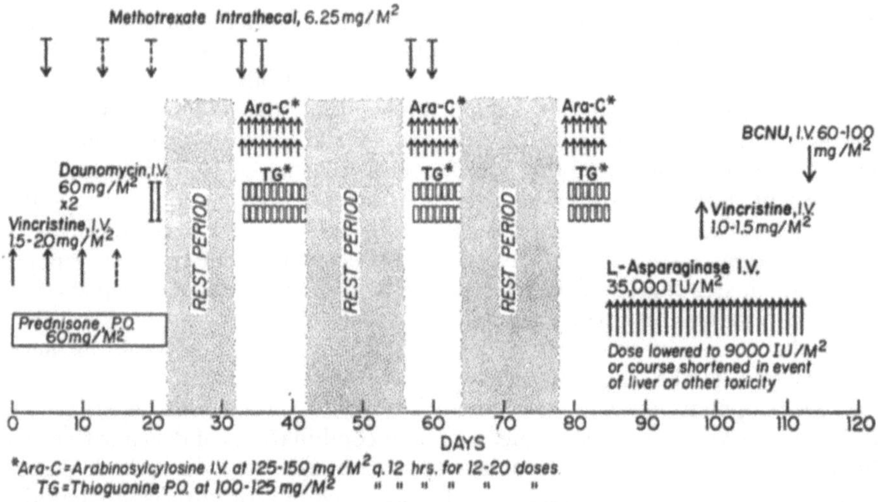


Fig. 1. Part I of "L-2" protocol for acute lymphoblastic leukemia presently being used at Memorial Hospital. As is emphasized in the text, there is considerable variability among patients regarding the amount of chemotherapy tolerated, and it is sometimes necessary to reduce the drug doses or frequency of administration because of toxicity. Thus not all patients have received the full regimen shown

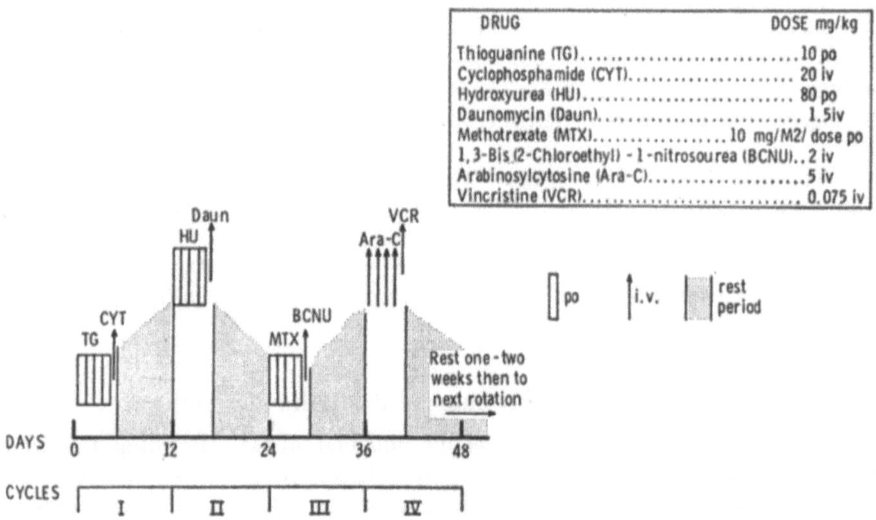


Fig. 2. Part II of "L-2" protocol for acute lymphoblastic leukemia. Not all patients can tolerate the treatment schedule shown, and it is often necessary to reduce the drug doses or extend the duration of treatment-free intervals to allow recovery of normal hematopoietic cells

The initial treatment consists of prednisone and vincristine; this drug combination has been shown empirically to induce remissions in approximately 90% of patients with relative safety since neither drug is very toxic to the normal hematopoietic cells (HENDERSON, 1969). Several decades of leukemic cells are usually killed, which is a sufficient reduction in the leukemic mass to release the normal stem cells from inhibition. Because of their faster proliferative rate, the normal precursors then repopulate the marrow before the surviving leukemic cells can do so, resulting in a "remission".

When the normal cells have recovered sufficiently, daunorubicin is given, while continuing prednisone, to further reduce the leukemic population. Probably several more decades of cells are killed, since this drug combination is also effective in inducing remissions (TAN et al., 1967; BERNARD et al., 1970; JONES et al., 1971; VIETTI et al., 1971). Daunorubicin, like most other cell cycle nonspecific agents (SKIPPER, 1971a), is quite toxic, and a substantial number of normal hematopoietic cells are also killed. However, by this time there has generally been enough recovery of the granulocytes and platelets to enable the patient to tolerate this insult with relatively little risk of fatal infection or hemorrhage.

Treatment is then interrupted to allow the normal cells to again repopulate the marrow. Upon resumption of therapy, a combination of *S* phase specific agents is used (SKIPPER, 1971a). Since the disease is usually already in remission at this time and there are too few leukemic cells left to make any kinetic measurements, it is not known for certain whether the surviving leukemic cells have a higher growth fraction and are proliferating faster than the original whole population. However, it is presumed that acute leukemia behaves similarly to other tumors and that the residual leukemic cells should at this stage be more vulnerable to *S* phase specific agents (CLARKSON and FRIED, 1971a). Over their measurable ranges, most if not all tumors grow in a Gompertzian fashion (i.e., growth slows progressively as the tumor mass increases) (GOMPERTZ, 1825; LAIRD, 1965; SCHABEL, 1969; SIMPSON-HERREN and LLOYD, 1970; SALMON, 1971; SKIPPER, 1971a). There is little reason to suppose that acute leukemia is different in this respect from other tumors, but the magnitude of cell kill and the time required before the surviving leukemic cells begin to grow at an accelerated rate is not known and undoubtedly varies in different cases.

It was elected to use arabinosylcytosine and 6-thioguanine at this stage, since this combination has been shown to be very effective in acute leukemia (GEE et al., 1969; CAREY, 1970), but possibly other *S* phase specific agents would be equally good or better. A combination of drugs is probably preferable to any single agent because of the lesser likelihood of development of drug resistance. In order to prevent any cells from completing *S* without having been exposed to (presumably) cytocidal drug concentrations, both drugs are given every 12 hours. It is of course impossible to determine the effectiveness of this component of the protocol since the patient is already in remission. However, evidence is developing that arabinosylcytosine and 6-thioguanine, when used as initial therapy in non-lymphoblastic forms of acute leukemia, are more effective if given every 12 hours rather than only once daily (CLARKSON et al., 1972b; DOWLING et al., 1972).

This drug combination is very toxic to normal hematopoietic precursors and stem cells, and since at this stage of the protocol the latter are usually still in a regenerative phase, they may also be more vulnerable to *S* phase specific drugs than after the marrow has become completely repopulated and the majority of stem cells have reverted to an inactive state. Thus one must be careful not to overtreat; while there is considerable individual variation, generally not more than 10 to 16 consecutive doses of arabinosylcytosine and 6-thioguanine can be safely tolerated, and even then the leukocyte and platelet counts may fall to very low levels. Since the maximum marrow depression usually occurs 10 to 14 days after interrupting treatment, the decision of when to stop must be partly anticipatory and is based largely on previous experience. Accurate data on leukemic cell kill are not yet available even when this combination is used as the initial treatment in nonlymphoblastic leukemia; however, a reasonable estimate is that on the average, each course of arabinosylcytosine and 6-thioguanine probably causes about a two decade reduction in the leukemic population, although this may vary appreciably (Clarkson et al., 1972b).

It is presumed that once remission is achieved, the growth fraction of the surviving cells increases significantly, but it is highly improbable that all the survivors begin to proliferate during the customary 5 to 8 day course of treatment (Clarkson and Fried, 1971a). A significant fraction undoubtedly persists in an extended $G_1$ phase for at least this long and hence remains unaffected by the drugs.

Thus, repeated courses of arabinosylcytosine and 6-thioguanine are given; a rest period is essential between each course to permit regeneration of the normal hematopoietic cells. During the rest periods, it is assumed that some of the previously dormant leukemic cells, which escaped being killed by the preceding course, will resume proliferating and become vulnerable to the next course of treatment. Since the leukemic cells remultiply during the treatment-free interval, this is kept as short as possible, consistent with sufficient recovery from hematotoxicity. Generally about three weeks must be allowed between each course for the normal cells to repopulate the marrow. There are no accurate data on doubling times of different leukemic populations, and this information is impossible to obtain during remission. The doubling time doubtless varies greatly from case to case, but it is probably seldom less than a week (Clarkson and Fried, 1971a). Regardless of the doubling time, providing the rest periods are not excessively long and the same drug combination is not repeated so often that the cells develop drug resistance, repeated courses of $S$ phase specific drugs interrupted by treatment-free intervals should progressively reduce the leukemic population, because the faster the surviving cells proliferate and the higher their growth fraction, the more readily should they be killed by the next course of therapy.

L-Asparaginase is started immediately after the last course of arabinosylcytosine and 6-thioguanine (Hill, 1967; Oettgen et al., 1967; Burchenal et al., 1970b; Clarkson et al., 1970d; Fairley, 1970; Mathé et al., 1970a; Tallal et al., 1970). The cell cycle specificity of L-asparaginase is not definitely established, but since it may be lethal only to proliferating cells, it is continued for a month on the presumption that most of the surviving cells will begin proliferating during this time. However, since the leukemic cells in a significant percentage of patients with lymphoblastic leukemia are not sensitive to L-asparaginase, one dose of vincristine is given midway through the course to prevent excessive proliferation of lymphoblasts in such patients.

Although it may cause other types of toxicity, L-asparaginase does not seriously damage normal hematopoietic cells and they usually recover during this period (Oettgen et al., 1970). A cell cycle nonspecific agent is given immediately at the end of the L-asparaginase course in as large a dose as can be tolerated in an attempt to kill residual dormant cells which may have survived the prior treatment. BCNU [1,3-*bis*(2-chloroethyl)-1-nitrosourea] was selected for this purpose since it is a highly effective cell cycle nonspecific agent and also because it has some effect against leukemic cells in the central nervous system (Skipper, 1971). However, there is as yet not much evidence regarding the effectiveness of BCNU in lymphoblastic leukemia, and it is quite possible that another nitrosourea, an alkylating agent, or a combination of the two might be more effective for the intended purpose.

Based on past experience with conventional chemotherapy, approximately half of patients with lymphoblastic leukemia can be expected to develop leukemia in the central nervous system (CNS) sometime in the course of their disease. Methotrexate is therefore given intrathecally on a prophylactic basis to try to eliminate any leukemic cells which have infiltrated the CNS; it is presumed this is most likely to occur when the disease is advanced and there are many leukemic cells circulating in the blood rather than after remission has been achieved. Several of the other drugs in the protocol which are given systemically, namely, prednisone, arabinosylcytosine, and BCNU, may also have some effect on leukemic cells in the CNS since all cross the blood-brain barrier to some degree. It is not yet known how vigorous or protracted chemotherapy must be to entirely prevent later development of CNS leukemia, but so far none of the previously untreated patients entered on the L-2 protocol have developed CNS leukemia (HAGHBIN et al., 1972). For the time being, we have elected not to use radiotherapy to the head or spine because of possible untoward delayed effects, but it should be noted that the best long-term results so far reported in preventing CNS leukemia have been with prophylactic radiation plus intrathecal methotrexate (PINKEL, 1971; SIMONE and PINKEL, 1971).

Figure 3 shows the estimated leukemic cell kill with Part I of the protocol. It is to be emphasized that the values shown are no more than reasonable guesses based on what might be expected on the average from past experience with each component of the protocol alone (CLARKSON and FRIED, 1971a). There are presently no methods to determine the true cell kill or doubling time during treatment-free intervals and these factors undoubtedly vary from case to case and during different stages of disease. Moreover, the problem of eradicating the long-term dormant cells has been ignored since there is no information about their behavior during intensive treatment.

On the assumption that a significant number of leukemic cells may survive Part I of the regimen, a second phase of less intensive treatment is then started. The basic design of Part II is a 4-day course of an *S* phase specific drug to kill any leukemic cells which have resumed dividing followed by a single dose of a cell cycle nonspecific agent to try to kill residual resting cells. To minimize development of drug resistance, the doses employed are as high as can be tolerated. Although it would be preferable to continue the *S* phase specific agents longer, generally no more than 4 consecutive days are tolerated at the doses used. Different drugs are used in rotation, again to avoid resistance; the choice is limited because only a few *S* phase specific agents are effective when taken orally, and this route of administration is of course desirable since treatment is carried out on an outpatient basis. (In some patients oral hydroxyurea was substituted for arabinosylcytosine).

There is as yet no way of knowing how long this therapy should be continued, but it is tentatively planned to treat the initial series of patients for 3 years. Possibly it might be preferable to eliminate Part II entirely and instead give several large doses of one or more cell cycle nonspecific agents shortly after completing Part I. However, since there is presently no means of determining the behavior of residual leukemic cells during remission, there is no way to choose which alternative is preferable except by trial and error. The results of the L-2 protocol to date are very encouraging, although there is as yet no proof that kinetic considerations are important in its design (HAGHBIN et al., 1971, 1972).

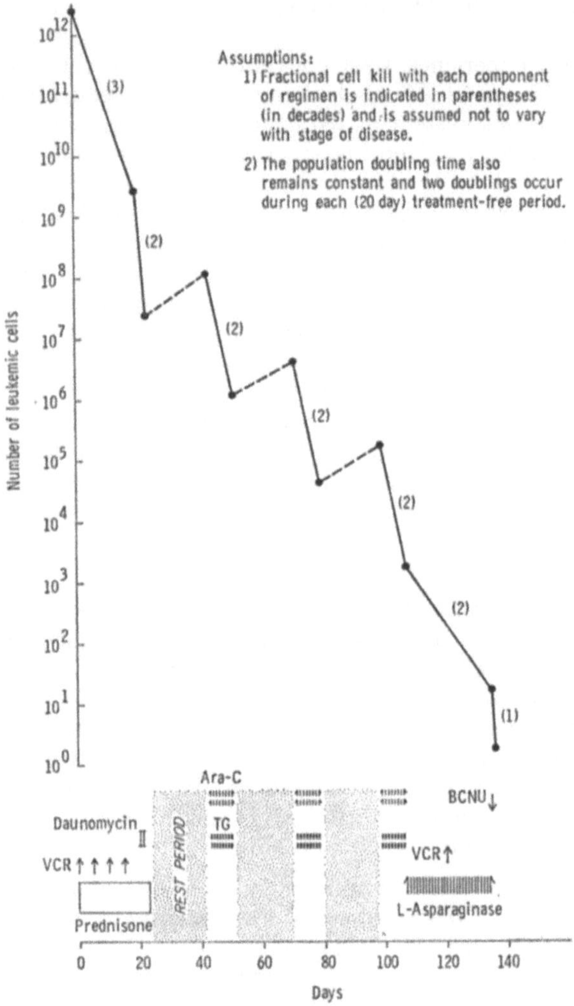


Fig. 3. Theoretical estimate of rate of reduction of leukemic population starting with $3 \times 10^{12}$ leukemic cells during Part I of "L-2" protocol. The values shown are considered to be reasonable average estimates of the rates of cell kill and remultiplication, although it is recognized that there is considerable individual variability and also that these rates undoubtedly change during the course of treatment rather than remain constant as has been assumed for the sake of simplicity

The treatment of nonlymphoblastic types of acute leukemia is much less well developed for two main reasons. (1) There is no safe and effective remission-induction regimen comparable to prednisone and vincristine, and it is therefore necessary to initiate treatment with drugs which are highly toxic to the normal hematopoietic cells at a time when the latter are usually already severely depleted by the disease (Gee et al., 1969; Henderson, 1969). This is very hazardous, and there is a high risk of fatal infection or hemorrhage. (2) Secondly, there are fewer drugs available which are effective in myeloblastic and related forms of acute leukemia, and it is thus much more difficult to design a good "remission consolidation" regimen after remission is achieved (i.e. one which will reliably result in a progressive further net reduction in the leukemic population). If estimates of cell kill similar to those in Fig. 3 are carried out for the best current treatment protocols for myeloblastic leukemia, the extent of kill is much less (CLARKSON et al., 1972b). Nevertheless, the treatment of nonlymphoblastic acute leukemia is improving, and it is not unreasonable to anticipate further improvements during the next few years (BERNARD et al., 1970; CROWTHER et al., 1970; FREIREICH et al., 1970; HOLLAND and GLIDEWELL, 1970; DOWLING et al., 1972).

There are still many gaps in our knowledge about the kinetic behavior of cells in acute leukemia. Some of the most important factors about which more information is needed are: the sizes and proliferative characteristics of the clonogenic fractions in different leukemic populations; the relative regenerative capacities and rates of growth of normal and leukemic cells following therapy; factors regulating cell division and possible ways to stimulate resting cells to go into cycle; the interrelationship between normal and leukemic cells (especially stem cells); and finally the mechanism of leukemic transformation and the reasons why leukemic cells fail to mature and respond properly to factors which regulate the production of normal cells. Techniques are now being developed which may help to answer some of these questions, and considerable improvements in treatment design can be anticipated when the information becomes more complete (BASERGA et al., 1971; BROWN and CARBONE, 1971; GREENBERG et al., 1971; LANDAU and SACHS, 1971a; METCALF, 1971b; MUELLER, 1971; PARDEE, 1971; TILL and McCULLOCH, 1971).

In the meantime, because of clinical necessity, it seems justified to attempt to integrate available kinetic information about acute leukemia with therapeutic conclusions derived from simpler experimental systems as well as with those arrived at empirically in the clinic in order to synthesize an overall logical plan of treatment. As new knowledge becomes available or deficiencies in current protocols become apparent, appropriate modifications can be made. The L-2 protocol represents a primitive attempt to use such a combined approach to design a comprehensive plan of treatment. Undoubtedly it can be improved and perhaps simplified considerably. Insofar as it is based on kinetic principles, they are only very general ones, and there has been no attempt to incorporate any fine strategic principles such as the exact temporal sequence in which the drugs might best be used. At the present time the available cytokinetic information is too incomplete to enable precision scheduling of drug administration.

## IV. Sequential Chemotherapy

There are beginning attempts to define specific drug effects with greater precision and to relate such information to the design of better treatment schedules (LAMPKIN et al., 1969, 1971a, 1971b; ERNST and KILLMANN, 1970, 1971; GAVOSTO, 1970; MAUER et al., 1970; STRYCKMANS et al., 1970). Although the experimental data are still limited and in many cases the therapeutic implications are not yet clear, several practical suggestions for more effective sequential drug administration have already been presented. For example, in lymphoblastic leukemia, prednisone has been shown to destroy both actively proliferating and resting leukemic cells, and probably also to reduce their rate of efflux from $G_1$ into $S$, whereas it has little effect on normal myeloblasts (LAMPKIN et al., 1969; ERNST and KILLMANN, 1970). Since the lethal effect of methotrexate is limited to $S$ phase cells, it has been suggested that it may be unwise to give methotrexate after corticosteroid therapy has been started since the antileukemic effects of the former may be reduced whereas its toxic effect on normal granulocytes will remain unchanged (Ernst and Killmann, 1970, 1971). Similarly, it has been suggested that vincristine should be expected to have greater antileukemic effect if given before rather than after corticosteroids (Ernst and Killmann, 1970), arabinosylcytosine (Lampkin et al., 1969), or methotrexate (Ernst and Killmann, 1971) have been started.

## V. Synchronization

Several investigators have attempted to synchronize leukemic blasts in the $S$ phase so that a higher proportion would be vulnerable to subsequent administration of $S$ phase-dependent drugs. Partial synchronization in $S$ has been reported following single doses of arabinosylcytosine or methotrexate (Ernst and Killmann, 1971; Lampkin et al., 1971a, 1971b). With the doses used, the most likely explanation is that these drugs slow the progression of cells through $S$, but are not immediately lethal; meanwhile other cells continue to enter $S$ from $G_1$ and likewise accumulate in $S$.

In one study it was found that after a single dose of arabinosylcytosine (5 mg/kg), partial synchronization in $S$ occurred in all patients 18 to 24 hours later (Lampkin et al., 1971a). At this time, a 12-hour infusion of arabinosylcytosine was begun, and the sequence was repeated until remission occurred. However, in an earlier report it was found that the time of maximum accumulation of cells in $S$ following a single dose of arabinosylcytosine varied between 24 and 96 hours (Lampkin et al., 1971b), and with this degree of variability it is unlikely that any standard schedule will be maximally effective in all patients. At the present time it is uncertain what schedule of arabinosylcytosine is most effective in acute leukemia (Frei and Carter, 1971), and the situation of course becomes much more complicated when drug combinations are used.

Because of individual variability, it seems unlikely that it will be possible to consistently achieve maximum synchronization with any single fixed chemotherapeutic schedule. Moreover, it is probably not reasonable to expect that a high degree of synchronization of leukemic blast cells can be accomplished in patients with any treatment schedule, since, except for the mitotic selection method which is obviously unsuitable *in vivo*, there is no good method for achieving complete synchrony of whole populations of mammalian cells even *in vitro* (Nias and Fox, 1971).

## VI. Recruitment of Dormant Cells

There have been a number of attempts to deliberately recruit dormant leukemic cells to begin active proliferation and thereby increase their vulnerability to cytotoxic drugs. These have included extracorporeal irradiation of the blood (Chan et al., 1969; Chan and Hayhoe, 1971); massive leukapheresis (Reich et al., 1971); partial exchange transfusions (Lampkin et al., 1971b); and treatment with various chemotherapeutic regimens (Clarkson, 1969; Clarkson et al., 1971b; Ernst and Killmann, 1971; Lampkin et al., 1971b; Ohara et al., 1971). While some degree of recruitment has sometimes been reported, the results in general have been inconsistent and unpredictable. Moreover, some experiments reporting successful recruitment can be interpreted otherwise. For example, if the effects of a drug are not immediately lethal but cause delay in the passage of cells through $S$ without interfering with their movement into $S$, cells will accumulate in this phase, thereby reducing the flow of post-mitotic cells into $G_1$ and decreasing the size of this latter compartment. In such cases, there may have been no recruitment at all of dormant cells, but simply depletion of the $G_1$ compartment by the continuing flow of cells into $S$ which would have occurred even in the absence of perturbation by the drug. The ability to cause true recruitment of long-term dormant leukemic cells is obviously of great importance, but successful achievement of this goal will probably have to await better understanding of the factors regulating initiation of DNA synthesis (BASERGA et al., 1971; MUELLER, 1971; PARDEE, 1971).

Since, as has been pointed out, the growth of tumors is usually Gompertzian, theoretical considerations would suggest that the growth fraction could be increased simply by reducing the leukemic mass sufficiently. However, the degree of reduction necessary and the time required for the dormant cells to begin proliferating are never known for any given leukemic population, and these factors undoubtedly vary greatly among different populations. As a practical matter it is probably preferable to drastically reduce the leukemic mass whenever possible (i.e. by at least several decades) prior to beginning treatment with drugs whose lethal effects are restricted to proliferating cells.

## B. Chronic Leukemias

The proliferative kinetics in chronic granulocytic leukemia are different than those in acute leukemia (GALBRAITH, 1969; OGAWA et al., 1970; WHANG-PENG et al., 1971). Although it is usually possible to achieve good control of the disease during its early stages, true remission is extremely rare [i.e. regrowth of normal hematopoietic cells and loss of leukemic cells containing the Philadelphia (*Ph'*) chromosome in the marrow] (NOWELL and HUNGERFORD, 1961; COURT-BROWN and TOUGH, 1963; FREI et al., 1964; MAURICE et al., 1971). Therapy causes only a slight prolongation of life at best, and there is as yet no indication that kinetic considerations have led to any advances in the treatment of this disease (GALTON, 1971; WHANG-PENG et al., 1971).

Aggressive chemotherapy, similar to that used in acute leukemia, has been tried in an attempt to eliminate the leukemic population (*Ph'*-positive cells), but this has rarely if ever succeeded (CLARKSON, 1970a, 1972a; GALTON, 1971). The major enigma in chronic granulocytic leukemia is the fate of the normal hematopoietic stem cells. Has the entire population mysteriously vanished or been universally transformed into *Ph'*-positive cells? Alternatively, are the normal stem cells still present but somehow defective, or do the leukemic cells merely have such an enormous proliferative advantage that they almost invariably overwhelm the normal cells, continuing to suppress them even after therapy has caused a drastic reduction in leukemic cells?

Whereas in some patients, all dividing marrow cells are *Ph'*-positive (NOWELL and HUNGERFORD, 1961; FREI et al., 1964; MCCULLOGH and TILL, 1972), in other cases both *Ph'*-positive and *Ph'*-negative cells have been demonstrated (FREI et al., 1964; CHERVENICK et al., 1971; GALTON, 1971; BAIKIE, 1972). However, even if two competing populations do in fact exist, it has proven extraordinarily difficult to tip the balance in favor of the normal one. Until this central enigma is resolved, it is doubtful whether real progress will be made towards curing the disease.

Similarly, most reports have failed to show significant prolongation of life in chronic lymphocytic leukemia (BOGGS et al., 1966; GALTON, 1971). However, HUGULEY (1972) has recently reported that some of the newer treatment regimens may lead to improved survival and that about 10% of patients may have complete remissions which are associated with especially long survival. Some advantage has been taken of the observations that the leukemic cells in this disease proliferate very slowly and are long-lived (SCHIFFER, 1968). Either by removing large quantities of the cells by leukapheresis (Curtis et al., 1972; Reich and Clarkson, 1972), or killing them by extracorporeal radiation of the blood (Cronkite, 1971), damage to the normal marrow is avoided and some therapeutic nebefit may be gained.

## C. Lymphomas

Some information is available on the kinetic behavior of different lymphomas (Cooper et al., 1966, 1968; Crowther et al., 1969; Peckham and Cooper, 1969, 1970; Engeset et al., 1971; Ohara et al., 1971). However, there has as yet been little attention given to using this information to improve the treatment of these diseases, and recent advances in the chemotherapy and radiotherapy of Hodgkin's disease and other lymphomas have been arrived at largely empirically (deVita et al., 1970; Lowenbraun et al., 1970; deVita, 1971; Johnson, 1971; Kaplan, 1971). Clinically the lymphomas vary greatly in their growth patterns and each pathologic designation may include a spectrum of tumors with diverse characteristics. When lymphosarcoma or reticulum cell sarcoma occurs in young individuals with extensive involvement of the marrow and blood, the kinetic behavior of the neoplastic cells appears to be similar to that of acute leukemic cells and they may respond well to the same type of intensive chemotherapy (Gee et al., 1970; Ohara et al., 1971). In older individuals, the growth patterns of lymphosarcoma and reticulum cell sarcoma are much more variable, and intensive chemotherapy is often contraindicated as it may do more harm than good.

There is still much to be learned about the kinetics of lymphomas before any general conclusions can be reached regarding possible relevance to therapeutic tactics. It seems quite possible that better appreciation of their proliferative behavior might lead to further improvements in treatment, but it is presently still uncertain whether or not differences in therapeutic responsiveness are related to cellular kinetic differences and if so to what extent.

## D. Multiple Myeloma

Improvement in the treatment of multiple myeloma has lagged behind that of the lymphomas (Alexanian et al., 1968, 1969; Hoogstraten et al., 1969; Lee et al., 1971). Patients responding favorably to chemotherapy, most commonly with Melphalan or cyclophosphamide plus prednisone, may have a modest prolongation of life, but like the chronic forms of leukemia, present-day therapy of disseminated myeloma falls far short of cure. It was recently reported that the colony forming capacity of one line of mouse myeloma cells was more than 70 times more sensitive to Melphalan than that of normal marrow progenitor cells, but comparable techniques have not yet been adapted to studying the differential sensitivity of human myeloma and hematopoietic stem cells (Ogawa et al., 1971).

Recently Salmon and his colleagues have provided an elegant demonstration of how precise knowledge of the kinetics of tumor cell proliferation might be used to develop more rational treatment (Salmon and Smith, 1970a, 1970b; Salmon, 1971; Salmon et al., 1971; Sullivan and Salmon, 1972). They have taken advantage of the fact that almost all populations of myeloma cells produce a monoclonal immunoglobulin which can be used as a specific tumor index substance or "marker". A highly sensitive "sandwich" radioimmunoassay was developed which is capable of measuring nanogram quantities of immunoglobulin produced by a few myeloma cells (Salmon and Smith, 1970a). In IgG myeloma, the mean synthetic rate of monoclonal protein is 14.5 (range 1.5 to 34) pg/myeloma cell per day, and the rate remains constant for several years whether or not the patient is receiving treatment. If the total body synthesis rate for the patient's monoclonal protein is divided by the average cellular rate, the total number of myeloma cells in the body can be determined.

Clinical manifestations of disease do not become apparent until more than $10^{11}$ myeloma cells are present, and patients with over $2 \times 10^{12}$ myeloma cells live only a short time; thus, during the clinical course from "early" diagnosis until death with advanced disease, only a little more than 4 doublings of the tumor cell population generally occur. Like other tumors, growth of myeloma follows Gompertzian kinetics, and the proliferative fraction decreases with progressive increase in tumor mass.

Patients having a good response to chemotherapy are estimated to have about a 2 decade reduction in the number of tumor cells (SULLIVAN and SALMON, 1972). Some patients, classified clinically as "nonresponders", actually may have a 50% reduction in tumor mass, and their survival is longer than those with less than 50% regression. Previous crude estimates based on electrophoretic patterns have been shown to underestimate the extent of tumor kill, and SALMON's technique should allow a much more accurate appraisal of the effect of chemotherapy.

Tumor regression during continuous Melphalan therapy is also Gompertzian with slowing of the regression rate as the tumor mass shrinks; the regression curve is in fact remarkably similar to that of regrowth on cessation of therapy. It has been suggested that this is because during drug-induced regression, the growth fraction increases until a new plateau of (lower) population size is reached with cell death due to treatment balanced by an increased birth rate due to a larger proliferative fraction (SULLIVAN and SALMON, 1972). Whereas these workers have tentatively concluded that the plateau phenomenon during remission does not reflect acquisition of drug resistance, there is no direct evidence for this, and resistance cannot yet be excluded as an explanation.

Using this "marker" technique for estimation of tumor mass, misinterpretation is possible if mutation occurs in the myeloma cells which results in an alteration in the specific "marker" immunoglobulin synthesis or a change in their proliferative rate. Mutant "subclones" are known to occur frequently in mouse myeloma (COFFINO et al., 1970) and have also been reported in human myeloma (HOBBS, 1971; SULLIVAN and SALMON, 1972).

SALMON'S work is so recent that there has not yet been time to determine its ultimate usefulness in improving treatment, but several tactical approaches have already been proposed. If the proliferative fraction of the tumor increases as the total population is reduced by a cell cycle stage nonspecific agent such as Melphalan, the residual cells should then be more sensitive to drugs active against proliferating cells. As in the case of L1210 and AK murine leukemias (SCHABEL 1968; SKIPPER, 1968; SKIPPER et al., 1969), the advanced hamster plasmacytoma cannot be cured with arabinosylcytosine alone, but it can be cured with the same drug if the total mass is first reduced by several decades with alkylating agents (GRISWOLD et al., 1970). It has recently been reported that during intermittent alkylating agent-prednisone treatment of 8 patients with myeloma, the flash $^3$H-thymidine labeling index of the myeloma cells characteristically increased progressively after each course of treatment (SALMON and SMITH, 1972). Once a high labeling index was attained, either vincristine or arabinosylcytosine (neither of which is usually effective in far-advanced myeloma) caused further significant regression in the total body tumor cell number. As has been mentioned, similar tactics have already been tried in acute leukemia, but the increment in labeling index following chemotherapy has been unpredictable and highly variable in different patients. It remains to be seen whether the results will prove more consistent in myeloma.

The ability to measure quantitatively a specific secretory product of neoplastic cells has been enormously helpful in guiding treatment of trophoblastic tumors and certain other tumors such as neuroblastomas. The development of precise methods for measuring the synthesis of myeloma protein to estimate tumor mass may potentially be of even greater value since myeloma is less responsive to treatment than choriocarcinoma. Furthermore, while the present chorionic gonadotrophin assay methods are not entirely specific for hormone produced by the tumor (BAGSHAWE, 1969), myeloma protein is produced exclusively by the myeloma cells and is thus a highly specific tumor index substance. Hopefully, specific index substances such as unique enzymes or other biochemical markers will be discovered for other tumors and quantitative assays developed to allow similar measurements of the effects of therapy.

## Solid Tumors

Human solid tumors vary strikingly in their response to treatment, but no simple cytokinetic explanation has been offered to account for their differing responsiveness. For example, there is presently no information as to how uterine choriocarcinoma and some of the childhood solid tumors which are very responsive to chemotherapy might differ in a kinetic sense from melanomas or other tumors which are usually extremely refractory to the same chemotherapeutic regimes. Similarly, no distinctive kinetic differences have been discovered between radiosensitive and radioresistant solid tumors. It is in fact very doubtful whether differences in kinetic behavior are sufficient to explain the great variability in sensitivity of different tumors to chemotherapy or radiation, and their variable responsiveness is more likely determined by other factors such as differences in sensitivity of individual cell types, location of the tumor, or possibly host defense mechanisms. Only limited information is yet available about the kinetics of human solid tumors, and since this suggests that they have many common kinetic features, they will be discussed as a group.

### A. Cytokinetic Considerations

The proliferation kinetics of solid tumors are more complex than those of diffusely disseminated hematologic neoplasms in which the majority of the tumor cells exist in a similar environment and are exposed to more or less the same supply of nutrients. An additional complication is that, in contrast to most human leukemias, some solid tumors such as carcinomas of the breast or colon may sometimes have a multicentric origin. No kinetic studies have been performed in such cases, but it would not be surprising if the different primary clones had different kinetic characteristics.

Like other tumors, the growth of solid tumors characteristically follows a Gompertzian pattern (LAIRD, 1965). The slower growth rate in large tumors is due mainly to a decreased growth fraction and/or increased cell loss, and the mean duration of the cell cycle of the proliferating cells usually remains fairly constant (FRINDEL et al., 1967; TANNOCK, 1968; SKIPPER, 1971a; LALA, 1972). This is in contrast to ascitic tumors in which the duration of the cell cycle frequently becomes longer as the number of tumor cells increases; the rate of cell loss may also increase (CLARKSON et al., 1965; LALA and PATT, 1966; WIEBEL and BASERGA, 1968; FRINDEL et al., 1969; TANNOCK, 1969; CHOQUET et al., 1970; SHEEHY et al.,

1972). Refined techniques employing $^{125}$I-iododeoxyuridine labeling of tumor cells have been developed to measure quantitatively the rate of cell loss due to migration or death in experimental tumors (HOFER and HOFER, 1971). Such precise measurements of cell loss are not available for human tumors, but estimates based on comparison between the actual and potential doubling times (as calculated from the cell cycle time and growth fraction) indicate that cell loss may be very extensive (STEEL, 1967; LAMERTON and STEEL, 1968; SHIRAKAWA et al., 1970).

In solid tumors the proliferative fraction is characteristically higher in the peripheral portions than in the center (HERMENS and BARENDSEN, 1967, 1969; SHIRAKAWA et al., 1970). TANNOCK (1968) studied a transplantable mouse tumor in which the viable tumor cells were in cords around blood vessels. The growth fraction of the tumor cells decreased progressively with increasing distance from the blood vessels, but the cell cycle time remained almost constant. There was a necrotic zone about 90 μm from the nearest vessel, and serial labeling studies indicated that cells from around the blood vessel migrated toward the necrotic region where they presumably died, probably as a result of impaired diffusion of oxygen and other nutrients.

Vascularization critically influences both the limitation and the rate of growth of solid tumors. Without being vascularized, most solid tumors are unable to grow larger than about 2 to 3 mm in diameter, after which simple diffusion of nutrients (and wastes) is insufficient to allow further expansion of their volume (GREENE, 1941). Even after a tumor has become vascularized, the tumor cells may proliferate faster than can the capillary endothelium, and the latter's proliferative rate may thus indirectly limit the tumor's growth (TANNOCK, 1970). Different human tumors may vary considerably in their dependence on endothelial cell proliferation; for example, brain tumors appear to be most dependent whereas chondrosarcomas may become extremely large and yet have only a sparse capillary network in which the endothelial cells are inactive (FOLKMAN, 1971).

FOLKMAN (1971) has recently isolated a "tumor-angiogenesis" factor (TAF) from both animal and human tumors which is mitogenic to endothelial cells and stimulates new capillary formation in animals; with the exception of the placenta, TAF has not been found in normal tissues. He has suggested that it might be possible to inhibit tumor growth and metastatic spread by "antiangiogenesis" therapy, perhaps by immunization against TAF if this factor does indeed prove to be the mediator of tumor neovascularization.

As in the case of animal solid tumors, the reported cell cycle durations of various human solid tumors (FRINDEL et al., 1968; BENNINGTON, 1969; SHIRAKAWA et al., 1970; YOUNG and DEVITA, 1970; DEVITA, 1971; TERZ et al., 1971) have not in most instances been sufficiently different to account for their huge variability in doubling times (STEEL and LAMERTON, 1966; ISRAEL and CHAHINIAN, 1969). The few very short cell cycle times which have been reported are based on fragmentary experimental data and require confirmation. The two major reasons for differences in growth rates appear to be variability in the size of the growth fraction and in the extent of cell loss. The latter may result from necrosis, exfoliation, death of differentiated end-cells, abnormal cell division, or migration (STEEL, 1967; TUBIANA, 1971). The rate of cell loss has generally been found to be greater in carcinomas than in sarcomas (DENEKAMP, 1970), and this may explain at least in part the observation that human epitheliomas usually have longer doubling times than do sarcomas (CHARBIT et al., 1971).

## B. Effects of Radiation and Chemotherapy

Due to the limited kinetic data available on human tumors and because of their complexity and variable growth rates, there has as yet been little success in devising improved treatment regimens based on any general kinetic principles (Bruce and Lin, 1969; deVita, 1971; Dutreix et al., 1971). A few attempts have been made, but the basic information about human tumor kinetics is so incomplete that these preliminary approaches must still be regarded as largely empirical. The perturbations in tumor growth caused by therapy compounds an already very complex situation, and it is quite understandable that no straightforward solutions for improved treatment regimens have yet been forthcoming.

The radiosensitivity of cells varies in relation to their position in the cell cycle. Different cell types vary in their radiosensitivity during different phases, but most cells are maximally sensitive during $G_2$ and mitosis and least sensitive during the latter part of $S$ (Terasima and Tolmach, 1961; Kim and Evans, 1964; Djordjevic and Tolmach, 1967; Elkind et al., 1968; Sinclair, 1968; Frindel and Tubiana, 1971). There is little information about the radiosensitivity of resting cells in different tumors, but in general resting cells are less vulnerable to radiation damage than cells in cycle although they have a reduced capacity for repairing the damage (Tubiana, 1971). Hypoxic cells in poorly vascularized regions are especially resistant (Thomlinson, 1968; Howes, 1969).

Radiotherapy of tumors is usually delivered in fractionated doses, and the modification of kinetics caused by the first dose(s) may influence the response to subsequent therapy. In addition to selectively killing cells in certain phases of the cell cycle, radiation retards the rate of progression through the cycle and thus perturbs the distribution of cells throughout the cycle. The cell cycle phase most affected differs depending on the type of cell, but in most cells delay is maximum in $S$ (Frindel and Tubiana, 1971). The age response for division delay is generally the inverse of that for survival; for example, cells in $S$ may have enhanced survival because of their delayed passage through $S$ which affords them a better opportunity to repair their damage. The perturbation in the cell cycle distribution, caused by the initial treatment, in turn results in a cyclic variation in sensitivity to subsequent doses of radiation, and the situation may be further complicated by recruitment of resting cells into the proliferative fraction as the population density is reduced and as hypoxic cells are reoxygenated (Elkind and Sutton, 1959; Frindel et al., 1966; Thomlinson and Craddock, 1967; Howes, 1969; Young and Fowler, 1969). Moreover, the rate at which sublethally damaged cells repair their lesions and recover their proliferative potential may vary in poorly vascularized and well oxygenated regions and further modify the tumor's response to continued therapy (Elkind and Sinclair, 1965; Suit and Urano, 1969).

Within several days to a week or more after a single large dose of irradiation, the surviving cells in most solid tumors have unchanged or shortened cell cycle times as compared to pretreatment values (Hermens and Barendsen, 1969; Denekamp, 1970; van Peperzeel, 1970; Tubiana, 1971). On the other hand, in both animal and human tumors, the volume doubling time may be significantly longer after irradiation or chemotherapy (Israel and Chahinian, 1969). Denekamp and Thomlinson (1971) have concluded that the slower doubling times after irradiation are more likely due to increased cell loss and a slow rate of removal of damaged cells than to a significant change in the growth fraction. However, they recognize the potential inaccuracies inherent in the methods employed for estimating these parameters following treatment. One difficulty is that the autoradiographic methods used fail to distinguish damaged cells or those with otherwise limited proliferative capacity from clonogenic cells, and it is of course only the latter which are of importance in the long-term evolution of the tumor.

By means of *in vitro* cloning techniques, it has been shown that the growth rate of surviving clonogenic cells may be significantly greater following irradiation as compared to untreated tumor cells, and that this faster growth rate may persist until the tumors are nearly repopulated (TUBIANA et al., 1968; BARENDSEN and BROERSE, 1969, 1970; TUBIANA. 1971). Similarly, the rate of tumor repopulation by clonogenic cells may be substantially increased after most of the cells have been killed by cyclophosphamide or other cytotoxic agents (GRISWOLD et al., 1968; SKIPPER, 1971b). The factors responsible for the faster growth rate of surviving clonogenic cells following treatment are not well understood but are probably somehow related to their reduced population density, enhanced supply of nutrients, and possibly to the liberation of growth stimulating substances from dying cells (MALAISE and TUBIANA, 1970; YATVIN et al., 1970). Whatever the mechanism(s), it is obvious that the rate at which clonogenic cells repopulate the tumor during intervals between treatment is of paramount importance in arriving at optimal treatment schedules. Unfortunately, largely because of formidable technical difficulties, there are as yet no quantitative data concerning the extent of clonogenic cell kill and rate of repopulation of human solid tumors with any form of treatment.

## C. Combined Methods of Treatment

If the exact temporal sequence of events were known, it would presumably be possible to develop more effective schedules for fractionated radiotherapy as well as better therapeutic programs combining ionizing radiation with chemotherapy. A number of cytotoxic drugs have been given in combination with irradiation, but most of these trials have been purely empirical and little attention has been paid to possible ways to exploit the kinetic effects caused by the therapeutic sequence.

Tumors that are radiosensitive but that have a high repopulating ability should be good targets for combination therapy. As has been pointed out, many of the cytotoxic drugs selectively kill cells in the $S$ phase of the cell cycle (which is generally the most radioresistant), whereas cells in $G_2$ and $M$ are usually most sensitive to radiation. Some enhancement of radiotherapeutic effect in human tumors has been reported following pretreatment with an 18-hour infusion of 5-fluorouracil; the radiation was given precisely 8 hours after stopping the infusion at which time the tumor cells were partially synchronized in $G_2$ (NITZE et al., 1971). Another potentially useful tactic would be to begin therapy with an $S$ phase specific drug after radiation had killed a large fraction of the tumor at a time when the surviving clonogenic cells had started rapid regrowth and hence become more vulnerable to such drugs.

Chemotherapy or radiotherapy following surgical removal of the majority of the tumor might be expected to achieve the same purpose. If 99% of the tumor could be resected, this would correspond to a complete remission in acute leukemia; however, as has been already noted, after a 2 decade reduction only 7 doublings are required for the tumor population to return to its original size. The surgical adjuvant chemotherapy (COHN et al., 1968; FISHER et al., 1968, 1970a) and radiotherapy (FISHER et al., 1970b) protocols which have been tried to date in breast cancer have either failed entirely or had very limited success in delaying tumor recurrence or prolonging life (FISHER, 1971). However, in comparison with the intensive regimens used in acute leukemia, the amount and duration of chemotherapy administered in these adjuvant protocols was clearly insufficient to even come close to achieving total destruction of residual tumor cells. Post-operative irradiation did in fact decrease the incidence of local and regional recurrences in the irradiated sites, but, as might be expected, failed to influence the growth of distant metastases or survival (FISHER et al., 1970b; FISHER, 1971). Prophylactic oophorectomy had no apparent beneficial effect (RAVDIN et al., 1970).

Trials of more intensive and protracted adjuvant chemotherapy are clearly indicated to try to completely eradicate disseminated metastatic foci, perhaps in conjunction with radiotherapy to help eliminate local disease. The value of combined therapy has already been reasonably well established in the case of several tumors, including retinoblastoma (REESE et al., 1958), WILMS' tumor (FARBER, 1961), and HODGKIN'S disease (HERSH et al., 1972). The primary tumor or other large bulky tumor masses are resected or greatly reduced by irradiation and then intensive chemotherapy is given to destroy residual local tumor and distant metastases. It is also encouraging that in a recent study of patients with metastatic testicular cancer, there was a significantly higher incidence of patients remaining free of disease when they were treated with surgery followed by repeated intensive courses of actinomycin D for a prolonged period than in those patients treated only by orchiectomy and retroperitoneal lymph node dissection (WHITMORE et al., 1972).

Ideally, use of combination therapy in an optimal temporal sequence requires precise knowledge of the repopulation kinetics of the clonogenic tumor cells. This information is not only extremely difficult to obtain in the case of human tumors, but it is probably not valid to draw general conclusions based on limited data, since the rate of repopulation undoubtedly varies considerably among different tumors and following different doses of radiation or other forms of treatment.

It is also important to understand more fully the kinetic perturbations in normal tissues which may be affected by the treatment (LAMERTON and STEEL, 1968; DUTREIX et al., 1971; LIPKIN, 1971). As in the case of tumors, some normal tissues are much more sensitive to irradiation and/or cytotoxic drugs than others. In normal tissues with a high turnover rate, the cells can compensate for cell loss by several mechanisms, such as shortening their cell cycle (CAIRNIE, 1967; LESHER, 1967; HANNA et al., 1969), increasing the number of cell generations before becoming committed to maturation (TARBUTT, 1969), or increasing their growth fraction (CAIRNIE et al., 1965). Migration of lymphoid or hematopoietic stem cells into and out of irradiated zones will also influence the amount of therapy that can be tolerated (LAJTHA et al., 1969; CROIZAT et al., 1970). In normal tissues with a slow turnover rate, such as the liver, the immediate changes resulting from irradiation are less obvious, but nevertheless the cumulative effects of continued treatment may cause serious and irreversible damage (TUBIANA, 1971). In planning antitumor therapy, it is essential to consider the tolerance of the normal tissues affected by the treatment, and this will in turn depend on the interplay of the multiple factors responsible for homeostasis and regeneration. Presumably these are as sensitive to alterations in treatment schedules as is the tumor, but until they are better defined, it is hardly possible to devise more advantageous treatment schedules to produce greater selective damage to the tumor.

## Future Developments

Several additional approaches to cancer therapy have been suggested which have not yet been dealt with, as there is presently insufficient evidence that they will prove to be reliable forms of treatment. However, since they are conceptually important, they will be discussed briefly; discussion will be restricted to those aspects which have some relationship to cytokinetic considerations.

### A. Immunotherapy

The current status of human tumor immunology has recently been reviewed by OETTGEN et al. (1971). Whereas no form of immunotherapy has yet been shown to be consistently effective in any human neoplastic disease, possible means of enhancing immunological defenses against cancer are becoming better defined. Since immune mechanisms are generally only capable of destroying relatively small numbers of tumor cells *in vivo*, the most favorable circumstances for immunotherapy would appear to be either very early in the course of the disease or else after the tumor population has first been greatly reduced by other forms of treatment. As with irradiation and many cytotoxic drugs, immune cytotoxic damage is dependent on position in the cell cycle; target cells in the middle of $S$ have been found to be most resistant to immune cytolysis (SHIPLEY, 1971).

Of possible relevance to cytokinetic considerations is that regular periodic changes in the cell membrane have recently been shown to occur during the cell cycle (BURGER, 1971; PARDEE, 1971). Important biochemical and functional alterations take place in cell surface properties, and architectural changes are reflected by differences in exposure of receptor sites for plant agglutinins. The agglutinin binding sites are exposed only during mitosis in normal cells, but are exposed throughout the cell cycle in polyoma-virus transformed cells (FOX et al., 1971). By covering the binding sites on transformed cells with monovalent concanavalin A, it has been found that the growth pattern of transformed fibroblasts can be restored to that of normal cells and, moreover, that the process is reversible (BURGER and NOONAN, 1970). The topographical distribution of H-2 antigens has been mapped on the surface of single cells by combined immunological and morphological techniques (STACKPOLE et al., 1971), and a link between H-2 antigens and hematopoietic regulation has been postulated (TILL and MCCULLOCH, 1971). If further work establishes and clarifies the importance of cell surface components in regulating cell division, this may open the way for manipulation of growth in neoplastic and/or normal cells by immunological means.

Immunoglobulin synthesis by human lymphoid cells in established cultures is limited to the late $G_1$ and early $S$ portions of the cell cycle (BUELL and FAHEY, 1969; TAKAHASHI et al., 1969), and stationary cultures produce less immunoglobulin than those growing exponentially (FAHEY et al., 1972). The state of differentiation also influences immunoglobulin synthesis. If mature plasma cells, which produce much more immunoglobulin than do primitive lymphoid cells in culture, are considered to be arrested in a functional $G_1$ condition, the given coding for the polypeptide chains of the antibody molecule may be continually transcribed and result in continuous production of immunoglobulin (FAHEY et al., 1972). During the course of differentiation, changes may also occur in the antigenic composition of the surface membranes of immunocompetent cells (TAKAHASHI et al., 1971).

Small immunocompetent lymphocytes, like lymphoid cells in stationary culture, might be considered to be in a $G_0$ phase or a very prolonged $G_1$ phase during which they are in a repressed state with respect to immunoglobulin synthesis as well as mitotic activity. Stimulation of such repressed cells *in vitro*, either with appropriate antigens or mitogens in the case of lymphocytes or by converting stationary lymphoid cultures to exponential growth by dilution in fresh medium, causes the cells to progress further into $G_1$ and to form immunoglobulin before passing through several cycles of cell division which are in turn characterized by increasing amounts of immunoglobulin synthesis (Saunders, 1969; Fahey et al., 1971).

Many of these events observed *in vitro* are paralleled by the immune response to antigenic stimulation *in vivo*. Clearer definition of the control processes and temporal sequence of events may in the future lead to development of ways to modify immune responses, possibly including those concerned with recognition and rejection of tumor cells.

## B. Inducing Tumor Cells to Differentiate

It is generally agreed that whatever might be the basic defect(s) responsible for neoplastic transformation, a cardinal characteristic of the neoplastic state is failure of normal differentiation. As in the case of normal cells, once neoplastic stem cells become committed to differentiation, albeit abnormal, they lose their capacity for unlimited proliferation (i.e. they are no longer clonogenic and are hence incapable of reproducing the tumor) (Clarkson and Fried, 1971a). If clonogenic tumor cells could be induced to differentiate, this would introduce a new approach to treatment.

Such an approach has been proposed in several neoplastic diseases such as neuroblastoma and acute myeloblastic leukemia. Preliminary observations suggest that it might sometimes be possible to force leukemic blast cells to differentiate *in vitro* with suitable inducing substances (Paran et al., 1970; Robinson and Pike, 1970; Landau and Sachs, 1971; Metcalf, 1971; Ichikawa, 1972; McCulloch and Till, 1972; Moore et al., 1972; Robinson et al., 1972). Trentin (1970) has provided evidence that the path of differentiation of normal hematopoietic stem cells is specified by the stromal microenvironments in which they reside. This interaction appears to be a short-range inductive mechanism, presumably similar to those operative in embryogenesis, but the communicating factors have not yet been isolated or characterized. Much further work is clearly necessary before it can be determined whether these observations might have any potential therapeutic significance.

## C. Control of Cell Division

The relative resistance of resting tumor cells to chemotherapy and radiotherapy has already been emphasized, and several possible ways have been mentioned as to how resting cells might be stimulated to reenter the division cycle and thereby become more vulnerable to these therapeutic modalities (e.g. reducing the tumor's population density, or decreasing the proportion of poorly nourished or hypoxic zones in solid tumors).

A large number of humoral growth stimulatory factors (Todaro et al., 1965; Rubin, 1966; Clarke et al., 1970; Robinson and Pike, 1970; Austin et al., 1971; Bürk, 1971; Greenberg et al., 1971; Holley, 1971; Landau and Sachs, 1971a, 1971b; Lipton et al., 1971; Metcalf et al., 1971, 1972; Paul et al., 1971; Stoker et al., 1971; Temin, 1971; Bradley et al., 1972) and inhibitory substances (Bullough, 1965; Bullough et al., 1967; Beierle, 1968; Holm-

BERG, 1968; BURNS, 1969; RYTOMAA, 1969; YEH and FISHER, 1969; DULBECCO, 1970; BICHEL, 1971; FROESE, 1971; METCALF, 1971; CHAN et al., 1972) have now been reported which have activity in various systems *in vitro* or *in vivo*. Recently progress has been made towards characterizing some of these substances (STANLEY and METCALF, 1969; HALPERN and RUBIN, 1970; AUSTIN et al., 1971; LANDAU and SACHS, 1971 a, 1971 b; LIPTON et al., 1971; ICHIKAWA, 1972; METCALF et al., 1972), and also towards defining the series of biochemical events that precede onset of DNA synthesis and mitosis when quiescent cells are stimulated to initiate cell division (DULBECCO and STOKER, 1970; BASERGA et al., 1971; COOPER, 1971; EPIFANOVA, 1971; MUELLER, 1971; TOBEY et al., 1971). In some instances differences have been reported between normal and neoplastic cells in their ability to produce stimulatory or inhibitory substances or in their response to these substances, although some of these reports are conflicting (SACHS, 1968; PARAN et al., 1969; RYTOMAA, 1969; ROBINSON and PIKE, 1970; GREENBERG et al., 1971; METCALF, 1971). It has also recently been found that cells transformed by oncogenic viruses (JAINCHILL and TODARO, 1970; SMITH et al., 1971) as well as cells derived from human solid tumors (SCHER and TODARO, 1971) will sometimes grow in medium lacking serum growth factors whereas normal cells will not. Some of the virus-transformed cells are "abortively transformed", since upon subsequent passage they no longer grow in factor-free medium and share no other properties of viral transformation (SCHER and NELSON-REES, 1971; SMITH et al., 1972).

These investigations are all in a early stage, and it is still unclear how relevant the effects observed *in vitro* are to regulation of cell growth *in vivo*. However, they are certain to reveal more about growth regulation and disturbances of control in tumor cells, and it is not unreasonable to suppose that future developments may uncover ways to influence the proliferative behavior of normal and neoplastic cells *in vivo*. For example, if quiescent tumor cells could be stimulated to divide while at the same time normal stem cells were inhibited, this would obviously give an enormous advantage in treating tumors with cell cycle-specific cytotoxic agents. Maintaining tumor cells in a $G_0$ state might be another approach, although this would appear to be a less reliable means of control since there would always be the danger that the cells would escape from inhibition.

## Conclusions

Clinical application of cell kinetic knowledge is only beginning, and it must be apparent that this review of the current state of the field has raised many questions but offered few solutions. Some primitive attempts have been made in a few diseases such as acute leukemia and multiple myeloma to use cell kinetic information to formulate better treatment schedules, but not enough is yet known about the kinetics of most human tumors to allow rational therapeutic application of kinetic principles.

Until recently, except for a few highly responsive tumors, the most one could anticipate in treating most inoperable tumors was temporary palliation, and therapeutic gains usually resulted in only a modest increase in survival time at best. Since there is now reason to believe that the newer intensive therapeutic regimens are nearing the goal of totally destroying the neoplastic populations in several disseminated tumors, it appears that we may be entering a new era of treatment – that of curative therapy. If this proves to be true, it becomes far more important to extend the knowledge gained from the few tumors so far treated successfully to those which are still refractory to present methods of treatment.

The clinical investigations necessary for further progress admittedly pose formidable technical and sometimes also ethical problems. Labeling experiments conducted *in vivo* and autoradiographic methods furnish much useful information, but reliable assays for clonogenic tumor and normal stem cells are urgently needed to be carried out in parallel with the labeling experiments to gauge the effectiveness of treatment. Sensitive clonogenic assays for various murine tumor cells and normal hematopoietic cells are already available, and it should not be impossible to develop suitable assays for human cells; ideally such assay systems should be capable of quantitating the clonogenic tumor and normal cells separately. Fuller understanding of the dormant state is greatly needed; hopefully when the key regulatory mechanisms become known, ways will be found to manipulate dormant cells to accomplish therapeutic goals. Another fundamental problem is cellular differentiation; if the clonogenic tumor cells could somehow be induced to differentiate, their proliferative ability would be self-limited.

Because of the enormous complexity of human tumors, understanding of basic mechanisms controlling cell division and differentiation will undoubtedly emerge from studies in simpler systems, and the clinical therapist must stay informed about the contributions of molecular biologists and other basic scientists and stand ready to use any new information that may be pertinent to the problems he faces.

## References

Alexanian, R., Bergsagel, D. E., Migliore, P. J., Vaughn, W. K., Howe, C. D.: Melphalan therapy for plasma cell myeloma. Blood **31**, 1—10 (1968).

Alexanian, R., Haut, A., Khan, A. U., Lane, M., McKelvey, E. M., Migliore, P. J., Stuckey, W. J., Jr., Wilson, H. E.: Treatment for multiple myeloma: combination chemotherapy with different melphalan dose regimes. J. Amer. med. Ass. **208**, 1680—1685 (1969).

Austin, P. E., McCulloch, E. A., Till, J. E.: Characterization of the factor in L-cell conditioned medium capable of stimulating colony formation by mouse marrow cells in culture. J. cell Physiol. **77**, 121—134 (1971).

Bagshawe, K. D.: Choriocarcinoma. The clinical biology of the trophoblast and its tumours. London: Edward Arnold Ltd. 1969.

Baikie, A. G.: What is a leukaemic remission: the evidence from cytogenetic studies. In: The nature of leukaemia. Proceedings of the International Cancer Conference, Sydney, 1972. Sydney, N.S.W.: V.C.N. Blight, Government Printer 1972.

Barendsen, G. W., Broerse, J. J.: Experimental radiotherapy of a rat rhabdomyosarcoma with 15 MeV neutrons and 300 kV X-rays. I. Effects of single exposures. Europ. J. Cancer **5**, 373—391 (1969).

Barendsen, G. W., Broerse, J. J.: Experimental radiotherapy of a rat rhabdomyosarcoma with 15 MeV neutrons and 300 kV X-rays. II. Effects of fractionated treatments, applied five times a week for several weeks. Europ. J. Cancer **6**, 89—109 (1970).

Baserga, R., Rovera, G., Farber, J.: Control of cellular proliferation in human diploid fibroblasts. In Vitro **7**, 80—87 (1971).

Beierle, J. W.: Cell proliferation: enhancement by extracts from cell surfaces of polyoma-virus-transformed cells. Science **161**, 798—799 (1968).

Bennington, J. L.: Cellular kinetics of invasive squamous carcinoma of the human cervix. Cancer Res. **29**, 1082—1088 (1969).

Bernard, J., Jacquiliat, C., Weil, M., Boiron, M., Tanzer, J.: Present results on daunorubicin. In: Recent results in cancer research. Advances in the treatment of acute (blastic) leukemias, vol. 30. Berlin-Heidelberg-New York: Springer 1970.

Bichel, P.: Autoregulation of ascites tumour growth by inhibition of the *G*-1 and the *G*-2 phase. Europ. J. Cancer **7**, 349—355 (1971).

Boggs, D. R., Sofferman, S. A., Wintrobe, M. M., Cartwright, G. E.: Factors influencing the duration of survival of patients with chronic lymphocytic leukemia. Am. J. Med. **40**, 243—254 (1966).

Bradley, T. R., Sumner, M. A., Fry, P. A.: Some factors influencing colony development of murine haemopoietic cells *in vitro*. In: The nature of leukaemia. Proceedings of the International Cancer Conference, Sydney, 1972. Sydney, N.S.W.: V.C.N. Blight, Government Printer 1972.

Brown, C. H., III, Carbone, P. P.: *In vitro* growth of normal and leukemic human bone marrow. J. nat. Cancer Inst. **46**, 989—1000 (1971).

Bruce, W. R., Bergsagel, D. E.: On the application of results from a model system to the treatment of leukemia in man. Cancer Res. **27**, 2646—2649 (1967).

Bruce, W. R., Lin, H.: An empirical cellular approach to the improvement of cancer chemotherapy. Cancer Res. **29**, 2308—2310 (1969).

Bruce, W. R., Meeker, B. E., Powers, W. E., Valeriote, F. A.: Comparison of the dose- and time-survival curves for normal hematopoietic and lymphoma colony-forming cells exposed to vinblastine, vincristine, arabinosylcytosine, and amethopterin. J. nat. Cancer Inst. **42**, 1015—1025 (1969).

Bruce, W. R., Meeker, B. E., Valeriote, F. A.: Comparison of the sensitivity of normal hematopoietic and transplanted lymphoma colony-forming cells to chemotherapeutic agents administered *in vivo*. J. nat. Cancer Inst. **37**, 233—245 (1966).

Bruce, W. R., Valeriote, F. A.: Normal and malignant stem cells and chemotherapy. In: The proliferation and spread of neoplastic cells. Baltimore: Williams and Wilkins Co. 1968.

Buell, D. N., Fahey, J. L.: Limited periods of gene expression in immunoglobulin-synthesizing cells. Science **164**, 1524—1525 (1969).

Bullough, W. S.: Mitotic and functional homeostasis: A speculative review. Cancer Res. **25**, 1683—1727 (1965).

Bullough, W. S., Laurence, E. B., Iversen, O. H., Elgjo, K.: The vertebrate epidermal chalone. Nature (Lond.) **214**, 578—580 (1967).

Burchenal, J. H.: Chemotherapy for leukemia and lymphoma. Postgrad. Med. **48**, 164—168 (1970a).

Burchenal, J. H.: Clinical evaluation and future prospects of asparaginase. In: Recent results in cancer research. Advances in the treatment of acute (blastic) leukemias, vol. 30. Berlin-Heidelberg-New York: Springer 1970b.

Burger, M. M.: Cell surfaces in neoplastic transformation. In: Current topics in cellular regulation, vol. 3. New York-London: Academic Press 1971.

Burger, M. M., Noonan, K. D.: Restoration of normal growth by covering of agglutinin sites on tumour cell surface. Nature (Lond.) **228**, 512—515 (1970).

Bürk, R. R., Williams, C. A.: Attempts to isolate $SV_{40}$ transformation factor. In: Growth control in cell cultures. Edinburgh-London: Livingstone 1971.

Burns, E. R.: On the failure of self-inhibition of growth in tumors. Growth **33**, 25—45 (1969).

Cairnie, A. B.: Cell proliferation studies in the intestinal epithelium of the rat: response to continuous irradiation. Radiat. Res. **32**, 240—264 (1967).

Cairnie, A. B., Lamerton, L. F., Steel, G. G.: Cell proliferation studies in the intestinal epithelium of the rat. Exp. cell. Res. **39**, 528—538, 539—553 (1965).

Carbone, P. P., Berard, C. W., Bennett, J. M., Ziegler, J. L., Cohen, M. L., Gerber, P.: Burkitt's tumor. Annals intern. Med. **70**, 817—832 (1969).

Carbone, P. P., Ziegler, J. L., Morrow, R., Kyalwazi, S., Brown, C. H., DeVita, V. T., Berard, C. W.: Burkitt's tumor: a comparative study in Africa and the United States. In: Recent results in cancer research. Normal and malignant cell growth, vol. 17. Berlin-Heidelberg-New York: Springer 1969.

Carey, R. W.: Comparative study of cytosine arabinoside (CA) therapy alone and combined with thioguanine (TG), mercaptopurine (MP) or daunomycin (DN) in acute myelocytic leukemia (AML). Proc. Amer. Assn. Canc. Res. **11**, 15 (1970).

Chan, B. W. B., Bullimore, J. A., Hayhoe, F. G. J.: Extracorporeal irradiation of the blood in acute myeloid leukaemia: a clinical and *in vitro* culture study. Brit. J. Haemat. **17**, 309 (1969).

Chan, B. W. B., Hayhoe, F. G. J.: Changes in proliferative activity of marrow leukemic cells during and after extracorporeal irradiation of blood. Blood **37**, 657—663 (1971).

Chan, S. H., Metcalf, D., Gunz, F. W.: Serum inhibitors of colony stimulating factor in leukaemia. In: The nature of leukemia. Proceedings of the International Cancer Conference, Sydney, 1972. Sydney, N.S.W.: V.C.N. Blight, Government Printer 1972.

Charbit, A., Malaise, E. P., Tubiana, M.: Relation between the pathological nature and the growth rate of human tumors. Europ. J. Cancer **7**, 307—315 (1971).

Chervenick, P. A., Ellis, L. D., Pan, S. F., Lawson, A. L.: Human leukemic cells: in vitro growth of colonies containing the Philadelphia (*Ph.*) chromosome. Science **174**, 1134—1135 (1971).

Choquet, C., Chavaudra, N., Malaise, E.: The influence of allogeneic inhibition and tumour age on the kinetics of L1210 leukaemia in vivo. Europ. J. Cancer **6**, 373—378 (1970).

Clarke, G. D., Stoker, M. G. P., Ludlow, A., Thornton, M.: Requirement of serum for DNA synthesis in BHK 21 cells: effects of density, suspension and virus transformation. Nature (Lond.) **227**, 798—801 (1970).

Clarkson, B. D.: Review of recent studies of cellular proliferation in acute leukemia. In: Human tumor cell kinetics, monograph no. 30. Bethesda: National Cancer Institute 1969.

Clarkson, B. D.: Clinical contribution of cytokinetics and cytogenetics to leukemia. Presented at Tenth International Cancer Congress, Houston, Texas (1970a).

Clarkson, B. D.: Unpublished observations 1972a.

Clarkson, B. D.: Acute Myelocytic Leukemia in Adults. Cancer **30**, 1572—1582 (1972b).

Clarkson, B. D., Fried, J.: Changing concepts of treatment in acute leukemia. In: Medical Clinics of North America, vol. 55. Philadelphia-London-Toronto: Saunders 1971a.

Clarkson, B. D., Fried, J., Strife, A., Sakai, Y., Ota, K., Ohkita, T.: Studies of cellular proliferation in human leukemia. III. Behavior of leukemic cells in three adults with acute leukemia given continuous infusions of $^3$H-thymidine for eight to ten days. Cancer **25**, 1237—1260 (1970b).

Clarkson, B. D., Fried, J., Strife, A., Sakai, Y., Ota, K., Ohkita, T., Masuda, R.: Studies of cellular proliferation in human leukemia. IV. Behavior of normal hematopoietic cells in three adults with acute leukemia given continuous infusions of $^3$H-thymidine. Cancer **26**, 1—19 (1970c).

Clarkson, B. D., Krakoff, I., Burchenal, J., Karnofsky, D., Golbey, R., Oettgen, H., Dowling, M., Lipton, A.: Clinical results of treatment with *E. coli* L-asparaginase in adults with leukemia, lymphoma, and solid tumors. Cancer **25**, 279—305 (1970d).

Clarkson, B. D., Ota, K., Ohkita, T., O'Connor, A.: Kinetics of proliferation of cancer cells in neoplastic effusions in man. Cancer **18**, 1189—1213 (1965).

Clarkson, B. D., Ohkita, T., Ota, K., Fried, J.: Studies of cellular proliferation in human leukemia. I. Estimation of growth rates of leukemic and normal hematopoietic cells in two adults with acute leukemia given single injections of tritiated thymidine. J. clin. Invest. **46**, 506—529 (1967).

Clarkson, B. D., Sakai, Y., Kimura, T., Ohkita, T., Fried, J.: Studies of cellular proliferation in human leukemia. II. Variability in rates of growth and cellular differentiation in acute myelomonoblastic leukemia and effects of treatment. In: The proliferation and spread of neoplastic cells. Baltimore: The Williams and Wilkins Company 1968.

Clarkson, B. D., Todo, A., Ogawa, M., Gee, T. S., Fried, J.: Consideration of the cell cycle in chemotherapy of acute leukemia. In: Recent results in cancer research. Current concepts in the management of lymphoma and leukemia. Berlin-Heidelberg-New York: Springer 1971b.

Coffino, P., Laskov, R., Scharff, M. D.: Immunoglobulin production: method for quantitatively detecting variant myeloma cells. Science (Washington) **167**, 186—188 (1970).

Cohn, I., Jr., Slack, N. H., Fisher, B.: Complications and toxic manifestations of surgical adjuvant chemotherapy for breast cancer. Surg. Gynecol. Obstet. **127**, 1201—1209 (1968).

Collins, V. P.: Time of occurrence of pulmonary metastasis from carcinoma of the colon and rectum. Cancer **15**, 387—395 (1962).

Collins, V. P., Loeffler, R. K., Tivey, H.: Observations on growth rates of human tumors. Amer. J. Roentgenol. **76**, 988—1000 (1956).

Cooper, E. H., Frank, G. L., Wright, D. H.: Cell proliferation in Burkitt's lymphoma. Europ. J. Cancer **2**, 377—384 (1966).

Cooper, E. H., Peckham, M. J., Millard, R. E., Hamlin, I. M. E., Gerard-Marchant, R.: Cell proliferation in human malignant lymphomas. Analysis of labelling index and DNA content in cell populations obtained by biopsy. Europ. J. Cancer **4**, 287—296 (1968).

Cooper, H. L.: Biochemical alterations accompanying initiation of growth in resting cells. In: The cell cycle and cancer. Dekker: New York 1971.

Court-Brown, W. M., Tough, I. M.: Cytogenetic studies in chronic myeloid leukemia. Advanc. Cancer Res. **7**, 351—381 (1963).

Croizat, H., Frindel, E., Tubiana, M.: Proliferative activity of the stem cells in the bone marrow of mice after single and multiple irradiation (total or partial body exposure). Inter. J. Radiat. Biol. **18**, 347—358 (1970).

Cronkite, E. P.: Extracorporeal irradiation of blood in the treatment of chronic lymphocytic leukemia. In: Recent results in cancer research. Current concepts in the management of leukemia and lymphoma, vol. 36. Berlin-Heidelberg-New York: Springer 1971.

Crowther, D., Hamilton Fairley, G., Sewell, R.: Significance of the changes in the circulating lymphoid cells in Hodgkin's disease. Brit. med. J. **2**, 473—477 (1969).

Crowther, D., Bateman, C. J. T., Vartan, C. P., Whitehouse, J. M. A., Malpas, J. S., Fairley, G. H., Scott, R. B.: Combination chemotherapy using L-asparaginase, daunorubicin, and cytosine arabinoside in adults with acute myelogenous leukemia. Brit. med. J. **4**, 513—517 (1970).

Curtis, J. E., Hersh, E. J., Freireich, E. J.: Leukapheresis therapy of chronic lymphocytic leukemia. Blood **39**, 163—175 (1972).

DENEKAMP, J.: Cellular proliferation kinetics of animal tumours. Cancer Res. **30**, 393—400 (1970).
DENEKAMP, J., THOMLINSON, R. H.: The cell proliferation kinetics of four experimental tumors after acute x-irradiation. Cancer Res. **31**, 1279—1284 (1971).
DEVITA, V. T.: Cell kinetics and the chemotherapy of cancer. Cancer Chemother. Rep. **2**, 23—33 (1971a).
DEVITA, V. T.: Chemotherapy of the lymphomas. In: Recent results in cancer research. Current concepts in the management of leukemia and lymphoma, vol. 36. Berlin-Heidelberg-New York: Springer 1971b.
DEVITA, V. T., SERPICK, A. A., CARBONE, P. P.: Combination chemotherapy in the treatment of advanced Hodgkin's disease. Ann. int. Med. **73**, 881—895 (1970).
DJORDJEVIC, B., TOLMACH, L. J.: X-ray sensitivity of HeLa $S3$ cells in the $G_2$ phase: comparison of two methods of synchronization. Biophys. J. **7**, 77—94 (1967).
DOWLING, M. D., GEE, T. S., LEE, B. J., CLARKSON, B. D., BURCHENAL, J. H.: Treatment of acute non-lymphoblastic leukemia with arabinosylcytosine (AraC) and 6-Thioguanine (TG) every 12 hours. Proc. Am. Assn. Cancer Res. **13**, 21 (1972).
DULBECCO, R.: Topoinhibition and serum requirement of transformed and untransformed cells. Nature (Lond.) **227**, 802—806 (1970a).
DULBECCO, R., STOKER, M.: Conditions determining initiation of DNA synthesis in 3T3 cells. Proc. nat. Acad. Sci. (Wash.) **66**, 204—210 (1970b).
DUTREIX, J., TUBIANA, M., WAMBERSIE, A., MALAISE, E.: The influence of cell proliferation in tumours and normal tissues during fractionated radiotherapy. Europ. J. Cancer **7**, 205—213 (1971).
ELKIND, M. M., SUTTON, H.: X-ray damage and recovery in mammalian cells in culture. Nature (Lond.) **184**, 1293—1295 (1959).
ELKIND, M. M., SINCLAIR, W. K.: Recovery in X-irradiated mammalian cells. In: Current topics in radiation research. Amsterdam: Holland 1965.
ELKIND, M. M., SAKAMOTO, K., KAMPER, C.: Age-dependent toxic properties of Actinomycin D and X-rays in cultured Chinese hamster cells. Cell Tissue Kinet. **1**, 209—224 (1968).
ENGESET, A., COOPER, E. H., BRENNHOVD, I., HOEG, K.: The thoracic duct lymph in Hodgkin's disease. II. Quantitative analysis of the cellular composition of the lymph. Int. J. Cancer **8**, 113—121 (1971).
EPIFANOVA, O. I.: Effects of hormones on the cell cycle. In: The cell cycle and cancer. New York: Dekker 1971.
ERNST, P., KILLMANN, S.: Perturbation of generation cycle of human leukemic blast cells by cytostatic therapy in vivo: effect of corticosteroids. Blood **36**, 689—696 (1970).
ERNST, P., KILLMANN, S.: Perturbation of generation cycle of human leukemic myeloblasts in vivo by methotrexate. Blood **38**, 689—705 (1971).
EVERSON, T. C., COLE, W. H.: Spontaneous regression of cancer. Philadelphia-London: Saunders 1966.
FAHEY, J. L., BUELL, D. N., SOX, H. C.: Proliferation and differentiation of lymphoid cells: studies with human lymphoid cell lines and immunoglobulin synthesis. Ann. N. Y. Acad. Sci. **190**, 221—234 (1971).
FAIRLEY, G. H.: Clinical experience with L-asparaginase in Britain. In: Recent results in cancer research. Advances in the treatment of acute (blastic) leukemias, Vol. 30. Berlin-Heidelberg-New York: Springer 1970.
FARBER, S.: Neuroblastoma. Am. J. Dis. Child. **60**, 749 (1940).
FARBER, S.: Current clinical and experimental studies in cancer chemotherapy. Cancer Chemother. Rep. **13**, 159—165 (1961).
FIALKOW, P. J., BRYANT, J. I., THOMAS, E. D., NEIMAN, P. E.: Leukaemic transformation of engrafted human marrow cells in vivo. Lancet **1**, 251—255 (1971).
FISHER, B.: Status of adjuvant therapy: results of the national surgical adjuvant breast project studies in oophorectomy, postoperative radiation therapy and chemotherapy. Cancer **28**, 1654—1658 (1971).
FISHER, B., RAVDIN, R. G., AUSMAN, R. K., SLACK, N. H., MOORE, G. E., NOER, R. J.: Surgical adjuvant chemotherapy in cancer of the breast: results of a decade of cooperative investigation. Ann. Surg. **168**, 337—356 (1968).
FISHER, B., MOORE, G. E., RAVDIN, R. G., AUSMAN, R. K., SLACK, N. H., NOER, R. J.: Surgical adjuvant chemotherapy in the treatment of breast cancer. In: Breast cancer: early and late. Thirteenth Annual Clinical Conference on Cancer, 1968, The University of Texas M. D. Anderson Hospital and Tumor Institute. Chicago: Year Book Medical Publishers 1970a.
FISHER, B., SLACK, N. H., CAVANAUGH, P. J., GARDNER, B., RAVDIN, R. G.: Postoperative radiotherapy in the treatment of breast cancer: results of the NSABD clinical trial. Ann. Surg. **172**, 711—732 (1970b).

FITZGERALD, P. H., ADAMS, A., GUNZ, F. W.: Chromosome studies in adult acute leukemia. J. nat. Cancer Inst. **32**, 395—417 (1964).
FOLKMAN, J.: Tumor angiogenesis: therapeutic implications. New Eng. J. med. **285**, 1182—1186 (1971).
FOX, T. O., PARDEE, A. B.: Animal cells: noncorrelation of length of $G_1$ phase with size after mitosis. Science **167**, 80—82 (1970).
FOX, T. O., SHEPPARD, J. R., BURGER, M. M.: Cyclic membrane changes in animal cells: transformed cells permanently display a surface architecture detected in normal cells only during mitosis. Proc. nat. Acad. Sci. **68**, 224—247 (1971).
FRAUMENI, J. F., JR.: Constitutional disorders of man predisposing to leukemia and lymphoma. In: Hematopoietic neoplasms, monograph no. 32. Bethesda: National Cancer Institute 1968.
FREI, E., III., CARTER, S. K.: Arabinosylcytosine: therapeutic trials in patients with neoplastic disease, unpublished.
FREI, E., III., TJIO, J. H., WHANG, J., CARBONE, P. P.: Studies of the Philadelphia chromosome in patients with chronic myelogenous leukemia. Ann. N. Y. Acad. Sci. **113**, 1073—1080 (1964).
FREIREICH, E. J., BODEY, G. P., HART, S., RODRIGUEZ, V., WHITECAR, J. P., FREI, E., III.: Remission induction in adults with acute myelogenous leukemia. In: Recent results in cancer research. Advances in the treatment of acute (blastic) leukemias, vol. 30. Berlin-Heidelberg-New York: Springer 1970.
FRINDEL, E., CHARRUYER, F., TUBIANA, M., KAPLAN, H. S., ALPEN, E. L.: Radiation effects on DNA synthesis and cell division in the bone-marrow of the mouse. Int. J. Radiat. Biol. **11**, 435—443 (1966).
FRINDEL, E., MALAISE, E., ALPEN, E., TUBIANA, M.: Kinetics of cell proliferation of an experimental tumour. Cancer Res. **27**, 1122—1131 (1967).
FRINDEL, E., MALAISE, E., TUBIANA, M.: Cell proliferation kinetics in five human solid tumours. Cancer **22**, 611—620 (1968).
FRINDEL, E., TUBIANA, M.: Radiobiology and the cell cycle. In: The cell cycle and cancer. New York: Dekker 1971.
FRINDEL, E., VALLERON, A. J., VASSORT, F., TUBIANA, M.: Proliferation kinetics of an experimental ascites tumour of the mouse. Cell Tissue Kinet. **2**, 51—65 (1969).
FROESE, G.: Regulation of growth in Chinese hamster cells by a local inhibitor. Exp. cell Res. **65**, 297—306 (1971).
GABUTTI, V., PILERI, A., TAROCCO, R. P., GAVOSTO, F., COOPER, E. H.: Proliferative potential of out-of-cycle leukaemic cells. Nature **224**, 375—376 (1969).
GALBRAITH, P. R.: Granulocyte kinetic studies in chronic myelogenous leukemia. Nat. Cancer Inst. Monogr. **30**, 121—134 (1969).
GALTON, D. A. G.: Management of the chronic leukaemias. In: Recent results in cancer research. Current concep's in the management of leukemia and lymphoma, vol. 36. Berlin-Heidelberg-New York: Springer 1971.
GARLAND, L. H., COULSON, W., WOLLIN, E.: The rate of growth and apparent duration of untreated primary bronchial carcinoma. Cancer **16**, 694—707 (1963).
GAVOSTO, F.: The proliferative kinetics of the acute leukaemias in relation to their treatment. Europ. J. clin. biol. Res. **15**, 1042—1047 (1970).
GAVOSTO, F., PILERI, A.: Cell cycle of cancer cells in man. In: The cell cycle and cancer. New York: Dekker 1971.
GEE, T. S., DOWLING, M. D., JR., CLARKSON, B. D.: Combination therapy with arabinosylcytosine (Ara-C) and 6-thioguanine (TG) in adult patients with the acute leukemic phase of lymphosarcoma (LSA) or reticulum cell sarcoma (RCS). XIII International Congress of Hematology, Munich, 1970.
GEE, T. S., YU, K.-P., CLARKSON, B. D.: Treatment of adult acute leukemia with arabinosyl cytosine and thioguanine. Cancer **23**, 1019—1032 (1969).
GILDEWELL, O. J., HOLLAND, J. F.: Clinical trials of the acute leukemia Group B in acute lymphocytic leukemia (ALL). In: The 5th international symposium on comparative leukemia research, Padova-Venice, Italy, September 13—17, 1971, p. 8.
GOMPERTZ, B.: On the nature of the function expressive of the law of human mortality, and on a new mode of determining the value of life contingencies. Phil. Trans. **115**, 513 (1825).
GOODELL, R., YOUNG, R., DEVITA, V.: Rapid *in vivo* kinetic studies in human acute leukemia (AL) by intramarrow double labelling (DL) with $^3$H and $^{14}$C thymidine (TdR). Proc. Amer. Assoc. Cancer Res. **11**, 31 (1970).
GREENBERG, P. L., NICHOLS, W. C., SCHRIER, S. L.: Granulopoiesis in acute myeloid leukemia and preleukemia. New Eng. J. Med. **284**, 1225—1232 (1971).
GREENE, H. S. N.: Heterologous transplantation of mammalian tumors. I. The transfer of rabbit tumors to alien species. J. exp. Med. **73**, 461—479 (1941).

GRISWOLD, D. P., SCHABEL, F. M., JR., WILCOX, W. S., SIMPSON-HERREN, L., SKIPPER, H. E.: Success and failure in the treatment of solid tumour. Cancer Chemother. Rep. **52**, 345—387 (1968).

GRISWOLD, D. P., JR., SIMPSON-HERREN, L., SCHABEL, F. M., JR.: Altered sensitivity of a hamster plasmacytoma to cytosine arabinoside (NSC-63878). Cancer Chemother. Rep. **54**, 337—346 (1970).

HAGHBIN, M., TAN, C., GEE, T., DOWLING, M., CLARKSON, B., SIDHU, J., SYKES, M., BURCHENAL, J., MURPHY, M. L.: Sequential intensive drug therapy in acute lymphoblastic leukemia (ALL) and leukosarcoma (LSA). Proc. Am. Assn. Cancer Res. **12**, 31 (1971).

HAGHBIN, M., TAN, C., GEE, T., DOWLING, M., CLARKSON, B., SIDHU, J., SYKES, M., MURPHY, M. L.: Intensive chemotherapy and prophylactic intrathecal methotrexate in acute lymphoblastic leukemia (ALL). Proc. Am. Assn. Cancer Res. **13**, 22 (1972).

HALPERN, M., RUBIN, H.: Proteins released from chick embryo fibroblasts in culture: I. Partial characterization of the proteins. Exp. cell. Res. **60**, 86—95 (1970).

HANNA, I. R. A., TARBUTT, R. G., LAMERTON, L. F.: Shortening of the cell-cycle time of erythroid precursors in response to anaemia. Brit. J. Haemat. **61**, 381—387 (1969).

HART, J. S., SHIRAKAWA, S., TRUJILLO, J., FREI, E., III.: The mechanism of induction of complete remission in acute myeloblastic leukemia in man. Cancer Res. **29**, 2300—2307 (1969).

HART, J. S., TRUJILLO, J. M., FREIREICH, E. J., GEORGE, S. L., FREI, E., III.: Cytogenetic studies and their clinical correlates in adults with acute leukemia. Ann. intern. Med. **75**, 353—360 (1971).

HENDERSON, E. S.: Treatment of acute leukemia. Sem. Hemat. **6**, 271—319 (1969).

HENDERSON, E. S., SAMAHA, R. J.: Evidence that drugs in multiple combination have materially advanced the treatment of human malignancies. Cancer Res. **29**, 2272—2280 (1969).

HERMENS, A. F., BARENDSEN, G. W.: Cellular proliferation patterns in an experimental rhabdomyosarcoma in the rat. Europ. J. Cancer **3**, 361—369 (1967).

HERMENS, A. F., BARENDSEN, G. W.: Changes of cell proliferation characteristics in a rat rhabdomyosarcoma before and after X-irradiation. Europ. J. Cancer **5**, 173—189 (1969).

HERSH, E. M., FREI, E., III., COLTMAN, C., LUCE, J.: Improved combination chemotherapy (MOPP) for remission induction and maintenance in advanced Hodgkin's disease. Amer. Soc. Clin. Oncol., Eighth Annual Scientific Meeting Program, Boston, Mass., May 3, 1972, abstract No. 28.

HILL, J. M., ROBERTS, J., LOEB, E., KAHN, A., MACLELLAN, A., HILL, R. W.: L-Asparaginase therapy for leukemia and other malignant neoplasms. J. Amer. med. Assn. **202**, 882—888 (1967).

HOBBS, J. R.: Modes of escape from therapeutic control in myelomatosis. Brit. med. J. **2**, 325 (1971).

HOFER, K. G., HOFER, M.: Kinetics of proliferation, migration, and death of L1210 ascites cells. Cancer Res. **31**, 402—408 (1971).

HOLLAND, J. F., GLIDEWELL, O.: Complementary chemotherapy in acute leukemia. In: Recent results in cancer research. Advances in the treatment of acute (blastic) leukemias, vol. 30. Berlin-Heidelberg-New York: Springer 1970.

HOLLAND, J. F., GLIDEWELL, O. J.: Progress in chemotherapy of acute leukaemia. In: The nature of leukaemia. Proceedings of the International Cancer Conference, Sydney, 1972. Sydney, N. S. W., V. C. N. Blight, Government Printer 1972.

HOLLEY, R. W., KIERNAN, J. A.: Studies of serum factors required by $_3T_3$ and $SV_3T_3$ cells. In: Growth control in cell cultures. Edinburgh-London: Livingstone 1971.

HOLMBERG, B.: A blockage in the *S*-phase of HeLa cells produced by a human tumor polypeptide. Europ. J. Cancer **4**, 475—480 (1968).

HOOGSTRATEN, B., COSTA, J., CUTTNER, J., FORCIER, R. J., LEONE, L. A., HARLEY, J. B., GLIDEWELL, O. J.: Intermittent melphalan therapy in multiple myeloma. J. Amer. med. Ass. **209**, 251—253 (1969).

HOWES, A. E.: An estimation of changes in the proportions and absolute numbers of hypoxic cells after irradiation of transplanted C3H mouse mammary tumors. Brit. J. Radiol. **42**, 441—447 (1969).

HUGULEY, C. M., JR.: Chronic myelocytic and chronic lymphocytic leukemia. Cancer **30**, 1583—1587 (1972).

ICHIKAWA, Y.: Differentiation of a cell line of myeloid leukemia. In: The nature of leukaemia. Proceedings of the International Cancer Conference, Sydney, 1972. Sydney, N. S. W.: V. C. N. Blight, Government Printer 1972.

ISRAEL, L., CHAHINIAN, P.: Evaluation of the survival gain in 22 measurable lung tumors treated with chemotherapy. An approach towards quantitative evaluation of cancer treatments in man. Europ. J. Cancer **5**, 631—637 (1969).

Iverson, U., Iversen, O. H., Bluming, A. Z., Ziegler, J. L., Kyalwasi, S.: Cell kinetics of African cases of Burkitt, lymphoma: a preliminary report. Europ. J. Cancer, 1972 in press.
Jainchill, J., Todaro, G. J.: Stimulation of cell growth in vitro by serum with and without growth factor. Relation to contact inhibition and viral transformation. Exp. cell Res. **59**, 137—146 (1970).
Jensen, M. K.: Chromosome studies in acute leukemia. III. Chromosome constitution of bone marrow cells in 30 cases. Acta med. Scand. **182**, 629—644 (1967).
Johnson, R. E.: The curative radiotherapy of lymphomas. In: Recent results in cancer research. Current concepts in the management of leukemia and lymphoma, vol. 36. Berlin-Heidelberg-New York: Springer 1971.
Jones, B., Holland, J. F., Morrison, A. R., Lee, S. L., Sinks, L. F., Cuttner, J., Rausen, A., Kung, F., Pluss, H. J., Haurani, F. I., Patterson, R. B., Blom, J., Burgert, E. O., Jr., Moon, J. H., Chevalier, L., Sawitsky, A., Albala, M. M., Forcier, R. J., Falkson, G., Gildewell, O. J.: Daunorubicin (NSC-82151) in the treatment of advanced childhood lymphoblastic leukemia. Cancer Res. **31**, 84—90 (1971).
Kaplan, H. S.: Radiation therapy with curative intent in the malignant lymphomas. In: Recent results in cancer research. Current concepts in the management of leukemia and lymphoma, vol. 36. Berlin-Heidelberg-New York: Springer 1971.
Keiser, G., Wagner, H. P., Frey-Wettstein, M.: Cytokinetic studies in two acute lymphoblastic leukemias. Helv. med. Acta. **34**, 155—169 (1968).
Killander, D.: Intercellular variations in generation time and amounts of DNA, RNA and mass in a mouse leukemia population in vitro. Exp. cell Res. **40**, 21—31 (1965).
Killander, D.: Intercellular variation in the amounts of DNA, RNA and mass in a leukemia and a fibroblast cell population in vitro. Europ. J. Cancer **3**, 309—314 (1967).
Killmann, S.: Acute leukemia: the kinetics of leukemic blast cells in man. Ser. Haemat. **1**, 38—102 (1968).
Killmann, S.: A biased view on the relapse and remission phase of acute myeloid leukaemia. In: The nature of leukaemia. Proceedings of the International Cancer Conference, Sydney, 1972. Sydney, N.S.W.: V.C.N. Blight, Government Printer 1972.
Kim, J. H., Evans, T. C.: Effects of X-irradiation on the mitotic cycle of Ehrlich ascites tumor cells. Radiat. Res. **21**, 129—143 (1964).
Kiossoglou, K. A., Mitus, W. J., Dameshek, W.: Chromosomal aberrations in acute leukemia. Blood **26**, 610—641 (1965).
Koop, C. E., Kiesewetter, W. B., Horn, R. C.: Neuroblastoma in childhood. Surgery **38**, 272—278 (1955).
Kubitschek, H. E., Bendigkeit, H. E., Loken, M. R.: Onset of DNA synthesis during the cell cycle in chemostat cultures. Proc. nat. Acad. Sci. (Wash.) **57**, 1611—1617 (1967).
Laird, A. K.: Dynamics of tumour growth: comparison of growth rates and extrapolation of growth curve to one cell. Brit. J. Cancer **19**, 278—291 (1965).
Lajtha, L. G.: Leukemic stem cell kinetics in experimental animals. The Vth International symposium on comparative leukemia Research, Padova-Venice, Italy, September 13—17, 1971.
Lajtha, L. G., Pozzi, L. V., Schofield, R., Fox, M.: Kinetic properties of haemopoietic stem cells. Cell Tissue Kinet. **2**, 39—49 (1969).
Lala, P. K.: Age-specific changes in the proliferation of Ehrlich ascites tumor cells grown as solid tumors. Cancer Res. **32**, 628—636 (1972).
Lala, P. K., Maloney, M. A., Patt, H. M.: Measurement of DNA-synthesis time in myeloid-erythroid precursors. Exp. cell Res. **38**, 626—634 (1965).
Lala, P. K., Patt, H. M.: Cytokinetic analysis of tumor growth. Proc. nat. Acad. Sci. (Wash.) **56**, 1735—1742 (1966).
Lamerton, L. F., Steel, G. G.: Cell population kinetics in normal and malignant tissues. Progr. biophys. molec. Biol. **18**, 247—283 (1968).
Lampkin, B. C., McWilliams, N. B., Mauer, A. M.: The advantage of cell synchronization in therapy of myeloid leukemias in children. In: Program — American society of hematology, p. 44. Fourteenth annual meeting, San Francisco, California, December 5—7, 1971a.
Lampkin, B. C., Nagao, T., Mauer, A. M.: Drug effect in acute leukemia. J. clin. Invest. **48**, 1124—1130 (1969).
Lampkin, B. C., Nagao, T., Mauer, A. M.: Synchronization and recruitment in acute leukemia. J. clin. Invest. **50**, 2204—2214 (1971b).
Landau, T., Sachs, L.: Characterization of the inducer required for the development of macrophage and granulocyte colonies. Proc. nat. Acad. Sci. (Wash.) **68**, 2540—2544 (1971).
Landau, T., Sachs, L.: Activation of a differentiation-inducing protein by adenine and adenine containing nucleotides. FEBS Let. **17**, 339—341 (1971b).
Lee, B. J., Pinsky, C., Miller, D. G.: The management of plasma cell neoplasms. In: The medical clinics of North America, vol. 55. Philadelphia-London-Toronto: Saunders 1971.

LESHER, S.: Compensatory reactions in intestinal crypt cells after 300 roentgens of cobalt-60 gamma irradiation. Radiat. Res. **32**, 510—519 (1967).
LI, M.C., HERTZ, R., SPENCER, D.B.: Effect of methotrexate therapy upon choriocarcinoma and chorioadenoma. Proc. Soc. exp. Biol. **93**, 361—366 (1956).
LIPKIN, M.: The proliferative cycle of mammalian cells. In: The cell cycle and cancer. New York: Dekker 1971.
LIPTON, A., KLINGER, I., PAUL, D., HOLLEY, R.W.: Migration of mouse 3T3 fibroblasts in response to a serum factor. Proc. nat. Acad. Sci. (Wash.) **68**, 2799—2801 (1971).
LOWENBRAUN, S., DEVITA, V.T., SERPICK, A.A.: Combination chemotherapy with nitrogen mustard, vincristine, procarbazine and prednisone in lymphosarcoma and reticulum cell sarcoma. Cancer **25**, 1018—1025 (1970).
MACMAHON, B., LEVY, M.A.: Prenatal origin of childhood leukemia. Evidence from twins. New Eng. J. Med. **270**, 1082—1085 (1964).
MALAISE, E., TUBIANA, M.: Etude *in vitro* de certains facteurs susceptibles d'influencer la croissance d'une ascite expérimentale. Comptes-Rendus de l'Académie de Sciences **270** D, 539—542 (1970).
MATHÉ, G., AMIEL, J.L., CLARYSSE, A., HAYAT, M., SCHWARZENBERG, L.: The place of the L-asparaginase in the treatment of acute leukemias. In: Recent results in cancer research. Advances in the treatment of acute (blastic) leukemias, vol. 30. Berlin-Heidelberg-New York: Springer 1970a.
MATHÉ, G., AMIEL, J.L., SCHWARZENBERG, L., SCHNEIDER, M., CATTAN, A., HAYAT, M., DE VASSAL, F., SCHLUMBERGER, J.R.: Methods and strategy for the treatment of acute lymphoblastic leukemia. In: Recent results in cancer research. Advances in the treatment of acute (blastic) leukemias, vol. 30. Berlin-Heidelberg-New York: Springer 1970b.
MAUER, A.M., FISHER, V.: Characteristics of cell proliferation in four patients with untreated acute leukemia. Blood **28**, 428—445 (1966).
MAUER, A.M., LAMPKIN, B.C., NAGAO, T.: Prospects for new directions in therapy of acute lymphoblastic leukemia. In: Hemopoietic cellular proliferation. New York: Grune & Stratton 1970.
MAURICE, P.A., ALBERTO, P., FERRIER, S., FREUND, M.: Leucémie myélocytaire chronique: «guerison» apparente depuis plus de 9 ans, consécutive à une hypoplasie médullaire thérapeutique. Schweiz. Med. Wschr. **101**, 1781—1782 (1971).
MAURO, F., MADOC-JONES, H.: Age responses of cultured mammalian cells to cytotoxic drugs. Cancer Res. **30**, 1397—1408 (1970).
MCCULLOCH, E.A., TILL, J.E.: Leukemia considered as defective differentiation: complementary *in vivo* and culture methods applied to the clinical problem. In: The nature of leukaemia. Proceedings of the International Cancer Conference, Sydney, 1972. Sydney, N.S.W.: V.C.N. Blight. Government Printer 1972.
METCALF, D.: Inhibition of bone marrow colony formation *in vitro* by dialysable products of normal and neoplastic haemopoietic cells. Aust. J. exp. biol. med. Sci. **49**, 351—363 (1971a).
METCALF, D.: The nature of leukaemia: neoplasm or disorder of haemopoietic regulation? Med. J. Aust. **2**, 739—746 (1971b).
METCALF, D., CHAN, S.H., GUNZ, F.W., VINCENT, P., RAVICH, R.B.M.: Colony-stimulating factor and inhibitor levels in acute granulocytic leukemia. Blood **38**, 143—152 (1971c).
METCALF, D., CHAN, S.H., STANLEY, E.R., MOORE, M.A.S., GUNZ, F.W., VINCENT, P.C.: Regulation of normal and leukaemic granulocytic cells by colony stimulating factor (CSF). In: The nature of leukaemia. Proceedings of the International Cancer Conference, Sydney, 1972. Australia: Sydney, N.S.W.: V.C.N. Blight, Government Printer, 1972.
MILLER, R.W.: Deaths from childhood cancer in sibs. New Eng. J. Med. **279**, 122—126 (1968).
MOORE, M.A.S., WILLIAMS, N., METCALF, D.: Characterisation of *in vitro* colony forming cells in acute and chronic myeloid leukaemia. In: The nature of leukaemia. Proceedings of the International Cancer Conference, Sydney, 1972. Sydney, N.S.W.: V.C.N. Blight, Government Printer 1972.
MUELLER, G.C.: Biochemical perspectives of the $G_1$ and $S$ intervals in the replication cycle of animal cells: a study in the control of cell growth. In: The cell cycle and cancer, vol. 1. New York: Dekker 1971.
NIAS, A.H.W., FOX, M.: Synchronization of mammalian cells with respect to the mitotic cycle. Cell Tissue Kinet. **4**, 375—398 (1971).
NITZE, H.R., VOSTEEN, K., GANZER, U.: Radiation treatment of human tumours following the in vivo synchronization of the cell cycle. Acta Otolaryng. **71**, 227—231 (1971).
NOWELL, P.C., HUNGERFORD, D.A.: Chromosome studies in human leukemia. II. Chronic granulocytic leukemia. J. nat. Cancer Inst. **27**, 1013—1021 (1961).
OETTGEN, H.F., OLD, L.J., BOYSE, E.A.: Human tumor immunology. In: The medical clinics of North America, vol. 55. Philadelphia-London-Toronto: Saunders 1971.

Oettgen, H. F., Old, L. J., Boyse, E. A., Campbell, H. A., Philips, F. S., Clarkson, B. D., Tallal, L., Leeper, R. D., Schwartz, M. K., Kim, J. H.: Inhibition of leukemias in man by L-asparaginase. Cancer Res. **27**, 2619—2631 (1967).
Oettgen, H. F., Stephenson, P. A., Schwartz, M. K., Leeper, R. D., Tallal, L., Clarkson, B. D., Golbey, R. B., Krakoff, I. H., Karnofsky, D. A., Burchenal, J. H.: The toxicity of *E. coli* L-asparaginase in man. Cancer **25**, 253—278 (1970).
Ogawa, M., Bergsagel, D. E., McCulloch, E. A.: Differential effects of melphalan on mouse myeloma (adj. PC-5) and hemopoietic stem cells. Cancer Res. **31**, 2116—2119 (1971).
Ogawa, M., Fried, J., Sakai, Y., Strife, A., Clarkson, B. D.: Studies of cellular proliferation in human leukemia. VI. The proliferative activity, generation time, and emergence time of neutrophilic granulocytes in chronic granulocytic leukemia. Cancer **25**, 1031—1049 (1970).
Ohara, K., Fried, J., Dowling, M. D., Bittar, E. S., Clarkson, B. D.: Studies of cellular proliferation in human leukemia. VII. Cytokinetic behavior of neoplastic cells in a patient with reticulum cell sarcoma in a leukemia phase. Cancer **28**, 862—885 (1971).
Paran, M., Ichikawa, Y., Sachs, L.: Feedback inhibition of the development of macrophage and granulocyte colonies. II. Inhibition by granulocytes. Proc. nat. Acad. Sci. (Wash.) **62**, 81—87 (1969).
Paran, M., Sachs, L., Barak, Y., Resnitzky, P.: *In vitro* induction of granulocyte differentiation in hematopoietic cells from leukemic and non-leukemic patients. Proc. nat. Acad. Sci. (Wash.) **67**, 1542—1549 (1970).
Pardee, A. B.: The surface membrane as a regulator of animal cell division. In Vitro **7**, 95—104 (1971).
Paul, D., Lipton, A., Klinger, I.: Serum factor requirements of normal and Simian virus 40-transformed 3T3 mouse fibroblasts. Proc. nat. Acad. Sci. (Wash.) **68**, 645—648 (1971).
Peckham, M. J., Cooper, E. H.: The pattern of cell growth in reticulum cell sarcoma and lymphosarcoma. Europ. J. Cancer **6**, 453—463 (1970).
Peckham, M. J., Cooper, E. H.: Proliferation characteristics of the various classes of cells in Hodgkin's disease. Cancer **24**, 135—146 (1969).
Pinkel, D.: Five-year follow up of "total therapy" of childhood lymphocytic leukemia. J. Amer. Med. Ass. **216**, 648—652 (1971).
Ravdin, R. G., Lewison, E. F., Slack, N. H., Dao, T. L., Gardner, B., State, D., Fisher, B.: Results of a clinical trial concerning the worth of prophylactic oophorectomy for breast carcinoma. Surg. Gynecol. Obstet. **131**, 1055—1064 (1970).
Reese, A. B., Hyman, G. A., Tapley, N. duV., Forrest, A. W.: The treatment of retinoblastoma by x-ray and triethylene melamine. Arch. Ophthal. **60**, 897—906 (1958).
Reich, L., Clarkson, B.: Unpublished observations 1972.
Reich, L., Ohara, K., Stoerzinger, P., Clarkson, B.: Effect of massive leukapheresis on proliferation in acute myeloblastic leukemia (AML). Proc. Amer. Assn. Cancer Res. **12**, 25 (1971).
Robinson, W. A., Entringer, M. A., Otsuka, A. L.: *In vitro* studies in acute granulocytic leukaemia in humans. In: The nature of leukaemia. Proceedings of the International Cancer Conference, Sydney, 1972. Sydney, N.S.W.: C.V.N. Blight, Government Printer 1972.
Robinson, W. A., Pike, B. L.: Leukopoietic activity in human urine. New Eng. J. Med. **282**, 1291—1297 (1970).
Rosen, P. J., Perry, S., Schabel, F. M., Jr.: Proliferative capacity of leukemic cells in AKR leukemia. J. nat. Cancer Inst. **45**, 1169—1178 (1970).
Rubin, H.: A substance in conditioned medium which enhances the growth of small numbers of chick embryo cells *in vitro*. Exp. cell Res. **41**, 138—148 (1966).
Rytomaa, T.: Granulocytic chalone and antichalone. In: In vitro, Vol. 4. Philadelphia: Williams and Wilkins 1969.
Sachs, L.: Feedback control of the development of hematopoietic cell clones *in vitro* and the mechanism of leukemogenesis. In: Canadian cancer conference 8. Canada: Pergamon 1968.
Salmon, S. E.: Immunoglobulin synthesis and tumor cell number and the natural history of multiple myeloma. Brit. med. J. **2**, 321 (1971a).
Salmon, S. E., McIntyre, C. R., Ogawa, M.: IgE Myeloma: total body tumor cell number and synthesis of IgE and DNA. Blood **37**, 696—705 (1971b).
Salmon, S. E., Smith, B. A.: Sandwich solid phase radioimmunoassays for the characterization of human immunoglobulins synthesized *in vitro*. J. Immunol. **104**, 665—672 (1970a).
Salmon, S. E., Smith, B. A.: Immunoglobulin synthesis and total body tumor cell number in IgG multiple myeloma. J. clin. Invest. **49**, 1114—1121 (1970b).
Salmon, S. E., Smith, B. A.: Induction of tumor-susceptibility to cycle-active agents in IgG multiple myeloma. Clin. Res. **20**, 570 (1972).

SANDBERG, A. A.: The chromosomes and causation of human cancer and leukemia. Cancer Res. **26**, 2064—2081 (1966).

SAUNDERS, E. F.: Maturation of hemolysin-producing cell clones. I. The kinetics of the induction period of an in vitro hemolysin response to erythrocyte antigen. J. exp. Med. **130**, 543—556 (1969).

SAUNDERS, E. F., LAMPKIN, B. C., MAUER, A. M.: Variation of proliferative activity in leukemic cell populations of patients with acute leukemia. J. clin. Invest. **46**, 1356—1363 (1967).

SAUNDERS, E. F., MAUER, A. M.: Reentry of nondividing leukemic cells into a proliferative phase in acute childhood leukemia. J. clin. Invest. **48**, 1299—1305 (1969).

SCHABEL, F. M., JR.: In vivo leukemic cell kill kinetics and "curability" in experimental systems. In: The proliferation and spread of neoplastic cells. Baltimore: Williams and Wilkins 1968.

SCHABEL, F. M., JR.: The use of tumor growth kinetics in planning "curative" chemotherapy of advanced solid tumors. Cancer Res. **29**, 2384—2389 (1969).

SCHABEL, F. M., JR., SKIPPER, H. E., TRADER, M. W., LASTER, W. R., SIMPSON-HERREN, L.: Spontaneous AK leukemia (lymphoma) as a model system. Cancer Chemother. Rep. **53**, 329—344 (1969).

SCHER, C. D., NELSON-REES, W. A.: Direct isolation and characterization of "flat" SV40-transformed cells. Nature (Lond.) **233**, 263—265 (1971).

SCHER, C. D., TODARO, G. J.: Selective growth of human neoplastic cells in medium lacking serum growth factor. Exp. cell Res. **68**, 479—481 (1971).

SCHIFFER, L. M.: Kinetics of chronic lymphocytic leukemia. Ser. Haemat. **1**, 3—23 (1968).

SHANKLIN, D. R., SOTELO-AVILA, C.: In situ tumors in fetuses, newborns and young infants. Biol. Neonat. **14**, 286—316 (1969).

SHEEHY, P. F., FRIED, J., WINN, R., CLARKSON, B. D.: Cell cycle changes in ovarian cancer after arabinosylcytosine (Ara-C). Proc. Amer. Assn. Cancer Res. **13**, 71 (1972).

SHIPLEY, W. U.: Immune cytolysis in relation to the growth cycle of Chinese hamster cells. Cancer Res. **31**, 925—929 (1971).

SHIRAKAWA, S., LUCE, J. K., TANNOCK, I. F., FRIE, E., III: Cell proliferation in human melanoma. J. clin. Invest. **49**, 1188—1199 (1970).

SIMONE, J., PINKEL, D.: Rationale and results of combination chemotherapy and cranial irradiation in acute lymphocytic leukemia. In: The 5th international symposium on comparative leukemia research, Padova-Venice, Italy, September 13—17, 1971.

SIMPSON-HERREN, L., LLOYD, H. H.: Kinetic parameters and growth curves for experimental tumor systems. Cancer Chemother. Rep. **54**, 143—174 (1970).

SINCLAIR, W. K.: Cyclic x-ray responses in mammalian cells *in vitro*. Radiat. Res. **33**, 620—643 (1968).

SKIPPER, H. E.: Cellular kinetics associated with "curability" of experimental leukemias. In: Perspectives in leukemia. New York: Grune and Stratton 1968.

SKIPPER, H. E.: The cell cycle and chemotherapy of cancer. In: The cell cycle and cancer. New York: Dekker 1971a.

SKIPPER, H. E.: Kinetic behaviour versus response to chemotherapy. J. Nat. Cancer Inst., in press.

SKIPPER, H. E., SCHABEL, F. M., JR., TRADER, M. W., LASTER, W. R., JR.: Response to therapy of spontaneous, first passage, and long passage lines of AK leukemia. Cancer Chemother. Rep. **53**, 345—366 (1969).

SMITH, H. S., GELB, L. D., MARTIN, M. A.: Detection and quantitation of simian virus 40 genetic material in abortively transformed BALB/3T3 clones. Proc. nat. Acad. Sci. (Wash.) **69**, 152—156 (1972).

SMITH, H. S., SCHER, C. D., TODARO, G. J.: Induction of cell division in medium lacking serum growth factor by SV40. Virology **44**, 359—370 (1971).

SPRATT, J. S., JR., SPRATT, T. L.: Rates of growth of pulmonary metastases and host survival. Ann. Surg. **159**, 161—171 (1964).

STACKPOLE, C. W., AOKI, T., BOYSE, E. A., OLD, L. J., LUMLEY-FRANK, J., DE HARVEN, E.: Cell surface antigens: serial sectioning of single cells as an approach to topographical analysis. Science **172**, 472—474 (1971).

STANLEY, E. R., METCALF, D.: Partial purification and some properties of the factor in normal and leukaemic human urine stimulating mouse bone marrow colony growth *in vitro*. Aust. J. exp. biol. med. Sci. **47**, 467—483 (1969).

STEEL, G. G.: Cell loss as a factor in the growth rate of human tumours. Brit. J. Cancer **3**, 381—387 (1967).

STEEL, G. G.: The cell cycle in tumours: an examination of data gained by the technique of labelled mitoses. Cell Tissue Kinet. **5**, 87—100 (1972).

STEEL, G. G., LAMERTON, L. F.: The growth rate of human tumours. Brit. J. Cancer **20**, 74—86 (1966).

Stoker, M. G. P., Clarke, G. D., Thornton, M.: Density dependent stimulation of thymidine incorporation in BHK21 cells by active material released from the same cells. J. cell. Physiol. **78**, 345—354 (1971).

Strychmans, P. A., Cronkite, E. P., Fache, J., Fliedner, T. M., Ramos, J.: DNA synthesis time of erythropoietic and granulopoietic cells in human beings. Nature (Lond.) **211**, 717—720 (1966).

Strychmans, P. A., Delalieux, G., Manaster, J., Socquet, M.: The potentiality of out-of-cycle acute leukemic cells to synthesize DNA. Blood **36**, 697—703 (1970).

Strychmans, P. A., Manaster, J., Socquet, M.: The effect of daunomycin on proliferation and survival of human leukemic blasts in vivo. In: Recent results in cancer research. Advances in the treatment of acute (blastic) leukemias, vol. 30. Berlin-Heidelberg-New York: Springer 1970.

Suit, H., Urano, M.: Repair of sublethal radiation injury in hypoxic cells of a C3H mouse mammary carcinoma. Radiat. Res. **37**, 423—434 (1969).

Sullivan, P. W., Salmon, S. E.: Kinetics of tumor growth and regression in IgG multiple myeloma. J. clin. Invest., in press.

Takahashi, M., Old, L. J., McIntire, K. R., Boyse, E. A.: Immunoglobulin and other surface antigens of cells of the immune system. J. exp. Med. **134**, 815—832 (1971).

Takahashi, M., Yagi, Y., Moore, G. E., Pressman, D.: Immunoglobulin production in synchronized cultures of human hematopoietic cell lines. I. Variation of cellular immunoglobulin level with generation cycle. J. Immunol. **103**, 834—843 (1969).

Tallal, L., Tan, C., Oettgen, H., Wollner, N., McCarthy, M., Helson, L., Burchenal, J., Karnofsky, D., Murphy, M. L.: *E. coli* L-asparaginase in the treatment of leukemia and solid tumors in 131 children. Cancer **25**, 306—320 (1970).

Tan, C., Tasaka, H., Yu, K. P., Murphy, L., Karnofsky, D. A.: Daunomycin, an antitumor antibiotic in the treatment of neoplastic disease. Clinical evaluation with special reference to childhood leukemia. Cancer **20**, 333—353 (1967).

Tannock, I. F.: The relation between cell proliferation and the vascular system in a transplanted mouse mammary tumour. Brit. J. Cancer **22**, 258—273 (1968).

Tannock, I. F.: A comparison of cell proliferation parameters in solid and ascites Ehrlich tumours. Cancer Res. **29**, 1527—1534 (1969).

Tannock, I. F.: Population kinetics of carcinoma cells, capillary endothelial cells, and fibroblasts in a transplanted mouse mammary tumor. Cancer Res. **30**, 2470—2476 (1970).

Tarbutt, R. G.: Cell population kinetics of the erythroid system in the rat. The response to protracted anaemia and to continuous X-irradiation. Brit. J. Haemat. **16**, 9—24 (1969).

Temin, H. M.: Stimulation by serum of multiplication of stationary chicken cells. J. cell Physiol. **78**, 161—170 (1971).

Terasima, T., Tolmach, L. J.: Changes in x-ray sensitivity of Hela cells during the division cycle. Nature (Lond.) **190**, 1210—1211 (1961).

Terz, J. J., Curutchet, P., Lawrence, W., Jr.: Analysis of the cell kinetics of human solid tumors. Cancer **28**, 1100—1110 (1971).

Thomlinson, R. H.: Change in oxygenation in tumors in relation to irradiation. In: Frontiers of radiation therapy and oncology, vol. 3. Basel: S. Karger 1968.

Thomlinson, R. H., Craddock, E. A.: The gross response of an experimental tumor to single doses of x-rays. Brit. J. Cancer **21**, 108—123 (1967).

Till, J. E., McCulloch, E. A.: Initial stages of cellular differentiation in the blood-forming system of the mouse. In: Developmental aspects of cell cycle. New York: Academic Press 1971.

Tobey, R. A., Petersen, D. F., Anderson, E. C.: Biochemistry of $G_2$ and mitosis. In: The cell cycle and cancer. New York: Dekker 1971.

Todaro, G. J., Lazar, G. K., Green, H.: The initiation of cell division in a contact-inhibited mammalian cell line. J. Cell Comp. Physiol. **66**, 325—333 (1965).

Todo, A.: Proliferation and differentiation of hematopoietic cells in hematology disorders. III. *In vivo* radioautographic study of leukemia including erythro-leukemia. Acta. Haemat. Jap. **31**, 947—966 (1968).

Trentin, J. J.: Influence of hematopoietic organ stroma (hematopoietic inductive microenvironments) on stem cell differentiation. In: Regulation of hematopoiesis. New York: Appleton-Century-Crofts 1970.

Tubiana, M.: Review article. The kinetics of tumor cell proliferation and radiotherapy. Brit. J. Radiol. **44**, 325—347 (1971).

Tubiana, M., Frindel, E., Malaise, E.: The application of radiobiologic knowledge and cellular kinetics to radiation therapy. Am. J. Roentgenol. **102**, 822—829 (1968).

van Peperzeel, H. A.: Patterns of tumour growth after irradiation. Groningen: Drukkerju van Denderen 1970.

VENDITTI, J. M.: Treatment schedule dependency of experimentally active antileukemic (L1210) drugs. Cancer Chemother. Rep. **2**, 35—59 (1971).
VIETTI, T. J., STARLING, K., WILBUR, J. R., LONSDALE, D., LANE, D. M.: Vincristine, prednisone and daunomycin in acute leukemia of childhood. Cancer **27**, 602—607 (1971).
WAGNER, H. P., COTTIER, H., CRONKITE, E. P.: Variability of proliferative patterns in acute lymphoid leukemia of children. Blood **39**, 176—186 (1972).
WHANG-PENG, J., PERRY, S., KNUTSEN, T. A., GART, J. J.: Cell cycle characteristics, maturation, and phagocytosis *in vitro* of blast cells from patients with chronic myelocytic leukemia. Blood **38**, 153—161 (1971).
WHITMORE, W., RAY, B., MOUNT, B.: Experience with retroperitoneal lymph node dissection and adjuvant chemotherapy in germinal testis tumors, in press.
WIEBEL, F., BASERGA, R.: Cell proliferation in newly transplanted Ehrlich ascites tumor cells. Cell Tissue Kinet. **1**, 273—289 (1968).
YATVIN, M. B., CROUSE, D. T., CLIFTON, K. H.: Studies on the mechanism of the stimulatory effect of lethally irradiated cells on tumour inocula. Proc. Soc. exp. Biol. (N. Y.) **133**, 1123—1128 (1970).
YEH, J., FISHER, H. W.: A diffusible factor which sustains contact inhibition of replication. J. cell Biol. **40**, 382—388 (1969).
YOUNG, J. M., FOWLER, J. F.: The effect of x-ray induced synchrony on two-dose cell survival experiments. Cell Tissue Kinet. **2**, 95—111 (1969).
YOUNG, R. C., DE VITA, V. T.: Cell cycle characteristics of human solid tumours *in vivo.* Cell Tissue Kinet. **3**, 285—290 (1970).
ZIEGLER, J. L., MORROW, R. H., JR., FASS, L., KYALWAZI, S. W., CARBONE, P. P.: Treatment of Burkitt's tumor with cyclophosphamide. Cancer **26**, 474—484 (1970).
ZUELZER, W. W., COX, D. E.: Genetic aspects of leukemia. Seminars in Hemat. **6**, 228—249 (1969).

## Chapter 9

# Metabolic Events in the Regulation of Cell Reproduction

ELTON STUBBLEFIELD and SANDRA MURPHREE

With 1 Figure

## Introduction

How the processes of growth and division are regulated in cells is one of the most fascinating problems of modern biology. Within the last two decades the research in this area of biology has undergone rapid change. The cell cycle is no longer regarded naively as a period of steady uniform growth between one cell division and the next. Instead, observations have led us to regard the growth and division of cells as a series of ordered chemical changes with precise temporal control mechanisms.

Before examining hypothetical control mechanisms for cell reproduction in detail we must first review our current concept of the cell replication cycle. The regulation mechanisms which have been studied will then be considered. These fall generally into two classes: (1) those which propose that the progress of cells through the replication process is limited by the availability of essential precursor molecules needed for the synthesis of DNA or some other essential macromolecule, and (2) those which propose that cell replication is a form of differentiation that can be repressed or activated by genetic control mechanisms. Both of these approaches to the problem have been examined to some extent, but the available evidence does not strongly support one viewpoint over the other. As we shall see, however, from a theoretical standpoint the latter explanation probably is more likely correct.

Although studies of cell replication have been made using cells from a wide variety of organisms, we shall limit our review largely to mammalian systems, in view of the medical orientation of this volume.

## The Cell Replication Cycle

The only obvious cytological phenomenon visible during the life cycle of somatic cells is mitosis. Until radioisotopes became available, the remainder of the cell replication cycle was referred to as the "resting phase". The modern era in cell cycle studies began with the publication of the pioneering work of HOWARD and PELC (1951). They exposed root meristems of the plant *Vicia faba* to radioactive phosphorus in the form of $NaH_2{}^{32}PO_4$ for periods up to 48 hours. The uptake of $^{32}P$ into DNA was monitored by autoradiography after ribonuclease treatment of slide preparations. After six hours, about 40% of the interphase nuclei were radioactive, while none of the cells in mitosis had radioactive chromosomes. Their results indicated that incorporation of $^{32}P$ into DNA took place in interphase rather than in mitosis, and further, that incorporation took place during only part of interphase. With longer periods of exposure to the isotope all of the cells became radioactive. In further experiments, HOWARD and PELC showed that in these cells only six hours out of a total interphase period of 30 hours was involved in DNA synthesis; this period was named the $S$ phase (synthesis phase). The period after mitosis but before the synthesis of DNA was called the first gap or $G_1$ phase, and the interphase period after the $S$ phase but before mitosis was called the second gap or $G_2$ phase. The experiment has been repeated many times since then in a variety of eukaryotic cells with similar results. Since about 1955 most studies have used isotopically labeled thymidine instead of $^{32}P$ because of the superior autoradiographic resolution obtainable with tritium and carbon 14.

The method of QUASTLER and SHERMAN (1959) has been applied extensively to determine the lengths of the different cell cycle phases in a variety of cells, both *in vivo* and *in vitro*. By measuring autoradiographically the percentage of radioactive mitotic cells at various times after the administration of a single brief exposure to tritiated thymidine, they were able to define more precisely the duration of the $G_1$, $S$, and $G_2$ phases of the cell cycle. CAMERON and GREULICH (1963) examined the renewing epithelia in adult mice and found that although the generation times varied from one cell type to another, the length of $S + G_2 +$ Mitosis was virtually constant at 10 hours in all of the cells. This was also seen by DEFENDI and MANSON (1963) in several tissue culture lines from humans, hamsters, and mice. Differences in generation times result mostly from variations in the length of the $G_1$ phase.

The length of the cell cycle has also been linked with the process of differentiation in mammalian cells. GAMOW and PRESCOTT (1970) studied the regulation of cell reproduction during embryogenesis and observed that the $G_1$ phase was very short or lacking until blastocyst formation. These authors suggested that regulation of the rate of cell reproduction is gradually imposed on various groups of cells during early differentiation of tissues in the embryonic cell mass. As the cells differentiate, they acquire a tissue specific $G_1$ phase of predetermined length. Cells that have ceased proliferation either for an extended period of time, or permanently (neurons and striated muscle cells) retire from the cell cycle in the $G_1$ phase (PRESCOTT, 1968). Two exceptions have been reported to this general rule in mammalian cells. GELFANT (1962) reported that cutting of the epidermis of the mouse ear specifically stimulated the cells to enter mitosis before the replication of DNA. Thus, the cells were apparently resting in the $G_2$ phase and mitosis could be initiated from the $G_2$ phase. In a later report DECOSSE and GELFANT (1968) observed that some ELD ascites tumor cells in mice are released from a noncycling $G_2$ state into mitosis after the administration of mouse antilymphocytic serum.

Studies of biochemical events in the cell cycle, other than DNA synthesis, were not generally possible until the development of methods for synchronization of cell cultures. As these technological advances were made in the last decade, information began to accumulate about specific molecular events in the replication cycle of cells. Synchronous populations of cells may be obtained in several ways (STUBBLEFIELD, 1968); each method has its advantages and limitations. [WHITMORE (1971) has listed certain general criteria by which various methods may be evaluated.] The oldest approach to gain wide use involved the chemical inhibition of DNA synthesis (RUECKERT and MUELLER, 1960) with drugs like methotrexate or 5-fluorodeoxyuridine, which could specifically block the synthesis of thymidine monophosphate and thereby prevent DNA synthesis. Cells would progress through the cell cycle until they reached the $S$ phase, where they would stop until rescued by the addition of exogenous thymidine to the medium by the investigator. The inhibition was quite reversible for about one generation time and so could be used to synchronize a growing culture at the start of the $S$ phase. A variety of other drugs work on this same principle (Sinclair, 1965; Galavazi et al., 1966; Pfeiffer and Tolmach, 1967; Xeros, 1962; Melnykovych et al., 1967). These drugs may produce unknown side effects (Cohen and Studzinski, 1967). Thus, results using these methods must be interpreted cautiously.

A second basic approach to cell synchronization involves the removal of mitotic cells from a growing culture and the use of these dividing mitotic cells to initiate a synchronous culture (Terasima and Tolmach, 1963). The principle disadvantage of this method is the small yield of mitotic cells in a culture. This has been overcome to some extent by the use of mitotic inhibitors such as colcemid to accumulate cells in mitosis (Stubblefield and Klevecz, 1965). So long as the colcemid treatment is not extended too long, the cells readily complete mitosis when the drug is removed and the ensuing cell cycles appear to be normal (Stubblefield et al., 1967).

The third general approach to cell synchrony has recently developed which will probably be the best in the long run. Based on the parameters of cell volume and density an entire population of cells may be fractionated according to their position in the cell cycle (Miller and Phillips, 1969). Such procedures are so new, however, that they have not yet seen extensive use in the study of metabolic events in the cell cycle.

Synchronization of yet another type has provided pertinent information. *In vivo* cell systems which are not actively dividing can be stimulated to do so in some cases by a variety of procedures. Lymphocytes obtained from the peripheral circulation can be stimulated to enter the mitotic cycle *in vitro* by treatment with phytohemagglutinin (Hungerford et al., 1959). Cells of the salivary gland can likewise be coaxed into the cell cycle by isoproterinol treatment (Barka, 1965). Liver parenchymal cells actively divide after partial hepatectomy (Bucher, 1963). Although such systems are not as precise as cell culture synchrony systems, they do provide information about the entry of cells from a nondividing state into active cell reproduction. The isoleucine deprivation experiments of Ley and Tobey (1970) may in some ways be similar to these systems, although the basis of their method is not yet understood.

## Biochemical Events in Cell Reproduction

The first clear evidence that a cultured cell is preparing to divide is the initiation of DNA replication in the nucleus. Once DNA synthesis is begun, the cell in most cases behaves as if it is following a preset program that will inevitably result in mitosis some ten hours later. We can readily assume that some molecular events led to the initiation of DNA synthesis, but specific delineation of these "triggering reactions" has been most elusive. Mueller et al. (1962) demonstrated that protein synthesis was essential for cells to make the transition from $G_1$ to $S$ phase, and likewise RNA synthesis has been implicated (Mueller and Kajiwara, 1966). But which specific protein and RNA molecules are involved has not been as readily uncovered. Of course, the RNA needed may be the messenger for the specific protein(s) needed. Thus, the search might be narrowed to seek that specific enzyme needed for the initiation of DNA replication. Since we already know that interference with the synthesis of DNA precursor molecules blocks DNA replication, it follows logically that the cell may regulate DNA synthesis in a similar way. This reasoning has led to an extensive study of the enzymes involved with deoxyribonucleotide production, especially the pyrimidine deoxyribonucleotide pathway.

## Enzyme Activities in the Cell Cycle

Thymidine kinase has been examined more extensively in synchronized mammalian cells than any other enzyme. STUBBLEFIELD and MUELLER (1965) synchronized HeLa cells with methotrexate and observed an increase in enzyme activity with the onset of the *S* phase. After division of the cells, enzyme activity per cell decreased by more than half. Similar results were reported by BRENT et al. (1965) in HeLa cells synchronized by selective detachment of mitotic cells. The level of thymidine kinase was low immediately after division ($G_1$ phase), rose during the *S* phase, and decreased rapidly during the subsequent division. The decrease in activity per cell was not completely accounted for by the increase in cell number. In L cells synchronized by mitotic selection, MITTERMAYER et al. (1968) observed a distinct periodicity in the activity of thymidine kinase during the cell cycle. Enzyme activity increased about the time of the onset of DNA synthesis to a maximum (6-fold increase) several hours after the peak of DNA synthesis. A rapid fall in enzyme activity coincided with the second synchronous mitosis. Similar results were also observed by STUBBLEFIELD and MURPHREE (1967) in colcemid synchronized Don-C cells. Thymidine kinase activity was high in cells blocked in metaphase by colcemid, but as soon as the cells divided, the activity dropped to low levels. Enzyme activity began to rise again after the cells entered the *S* phase, and continued to increase until the cells entered the second wave of mitosis.

MITCHISON (1969) has classified the patterns of enzyme synthesis into two groups, depending on whether or not synthesis is continuous during the cell cycle, and each of these groups has been further subdivided into two categories. If the enzyme is stable and synthesized discontinuously, the pattern of activity resembles the synthesis of DNA in higher cells and is called a "step" pattern. A" peak" enzyme is also synthesized discontinously, but is unstable, and the activity decreases because of the inactivation or breakdown of the enzyme. Of the enzymes that are formed continuously, the simplest pattern of activity is an "exponential" curve. The "linear" enzyme is also synthesized at a constant rate but when a characteristic point in the cycle is reached, the rate of synthesis of the enzyme suddenly doubles. By this classification scheme, thymidine kinase is clearly a "peak" enzyme, with synthesis beginning in the *S* phase and the peak occurring in the $G_2$ phase. Thymidine kinase is not an essential enzyme for the cell and numerous mutant cell lines have been isolated lacking this enzyme (KIT et al., 1963; LITTLEFIELD, 1964). On the other hand, more is known about the control of this enzyme than any of the others, and we shall return to this point later.

Among those enzymes actually needed by the cell to make deoxyribonucleotides, several which have been studied are listed in Table 1 along with their corresponding references. All appear to be peak enzymes with fluctuations similar to those seen for thymidine kinase. Of most importance, from the standpoint of a control mechanism, is a determination of the point in the cell cycle where the enzyme activity rises. This is difficult to ascertain in those synchrony systems utilizing inhibitors of the synthesis of DNA, so only those systems using mitotic selection to synchronize the cells can be considered. These cases are plotted in Fig. 1 for those enzymes directly involved in pyrimidine deoxyribonucleotide synthesis in Don-C Chinese hamster fibroblasts. With a single exception, enzyme activity begins to rise after DNA synthesis begins, and they all begin to increase at about the same point in time. The one exception is the enzyme ribonucleotide reductase, which clearly rises at the beginning of the *S* phase. This might point to the enzyme ribonucleotide reductase as a possible control enzyme in the initia-

Table 1. *Enzymes involved in deoxyribonucleotide production which have been studied in synchronized mammalian cells*

| Enzyme | Cell Type | Synchronization Method | Ref. |
|---|---|---|---|
| Ribonucleotide reductase | Mouse L-cells | Methotrexate DNA block | TURNER et al. (1968) |
| Ribonucleotide reductase | Chinese hamster Don-C | Colcemid mitotic selection | MURPHREE et al. (1969) |
| Deoxycytidylate deaminase | Mouse L-cells | Mitotic selection | MITTERMAYER et al. (1968) |
| Deoxycytidylate deaminase | Human HeLa | Mitotic selection | GELBARD et al. (1969) |
| Deoxycytidylate deaminase | Chinese hamster Don-C | Colcemid mitotic selection | MURPHREE (1972) |
| Deoxycytidylate kinase | Chinese hamster Don-C | Colcemid mitotic selection | MURPHREE (1972) |
| Thymidylate synthetase | Chinese hamster Don-C | Colcemid mitotic selection | CONRAD (1971) |
| Thymidylate kinase | Human HeLa | Mitotic selection | BRENT et al. (1965) |

tion of DNA synthesis, but of course it does not prove any cause-effect relationship. It is, of course, extremely interesting that this enzyme appears first, since it is probably the source of all deoxyribonucleotides made by the cell (MOORE and HURLBERT, 1966).

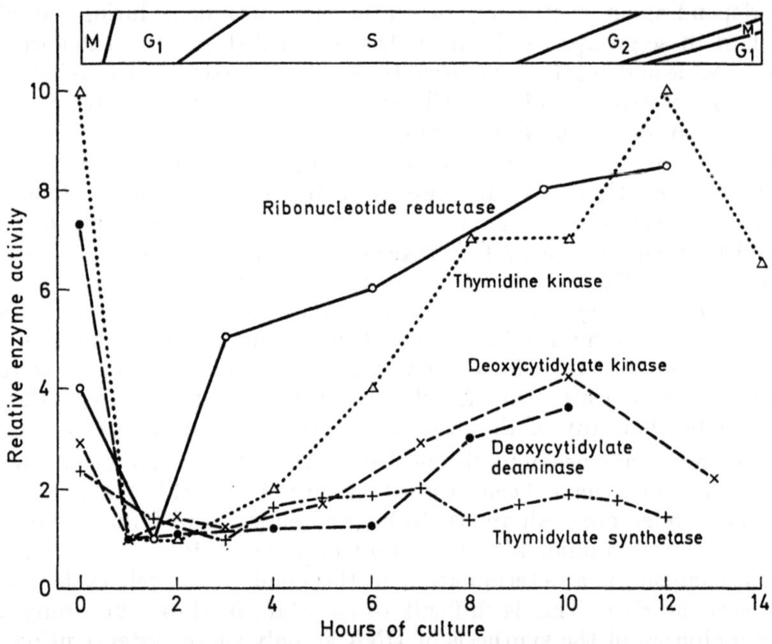


Fig. 1. Fluctuations in the activities of five enzymes involved in pyrimidine deoxyribonucleotide synthesis during the cell reproduction cycle of Don-C fibroblasts. The cultures were synchronized by mitotic selection after a brief colcemid block. The progress of the cells through the phases of the cell cycle and the degradation of synchrony is indicated at the top of the chart. The enzyme activity values were normalized to a minimal value of 1.0, which in all cases occurs in the $G_1$ or early $S$ phase. The activity of ribonucleotide reductase rises at the beginning of the $S$ phase, while the rest of the enzyme activities increase later. The data for this figure were calculated from information published in the references listed in the text and in Table 1

All of these enzymes fall to low levels of activity during the $G_1$ phase of the cell cycle, for reasons that are not well understood. In some cases enzyme levels are maintained in colcemid-blocked metaphase cells, where transcription and translation are minimal (STUBBLEFIELD and MURPHREE, 1967). As soon as the colcemid is removed and the cells are allowed to divide, the enzyme activities drop to a low level. In some cases there is evidence indicating the lack of an inhibitor of enzyme activity in these $G_1$ cells (MURPHREE et al., 1969), so we presume that the enzyme protein is degraded or the enzyme is dissociated into subunit components. In none of these cases has it been technically possible to measure the amount of enzyme protein present. The antibody procedure demonstrated by KLEVECZ (1969) in a study of lactate dehydrogenase should be possible with some of these enzymes, and it is anticipated that this will be done in the near future.

If a necessary enzyme were to act as a limiting control of DNA synthesis, then it should be totally absent during the $G_1$ phase. Although the enzymes in Fig. 1 are low in $G_1$, they are still present in measureable activities. However, it must be remembered that the synchrony systems used in these studies are not perfect, and some contamination of $G_1$ cells with cells from other stages occurs. These contaminating cells may be the source of the measured enzyme in these cases.

Although the enzyme thymidine kinase is not an essential enzyme, it follows the same pattern as most of the enzymes shown in Fig. 1. The product of this enzyme, thymidine monophosphate (TMP), is also the product of the enzyme thymidylate synthetase. The synthesis of TMP by the cell can be regulated *in vitro* by the drugs methotrexate and 5-fluorodeoxyuridine (5-FUdR). Both have a definite influence on the rise of enzymatic activity of thymidine kinase in the cell cycle (STUBBLEFIELD and MURPHREE, 1967). In the presence of methotrexate added at 2 hours ($G_1$), when enzyme activity is lowest, the enzyme increases at a rate about 50% over the control rates. Contrarywise, 5-FUdR, which is phosphorylated as a thymidine analog, has the effect of inhibiting the rise in enzyme activity. This behavior can be explained if one assumes that the synthesis of the enzyme is regulated by the size of the TMP pool in the cell. With methotrexate treatment, the TMP pool disappears as the $S$ phase begins in the cell replication cycle, and thymidine kinase activity rises rapidly as all available TMP is used up. In the case of 5-FUdR treatment, the TMP pool also vanishes, but in this case the nucleotide of 5-FUdR mimics the action of TMP in the repression system for this enzyme, and thymidine kinase activity does not increase rapidly. In such a regulation system one would expect to find a specific repressor for the operator controlling the gene making the messenger RNA for this enzyme, and TMP (the corepressor) should interact with the repressor and regulate its binding to the operator (JACOB and MONOD, 1961). Contrary to all expectation, however, blockage of DNA synthesis by excess thymidine (which blocks the formation of deoxycytidine) does not suppress the synthesis of thymidine kinase, but rather stimulates the synthesis of this enzyme (STUBBLEFIELD and MURPHREE, 1967). Surely there would be an expanded TMP pool in this case, which should repress the operon and prevent enzyme synthesis. The stimulatory effect is abolished by the addition of a small amount of deoxycytidine, however, so the repression mechanism can be explained if both TMP and deoxycytidine monophosphate are needed simultaneously as corepressors to activate the repressor. Similar studies are needed for such enzymes as thymidylate synthetase and ribonucleotide reductase before we draw any solid conclusions about how the repression mechanism may operate.

It does seem reasonable to suppose that the synthesis of the enzymes in Fig. 1, which begin to increase after $S$ phase begins, are all regulated by the sizes of the deoxyribonucleotide pools; as these pools fall in early $S$ phase, enzyme synthesis is turned on to continue for the rest of the cell cycle. On the other hand, ribonucleotide reductase activity may be regulated in some other way, since it is present in elevated levels as DNA synthesis begins.

The enzyme DNA polymerase has been examined in several cell lines (GOLD and HELLEINER, 1964; TURNER, 1968; FRIEDMAN, 1970). Although there is considerable argument about the distribution of this enzyme in the nuclear and cytoplasmic compartments of the cell, the enzyme seems to be present in ample quantities at all phases of the cell cycle. Our own unpublished studies in Chinese hamster cells also support this conclusion.

## RNA in the Cell Cycle

An entirely different approach to the regulation mechanism in the cell cycle has been a study of the heterogeneous nuclear RNA found in cells. Nine different species of low molecular weight nuclear RNA (LMN-RNA) can be demonstrated in human lymphocytes by polyacrylamide gel electrophoresis (HOWARD and STUBBLEFIELD, 1972). These are distinctly different from ribosomal, transfer, or messenger RNA. Upon treatment of these cells *in vitro* with phytohemagglutinin, most of them transform into lymphoblasts and reenter the cell replication cycle. In doing so, a new LMN-RNA species is synthesized and the synthesis of all of the remaining species is greatly accelerated (HOWARD and STUBBLEFIELD, 1972). No function has yet been ascribed to any of these LMN-RNA's, but the appearance of a new one during lymphocyte stimulation suggests that these molecules should be examined as potentially part of a control mechanism for the initiation of cell replication.

The methylation of transfer RNA (tRNA) has also been examined in synchronized cell cultures (TIDWELL and STUBBLEFIELD, 1971) and in the regenerating rat liver system (TIDWELL, 1970). In the latter system it was shown that a rapid increase in the rate of tRNA methylation immediately preceded an increase in the rate of tRNA synthesis, which came a few hours before the initiation of DNA synthesis in these cells. Thus, the existing pool of tRNA was first heavily methylated, and then the pool was diluted with newly synthesized unmethylated tRNA. There is some evidence suggesting that methylation of a tRNA molecule may be important to its functioning in translation (GEFTER and RUSSELL, 1969). Thus, one can imagine a control mechanism where certain proteins essential to the initiation of DNA synthesis can only be made when certain specific (initiator) tRNA molecules bearing a unique codon are methylated.

We examined this same potential mechanism in synchronized Chinese hamster fibroblasts where better synchrony was available (TIDWELL and STUBBLEFIELD, 1971). Here tRNA synthesis was almost constant throughout the cell cycle. The level of tRNA methylation which existed in $G_1$ increased about 50% during early $S$ phase and then dropped to a low level in $G_2$. When we hydrolyzed the tRNA to see which bases were methylated, we found most of the methyl had been added to guanine and adenine, and none to uridine. Cytidine methylation was moderate in the $G_1$ and $S$ phases, but it was drastically reduced in the $G_2$ phase. Of course, the significance of these fluctuations in tRNA methylase is unknown, but they serve to illustrate the complexity of the metabolic system in which we are searching for the control mechanism which regulates reproduction of the cell.

## DNA-Binding Proteins

SALAS and GREEN (1971) and FOX and PARDEE (1971) have recently reported preliminary studies on an interesting fraction of cellular proteins which have an affinity for DNA and can therefore be isolated by absorption on DNA-cellulose columns. By comparing the kinds of proteins which were made by cells in different phases of the cell cycle or in active growth and nongrowing conditions, they were able to show differences in the spectrum of proteins synthesized in cells in the different states. How these proteins function in growth regulation is not yet known, but it is possible that they may represent general or specific repressors of genetic activities that characterize the different phases of the cell cycle. BASERGA and STEIN (1971), reach essentially this same conclusion by a different logic in considering the probable role of nuclear acidic proteins in cell proliferation.

In studies of DNA replication in isolated cell nuclei, FRIEDMAN and MUELLER (1968) demonstrated the need for a cytoplasmic factor, possibly a protein, for optimal synthesis of DNA. A similar factor was also found by THOMPSON and McCARTHY (1968), and in both cases it would appear that DNA synthesis is under positive control, i.e. the (protein) factor is needed for DNA synthesis to continue. That this idea is basically correct has been elegantly shown by RAO and JOHNSON (1970). By fusing cells together that were in different stages of the cell cycle they were able to analyze the effects of $S$ phase cells on $G_1$ and $G_2$ cells. Their study clearly shows that $S$ phase cells induce DNA synthesis in $G_1$ cells, but not $G_2$ cells. We may then conclude that $G_1$ cells do not contain inhibitors of DNA synthesis, but rather that $S$ phase cells contain factors that promote DNA synthesis in $G_1$ nuclei. The $G_2$ and $S$ phase nuclei and cytoplasms had no observable effect on one another, nor did $G_2$ cells fused with $G_1$ cells have any effect on the entry of the $G_1$ nucleus into $S$ phase. The $G_2$ cell therefore contains no inhibitors or promoters of DNA synthesis. That the $S$ phase cell does not cause reinitiation of DNA synthesis in the $G_2$ nucleus is interesting, since the phenomenon of endoreduplication (LEVAN and HAUSCHKA, 1953) in cultured cells indicates that such a mistake is occasionally made.

## Conclusions

Although it does not seem likely that replication is controlled by enzymatic fluctuations which regulate precursor pools needed for DNA synthesis, it is still important for us to learn how these enzymes are regulated. It may then prove possible to greatly increase the effectiveness of antimetabolite drugs used in chemotherapy by shutting off the synthesis of the normal endogenous precursors with which the drug is in competition.

The possibility that ribonucleotide reductase is involved in regulating DNA synthesis clearly needs further study. The resolution of the experiments conducted so far does not permit us to determine whether the enzyme appears in elevated levels before or simultaneous with the beginning of the $S$ phase. Probably a more direct approach would be to carefully measure the sizes of the deoxyribonucleotide pools in highly synchronized cell cultures. The studies of NORDENSKJÖLD et al. (1970) represent an initial approach to this problem; however, the synchrony system which they employed (cultivation in low serum medium) was not adequate to determine the absence of deoxyribonucleotide pools in the $G_1$ phase, since there were always $S$ phase cells present in their mouse embryo cultures. As was pointed out by WATSON (1971) the pools are obviously adequate in the $G_2$ phase of the cell cycle, so there must exist in the cell some other mechanism to prevent DNA synthesis in the $G_2$ phase. It is still a possibility that the availability of precursor molecules for DNA replication is involved in the regulation of the initiation of the $S$ phase.

How a cytoplasmic factor might promote DNA replication is the subject of intense interest at the moment. It appears to be a protein, but whether its role is enzymatic (e.g. a nuclease or ligase) or a genetic repressor is not known. An excellent discussion of the latter possibility has been presented by Mueller (1971). It is possible that in eukaryotic cells replication is regulated by genetic control mechanisms quite analogous to those discovered in prokaryotic cells (Watson, 1971). At this time it seems more likely, however, that eukaryotic cells are sufficiently more complex to require additional control mechanisms not found in prokaryotes. We do not yet know how cellular differentiation is regulated, but once we do, we may find that replication is simply a form of differentiation controlled by a similar mechanism.

## References


Barka, T.: Stimulation of DNA synthesis by isoproterenol in the salivary gland. Exp. cell Res. **39**, 355—364 (1965).

Baserga, R., Stein, G.: Nuclear acidic proteins and cell proliferation. Fed. Proc. **30**, 1752—1759 (1971).

Brent, T. P., Butler, J. A. V., Crathorn, A. A.: Variations in phosphokinase activities during the cell cycle in synchronous populations of HeLa cells. Nature (Lond.) **207**, 176—177 (1965).

Bucher, N. L. R.: Regeneration of mammalian liver. Int. Rev. Cytol. **15**, 245—300 (1963).

Cameron, I. L., Greulich, R. C.: Evidence for an essentially constant duration of DNA synthesis in renewing epithelia of the adult mouse. J. cell Biol. **18**, 31—40 (1963).

Cohen, L. S., Studzinski, G. P.: Correlation between cell enlargement and nucleic acid and protein content of HeLa cells in unbalanced growth produced by inhibitors of DNA synthesis. J. cell. Physiol. **69**, 331—340 (1967).

Conrad, A. H.: Thymidylate synthetase activity in cultured mammalian cells. J. biol. Chem. **246**, 1318—1323 (1971).

deCosse, J. J., Gelfant, S.: Noncycling tumor cells: Mitogenic response to antilymphocytic serum. Science **162**, 698—699 (1968).

Defendi, V., Manson, L. A.: Analysis of the life-cycle in mammalian cells. Nature (Lond.) **198**, 359—361 (1963).

Friedman, D. L.: DNA polymerase from HeLa cell nuclei: Levels of activity during a synchronized cell cycle. Biochem. biophys. Res. Commun. **39**, 100—109 (1970).

Friedman, D. L., Mueller, G. C.: A nuclear system for DNA replication from synchronized HeLa cells. Biochim. biophys. Acta (Amst.) **161**, 455—468 (1968).

Fox, T. O., Pardee, A. B.: Proteins made in the mammalian cell cycle. J. biol. Chem. **246**, 6159—6165 (1971).

Galavazi, G., Schenk, H., Bootsma, D.: Synchronization of mammalian cells *in vitro* by inhibition of the DNA synthesis. I. Optimal conditions. Exp. cell Res. **41**, 428—437 (1966).

Gamow, E. I., Prescott, D. M.: The cell life cycle during early embryogenesis of the mouse. Exp. cell Res. **59**, 117—125 (1970).

Gefter, M. L., Russell, R. L.: Role of modifications in tyrosine transfer RNA: A modified base affecting ribosome binding. J. molec. Biol. **39**, 145—157 (1969).

Gelbard, A. S., Kim, J., Perez, A.: Fluctuations in deoxycytidine monophosphate deaminase activity during the cell cycle in synchronous populations of HeLa cells. Biochim. biophys. Acta (Amst.) **182**, 564—566 (1969).

Gelfant, S.: Initiation of mitosis in relation to the cell division cycle. Exp. cell Res. **26**, 395—403 (1962).

Gold, M., Helleiner, C. W.: Deoxyribonucleic acid polymerase in L-cells. I. Properties of the enzyme and its activity in synchronized cell cultures. Biochim. biophys. Acta (Amst.) **80**, 193—203 (1964).

Hungerford, D. A., Donnelly, A. J., Nowell, P. C., Beck, S.: The chromosome constitution of a human phenotypic intersex. Amer. J. Human Genet. **11**, 215—236 (1959).

Howard, A., Pelc, S. R.: Nuclear incorporation of $P^{32}$ as demonstrated by autoradiographs. Exp. cell Res. **2**, 178—187 (1951).

Howard, E. F., Stubblefield, E.: Low molecular weight nuclear RNA in phytohemagglutinin-treated and untreated human lymphocytes. Exp. cell Res. **70**, 460—462 (1972).

Jacob, F., Monod, J.: Genetic regulatory mechanisms in the synthesis of proteins. J. molec. Biol. **3**, 318—356 (1961).

Kit, S., Dubbs, D. R., Pickarski, L. J., Hsu, T. C.: Deletion of thymidine kinase activity from L-cells resistant to bromodeoxyuridine. Exp. cell Res. **31**, 297—312 (1963).

Klevecz, R. R.: Temporal order in mammalian cells. I. The periodic synthesis of lactate dehydrogenase in the cell cycle. J. cell Biol. **43**, 207—219 (1969).

LEVAN, A., HAUSCHKA, T. S.: Endomitotic reduplication mechanisms in ascites tumors of the mouse. J. nat. Cancer Inst. **14**, 1—43 (1953).
LEY, K. D., TOBEY, R. A.: Regulation of initiation of DNA synthesis in Chinese hamster cells. II. Induction of DNA synthesis and cell division by isoleucine and glutamine in $G_1$-arrested cells in suspension culture. J. cell Biol. **47**, 453—459 (1970).
LITTLEFIELD, J. W.: Selection of hybrids from matings of fibroblasts in vitro and their presumed recombinants. Science **145**, 709—710 (1964).
MELNYKOVYCH, G., BISHOP, C. F., SWAYZE, M. A. B.: Fluctuation of alkaline phosphatase activity in synchronized heteroploid cell cultures: Effects of prednisolone. J. cell. Physiol. **70**, 231—236 (1967).
MILLER, R. G., PHILLIPS, R. A.: Separation of cells by velocity sedimentation. J. cell. Physiol. **73**, 191—202 (1969).
MITCHISON, J. M.: Enzyme synthesis in synchronous cultures. Science **165**, 657—663 (1969).
MITTERMAYER, C., BOSSELMANN, R., BREMERSHOV, V.: Initiation of DNA synthesis in a system of synchronized L-cells: Rhythmicity of thymidine kinase activity. Euro. J. Biochem. **4**, 487—489 (1968).
MOORE, E. C., HURLBERT, R. B.: Regulation of mammalian deoxyribonucleotide biosynthesis by nucleotides as activators and inhibitors. J. biol. Chem. **241**, 4802—4809 (1966).
MUELLER, G. C.: Biochemical perspectives of the $G_1$ and $S$ intervals in the replication cycle of animal cells: A study in the control of cell growth. In: The cell cycle and cancer **1**, 269—307. New York: Marcel Dekker 1971.
MUELLER, G. C., KAJIWARA, K.: Actinomycin D and *p*-fluorophenylalanine, inhibitors of nuclear replication in HeLa cells. Biochim. biophys. Acta (Amst.) **119**, 557—565 (1966).
MUELLER, G. C., KAJIWARA, K., STUBBLEFIELD, E., RUECKERT, R. R.: Molecular events in the reproduction of animal cells. I. The effect of puromycin on the duplication of DNA. Cancer Res. **22**, 1084—1090 (1962).
MURPHREE, S. A.: Temporal variation of enzyme activity and adenosine nucleotide pools during the cell cycle of mammalian cells in culture. Ph. D. Thesis. The University of Texas Graduate School of Biomedical Sciences, Houston, Texas, U.S.A. (1972).
MURPHREE, S. A., STUBBLEFIELD, E., MOORE, E. C.: Synchronized mammalian cell cultures. III. Variation of ribonucleotide reductase activity during the replication cycle of Chinese hamster fibroblasts. Exp. cell Res. **58**, 118—124 (1969).
NORDENSKJÖLD, B. A., SKOOG, L., BROWN, N. C., REICHARD, P.: Deoxyribonucleotide pools and deoxyribonucleic acid synthesis in cultured mouse embryo cells. J. biol. Chem. **245**, 5360—5368 (1970).
PFEIFFER, S. E., TOLMACH, L. J.: Inhibition of DNA synthesis in HeLa cells by hydroxyurea. Cancer Res. **27**, 124—129 (1967).
PRESCOTT, D. M.: Regulation of cell reproduction. Cancer Res. **28**, 1815—1820 (1968).
QUASTLER, H., SHERMAN, F. G.: Cell population kinetics in the intestinal epithelium of the mouse. Exp. cell Res. **17**, 420—438 (1959).
RAO, P. N., JOHNSON, R. T.: Mammalian cell fusion: Studies on the regulation of DNA synthesis and mitosis. Nature (Lond.) **225**, 159—164 (1970).
RUECKERT, R. R., MUELLER, C. G.: Studies on unbalanced growth in tissue culture. I. Induction and consequences of thymidine deficiency. Cancer Res. **20**, 1584—1591 (1960).
SALAS, J., GREEN, H.: Proteins binding to DNA and their relation to growth in cultured mammalian cells. Nature (Lond.) **229**, 165—169 (1971).
SINCLAIR, W. K.: Hydroxyurea: Differential lethal effects on cultured mammalian cells during the cell cycle. Science **150**, 1729—1731 (1965).
STUBBLEFIELD, E.: Synchronization methods for mammalian cell cultures. In: Methods in cell physiology **3**, 25—43. New York: Academic Press 1968.
STUBBLEFIELD, E., KLEVECZ, R.: Synchronization of Chinese hamster cells by reversal of colcemid inhibition. Exp. cell Res. **40**, 660—664 (1965).
STUBBLEFIELD, E., KLEVECZ, R., DEAVEN, L.: Synchronized mammalian cell cultures. I. Cell replication cycle and macromolecular synthesis following brief colcemid arrest of mitosis. J. cell. Physiol. **69**, 345—354 (1967).
STUBBLEFIELD, E., MUELLER, G. C.: Thymidine kinase activity in synchronized HeLa cell cultures. Biochem. biophys. Res. Commun. **20**, 535—538 (1965).
STUBBLEFIELD, E., MURPHREE, S. A.: Synchronized mammalian cell cultures. II. Thymidine kinase activity in colcemid synchronized fibroblasts. Exp. cell Res. **48**, 652—656 (1967).
TERASIMA, T., TOLMACH, L. J.: Growth and nucleic acid synthesis in synchronously dividing populations of HeLa cells. Exp. cell Res. **30**, 344—362 (1963).
THOMPSON, L. R., MCCARTHY, B. J.: Stimulation of nuclear DNA and RNA synthesis by cytoplasmic extracts *in vitro*. Biochem. biophys. Res. Commun. **30**, 166—172 (1968).
TIDWELL, T.: The methylation of transfer ribonucleic acid during regeneration of the liver. J. cell Biol. **46**, 370—378 (1970).

TIDWELL, T., STUBBLEFIELD, E.: Methylation and synthesis of transfer ribonucleic acid in synchronized Chinese hamster fibroblasts. Exp. cell Res. **64**, 350—354 (1971).
TURNER, M. K., ABRAMS, R., LIEBERMAN, I.: Levels of ribonucleotide reductase activity during the division cycle of the L cell. J. biol. Chem. **243**, 3725—3728 (1968).
WATSON, J. D.: The regulation of DNA synthesis in eukaryotes. Advanc. cell Biol. **2**, 1—46 (1971).
WHITMORE, G. F.: Natural and induced synchronous cultures. In Vitro **6**, 276—285 (1971).
XEROS, N.: Deoxyriboside control and synchronization of mitosis. Nature (Lond.) **194**, 682—683 (1962).

Chapter 10

# Site of Action of Cytotoxic Agents in the Cell Life Cycle

H. MADOC-JONES and F. MAURO

With 3 Figures

## Introduction

In the past decade a considerable interest in the mechanisms of action of cytotoxic agents at the cellular level has been generated. The work of BRUCE (1966) and his collaborators (BRUCE et al., 1966, 1969) comparing rapidly dividing transplantable murine lymphoma cells with essentially "resting" normal bone marrow cells, both of which form colonies in the spleen, showed that some lethal agents may be regarded as cell cycle specific, or even phase specific within the cycle, while others act on resting noncycling cells to the same extent as on cycling cells. This *in vivo* work was augmented by the demonstration *in vitro* that cells in the "stationary phase" of the growth cycle may be relatively inert to some of the agents which act preferentially on proliferating exponential phase cultured cells (BHUYAN et al., 1962; MADOC-JONES and BRUCE, 1967; HAHN, 1969; HRYNIUK et al., 1969; BORSA and WHITMORE, 1969). The obvious application of this type of work to the problem of designing treatment schedules for malignant disease (*vide* SCHABEL et al., 1965; BASERGA, 1965; SKIPPER et al., 1967; SCHABEL, 1968; for example) spurred much research towards defining which agents exert their lethal effect at which phase of the cell generation cycle, that is in $G_1$, $S$, $G_2$, or $M$ as defined in previous chapters of this volume.

The determination of variations in the sensitivity to cytotoxic agents of cells as they pass through the cell division cycle became possible after the development of cell synchronization techniques. These have been reviewed recently by STUBBLEFIELD (1968) and SINCLAIR (1969). Chief among the various methods utilized in the investigations summarized below are: the mitotic cell selection technique of TERASIMA and TOLMACH (1963), the reversible blocking at the entry into the $S$ phase by 5-fluorodeoxyuridine or methotrexate (RUECKERT and MUELLER, 1960), the $S$ phase blocking and killing effect of hydroxyurea (SINCLAIR, 1965) and the excess thymidine block (XEROS, 1962). For estimation of the lethal effect of an agent, cells plated into petri dishes are synchronized and then treated at various times thereafter with a given agent (for a given length of time for chemical agents of long half-life). The dishes are then incubated for a week or so under appropriate conditions to allow the growth of surviving cells into macroscopic colonies after the method of PUCK et al. (1956). The surviving fraction of cells is then plotted against the time in the cell cycle at which the cells were exposed to the agent (marked out by labeling replicate cell cultures in the $S$ phase with radioactively-tagged thymidine and by observing rounded up cells in mitosis). Such a plot has been called an age-response of a cell line to a given lethal agent (ELKIND and WHITMORE, 1967). Because no synchronization technique affords more than a partial synchrony, at a given time, the cells being treated are spread throughout a number of phases of the cycle, although one or more phase may predominate. This is an important consideration in the interpretation of such an age-response. Thus, it is impossible from such experiments alone, to distinguish between a truly phase specific age-response where only one phase is susceptible, as compared with a differential age-response where many or all phases are susceptible but to a different degree. In fact, only certain inhibitors of DNA synthesis (methotrexate and 5-fluorodeoxyuridine excepted) appear to be truly phase specific. The term "age-response" might equally well be used to refer to the reversible blocking or the delay (partial blocking at a given moment in time) of cells at a given point in the cycle.

Both types of age-response (lethal and blocking) have now been determined for a large number of agents as collated in Table 1. The experiments summarized in Table 1 have been performed on many different cultured cell lines. Because there appears to be a remarkable general level of agreement between results from different cell lines (and different workers), for simplicity's sake, each individual cell line is not cited; they may be found in the references listed in Table 1, and many of them, at a glance, in an earlier edition of Table 1 in MAURO and MADOC-JONES (1970). Chief among them are HeLa S3, Chinese hamster V79, Chinese hamster CHO, and mouse L cells. It should be pointed out that the activity of a drug and possibly the cellular response may be affected by the particular medium and/or serum supplement in which tests are performed (MADOC-JONES and MAURO, 1968, for example). There are too many agents recorded to describe each in detail but, fortunately, and most interestingly, it turns out that the agents known to have a common biochemical mode of action (mitotic arrest agents, inhibitors of DNA synthesis, for example) elicit distinctive patterns of lethal age-response and sometimes of blocking age-response (Table 1). Therefore, the age-response to various agents comprising such a group will be described together. This interesting finding is consistent with but does not prove the hypothesis that the known biochemical action is causally related to the lethal (or blocking) action for the various classes of drug. Insofar as possible, the many references in Table 1 will not be repeated in the text. Only agents whose lethal age-responses have been described are cited in Table 1. Thus, not included are the effect of high concentrations of thymidine (XEROS, 1962), that of *p*-fluorophenylalanine (KISHIMOTO and LIBERMAN, 1964; MUELLER and KAJIWARA, 1966) and that of $\gamma$-chlordane (BRUBAKER et al., 1970), a pesticide.

The grouping of agents according to their known biochemical actions is in no way meant to imply that a given drug has only one biochemical mode of action or that the biochemical mode of action under which the drug is listed is necessarily related to its lethal or blocking action on cells. In fact, a single agent may have various biochemical, chromosomal, or mitotic effects which may not be related to their effect on cell viability. Furthermore, such effects may take place at different dose levels, further complicating the rational for a possible therapeutic application. Such problems will be illustrated below by considering two mitotic poisons (vinblastine and vincristine) and one inhibitor of DNA synthesis (methotrexate) in greater detail. Finally, the relevance of these cellular age-responses to the planning of treatment schedules will be discussed briefly.

## Age-Responses to Various Agents

*Mitotic Arrest Agents.* While, by definition, mitotic agents arrest cells in mitosis at the metaphase stage thereby leading to cell lysis as recorded by time-lapse cinematography (L. J. TOLMACH and associates, unpublished results) it came as somewhat of a surprise to find that when cells are subjected to high concentrations of these agents for 3-hour periods only, they are most sensitive to the lethal action when exposed to the agents in the $S$ phase of the cycle (Table 1). Indeed, with the exception of vinblastine, the mitotic arrest agents have little irreversible effect on mitotic cells, even at high concentration, provided that the exposure to the agent is limited to a short period. It has been suggested that this sensitivity is due to the availability of spindle binding sites as the spindle protein is laid down in the $S$ phase prior to mitosis (MADOC-JONES and MAURO, 1968).

The complexity of action of the Vinca alkaloids will be elaborated on below.

*Chemical Mutagens.* Two such agents, hydroxylamine and nitrous acid, have their most marked lethal effect also on cells in the $S$ phase.

*Alkylating Agents.* Both the mono- and bi-functional alkylating agents so far investigated (Table 1) are lethally most effective on cells at mitosis and in most cases at the $G_1/S$ transition[1] as well. Not enough is known of their blocking actions to establish whether there is a definite pattern or not.

*Inhibitors of DNA Synthesis.* Those investigated (Table 1) will kill cells exposed in the $S$ phase. Cytosine arabinoside, 5-azacytidine, hydroxyurea, and pederine appear to be the one group of truly phase specific agents and kill only cells in the $S$ phase as indicated by the inactivation kinetics of the dose-survival curves and other evidence (see Ref. in Table 1). 5-Fluorodeoxyuridine and streptozotocin appear to be exceptions in that they have been reported to kill cells in all phases. The complex case of methotrexate will be considered more fully below. All members of this group so far investigated have a clear blocking action at the $G_1/S$ transition and some at the $S/G_2$ transition as well (Table 1).

*Inhibitors of RNA Synthesis.* Both actinomycin D and nogalamycin preferentially kill cells exposed at mitosis and again at the $G_1/S$ transition. Chromomycin succinate shows a preferential lethal action early in the $S$ phase (which may not be very different from a $G_1/S$ transition effect) but not at mitosis.

*Inhibitors of Protein Synthesis.* These agents elicit lethal age-responses characterized by a preferential action at the $G_1/S$ transition. It is interesting to note that this $G_1/S$ transition point is especially vulnerable to a number of different types of agent including inhibitors of protein or RNA synthesis, alkylating agents, and x-irradiation.

*Miscellaneous Inhibitors.* The remaining group of agents in Table 1 are included for the sake of completeness and will not be discussed, since no further patterns of age-response are yet apparent. The age-responses of x-irradiation and ultraviolet light are, of course, well known.

*Mechanism of Action of Vinblastine and Vincristine.* The mechanism of action of these two agents will be discussed to illustrate how two drugs, whose molecular structure differs only by two H atoms, may differ so markedly in the details of their action, a fascinating problem of molecular pharmacology. The lethal age-response of HeLa to these two *Vinca* alkaloids is shown in Fig. 1. In these experiments, cells were exposed for three hours to the drug, at a concentration of $3 \times 10^{-7}$ M for vinblastine and $10^{-7}$ M for vincristine. These concentrations are about ten times those required to produce arrest in metaphase by continuous exposure to the drug. The lethal effect of vinblastine is most evident at two distinct

1 The term $G_1/S$ transition refers to populations of cells distributed in the late part of $G_1$ and the early part of $S$ phase, and does not necessarily imply the definition of specific border regions (similarly, "$S/G_2$ transition").

Table 1. *Summary of in vitro age-responses to various agents*

| Agent | Phase of block in progression | Ref. | Phase of greatest lethal sensitivity | Ref. |
|---|---|---|---|---|
| Mitotic poisons: | | | | |
| Colchicine | $M$ | LUDFORD (1936) | $S$ | MAURO and MADOC-JONES (1970) |
| Demecolcin (Colcemid) | $M$ | GELFANT (1963) | $S$ | MAURO and MADOC-JONES (1970) |
| Griseofulvin (Grifulvin) | $M$ | DUSTIN (1963) | $S$ | MAURO and MADOC-JONES (1970) |
| Vinblastine sulfate (Velban) | $M$ | PALMER et al. (1960)<br>CUTTS (1961)<br>BRUCHOVSKY et al. (1965)<br>MALAWISTA et al. (1968) | $S$, late-$G_1$, $M$ | MADOC-JONES and MAURO (1968) |
| Vincristine sulfate (Oncovin) | $M$ | CARDINALI and MEHROTA (1963) | $S$ | MADOC-JONES and MAURO (1968) |
| Chemical mutagens: | | | | |
| Hydroxylamine-HCl | ? | | $S$ | MAURO and MADOC-JONES (1970) |
| Potassium nitrate (nitrous acid) | ? | | $S$ | MAURO and MADOC-JONES (1970) |
| Monofunctional alkylating agents: | | | | |
| Ethylmethanesulfonate | ? | | $M$, $G_1$ | HAHN, G.M. (pers. comm.) |
| Methylmethanesulfonate | Delay | FOX and FOX (1967) | $M$, $G_1$ | FOX and FOX (1967)<br>NIAS et al. (1970)<br>HAHN, G.M. (pers. comm.) |
| Bifunctional alkylating agents: | | | | |
| 1,3-bis(2-chloroethyl)-1-nitrosourea (BCNU) | Delay | BARRANCO and HUMPHREY (1971) | $G_1/S$ | BARRANCO and HUMPHREY (1971)<br>BHUYAN et al. (1972) |
| Chlorambucil | ? | | $M$, $G_1$ | BHUYAN et al. (1972) |
| 1-(2-chloroethyl)-3-cyclohexyl-1-nitrosourea (CCNU) | ? | | $M$, $G_1$ | BHUYAN et al. (1972) |
| Dimethylmyleran | ? | | $M$ | SCHINDLER, R. (pers. comm.) |
| Mechlorethamine-HCl (nitrogen mustard) | $G_2$ | CASPERSSON et al. (1963) | $M$, $G_1/S$ | SAKAMOTO and ELKIND (1969)<br>MAURO and MADOC-JONES (1970) |
| Methylenedimethanesulfonate | ? | | $G_1/S$ | NIAS, A. H. W. (pers. comm.) |
| Mitomycin C | $S/G_2$ and/or delay | NOWELL (1964)<br>DOI et al. (1967) | $M$, $G_1$ and/or $G_2$ | NOWELL (1964)<br>DJORDJEVIC and KIM (1968)<br>OHARA, H. and TERASIMA, T. (pers. comm.) |
| Phenylalanine mustard | ? | | $M$, $G_1$ | BHUYAN et al. (1972) |

| | | | | |
|---|---|---|---|---|
| Sulfur mustard (mustard gas) | Delay | MAURO et al. (1968) | $M$ and/or $G_1/S$ | WALKER and HELLEINER (1963)<br>MAURO and ELKIND (1968)<br>ROBERTS et al. (1968)<br>MAURO and MADOC-JONES (1970) |
| Tris(1-aziridinyl)phosphine sulfide (Thio-TEPA) | ? | | $M$, $G_1$ | BHUYAN et al. (1972) |
| Uracil mustard | ? | | $M$, $G_1/S$ | MAURO and MADOC-JONES (1970) |
| Inhibitors of DNA synthesis: | | | | |
| Adriamycin | ? | | $S$ | KIM and KIM (1972) |
| Arabinosylcytosine (Cytosar) | $G_1/S$, $S/G_2$ | BREMERSKOV et al. (1970)<br>KARON and SHIRAKAWA (1970) | $S$ | KARON and FISHER (1968)<br>YOUNG and FISHER (1968)<br>BREMERSKOV et al. (1970)<br>BHUYAN et al. (1972) |
| 5-Azacytidine | $S/G_2$ | LI et al. (1970) | $S$ | LI et al. (1970)<br>BHUYAN et al. (1972) |
| Daunomycin | ? | | $S$ | KIM et al. (1968) |
| 5-Fluorodeoxyuridine | $G_1/S$ | RUECKERT and MUELLER (1960)<br>LITTLEFIELD (1962) | $S$, $G_1$, $G_2$ | LOZZIO (1969)<br>BHUYAN et al. (1972) |
| 5-Fluorouracil | ? | | All phases | BHUYAN et al. (1972) |
| 5-Hydroxy-2-formylpyridine thiosemicarbazone | ? | | $S$ | BHUYAN et al. (1972) |
| Hydroxyurea | $G_1/S$ | SINCLAIR (1965, 1967)<br>KIM et al. (1967)<br>PFEIFFER and TOLMACH (1967)<br>BACCHETTI and WHITMORE (1969) | $S$ | SINCLAIR (1965, 1967)<br>KIM et al. (1967)<br>PFEIFFER and TOLMACH (1967)<br>BACCHETTI and WHITMORE (1969)<br>MAURO and MADOC-JONES (1970) |
| Methotrexate (amethopterin) | $G_1/S$ | RUECKERT and MUELLER (1960) | $S$, early-$G_1$, $G_1/S$ | MAURO (this paper) |
| Neocarzinostatin | | | $M$, $G_1$, $G_2$ | BHUYAN et al. (1972) |
| Pederine | ? | | $S$ | MAURO and MADOC-JONES (1970) |
| Sodium campothecin | ? | | $S$ | BHUYAN et al. (1972) |
| Streptozotocin | ? | | All phases | BHUYAN et al. (1972) |
| Tubercidin | ? | | $G_1/S$ | BHUYAN et al. (1972) |
| Inhibitors of RNA synthesis: | | | | |
| Actinomycin D (Lyovac, Cosmegen) | $G_1/S$, $S/G_2$, $G_2$ | KISHIMOTO and LIBERMAN (1964)<br>BASERGA et al. (1965)<br>TOBEY et al. (1966)<br>EPIFANOVA et al. (1969) | x-ray-like | BACCHETTI and WHITMORE (1967, 1969)<br>ELKIND et al. (1969)<br>ELKIND and KANO (1970)<br>MAURO and MADOC-JONES (1970)<br>BHUYAN et al. (1972) |

Table 1 (continued)

| Agent | Phase of block in progression | Ref. | Phase of greatest lethal sensitivity | Ref. |
|---|---|---|---|---|
| Chromomycin succinate | ? | | Early-$S$ | FUJIWARA (1967) |
| Nogalamycin | ? | | $M$, $G_1/S$ | MAURO and MADOC-JONES (1970) |
| Inhibitors of protein synthesis: | | | | |
| Cycloheximide | $G_2$ | BACCHETTI and SINCLAIR (1970) | $G_1/S$ | MAURO and MADOC-JONES (1970) |
| Pactamycin | ? | | $S$ | BHUYAN et al. (1972) |
| Puromycin | $G_2/M$ | KISHIMOTO and LIBERMAN (1964)<br>TOBEY et al. (1966)<br>EPIFANOVA et al. (1969) | $G_1/S$ | MAURO and MADOC-JONES (1970) |
| Sparsomycin | ? | | $S$ | BHUYAN et al. (1972) |
| Streptovitacin A | ? | | $G_1/S$ | MAURO and MADOC-JONES (1970) |
| Corticosteroids: | | | | |
| Hydrocortisone Na-succinate | ? | | None | DAWSON, K. B. and MAURO, F. (unpubl. data) |
| Methyl hydrazine derivatives: | | | | |
| Natulan | ? | | $G_1/S$ | DAWSON, K. B. and MAURO, F. (unpubl. data) |
| Miscellaneous, unclassified: | | | | |
| Bleomycin | $G_2$ | BARRANCO and HUMPHREY (1971)<br>TOBEY (1972) | $M$, $G_2$ | TERASIMA and UMEZAWA (1970)<br>BARRANCO and HUMPHREY (1971) |
| Ellipticine | ? | | $M$, $G_1$ | BHUYAN et al. (1972) |
| Formycin | ? | | $M$, $G_2$ | KUNIMOTO et al. (1967) |
| ICRF 159 | $G_2/M$ | SHARPE et al. (1970) | $G_1/S$ | DAWSON, K. B. and MAURO, F. (unpub.) |
| Phleomycin | $G_2/M$ | DJORDJEVIC and KIM (1967)<br>KUNIMOTO et al. (1967) | Mid-$G_1$, $S/G_2$ | DJORDJEVIC and KIM (1967)<br>KUNIMOTO et al. (1967) |
| Pseudourea | ? | | $S$ | BHUYAN et al. (1972) |
| Physical agents: | | | | |
| Heat shock | $M$ | WESTRA and DEWEY (1971) | $S$, $M$ | WESTRA and DEWEY (1971) |
| Ultraviolet light | Delay | DOMON and RAUTH (1968)<br>TODD et al. (1969) | $S$ | SINCLAIR and MORTON (1965)<br>RAUTH and WHITMORE (1966)<br>DJORDJEVIC and TOLMACH (1967)<br>HAN and SINCLAIR (1969) |
| x-radiation | Delay | ELKIND and WHITMORE (1967) | $M$, $G_1/S$ | SINCLAIR (1968) |

positions in the cell cycle, corresponding to late $G_1$ and to the $S$ phase. Furthermore, cells in mitosis are also very sensitive to the lethal effect of vinblastine, but not to that of vincristine (short three hour exposure in both cases) as suggested but not clearly indicated in Fig. 1 but confirmed by other experiments (unpublished results). All these fluctuations in survival have been shown to be characterized by changes in both shape and shoulder width of the dose-survival curve at different positions in the cell cycle. In particular, the dose-survival curve for cells treated with vinblastine at the $G_1/S$ transition point of relative resistance is characterized by a very wide shoulder (MADOC-JONES and MAURO, 1968).

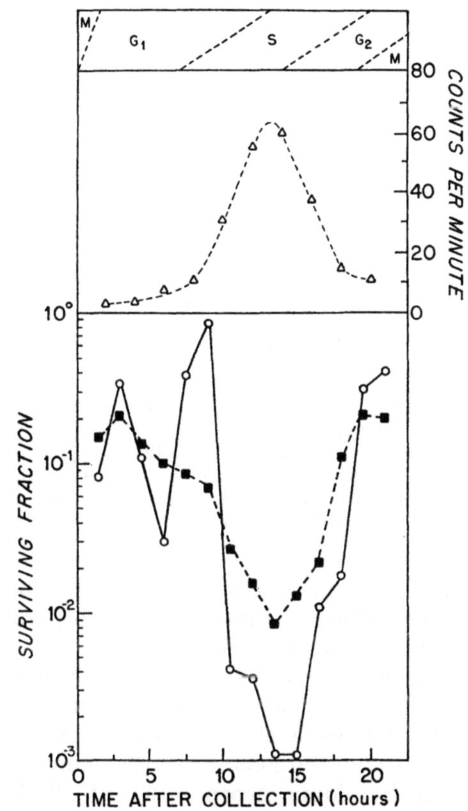


Fig. 1. Age-response of HeLa cells to vinblastine and vincristine. Lower figure (left ordinate): survival of synchronous cells exposed to 0.3 μg/ml of vinblastine (circles) or 0.1 μg/ml of vincristine (squares) at different times in the mitotic cycle. Duration of exposure was 3 h. The abscissa refers to the time at which exposure began after collection of mitotic cells. Cell multiplicity was about 2. Upper figure (right ordinate): rate of DNA synthesis measured by incorporation of $^{14}C$-thymidine in a 20 min pulse at different times in the cycle. The box at the top of the figure indicates the approximate distribution of cells in the different phases of the cycle

The action of vinblastine is especially complex. Cells treated in the late-$G_1$ sensitive phase were shown by repeated microscopic observation and by time-lapse cinematography to undergo lysis in interphase a few hours after treatment, well in advance of the next mitosis; that is, they die an interphase death (MADOC-JONES and MAURO, 1968). In contrast, cells treated with vinblastine or vincristine in the sensitive $S$ phase (for 3 h) proceed to mitosis without any delay and accumulate there as illustrated in Fig. 2 (for vinblastine only). Time-lapse cinematography again showed that after about 12 h in metaphase-arrest the cells begin to lyse (unpublished data). If either of the two drugs were added in early $G_1$ or $G_2$ at low concentration and left in the culture dishes to give a continuous exposure, then the cells also accumulated in mitosis, after a short delay as shown for vinblastine in Fig. 2.

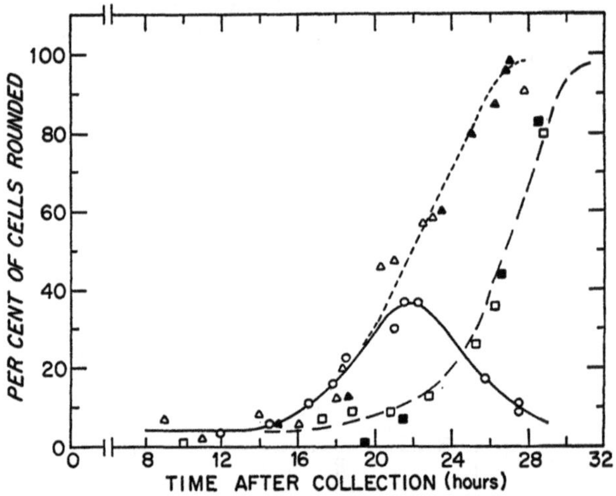


Fig. 2. Arrest of synchronous HeLa cells in mitosis after exposure to vinblastine. The percent of the total number of cells which are rounded up (in the next mitosis) is shown as a function of time after collection of mitotic cells. Open circles: control untreated cells. Open triangles: cells exposed (0.3 μg/ml) between 6 and 9 h after collection (late-$G_1$ surviving interphase). Closed triangles: cells exposed (0.3 μg/ml between 12 and 15 h (mid-$S$). Open squares: continuous exposure (0.03 μg/ml) commencing at 3 h (early-$G_1$). Closed squares: continuous exposure (0.03 μg/ml) commencing at 18 h ($G_2$)

In other, unpublished experiments, we investigated the effect of these two drugs on the rate of DNA synthesis as measured by incorporation of $^{14}$C-thymidine in a 20 min pulse, at different times through the cycle. The results showed that vinblastine, at the same concentration as that used for the lethal effect ($3 \times 10^{-7}$ M) 3 h exposure) had no effect on thymidine incorporation except when the cells were exposed at the initial part of the $S$ phase, where the incorporation was reduced to about 75% of that of the control culture. Vincristine, at lethal concentrations, did not depress thymidine incorporation at all. The various effects of these two drugs at different concentrations are shown in Table 2, compiled from our experiments and those of CREASEY and MARKIW (1964), CLINE (1968), and WAGNER and ROIZMAN (1968). The difference by a factor of 50 to 200 in drug concentration necessary to induce mitotic arrest as compared with a minimal depression of DNA synthesis is in agreement with recent work of PLAGEMANN (1970) on rat hepatoma cells.

Table 2 gives only an approximate indication of the relative drug concentrations at which the different effects take place, since the various authors use different cell systems and different exposure times; it serves to illustrate the important principle that a given drug may elicit different biochemical or cellular end-points at widely different concentrations. These considerations suggest that the general picture of the chemotherapeutic mechanism of these agents is far more complex than is frequently assumed and show how difficult it is to link a known biochemical action to a lethal effect.

Table 2. *Various effects of vinblastine and vincristine at different concentrations*

| Type of Effect | Relative concentration necessary to obtain the effect indicated | |
|---|---|---|
| | Vinblastine | Vincristine |
| Reversible mitotic arrest (continuous exposure) | 3 | 1 |
| Lethality, about 20% colony survival of asynchronous cells (discrete 3 h exposure) | 30 | 10 |
| DNA synthesis, about 75% of control[a] (thymidine incorporation) | 30 | — |
| RNA synthesis, about 75% of control (uridine incorporation) | 50 to 200 | 50 to 200 |

[a] Only for cells treated at the beginning of the *S* phase.

*Mechanism of Action of Methotrexate.* The action of this drug serves to illustrate just how complex a metabolic inhibitor can be. It is a folic acid antagonist (like many compounds related to aminopterin), an inhibitor of DNA synthesis consequent upon the inhibition of folate enzymes (NICHOL and WELCH, 1960; OSBORN et al., 1958) leading to a cessation of the biosynthesis not only of deoxythymidine monosphate but also of purine nucleotides (BALIS and DANCIS, 1955; WELLS and WINZLER, 1959). Its action can be prevented by an appropriate concentration of Leucovorin, a synthetic preparation of citrovorum factor, identical to folinic acid (BURCHENAL and BABCOCK, 1951). The mode of death induced by this drug is not well understood (SARTORELLI and LEPAGE, 1958; ROBERTS and HALL, 1967; HRYNIUK et al., 1969) but at least one mode is thought to be similar to "thymineless

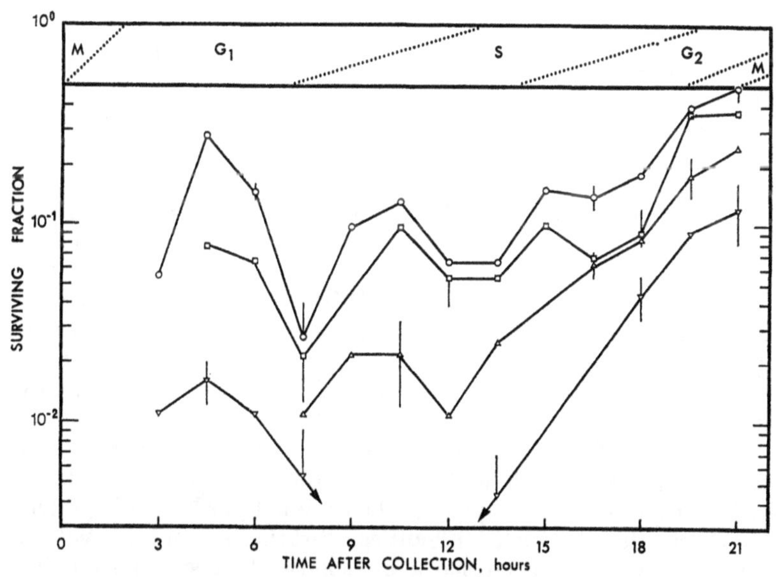


Fig. 3. Age-response of HeLa cells to methotrexate. Synchronous cells have been exposed for 3 h (in presence of $2.5 \times 10^{-5}$ M deoxyadenosine) at different times in the mitotic cycle. Circles: 2 μg/ml methotrexate. Squares: 3 μg/ml. Triangles: 4 μg/ml. Inverted triangles: 6 μg/ml. The abscissa refers to the time at which exposure began after collection of mitotic cells. The box at the top of the figure indicates the approximate distribution of cells in the different phases of the cycle. Vertical bars denote standard errors of the means

death" in bacteria (RUECKERT and MUELLER, 1960; DEMARS and HOPPER, 1960). Recently, WHITMORE and coworkers have shown that addition of purines in suitable concentration augments the lethal effectiveness of methotrexate, whereas certain concentrations of thymidine protect against its lethal action (WHITMORE et al., 1969; BORSA and WHITMORE, 1969). In recent experiments by one of us (F. M.), described below, HeLa cells were grown in a medium, supplemented with deoxyadenosine at a concentration between $4 \times 10^{-5}$ and $4 \times 10^{-6}$ M, at which a plateau of maximal effectiveness of methotrexate is reached. In this regard these experiments agree with those of BORSA and WHITMORE (1969) working with mouse L cells. The lethal age-response of HeLa cells collected at mitosis and exposed to methotrexate for 3 hour periods at various times in the cycle is shown in Fig. 3. The cell survival is lowest in early $G_1$, at the $G_1/S$ transition, and again at mid-$S$. An analysis of these variations in survival in terms of the parameters of the dose-survival curves show opposite tendencies in slope and shoulder-width, i.e. as the slope becomes steeper, the shoulder-width increases. The fine structure of this age-response is too complex to interpret at present, though it probably reflects fluctuations in enzyme activity known to occur through the cycle (MITCHISON, 1969). It appears to include a mid-$S$ phase sensitivity characteristic of DNA synthesis inhibitors together with a superimposed early $G_1$ and a $G_1/S$ transition sensitivity. The apparent resistance of mid-$G_1$ cells (Fig. 3) is of interest, because stationary phase cultures have been shown to be relatively resistant as compared with logarithmically growing cells (HRYNIUK et al., 1969; BORSA and WHITMORE, 1969) suggesting that the so-called "$G_0$" phase of resting cells may be analogous to the mid $G_1$ phase in this respect.

## Application of Age-Responses to the Design of Chemotherapeutic Regimes

Having summarized the various age-responses in Table 1 and having discussed in detail the two *Vinca* alkaloids and methotrexate, *in vitro*, we pass now to a consideration of possible chemotherapeutic applications of these kinds of data. First, it was necessary to show that similar age-responses obtain under *in vivo* conditions as under *in vitro*. Recently, synchronization methods using hydroxyurea for a number of *in vivo* animal cell systems have been described (MAURO and MADOC-JONES, 1969; PHILIPS et al., 1969; RAJEWSKY, 1970; GILLETTE et al., 1970).

The lethal age-responses of murine lymphoma cells *in vivo* to x-rays, vinblastine, vincristine and hydroxyurea were shown to be exactly analogous to those of cultured cells (MADOC-JONES and MAURO, 1970). However, to apply such data to the design of chemotherapeutic regimens in the most effective way would require knowledge of cell population kinetics for each cell-tumor system, which in most cases is simply not available. Fundamental differences may exist between the cell population kinetics of disseminated and solid tumors, of spontaneous and transplanted tumors, and of laboratory rodent and human tumors as has been stressed particularly by STEEL (1970) and MENDELSOHN and DETHLEFSEN (in press) *inter alia*. The responses of non-cycling cells have not yet been adequately investigated. However, despite such difficulties, certain elementary yet important conclusions can be drawn from the age-response data summarized in Table 1.

With the singular exception of hydrocortisone, which appears to affect cells equally wherever they are in the cycle at the time of treatment (Table 1, in agreement with the *in vivo* classification of BRUCE, 1966), all chemical agents (as well as radiation, including heat) elicit definitive lethal age-responses; that is, cells vary in their sensitivity to the lethal action of chemical agents according to which phase of the cell cycle the cells are in at the time of treatment. Most of the agents also cause a blocking response at one or more points in the cycle which may be next to or separated from the phase of lethal sensitivity (Table 1). It follows therefore (with the one exception) that when an asynchronous population of cells is treated with any agent listed in Table 1, the surviving cell population must have a distribution skewed in favor of one or more phases of the cycle; that is, it will be partially synchronized. In addition, the same cells may be partially synchronized by a reversible blocking age-response, causing cells to pile up at the block. When the block occurs just before the phase of lethal sensitivity, a particularly effective double synchronizing action will result, as in the case of hydroxyurea which has been exploited as a synchronizing agent both *in vitro* and *in vivo* for this very reason.

Because of the induction of a state of partial synchronization by almost any cytotoxic drug, it follows that, ideally, the timing of a second and subsequent dose fractions should be of crucial importance; this is still a truism even in the absence of requisite cell kinetic data needed to predict exactly when the doses should be given.

Because many of the agents cause a block in progression as well as a lethal effect, and at doses lower than those required for a lethal effect, it follows that a given cytotoxic drug will protect a part of the cell population against its own lethal action. In such a case, cure by single drug therapy would be theoretically unlikely.

If a combination of agents is to be used at a given moment in time against an asynchronous logarithmic phase cell population, the drugs could be chosen from the different age-response types listed in Table 1. One would choose a drug that "kills" cells in $G_1$, a second drug to act on cells at the $G_1/S$ transition, a third for $S$ phase cells, and even one for $G_2$ cells, as well as one for cells at mitosis. It is interesting to note that when the VAMP program was formulated it was thought that vincristine would affect cells in mitosis, methotrexate cells in the $S$ phase with a possible additive nonoverlapping effect; now it appears that both will act on $S$ phase cells predominantly, to give a considerable degree of "double" or "over kill". This argument would be even stronger regarding a combination of, say, hydroxyurea and vincristine.

If a two-drug combination is being planned, the neatest approach would be to choose an agent causing a block just before the phase of its lethality, and then pick a second drug with a lethal action at the point of the block in progression caused by the first drug, at which surviving cells would be piling up. For example, hydroxyurea or cytosine arabinoside could be followed by an agent acting predominantly at the $G_1/S$ transition, such as an inhibitor of protein or DNA synthesis, or an alkylating agent, or even ionizing radiation (see, for example, cytosine arabinoside plus BCNU in Tyrer et al., 1967).

Finally, although adequate cell kinetic data are unavailable, it is possible to make computer predictions based upon age-response data as to the effect of various dose regimens in combination drug therapy for "model cell systems" as pioneered by Steward and Hahn (1971) which may be of great usefulness in suggesting new regimes for experimental trial.

## References


Bacchetti, S., Sinclair, W. K.: The relation of protein synthesis to radiation-induced division delay in Chinese hamster cells. Radiat. Res. **44**, 788—806 (1970).

Bacchetti, S., Whitmore, G. F.: Actinomycin D and X-ray sensitivity in synchronized mouse L-cells. Radiat. Res. **31**, 577—578 (1967).

Bacchetti, S., Whitmore, G. F.: The action of hydroxyurea on mouse L-cells. Cell Tissue Kinet. **2**, 193—211 (1969a).
Bacchetti, S., Whitmore, G. F.: Actinomycin D: Effects on mouse L-cells. Biophys. J. **9**, 1427—1455 (1969b).
Balis, M. E., Dancis, J.: Effects of amethopterin on nucleic acid synthesis in leukemic spleen breis. Cancer Res. **15**, 603—608 (1955).
Barranco, S. C., Humphrey, R. M.: The effects of 1,3-*bis*(2-chloroethyl)-1-nitrosourea on survival and cell progression in Chinese hamster cells. Cancer Res. **31**, 191—195 (1971a).
Barranco, S. C., Humphrey, R. M.: The effects of bleomycin on survival and cell progression in Chinese hamster cells *in vitro*. Cancer Res. **31**, 1218—1223 (1971b).
Baserga, R.: The relationship of the cell cycle to tumor growth and control of cell division: A review. Cancer Res. **25**, 581—595 (1965).
Baserga, R., Estensen, R. D., Petersen, R. O.: Inhibition of DNA synthesis in Ehrlich ascites cells by actinomycin D, II. The presynthetic block in the cell cycle. Proc. nat. Acad. Sci. (Wash.) **54**, 1141—1148 (1965).
Bhuyan, B. K., Reuis, H. E., Smith, C. G.: A collagen plate assay for cytotoxic agents. II. Biological studies. Cancer Res. **22**, 1131—1136 (1962).
Bhuyan, B. K., Scheidt, L. G., Fraser, T. J.: Cell cycle phase specificity of antitumor agents. Cancer Res. **32**, 398—407 (1972).
Borsa, J., Whitmore, G. F.: Cell killing studies on the mode of action of methotrexate on L-cells *in vitro*. Cancer Res. **29**, 737—744 (1969).
Bremerskov, V., Kaden, P., Mittermayer, C.: DNA synthesis during the life cycle of L-cells: Morphological, histochemical and biochemical investigations with arabinosylcytosine and thioarabinosylcytosine. Europ. J. Cancer **6**, 379—392 (1970).
Brubaker, P. E., Flamm, W. G., Berheim, W. J.: Effect of $\gamma$-chlordane on synchronized lymphoma cells and inhibition of cell division. Nature (Lond.) **226**, 548—549 (1970).
Bruchovsky, N., Owen, A. A., Becker, A. J., Till, J. E.: Effects of vinblastine on the proliferative capacity of L-cells and their progression through the division cycle. Cancer Res. **25**, 1232—1237 (1965).
Bruce, W. R.: The action of chemotherapeutic agents at the cellular level and the effects of these agents on hematopoietic and lymphomatous tissue. Can. Cancer Conf. **7**, 53—64 (1966).
Bruce, W. R., Meeker, B. E., Valeriote, F. A.: Comparison of the sensitivity of normal hematopoietic and transplanted lymphoma colony-forming cells to chemotherapeutic agents administered *in vivo*. J. nat. Cancer Inst. **37**, 233—245 (1966).
Bruce, W. R., Meeker, B. E., Powers, W. E., Valeriote, F. A.: Comparison of the dose- and time-survival curves for normal hematopoietic and lymphoma colony-forming cells exposed to vinblastine, vincristine, arabinosylcytosine, and amethopterin. J. nat. Cancer Inst. **42**, 1015—1023 (1969).
Burchenal, J. H., Babcock, G. M.: Prevention of toxicity of massive doses of A-methopterin by citrovorum factor. Proc. Soc. exp. Biol. (N. Y.) **76**, 382—384 (1951).
Cardinali, G., Mehrota, T. N.: Comparative studies on the stathmokinetic effect of vincristine (VCR), vinblastine (VLB), and colchicine. Proc. Amer. Assoc. Cancer Res. **4**, 10—11 (1963).
Caspersson, T., Faber, S., Foley, G. E., Killander, D.: Cytochemical observations on the nucleolus-ribosome system: Effects of actinomycin D and nitrogen mustard. Exp. cell Res. **32**, 529—552 (1963).
Cline, M. J.: Effect of vincristine on synthesis of ribonucleic acid and protein in leukemic leukocytes. Brit. J. Haemat. **14**, 21—29 (1968).
Creasey, W. A., Markiw, M. E.: Biochemical effects of the *Vinca* alkaloids, II. A comparison of the effects of colchicine, vinblastine and vincristine on the synthesis of ribonucleic acid in Ehrlich ascites carcinoma cells. Biochim. Biophys. Acta (Amst.) **87**, 601—609 (1964).
Cutts, J. H.: The effect of vincaleukoblastine on dividing cells *in vivo*. Cancer Res. **21**, 168—172 (1961).
Demars, R. L., Hooper, J. L.: A method for selecting for auxotrophic mutants of HeLa cells. J. exp. Med. **111**, 559—572 (1960).
Djordjevic, B., Kim, J. H.: Lethal effect of phleomycin in different stages of the division cycle of HeLa cells. Cancer Res. **27**, 2255—2261 (1967).
Djordjevic, B., Kim, J. H.: Different lethal effects of mitomycin C and actinomycin D during the division cycle of HeLa cells. J. cell Biol. **38**, 477—483 (1968).
Djordjevic, B., Tolmach, L. J.: Responses of synchronous populations of HeLa cells to ultraviolet irradiation at selected stages of the generation cycle. Biophys. J. **32**, 327—347 (1967).
Doi, O., Takai, S., Aoki, Y., Higashi, H., Kosaki, G.: Effects of mitomycin C on HeLa cells at various stages of the division cycle. Gann **58**, 125—127 (1967).

DOMON, M., RAUTH, A.: Ultraviolet irradiation of mouse L-cells: Effects of DNA synthesis and progression through the cell cycle. Radiat. Res. **35**, 350—368 (1968).

DUSTIN, P.: New aspects of the pharmacology of antimitotic agents. Pharmacol. Rev. **15**, 449—480 (1963).

ELKIND, M. M., KANO, E.: Actinomycin D and radiation fractionation studies in asynchronous and synchronized Chinese hamster cells. Radiat. Res. **44**, 484—497 (1970).

ELKIND, M. M., WHITMORE, G. F.: The radiobiology of cultured mammalian cells, Chapter 7. New York: Gordon & Breach 1967.

ELKIND, M. M., SAKAMOTO, K., KAMPER, C.: Age-dependent toxic properties of actinomycin D and X-rays in cultured Chinese hamster cells. Cell Tissue Kinet. **1**, 209—224 (1968).

EPIFANOVA, O. I., SMOLENSKAYA, I. N., SEVESTYANOVA, M. V., KURDYUMOVA, A. G.: Effect of actinomycin D and puromycin on the mitotic cycle in synchronized cell cultures. Exp. cell Res. **58**, 401—410 (1969).

FOX, M., FOX, B. W.: Effect of methyl methanesulfonate on the growth of P388 lymphoma cells *in vitro* and on their rate of progress through the cell cycle. Cancer Res. **27**, 1805—1812 (1967).

FUJIWARA, Y.: Role of RNA synthesis in DNA duplication of synchronized populations of cultured mammalian cells. J. cell. comp. Physiol. **70**, 291—300 (1967).

GELFANT, S.: Inhibition of cell division. A critical and experimental analysis. Int. Rev. Cytol. **14**, 1—39 (1963).

GILLETTE, E. L., WITHERS, H. R., TANNOCK, I. F.: The age sensitivity of epithelial cells of mouse small intestine. Radiology **96**, 639—643 (1970).

HAHN, G. H.: Radiochemotherapy of cell cultures containing cycling and non-cycling cells. Front. Radiation Ther. Onc. **4**, 17—23 (1969).

HAN, A., SINCLAIR, W. K.: Sensitivity of synchronized Chinese hamster cells to ultraviolet light. Biophys. J. **9**, 1171—1192 (1969).

HRYNIUK, W. M., FISHER, G. A., BERTINO, J. R.: *S*-phase cells of rapidly growing and resting populations: Differences in response to methotrexate. Molec. Pharmacol. **5**, 557—564 (1969).

KARON, M., SHIRAKAWA, S.: Effect of 1-beta-D-arabinofuranosylcytosine on cell cycle passage time. J. nat. Cancer Inst. **45**, 861—867 (1970).

KIM, J. H., GELBARD, A. S., PEREZ, A. G.: Action of hydroxyurea on the nucleic acid metabolism and viability of HeLa cells. Cancer Res. **27**, 1301—1305 (1967).

KIM, J. H., GELBARD, A. S., DJORDJEVIC, B., KIM, S. H., PEREZ, A. G.: Action of daunomycin on the nucleic acid metabolism and viability of HeLa cells. Cancer Res. **28**, 2437—2442 (1968).

KIM, S. H., KIM, J. H.: Lethal effect of adriamycin on the division cycle of HeLa cells. Cancer Res. **32**, 323—325 (1972).

KISHIMOTO, S., LIBERMAN, I.: Synthesis of RNA and protein required for the mitosis of mammalian cells. Exp. cell Res. **36**, 92—101 (1964).

KUNIMOTO, T., HORI, M., UMEZAWA, H.: Modes of action of phleomycin, bleomycin and formycin on HeLa S3 cells in synchronized culture. J. Antibiotics (Tokyo) **20**, 277—281 (1967).

LI, L. H., OLIN, E. S., FRASER, T. S., BHUYAN, B. K.: Phase specificity of 5-azacytidine against mammalian cells in tissue culture. Cancer Res. **30**, 2770—2775 (1970).

LITTLEFIELD, J. W.: DNA synthesis in partially synchronized L cells. Exp. cell Res. **26**, 318—323 (1962).

LOZZIO, C. B.: Lethal effects of fluorodeoxyuridine on cultured mammalian cells at various stages of the cell cycle. J. cell Physiol. **74**, 57—62 (1969).

LUDFORD, R. J.: The action of toxic substances upon the division of normal and malignant cells *in vitro* and *in vivo*. Arch. Exp. Zellforsch. **18**, 411—441 (1936).

MADOC-JONES, H., BRUCE, W. R.: Comparison of the sensitivity of L cells in exponential and stationary phase to 5-fluorouracil. Nature (Lond.) **215**, 302—303 (1967).

MADOC-JONES, H., MAURO, F.: Interphase action of vinblastine and vincristine; Differences in their lethal action through the mitotic cycle of cultured mammalian cells. J. cell Physiol. **72**, 185—196 (1968).

MADOC-JONES, H., MAURO, F.: Age-responses to x-rays, *Vinca* alkaloids, and hydroxyurea of murine lymphoma cells synchronized *in vivo*. J. nat. Cancer Inst. **45**, 1131—1143 (1970).

MALAWISTA, S. E., SATO, H., BENSCH, K. G.: Vinblastine and griseofulvin reversibly disrupt the living mitotic spindle. Science **160**, 770—772 (1968).

MAURO, F., ELKIND, M. M.: Differences in survival variations during the growth cycle of cultured Chinese hamster cells treated with X-rays and sulfur mustard. Cancer Res. **28**, 1150—1155 (1968).

Mauro, F., Elkind, M. M., Sakamoto, K.: Comparison of survival kinetics and modifications of lethal damage in cultured Chinese hamster cells exposed to sulfur mustard and X-rays. Cancer Res. **28**, 1143—1149 (1968).
Mauro, F., Madoc-Jones, H.: Age-response to X-irradiation of murine lymphoma cells synchronized *in vivo*. Proc. nat. Acad. Sci. U.S. **63**, 666—691 (1969).
Mauro, F., Madoc-Jones, H.: Age-responses of cultured mammalian cells to cytotoxic drugs. Cancer Res. **30**, 1397—1408 (1970).
Mendelsohn, M. L., Dethlefsen, L. A.: Cell kinetics of breast cancer: The turnover of nonproliferating cells. In: Griem, M. L., Jensen, E. V., Ultmann, J. E., Wissler, R. W. (Eds.): Breast Cancer: a challenging problem. Recent results in cancer research. Berlin-Heidelberg-New York: Springer (in press.).
Mitchison, J. M.: Enzyme synthesis in synchronous cultures. Science **165**, 657—663 (1969).
Mueller, G. C., Kajiwara, K.: Actinomycin D and *p*-fluorophenylalanine inhibition of nuclear replication in HeLa cells. Biochim. biophys. Acta (Amst.) **119**, 557—565 (1966).
Nias, A. H. W., Fox, M., Fox, B. W.: Kinetics of a drug sensitive clone of HeLa cells. Cell Tissue Kinet. **3**, 207—215 (1970).
Nichol, C. A., Welch, A. D.: On the mechanism of action of aminopterin. Proc. Soc. exp. Biol. (N. Y.) **74**, 403—411 (1950).
Nowell, P. C.: Mitotic inhibition and chromosome damage by mitomycin in human leukocyte culture. Exp. cell Res. **33**. 445—449 (1964).
Osborn, M. J., Freeman, M., Huennekens, F. M.: Inhibition of dihydrofolate reductase by aminopterin and amethopterin. Proc. Soc. exp. Biol. (N. Y.) **97**, 429—431 (1958).
Palmer, C. G., Livergood, D., Warren, A. K., Simpson, P. J., Johnson, I. S.: The action of vincaleukoblastine on mitosis *in vitro*. Expt. cell Res. **20**, 198—201 (1960).
Pfeiffer, S. E., Tolmach, L. J.: Inhibition of DNA synthesis in HeLa cells by hydroxyurea. Cancer Res. **27**, 124—129 (1967).
Philips, F. S., Sternberg, S. S., Lenaz, L.: Susceptibility of intestinal crypt epithelium to hydroxyurea and other antitumor agents. In: Fry, R. J. M., Griem, M. L., Kirsten, W. H. (Eds.): Normal and malignant cell growth. Recent results in cancer research, Vol. 12, pp. 104—108. Berlin-Heidelberg-New York: Springer 1969.
Plagemann, P. G. W.: Vinblastine sulfate: Metaphase arrest, inhibition of RNA synthesis, and cytotoxicity, in Novikoff rat hepatoma cells. J. nat. Cancer Inst. **45**, 589—595 (1970).
Puck, T. T., Marcus, P. I., Cieciura, S. J.: Clonal growth of mammalian cells *in vitro*. Growth characteristics of colonies of single HeLa cells with and without "feeder" layer. J. exp. Med. **103**, 273—284 (1956).
Rajewsky, M. F.: Synchronization *in vivo:* Kinetics of a malignant cell system following temporary inhibition of DNA synthesis with hydroxyurea. Exp. cell Res. **60**, 269—276 (1970).
Rauth, A. M., Whitmore, G. F.: The survival of synchronized L cells after ultraviolet irradiation. Radiat. Res. **28**, 84—95 (1966).
Roberts, D., Hall, T. C.: Dihydrofolate reductase activity and deoxynucleoside incorporation into DNA of human leukocytes. Cancer **20**, 905—910 (1967).
Roberts, J. J., Brent, T. P., Crathorn, A. R.: The mechanism of the cytotoxic action of alkylating agents on mammalian cells. In: Campbell, P. N. (Ed.): The interaction of drugs and subcellular components in animal cells, pp. 5—27. Boston: Little, Brown & Co. 1968.
Rueckert, R. R., Mueller, G. C.: Studies on unbalanced growth in tissue culture. 1. Induction and consequences of thymidine deficiency. Cancer Res. **20**, 1584—1591 (1960).
Sakamoto, K., Elkind, M. M.: X-rays and nitrogen mustard: Independent action in Chinese hamster cells. Biophys. J. **9**, 1115—1130 (1969).
Sartorelli, A. C., LePage, G. A.: Effects of Amethopterin on the purine biosynthesis of susceptible and resistant TA3 ascites cells. Cancer Res. **18**, 1336—1339 (1958).
Schabel, F. M.: *In vivo* leukemic cell kill kinetics and "curability" in experimental systems. In: The Proliferation and spread of neoplastic cells, pp. 379—408. Baltimore: Williams & Wilkins 1968.
Schabel, F. M., Skipper, H. E., Trader, M. W., Wilcox, W. S.: Experimental evaluation of potential anticancer agents. XIX. Sensitivity of nondividing leukemic cell populations to certain classes of drugs *in vivo*. Cancer Chemother. Rep. **48**, 17—30 (1965).
Sharpe, H. B. A., Field, E. O., Hellmann, K.: Mode of action of the cytostatic agent "ICRF 159". Nature (Lond.) **226**, 524—526 (1970).
Sinclair, W. K.: Hydroxyurea: Differential lethal effects on cultured mammalian cells during the cell cycle. Science **150**, 1729—1731 (1965).
Sinclair, W. K.: Hydroxyurea: Effects on Chinese hamster cells grown in culture. Cancer Res. **27**, 297—308 (1967).

SINCLAIR, W.K.: Cyclic X-ray responses in mammalian cells *in vitro*. Radiat. Res. **33**, 620—643 (1968).
SINCLAIR, W.K.: Methods and criteria of mammalian cell synchrony. In: FRY, R.J.M., GRIEM, M.L., KIRSTEN, W.H. (Eds.): Normal and malignant cell growth. Recent results in cancer research, Vol. 17, pp. 90—103, Berlin-Heidelberg-New York: Springer-Verlag 1969.
SINCLAIR, W.K., MORTON, R.A.: X-ray and ultraviolet sensitivity of synchronized Chinese hamster cells at various stages of the cell cycle. Biophys. J. **5**, 1—25 (1965).
SKIPPER, H.E., SCHABEL, F.M., WILCOX, W.S.: Experimental evaluation of potential anti-cancer agents. XXI. Scheduling of arabinosylcytosine to take advantage of its *S*-phase specificity against leukemia cells. Cancer Chemother. Rep. **51**, 125—165 (1967).
STEEL, G.G.: The kinetics of cell proliferation in tumours. In: Time and dose relationships in radiation biology as applied to radiotherapy, Brookhaven National Laboratory Publication BNL 50503 (C-57), pp. 130—140. Upton, New York (1970).
STEWARD, P.G., HAHN, G.M.: The application of age response functions to the optimization of treatment schedules. Cell Tissue Kinet. **4**, 279—291 (1971).
STUBBLEFIELD, E.: Synchronization methods for mammalian cell cultures. In: PRESCOTT, D.M. (Ed.): Methods in cell physiology, New York: Academic Press 1968, pp. 25—43.
TERASIMA, T., TOLMACH, L.J.: Variations in several responses of HeLa cells to X-irradiation during the division cycle. Biophys. J. **3**, 11—33 (1963).
TERASIMA, T., UMEZAWA, H.: Lethal effects of bleomycin on cultured mammalian cells. J. Antibiotics **23**, 300—304 (1970).
TOBEY, R.A.: Arrest of Chinese hamster cells in G2 following treatment with the anti-tumor drug bleomycin. J. cell. Physiol. **79**, 259—266 (1972).
TOBEY, R.A., PETERSEN, D.F., ANDERSON, E.C., PUCK, T.T.: Life cycle analysis of mammalian cells. III. The inhibition of division in Chinese hamster cells by puromycin and actinomycin. Biophys. J. **6**, 567—581 (1966).
TODD, P., COOHILL, T.P., HELLWELL, A.B., MAHONEY, J.A.: Post-irradiation properties of cultured Chinese hamster cells exposed to ultraviolet light. Radiat. Res. **38**, 321—339 (1969).
TYRER, D.D., KLINE, I., VENDITTI, J.M., GOLDIN, A.: Separate and sequential chemotherapy of mouse leukemia L1210 with 1-$\beta$-D-arabinofuranosylcytosine hydrochloride and 1,3-*bis*-(2-chloroethyl)-1-nitrosourea. Cancer Res. **27**, 873—879 (1967).
WAGNER, E.K., ROIZMAN, B.: Effect of the *Vinca* alkaloids on RNA synthesis in human cells *in vitro*. Science **162**, 569—570 (1968).
WALKER, I.G., HELLEINER, C.W.: The sensitivity of cultured mammalian cells in different stages of the division cycle to nitrogen and sulfur mustard. Cancer Res. **23**, 734—739 (1963).
WELLS, W., WINZLER, R.J.: Metabolism of human leukocytes *in vitro* III. Incorporation of formate-$^{14}$C into cellular components of leukemic human leukocytes. Cancer Res. **19**, 1086—1090 (1959).
WESTRA, A., DEWEY, W.C.: Variation in sensitivity to heat shock or X-rays during the cell cycle of Chinese hamster cells *in vitro*. Abstract to the Joint Meeting of the British Association for Radiation Research and the Netherlands Radiobiological Society, Oxford (1971).
WHITMORE, G.F., BORSA, J., BACCHETTI, S., GRAHAM, F.: Mammalian cell killing by inhibitors of DNA synthesis. In: FRY, R.J.M., GRIEM, M.L., KIRSTEN, W.H. (Eds.): Normal and Malignant Cell Growth. Recent results in cancer research, Vol. 17. pp. 109—117. New York: Springer-Verlag 1969.
YOUNG, R.S.K., FISHER, G.A.: The action of arabinosylcytosine on synchronously growing populations of mammalian cells. Biochem. biophys. Res. Comm. **32**, 23—29 (1968).
XEROS, N.: Deoxyriboside control and synchronization of mitosis. Nature (Lond.) **194**, 682—683 (1962).

Chapter 11

# Pharmacokinetic Models for Antineoplastic Agents

DANIEL S. ZAHARKO and ROBERT L. DEDRICK

With 4 Figures

## Introduction

The action of most drugs is the result of a series of interactive processes relating to: (a) the physical and chemical properties of the drug, (b) the manner and site of administration, (c) the nature of the drug's absorption, distribution, and metabolism, and (d) the interaction of the drug with cellular processes. No exploitable unique biochemical processes have been discovered which make neoplastic cells more sensitive to chemotherapeutic agents than dividing normal cells. The selectivity of most antineoplastic agents depends, in part at least, upon particular differences in cell growth kinetics and pharmacologic effects of drug exposure.

In this chapter, concepts of pharmacokinetics which generally lead to quantitative expressions of drug exposure in whole animals will be discussed. Other chapters will deal in some detail with drug distribution, metabolism, and factors relating drug exposure to chemotherapeutic effect.

## The Utility of Pharmacokinetics

Experiences in other areas of pharmacology [antimalarial, central nervous system (CNS) and antibiotic drugs], suggest that a thorough study and quantitation of physiological disposition of drugs expedites the selection of clinically effective agents (SHANNON, 1945; BRODIE, 1964a; KRÜGER-THIEMER et al., 1965, 1966). BRODIE (1964a) recommends that such studies should be extented to man as soon as practically possible, since large unpredictable differences in metabolism of most drugs exist between animals and man. No one experienced in comparative toxicology will dispute that extrapolation of findings from animals directly to man can be extremely dangerous, however, even more dangerous is the refusal to extrapolate at all. There are certainly differences among experimental animals, between experimental animals and man, and among different individuals of the same species, but there are also many similarities. Knowledge of similarities and proper accounting for differences can lead to rational pharmacokinetic models. Such models enable an investigator to rapidly synthesize many observations and quantitatively describe the time-course of drug concentrations at various tissue loci. Pharmacokinetic considerations of findings in experimental animals should help the clinician in his first approach to patient treatment with new drugs and perhaps assist in improving treatment with older effective drugs, as more kinetic information is gathered concerning their pharmacology in humans. For example, when the effect of an antineoplastic drug is exerted during a certain cell cycle phase at a certain effective concentration, then the timing of dose and schedule to achieve this effective concentration is critical and dependent on drug distribution and elimination kinetics. For nonphase-specific agents it is important that the timing of dose and schedule allows for periods of noneffective drug concentration during which normal cells can recover (SHACKNEY, 1970; SKIPPER et al., 1970; JUSKO, 1971).

Detailed kinetic considerations of protein binding, excretion rates, tissue uptakes, and metabolism of drugs should also provide organic chemists with information for design and synthesis of drugs with the appropriate physical and chemical properties to achieve appropriate concentrations at tumor sites relative to normal tissues.

Kinetic studies of normal tissues *in vivo* should help to improve understanding of drug tissue interactions in tumors that arise embryologically from similar tissues.

Lastly, but perhaps most important, is the test of the completeness of one's knowledge about a drug's disposition. Model building forces one to define relevant factors in an operational way. The process of building a kinetic model to describe the *in vivo* time-course of a drug pinpoints areas where knowledge is incomplete and in which fruitful research might be pursued.

## Model Types and Kinetic Principles

A pharmacokinetic model consists of a set of differential equations relating phenomena such as protein binding, excretion rates, tissue uptake rates and metabolic rates. The equations can be written in the context of a classical compartmental model and the parameters adjusted by statistical considerations to best fit available data. Alternatively, the equations can be written to describe physical, chemical, and physiological processes which would be expected from past experience to influence drug disposition, or a combination of the above two processes can be used.

Models can be simple or complex depending upon the purpose of the model, the nature of the drug and the type of animal considered. We will briefly describe a range of models from the simple physiologically unrealistic to the more physiologically realistic, but naturally more complex, and attempt to relate their strengths and weaknesses to chemotherapeutic utility.

### A. One Compartment Model (Fig. 1)

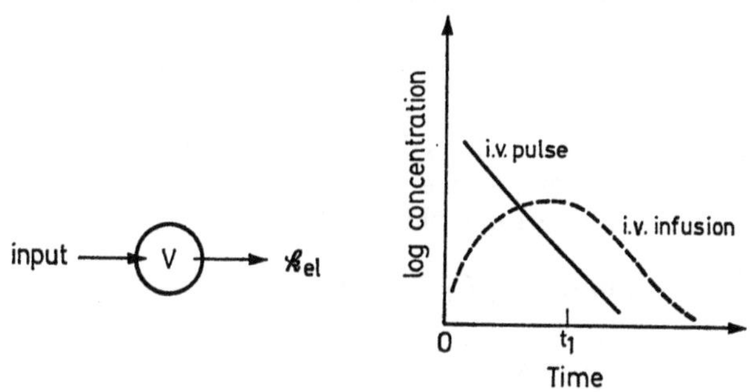


a b

Fig. 1. a Schematic diagram of one-compartment open model; b solid line, a typical solution for a pulse i.v. injection into a single compartment; dashed line, a typical solution for a constant infusion from time zero to $t_1$ into a single compartment

The changing concentration that occurs in the compartment may be expressed by a differential equation:

$$\frac{dC}{dt} = \text{input} - k_{el}C \quad (1)$$

The solution to Eq. (1) gives the concentration, $C$, of a drug in volume $V$ at any time. The constant $k_{el}$, the elimination rate constant, presents a composite of the mechanisms which remove drug, e.g. renal excretion and metabolism. Figure 1b illustrates typical solutions. The rate of rise and level of plateau for a constant infusion (dashed line) are functions of both the input and the elimination rates. Once $k_{el}$ is determined, solution of the equation at any time under a variety of inputs can predict the expected concentration. The elimination process is often first order so that $k_{el}$ does not change as the dose is changed. However, occasionally a saturable elimination process exists. In this case, the rate constant might be represented by $k_{el} = a/b+C$ where $a$ represents maximum rate and $b$ represents the concentration at one-half maximum rate. Other expressions may be required to adequately describe composite elimination mechanisms.

This model describes the body as a single well-mixed compartment. The assumption to chemotherapists is that all tissues experience the same changing drug concentration with time. RIEGELMAN et al. (1968) discuss the unrealistic nature of this assumption and show that a two compartment model, at least, is necessary to describe the plasma concentration of most drugs with time.

## B. Two Compartment Open Model (Fig. 2)

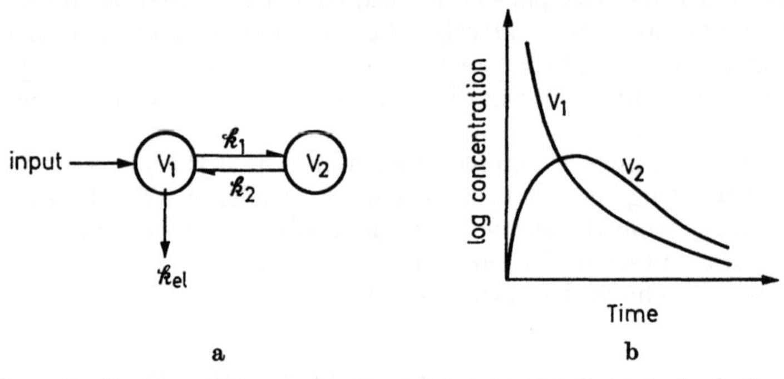


Fig. 2. a Schematic diagram of two-compartment open model; b typical solution for a pulse i.v. injection into compartment $V_1$

The rate of change of drug concentration in compartment $V_1$ (often called the central compartment) depends not only upon input and elimination rates of compartment $V_1$, but also upon the drug's distribution into another compartment $V_2$ (often called the peripheral compartment).

The differential equations describing this model are:

$$\frac{dC_{V_1}}{dt} = \text{input} - k_1 C_{V_1} + k_2 C_{V_2} - k_{el} V_1 \quad (2)$$

$$\frac{dC_{V_2}}{dt} = k_1 C_{V_1} - k_2 C_{V_2} \quad (3)$$

The rate constants $k_1$ and $k_2$ quantitate the instantaneous rate of drug flow between compartment $V_1$ and compartment $V_2$. Once the rate constants *(k's)* are determined [usually by statistical fit of the assumed model to plasma and urinary excretion data (BERMAN, 1956)], then the equations can be solved simultaneously for a variety of inputs to give expected concentrations with time. A typical solution for a pulse i.v. injection is illustrated in Fig. 2b.

## C. Multicompartment Models (Fig. 3)

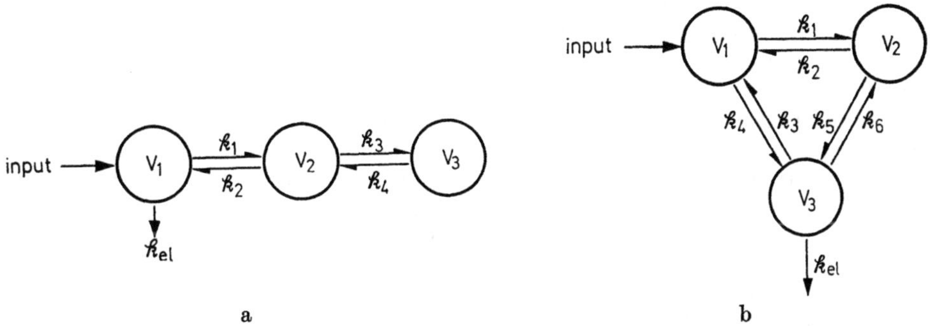


Fig. 3. Schematic diagrams to illustrate two possible three-compartment models

A variety of combinations of compartments is possible. Two illustrations are given in Fig. 3. The differential equations for these models can be easily written as previously described. Difficulties arise in selecting appropriate and meaningful compartments and then solving for rate constants so that the model not only fits plasma and urinary data, but also can be interpreted to assist in a better understanding of drug localization. Loo et al. (1968) have compared the use of two and three compartment models in describing the kinetics of 5-(3,3-dimethyl-1-triazeno)imidazole-4-carboxamide (DIC) in dogs. For readers interested in further details, such models are discussed in some detail by TEORELL (1937), BERMAN (1963), KRÜGER-THIEMER (1968), LEVY (1968), GIBALDI (1971), and WAGNER (1971).

In the classical approach to pharmacokinetic modeling described above, the parameters (rate constants and compartments) are not specifically identified with individual physiological or anatomical concepts. Instead, they are statistically functional in the sense that they are best estimates of parameters necessary to simulate plasma concentration and urinary excretion data within the context of the model chosen. Some literature exists on correlating pharmacological response with pharmacokinetic models (WAGNER, 1968; LEVY et al., 1969); however, direct application of classical pharmacokinetic models to problems in cancer chemotherapy is limited. BROCK et al. (1971) have used similar models in the analysis of the effects of cyclophosphamide in animals and man. The above models make no attempt to generally predict drug concentration at an arbitrary anatomic site, and they do not provide a ready mechanism for incorporation of known or measurable physiological, anatomical, and biochemical information. They do provide a means of predicting the plasma drug concentration with time following a variety of doses, schedules, and routes of administration.

Extensive information exists on many aspects of physiology and drug-tissue interactions which is not usually used in the kinetic compartmental models described above. Such information includes blood flow rates to various organs, organ sizes, binding to tissue and plasma proteins, lipid solubility, and membrane permeability. The above models are valuable when the description and prediction of plasma concentration and urinary excretion of a drug is desired. However, it is well documented that a drug may have high intrinsic activity in an isolated *in vitro* system, but exert little biological effect *in vivo* because the drug's physico-chemical characteristics do not permit it to reach its site of action (BRODIE, 1964). BAKER (1968), with folic acid analogs, verified this principle with at least some antineoplastic agents. Much evidence exists in the chemotherapeutic literature for the need to consider drug-tissue interactions (SPITZY, 1958; WHELAN, 1964; HAKALA, 1965; GOLDMAN et al., 1968; KESSEL et al., 1968).

More comprehensive knowledge concerning drug-tissue interactions *in vivo* would be helpful in predicting effects. Although tissue drug concentrations in man are difficult to obtain experimentally, tissue concentrations are (or will be) readily obtainable in experimental animals as new microanalytical techniques are developed. By analogy to the extrapolation of basic biochemical mechanisms from bacteria and animals to man, there are certain basic physico-chemical interactions of drugs with tissues of experimental animals that can be extrapolated to man. We are not referring here to drug metabolism, where genetic differences among species are known to occur, but to such things as diffusion, other forms of transport, lipid solubility, and protein binding.

Attempts to use the existing wealth of anatomical, biochemical, and physiological information to construct more meaningful antineoplastic model systems have been made (BISCHOFF et al., 1970; SHACKNEY, 1971; SKIPPER et al., 1971). With respect to the pharmacokinetic aspect of these types of models, the compartments and rate constants have a physiological basis in addition to a drug data basis. They offer, therefore, a unique opportunity to "scale up" phenomena from one species to another. For example, extensive studies of the pharmacological disposition of methotrexate in mice permitted prediction of plasma and several tissue drug concentrations in rats, dogs, monkeys, humans, and even sting rays, when the mouse model parameters were adjusted appropriately on the basis of known or measured physiological and pharmacological differences among the species (BISCHOFF et al., 1971; ZAHARKO et al., 1971, 1972).

The development of a physiological model is illustrated by the work with methotrexate in several species. Figure 4a shows a model that successfully predicts plasma and tissue concentrations and urinary and fecal excretion over a wide range of doses (BISCHOFF et al., 1971).

Mathematical development of this model is based on mass balance equations for each compartment. For illustrative purposes, the mass balance for the kidney is:

$$\underbrace{V_K \frac{dC_K}{dt}}_{\text{Accumulation of drug in kidney}} = \underbrace{Q_K C_P}_{\text{Rate of inflow with blood}} - \underbrace{Q_K \frac{C_K}{R_K}}_{\text{Rate of outflow with blood}} - \underbrace{k_K \frac{C_K}{R_K}}_{\text{Clearance by kidney}}$$

where $V$ = organ weight, g; $C$ = concentration, μg/g or μg/ml; $t$ = time, min; $Q$ = flow rate, ml/min; $R$ = equilibrium tissue-to-plasma distribution ratio; $k$ = clearance, ml/min, and the subscripts $K$ and $P$ refer to kidney and plasma.

The full set of equations is solved on a digital computer to provide predictions of drug concentration in each compartment as a function of time after an arbitrary dose. Figure 4b shows typical results. The solid lines are model predictions; the symbols represent experimental data.

Complications such as metabolism and resistance to drug transfer by cell membranes can be included when sufficient data are available. The identification of each compartment with an anatomic rather than functional space permits incorporation of concepts from physiology, membrane transport, and enzyme

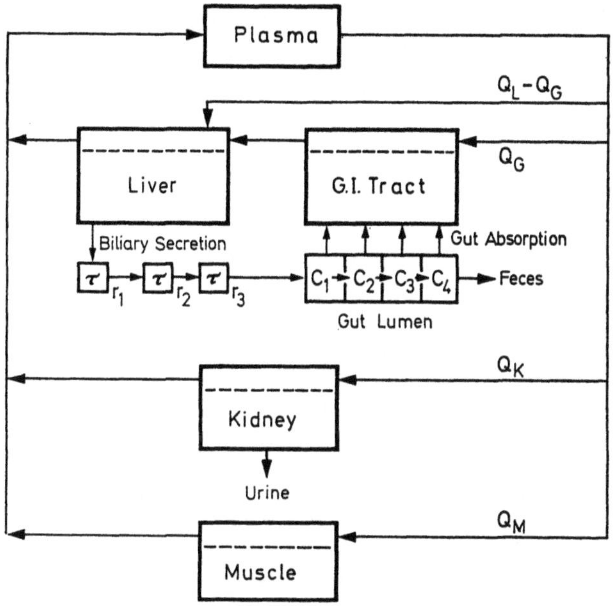


Fig. 4a

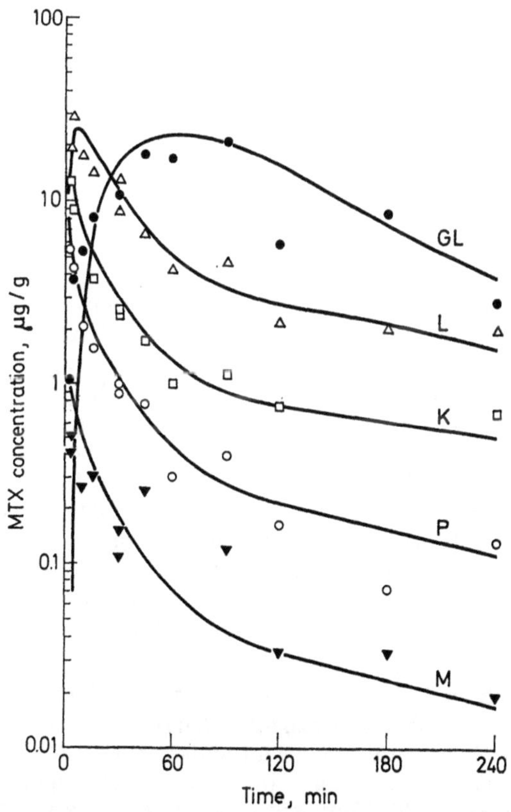


Fig. 4b

Fig. 4. a Body compartments important in methotrexate distribution; b results for i.v. injection of 3 mg/kg in a mouse. Solid lines represent model predictions; symbols represent experimental data. Key: *GL* (●), small intestine; *L* (△), liver; *K* (□), kidney; *P* (○), plasma; *M* (▼), muscle kinetics at the local site. Information on sensitivity of cells to their local environment may provide a reasonable basis for optimization of therapy.

Furthermore, attempts may be made to correlate metabolism, transport and cell response *in vivo* with measurements made *in vitro*. The deamination of cytosine arabinoside by pyrimidine nucleoside deaminase in human liver, kidney, and heart has been successfully modeled in this way (Dedrick et al., 1972).

## Prediction by Models

It is hoped that the impression has not been given that experimental animals are capable of predicting entirely pharmacologic events in man. Pharmacokinetic models are operational descriptions of natural processes which have a certain amount of intrinsic uncertainty and, therefore, are not always precisely predictable. The mathematically correct solution may not always represent the biological solution. To illustrate this point, consider the expected answers to the following question by a mathematically oriented child, as contrasted with a biologically oriented child: "How long will it take for a man to run one mile if he can run 100 yards in 10 sec?" It is well known that the four-minute mile is quite a biological achievement, whereas the straight mathematical extrapolation of 2.9 min would be a biological miracle. The point is that biological principles and experiences must be utilized to the fullest extent in order to solve biological problems (Skellum, 1969). Those who would construct mathematical models to help solve the complicated problems of neoplasia must constantly keep this in mind. Desirable pharmacokinetic models start with provisional working concepts and are progressively improved as new findings are made. The provisional working concepts should use as much relevant background information as possible.

## Problems of Variability

Kinetic models usually apply to the average animal. Most investigators are quite aware of the many differences that exist in physiologic and biochemical occurrences among different species with respect to drug disposition. Pharmacologists are becoming aware of the wide differences that can exist within such a heterogenous species as man (Brodie, 1964b; Brock et al., 1971). To be ultimately successful in their application to neoplastic treatment, human pharmacologic models must account for and quantitate the effect of individual differences that are known to exist. For example, it would be a simple mathematical matter to adjust a parameter to allow for lower metabolism or lower kidney clearance of a drug. That such factors are important has been discussed by Condit (1971) for the antineoplastic agent methotrexate and by Jelliffe et al. (1970) who used pharmacokinetics and analysis of individual differences to devise improved digitoxin therapy.

Other factors such as drug interactions and their effects on drug kinetics are now being explored with chemotherapeutic drugs. Tissue transport of structural analogs is altered by their simultaneous administration (Lichtenstein and Goldman, 1970); metabolism and toxicity of antineoplastic agents may be affected by antibiotics (Vogler, 1966; Bruckner, 1969; Zaharko, 1969). Certainly, the effectiveness of combination chemotherapy is well established (Venditti and Goldin, 1964; Henderson and Samaha, 1969; Devita, 1970), but a thorough understanding of the basis is still lacking.

## References


BAKER, B. R.: Tissue-specific irreversible inhibitors of dihydrofolic reductase. Accounts of chem. Res. **2**, 129—136 (1969).

BERMAN, M.: A postulate to aid in model building. J. theor. Biol. **4**, 229—236 (1963).

BERMAN, M., SCHOENFELD, R.: Invariants in experimental data on linear kinetics and the formulation of models. J. appl. Physics. **27**, 1361—1370 (1956).

BISCHOFF, K. B., DEDRICK, R. L.: Generalized solution to linear two-compartment model for drug distribution. J. theor. Biol. **29**, 63—83 (1970).

BISCHOFF, K. B., DEDRICK, R. L., ZAHARKO, D. S.: Preliminary model for methotrexate pharmacokinetics. J. pharm. Sci. **59**, 149—154 (1970).

BISCHOFF, K. B., DEDRICK, R. L., ZAHARKO, D. S., LONGSTRETH, J. A.: Methotrexate pharmacokinetics. J. pharm. Sci. **60**, 1128—1133 (1971).

BROCK, N., GROSS, R., HOHORST, H. J., KLEIN, H. D., SCHNEIDER, B.: Activation of cyclophosphamide in man and animals. Cancer **27**, 1512—1529 (1971).

BRODIE, B. B.: Physicochemical factors in drug absorption. In: Absorption and distribution of drugs. Baltimore: Williams and Wilkins 1964a.

BRODIE, B. B.: Distribution and fate of drugs; therapeutic implications. In: Absorption and distribution of drugs. Baltimore: Williams and Wilkins 1964b.

BRUCKNER, H.: Evaluation of the influence of antibiotics on the toxicity of antitumor drugs. Fed. Proc. **28**, 263 (1969).

CONDIT, P. T.: Chemotherapy of neoplastic disease with folate antagonists. In: Folate antagonists as chemotherapeutic agents. N. Y. Acad. Sci. **186**, 475—485 (1971).

DEDRICK, R. L., FORRESTER, D. D., HO, D. H.: *In vitro - in vivo* correlation of drug metabolism—deamination of 1-β-D-arabinofuranosylcytosine. Biochem. Pharmacol. **21**, 1—16 (1972).

DEVITA, V. T., SERPICK, A. A., CARBONE, P. P.: Combination chemotherapy in treatment of advanced HODGKIN's disease. Ann. intern. Med. **73**, 881—895 (1970).

GIBALDI, M.: Pharmacokinetic aspects of drug metabolism. Ann. N. Y. Acad. Sci. **179**, 19—31 (1971).

GOLDMAN, I. D., LICHTENSTEIN, N. S., OLIVERIO, V. T.: Carrier mediated transport of the folic acid analogue methotrexate in the L1210 leukemia cell. J. biol. Chem. **243**, 5007—5017 (1968).

HAKALA, M. T.: On the role of drug penetration in amethopterin resistance of sarcoma-180 cells *in vitro*. Biochim. biophys. Acta (Amst.) **102**, 198—209 (1965).

HENDERSON, E. S., SAMAHA, R. J.: Evidence that drugs in multiple combinations have materially advanced the treatment of human malignancies. Cancer Res. **29**, 2272—2280 (1969).

JELLIFFE, R. W., BUELL, J., KALABA, R., SRIDHAR, R., ROCKWELL, R., WAGNER, J.: An improved method of digitoxin therapy. Ann. intern. Med. **72**, 453—464 (1970).

JUSKO, W. J.: Pharmacodynamics of chemotherapeutic effects: Dose-time-response relationships for phase-nonspecific agents. J. pharm. Sci. **60**, 892—895 (1971).

KESSEL, D., HALL, T. C., ROBERTS, D.: Modes of uptake of methotrexate by normal and leukemic human leucocytes *in vitro* and their relation to drug response. Cancer Res. **28**, 564—570 (1968).

KRÜGER-THIEMER, E.: Pharmacokinetics and dose-concentration relationships. In: Physicochemical aspects of drug action. New York: Pergamon 1968.

KRÜGER-THIEMER, E., BUNGER, P.: The role of the therapeutic regimen in dosage design. Chemotherapia **10**, 61—73 (1965—1966).

LEVY, G., GIBALDI, M., JUSKO, W. J.: Multicompartment pharmacokinetic models and pharmacologic effects. J. pharm. Sci. **58**, 422—424 (1969).

LICHTENSTEIN, N. S., GOLDMAN, I. D.: Riboflavin-methotrexate interactions. Biochem. Pharmacol. **19**, 1229—1239 (1970).

LOO, T. L., TANNER, B. B., HOUSEHOLDER, B. E., SHEPARD, B. J.: Some pharmacokinetic aspects of 5-(dimethyltriazeno) imidazole-4-carboxamide in the dog. J. pharm. Sci. **57**, 2126—2131 (1968).

RIEGELMAN, S., LOO, J. C. K., ROWLAND, M.: Shortcomings in pharmacokinetic analysis by conceiving the body to exhibit properties of a single compartment. J. pharm. Sci. **57**, 117—123 (1968).

SHACKNEY, S. E.: A computer model for tumor growth and chemotherapy, and its application to L1210 leukemia treated with cytosine arabinoside. Cancer Chemother. Rep. **54**, 399—429 (1970).

SHANNON, J. A.: The study of antimalarials and antimalarial activity in the human malarials. Harvey Lectures **41**, 43—49 (1945—1946).

SKELLUM, J. G.: Models, inference, and strategy. Biometrics **25**, 457—475 (1969).

SKIPPER, H. E., SCHABEL, F. M., MELLETT, L. B., MONTGOMERY, J. A., WILKOFF, L. J., LLOYD, H. H., BROCKMAN, R. W.: Implications of biochemical, cytokinetic, pharmacologic, and

toxicologic relationships in the design of optimal therapeutic schedules. Cancer Chemother. Rep. **54**, 431—450 (1970).
Spitzy, K. H., Hitzenberger, G.: The distribution volume of some antibiotics. In: Antibiotics annual. New York: Medical Encyclopedia Inc. 1958.
Teorell, T.: Kinetics of distribution of substances administered to the body. Arch. int. Pharmacodyn. **57**, 205—225 (1937).
Venditti, J. M., Goldin, A.: Drug synergism in antineoplastic chemotherapy. In: Advances in chemotherapy. New York: Academic 1964.
Vogler, W. R., Basin, J. A., Huguley, C. M., Palmer, H. G., Lowrey, M. E.: Metabolic and therapeutic effects of allopurinol in patients with leukemia and gout. Amer. J. Med. **40**, 548—559 (1966).
Wagner, J. G.: Kinetics of pharmacologic response. J. theor. Biol. **20**, 173—201 (1968).
Wagner, J. G.: Biopharmaceutics and relevant pharmacokinetics. Hamilton: Hamilton 1971.
Whelan, J. P. F., McFadzean, J.: The debatable significance of serum levels of chemotherapeutic agents. In: Absorption and distribution of drugs. Baltimore: Williams and Wilkins 1964.
Zaharko, D. S., Bruckner, H., Oliverio, V. T.: Antibiotics alter methotrexate metabolism and excretion. Science **166**, 887—888 (1969).
Zaharko, D. S., Dedrick, R. L., Bischoff, K. B., Longstreth, J. A., Oliverio, V. T.: Methotrexate tissue distribution: prediction by a mathematical model. J. nat. Cancer Inst. **46**, 775—784 (1971).
Zaharko, D. S., Dedrick, R. L., Oliverio, V. T.: Prediction of the distribution of methotrexate in the sting ray by use of a model developed in mice. Comp. Biochem. Physiol. **42 A**, 183—194 (1972).

Chapter 12

# Absorption, Distribution, and Excretion of Antineoplastic and Immunosuppressive Agents

VINCENT T. OLIVERIO

With 3 Figures

## Introduction

The general principles of pharmacological disposition apply almost universally to compounds which are foreign to the mammalian organism, including antineoplastic and immunosuppressive agents. Thus, the interrelated mechanisms of absorption, binding, distribution, metabolism, and excretion are the chief factors that determine the effective concentration of a drug at a receptor site (Fig. 1).

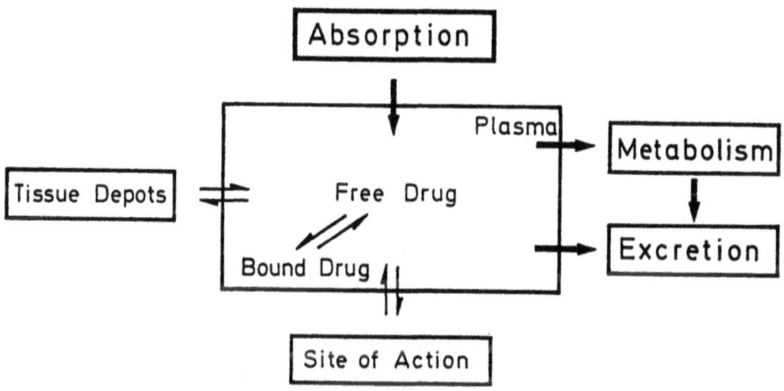


Fig. 1. Factors influencing concentration of active (unbound) drug in plasma and other tissues

In this chapter, a brief consideration is given to those processes which regulate the response of an organism to several commonly used antineoplastic and immunosuppressive agents. Excluded is the more complex process of metabolism since this aspect of pharmacological disposition is considered in some detail in two later chapters, and also in the chapters dealing with individual agents.

## Cell Membrane Barriers

Of importance to an understanding of the pharmacological processes listed above is some knowledge of the modes of passage of drugs across cell membrane barriers when entering the body, entering intracellular sites of action, or during removal by excretion mechanisms (GOLDSTEIN et al., 1969; SCHANKER, 1962, 1964, 1971). These barriers are similar to one another and resemble very closely a typical cell membrane (Fig. 2), which by virtue of its bimolecular lipid layer, containing pores, and a monomolecular protein layer, is capable of accepting nonpolar (lipid soluble) substances and excluding polar molecules. Thus, drugs appear to cross membranes either by filtration through pores, by simple diffusion, or by special transport mechanisms.

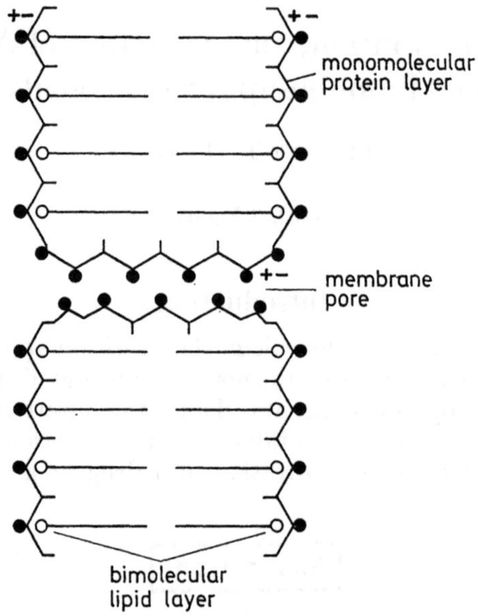


Fig. 2. Schematic diagram of a cell membrane

## A. Simple Diffusion

Most drugs enter cells by dissolving in the lipid membrane and diffusing across, under the influence of a concentration gradient, to the aqueous phase. Nonpolar drugs pass through the membrane more freely than polar compounds. The ease with which a drug can pass through a membrane is generally well-correlated with its partition coefficient between the aqueous phase and the lipid phase of the membrane. Quantitative comparisons of partition coefficients have been made. Using a lipid solvent (e.g. chloroform, ether, octanol, or olive oil) and water adjusted to physiological pH, the partition coefficient *(Ca)* of a substance, HA, is defined as the ratio of the concentrations in two phases at equilibrium.

$$Ca = \frac{[\text{HA}] \text{ in organic solvent}}{[\text{HA}] \text{ in aqueous solvent}}$$

For a pure chemical substance, *Ca* is a physical constant. In general, the greater the partition coefficient, the greater the affinity for lipid membranes, and the more rapidly the absorption of a drug across cell membranes occurs.

Many drugs contain acidic or basic groups (or both) which may be ionized in aqueous solution. The nonionized neutral form of these compounds is usually the most lipid soluble form and diffuses most readily across cell membranes, because cell membranes are preferentially permeable to lipid soluble, nonionized forms of weak acids or bases. At equilibrium the concentration of the nonionized form is identical on both sides of the membrane. The degree of ionization, which varies with pH, or the relative proportion of the nonionized to the ionized species of a drug is given by the dissociation constant and is expressed for both acids and bases as pKa. The pKa can be calculated from the HENDERSON-HASSELBACH equation as follows:

$$pKa = pH + \log \frac{[HA]}{[H^+][A^-]}$$

The pKa of a basic drug is 14-pKb. The larger the pH of the solution the greater is the degree of ionization of acidic drugs and the smaller is the degree of ionization of basic drugs.

## B. Filtration

The membranes of the blood capillaries and the glomeruli of the kidneys appear to have pores of sufficient size to permit the passage of relatively large size (up to 40 Å) molecules. Generally, however, penetration of cell membranes by pore filtration is limited to drug molecules whose equivalent pore radius is less than 4 Å. The filtration of a compound may be prevented by binding to plasma proteins which results in larger molecules which are unable to pass through the pores. Passage through pores of membranes is usually regulated by a combination of hydrostatic pressure and electrostatic, osmotic, and concentration gradients.

## C. Specialized Transport

For a number of drugs, simple filtration or diffusion does not account for their passage across membranes. Special transport mechanisms have been postulated for these compounds, such as "carrier-mediated transport". This latter mechanism postulates the formation of a complex with a carrier in the membrane which is lipid-soluble and able to cross the membrane. On the other side the complex dissociates and the transported drug is released. When a substrate molecule is moved against a concentration gradient, energy is required and the process is termed "active transport". Active transport processes are sensitive to metabolic inhibitors which impair the production of cellular energy. The carrier-mediated transport process can be saturated by high concentrations of substrate molecules. In the transport of natural metabolites, the carrier molecules show specificity for a particular type of chemical structure. Quite often, however, a foreign molecule will compete for or be transported by a carrier mechanism, especially when its chemical structure is similar to that of the natural structure. This has been established for the antimetabolites methotrexate (MTX) and 5-fluorouracil (5-FU), both immunosuppressive and antineoplastic agents with wide clinical application.

Methotrexate (Fig. 3), a structural analog of the naturally occurring coenzyme precursor folic acid, contains two carboxyl groups in its glutamic acid moiety. The pKa values of these groups have been estimated to be 4.8 and 5.5 (LIEGLER et al., 1969). At physiological pH these groups would be expected to be completely

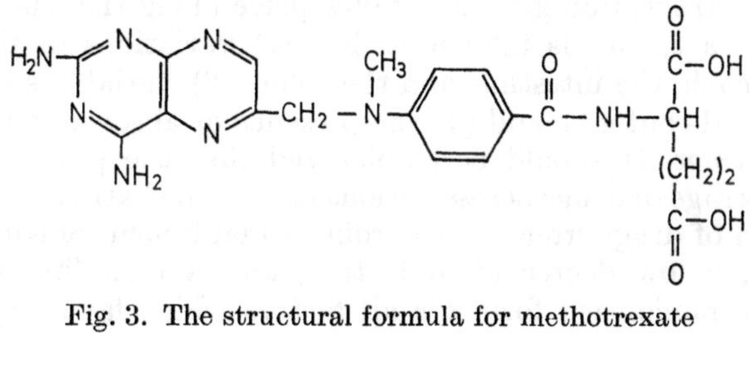

Fig. 3. The structural formula for methotrexate

ionized, while the pteridine amino groups are probably non-ionized. Studies of MTX transport *in vitro* in mammalian cells, particularly in L1210 murine leukemia cells, indicate that this moderately weak organic acid satisfies the criteria for a carrier-mediated transport model (GOLDMAN et al., 1968). The transport of this drug in the L1210 cell shares at least in part the same transport mechanism as folic and folinic acids. The efficacy of this lipophobic agent as a chemotherapeutic agent has been attributed to its high affinity for dihydrofolic acid reductase, thus preventing the reduction of folic acid to its tetrahydrofolate forms (BERTINO, 1963). Therefore, the rate of entry of this drug into the cancer cell is a crucial factor in the rate at which dihydrofolic acid reductase is inactivated. Data of KESSEL and HALL (1967) and GOLDMAN et al. (1968) indicate that the molecular configuration necessary for binding to dihydrofolate reductase is distinct from the configuration which determines the affinity for the transport system.

An active renal tubular transport mechanism has also been described for methotrexate (LIEGLER et al., 1969) and is discussed in the section on drug excretion.

The halogenated pyrimidine, 5-fluorouracil, has been shown to be actively transported across a membrane barrier (SCHANKER, 1964). In this case, the intestinal epithelium of rats served as the model, and 5-FU was actively transported across this membrane by the process which transports the natural pyrimidines uracil and thymine.

Thus, the rate and extent of passage (or absorption) of drugs across a variety of cell membrane barriers are markedly influenced by (a) solubility in aqueous media, (b) the lipid/aqueous partition coefficient, and (c) the degree of ionization. The relative importance of these factors is determined primarily by the chemical structural characteristics of the foreign molecules.

With few exceptions, a drug must first enter the blood in order to distribute throughout the body and exert its action. It will reach organs and tissues at a rate determined by blood flow. The effective concentration at the reactive site will depend not only on the relative rates of absorption, binding, distribution, metabolism, and excretion, but also on the physical-chemical factors discussed above and the interaction of the drug with other tissue components. A number of routes exist by which a drug can enter the circulatory system. These are discussed below with certain general considerations.

## Drug Routes of Administration

### A. Oral Route

Drugs in most clinical situations are given by mouth, the most convenient, and perhaps the most economical route. This route of administration is used particularly for drugs of low aqueous solubility which are not irritating to the gastrointestinal tract or subject to hydrolysis or the destructive action of digestive enzymes. Absorption generally takes place along the whole length of the gastrointestinal tract, and is influenced by: (1) variations in the transit time through the stomach, the intestine, and the colon, (2) variations in the pH of the gastric or intestinal contents, and (3) the presence or absence of foodstuffs in the gastrointestinal tract. It should be emphasized that the principles cited above governing the passage of drugs across various membrane barriers are also operative in the absorption of drugs from the gastrointestinal lumen. Small molecular size, water solubility, a low degree of ionization, and a high lipid/water partition coefficient of the nonionized form are all factors which favor rapid absorption.

Drugs absorbed across the membranes of the gastrointestinal tract are carried in the portal vein to the liver. Here they may be exposed to the action of various enzyme systems, resulting in some instances in less potent or more active substances, and may also be secreted into the bile. The concentrative transfer from blood to bile of large lipid-insoluble molecules such as methotrexate (MTX) probably occurs by specialized transport processes resembling the mechanism of transport of organic acids across the kidney tubule. Drugs appearing in the bile may be excreted directly from the gastrointestinal tract or reabsorbed by the small intestine. The latter process is referred to as entero-hepatic recirculation, and is of potential importance in prolonging the action of a drug.

Some dramatic examples of species differences in the oral absorption of such drugs as sulfanilamide, 6-azauridine, thiopental, pentobarbital, and thalidomide have been cited (RALL, 1968), but similar data for antineoplastic and immunosuppressive drugs are not readily available.

In at least one well documented study (HENDERSON et al., 1965b), the size of a dose of an antitumor drug has been shown to influence its extent of absorption. In man, oral doses of 0.1 mg/kg of MTX were rapidly and completely absorbed from the gastrointestinal tract. This was evidenced by plasma levels of the drug which were essentially identical to plasma levels achieved after intravenous injection of the same dose. Large oral doses of 10 mg/kg, however, were slowly and incompletely absorbed as evidenced by plasma levels which were lower than if the same dose had been given intravenously. Thus, for MTX, absorption from the gastrointestinal tract of man appears to be a saturable process. In mice, MTX bile to plasma ratios of 300/1 have been reported (BISCHOFF et al., 1970), but no saturation of drug transport into the bile was observed over a wide range of doses (ZAHARKO, 1972).

Another important variable regulating absorption after oral administration is the rate at which a drug goes into solution. For many drugs, including a number of antineoplastic and immunosuppressive agents, this is determined by the different dosage forms. Generally, oral dosage forms that allow the release of drugs most rapidly can be placed in the following decreasing order: aqueous solution, suspension, powder, compressed tablet, and coated tablet. Particle size of a drug also markedly influences its rate of dissolution (LEVY and BARR, 1972).

Sublingual administration followed by absorption through the oral mucosa is occasionally used with some drugs (BECKETT and HOSSIE, 1971), but this route is not generally preferred for antitumor and immunosuppressive agents. These agents are likewise not generally given by rectum, although this route is often employed for other types of drugs. While the absorption from the colon is less rapid than from the small intestine, the absorption mechanisms are essentially identical (SCHANKER, 1971).

## B. Parenteral Route

Drugs which are not absorbed through membrane barriers, as well as those which undergo degradation in the gastrointestinal tract or rapid biotransformation in the liver to less active or more toxic compounds, may be introduced into the blood stream by intravenous injection. Prompt high drug levels result and gastrointestinal absorption is not a factor modifying the pharmacological response unless a high degree of enterohepatic circulation is present due to rapid biliary excretion. This route also permits a greater proportion of administered drug to reach potential target tissues prior to being exposed to the biotransformation activity of various enzyme systems of the liver. This is also the route of choice when (a) a rapid response is required, (b) the patient is unconscious or unable to swallow, and (c) the drug cannot be retained because of vomiting. Another advantage is that the rate of injection can be controlled or stopped if untoward effects are encountered. In many instances it is desirable to administer the drug by a slow constant infusion so as to maintain a sustained plasma level of drug for therapeutic effect with the least toxicity. The disadvantages of intravenous injection (including the intra-arterial route) are associated with the development of infection, potential anaphylactic reactions, the formation of emboli, precipitous drop in blood pressure, cardiac arrhythmia or arrest, and local irritation. Intra-arterial injections have primarily been used with diagnostic radiopaque drugs and for regional perfusion of malignant neoplasms by such agents as 5-fluorouracil, methotrexate, phenylalanine mustard, nitrogen mustard, and actinomycin D (STRAWITZ, 1972; SULLIVAN and SEMEL, 1972).

Subcutaneous or intramuscular injections are often used to achieve a systemic action of a drug (SCHOU, 1971). Larger amounts of drug solution can be given intramuscularly than subcutaneously with usually less pain and local irritation and more rapid absorption. The latter is facilitated by greater spreading of the injected drug and better blood flow to the muscle as compared to subcutaneous tissues. Both the intramuscular and subcutaneous routes are commonly used with depot forms of various drugs when it is desirable to prolong the rate of entry into the blood and maintain sustained drug levels. In this regard, the depot form of arabinosyl cytidine (ara-C), 1-$\beta$-D-arabinofuranosylcytosine-5′-palmitate (palmoyl-ara-C), is currently undergoing clinical trial in an effort to prolong the plasma and tissue levels of the active parent compound, which is rapidly inactivated *in vivo* by deaminase enzymes to uracil arabinoside (FREI, 1972).

### C. Percutaneous Route

Drugs may be applied to the surface of the skin in the form of ointments, to produce a local effect or a systemic effect, usually after unpredictable absorption. Highly lipid-soluble drugs are usually rapidly absorbed through the keratinized epidermal layer of the skin (KATZ and POULSEN, 1971). Drugs applied to damaged skin surfaces may be very rapidly absorbed, as would be expected with any damaged membrane barrier. The rate of penetration through the skin is determined by the lipid/aqueous partition coefficients, with water-soluble highly ionized molecules being largely excluded. The topical route of administration is commonly used clinically with 5-FU for the treatment of actinic keratosis (SHELLEY, 1970). The drug is commonly employed as a 2% solution in polyethylene glycol and primarily acts locally with little evidence of absorption systemically.

### D. Other Routes

Certain drugs are sometimes administered in forms that are absorbed through the membranes of the vagina, urethra, conjunctiva, nose and oropharynx. Anesthetic gases and certain sympathomimetic drugs are rapidly absorbed through the mucous membranes of the latter to produce their systemic effects. These routes of drug administration have not been generally employed for antineoplastic and immunosuppressive agents.

## Drug Distribution

After a drug has been absorbed or injected intravascularly, it is distributed through the body by the blood stream. The initial distribution or localization in the target site and in other organs and tissues of the body is regulated by blood flow, available binding sites, and its physical chemical properties (solubility, etc.). The drug may remain in the plasma, usually bound to plasma proteins; it may permeate freely through cell membranes and become distributed throughout the body water; it may be distributed largely to extracellular water because of its inability to penetrate cell membranes. The effective concentration of drug at the reactive site is related to its concentration in the plasma and the duration of time that an effective level is maintained. This is the $C \times t$ (concentration times time) constant which is markedly affected by dose level and dose schedule. The latter can be manipulated to influence rates of drug absorption across membrane barriers and rates of elimination (loss), which in turn are affected by interacting processes of plasma and/or tissue binding, metabolism, and excretion. In some cases, a drug will localize selectively in fatty tissue or in particular cellular constituents of an organ such as the liver, because of affinity for specific binding sites. Tissue binding of drugs usually occurs with proteins, phospholipids, or nucleoproteins and is generally reversible. The passage of some drugs across the "blood-brain barrier" or the placental barrier constitutes special aspects of drug distribution but is of considerable importance in the clinical use of antineoplastic agents. The properties of these special membrane barriers and their influence on drug distribution are considered in a separate chapter.

## A. Plasma Protein Binding

In the blood a drug may be bound to plasma proteins. While several kinds of plasma proteins will interact with drug molecules, albumin, the principal protein of plasma, accounts for most drug binding (SETTLE et al., 1971; KEEN, 1971). The binding to plasma protein is usually reversible and involves ionic, hydrogen, and van der Waal's bonds. The extent of binding depends on the particular drug. Extensive binding to plasma proteins may in effect serve as a large storage depot for drugs and in some cases be used to advantage when prolonged low plasma levels of drug must be maintained after a single dose. The coadministration or presence of several drugs in the blood, especially molecules with similar structural characteristics, may have a profound effect on distribution of each drug because of competition for the same binding sites on plasma protein. Methotrexate binding to primarily the albumin fraction of human plasma is reduced from approximately 70% to 40% by coadministration of organic acids such as salicylic acid or sulfisoxazole at MTX therapeutic plasma concentrations ranging between 90 and 200 μg/ml (LIEGLER, 1969).

The interaction of such factors as (a) pH differences on either side of a cell lipid membrane, (b) differences in degrees of drug binding to protein of plasma or to other cellular components of tissues, and (c) differences in active transport processes, generally determines the distribution of drugs in the body and accounts for the fact that drugs may become more concentrated in some tissues than in others (SCHANKER, 1962, 1964).

An experimental approximation of the extent to which a drug is concentrated in or on the nonaqueous phases (compartments) of the body can be made by measuring the apparent volume of distribution, $V_D$, or the fluid volume in which a drug seems to be dissolved (GOLDSTEIN et al., 1969).

$$V_D = \frac{\text{total amount of drug in body (mg/kg)}}{\text{conc. in plasma water (mg/l)}}$$

After allowing sufficient time for the drug to distribute and "equilibrate" following its administration, without regard to factors of metabolism, binding, and excretion, the $V_D$ can be determined. Since most drugs never reach a distribution plateau, because of the combined processes of metabolism, binding, and excretion that contribute to continual decline in plasma drug levels, the $V_D$ is determined by extrapolating the eventual stable rate of decline back to the time of injection on a semilogarithmic scale.

$V_D$ may correspond to one or another of the water compartments of the body (plasma 4%, interstitial 13%, intracellular 41%) or it may be larger. If much larger, the drug is undoubtedly highly bound to plasma proteins and/or cellular components, or concentrated in the fat of adipose tissue. A large $V_D$ is invariably associated with a relatively slow elimination of drug from the body; the concentration of freely diffusable molecules is low, and only small numbers of them are "available" at any given time to metabolizing enzymes or to excretory mechanisms.

### B. Redistribution

Following drug absorption and initial distribution in body fluids and tissues, the processes of metabolism and excretion become important factors in terminating the drug's effect by removing it from the blood and from tissue areas of high concentration and low affinity where storage may be temporary. However, in some cases, termination of drug effect may result following its redistribution to other tissue sites of high binding affinity and low blood flow, such as bone (FOREMAN, 1971) and adipose tissue (MARK, 1971). Pharmacological studies with MTX and its halogenated congener, dichloromethotrexate (DCM), indicate that these carcinostatic agents are redistributed in the body by processes of enterohepatic recirculation and metabolism (OLIVERIO and ZAHARKO, 1971). Redistribution has been less well studied for other antineoplastic and immunosuppressive agents, but it is reasonable to expect that factors affecting this process are similar to those described for agents such as thiopental (SHARPLESS, 1970; MARK, 1971).

## Drug Excretion

The most important route of excretion for drugs and drug metabolites is the kidney (WEINER, 1971). Some drugs are secreted into the bile, but are then generally reabsorbed from the intestine and become involved in an enterohepatic circulation (SMITH, 1971). Both MTX and DCM undergo enterohepatic circulation, but in the case of the latter compound, its metabolite, 7-OH DCM, is not extensively reabsorbed in the gut after biliary excretion and thus appears in the stool (OLIVERIO and ZAHARKO, 1971). In general, excluding the excretion of large molecules into the bile, the hepatic handling of drugs follows similar rules to that of the kidney, except that there are very significant anatomical differences. Excretion through the intestine, and sometimes the lungs, salivary fluid, sweat, and milk (RASMUSSEN, 1971), accounts for the other routes of excretion. In this regard both nitrogen mustard (OCHOA and HIRSCHBERG, 1967) and procarbazine (OLIVERIO, 1972) are extensively biotransformed with a significant proportion of the excretory products appearing in the expired air. Recently, JOHNS et al. (1972) reported that after oral dosage in a lactating patient with choriocarcinoma, MTX was excreted in milk at low, but readily detectable levels.

Renal function is primarily governed by glomerular filtration, tubular secretion, and tubular reabsorption. The rate at which a drug is filtered by the glomeruli depends on its molecular weight and on its concentration as the unbound form in plasma. Plasma protein binding will retard the rate of filtration. Classic examples of drugs which are excreted by pure glomerular filtration include inulin and creatinine. Very few, if any, common drugs, including the antineoplastic and immunosuppressive agents, approach this ideal mechanism for renal clearance. Drugs which are filtered by the glomeruli may be reabsorbed later from the tubule. As with absorption of drugs through other membranes, tubular resorption is markedly affected by the lipid/water partition coefficient. For ionizing drugs this depends on the pH of the urine. Thus, basic drugs are more readily excreted in acid urine, and acidic compounds in alkaline urine. Renal tubular secretion involves the concentration of both acidic and basic drugs by the cells of the proximal convoluted tubules of the kidney and secretion into the lumen across a large concentration gradient. Importantly, the tubules act on unbound drug, shift the equilibrium, and thus appear capable of "unbinding" drugs from plasma protein. The rate at which the renal tubular secretion of a drug proceeds is essentially independent of its plasma binding.

As a moderately weak organic acid, MTX is not only filtered by the kidney glomeruli, but is also actively secreted by the renal tubules (LIEGLER et al., 1969). Weak organic acids such as salicylate, para-aminohippurate, and to a lesser extent, sulfisoxazole, when administered simultaneously with MTX, suppress its renal clearance. MTX is insoluble in most lipid solvents at body pH but is highly soluble in water as the sodium salt. Similarly to most lipid insoluble drugs, it is primarily excreted in the urine in the unaltered form (HENDERSON et al., 1965a, 1965b). On the other hand, lipid soluble antineoplastic agents such as busulfan (NADKARNI et al., 1959; PENG, 1959; VODOPICK et al., 1969), cyclophosphamide (HILL et al., 1972), 1,3-*bis*(2-chloroethyl)-1-nitrosourea (DEVITA et al., 1967), 1-(2-chloroethyl)-3-cyclohexyl-1-nitrosourea (CCNU) (OLIVERIO et al., 1970), methyl CCNU (SPONZO et al., 1972), and procarbazine (OLIVERIO, 1972) are excreted in the urine primarily as biotransformation products. The latter metabolic changes facilitate excretion and the products are more polar and less lipid soluble. The above relationships between solubility characteristics, biotransformation, and excretion by the kidney are not so clearly correlated for those antimetabolites (5-fluorouracil, 6-mercaptopurine, ara-C) that can undergo anabolic transformation *in vivo*, and for higher molecular weight carcinostatic agents, such as the plant alkaloids, vincristine and vinblastine.

## Conclusions

In this chapter the folate antagonist methotrexate has served as the primary model to illustrate the general principles governing the absorption, distribution, and excretion of antineoplastic and immunosuppressive agents. As a class of antineoplastic agents, the folate antagonists have probably been the most extensively studied as pertains to pharmacological disposition. As acidic molecules, however, they are not truly representative of that large group of tumor and immunosuppressive agents that are basic compounds. Despite this difference, the general principles of pharmacological disposition described above apply equally well to both classes of drug molecules.

## References

BECKETT, A. H., HOSSIE, R. D.: Buccal absorption of drugs. In: BRODIE, B. B., GILLETTE, J. R. (Eds.): Concepts in biochemical pharmacology, Part. 1 pp. 25—46. Berlin: Springer 1971.

BERTINO, J. R.: The mechanism of action of the folate antagonists in man. Cancer Res. **23**, 1286—1306 (1963).

BISCHOFF, K. B., DEDRICK, R. L., ZAHARKO, D. S.: Preliminary model for methotrexate pharmacokinetics. J. pharm. Sci. **59**, 149—154 (1970).

DeVita, V.T., Denham, C., Davidson, J.D., Oliverio, V.T.: The physiological disposition of the carcinostatic 1,3-*bis*(2-chloroethyl)-1-nitrosourea (BCNU) in man and animals. Clin. Pharmacol. Ther. 8, 566—577 (1967).
Foreman, H.: Translocation of drugs into bone. In: Brodie, B.B., Gillette, J.R. (Eds.): Concepts in biochemical pharmacology, Part 1. pp. 249—257. Berlin: Springer 1971.
Frei, E., III: Personal communication (1972).
Goldman, I.D., Lichtenstein, N.S., Oliverio, V.T.: Carrier-mediated transport of the folic acid analogue, methotrexate, in the L1210 leukemia cell. J. biol. Chem. **243**, 5007—5017 (1968).
Goldstein, A., Aronow, L., Kalman, S.M.: Principles of drug action. pp. 106—205. New York: Harper and Row 1969.
Henderson, E.S., Adamson, R.H., Denham, C., Oliverio, V.T.: The metabolic fate of tritiated methotrexate. I. Absorption, excretion and distribution in mice, rats, dogs and monkeys. Cancer Res. **25**, 1008—1017 (1965a).
Henderson, E.S., Adamson, R.H., Oliverio, V.T.: The metabolic fate of tritiated methotrexate. II. Absorption and excretion in man. Cancer Res. **25**, 1018—1024 (1965b).
Hill, D.L., Laster, R., Jr., Struck, R.F.: Enzymatic metabolism of cyclophosphamide and nicotine and production of a toxic cyclophosphamide metabolite. Cancer Res. **32**, 658—665 (1972).
Johns, D.G., Rutherford, L.D., Leighton, P.C., Vogel, C.L.: Secretion of methotrexate into human milk. Amer. J. Obstet. Gynec. **112**, 978—980 (1972).
Katz, M., Poulsen, B.J.: Absorption of drugs through the skin. In: Brodie, B.B., Gillette, J.R. (Eds.): Concepts in biochemical pharmacology, Part 1, pp. 103—174. Berlin: Springer 1971.
Keen, P.: Effect of binding to plasma proteins on the distribution, activity and elimination of drugs. In: Brodie, B.B., Gillette, J.R. (Eds.): Concepts in biochemical pharmacology. Part 1. pp. 213—233. Berlin: Springer 1971.
Kessel, D., Hall, T.C.: Amethopterin transport in Ehrlich ascites carcinoma and L1210 cells. Cancer Res. **27**, 1539—1543 (1967).
Levy, G., Barr, W.H.: The basis for selection of the dosage form and source of drug. Rational Drug Ther. **6**, 1—7 (1972).
Liegler, D.G., Henderson, E.S., Hahn, M.A., Oliverio, V.T.: The effect of organic acids on renal clearance of methotrexate in man. Clin. Pharmacol. Ther. **10**, 849—857 (1969).
Mark, L.C.: Translocation of drugs and other exogeneous chemicals into adipose tissue. In: Brodie, B.B., Gillette, J.R. (Eds.): Concepts in biochemical pharmacology, Part 1. pp. 258—275. Berlin: Springer 1971.
Nadkarni, M.V., Trams, E.G., Smith, P.K.: Preliminary studies on the distribution and fate of TEM, TEPA and Myleran in the human. Cancer Res. **19**, 713—718 (1959).
Ochoa, M., Jr., Hirschberg, E.: Alkylating agents. In: Schnitzer, R.J., Hawking, F. (Eds.): Experimental chemotherapy, vol. V, Part II, pp. 1—132. New York: Academic Press 1967.
Oliverio, V.T.: Derivatives of triazenes and hydrazines. In: Holland, J.F., Frei, E., III (Eds.): Cancer medicine. pp. 806—817. Philadelphia: Lea and Febiger 1973.
Oliverio, V.T., Vietzke, W.M., Williams, M.K., Adamson, R.H.: The absorption, distribution, excretion, and biotransformation of the carcinostatic 1-(2-chloroethyl)-3-cyclohexyl-1-nitrosourea in animals. Cancer Res. **30**, 1330—1337 (1970).
Oliverio, V.T., Zaharko, D.S.: Tissue distribution of folate antagonists. Ann. N. Y. Acad. Sci. **186**, 387—399 (1971).
Peng, C.T.: Distribution and metabolic fate of $S^{35}$-labeled myleran (Busulfan) in normal and tumor-bearing rats. J. Pharmacol. exp. Ther. **120**, 229—238 (1959).
Rall, D.P.: Role of pharmacological disposition in drug action. In: Tedeschi, D.H., Tedeschi, R.E. (Eds.): Importance of fundamental principles in drug evaluation. pp. 173—182. New York: Raven Press 1968.
Rasmussen, F.: Excretion of drugs by milk. In: Brodie, B.B., Gillette, J.R. (Eds.): Concepts in biochemical pharmacology, Part 1. pp. 390—402. Berlin: Springer 1971.
Schanker, L.S.: Absorption of drugs from the gastrointestinal tract. In: Brodie, B.B., Gillette, J.R. (Eds.): Concepts in biochemical pharmacology, Part 1. pp. 9—24. Berlin: Springer 1971.
Schanker, L.S.: Passage of drugs across body membranes. Pharmacol. Rev. **14**, 501—530 (1962).
Schanker, L.S.: Physiological transport of drugs. In: Harper, N.J., Simmonds, A.B. (Eds.): Advances in drug research. pp. 71—106. London: Academic Press 1964.
Schou, J.: Subcutaneous and intramuscular injection of drugs. In: Brodie, B.B., Gillette, J.R. (Eds.): Concepts in biochemical pharmacology, Part 1, pp. 47—66. Berlin: Springer 1971.

SETTLE, W., HEGEMAN, S., FEATHERSTONE, R. M.: The nature of drug-protein interaction. In: BRODIE, B. B., GILLETTE, J. R., (Eds.): Concepts in biochemical pharmacology, Part 1. pp. 175—186. Berlin: Springer 1971.
SHARPLESS, S. K.: Hypnotics and sedatives. In: GOODMAN, L. S., GILMAN, A. (Eds.): The pharmacological basis of therapeutics. pp. 98—120. New York: Macmillan 1970.
SHELLEY, W. B.: Drugs and their use in dermatology. In: RABINOWITZ, J. L., MYERSON, R. M. (Eds.): Topics in medicinal chemistry, vol. 3, pp. 285—331. New York: John Wiley and Sons 1970.
SMITH, R. L.: Excretion of drugs in bile. In: BRODIE, B. B., GILLETTE, J. R. (Eds.): Concepts in biochemical pharmacology. Part 1. pp. 354—389. Berlin: Springer 1971.
SPONZO, R. W., DEVITA, V. T., OLIVERIO, V. T.: Physiologic disposition of 1-(2-chloroethyl)-3-cyclohexyl-1-nitrosourea (CCNU) and 1-(2-chloroethyl)-3-(4-methylcyclohexyl)-1-nitrosourea (MeCCNU) in man. Cancer **31**, 1154—1159 (1973).
STRAWITZ, J. G.: Cancer chemotherapy using isolation perfusion. In: BRODSKY, I., KAHN, S. B., MOYER, J. H. (Eds.): Cancer chemotherapy II. The twenty-second Hahnemann symposium, pp. 443—451. New York: Grune and Stratton 1972.
SULLIVAN, R. D., SEMEL, C. J.: Arterial infusion cancer chemotherapy for solid tumors. In: BRODSKY, I., KAHN, S. B., MOYER, J. H. (Eds.): Cancer chemotherapy II. The twenty-second Hahnemann symposium, pp. 453—458. New York: Grune and Stratton 1972.
VODOPICK, H., HAMILTON, H. E., JACKSON, H. L., PENG, C. T., SHEETS, R. F.: Metabolic fate of tritiated busulfan in man. J. Lab. clin. Med. **73**, 266—276 (1969).
WEINER, I. M.: Excretion of drugs by the kidney. In: BRODIE, B. B., GILLETTE, J. R. (Eds.): Concepts in biochemical pharmacology, Part 1. pp. 328—353. Berlin: Springer 1971.
ZAHARKO, D. S.: Personal communication (1972).

Chapter 13

# Transport of Antineoplastic Agents

M. T. HAKALA

## Introduction

Before an agent can damage a cancer cell, it must be able to pass through the outer cell membrane, also called the plasma membrane. An exception to this rule would be provided by a "membrane-active" compound, which would affect the plasma membrane only and by so doing cause cell death. Antibacterial agents of this type do exist (HAMILTON, 1970). One may speculate that highly lipid soluble compounds could be localized in plasma membranes of mammalian cells and thereby seriously alter cellular metabolism. However, most of the antineoplastic agents whose mode of action is understood appear to act somewhere within the cell. A notable exception is provided by asparaginase, which, without entering the cells, causes a critical deficiency of asparagine by cleaving it extracellularly to aspartic acid (BROOME, 1968; SUOLINNA et al., 1971).

The interior of mammalian cells is a heterogenous entity composed of various subcellular compartments with different enzymatic compositions and consequently different functions. Compartments such as the nucleus, mitochondria, lysosomes, and Golgi apparatus are all surrounded by membranes, each different from the other. Thus, depending on the site of action of an antimetabolite, it might have to pass not only through the plasma membrane, but through an intracellular membrane as well. It is known, e. g., that tetracycline becomes localized specifically in the mitochondria of mammalian tissues (DUBUY and SHOWACRE, 1961).

It is generally agreed that all biological membranes are structures composed of proteins and lipids and that these structures may differ in different tissues. Analysis of red cell membranes of 17 mammalian species revealed that they were similar in composition, consisting of 70 lipoid molecules for each protein molecule, most of them in a bound form (PARPART and BALLENTINE, 1952). The lipid: protein ratio for a plasma membrane preparation of liver cells and human erythrocytes was reported as 2:3 (MADDY, 1966; BENEDETTI and EMMELOT, 1968) and for bovine mitochondrial membrane as 1:3 (DEWEY and BARR, 1970). The lipid component consists mainly of phospholipid and cholesterol, although the cholesterol content of mitochondrial membranes is very much lower than of erythrocyte or liver cell plasma membranes. There is no doubt that the specific structures and/or compositions of the plasma membranes of cells from different tissues are different and are likely to provide tissue selectivity even for compounds that enter the cells purely by diffusion.

In a neutral environment, the cells carry a net negative charge and the inner surface of the cell membrane is more negative than the outer surface, with a pH gradient of about 0.1. The negative charge of the cells is the net result of a number of acidic and basic groups on the cell surface, among them the carboxyl groups of sialic acid. The spatial arrangement of these charged groups on the cell surface is not known, but this arrangement may play an important role in the passage of charged molecules across the membranes (WEISS and HAKALA, 1971).

From a purely practical point of view the main question which needs to be answered concerning the cellular uptake of an antineoplastic agent is whether, at tolerable drug levels, this uptake is rapid enough to allow the drug to reach its site of action in the target cell in time to prevent cell division. An understanding of the factors which underlie a slow or rapid uptake of a drug may provide basic information useful for designing new drugs.

## Modes of Cellular Uptake

The passage of molecules through plasma membranes proceeds by one of the following ways:

1. Passive transfer or simple diffusion
2. Facilitated diffusion
3. Active transport
4. Pinocytosis

Only in a few cases is the actual mechanism of the uptake of antineoplastic agents fully understood. The uptake of structural analogs of normal metabolites proceeds usually by the same mechanism as the uptake of the corresponding metabolite. However, passive permeation is particularly important for compounds for which a specific transport mechanism is missing. In the case of passive permeation the membrane behaves as an inert boundary and the rate of uptake is directly proportional to the extracellular concentration of the compound. Small molecules diffuse through the membrane faster than large ones, and due to the high lipid content of the membranes the lipid solubility greatly affects the rate of uptake. Early studies demonstrated how the passage of molecules through biological membranes increased with increasing lipid/water partition coefficient. For a comprehensive review see WARTIOVAARA and COLLANDER (1960). Water solvent systems, which are usually used in biological tests, pose limitations with respect to the study of highly lipophilic compounds. This limitation was overcome in a test system, which concerned penetration of human skin, by applying the dry, lipid-soluble compounds directly on a piece of skin (2 to 3 mg/0.2 $cm^2$), which was constantly bathed underneath by circulating saline (MARZULLI et al., 1965). These studies confirmed, what had earlier been predicted (BOOIJ and BUNGENBERG DEJONG, 1956), namely, that the most lipophilic compounds hardly penetrated the skin at all. PENNISTON et al. (1969), presented a nonsteady state mathematical model to explain this parabolic permeation behavior of molecules by diffusion. As pointed out by these authors, it indeed makes sense that permeability must first increase with the increasing lipid/water partition coefficient, reach a maximum and thereafter decrease. When the coefficient approaches zero, the compound would be so hydrophilic as to be unable to enter a lipid barrier; as the coefficient approaches infinity the compound would become so lipophilic as to be unable to return to an aqueous phase from the first lipid barrier that it meets. According to this theory there will be, for each group of compounds, an intermediate value for the lipid/water partition coefficient (0.1 to 10), which will coincide with the optimal rate of passage through a biological membrane.

It is only the unionized form of weak acids and bases which diffuses through the plasma membranes of cells. However, the net negative charge on the cell surface creates an attraction for positively charged compounds as opposed to negatively charged ones and results in a generally faster rate of uptake of positively charged compounds. An example of charge effect is provided by comparing the uptake of methotrexate and 4,4′-diacetyl-diphenyl-urea-*bis*-guanylhydrazone (DDUG) by Sarcoma 180 cells *in vitro* (HAKALA, 1965a, 1971). These compounds have about the same molecular weight and both are rapidly bound within the cells, methotrexate to dihydrofolate reductase and DDUG to the nucleus and mitochondria. Methotrexate carries two negative and DDUG two positive charges. DDUG is taken up by simple diffusion and methotrexate by facilitated diffusion, yet DDUG is taken up 40-times faster than methotrexate. The rate of uptake of methotrexate was doubled when the negative charges were reduced by lowering the pH of the incubation medium to 5.5 (HAKALA, 1965b). Indirect evidence for the role of charge in uptake was also provided by RYSER and HANCOCK (1965). They demonstrated a 50-fold increase in the rate of uptake of albumin by Sarcoma 180 cells in monolayer cultures in the presence of polyornithine, which is a polycation and thus neutralizes the negative charges of the albumin molecule.

Due to the higher level of negativity of the cell interior as compared with the outer surface of the cells, it is to be expected that even at equilibrium the intra-extracellular molar concentrations of diffusible, charged compounds cannot be equal. For negatively charged compounds one should observe a concentration gradient in favor of the extracellular environment, while for positively charged compounds the opposite would be true.

Plasma membranes of somatic cells can by no means be considered to be rigid structures. Indicative of their nonrigidity is the ameboid movement of single mammalian cells. Thus, one can assume that membranes are dynamic, fluid structures, with a fixed state only at death. This fluidity provides the cells with the capacity for pinocytosis, which enables the cells to take up large molecules. Even particles such as asbestos, carmin crystals, and latex droplets have been shown to be engulfed by mammalian cells in *in vitro* cultures (BENSCH et al., 1959; OVERMAN, 1961; DOURMASHKIN and DOUGHERTY, 1961). The uptake of large molecules of proteins, nucleic acids, and even chromosomes also proceeds by pinocytosis (for review see HOLTER, 1959).

It is generally agreed that there are two parameters which distinguish active transport from facilitated diffusion. These are the uptake against an electrochemical concentration gradient and the need for energy in the case of active transport. Common characteristics for the two processes are the saturability, specificity, and inhibition by analogs, as well as by enzyme poisons. The question of temperature dependence may sometimes be confusing. While a low activation energy ($Q_{10}$ of about 2) undoubtedly indicates facilitated or simple diffusion, a high $Q_{10}$ alone does not provide proof of active transport. This is especially true when the uptake is linked to cellular metabolism of the permeant. In such a case it may be the intracellular metabolism which is more dependent on temperature than the membrane passage, leading to slowing down of the net uptake at low temperatures. A more definite criterion for active transport is the uptake against a concentration gradient. However, as was mentioned above, even in the case of diffusion a positively charged molecule is expected to accumulate within the cells. In this regard, one must also consider the fate of the compound inside the cells. Thus, uptake against a concentration gradient, strictly speaking, means a concentration gradient of free, unaltered permeant. There are several examples of uptake of antineoplastic agents, which at first sight seem to indicate uptake against a concentration gradient and thus suggest active transport. Examples of this sort are the uptake of methotrexate, DDUG, purines, pyrimidines, and their nucleosides. In only a few of these cases has the presence of excess unaltered permeant within the cells been demonstrated. Thus, e. g., methotrexate immediately forms a complex with the cytoplasmic dihydrofolate reductase and DDUG is tightly bound by the nucleus and mitochondria. Purines, on the other hand, are rapidly converted by the intracellular phosphoribosyltransferases to nucleoside 5′-monophosphates. The nucleosides of purines and pyrimidines react avidly with the corresponding kinases and accumulate again mainly as triphosphates.

Only rarely can one observe a real accumulation of free unaltered permeant within the cells. This is true for most of the amino acids, which can reach 10 to 15 times greater intracellular than extracellular concentrations. However, even in this case the uptake process is considered by some authors to represent only "facilitated diffusion" and not active transport, the concentration gradient being influenced by ion fluxes. It is generally agreed that the only cases which represent a primary active uptake process are the transport of $K^+$ and $Na^+$, which are dependent on the membrane ATPase.

Even though the plasma membranes of liver cells are known to be the reservoirs of more than twenty enzymes (EMMELOT and BOS, 1966), the role of these enzymes as structural parts of the membranes is not understood. Thus, apart from the localization of blood group substances on the outer surfaces of erythrocyte membranes, and ATPase, a lipoprotein responsible for $Na^+$-$K^+$-transport on their inner surfaces, there is little precise information about the localization and distribution of other structural or functional entities in the cell membrane. The exact localization, for example, of antigenic proteins and their role as either functional or structural components of the membrane is not known.

Several proteins believed to be involved in transport of amino acids and sugars have been isolated from bacterial membranes using osmotic shock (KOTYK, 1970). However, caution must be exercised in relating the data concerning bacterial membrane systems to mammalian cells. Bacteria are surrounded by a cell wall composed of several layers. Furthermore, because of the absence in bacteria of several specialized organelles which are present in mammalian cells, the bacterial membranes possess the capabilities of carrying out the functions of missing organelles in addition to their function as a plasma membrane. Any comparisons of bacterial and mammalian transport processes must keep these facts in mind. Isolation of a glucose-binding protein from membranes of human red blood cells has also been reported, but the role of this protein in glucose transport needs clarification (BOBINSKI and STEIN, 1966).

## Effect of Cell Size and Cell Generation Time

Mammalian cell cultures provide an ideal tool for basic research on permeability processes at the cellular level. One serious drawback in the use of cell cultures is the uncertainty of their identity with the tissue of origin. Even though the results obtained in cell culture cannot be directly applied to the situation *in vivo*, cell cultures offer several advantages, the most important being the controllability of the extracellular environment. Even studies on ascites cells in the intraperitoneal cavity of a mouse are complicated by the often unpredictable degree of excretion and metabolism of the compound, which can cause rapid changes in the extracellular environment. On the other hand, when cells are removed from their *in vivo* environment and transferred into a more or less ideal salt solution or tissue culture medium, they are traumatized, as revealed by generally poor long-term survival. Results of such experiments cannot be translated to the *in vivo* situation without reservation. This concerns especially cellular material which has been exposed to an osmotic shock to remove contaminating erythrocytes. Osmotic shock is an effective means of altering the influx and efflux pattern of cells. When using such a technique, comparison of two cell lines with respect to drug uptake is jeopardized because the cells may differ in their resistance to the osmotic shock rather than in uptake *per se*. Established cultures of mammalian cells when used for permeability studies in their "normal" environment, i. e. in the culture medium in which they replicate, are devoid of these drawbacks. Moreover, the permeability data can in this case be directly related to and evaluated with findings concerning the growth inhibitory potency of the same compound in an identical environment.

## A. Cell Size

A compound might pass through the plasma membranes of different cells with identical speed. Yet one might find a faster increase in the intracellular concentration of the compound in one cell than in another. An explanation which is usually overlooked, could be difference in cell size. For example, the average diameter of Sarcoma 180 cells is 19 μ (HAKALA, 1965a), that of L1210 only 9 μ (SIROTNAK et al., 1968) and, therefore, the cell surface area per unit weight is 2-times larger in L1210 than in Sarcoma 180 cells. One can clearly see, that a compound with the same rate of influx through the plasma membranes of both cells, when measured per unit surface area, would enter L1210 cells about 2-times faster than Sarcoma 180 cells when measured on a per unit weight basis. If the uptake of an agent proceeds by diffusion it would also mean that in identical conditions 2-times higher extracellular concentration of the agent would be required in Sarcoma 180 than in L1210 cells for the same uptake per unit weight. The diameters of other mammalian cells vary in wider limits than shown by Sarcoma 180 and L1210 cells, e. g. lymphocytes 9 to 12 μ, plasmocytes 14 to 20 μ, monocytes 16 to 22 μ and megakaryocytes 100 μ, while muscle and nerve cells are very long and cylindrical. The difference in cell size can well be one of the major factors in determining selective action of drugs *in vivo*.

## B. Cell Generation Time

Ordinarily it is thought that inhibitors of cell multiplication act first on the rapidly dividing cells of a population. This is usually true and logical from the point of view that cells which multiply faster must also synthesize all of the cell constituents more rapidly and therefore need more raw materials and energy than more slowly proliferating cells. When the synthesis of macromolecules, such as DNA, is the target of the inhibitor, then indeed the multiplying cell is damaged, while the nonreplicating cell is not.

It might be useful, however, to consider that in some cases the rapidly multiplying cell might escape the inhibitor, while the slowly multiplying cell would not. This would apply if an antineoplastic agent is taken up so slowly that it cannot keep up with the rapid increase in cell mass, every cell division meaning a doubling of the mass including membranes and target enzyme. If it would require, e. g., longer than 10 hours for an agent to reach the necessary intracellular concentration, then the rapidly multiplying cells such as L1210 and P-815, with a generation time of 10 to 12 hours, might be able to escape the agent, while the cells with a generation time of 20 hours or longer would be affected. One may suggest that even a partial block at the target site may slow down the cellular multiplication and give more time for the drug to be taken up. Whether such a "multi-step" process plays a role in aiding the slowly penetrating substances is a hypothetical question.

# Uptake of Individual Agents

## A. Steroids

There is much evidence which shows that steroids are bound to membranes, cytoplasmic proteins, or nuclei. However, direct information on their mode of passage through plasma membranes is still missing. Since the binding of steroids is to a certain degree relevant to their uptake it has been included in the present discussion.

### I. Cholesterol

As mentioned previously, cholesterol is one of the lipoid compounds which are structural elements of the plasma membranes. The cellular uptake of cholesterol, namely, passage through the plasma membrane is not understood. The existing evidence at this time suggests a purely physical adsorption of the compound on the cell surface. This was shown by ROTHBLAT et al. (1968) when they found no difference between the binding of 7α-$^{3}$H-cholesterol to viable and nonviable (30 min at 60°) L-5178Y cells *in vitro*. In general, the adsorption increased with increasing concentration of free cholesterol and was dependent on the presence of serum protein. Using delipidized rabbit serum, these investigators were able to demonstrate a striking inhibition of cholesterol adsorption by certain phospholipids, sphingomyelin being the most effective.

### II. Corticosteroids

Cortisol has been shown to be bound not only to plasma membranes, but also to supernatant proteins. When the high speed supernatant of P1798 mouse lymphosarcoma cells was incubated at 4° with 1,2-$^{3}$H-cortisol, it became bound to a protein fraction (HOLLANDER and CHIU, 1966). The binding was reduced in the presence of cortisone and corticosterone suggesting a common cytoplasmic binding site for all three steroids. It is of interest also that the supernatant of a corticoid-sensitive tumor in a cell-free system had a capacity to bind and retain significantly more cortisol than the supernatant of a resistant tumor. Adrenalectomy was shown to cause an increase in the binding of a synthetic glucocorticoid in sensitive cells (KIRKPATRICK et al., 1972). These authors also observed large differences in the binding capacity in different tissues of the same animal. Recently, one of the four macromolecules of liver cytoplasm that binds cortisol was shown to be identical with the major protein involved in the binding of the carcinogen 3-methylcholanthrene (SINGER and LITWACK, 1971). Another study using HeLa cells and 2,3-$^{3}$H-hydrocortisone, revealed the hormone in nuclei (60%) and cytoplasm (40%) after 48 hours incubation (BER and GRIFFIN, 1967). The major portion (65 to 90%) of the hormone found in these fractions was acid-soluble.

Incubation of isolated plasma membranes of rat liver with $^{3}$H-cortisol (75 min at 37°) also resulted in binding (GRAHAM and GREEN, 1969). Prior removal of unesterified cholesterol from these membrane preparations increased not only the binding of cortisol, but also that of corticosterone. In contrast, this treatment decreased the binding of deoxycorticosterone, progesterone, testosterone, and diethylstilbestrol. Thus, plasma membrane cholesterol plays an important role in regulating the membrane binding of steroids. It should be noted that with the exception of the glucocorticoids, the major role of liver in taking up steroids is their detoxication. The mechanism by which these molecules pass through the plasma membrane is unknown. The binding of steroids by these membranes may represent the first step in the uptake process. One difference between mitochondrial and plasma membranes is the much lower content of cholesterol in the mitochondrial membranes. Thus, it is of interest that the enrichment of mitochondrial membranes with cholesterol resulted in reduced binding of corticosterone and increased binding of testosterone (Graham and Green, 1969). Thus, in both types of membranes, cholesterol has similar regulatory properties regarding the binding of steroid hormones. These authors concluded that the effect of membrane cholesterol on the binding of steroid hormones by the membranes is consistent with the view that a specific arrangement of cholesterol-OH groups is required for steroid uptake.

That corticosteroids have an effect on plasma membranes was indirectly demonstrated by Ballard and Tomkins (1969) using suspension cultures of a Morris hepatoma. These authors observed adhesion of cells to glass in the presence of 0.1 μM cortisol, 10 μM progesterone, or 10 μM corticosterone. It was suggested that these steroids probably induced the synthesis of a cell surface factor, most likely a basic protein. There are numerous reports on the effects of corticosteroids on the uptake of precursors of DNA, RNA, and protein, as well as on the uptake of sugars. In certain tissues these effects appear to be indirect and are not due to interference by the steroids at the plasma membrane level, but rather reflect alterations in intracellular synthetic processes.

## III. Estradiol

Studies on the uptake and binding of $^3$H-estrogen (0.02 μM) in the cytoplasm of isolated rat uteri revealed a rapid saturation (5 min) of the 8 S protein by the hormone and subsequent appearance of estradiol in the nucleus (Giannopoulos and Gorski, 1971a). This sequence of events is associated with the stimulation of nucleolar RNA synthesis caused by estrogen. In rat uterus, after administration *in vivo* or incubation *in vitro*, $^3$H-estradiol was found in bound form mainly in the nuclear fraction. Depending on the method of isolation of the protein it appeared in 8 S, 6 S, 5 S or 4 S forms (Giannopoulos and Gorski, 1971b). The complex of all of these proteins with estradiol had the same dissociation constant ($2$ to $4 \times 10^{-10}$ M) suggesting that the same binding site was involved. It appears that estradiol is transferred from cytoplasm to the nucleus as a protein-estradiol complex. The estrogen binding protein has been purified from calf uterus; the 8 S form was shown to have a molecular weight of 238,000 and the 4 S form 61,000, the 8 S probably being a tetramer of the 4 S form. The dissociation constants of the protein-estradiol complexes were of the order of $3$ to $6 \times 10^{-10}$ M at 4°, suggesting that the binding proteins in calf and rat uterus may be identical. The affinity for 17β-hydroxy estradiol was greater than that for estrone or estriol, and no significant binding of cortisol, progesterone, deoxycorticosterone, or testosterone was observed (Puca et al., 1971).

An interesting correlation was reported for the binding capacity of 6,7-$^3$H-estradiol in hormone responsive and nonresponsive rat tumors (Mobbs, 1966). The responsive tumor accumulated 4- to 10-times more of the hormone than the nonresponsive one. Similar correlation was observed in human breast cancer tissue with regard to accumulation of $^3$H-hexestrol (Folca et al., 1961). The responsive tumors concentrated up to 10-times more of the hormone than nonresponsive ones. The relatively long uptake time (4 h) for 6,7-$^3$H-estradiol was compared in hamster kidney tumors *in vivo*, dependent on, independent of, or nonresponsive to estrogen (Steggles and King, 1968). The dependent tumor took up about 10-times more than the independent neoplasm and the nonresponsive tumor less than the independent one. The results were interpreted as indicating large differences in the amounts of estrogen receptor proteins in these tumors. In rat mammary carcinoma two types of estradiol binding proteins were demonstrated (McGuire and Julian, 1971). One, which occurred only in the hormone-dependent tumors, had a dissociation constant of $1.2 \times 10^{-10}$ M and failed to bind nonestrogenic steroids. The other, which was present in both dependent and independent tumors, bound estradiol much less firmly ($K_D = 10^{-7}$ M).

The general consensus is, that the extent of estradiol uptake depends on the amount of the receptor protein which binds the hormone into a hormone-receptor complex in the cytoplasm and carries it to the nucleus. The receptor protein appears to be low or absent in tumors nonresponsive to hormone therapy. The actual mode of cellular uptake of estradiol is unknown.

## B. Purine and Pyrimidine Bases

When considering the mode of uptake of purine and pyrimidine analogs, one must keep in mind the fate of these agents within cells. As is well established, to inhibit target tissue, enzymes must be present to convert the analogs to their phosphorylated forms, which do not diffuse out of cells. In mammalian tissues there are two distinct enzymes responsible for the conversion of purine bases to their nucleotides, namely, adenine phosphoribosyltransferase (E. C. 2.4.2.7) and hypoxanthine-guanine phosphoribosyltransferase (E. C. 2.4.2.8). Thus, for example, for 6-mercaptopurine to be an effective cytotoxic agent, the target tissue must contain hypoxanthine-guanine phosphoribosyltransferase, which converts it to 6-thioIMP, the active inhibitory form. Indeed, cells and tissues deficient in this enzyme are resistant to 6-mercaptopurine, and cross-resistant to 6-thioguanine and 8-azaguanine. The conversion of pyrimidine bases to their nucleotides may proceed either through orotate phosphoribosyltransferase (E. C. 2.4.2.10) or, after being converted to nucleosides by one of the two pyrimidine nucleoside phosphorylases, through one of three distinct nucleoside kinases (for review see Hakala, 1973).

The mechanism by which analogs of purine and pyrimidine bases pass through plasma membranes is poorly understood; however, some evidence is available to indicate that the uptake of analogs proceeds by the same mechanisms employed for the natural bases. The uptake of physiological bases is relatively well understood having been studied in blood cells, in mammalian cells in culture, and in intestinal epithelium.

### I. Purines (Table 1)

In human red cells the uptake of uric acid ($K_m = 2.8$ mM) was shown to be slow, nonconcentrative (I (intracellular concentration)/E (extracellular concentration) = 0.55) and to be inhibited by hypoxanthine ($K_i = 0.3$ mM), adenine, and guanine, as well as by several nonphysiological purines such as 8-azaguanine, 6-chloropurine, 6-mercaptopurine, and 2,6-diaminopurine (Overgaard-Hansen and Lassen, 1959; Lassen and Overgaard-Hansen, 1962a, b; Lassen, 1962). In these cells, which do not metabolize or accumulate hypoxanthine, its uptake was rapid and proceeded by a two-component system, one saturable ($K_m = 0.4$ mM) and the other nonsaturable (Lassen, 1967). These studies suggested that human erythrocytes utilize a common mechanism for the uptake of purine bases, whether they are of the uric acid, adenine, hypoxanthine, or guanine type. Canine erythrocytes differed from human erythrocytes in that uric acid uptake was less sensitive to inhibition by hypoxanthine (Harvey and Christensen, 1964). In red cells of

Table 1. Uptake of purine bases by mammalian cells[a]

| Compound | Test system | Remarks | Ref. |
|---|---|---|---|
| Uric acid | Human Erythrocytes | $Q_{10}$ 2.2; $K_m = 2.8$ mM; I/E at equilibrium 0.55; Inhibitors: G, 8-AzaG, A, 6-ClP, 6-MP, P, Hx, 2,6-DAP; $K_i$ for Hx = 0.3 mM. | OVERGAARD-HANSEN and LASSEN, 1959; LASSEN, 1962; LASSEN and OVERGAARD-HANSEN 1962a, b |
| Uric acid | Canine Erythrocytes | Slight inhibition by Hx; | HARVEY and CHRISTENSEN (1964) |
| Uric acid | Red cells of Dalmatian coach hound | Uptake not mediated; no inhibition by Hx | |
| Hypoxanthine | Human Erythrocytes | $K_m = 0.4$ mM; I/E at equilibrium = 1.3; two-component system; Hx not metabolized | LASSEN (1967) |
| Adenine | Rabbit Neutrophils | $Q_{10} = 2.3$; two-component system; low $K_m$ at 0.013 to 5 mM; high $K_m$ at 5 to 73 mM; not inhibited by AR | HAWKINS and BERLIN (1969) |
| Hypoxanthine | Rabbit Neutrophils | Velocity: G > A > Hx | HAWKINS and |
| Guanine | Rabbit Neutrophils | >>> X | BERLIN (1969) |
| 8-Azaguanine | Mouse L1210 leukemic cells | Diffusion | DAVIDSON (1958) |
| 6-Mercaptopurine | L1210 cells | Diffusion | |
| Hypoxanthine | L1210 cells, sensitive and resistant to 8-AzaG | 10-times faster in sensitive than in resistant cells; inhibited by 6-MP | DAVIDSON (1958) |
| 6-Mercaptopurine | J128 cells *in vitro* | Uptake inhibited by A, Hx, and AICA | VANDEVOORDE and HANSEN (1967) |
| 6-Mercaptopurine | Normal Human Leukocytes | Diffusion | KESSEL and HALL (1967) |
| Hypoxanthine | Human Fibroblasts | Uptake dependent on Hx-G phosphoribosyltransferase | ROSENBLOOM et al. (1967) |
| Adenine | Ehrlich ascites cells | Diffusion | JACQUEZ and GINSBERG (1960) |
| Adenine | Sarcoma 180 cells *in vitro* | $K_m = 0.14$ mM | HAKALA, unpublished |
| Adenine | Sarcoma 180 cells deficient in A-phosphoribosyltransferase | $K_m = 0.15$ mM; velocity of uptake 1/13th of that in S-180 cells | HAKALA, unpublished |
| Hypoxanthine | Sarcoma 180 cells *in vitro* | $K_m = 0.05$ mM; $V_{max}$ equal to 1/5th of that for A | HAKALA, unpublished |
| 6-Mercaptopurine | Ehrlich ascites cells sensitive and resistant to 6-MP | Uptake impaired in resistant cells; not due to deficiency of Hx-G phosphoribosyltransferase | PATERSON (1962) |
| 6-Thioguanine | Sarcoma 180 cells sensitive and resistant to 6-TG | Diffusion | BIEBER and SARTORELLI (1964) |
| 2,6-Diaminopurine | Mouse L-cells sensitive to 2,6-DAP | $Q_{10} = 1.83$; saturable process; at 4° no difference from resistant cells | BLAIR and HEBERT (1970) |
| 2,6-Diaminopurine | L-cells resistant to 2,6-DAP | Uptake linear, diffusion; these cells deficient in A-phosphoribosyltransferase | BLAIR and HEBERT (1970) |
| Hypoxanthine | Small intestine of rat *in vitro* | At equilibrium serosal/mucosal = 0.9; inhibition by U and T; not active transport | SCHANKER et al. (1963) |

[a] The following abbreviations are used: G, guanine; 8-AzaG, 8-azaguanine; A, adenine; 6-ClP, 6-chloropurine; 6-MP, 6-mercaptopurine; P, purine; Hx, hypoxanthine; 2,6-DAP, 2,6-diaminopurine; AR, adenosine; X, xanthine; AICA, 4(5)-aminoimidazole carboxamide; 6-TG, 6-thioguanine; U, uracil; T, thymine.

the Dalmatian coach hound, the difference was still more pronounced, in that hypoxanthine did not cause any interference with the uptake of uric acid.

The $Q_{10}$ for adenine uptake in rabbit neutrophils was rather low (2.26) and the uptake seemed to consist of two saturable processes, one operative below 5 mM adenine and the other above this level (HAWKINS and BERLIN, 1969). Comparison of the rate of uptake of different purine bases revealed it to be in the following order: guanine> adenine> hypoxanthine>>> xanthine. No conclusion as to the mode of uptake was reached; however, lack of inhibition of adenine uptake by a 100-fold greater concentration of adenosine indicated that the specificity of the uptake of purine bases was different from that of nucleosides. In Ehrlich ascites cells, the uptake of adenine was found to be linear over a concentration range of from 0.1 to 10 mM and to be 5-times faster at 37° than at 4° (JACQUEZ and GINSBERG, 1960); the mode of uptake was thus described as simple diffusion. In Sarcoma 180 cells grown *in vitro*, the uptakes of adenine and hypoxanthine at 36° were found to be saturable processes with apparent $K_m$ values of 0.14 and 0.05 mM and $V_{max}$ values 0.21 and 0.04 nmole/min/mg cells, respectively (HAKALA, unpublished). The velocity of uptake was dependent on the activity of the corresponding PRPP transferase. Thus, in a subline of Sarcoma 180 cells with 1/40th the activity of adenine PRPP transferase, the velocity of adenine uptake was reduced 13-fold; at the same time the $K_m$ value for the uptake was unaltered. Compounds such as $N^6$-isopentenyladenosine and *p*-nitrobenzylthioguanosine, which are potent inhibitors of nucleoside uptake (see below), had no effect on the uptake of adenine.

A number of cell systems sensitive and resistant to purine analogs have been studied with respect to the cellular uptake of the analogs. Thus, in mouse Sarcoma 180 cells, the uptake of 6-thioguanine and 6-mercaptopurine did not differ, whether cells were susceptible or insensitive to 6-thioguanine (BIEBER and SARTORELLI, 1964). The mode of uptake was described as diffusion. Similarly, in L1210 leukemic cells, sensitive and resistant to 8-azaguanine, the uptake of 8-azaguanine and 6-mercaptopurine proceeded by diffusion (DAVIDSON, 1958). The uptake of hypoxanthine, which entered the sensitive cells 10-times more rapidly than the resistant ones, was inhibited by 6-mercaptopurine. In Ehrlich ascites cells resistant to 6-mercaptopurine the uptake of this compound seemed to be impaired, with no difference existing in intracellular activity of hypoxanthine-guanine phosphoribosyltransferase (PATERSON, 1962). In contrast, human fibroblast cells deficient in this enzyme were able to take up adenine, but not hypoxanthine (ROSENBLOOM et al., 1967). An interesting study employing mouse fibroblasts (L-cells) demonstrated that the uptake of 2,6-diaminopurine at 37° was 5 to 6 times faster in sensitive than in resistant cells that were deficient in adenine phosphoribosyltransferase (BLAIR and HEBERT, 1970). At 4° both cells took up the analog equally and by diffusion, leading to the conclusion that the uptake of 2,6-diaminopurine by insensitive cells at 37° was the result of diffusion and that sensitive and resistant cells did not differ with respect to uptake *per se*. Thus it appears that in most mammalian cells studied, the uptake of purines and their analogs proceeds by diffusion, which, at physiological temperatures, is coupled to the intracellular metabolism of the permeant.

An entirely different experimental system, namely, rat small intestine *in vitro*, revealed that the penetration of hypoxanthine from the mucosal to the serosal side was inhibited by both uracil and thymine and that the serosal to mucosal ratio never exceeded 0.9 (SCHANKER et al., 1963). These observations were interpreted to indicate a common facilitated diffusion process for purine and pyrimidine bases.

## II. Pyrimidines (Table 2)

Studies on the uptake of thymine, uracil, and 5-fluorouracil in Ehrlich ascites cells led to the conclusion that these bases were taken up by diffusion, and that thymine was taken up about 3 times faster than uracil and 5-fluorouracil (JACQUEZ, 1962a).

Table 2. Uptake of pyrimidine bases by mammalian cells[a]

| Compound | Test system | Remarks | Ref. |
|---|---|---|---|
| Thymine<br>Uracil<br>5-Fluorouracil | Ehrlich ascites cells *in vitro* | Diffusion; T taken up 3 times faster than U and FU | JACQUEZ (1962a) |
| Uracil | Small intestine of rat *in vitro* | At equilibrium serosal/mucosal = 4.7; U not metabolized; potent inhibitors: T, FU, BrU and Hx; poor inhibitors: C, A, 6-AzaU and 6-AzaT; uptake saturable | SCHANKER and JEFFREY (1961, 1962); SCHANKER and TOCCO (1962); SCHANKER et al. (1963) |
| Thymine | Rat small intestine *in vitro* | At equilibrium serosal/mucosal = 2.8; inhibited competitively by U; strong inhibitor: Hx; poor inhibitors: C, 6-AzaT and 6-AzaU | SCHANKER and TOCCO (1960) |
| Cytosine | Rat small intestine *in vitro* | At equilibrium serosal/mucosal = 0.82 | SCHANKER and JEFFREY (1962) |
| 5-Fluorouracil | Rat small intestine *in vitro* | At equilibrium serosal/mucosal = 4.5; FU not metabolized; uptake saturable | SCHANKER and JEFFREY (1961) |
| 5-Bromouracil | Rat small intestine *in vitro* | At equilibrium serosal/mucosal = 3.0; BrU not metabolized; uptake saturable | SCHANKER and JEFFREY (1961) |
| 5-Fluorouracil | Human normal leukocytes | Diffusion | KESSEL and HALL (1967) |

[a] The following abbreviations are used: T, thymine; U, uracil; FU, 5-fluorouracil; BrU, 5-bromouracil; Hx, hypoxanthine; C, cytosine; A, adenine; 6-AzaU, 6-azauracil; 6-AzaT, 6-azathymine.

Using rat small intestine *in vitro*, it was found that at steady state the serosal to mucosal distribution ratio for pyrimidines decreased in the order of uracil (4.7), 5-fluorouracil (4.5), 5-bromouracil (3.0), thymine (2.8), and cytosine (0.82) (SCHANKER and TOCCO, 1960, 1962; SCHANKER and JEFFREY, 1961, 1962). No metabolic alteration of uracil, 5-fluorouracil, or 5-bromouracil was noted in this system. The most potent inhibitors of uracil uptake were thymine, 5-fluorouracil, 5-bromouracil, and hypoxanthine. Xanthine, uric acid, cytosine, 6-azauracil, 6-azathymine, guanine, and adenine were poor inhibitors. In agreement with these observations, the uptake of thymine was inhibited competitively by uracil and markedly by hypoxanthine. It was concluded that purine and pyrimidine bases share a common transport system through the intestinal mucosa.

## C. Purine and Pyrimidine Nucleosides

As in the case of analogs of purine and pyrimidine bases, the nucleoside analogs must also be converted to the corresponding nucleotides to be active as antineoplastic agents. For purine nucleosides, there are three different kinase enzymes, one for adenosine, one for deoxyadenosine and deoxyguanosine, and the third, whose existence was long disputed, for inosine and guanosine. For pyrimidine nucleosides there are also three kinase enzymes, one for uridine and cytidine, another for thymidine and deoxyuridine, and the third for deoxycytidine. An interesting overlap of substrate specificity is observed between the purine and pyrimidine enzymes. Thus, deoxyadenosine-deoxyguanosine kinase acts also on cytidine, and deoxyadenosine and deoxyguanosine are substrates for deoxycytidine kinase. It is possible that the latter enzyme actually is the physiological kinase for deoxyadenosine and deoxyguanosine as judged by $K_m$ values, which are lower for this enzyme than for the enzyme usually identified as deoxyadenosine-deoxyguanosine kinase (for review see HAKALA, 1973).

The uptake of natural nucleosides has been studied more extensively than that of free bases. Only a few investigations exist that are concerned with the uptake of nucleoside analogs. Again it appears that the uptake of the nucleoside analogs proceeds by the same basic mechanisms as those of their natural counterparts, whose uptake will be considered in detail.

The uptake of purine nucleosides by erythrocytes has been of special interest since it is known that these cells lack the ability both to synthesize purine nucleotides *de novo* and to convert IMP to AMP (LOWY et al., 1962). Thus, inosine and guanosine, which are taken up rapidly, serve, after being converted to free purines, as precursors of GTP only. On the other hand, adenosine, which is also taken up rapidly, serves mainly as a precursor of ATP (LOWY and WILLIAMS, 1966), but after deamination to inosine and its further conversion to hypoxanthine, adenosine can be the source of guanine nucleotides as well.

In canine erythrocytes the $K_m$ for adenosine uptake, which appears to proceed by facilitated diffusion, was 0.25 mM, and the heat of activation 15.6 kcal per mole (KÜBLER and BRETSCHNEIDER, 1964). The uptake was competitively inhibited by inosine employed at mM levels and by persantin (dipyridamole) at the 0.1 μM level. The effect of persantin is of interest because this compound potentiated 40-fold the dilating effect on coronary vessels of adenosine administered i. v. It appears that persantin prolongs the presence of adenosine in the plasma by preventing its otherwise rapid uptake into the erythrocytes. The uptake of uridine ($K_m = 0.7$ or 3 mM), thymidine and cytidine ($K_m = 1.1$ mM) by human erythrocytes, which do not metabolize these nucleosides, was shown to be inhibited at μM levels by a totally unrelated nucleoside, *p*-nitrobenzylthioguanosine, which became firmly bound to these cells (PATERSON and SIMPSON, 1966; OLIVER and PATERSON, 1971; PATERSON and OLIVER, 1971). The uptake of uridine was also competitively inhibited by formycin B ($K_i = 0.32$ mM). *p*-Nitrobenzylthioguanosine, which had no effect on the uptake of free bases, was also a potent inhibitor of the uptake of inosine and guanosine by human erythrocytes. The uptake of all of these nucleosides is considered to proceed by facilitated diffusion.

Studies on the uptake of purine nucleoside analogs by erythrocytes include those on tubercidin, 7-deazainosine, and 6-methylmercaptopurine ribonucleoside. Tubercidin, an adenosine analog, was shown to be taken up rapidly, being converted mainly to the triphosphate (SMITH et al., 1970). The inosine analog, 7-deazainosine, was taken up by human erythrocytes at a rate only 1/100 of that of tubercidin. This difference probably reflects the low level or absence of inosine kinase in erythrocytes and the resistance of 7-deazainosine to phosphorolysis. Another adenosine analog, 6-methylmercaptopurine ribonucleoside, is also taken up by human erythrocytes ($K_m = 0.47$ mM) and phosphorylated to its 5′-monophosphate only (LOO et al., 1969). The energy of activation for this uptake was 6.5 kcal per mole and the $Q_{10} = 1.4$. The uptake of 6-methylmercaptopurine ribonucleoside was competitively inhibited by adenosine, deoxyadenosine, and $N^6$-methyladenosine with $K_i$ values of 2.1 to 7.8 mM.

Novikoff heptatoma cells in culture have found wide use in studies of nucleoside uptake. Thus, it was shown that 80 to 90% of thymidine taken up by these cells was rapidly converted to thymidine triphosphate (GENTRY et al., 1965). Uptake of uridine ($K_m = 0.013$ mM) by these cells was shown to be competitively inhibited by such unrelated compounds as adenosine ($K_i = 0.13$ mM), persantin ($K_i = 4$ μM) and phenethyl alcohol ($K_i = 3.5$ mM) (PLAGEMANN and ROTH, 1969). It was concluded that the uptake of uridine was independent of the action of uridine kinase; this was corroborated by the absence of uridine kinase activity in isolated plasma membrane fractions of these cells. Even though uridine kinase was not instrumental in the actual uptake process it was shown to affect the uptake into the nucleotide pool (PLAGEMANN et al., 1969). Thus, during the cell cycle the activity of this enzyme was shown to vary up to 10-fold, causing corresponding variation in the rate of uridine entry into the nucleotide pool. A similar dependence of uptake on uridine kinase activity was observed in human lymphocytes transformed by phytohemagglutinin; these cells showed 20-fold increases in uridine kinase and in the incorporation of uridine into the nucleotide pool (LUCAS, 1967; HANSEN and STEIN, 1968). Further studies using Novikoff hepatoma cells have indicated that uridine and cytidine ($K_m = 23$ μM) may share a common transport process which is distinct from that for adenosine ($K_m = 8.8$ μM), inosine ($K_m = 11$ μM), or guanosine ($K_m = 12$ μM) (PLAGEMANN, 1971). These conclusions were based on the $K_m/K_i$ ratios for mutual inhibitions of uptake. The ratio was equal to 1.0 within each specific system, but varied up to 600-fold from one system to another. Heat treatment (5 min, 47.5°) of these cells, which resulted in different degrees of inactivation of each transport process, was considered as additional evidence for separate processes. The specificity of the "separate" uptake processes, however, resembles the specificity for the kinase enzymes involved and, therefore, the mutual inhibitions as well as the heat inactivations may be the result of different intracellular metabolism of these nucleosides rather than effects on their membrane passage. A common uptake process for all purine and pyrimidine nucleosides is suggested by the data of PLAGEMANN (1971), which shows similar competitive inhibitions exerted on the uptake of every nucleoside by thymidine ($K_i = 0.26$ to 0.56 mM), persantin ($K_i = 2.4$ to 5.8 μM) and phenethyl alcohol ($K_i = 1.6$ to 3.6 mM).

Studies concerned with the uptake of pyrimidine nucleoside analogs have been performed using mouse tumor systems. The uptake of 5-fluorouridine by P-388 mouse leukemia cells deficient in uridine phosphorylase and uridine kinase had a $K_m$ of 2.5 mM and $Q_{10}$ of 1.3 (KESSEL et al., 1971). The uptake was considered to be facilitated diffusion and was inhibited competitively by deoxycytidine and uridine, but not by adenosine or 5-fluorouracil. The uptake of 5-fluorouridine, 5-fluorodeoxyuridine, arabinosyl-5-fluorouracil and the corresponding natural nucleosides by Ehrlich ascites cells appeared to proceed by passive or facilitated diffusion (JACQUEZ, 1962). In L1210 cells lacking deoxycytidine deaminase and deoxycytidine kinase, the uptake of deoxycytidine ($K_m = 7.5$ mM) and arabinosylcytosine appeared to be by facilitated diffusion (KESSEL and SHURIN, 1968). The uptake of deoxycytidine by these cells was inhibited by purine and pyrimidine nucleosides and noncompetitively by persantin (KESSEL and HALL, 1970).

In Sarcoma 180 cells *in vitro*, the uptake of adenosine was more rapid than that of any other nucleoside (HAKALA et al., 1973). After 15 min at 10 μM 8-$^{14}$C-adenosine, the I/E ratio for $^{14}$C was 125, but less than 0.5% of the cellular $^{14}$C was in the form of unaltered adenosine. The maximal velocities and the $K_m$ values for the uptake decreased in the following order: ribosylpurines > ribosylpyrimidines > deoxyribosylpurines > deoxyribosylpyrimidines. There was no correlation between the $K_m$ values for the uptake and the $K_m$ values for the corresponding kinases, while the activity of the kinases determined the velocity of uptake. This was clearly demonstrated in two sublines of Sarcoma 180 cells which differed 20,000-fold with respect to adenosine kinase activity (DIVEKAR et al., 1972). In these cells the velocity of uptake of $N^6$-($\triangle^2$-isopentenyl)adenosine differed 40-fold while the $K_m$ values were not significantly different. Several $N^6$-substituted adenosine analogs were potent inhibitors of the uptake of all the natural purine and pyrimidine nucleosides (HAKALA et al., 1971; HAKALA and KENNY, 1972). The uptake of deoxyribonucleosides was generally less sensitive to inhibition than the uptake of ribonucleosides and $N^6$-substituted deoxyadenosine was a much more potent inhibitor than the corresponding $N^6$-substituted adenosine. Studies on Sarcoma 180 cells indicate that deoxyribose and pyrimidine moieties increase the affinity of the nucleoside for the plasma membrane as compared with ribose and purine moieties, respectively.

In several cellular systems, diverse organic compounds which had no effect on intracellular enzymes, had profound effects on the uptake of extracellular nucleosides. Among these are *p*-nitrobenzylthioguanosine, persantin, phenethylalcohol, mercaptopyridethylbenzimidazole (BUCKNALL and CARTER, 1967; NAKATA and BADER, 1969), streptovaricin D (TAN and MCAUSLAN, 1971), and dimethylsulfoxide (COLLINS and ROBERTS, 1971). The general conclusion appears to be that the purine and pyrimidine nucleosides are taken up by mammalian cells by a common facilitated diffusion process not involving nucleoside kinases, even though the activity of these enzymes affects the rate and extent of uptake. The inhibition of nucleoside passage through plasma membranes by unrelated nucleosides, as well as by diverse organic compounds, suggests that caution must be exerted in interpreting results of studies designed to measure effects on the incorporation of precursor nucleosides into DNA and RNA.

## D. Purine and Pyrimidine Nucleotides

ROLL et al. (1956) showed that the incorporation of 2′ and 3′ isomers of AMP and GMP into visceral nucleic acids was preceded by extensive dephosphorylation. Studies in other cellular systems have also demonstrated that nucleoside phosphates *per se* are unable to penetrate plasma membranes, and are first cleaved to the corresponding nucleosides and taken up as such. The presence of 5′-nucleotidase in plasma membranes of liver cells has been demonstrated (SONG et al., 1969) and, therefore, the cleavage of the phosphate can occur at the cell membrane. However, in human blood the cleavage of AMP to adenosine was believed to occur in the plasma (KÜBLER and BRETSCHNEIDER, 1964; HOLMSEN and ROZENBERG, 1968). In human platelets, dog erythrocytes and Ehrlich ascites cells (LEIBMAN and HEIDELBERGER, 1955), 2′-, 3′-, and 5′-AMP have been shown to be taken up in the form of adenosine. Other nucleotides such as 2′-, 3′-, and 5′-CMP, UMP, and GMP are similarly cleaved before entering Ehrlich ascites cells. Also the passage of 5′-TMP, 5′-CMP, and 5′-UMP through the small intestine of the rat or the golden hamster was associated with a cleavage to the corresponding nucleoside (WILSON and WILSON, 1954, 1958). It is likely that the uptake of the 5′-phosphate of tubercidin by human erythrocytes also involved prior breakdown to tubercidin, as judged by the much slower (1/30th) passage of the nucleotide as compared with tubercidin itself (SMITH et al., 1970). Lack of affinity of a nucleotide for the nucleoside uptake process was indicated by showing that CMP had no effect on the uptake of arabinosylcytosine in L1210 cells (KESSEL and SHURIN, 1968). In contrast, in Sarcoma 180 cells the uptake of 5'-AMP-8-$^{14}$C resembled that of adenosine with respect to both kinetics and inhibitor specificity, indicating its cleavage to adenosine prior to membrane passage (HAKALA, unpublished).

Indirect evidence, however, suggests that certain types of nucleotides pass the plasma membrane intact. One of these is cyclic AMP which, on the basis of its biological effects, must be assumed to be taken up as such (for pertinent references see JOST and RICKENBERG, 1971). Such a conclusion was reached in studies of several cell lines in culture (RYAN and HEIDRICK, 1968; HEIDRICK and RYAN, 1970). The growth of these cells was inhibited by 0.12 and 0.3 mM cyclic AMP, whereas similar concentrations of adenosine or 5'-AMP had no effect. However, recent studies on Novikoff rat hepatoma cells in culture (SCHRÖDER and PLAGEMANN, 1971) revealed no direct uptake of cyclic AMP. Labeled cyclic AMP entered the cells only after being degraded to adenosine in the surrounding medium.

A nucleotide antimetabolite, *bis*(thioinosine) 5',5''-phosphate also appeared to be taken up by H. Ep. cells which were incapable of converting 6-mercaptopurine to 6-thioinosinic acid (MONTGOMERY et al., 1963). This was indicated by inhibition of the growth of these cells by the nucleotide analog. Similarly, by comparing the inhibition of sensitive and resistant P815 mouse leukemia cells, it was concluded that the N$^4$-octanoyl derivative of 3',5'-cyclic phosphate of 1-$\beta$-D-arabinofuranosylcytosine entered these cells (KREIS and WECHTER, 1972). Another nucleotide analog, 9-$\beta$-D-arabinofuranosyladenine 5'-monophosphate, was reported to penetrate into L-cells in small amounts as the intact nucleotide (PLUNKETT et al., 1973).

## E. Folate Analogs

The folate analog studied most thoroughly with respect to cellular uptake is amethopterin, (4-amino, $N^{10}$-methylfolate), also called methotrexate (MTX). This compound is tightly bound to dihydrofolate reductase (DFR, 5,6,7,8-tetrahydrofolate:NADP-oxidoreductase, E. C. 1.5.1.3) (WERKHEISER, 1961) due to the 2,4-diamino structure (ZAKRZEWSKI, 1963a, 1963b). Therefore, as long as DFR is available, no free MTX can be detected within the cells. This finding provided an excellent tool for studying the initial rate of influx of MTX into cells and was first taken advantage of in the Sarcoma 180 cell system *in vitro* (HAKALA, 1965a, b). The analytical methods used in studies of uptake have included titration with DFR of the MTX liberated from cellular DFR by heat (HAKALA, 1965a, b), microbiological assay (DIVEKAR et al., 1967; BRAGANCA et al., 1967), spectrophotometric assay (JACQUEZ, 1966) and later, tritiated MTX. While the biological methods were tedious, their use guarded against some misinterpretations which occurred with the use of labeled drug (GOLDMAN et al., 1968; LICHTENSTEIN and GOLDMAN, 1970). The use of biological methodology, on the other hand, is limited by the concentrations of MTX that can be studied with confidence because of the generally rather low cellular DFR content. In the case of Sarcoma 180 cells this limitation was overcome by taking advantage of cell lines resistant to MTX that contained greatly elevated levels of DFR (up to 700 mμmoles per g dry weight), and did not differ with respect to the plasma membrane passage of MTX (HAKALA, 1965a, b). An exact comparison of the MTX uptake data reported in the literature is impossible. This is due in small part to variations in methodology and to the use of different units of measurement. More serious difficulties arise from the fact that many MTX uptake studies do not distinguish the initial velocity of uptake from the saturation of cellular DFR. At a state of saturation the data no longer reflect the actual influx velocity, the true values necessarily being greater than those reported. This limitation applies especially to most of the data on human cells, which contain only traces of DFR (HALL et al., 1966; KESSEL et al., 1968a, b). The only data that report the actual influx velocities concern Sarcoma 180, the L1210 leukemia, and rabbit reticulocytes (HAKALA, 1965a; GOLDMAN et al., 1968; BOBZIEN and GOLDMAN, 1972). Unfortunately, even these studies differ with respect to conditions used, as is discussed below.

## I. Concentration Versus Uptake

The rate of influx of MTX in Sarcoma 180 cells was found to be directly proportional to the extracellular concentration of drug from 0.3 to 300 μM MTX (HAKALA, 1965a). These data indicate either a simple diffusion process or one saturable above 300 μM MTX. In these studies the rate of uptake was so slow that when cells were incubated in a medium containing 1 μM MTX, more than an hour was estimated to be required to saturate all of the DFR in the sensitive Sarcoma 180 cells. The rate of uptake was therefore clearly the limiting factor for the cytotoxic effect of MTX in these neoplastic cells. In Ehrlich ascites cells the uptake of mM levels of MTX resembled diffusion, with a rate constant 1/10th that for Sarcoma 180 cells (JACQUEZ, 1966).

An uptake process which was saturable at 10 μM MTX was reported for L5178Y cells (FISCHER, 1962). A saturable process has also been reported for L1210 cells within 0.5 to 9 μM MTX with a $K_m$ of 0.4 μM (SIROTNAK et al., 1968) or 3 to 10 μM (GOLDMAN et al., 1968), and in Yoshida sarcoma cells (DIVEKAR et al., 1967). An uptake process which roughly resembled a Michaelis-Menten relationship with a $K_m$ of 1.4 μM was also observed in rabbit reticulocytes (BOBZIEN and GOLDMAN, 1972). Large differences have been noted between cell lines with respect to the velocity of uptake of MTX (see below).

## II. Intracellular Accumulation of Free Methotrexate

In order to interpret the mode of uptake of MTX it is essential to know the concentration of free MTX in cell water in the steady state, as opposed to MTX bound by DFR and thus not available for free exchange. Only few studies provide clear documentation of these factors. The studies in the Sarcoma 180 cell system, which included simultaneous determination of free and bound MTX, as well as of free DFR (if any), showed that even at a steady state, when all of the DFR was saturated by MTX, the free intracellular MTX remained less than 1/10th that of the extracellular concentration at 30 to 100 μM MTX. Lack of intracellular accumulation of MTX was also noted in human granulocytes; the total intracellular MTX (free + bound) remained far below (1/5th to 1/30th) the extracellular MTX concentration at 0.2 to 200 μM (KESSEL et al., 1968b). Also, small human lymphocytes never contained more than 1/40th of the extracellular MTX level. In rabbit reticulocytes, free intracellular MTX (with 15 μM MTX) was only 20% of the expected level for equilibrium in a passive system (BOBZIEN and GOLDMAN, 1972). At steady state L1210 leukemia cells also had free intracellular concentrations of MTX below extracellular levels, namely, 0.75 μM at 1 μM MTX and 5 μM at 10 μM MTX (GOLDMAN et al., 1968). If the divalent anionic nature of MTX is taken into account, low intracellular/extracellular ratios for equilibrium in a diffusion system can be predicted. Even taking this factor into consideration, it appears that in most of the cell systems cited above, the influx of MTX proceeds downhill. In this regard it is of interest that glutamic acid, which also has two negative charges and is believed by some to be taken up by facilitated diffusion (others believe active transport is involved), was found at a 13 to 19 mM level in Sarcoma 180 cell water, in a steady state with 9 mM extracellular glutamic acid (HAKALA et al., in press).

A number of other observations suggest that MTX uptake involves influx against a concentration gradient. In most of these studies the simultaneous determination of bound intracellular MTX was not carried out. Thus, L1210 cells were reported to accumulate free MTX 8-times above the extracellular level (SIROTNAK et al., 1968). Similarly, L5178Y cells at equilibrium were said to contain 2- to 3-times the level present in the medium and only a fraction of this was bound (FISCHER, 1962). Sensitive Yoshida sarcoma cells of the rat were reported to contain free aminopterin at 2.4-times the 0.9 μM level outside (DIVEKAR et al., 1967), and renal cortical slices of rabbit appeared to accumulate MTX above the extracellular level (RUBIN et al., 1967).

## III. Energetics of Methotrexate Uptake

In most studies the uptake of MTX has been found to be highly dependent on temperature. In the Sarcoma 180 cell system, at 10 to 40°, an activation energy of 30.5 kcal/mole and a $Q_{10}$ of 6.2 were found (HAKALA, 1965b). Similar values were found for L1210 cells at 23 to 40°, namely, 35.2 kcal/mole and a $Q_{10}$ of 6.9 (GOLDMAN et al., 1968). Another study employing L1210 leukemic cells indicated a $Q_{10}$ of 15 (KESSEL, 1969), and in Yoshida sarcoma cells the $Q_{10}$ for aminopterin was 2.0 at 25 to 35° (DIVEKAR et al., 1967). In human granulocytes, but not in small lymphocytes, MTX uptake was also quite dependent on temperature (KESSEL et al., 1968b).

At least part of the high energy requirement for MTX uptake is due to the very unfavorable properties of the MTX molecule for plasma membrane passage. Thus, MTX is poorly lipid soluble (HAKALA, 1965b) and has a net negative charge at physiological pH, the mean pK being 5.2. The importance of charge was made clear by showing that the rate of uptake of MTX in Sarcoma 180 cells more than doubled as a consequence of lowering the extracellular pH to 5.5 (HAKALA, 1965b).

## IV. Methotrexate Efflux

In both Sarcoma 180 and L1210 cells the efflux of MTX appeared to be more rapid than the influx (HAKALA, 1965b; GOLDMAN et al., 1968). Furthermore, it appears that inhibitors of energy metabolism, such as 2,4-dinitrophenol (HAKALA, 1965b) and sodium azide (GOLDMAN, 1969), inhibit mainly the efflux leading to an increased net uptake rate, as well as to an increased intracellular concentration of free MTX at steady state (see below).

## V. Inhibitors of Energy Metabolism

The inhibitor of energy metabolism 2,4-dinitrophenol, at a level of 0.1 to 1 mM, increased the net rate of uptake of MTX by 50 to 140% in Sarcoma 180 cells and altered the steady state intra: extra cellular ratio of free MTX from less than 0.1 to 1.0 (HAKALA, 1965b). In L1210 cells, stimulation of MTX uptake by 2,4-dinitrophenol was also seen (GOLDMAN, 1971a), while in both normal and leukemic human leukocytes, 1 mM 2,4-dinitrophenol had no effect (KESSEL et al., 1968b), and in Yoshida sarcoma cells 2,4-dinitrophenol had no effect on the extent of aminopterin uptake (DIVEKAR et al., 1967). In contrast, in rabbit kidney cortex slices 1 mM 2,4-dinitrophenol and 100 μM iodoacetic acid inhibited MTX uptake by about 50% (RUBIN et al., 1967).

Another metabolic poison, sodium azide, had no effect on MTX uptake in Sarcoma 180 cells at a concentration of 1 mM (HAKALA, 1965b), while in L1210 cells sodium azide at 10 mM caused a 4-fold increase in the steady state level of intracellular MTX (GOLDMAN, 1969). The effect of sodium azide was prevented by including an energy source in the electrolyte incubation medium. This finding may explain the lack of effect of sodium azide in Sarcoma 180 cells which were incubated in cell culture medium containing 5.5 mM glucose. The inhibitor of SH groups, *p*-chloromercuribenzoate, at a level of 100 μM had no effect on MTX uptake in Sarcoma 180 (HAKALA, 1965b), but was a potent inhibitor of the same process in L1210 cells (GOLDMAN et al., 1968). In rabbit kidney cortex slices, 100 μM mercuric chloride had only slight effect on MTX uptake (RUBIN et al., 1967).

## VI. Effects of other Inhibitors

In Sarcoma 180 tumor cells the influx of 5 μM MTX was inhibited almost 50% by 27 μM riboflavin (HAKALA, 1965b), while in L1210 cells the uptake of $^{3}$H-MTX was reported to be greatly stimulated by riboflavin-5′-phosphate (GOLDMAN et al., 1968). The latter was due to a photochemical breakdown of $^{3}$H-MTX in the presence of the flavin (LICHTENSTEIN and GOLDMAN, 1970). Such a breakdown of folic acid in the presence of riboflavin-5′-phosphate was observed earlier by ROBERTS (1961). The breakdown product was not bound to DFR and was taken up more rapidly than MTX. Riboflavin-5′-phosphate was actually found to be a competitive inhibitor of MTX uptake in L1210 cells with a $K_i$ of 0.34 mM; such inhibition was possibly due to the phosphate group (see below). With Sarcoma cells, 100 to 200 μM folinic acid inhibited the uptake of 10 to 20 μM MTX by 50 to 70% (HAKALA, 1965b, 1969). The latter inhibition was not strictly competitive and 100 μM folic and dihydrofolic acids had no effect on MTX uptake. In L1210 cells, 5-methyltetrahydrofolate, folinic acid, and folic acid were shown to be competitive inhibitors of MTX uptake with $K_i$ values of 1 μM, 3 to 5 μM, and 0.2 to 0.26 mM, respectively (GOLDMAN et al., 1968; GOLDMAN, 1971b). Thus, in L1210 cells, folinic acid appears to have an affinity for the uptake process equal to that of MTX. Indeed, it had been shown earlier in both L1210 and Ehrlich ascites cells that folinic acid inhibited $^{3}$H-MTX uptake as effectively as unlabeled MTX (KESSEL and HALL, 1967b). In another study using L1210 leukemic cells, the uptake of labeled folinic acid had a $K_m$ of 2.5 μM and was competitively inhibited by MTX with a $K_i$ of 7.7 μM (NAHAS et al., 1969). Another study, which also employed L1210 cells, revealed 40% and 65% inhibition of MTX uptake by 1000-fold higher concentrations of folic and dihydrofolic acids, respectively (SIROTNAK et al., 1968). Folic acid was also a poor inhibitor of aminopterin uptake in Yoshida sarcoma cells (DIVEKAR et al., 1967) and of MTX in rabbit kidney cortex slices (RUBIN et al., 1967). In the latter system, folinic acid had no effect on MTX uptake.

There are conflicting reports on the effect of glucose or pyruvate on MTX uptake. In L1210 cells these metabolites were shown to decrease the rate of influx of MTX (GOLDMAN, 1969), while in human leukocytes (KESSEL et al., 1968b) and in rabbit kidney slices (RUBIN et al., 1967), no effect of glucose was noted. Serum, on the other hand, has been shown to decrease the rate of MTX uptake in human leukocytes (KESSEL et al., 1968b), as did human serum albumin in Ehrlich ascites cells (GOLDMAN, 1971a). The inhibitory effect of serum on MTX uptake is probably due to the binding of MTX to serum albumin (HENDERSON et al., 1965). Organic phosphates and inorganic anions such as nitrate, sulfate, and phosphate were also reported to inhibit MTX uptake in Ehrlich ascites cells (GOLDMAN, 1971a).

## VII. Uptake of other Folate Analogs

The rates of uptake of aminopterin, MTX, and dichloromethotrexate into Sarcoma 180 cells were equal, yet the concentrations producing 50% inhibition of growth required the following ratio 1:4:10 (Hakala, 1969). Studies with L1210 and Ehrlich ascites cells showed that aminopterin and dichloromethotrexate reduced the uptake of $^3$H-MTX and unlabeled MTX equally well (Kessel and Hall, 1967b). Similarly, in rabbit kidney cortex slices dichloromethotrexate, 3-bromomethotrexate and triamterene were as effective as unlabeled MTX in reducing the uptake of $^3$H-MTX (Rubin et al., 1967). In human white blood cells, triamterene increased the uptake of MTX by 3-fold (Hall et al., 1966).

## VIII. Comparison of Cells with Respect to Methotrexate Uptake

Table 3 provides only a rough comparison between different cell lines because the data reflect not only the rate of influx, but also the content of DFR in these cells. Even so, the comparison reveals enormous differences between cells with respect to MTX uptake. The 25-times more rapid rate of MTX uptake by L1210 cells, as compared to Sarcoma 180 cells, is partially due to the smaller size of the

Table 3. Comparison of the rates of uptake of methotrexate (MTX) by mammalian cells

| Species | Cell type | Reported data on the rate of MTX uptake | Relative rate | Ref. |
|---|---|---|---|---|
| Mouse | Sarcoma 180 | At 1 μM MTX influx rate = 0.4 μmole/h/kg cell pellet[a] = 0.04 mμmole/min/g dry weight | 1.0 | Hakala (1965a, b) |
| | L1210 leukemia | At 1 μM MTX influx rate = 1 mμmole/min/g dry weight | 25.0 | Goldman et al. (1968) |
| | | $V_{max}$ = 5.6 mμmoles/min/g dry weight | | |
| | L1210 leukemia | $V_{max}$ = 4.5 mμmoles/min/g dry weight | 20.0 | Sirotnak et al. (1968) |
| | P288 lymphoma | Similar to L1210 leukemia | 20.0 | Kessel et al. (1965) |
| | P1534 lymphoma | 1/13th of the rate in L1210 leukemia | 2.0 | Kessel (1969) |
| | Ehrlich carcinoma | At 20° half the rate in L1210 leukemia | 10.0 | Kessel and Hall (1967) |
| | Ehrlich carcinoma | At mM MTX 1/10th of that in Sarcoma 180 | 0.1 | Jacquez (1966) |
| Rat | Yoshida sarcoma | 10-Times faster than in Sarcoma 180 | 10.0 | Divekar et al. (1967) |
| Rabbit | Reticulocytes | $V_{max}$ 1/20th that in L1210 leukemia | 0.20 | Bobzien and Goldman (1972) |
| Human | Granulocytes | 0.012 mμmole/min/g dry weight | 0.30 | Kessel et al. (1968a, b) |
| | Acute myelocytic leukemia | 24 mμmoles/15 min/kg wet weight[a] | 0.25 | |
| | Small lymphocytes | 6 mμmoles/15 min/kg wet weight[a] | 0.055 | |
| | Chronic lymphocytic leukemia | Same as small lymphocytes | 0.055 | |

[a] Dry weight estimated as 18% of wet weight (Hakala, 1965a).

L1210 cells. Thus, the ratio of cell surface to volume of the L1210 leukemia is 2.5-times that of Sarcoma 180 (HAKALA, 1969). Other factors that most likely are partially responsible for the difference are experimental conditions. For example, while MTX uptake by L1210 cells was studied in suspensions in inorganic buffers devoid of an energy source, Sarcoma 180 cells were incubated as monolayers on glass in their "physiological environment," i. e. in cell culture medium containing salts, glucose, amino acids, vitamins, and 10% serum. The latter conditions allowed direct correlation of uptake data with measurements of cytotoxicity of MTX. The cell culture medium contains several ingredients which have been shown to decrease MTX uptake, such as riboflavin, glucose, and serum (HAKALA, 1965b, KESSEL et al., 1968b; GOLDMAN, 1969). An additional factor which may have increased the difference between the two cell lines is the deletion of intracellular reduced folates from Sarcoma 180 cells prior to their use for MTX uptake studies. This was not done with L1210 leukemic cells, and accumulated intracellular reduced folates have been shown to increase the rate of influx of MTX by hetero-exchange (GOLDMAN, 1971b). It is doubtful, however, that even the sum of these multiple factors could be responsible for the 25-fold difference in the rate of uptake of MTX by these cells. Indeed, it is of interest that the 50% growth inhibitory concentrations of MTX under conditions of cell culture were $1.7 \times 10^{-8}$ M for the L1210 leukemia (GRINDEY and NICHOL, 1972) and $5.4 \times 10^{-8}$ M for Sarcoma 180 (HAKALA et al., 1961), i. e., Sarcoma 180 cells were 3-times more resistant to MTX. It appears that the rate of uptake of MTX plays a critical role in determining the inherent sensitivity of cells to MTX. Thus, the difference in MTX sensitivity of L1210 and Sarcoma 180 cells *in vivo*, most likely is due to the difference in the rate of uptake of MTX. L1210 cells are sensitive to MTX therapy in spite of the fact that their DFR content (10 mμmoles/g dry weight) is 5-times greater than that of Sarcoma 180 cells (2 mμmoles/g dry weight). These findings appear operative at the level of man, since the uptake of MTX in human leukemic cells responsive to MTX therapy (i. e., acute myelocytic leukemia) appears faster than in naturally unresponsive neoplastic cells (i. e., chronic lymphocytic leukemia). An effective uptake of MTX by the target cells is essential for successful chemotherapy with the agent because of its rapid disappearance and low blood levels (about 0.2 μM) during human chemotherapy (HENDERSON et al., 1965). In view of these data, it must be concluded that plasma membranes of mammalian cells, even within one species, differ greatly with respect to MTX passage.

## IX. The Mode of Uptake of Methotrexate

The foregoing discussion described not only a large variation between data, but also a variation in interpretation of data. Thus, MTX uptake has been considered to be (a) a passive diffusion, (b) facilitated diffusion, and (c) an active transport. In Sarcoma 180 cells the MTX uptake system is relatively simple, consisting of influx, efflux, binding to DFR, and release. By far the fastest step was the binding to DFR; the velocities of the different processes being in the general order of: binding $\gg$ efflux $>$ influx $\gg$ release from DFR (HAKALA, 1965b). Even though the high energy of activation indicated active transport, this conclusion was not substantiated by the low levels of intracellular free MTX at steady state. The strongest evidence for a facilitated diffusion process was provided by the inhibition of uptake by folinic acid; however, saturability of the uptake process was not observed. A membrane carrier system has been suggested for L5178Y (FISCHER, 1962), Yoshida sarcoma (DIVEKAR et al., 1967) and L1210 cells (SIROTNAK et al., 1968; GOLDMAN et al., 1968). Such a system has been further elaborated using L1210 leukemic cells (GOLDMAN, 1971a), and is thought to be shared by folic and folinic acids.

### X. Dihydrofolic Acid Reductase Inhibitors with Improved Uptake

The mode of action of MTX involves inhibition of DFR. As mentioned before, MTX is a potent inhibitor of this enzyme, but the passage of this agent through the plasma membrane appears to be the factor limiting its effectiveness. Therefore, the search for potent DFR inhibitors with properties that provide better membrane passage should continue. It is the 2,4-diamino portion of the molecule which is critical for binding to DFR (ZAKRZEWSKI, 1963a, b) and therefore must be retained to inhibit this target enzyme. Elimination of the negatively charged glutamate moiety resulted in a compound which was taken up by L1210 cells 1/5th as fast as MTX, and by P-1534 cells somewhat faster than MTX (KESSEL, 1969). A 2,4-diamino-6-methylpyrimidine with a strongly lipophilic adamantyl group at the 5-position was found to be more cytotoxic than MTX, even though the $K_i$ value for DFR was 60-times greater than that for MTX (HO et al., 1972). This suggests an improved uptake of this less negatively charged and more lipophilic molecule by mammalian cells, as compared with MTX. It remains to be seen whether this analog utilizes the folate-folinic acid transport system when passing through plasma membranes.

## F. Alkylating Agents

Nitrogen mustards, both aliphatic and aromatic, are clinically useful antitumor agents. They form irreversible, covalent bonds with cellular material by alkylating amino, carboxyl, and sulfhydryl groups of proteins, phosphate groups of phospholipids, and nucleic acids, and the ring nitrogens of purine and pyrimidine nucleotides. The alkylation of nucleic acids is thought to be responsible for the antitumor effect.

### I. Nitrogen Mustard (HN2)

In murine leukemia L1210 cells *in vitro*, HN2 was shown to be taken up quite rapidly. It accumulated in the cells (cell/medium ratio was about 10 after 10 min at 10 μM HN2) largely in a nondiffusible form. Cellular binding was shown to be dependent on temperature (KESSEL et al., 1969). In Ehrlich ascites cells, the $Q_{10}$ for HN2 uptake was about 2 and the cell/medium ratio was equal or smaller than 1.0. Intracellular drug was present predominantly in bound form (WOLPERT and RUDDON, 1969). Homogenates and intact cells bound the drug equally and binding in both systems was dependent on temperature. These authors interpret HN2 uptake as a mediated transport system. Treatment of rat ascites hepatoma cells with Tween 80 increased the rate of cellular uptake of HN2 by 50 to 100% (YAMADA et al., 1963). This suggests that the intact plasma membrane is a real barrier for the uptake of HN2.

In L5178Y cells, HN2 was shown to be taken up by a saturable process with a $K_m$ of 0.13 to 0.22 mM (GOLDENBERG et al., 1970). The uptake was competitively inhibited by the hydrolysis product of HN2 [i. e. 2-*bis*(hydroxyethyl)methylamine] with a $K_i$ of 54 μM, and by ethanolamine, hemicholinium-3, and by choline with a $K_i$ of 0.15 mM (GOLDENBERG et al., 1971). Thus, HN2 seems to employ the membrane carrier system which normally is utilized by choline. This was confirmed by demonstrating mutual inhibitions. Thus, choline uptake by L5178Y cells ($K_m = 25$ μM) was inhibited by HN2 ($K_i = 89$ μM). The cellular supernatant contained 7 to 10-times more drug than the membrane fraction and the total intracellular concentration of the drug was greater than that of the medium. However, these studies did not reveal the fraction of free unaltered drug present, if any. In L5178Y cells, the uptake of HN2 is considered to be an active, carrier mediated process.

There appears to be no doubt that HN2 employs the uptake mechanism for choline. Therefore, it is of interest to compare what is known about choline uptake by various tissues. Choline was shown to be taken up rapidly by Ehrlich ascites cells. The process was considered to represent diffusion and 75% of the choline which accumulated in the cells was in the form of phosphorylcholine (SUNG and JOHNSTONE, 1965). In Novikoff hepatoma cells *in vitro*, the passage of choline through the plasma membrane was shown to be rate-limiting for intracellular phosphorylation (PLAGEMANN and ROTH, 1969). In rat kidney cortex slices, choline uptake appeared to proceed by active transport resulting in accumulation of betaine (SUNG and JOHNSTONE, 1965). The uptake of choline by human erythrocytes has been described as simultaneous simple diffusion and facilitated diffusion with a $K_m$ of 20 μM (ASKARI, 1966), or as active transport dependent on $Na^+$ ($K_m = 30$ μM) (MARTIN, 1968). In each case, the compound found in erythrocytes was unaltered choline (ASKARI, 1966).

In giant axons of *Loligo*, the uptake of choline consisted of two components, diffusion and a saturable system ($K_m = 0.10$ mM) (HODGKIN and MARTIN, 1965). The uptake was temperature dependent ($Q_{10} = 2.0$) and was inhibited by hemicholinium-3 ($K_i = 20$ μM) and by acetylcholine ($K_i = 0.10$ mM). An active uptake of choline was reported for mouse cerebral cortex slices ($K_m = 0.23$ mM) (SCHUBERTH et al., 1966, 1967). Choline within the slices was unaltered and the accumulation depended on the presence of $Na^+$ in the medium. A facilitated diffusion of choline has been reported in nerve endings of rat cerebral cortex ($K_m = 40$ to 80 μM) (POTTER, 1968) and in synaptic nerve endings of guinea pig ($K_m = 83$ μM) (DIAMOND and KENNEDY, 1969). The cellular material was mainly (60 to 80%) unaltered choline; this uptake was also dependent on $Na^+$ (POTTER, 1968) and was inhibited by hemicholinium ($K_i = 19$ μM, 40 μM) and by acetylcholine ($K_i = 90$ μM).

### II. Other Alkylating Agents

Few studies with alkylating agents other than HN2 have been carried out to measure cellular uptake. However, it is clear that compounds such as chlorambucil, melphalan, and cyclophosphamide are taken up by a mechanism different from the choline system involved in the uptake of HN2. This conclusion is justified on the basis of the lack of effect of other alkylating agents on the uptake of HN2 (GOLDENBERG et al., 1970).

In L1210 cells *in vitro*, busulfan was shown to be taken up by a rapid, temperature-insensitive process which never led to intracellular accumulation of the drug (KESSEL et al., 1969). Chlorambucil became attached to plasma proteins and to the membranes of human erythrocytes, causing lysis at neutral pH and at physiological temperatures. This adsorption appeared not to involve alkylation, but resulted in stabilization of the drug (LINFORD et al., 1969).

## G. Guanylhydrazones and Phthalanilides

### I. Methylglyoxal-*bis*-Guanylhydrazone (CH3-G)

$CH_3$-G, a clinically useful agent against myelogenous leukemia, was shown to form a complex with DNA isolated from Sarcoma 180 cells (SARTORELLI et al., 1965). The uptake of $CH_3$-G has been compared in normal and leukemic human leukocytes, in HeLa and L1210 cells, and in erythrocytes of several species (FIELD et al., 1964). Human and rabbit erythrocytes differed from all of the other cells by not accumulating the compound against a concentration gradient. The uptake appeared to be a saturable process ($K_m = 50\ \mu M$). It was energy dependent as indicated by temperature dependence and inhibition by metabolic poisons. $CH_3$-G seems to share the membrane carrier for spermine, spermidine, and putrescine, all of which inhibited $CH_3$-G uptake. The carrier was specific for compounds with 2 amino groups separated from each other by at least 4 atoms. The best inhibitors of the $CH_3$-G uptake process were *p*- and *o*-phenylene-*bis*-guanylhydrazones.

In a separate study with L1210 leukemic cells, the uptake of $CH_3$-G appeared to proceed by facilitated diffusion with a $K_m$ of 40 $\mu$M (DAVE et al., 1971). Spermidine was shown to competitively inhibit the uptake with a $K_i$ of 10 $\mu$M. However, spermidine, when added later, could not displace cellular $CH_3$-G. This suggests that spermidine did, indeed, compete with $CH_3$-G at the cell surface and not for the intracellular binding sites (DAVE and CABALLES, 1973).

## II. 4,4′-Diacetyl-Diphenyl-Urea-*bis* Guanylhydrazone (DDUG)

This compound, which has shown antineoplastic activity in certain rodent tumor systems, was found to be taken up very rapidly by Sarcoma 180 cells *in vitro* (HAKALA, 1971). It accumulated in nuclei and mitochondria of sensitive and resistant Sarcoma 180 cells in a tightly bound form. The cellular drug could be extracted only by lipid solvents in the presence of phosphate and the binding was thought to involve cellular phospholipids. The uptake itself appeared to proceed by diffusion as judged by the linear relationship of uptake velocity and extracellular drug concentration and by the relatively low energy of activation (10 kcal/mole).

The uptake of DDUG thus is totally different from the uptake of another guanylhydrazone, $CH_3$-G (see above). Indeed, $CH_3$-G had no effect on the uptake of DDUG (HAKALA, 1971). The only compounds which were found to inhibit DDUG uptake were the terephthalanilide [2-chloro-4′,4″-di(2-imidazolin-2-yl)-terephthalanilidedihydrochloride; NSC 38280] and Janus Green B, a mitochondrial stain. These inhibitions were thought to reflect mainly the similarities in cellular binding of these compounds rather than membrane passage. The anionic sites at the cell surface seem to affect the sensitivity of cells to the positively charged DDUG. This was shown by the finding that ribonuclease and neuraminidase, both of which remove anionic groups, made the sensitive cells more resistant to DDUG (WEISS and HAKALA, 1971).

With L1210 cells, *in vivo* and *in vitro,* DDUG was also taken up by rapid diffusion (DAVE and MIHICH, 1972). The main difference between the L1210 and Sarcoma 180 cell systems appeared to be more rapid uptake by the L1210. This may be due to the smaller size of L1210 leukemic cells.

## III. Phthalanilides

The substituted phthalanilides are a class of chemotherapeutic agents highly effective against certain types of rodent leukemias and lymphomas (BENNETT, 1965). One of these derivatives, 2-chloro-4′,4″-di(2-imidazolin-2-yl) terephthalanilide (NSC 60339), was found to be bound primarily in the nucleus and mitochondria of both sensitive and resistant P-388 leukemic cells (YESAIR et al., 1966) and to form drug-lipid complexes in a variety of tissues. The amount of bound drug was shown to be related to the drug response, while the intracellular concentration of free drug was not (YESAIR et al., 1967).

No direct information is available on the mode of plasma membrane passage of the phthalanilides. It is of interest that a terephthalanilide (NSC 38280) was a potent inhibitor of DDUG uptake in sensitive Sarcoma 180 cells (HAKALA, 1971). Cells which were resistant to DDUG, due to restricted plasma membrane passage, were cross resistant to this phthalanilide, which in these cells had little effect on DDUG uptake. Thus, there appears to be a definite similarity between DDUG and terephthalanilides, not only with respect to the intracellular binding, but with respect to plasma membrane passage as well.

## Conclusions

The foregoing discussion on the plasma membrane passage of antineoplastic agents has been limited largely to mammalian cells and tissues. This was a choice intended to focus on aspects more relevant to human cancer chemotherapy.

Interesting general features of the uptake of antineoplastic agents are apparent. One finds that the antimetabolites utilize the processes intended for normal metabolites. This is true for analogs of purines and pyrimidines and their nucleosides. Similarly, folate analogs utilize the uptake system intended for folate and tetrahydrofolates. Most surprisingly, nitrogen mustard was shown to utilize the uptake system which nature intended for choline, and methylglyoxal-*bis*-guanylhydrazone the system intended for spermidine.

Many of the antineoplastic agents become bound to cellular material and accumulate in that form, e. g. steroids, antifolates, alkylating agents, *bis*-guanylhydrazones, and phthalanilides. In contrast, the uptake of the analogs of purine and pyrimidine bases and their nucleosides is largely associated with their intracellular conversion to nucleotides. Thus, the extent of uptake of most antineoplastic agents is determined either by the availability of intracellular binding sites or by the activity of "salvage enzymes". More work is needed to clarify the relationship between the intracellular fate of the compound and the velocity of its passage through the plasma membrane. It appears that in many cases plasma membrane passage is the rate-limiting step for intracellular conversion or binding; this certainly applies to methotrexate. However, there may be situations in which the intracellular conversion or binding of a compound is the rate-limiting step and can, thereby, affect membrane passage. The latter possibility seems, indeed, to apply for purines, pyrimidines, and their nucleosides. It is clear that the plasma membranes of cells and tissues vary greatly with respect to their permeability characteristics. This variation most certainly is a major factor in determining the natural selectivity of action of antineoplastic agents.

## References


ASKARI, A.: Uptake of some quaternary ammonium ions by human erythrocytes. J. gen. Physiol. **49**, 1147—1160 (1966).

BALLARD, P. L., TOMKINS, G. M.: Hormone induced modification of the cell surface. Nature (Lond.) **224**, 344—345 (1969).

BENEDETTI, E. L., EMMELOT, P.: Structure and function of plasma membranes isolated from liver. In: DALTON, A. J., HAGUENAU, F. (Eds.): Ultrastructure in biological systems, vol. 4, The Membranes. pp. 33—120. New York: Academic Press (1968).

BENNETT, L. L., Jr.: Phthalanilides and some related dibasic and polybasic compounds: A review of biological activities and modes of action. Progr. exp. Tumor Res. **7**, 259—325 (1965).

BENSCH, K. G., SIMBONIS, S., HILL, R. B., KING, D. W.: Phagocytosis and cell division. Nature (Lond.) **183**, 476—477 (1959).

Ber, R., Griffin, M.J.: Location of hydrocortisone in dividing HeLa S3 cells. Fed. Proc. **26**, 616 (1967).
Bieber, A.L., Sartorelli, A.C.: The metabolism of thioguanine in purine analog resistant cells. Cancer Res. **24**, 1210—1215 (1964).
Blair, D.G.R., Hebert, G.J.: Uptake of 2,6-diaminopurine-2-$C^{14}$ by 2,6-DAP-sensitive and -resistant L strain mouse cells grown on plastic discs. Canad. J. Physiol. Pharmacol. **48**, 791—800 (1970).
Bobinski, H., Stein, W.D.: Isolation of a glucose-binding component from human erythrocyte membranes. Nature (Lond.) **211**, 1366—1368 (1966).
Bobzien, W., Goldman, I.D.: The mechanism of methotrexate transport in rabbit reticulocytes. J. clin. Invest. **51**, 1688—1696 (1972).
Booij, H.L., Bungenberg De Jong, H.G.: Biocolloids and their interactions. Protoplasmatologia I **2**, 142. Springer: Wien 1956.
Braganca, B.M., Divekar, A.Y., Vaidya, N.R.: Defective transport of aminopterin in relation to development of resistance in Yoshida sarcoma cells. Biochim. biophys. Acta (Amst.) **135**, 937—946 (1967).
Broome, J.D.: Studies on the mechanism of tumor inhibition by L-asparaginase. J. exp. Med. **127**, 1055—1072 (1968).
Bucknall, R.M., Carter, S.B.: A reversible inhibitor of nucleic acid synthesis. Nature (Lond.) **213**, 1099—1101 (1967).
Collins, F.D., Roberts, W.K.: The effect of dimethyl sulfoxide on nucleoside transport in L-cells. Biochim. biophys. Acta (Amst.) **233**, 459—464 (1971).
Dave, C., Caballes, L.: Studies on the uptake of methylglyoxal-bis(guanylhydrazone) and spermidine in mouse leukemia L1210 sensitive and resistant to $CH_3$-G. Fed. Proc. **32**, 736 (1973).
Dave, C., Mihich, E.: Uptake and intracellular distribution of 4,4′-diacetyldiphenylurea-bis-(guanylhydrazone) in sensitive and resistant leukemia L1210 cells. Biochem. Pharmacol. **21**, 2681—2695 (1972).
Dave, C., Ehrke, J., Soucek, J., Mihich, E.: Differences in the action of methylglyoxal-*bis*-guanylhydrazone, 4,4′-diacetyl-diphenyl-urea-*bis*-guanylhydrazone and related analogs. Fed. Proc. **30**, 628 (1971).
Davidson, J.R.: Permeability of resistant L1210 leukemia cells to 8-azaguanine and 6-mercaptopurine. Proc. Amer. Ass. Cancer Res. **2**, 290 (1958).
Dewey, M.M., Barr, L.: Some considerations about the structure of cellular membranes. In: Bonner, F., Kleinzeller, A. (Eds.): Current topics in membrane transport, vol. 1, pp. 1—33. New York: Academic Press 1970.
Diamond, I., Kennedy, E.P.: Carrier-mediated transport of choline into synaptic nerve endings. J. biol. Chem. **244**, 3258—3263 (1969).
Divekar, A.Y., Fleysher, M.H., Slocum, H.K., Kenny, L.N., Hakala, M.T.: Changes in Sarcoma 180 cells associated with drug-induced resistance to adenosine analogs. Cancer Res. **32**, 2530—2537 (1972).
Divekar, A.Y., Vaidya, N.R., Braganca, B.M.: Active transport of aminopterin in Yoshida sarcoma cells. Biochim. biophys. Acta (Amst.) **135**, 927—936 (1967).
Dourmashkin, R.R., Dougherty, R.M.: Phagocytosis of crystalline particles by cells grown in tissue culture. Exp. Cell Res. **25**, 480—484 (1961).
DuBuy, H.G., Showacre, J.L.: Selective localization of tetracycline in mitochondria of living cells. Science **133**, 196—197 (1961).
Emmelot, P., Bos, C.J.: Studies on plasma membranes. I. Chemical composition and enzyme content of plasma membranes from rat liver. Biochim. biophys. Acta (Amst.) **90**, 126—145 (1966).
Field, M., Block, J.B., Oliverio, V.T., Rall, D.P.: Cellular accumulation of methylglyoxal-*bis*-guanylhydrazone *in vitro*. I. General characteristics of cellular uptake. Cancer Res. **24**, 1939—1946 (1964).
Fischer, G.A.: Defective transport of amethopterin as a mechanism of resistance to the antimetabolite. Biochem. Pharmacol. **11**, 1233—1237 (1962).
Folca, P.J., Glascock, R.F., Irvine, W.T.: Studies with tritium-labeled hexoestrol in advanced breast cancer. Comparison of tissue accumulation of hexoestrol with response to bilateral adrenalectomy and oophorectomy. Lancet **2**, 796—798 (1961).
Gentry, G.A., Morse, P.A., Ives, D.H., Gebert, R., Potter, V.R.: Pyrimidine metabolism in tissue culture cells derived from rat hepatomas. II. Thymidine uptake in suspension cultures derived from Novikoff hepatomas. Cancer Res. **25**, 509—516 (1965).
Giannopoulos, G., Gorski, J.: Estrogen receptors. Quantitative studies on transfer of estradiol from cytoplasmic to nuclear binding sites. J. biol. Chem. **246**, 2524—2529 (1971a).
Giannopoulos, G., Gorski, J.: Estrogen-binding protein of the rat uterus. Different molecular forms associated with nuclear uptake of estradiol. J. biol. Chem. **246**, 2530—2536 (1971b).

GOLDENBERG, G. J., VANSTONE, C. L., BIHLER, I.: Transport of nitrogen mustard on the transport carrier for choline in L5178Y lymphoblasts. Science **172**, 1148—1149 (1971).
GOLDENBERG, G. J., VANSTONE, C. L., ISRAELS, L. G., ILSE, D., BIHLER, I.: Evidence for a transport carrier of nitrogen mustard in nitrogen mustard-sensitive and -resistant L5178Y lymphoblasts. Cancer Res. **30**, 2285—2291 (1970).
GOLDMAN, I. D.: Transport energetics of the folic acid analog, methotrexate, in L1210 leukemia cells. J. biol. Chem. **244**, 3779—3785 (1969).
GOLDMAN, I. D.: The characteristics of the membrane transport of amethopterin and the naturally occurring folates. Ann. N. Y. Acad. Sci. **186**, 400—422 (1971a).
GOLDMAN, I. D.: A model system for the study of heteroexchange diffusion: methotrexate-folate interactions in L1210 leukemia and Ehrlich ascites tumor cells. Biochim. biophys. Acta (Amst.) **233**, 624—634 (1971b).
GOLDMAN, I. D., LICHTENSTEIN, N. S., OLIVERIO, V. T.: Carrier transport of the folic acid analogue, methotrexate, in the L1210 leukemia cell. J. biol. Chem. **243**, 5007—5017 (1968).
GRAHAM, J. M., GREEN, C.: The binding of hormones and related compounds by normal and cholesterol-depleted plasma membranes of rat liver. Biochem. Pharmacol. **18**, 493—502 (1969).
GRINDEY, G., NICHOL, C. A.: Interaction of drugs inhibiting different steps in the synthesis of DNA. Cancer Res. **32**, 527—531 (1972).
HAKALA, M. T.: On the role of drug penetration in amethopterin resistance of S-180 cells *in vitro*. Biochim. biophys. Acta (Amst.) **102**, 198—209 (1965a).
HAKALA, M. T.: On the nature of permeability of S-180 cells to amethopterin *in vitro*. Biochim. biophys. Acta (Amst.) **102**, 210—225 (1965b).
HAKALA, M. T.: Biochemical basis of resistance to folic acid antagonists. FEBS Symp. **16**, 31—47 (1969).
HAKALA, M. T.: Uptake and distribution of 4,4′-diacetyl-diphenyl-urea-*bis*-guanylhydrazone in sensitive and resistant Sarcoma 180 cells *in vitro*. Biochem. Pharmacol. **20**, 81—95 (1971).
HAKALA, M. T.: Enzyme changes in resistant tissues. In: MIHICH, E. (Ed.): Drug resistance and selectivity: biochemical and cellular basis. pp. 263—298. New York: Academic Press 1973.
HAKALA, M. T., CHHEDA, G. B., KENNY, L. N.: Kinetics and specificity of uptake of 8-$^{14}$C-purine and 2-$^{14}$C-pyrimidine nucleosides in Sarcoma 180 cells *in vitro*. Abstracts, Am. Chem. Soc. Meeting, Chicago, August 1973, Biol. No. 233 (1973).
HAKALA, M. T., KENNY, L. N.: Common mechanism for the passage of purine and pyrimidine nucleosides through the plasma membrane of Sarcoma 180 cells. Fed. Proc. **31**, 475 (1972).
HAKALA, M. T., KENNY, L. N., SLOCUM, H. K.: Inhibition of adenosine uptake by $N^6$-($\Delta^2$-isopentenyl) adenosine and kinetin riboside. Fed. Proc. **30**, 697 (1971).
HAKALA, M. T., SUOLINNA, E. M., KENNY, L. N., TRITSCH, G.: Biochim. biophys. Acta (Amst.), in press.
HALL, T. C., ROBERTS, D., KESSEL, D.: Methotrexate and folate reductase in human cancer. Europ. J. Cancer **2**, 135—142 (1966).
HAMILTON, W. A.: The mode of action of membrane-active antibacterials. Fed. Europ. biochem. Soc. **20**, 71 (1970).
HANSEN, P., STEIN, H.: On the synthesis of RNA in lymphocytes stimulated by phytohemagglutinin. I. Induction of uridine kinase and the conversion of uridine to UTP. Europ. J. Biochem. **4**, 401—406 (1968).
HARVEY, A. M., CHRISTENSEN, H. N.: Uric acid transport system. Apparent absence in erythrocytes of the Dalmatian coach hound. Science **145**, 826—827 (1964).
HAWKINS, R. A., BERLIN, R. D.: Purine transport in polymorphonuclear leukocytes. Biochim. biophys. Acta (Amst.) **173**, 324—337 (1969).
HEIDRICK, M. L., RYAN, W. L.: Cyclic nucleotides on cell growth *in vitro*. Cancer Res. **30**, 376—378 (1970).
HENDERSON, E. S., ADAMSON, R. H., OLIVERIO, V. T.: The metabolic fate of tritiated methotrexate. II. Absorption and excretion in man. Cancer Res. **25**, 1018—1024 (1965).
HO, Y. K., HAKALA, M. T., ZAKRZEWSKI, S. F.: 5-(1-Adamantyl) pyrimidines as inhibitors of folate metabolism. Cancer Res. **32**, 1023—1028 (1972).
HODGKIN, A. L., MARTIN, K.: Choline uptake by giant axons of *Loligo*. J. Physiol. (Lond.) **179**, 26P—27P (1965).
HOLLANDER, N., CHIU, Y. W.: *In vitro* binding of cortisol[1-2-$H^3$] by a substance in the supernatant fraction of P1798 mouse lymphosarcoma. Biochem. biophys. Res. Comm. **25**, 291—297 (1966).
HOLMSEN, H., ROZENBERG, M. C.: Adenine nucleotide metabolism of blood platelets. I. Adenosine kinase and nucleotide formation from exogenous adenosine and AMP. Biochim. biophys. Acta (Amst.) **155**, 326—341 (1968).
HOLTER, H.: Pinocytosis. Int. Rev. Cytol. **8**, 481—504 (1959).

JACQUEZ, J.A.: Permeability of Ehrlich (ascites) cells to uracil, thymine, and fluorouracil. Proc. Soc. exp. Biol. (N.Y.) **109**, 132—135 (1962a).
JACQUEZ, J.A.: Transport and enzymic splitting of pyrimidine nucleosides in Ehrlich cells. Biochim. biophys. Acta (Amst.) **61**, 265—277 (1962b).
JACQUEZ, J.A.: Permeability of Ehrlich ascites cells to folic acid, aminopterin and amethopterin. Cancer Res. **26**, 1616—1624 (1966).
JACQUEZ, J.A., GINSBERG, F.: Permeability of Ehrlich ascites cells to adenine. Proc. Soc. exp. Biol. (N. Y.) **105**, 478—480 (1960).
JOST, J.P., RICKENBERG, H.V.: Cyclic AMP. Ann. Rev. Biochem. **40**, 741—774 (1971).
KESSEL, D.: A comparison of 4-amino, $N^{10}$-methylpteroic acid and methotrexate transport by mouse leukemic cells. Molec. Pharmacol. **5**, 21—25 (1969).
KESSEL, D., BOTTERILL, V., HALL, T.C.: Stimulation by pteridines of the uptake of amethopterin by human lymphocytes. Biochem. Pharmacol. **17**, 1727—1733 (1968a).
KESSEL, D., BRUNS, R., HALL, T.C.: Determinants of responsiveness to 5-fluorouridine in transplantable murine leukemias. Molec. Pharmacol. **7**, 117—121 (1971).
KESSEL, D., HALL, T.C.: Studies on drug transport by normal human leukocytes. Biochem. Pharmacol. **16**, 2395—2403 (1967a).
KESSEL, D., HALL, T.C.: Amethopterin transport in Ehrlich ascites carcinoma and L1210 cells. Cancer Res. **27**, 1539—1543 (1967b).
KESSEL, D., HALL, T.C.: Effects of persantin on deoxycytidine transport by murine leukemia cells. Biochim. biophys. Acta (Amst.) **211**, 88—94 (1970).
KESSEL, D., HALL, T.C., ROBERTS, D.: Modes of uptake of methotrexate by normal and leukemic human leukocytes *in vitro* and their relation to drug response. Cancer Res. **28**, 564—570 (1968b).
KESSEL, D., HALL, T.C., ROBERTS, D., WODINSKY, I.: Uptake as a determinant of amethopterin response in mouse leukemias. Science **150**, 752—754 (1965).
KESSEL, D., MYERS, M., WODINSKY, I.: Accumulation of two alkylating agents, nitrogen mustard and busulfan, by murine leukemia cells *in vitro*. Biochem. Pharmacol. **18**, 1229—1234 (1969).
KESSEL, D., SHURIN, S.B.: Transport of two non-metabolizable nucleosides, deoxycytidine and arabinosylcytosine in a subline of L1210 murine leukemia. Biochim. biophys. Acta (Amst.) **163**, 179—187 (1968).
KIRKPATRICK, A.F., KAISER, N., MILHOLLAND, R.J., ROSEN, F.: Glucocorticoid-binding macromolecules in normal tissues and tumors. Stabilization of the specific binding component. J. biol. Chem. **247**, 70—74 (1972).
KOTYK, A.: Present situation in the identification of membrane transport proteins of single cells. Fed. Europ. biochem. Soc. **20**, 99—108 (1970).
KREIS, W., WECHTER, W.J.: Biological activity of 3′,5′-cyclic phosphates of 1-$\beta$-D-arabinofuranosylcytosine (ara-C). Proc. Am. Ass. Cancer Res. **13**, 62 (1972).
KÜBLER, W., BRETSCHNEIDER, H.J.: Kompetitive Hemmung der katalysierten Adenosin-Diffusion als Mechanismus der coronarerweiternden Wirkung eines Pyrimidopyrimidin-Derivates. Arch. ges. Physiol. **280**, 141—157 (1964).
LASSEN, U.V.: Asymmetry of uric acid transport through the human erythrocyte membrane induced by hypoxanthine. Biochim. biophys. Acta (Amst.) **57**, 123—129 (1962).
LASSEN, U.V.: Hypoxanthine transport in human erythrocytes. Biochim. biophys. Acta (Amst.) **135**, 146—154 (1967).
LASSEN, U.V., OVERGAARD-HANSEN, K.: Hypoxanthine as inhibitor of uric acid transport in human erythrocytes. Biochim. biophys. Acta (Amst.) **57**, 111—117 (1962a).
LASSEN, U.V., OVERGAARD-HANSEN, K.: Purine derivatives as inhibitors of uric acid transport into human erythrocytes. Biochim. biophys. Acta (Amst.) **57**, 118—122 (1962b).
LEIBMAN, K.C., HEIDELBERGER, C.: The metabolism of $^{32}$P-labeled ribonucleotides in tissue slices and cell suspensions. J. biol. Chem. **216**, 823—830 (1955).
LICHTENSTEIN, N.S., GOLDMAN, I.D.: Riboflavin-methotrexate interactions. Photochemical reaction and competition for transport in the L1210 mouse leukemia cell. Biochem. Pharmacol. **19**, 1229—1239 (1970).
LINFORD, J.H., HRYNIUK, W., ISRAELS, L.G.: Adsorption to human red blood cells of chlorambucil and other biological alkylating agents. Biochem. Pharmacol. **18**, 2723—2735 (1969).
LOO, T.L., WANG-HO, D.H., BLOSSOM, D.R., SHEPARD, B.J., FREI, E. III: Cellular uptake of purine antimetabolites *in vitro*. I. Uptake of methylmercaptopurine riboside by human red blood cells. Biochem. Pharmacol. **18**, 1711—1725 (1969).
LOWY, B.A., WILLIAMS, M.K.: Studies on the metabolism of adenosine and adenine in stored and fresh human erythrocytes. Blood **27**, 623—628 (1966).
LOWY, B.A., WILLIAMS, M.K., LONDON, I.M.: Enzymatic deficiencies of purine nucleotide synthesis in the human erythrocytes. J. biol. Chem. **237**, 1622—1625 (1962).

LUCAS, Z. J.: Pyrimidine nucleotide synthesis: Regulatory control during transformation of lymphocytes *in vitro*. Science **156**, 1237—1240 (1967).

MADDY, A. H.: The properties of the protein of the plasma membrane of ox erythrocytes. Biochim. biophys. Acta (Amst.) **117**, 193—200 (1966).

MARTIN, K.: Concentrative accumulation of choline by human erythrocytes. J. gen. Physiol. **51**, 497—516 (1968).

MARZULLI, F. N., CALLAHAN, J. F., BROWN, D. W. C.: Chemical structure and skin penetrating capacity of a short series of organic phosphates and phosphoric acid. J. invest. Dermatol. **44**, 339—344 (1965).

MCGUIRE, W. L., JULIAN, J. A.: Comparison of macromolecular binding of estradiol in hormone-dependent and hormone-independent rat mammary carcinoma. Cancer Res. **31**, 1440—1445 (1971).

MOBBS, B. G.: The uptake of tritiated estradiol by 9,10-dimethyl-1,2-benzanthracene-induced mammary tumors of the rat. J. Endocrinol. **36**, 409—414 (1966).

MONTGOMERY, J. A., DIXON, G. J., DULMAGE, E. A., THOMAS, H. J., BROCKMAN, R. W., SKIPPER, H. E.: Inhibition of 6-mercaptopurine-resistant cancer cells in culture by *bis*(thioinosine) 5',5''-phosphate. Nature (Lond.) **199**, 769—772 (1963).

NAHAS, A., NIXON, P. F., BERTINO, J. R.: Uptake of 5-formyltetrahydrofolate by L1210 mouse leukemia cells and its effect on uptake of methotrexate. Proc. Amer. Assoc. Cancer Res. **10**, 64 (1969).

NAKATA, Y., BADER, J. P.: The uptake of nucleosides by cells in culture. II. Inhibition by 2-mercapto-1-($\beta$-4-pyridethyl)benzimidazole. Biochim. biophys. Acta (Amst.) **190**, 250—256 (1969).

OLIVER, J. M., PATERSON, A. R. P.: Nucleoside transport. I. A mediated process in human erythrocytes. Canad. J. Biochem. **49**, 262 (1971).

OVERGAARD-HANSEN, K., LASSEN, U. V.: Active transport of uric acid through the human erythrocyte membrane. Nature (Lond.) **184**, 553—554 (1959).

OVERMAN, J. R.: Ingestion of latex particles by chicken fibroblasts in tissue culture. Proc. Soc. exp. Biol. Med. **107**, 895—900 (1961).

PARPART, A. K., BALLENTINE, R.: Molecular anatomy of red cell membrane. In: Modern trends in physiology and biochemistry. New York: Academic Press 1952.

PATERSON, A. R. P.: Resistance to 6-mercaptopurine II. The synthesis of thioinosinic acid in a resistant subline of the Ehrlich ascites carcinoma. Canad. J. Biochem. **40**, 195—206 (1962).

PATERSON, A. R. P., OLIVER, J. M.: Nucleoside transport II. Inhibition by *p*-nitrobenzylthioguanosine and related compounds. Canad. J. Biochem. **49**, 271—274 (1971).

PATERSON, A. R. P., SIMPSON, A. I.: Inhibitors of nucleoside metabolism. Canad. J. Biochem. **44**, 1423—1433 (1966).

PENNISTON, J. T., BECKETT, L., BENTLEY, D. L., HANSCH, C.: Passive permeation of organic compounds through biological tissue: A nonsteady state theory. Molec. Pharmacol. **5**, 333—341 (1969).

PLAGEMANN, P. G. W.: Nucleoside transport by Novikoff rat hepatoma cells growing in suspension culture. Specificity and mechanism of transport reactions and relationship to nucleoside incorporation into nucleic acids. Biochim. biophys. Acta (Amst.) **233**, 688—701 (1971).

PLAGEMANN, P. G. W., ROTH, M. F.: Permeation as the rate limiting step in the phosphorylation of uridine and choline and their incorporation in macromolecules by Novikoff hepatoma cells. Competitive inhibition by phenethyl alcohol, persantin and adenosine. Biochem. **8**, 4782—4789 (1969).

PLAGEMANN, P. G. W., WARD, G. A., MAHY, B. W. J., KORBECKI, M.: Relationship between uridine kinase activity and rate of incorporation of uridine into acid soluble pool and into RNA during growth cycle of rat hepatoma cells. J. cell. Physiol. **73**, 233—250 (1969).

PLUNKETT, W., LAPI, L., ORTIZ, P., COHEN, S. S.: Cellular penetration and metabolism of 9-$\beta$-D-arabinofuranosyl adenine 5'-monophosphate (araAMP). Proc. Am. Ass. Cancer Res. **14**, 32 (1973).

POTTER, L. T.: Uptake of choline by nerve endings isolated from the rat cerebral cortex. In: CAMPBELL, P. N. (Ed.): The interaction of drugs and subcellular components in animal cells, p. 293. Boston: Little, Brown and Co. 1968.

PUCA, G. A., NOLA, E., SICA, V., BRESCIANI, F.: Estrogen-binding proteins of calf uterus. Partial purification and preliminary characterization of two cytoplasmic proteins. Biochemistry **10**, 3769—3780 (1971).

ROBERTS, D. W.: Cleavage of folic acid by hydrogen peroxide. Biochim. biophys. Acta (Amst.) **54**, 572—574 (1961).

ROLL, P. M., WEINFELD, H., CARROLL, E., BROWN, G. B.: The utilization of nucleotides by the mammal IV. Triply labeled purine nucleotides. J. biol. Chem. **220**, 439—454 (1956).

Rosenbloom, F.M., Kelley, W.N., Henderson, J.F., Seegmiller, J.E.: Lyon hypothesis and X-linked disease. Lancet 2, 305—306 (1967).
Rothblat, G.H., Buchko, M.K., Kritchevsky, D.: Cholesterol uptake by L5178Y cells: Studies with delipidized serum. Biochim. biophys. Acta (Amst.) 164, 327—338 (1968).
Rubin, R.C., Henderson, E.S., Owens, E.S., Rall, D.P.: Uptake of methotrexate-$H^3$ by rabbit kidney slices. Cancer Res. 27, 553—557 (1967).
Ryan, W.L., Heidrick, M.L.: Inhibition of cell growth *in vitro* by adenosine 3′,5′-monophosphate. Science 162, 1484—1485 (1968).
Ryser, H.J.P., Hancock, R.: Histones and basic polyamino acids stimulate the uptake of albumin by tumor cells in culture. Science 150, 501—503 (1965).
Sartorelli, A.C., Iannotti, A.I., Booth, B.A., Schneider, F.H., Bertino, J.R., Johns, D.G.: Complex formation with DNA and inhibition of nucleic acid synthesis by methylglyoxal *bis*(guanylhydrazone). Biochim. biophys. Acta (Amst.) 103, 174—176 (1965).
Schanker, L.S., Jeffrey, J.J.: Active transport of foreign pyrimidines across the intestinal epithelium. Nature (Lond.) 190, 727—728 (1961).
Schanker, L.S., Jeffrey, J.J.: Structural specifity of the pyrimidine transport process of the small intestine. Biochem. Pharmacol. 11, 961—966 (1962).
Schanker, L.S., Jeffrey, J.J., Tocco, D.J.: Interaction of purines with the pyrimidine transport process of the small intestine. Biochem. Pharmacol. 12, 1047—1053 (1963).
Schanker, L.S., Tocco, D.J.: Active transport of some pyrimidines across the rat intestinal epithelium. J. Pharmacol. exp. Ther. 28, 115—121 (1960).
Schanker, L.S., Tocco, D.J.: Some characteristics of the pyrimidine transport process of the small intestine. Biochim. biophys. Acta (Amst.) 56, 469—473 (1962).
Schröder, J., Plagemann, P.G.W.: Growth of Novikoff rat hepatoma cells in suspension culture in the presence of adenosine 3′,5′-cyclic monophosphate. J. Natl. Cancer Inst. 46, 423—429 (1971).
Schuberth, J., Sundwall, A., Sörbo, B.: Relation between $Na^+$-$K^+$ transport and the uptake of choline by brain slices. Life Sci. 6, 293—295 (1967).
Schuberth, J., Sundwall, A., Sörbo, B., Lindell, J.O.: Uptake of choline by mouse brain slices. J. Neurochem. 13, 347—352 (1966).
Singer, S., Litwack, G.: Identity of corticosteroid binder I with the macromolecule binding 3-methyl cholanthrene in liver cytosol *in vivo*. Cancer Res. 31, 1364—1368 (1971).
Sirotnak, F.M., Kurita, S., Hutchison, D.J.: On the nature of a transport alteration determining resistance to amethopterin in the L1210 leukemia. Cancer Res. 28, 75—80 (1968).
Smith, C.G., Reineke, L.M., Burch, M.R., Shefner, A.M., Muirhead, E.E.: Studies on uptake of tubercidin by blood cells and its distribution in whole animals. Cancer Res. 30, 69—75 (1970).
Song, C.S., Kappas, A., Bodansky, O.: 5′-Nucleotidase of plasma membranes of the rat liver: Studies on subcellular distribution. Ann. N. Y. Acad. Sci. 166, 565—573 (1969).
Steggles, A.W., King, R.J.B.: The uptake of [6,7-$^3$H] oestradiol by estrogen dependent and independent hamster kidney tumors. Eur. J. Cancer 4, 395—401 (1968).
Sung, C.P., Johnstone, R.M.: Evidence for active transport of choline in rat kidney cortex slices. Canad. J. Biochem. 43, 1111—1118 (1965).
Suolinna, E.M., Tritsch, G., Hakala, M.T.: Asparagine and glutamine metabolism in Sarcoma 180 cells *in vitro*. Proc. Amer. Ass. Cancer Res. 12, 29 (1971).
Tan, K.B., McAuslan, B.R.: Inhibition of nucleoside incorporation into Hela cells by streptovaricin. Biochem. biophys. Res. Comm. 42, 230—236 (1971).
Vandevoorde, J.P., Hansen, H.J.: Inhibition of J128 cell culture by 6-mercaptopurine and 9-alkylated derivatives of 6-mercaptopurine. Proc. Amer. Ass. Cancer Res. 8, 70 (1967).
Wartiovaara, V., Collander, R.: Permeabilitätstheorien. In: Protoplasmatologia: Handbuch der Protoplasmaforschung, vol. II, C. 8d. Vienna: Springer 1960.
Weiss, L., Hakala, M.T.: The anionic nature of Sarcoma 180 cell surfaces, and sensitivity to 4,4′-diacetyl-diphenyl-urea-*bis*-guanylhydrazone. Cancer Res. 31, 1369—1372 (1971).
Werkheiser, W.C.: Specific binding of 4-amino folic acid analogues by folic acid reductase. J. biol. Chem. 236, 888—893 (1961).
Wilson, T.H., Wilson, D.W.: Intestinal absorption *in vitro* of uridylic and thymidylic acids. Biochim. biophys. Acta (Amst.) 22, 587 (1956); J. Physiol. 123, 116 (1954).
Wilson, T.H., Wilson, D.W.: Studies *in vitro* of digestion and absorption of pyrimidine nucleotides by the intestine. J. biol. Chem. 233, 1544—1547 (1958).
Wolpert, M.K., Ruddon, R.W.: A study on the mechanism of resistance to nitrogen mustard (HN2) in Ehrlich ascites tumor cells: Comparison of uptake of HN2-$^{14}$C into sensitive and resistant cells. Cancer Res. 29, 873—879 (1969).
Yamada, T., Iwanami, Y., Baba, T.: The transport of $^{14}$C-labeled nitrogen mustard *N*-oxide through cellular membrane treated with Tween-80 *in vitro*. Gann 54, 171—176 (1963).

YESAIR, D. W., KOHNER, F. A., ROGERS, W. I., BARONOWSKY, P. E., KENSLER, C. J.: Relationship of phthalanilide-lipid complexes to uptake and retention of 2-chloro-4′,4″-di(2-imidazolin-2-yl)terephthalanilide (NSC 60339) by sensitive and resistant P388 leukemia cells. Cancer Res. **26**, 202—207 (1966).
YESAIR, D. W., ROGERS, W. I., BARONOWSKY, P. E., WODINSKY, I., THAYER, P. S., KENSLER, C. J.: Relationship of uptake and binding of an antileukemic phthalanilide to its biochemical and chemotherapeutic effects on P388 lymphocytic leukemia cells. Cancer Res. **27**, 314—321 (1967).
ZAKRZEWSKI, S. F.: The mechanism of binding of folate analogues by folate reductase. J. biol. Chem. **238**, 1485—1490 (1963a).
ZAKRZEWSKI, S. F.: Relationship between basicity of certain folate analogues and their affinities for folate reductase. J. biol. Chem. **238**, 4002—4004 (1963b).

Chapter 14

# Metabolism of Cancer Chemotherapeutic Agents via Pathways Utilized by Endogenous Substrates

DAVID G. JOHNS

With 7 Figures

## Introduction

Cancer chemotherapeutic agents, like other classes of xenobiotics, undergo a variety of metabolic transformations, both anabolic and catabolic in type. The former group of reactions includes such transformations as conversion of purine and pyrimidine analogs, to their pharmacologically active nucleotide forms and incorporation of the latter into nucleic acids. Because of their immediate relevance to the antitumor activity of these agents, and also to mechanisms of acquired resistance to continued therapy, such anabolic conversions have received great attention from investigators in the field of cancer chemotherapy. The catabolic reactions which these drugs undergo, on the other hand, usually result in a partial or complete loss of antitumor activity; the practical impetus toward the study of the latter group of reactions has been the possibility of developing specific inhibitors of such catabolic inactivation, thus increasing the potency and duration of action of the parent form of the drug.

Drugs with cancer chemotherapeutic activity encompass a variety of chemical structures and are susceptible to biological alteration by enzyme systems located in soluble, microsomal, and mitochondrial subcellular fractions. Not all antitumor agents are acted upon by drug-metabolizing enzymes; some of these compounds are unstable in aqueous solutions and undergo rapid spontaneous decomposition, while others undergo no detectable change *in vivo*. In addition, examples are now available of antitumor agents which, while not susceptible to alteration by the mammalian host, are catabolized by the bacterial flora of the intestinal tract during enterohepatic circulation.

While compounds with antitumor activity comprise a variety of chemical structures, this class of pharmacological agents is made up of an unusually large proportion of compounds which are analogs and isomers of physiological compounds. The early demonstration (1948–1953) that aminopterin and 6-mercaptopurine, analogs of pteroylglutamate and hypoxanthine, respectively, possess significant activity in clinical cancer, provided the impetus for the development of a host of other analogs of naturally occurring purines, pyrimidines, and coenzymes; those which have survived clinical trials to become antitumor agents with well-established clinical usefulness include methotrexate, 5-fluorouracil, cytosine arabinoside, 6-mercaptopurine, and 6-thioguanine. Analogs of theoretical interest or of potential, but not yet established clinical value include dichloromethotrexate, 5-azacytidine, 6-azauridine, and 6-methylthiopurine ribonucleoside. Finally, as by-products of this effort to devise analogs and isomers of naturally occurring compounds are agents with other useful pharmacological activity; among these are allopurinol and the immunosuppressive agent azathioprine; the latter drug possesses significant antitumor activity (RUNDLES et al., 1961), although it is not used routinely for this purpose.

The significance of this development from the point of view of drug metabolism is that many of these agents, because of their close resemblance to naturally occurring compounds, undergo the same anabolic and catabolic conversions as do their parent compounds. Not significantly different in chemical and physical properties from normal body constituents, and possessing, in most cases, poor lipid solubility, they are apparently not recognized as foreign compounds or xenobiotics by the usual drug-metabolizing enzyme systems, and tend rather to undergo transformations catalyzed by the enzymes of purine, pyrimidine, and pteridine anabolism and catabolism. Thus, cancer chemotherapeutic agents can, from the point of view of drug metabolism, be conveniently divided into two classes: those agents which are recognized as foreign by the microsomal drug-metabolizing enzyme systems and which follow the usual metabolic pathways for xenobiotics, and those which are not so recognized and which are either not metabolized or which undergo conversion by enzyme systems operative in physiological metabolic pathways. This review will be concerned with the metabolism of the latter group of drugs; metabolism of those antitumor agents which utilize the microsomal drug-metabolizing enzyme system will be discussed in the accompaning chapter (GUARINO, 1973).

Most of the drugs to be discussed in these two chapters are also discussed in the chapters devoted to specific agents; the present review is not an exhaustive compilation of the metabolic alterations undergone by these agents, but rather will list specific reactions and agents to illustrate general principles. Since the number of agents with demonstrable antitumor activity in experimental systems now runs to many thousands, emphasis will here be placed mainly on drugs with proven or potential clinical usefulness in human cancer. Of previous reviews of this area, the most comprehensive is that of MANDEL (1959); in a more recent survey, this author has discussed the metabolism and mode of action of selected agents (MANDEL, 1971). A number of the catabolic reactions which these agents undergo has recently been summarized by ADAMSON (1971). In addition, metabolic alterations undergone by antitumor agents have been surveyed in the course of reviews on the basic and clinical pharmacology of these drugs (OLIVERIO and ZUBROD, 1965; SARTORELLI and CREASEY, 1969; HEIDELBERGER, 1967; STOCK, 1967; YOUNG and BURCHENAL, 1971).

## Folate Antagonists

The folate antagonist aminopterin (4-amino-4-deoxypteroylglutamate) (Fig. 1) was the first antimetabolite shown to produce a remission in acute leukemia (FARBER et al., 1948). Following this initial finding, several hundred folate antagonists have been synthesized and tested for antitumor activity (MEAD et al., 1968). Of these agents, the antifolate currently in general clinical use is methotrexate (4-amino-4-deoxy-$N^{10}$-methylpteroylglutamate), while several other compounds of this class currently have the status of experimental clinical agents. The mechanism of action of the clinically important folate antagonists is generally felt to be inhibition of dihydrofolate reductase, the enzyme which catalyzes the generation of tetrahydrofolate, a cofactor utilized in the biosynthesis of thymidylate and also of purine nucleotides and certain amino acids.

Of the clinically important antifolates, only 3′,5′-dichloromethotrexate undergoes significant metabolic alteration in man and most experimental animals (DAVIDSON and OLIVERIO, 1965; LOO and ADAMSON, 1962); the product is 3′,5′-dichloro-7-hydroxymethotrexate (LOO and ADAMSON, 1965). In rabbit and guinea pig, but not in most other mammalian species, the nonhalogenated compounds

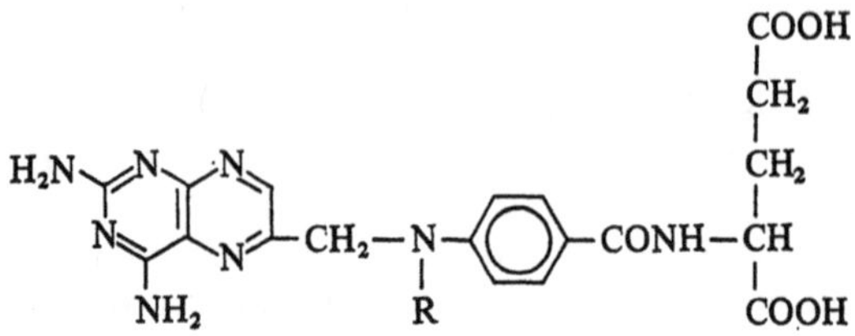

Aminopterin (R = H)
Methotrexate (R = $CH_3$)

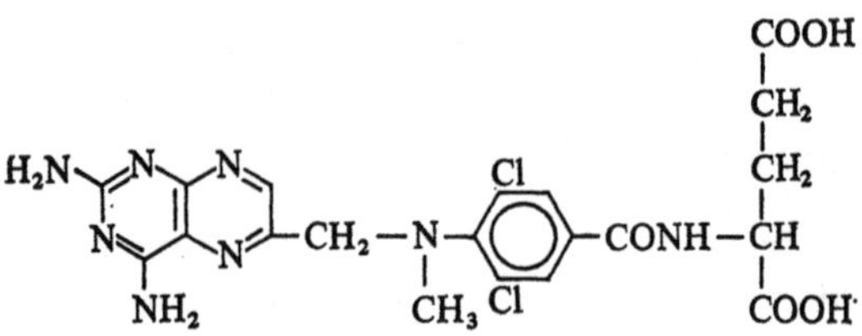

3′,5′-Dichloromethotrexate

**Fig. 1. Folate antagonists of clinical importance**

methotrexate and aminopterin also undergo hydroxylation, (REDETZKI et al., 1966; JOHNS et al., 1966a). The 7-hydroxy antifolates are much less effective inhibitors of dihydrofolate reductase than are the parent compounds, and the toxicity of methotrexate and aminopterin is much less in those species which are able to carry out this conversion (MINNICH et al., 1950; REDETZKI et al., 1966). It is unlikely, however, that the susceptibility to enzymatic inactivation is the sole explanation for the species differences in toxicity observed among the antifolates. The dog, for example, is unable to metabolize either methotrexate or dichloromethotrexate, but nevertheless exhibits twelve fold greater tolerance to the latter compound (RALL et al., 1959).

The enzyme carrying out the 7-hydroxylation of 4-aminofolates is hepatic aldehyde oxidase (EC 1.2.3.1), a molybdoflavoprotein present in the soluble supernatant fraction from mammalian liver homogenates (JOHNS et al., 1965). The range of substrate activity of this enzyme is extremely wide, and its natural substrate has not been unequivocally identified, although the physiological compounds pyridoxal and *N*-methylnicotinamide both show substrate activity and may occupy this role (KNOX, 1946; STANULOVIĆ and CHAYKIN, 1971). The enzyme from rabbit liver is extremely active and shows low specificity for *N*-heterocyclic substrates. The ability to utilize such substrates, in other mammalian species, appears to depend not only on the molecular configuration of the *N*-heterocyclic moiety of the substrate, but also on its general lipid solubility. For example, the aldehyde oxidase from rat liver has almost no ability to 7-hydroxylate methotrexate, but can readily hydroxylate derivatives of methotrexate with greater lipid solubility, such as methotrexate: diethyl ester (WOLPERT et al., 1972) and 3′,5′-dichloromethotrexate (JOHNS et al., 1965). These observations would appear to be compatible with the presence of a hydrophobic area in close juxtaposition to the binding site of the enzyme.

ADAMSON et al. (1962) have shown that rapidly growing "multiple deviation" rat liver tumors possess little or no ability to oxidize and inactivate dichloromethotrexate, while the activity in minimal deviation hepatomas is comparable to that of normal liver. Since primary hepatoma in man is responsive to antifolates (GEDDES and FALKSON, 1970), dichloromethotrexate has been used in the treatment of this tumor in an attempt to take advantage of this difference in enzyme levels and thus of the possibility of greater selective toxicity against tumor tissue with its lesser ability to inactivate the drug, than against surrounding normal liver. To date, however, no therapeutic advantage has been noted in the use of dichloromethotrexate over methotrexate in the treatment of this type of neoplastic disease (VOGEL et al., 1972).

Although methotrexate does not undergo 7-hydroxylation in most mammalian species, an alternative metabolic pathway, cleavage to yield 2,4-diamino-$N^{10}$-methylpteroic acid and glutamate, has been shown to have quantitative significance in the mouse and rat (ZAHARKO et al., 1969; VALERINO et al., 1972). The cleavage appears to be due to the action of bacterial peptidases, and takes place during the enterohepatic circulation of the drug. The cleavage reaction is not a major pathway in man, although trace amounts of urinary metabolites with the same chromatographic properties as 2,4-diamino-$N^{10}$-methylpteroic acid have been noted after administration of tritium-labeled drug to human subjects (JOHNS et al., 1964).

Studies on the metabolism of antifolates other than the 2,4-diaminopteridine class have not been extensive. FÖLSCH and BERTINO (1970), however, have reported an interesting example of hydrolytic cleavage and inactivation of a substituted 4,6-diaminotriazine folate antagonist by an enzyme present in mouse serum, but not in the serum of other species examined, including humans. These authors point out that, because of this rapid inactivation of the drug, mouse tumor systems would be inappropriate for determining the antineoplastic activity of compounds of this class.

## Thiopurines

### A. 6-Mercaptopurine

6-Mercaptopurine (6-MP) was the first member of the now extensive thiopurine series (Fig. 2) which was found to have useful antineoplastic activity in humans (BURCHENAL et al., 1953). This group of agents now includes 6-thioguanine, azathioprine, 6-methylthiopurine riboside, and a number of other purine analogs of experimental and clinical interest. The parent compound 6-MP is still in general clinical use as a component of the combination drug protocols used in the treatment of acute leukemia of childhood, in remission maintenance, and as an immunosuppressive agent.

6-MP is converted *in vivo* to 6-thiouric acid, 6-methylsulfinyl-8-hydroxypurine, and free sulfate; a significant fraction of the drug is excreted unchanged (ELION et al., 1954; HAMILTON and ELION, 1954; ELION, 1967). The enzyme responsible for the conversion of 6-MP to 6-thiouric acid is xanthine oxidase; the reaction appears to proceed *via* 6-mercapto-8-hydroxypurine (ELION et al., 1954, 1959; LOO et al., 1959). Successful attempts have been made to slow the catabolism of 6-MP by the administration of the xanthine oxidase inhibitor allopurinol, and thus to increase the fraction of the drug available for anabolism to the active nucleotide forms (RUNDLES et al., 1963; ELION et al., 1963a). In a typical experiment in a human subject, a dose of 150 mg of 6-MP was excreted as 7.2%

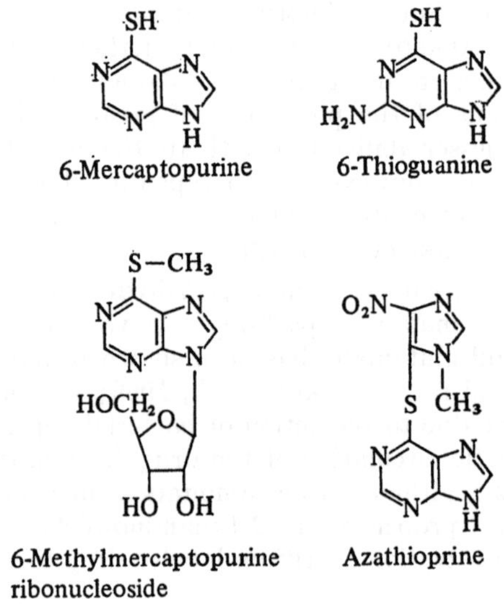


Fig. 2. Thiopurines with clinically useful antineoplastic or immunosuppressive activity

unchanged drug and 26.5% as thiouric acid in 24 hours; after a dose of 300 mg of allopurinol, the 24 hour excretion was 29.2% as 6-MP and only 3.8% as thiouric acid. Unexpectedly, the combination of 6-MP with allopurinol resulted in an improvement not only in the potency of 6-MP, but also in its therapeutic index in adenocarcinoma 755 in mice (ELION et al., 1963a).

6-MP, like other thiopurines, must undergo anabolic conversion to nucleotide forms in order to exert its antineoplastic activity; the conversion to the monophosphate is catalyzed by the enzyme guanine:hypoxanthine phosphoribosyltransferase (IMP:pyrophosphate phosphoribosyltransferase; EC 2.4.2.8). The anabolite 6-thioinosinic acid, inhibits a number of enzymes of purine nucleotide interconversion. Evidence exists, however, that significant amounts of 6-methylthiopurine ribonucleotide and thioguanylic acid also arise from 6-MP, and may contribute to its antineoplastic activity (ALLAN et al., 1966; SCANNELL and HITCHINGS, 1966; MIECH et al., 1969). The inability to convert 6-MP to its nucleotide form because of a decrease in the level of guanine:hypoxanthine phosphoribosyltransferase is a known mechanism of resistance to the drug in experimental tumor systems (BROCKMAN, 1963). In man, however, the mechanism of resistance to 6-MP is not well established; of fifteen leukemia patients clinically resistant to 6-MP who were studied by DAVIDSON and WINTER (1964), only one showed a decrease in the level of the enzyme when compared to previously untreated patients and to normal controls.

## B. 6-Thioguanine

6-Thioguanine (6-TG), although it has not to date gained the widespread clinical acceptance of 6-MP, has significant antitumor activity in several types of human neoplastic disease, and is still under active clinical study, particularly in combination with 1-β-D-arabinosylcytosine (ara-C). Like other thiopurines, 6-TG is multi-faceted in its action, and inhibits PRPP-amidotransferase, IMP dehydrogenase, and ATP:GMP phosphotransferase (MIECH et al., 1967). These multiple inhibitory activities combine to result in a general inhibition of formation of guanine nucleotides. In addition, a significant fraction of administered 6-TG is incorporated into DNA in the place of the normal guanine component, and this latter property appears to correlate well with the drug's cytotoxic effects (LEPAGE and WHITECAR, 1971).

Like other thiopurines, 6-TG must undergo conversion to nucleotides in order to exert its biological effects. Enhanced activity of a particulate alkaline phosphohydrolase which cleaves the 6-TG nucleotide may be responsible for resistance to the drug in some cell lines (WOLPERT et al., 1971). The enzyme was inhibited by EDTA and cyanide. The activity was present in all cell fractions, but was greatest in the crude nuclear fraction obtained by centrifugation at 1000 × g. This would appear to be one of the few examples known of enhanced catabolism of an antitumor agent being responsible for resistance to the drug.

In man, 6-TG is excreted to a small extent as the unchanged drug during early time-periods. The major excretion products, however, are 6-thiouric acid and 6-methylTG (2-amino-6-methylthiopurine), plus a small percentage of inorganic sulfate (LEPAGE and WHITECAR, 1971); the 6-thiouric acid presumably arises *via* 6-thioxanthine, since 6-TG, unlike 6-MP, is apparently not a substrate for xanthine oxidase (MOORE and LEPAGE, 1958).

## C. 6-Methylthiopurine (6-MMP) and 6-MMP Ribonucleoside

The metabolic fate of 6-methylthiopurine (6-MMP) differs significantly from that of its parent compound, 6-MP; with 6-MP, thiouric acid is a major metabolite, whereas with 6-MMP, 6-thiouric acid is excreted in only trace amounts, with a significant amount of the drug being excreted as glucuronyl and sulfinyl derivatives of 6-methylthio-8-hydroxypurine (ELION et al., 1963b; REMY, 1963) and as free sulfate. 6-MMP has relatively low substrate activity for xanthine oxidase, and the enzyme mainly responsible for 8-hydroxylation appears, at least in the rabbit, to be hepatic aldehyde oxidase (EC 1.2.3.1) rather than xanthine oxidase (EC 1.2.3.2) (LOO et al., 1967).

In addition to the latter catabolic pathway, *S*-demethylation of 6-MMP by a hepatic microsomal preparation to yield 6-MP has been demonstrated *in vitro* (MAZEL et al., 1964). In *in vivo* studies in man, and also the rat and mouse, trace amounts of free 6-MP have been detected in the urine after administration of 6-MMP (SARCIONE and STUTZMAN, 1960; ELION et al., 1963b), and the administration of the xanthine oxidase inhibitor, allopurinol, which blocks the conversion of 6-MP to 6-thiouric acid, causes a significant increase in the antineoplastic activity of both 6-MP and 6-MMP (ELION et al., 1963a). It is likely that this conversion of 6-MMP to 6-MP accounts for the biological activity of 6-MMP, although the mechanism and the quantitative importance of the conversion are still unclear.

6-MMP, unlike 6-MP, is not a substrate for purine nucleotide pyrophosphorylase, and appears to undergo little if any direct conversion to the nucleotide form

(BENNETT et al., 1965). The riboside of 6-MMP, 6-MMPR, has been prepared synthetically, however, and is of interest because of its lack of susceptibility, unlike most thiopurine ribosides, to phosphorylytic cleavage. 6-MMPR can, however, function as a substrate for adenosine kinase, and undergo conversion to the biologically active nucleotide (CALDWELL et al., 1966; SCHNEBLI et al., 1967). Resistance to 6-MMPR arising from a loss of this ability to convert the compound to the nucleotide form has been described by CALDWELL et al. (1967). 6-MMPR-nucleotide is also formed from 6-MP; its route of formation is thought to be the direct *S*-methylation of 6-MP ribonucleotide (ALLAN et al., 1966).

*In vivo* studies confirm the *in vitro* observation that 6-MMPR is not susceptible to either phosphorylytic or hydrolytic cleavage; the major excretion products are the unchanged ribonucleoside and its 5′-mononucleotide (LOO et al., 1968).

## D. Azathioprine

Azathioprine (Imuran), an *S*-substituted nitroimidazolyl derivative of 6-MP, is one of a series of *S*-alkylthiopurines prepared in an effort to protect the sulfur of 6-MP from oxidation *in vivo*, and the purine moiety from hydroxylation by xanthine oxidase. The electron-attracting nature of the nitroimidazolyl group makes the bond between it and the sulfur relatively labile, in contrast to the analogous bond of the *S*-methyl and *S*-propyl derivatives (ELION et al., 1963b). Azathioprine has a significant antineoplastic activity (ELION et al., 1961; RUNDLES et al., 1961). Its major clinical application, however, has been as an immunosuppressive agent, and for this purpose it is superior to its parent compound, 6-MP.

Azathioprine, in contrast to *S*-methyl and *S*-propylthiopurine, is subject under physiological conditions to nonenzymatic *S*-dealkylation, by means of thiolysis by compounds such as glutathione and cysteine (BRESNICK, 1959; CHALMERS et al., 1967). In addition, the compound is a very rapidly oxidized substrate for hepatic aldehyde oxidase; the product of the latter reaction is 8-hydroxyazathioprine (CHALMERS et al., 1969). The relative importance *in vivo* of the nonenzymic *S*-dealkylation and the enzyme-catalyzed 8-hydroxylation reactions has not been assessed. The pharmacological importance of the 8-hydroxylation reaction, as pointed out by CHALMERS (1969), lies in the possibility that if 8-hydroxylation precedes thiolysis, catabolism of the fraction of the administered drug utilizing this pathway could take place without release of free 6-MP.

*In vivo*, the excretion products observed after the administration of azathioprine are the same as those seen after 6-MP, i. e., free 6-MP, 6-thiouric acid, and sulfate. In the mouse, a considerable fraction of administered azathioprine is excreted in the urine unchanged, but in man only a trace of unchanged drug is observed (ELION et al., 1963b).

Recent studies (ELION, 1970) have been concerned with the fate of the nitroimidazolyl moiety of azathioprine. A small amount of the 5-thiol of 1-methyl-4-nitroimidazole is excreted in the urine; several other metabolites are detectable, including the corresponding 5-amino compound (ELION, 1970). The contribution of the nitroimidazolyl moiety of azathioprine to the total immunosuppressive activity of the drug is unknown. It would appear possible that the superiority of azathioprine over 6-MP as an immunosuppressive agent might be due, not to the presence of the imidazolyl moiety per se, but to differences in the pharmacokinetics of 6-MP when given as the free drug or in a "slowrelease" form such as azathioprine.

## E. Formycin A and B

The Formycins (Fig. 3), naturally occurring purine analogs obtained from cultures of *Nocardia* and *Streptomyces*, have been studied by UMEZAWA et al. (1965), CALDWELL et al. (1967, 1969), and SHEEN et al. (1968, 1970). Formycin A and B are isomers of adenosine and inosine, respectively, with the 8-carbon and 9-nitrogen of the purine skeleton interchanged, giving a pyrazolo(4,3-d)pyrimidine

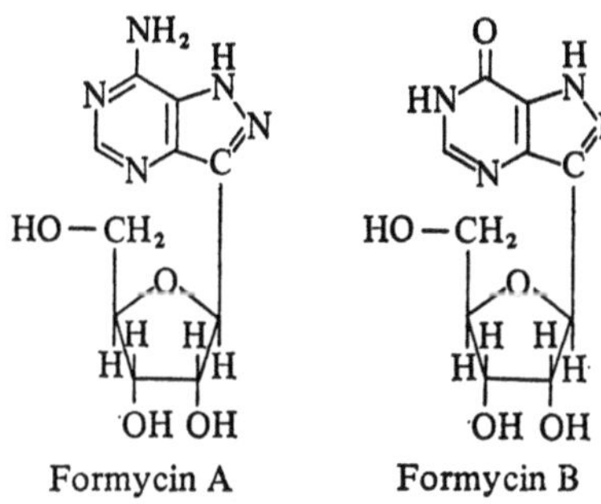


Fig. 3. Formycin A and B

structure. Formycin A shows significant antineoplastic activity in experimental systems, while Formycin B has antibacterial and antiviral activity, but lacks antineoplastic activity. The Formycins lack the clinical importance of the other purine analogs discussed in this section, but are included in the present survey because of several interesting and unusual aspects of their metabolism.

Formycin A is converted by adenosine kinase to the 5′-triphosphate; cells which lack this enzyme are resistant to the drug (CALDWELL, 1967, 1969). The compound is converted by adenosine deaminase to Formycin B, which is oxidized to the 5-hydroxy derivative by hepatic aldehyde oxidase (SHEEN et al., 1970). The latter reaction is the only known example of a purine nucleoside or nucleoside analog acting as a substrate for aldehyde oxidase; the naturally occurring riboside to which Formycin B corresponds, inosine, lacks substrate activity for this enzyme. SHEEN et al. (1970) have suggested that this difference in substrate activity arises because, as a consequence of the greater length of the C-C bond as compared to the N-C bond, the ribose moiety can rotate freely in Formycin B but not in inosine, and that as a result, Formycin B can assume configurations not possible with the corresponding purine nucleosides. Evidence against this interpretation, however, would seem to be provided by studies with the purine analog 9-butylazathioprine. This compound, in which a simple aliphatic chain rather than ribose is present at the 9-position, also lacks substrate activity for aldehyde oxidase, while the parent compound, azathioprine, is rapidly oxidized (CHALMERS et al., 1969). An alternative explanation would appear to be that the 9-nitrogen of purine bases acts as a necessary attachment site for the enzyme before oxidation can take place at the neighboring 8-carbon, and that consequently 9-substituted purine ribosides lack substrate activity. In Formycin B, however, the corresponding attachment to enzyme takes place at either the 4- or the 6-nitrogen of the 6-membered ring, with oxidation consequently taking place at C-5, i. e. Formycin B binds to aldehyde oxidase with a reverse orientation to that seen with conventional purine substrates. A similar reversal in orientation of binding of a pyrazolo-pyrimidine and its isomeric purine was postulated to be a possible explanation for the anomalous properties of allopurinol as a substrate and inhibitor for xanthine oxidase (BAKER et al., 1968).

## 5-Fluorouracil and Related Fluoropyrimidines

5-Fluorouracil (Fig. 4) was synthesized by DUSCHINSKY et al. (1957) in an attempt to take therapeutic advantage of early observations that uracil may be utilized preferentially for nucleic acid biosynthesis in tumors (RUTMAN et al., 1954)

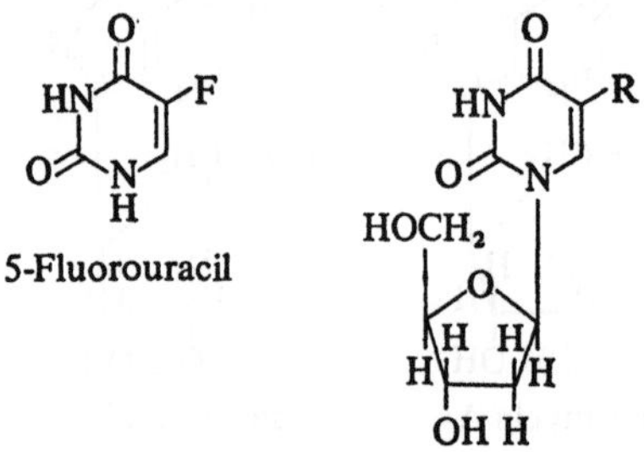


5-Fluorouracil

Fluorodeoxyuridine (R = F)
Iododeoxyuridine (R = I)

Fig. 4. Halogenated pyrimidines of clinical importance

and of the report by HAKALA et al. (1956) of the tumor-inhibitory activity of the pyrimidine analog 6-azauracil. A considerable literature has accumulated on the clinical utility of 5-fluorouracil; it is at the present time an established agent in the treatment of tumors of the colon, rectum, and breast, and is of experimental interest in a number of other forms of neoplastic disease.

5-Fluorouracil undergoes rapid biotransformation, utilizing both anabolic and catabolic pathways. The compound is readily converted to both ribosyl and deoxyribosyl derivatives, with significant amounts of the former being incorporated into RNA. The primary site of action of the drug lies, however, in the inhibition of DNA rather than RNA synthesis, and appears to consist of the inhibition by 5-fluoro-2′-deoxyuridine 5′-phosphate of the formation of thymidylate from deoxyuridylate, a reaction catalyzed by the enzyme thymidylate synthetase (REYES and HEIDELBERGER, 1965).

5-Fluorouracil is rapidly catabolized by the same pathway as that utilized by uracil (CHAUDHURI et al., 1959; MUKHERJEE and HEIDELBERGER, 1960). The enzyme concerned is present in the supernatant fraction of mammalian liver homogenates, is NADPH-dependent, and can utilize 5-fluorouracil or thymine as substrates. The product, dihydrouracil when uracil is used as substrate, undergoes a hydrolytic cleavage to $\beta$-ureidopropionic acid and thence to $\beta$-alanine and $CO_2$ (CANELLAKIS, 1956). There appears to be an inverse relationship between these catabolic reactions and the anabolic pathway to uridine and uridylate; tissues with high levels of the enzymes catalyzing the latter anabolic reactions have diminished or no ability to catalyze the catabolism of uracil, and vice versa (CANELLAKIS, 1957). With 5-fluorouracil, the same catabolic pathways are utilized, with the major catabolic products being $\alpha$-fluoro-$\beta$-alanine in man, and the latter compound plus its precursor, $\alpha$-fluoroureidopropionic acid, in the mouse (MUKHERJEE and HEIDELBERGER, 1960). Thymine and uracil increase the toxicity of 5-fluorouracil in mice, presumably by alternate substrate inhibition of the enzyme which reduces the drug. A variety of attempts have been made to slow the enzymic catabolism of 5-fluorouracil and thus to enhance its potency: a recent study of this type utilizing the pyrimidine reductase inhibitor 5-cyanouracil is reported by GENTRY et al. (1971).

Unlike 5-FU, the 5-trifluoromethyl analogs of uracil do not undergo ring cleavage (HEIDELBERGER et al., 1965). 5-Trifluoromethyl-2′-deoxyuridine is cleaved to yield the free base, and the latter is converted to 5-carboxyuracil, but is not further degraded.

Since the form of 5-FU which is active in the inhibition of DNA synthesis is the deoxynucleotide, numerous attempts have been made to increase the therapeutic efficacy by the administration of anabolites of 5-FU rather than the free base. These studies were stimulated by early clinical reports of possible greater therapeutic effectiveness of 5-fluoro-2′-deoxyuridine (FUdR) as compared to its parent compound 5-FU in the treatment of tumors of colon, rectum, and breast; more recent studies with greater numbers of patients appear to indicate, however, that the two forms of the drug are approximately equal in their therapeutic efficacy (Eastern Cooperative Group in Solid Tumor Chemotherapy, 1967).

FUdR is readily cleaved *in vivo*; the nucleoside phosphorylase which catalyzes the reaction is present in the high-speed supernatant fraction from Ehrlich ascites cells and from liver, and can utilize a number of other nucleoside substrates, including 5-fluorouridine (5-FUR) and 2′-deoxyuridine. Uridine is a competitive inhibitor of the cleavage reaction, but 3′- and 3′,5′-acetyl derivatives of FUdR are not. The latter compounds, however, were degraded when liver homogenates containing microsomal deacetylase activity were added to the supernatant fraction (BIRNIE et al., 1963).

The fluoropyrimidines, 2-hydroxy- and 4-hydroxy-5-fluoropyrimidine, appear to possess antitumor activity *in vivo* by virtue of their conversion to 5-fluorouracil (BUDĚŠÍNSKÝ et al., 1962, 1965; SARTORELLI and CREASEY, 1967). The enzymes responsible for the oxidation are aldehyde oxidase in the case of 2-hydroxy-5-fluoropyrimidine, and xanthine oxidase in the case of 4-hydroxy-5-fluoropyrimidine (JOHNS et al., 1966b); the antineoplastic effects of 4-hydroxy-5-fluoropyrimidine in the Sarcoma 180 ascites cell system *in vivo* were abolished by the simultaneous administration of the xanthine oxidase inhibitor allopurinol (SARTORELLI and CREASEY, 1967). The use of these precursor forms of 5-fluorouracil appears to offer no therapeutic advantage over fluorouracil itself. The reactions are of interest, however, as examples of drug-catabolizing enzymes participating in the conversion of an antineoplastic agent from an inactive to an active form.

## Iododeoxyuridine

Iododeoxyuridine (IUdR) (Fig. 4) has significant activity in several experimental tumor systems (PRUSOFF, 1959). Its main clinical application, however, has been in the topical treatment of keratitis caused by herpes simplex and vaccinia viruses (KAUFMAN, 1962). The compound undergoes anabolic conversion to nucleotide forms, and competitively inhibits the incorporation of thymidine into DNA. In addition, incorporation of IUdR into DNA appears to render the cell more susceptible to radiation damage. The main catabolic pathway for IUdR is enzymatic cleavage to 5-iodouracil, followed by deiodination of the latter, with a large fraction of the administered iodine being excreted as free iodide (PRUSOFF, 1970). The corresponding cytidine derivative is rapidly deaminated *in vivo* to yield IUdR (CALABRESI et al., 1963).

## 1-β-D-Arabinosylcytosine

1-β-D-Arabinosylcytosine (ara-C; cytosine arabinoside) (Fig. 5) is of clinical value in the treatment of several types of human neoplastic disease. As with most pyrimidine and purine analogs with antineoplastic potency, ara-C requires phosphorylation to express this activity. Ara-C, as the triphosphate, is an inhibitor of

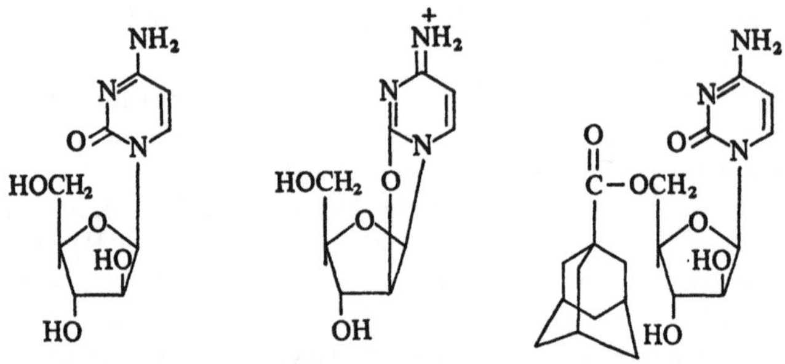


Fig. 5. 1-β-D-Arabinosylcytosine (ara-C) and related compounds

DNA synthesis, and thus exerts its effects primarily during the *S*-phase of the cell cycle. Inhibition of DNA polymerase by ara-C is one means by which the drug inhibits DNA synthesis. The drug is also incorporated into both DNA and RNA; irreversible inhibition of cell growth appears to correlate well with the latter process, and particularly with the incorporation of ara-C into 2 to 7S RNA (Chu, 1971).

Phosphorylation of ara-C to yield the active form of the drug is carried out by deoxycytidine kinase (CdR kinase), an enzyme found in thymus and other lymphoid tissues. CdR is the kinetically preferred substrate, with a Michaelis constant of $5.3 \times 10^{-6}\,M$ while ara-C has a Michaelis constant of $4.1 \times 10^{-5}\,M$; other substrates for CdR kinase are GdR and AdR. The enzyme activity is subject to complex regulation by a number of nucleotides and nucleosides. Durham and Ives (1969) have suggested that the rate of phosphorylation of ara-C to ara-CMP determines the toxicity of the drug, rather than the rate of its inactivation by conversion to ara-U. These authors point out that ara-C is much more toxic in the mouse than in the rat; although the mouse has a higher deaminase level than the rat, it also phosphorylates ara-C more efficiently.

The enzyme which inactivates ara-C, pyrimidine nucleoside deaminase or cytosine nucleoside deaminase, has been subjected to intensive study. The enzyme is extremely active in man; Camiener (1965) has calculated that the pyrimidine nucleoside deaminase present in human liver could deaminate more than 5 g of ara-C per hour. Most other species have much lower levels of the enzyme; from the point of view of selection of a model animal system for the study of the pharmacology of this drug, the rhesus monkey has an enzyme level comparable to that of man, while the squirrel monkey has a much lower level, one-fifth to one-half that seen in man.

The pyrimidine nucleoside deaminase activity of mouse kidney has been studied by Creasey (1963) and by Tomchick et al. (1968); the enzymes studied by these two groups do not appear to be identical, however, since that studied by Creasey was stabilized by glutathione, and nucleotides as well as nucleosides could be used as substrates, whereas neither of these properties was demonstrable with the enzyme studied by the latter group.

The pyrimidine nucleoside deaminase of human liver has been described by CAMIENER (1967a). No cofactor requirements were detected, and the enzyme appeared to be a simple aminohydrolase. Preincubation with *p*-chloromercuribenzoate destroyed the activity, indicating possible involvement of reduced sulfhydryl groups in the catalytic activity. In an interesting structure-activity study with the human enzyme, CAMIENER (1967b) has observed that a 2-keto group and an unsubstituted N-3 ring nitrogen are required for substrate activity.

A number of investigators have studied the effect of various pyrimidine analogs as inhibitors of the enzyme, for possible use in prolonging the activity of the drug *in vivo* by inhibiting its deamination. The most useful compound of this type appears to be tetrahydrouridine (CAMIENER, 1969); this compound inhibits pyrimidine nucleoside deaminase from human liver, rhesus monkey liver, mouse kidney, and bacterial sources. The inhibition appears to be "partial noncompetitive" or "regulatory" in type, i. e. enzyme present in the EI complex is still catalytically active, but the reaction rate is about one-fourth that seen with the uninhibited enzyme. Preincubation of inhibitor with enzyme was required for maximal inhibition. Because of the complex nature of the inhibition, the dissociation constant of the EI complex could not be determined accurately; it was estimated to be between $10^{-4}$ and $10^{-5}$ *M*. Other tetrahydropyrimidine nucleosides were also effective inhibitors, but the dihydro compounds were much less effective. *In vivo*, tetrahydrouridine was found to be active in slowing the deamination of ara-C in the monkey (MULLIGAN and MELLETT, 1970).

Another interesting approach to the problem of the rapid *in vivo* inactivation of ara-C is the use of ara-C precursor compounds such as 5′-adamantoyl-ara-C (NEIL et al., 1970) and O[2], 2′-anhydrocytidine-3′-phosphate (NAGYVARY, 1969). The latter compound appears not to be subject to deamination by pyrimidine nucleoside deaminase, but to be slowly hydrolyzed to yield ara-C, thus acting as a "slow-release" form of the drug.

## Hydroxyurea

Hydroxyurea (Fig. 6) is an inhibitor of the enzyme ribonucleoside diphosphate reductase (ELFORD, 1968), and is used at high dosage levels in the management of chronic granulocytic leukemia and occasionally in the treatment of other types of neoplastic disease.

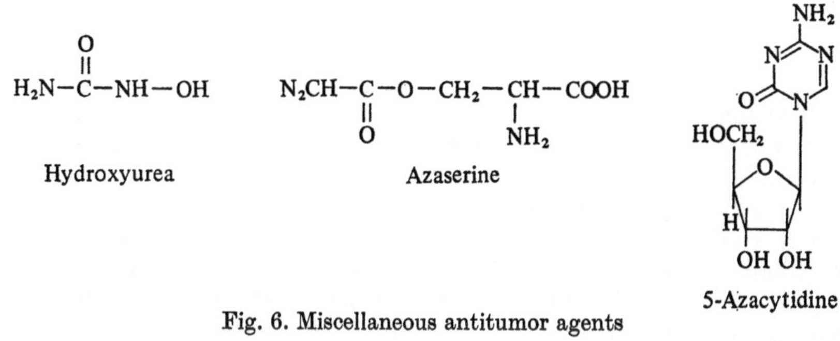


Fig. 6. Miscellaneous antitumor agents

The conversion of hydroxyurea to urea was reported by ADAMSON et al. (1965), and the enzyme system responsible for the conversion has been studied by COLVIN and BONO (1970). Activity was greatest in the mitochondrial fraction from mouse liver homogenates, but was present to a lesser extent in other subcellular fractions. The enzyme activity utilized either NADH or NADPH as electron donor, and was stimulated by added FAD. A slow rate of nonenzymic conversion of hydroxyurea to urea could be detected in the presence of ferrous ion; these investigators suggest, therefore, that the distribution of activity among several subcellular fractions might indicate that the conversion can be catalyzed by several ferrous iron-containing proteins, rather than being carried out by a single enzyme.

In man, conversion of hydroxyurea to acetohydroxamic acid has been reported (Fishbein and Carbone, 1963).

## Vinca Alkaloids

Although the Vinca alkaloids, vinblastine and vincristine (Fig. 7), are in general clinical use in the treatment of acute leukemia and of lymphomas, and considerable information is available on their mode of action at the molecular level (Sartorelli and Creasey, 1969), many aspects of their pharmacology are little understood. Radioactive tracer studies have been technically difficult because the available methods of tritium-labeling result in partial reduction and degradation of these complex molecules, with resulting difficulties in isolating the pure tritium-labeled compound from the resulting mixture, while the introduction of a carbon-14 label has, to date, posed insoluble synthetic problems.

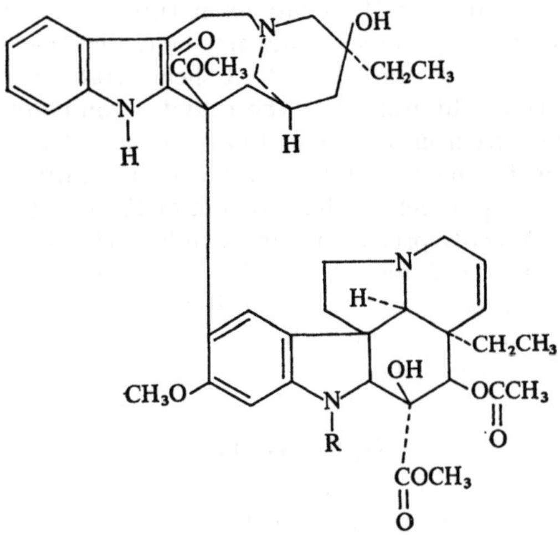


Vincristine (R = CHO)
Vinblastine (R = $CH_3$)

Fig. 7. Clinically useful vinca alkaloids

In early studies with tritium-labeled vinblastine prepared by the Wilzbach method, Beer and Richards (1964) found some 20% of an administered dose in the range 1.0 to 1.6 mg/kg to be excreted in 24 hours in the bile in rats; little radioactivity appeared in the urine. More than 90% of the biliary radioactivity consisted of vinblastine metabolites, of which at least six could be distinguished.

In more recent studies with tritium-labeled vinblastine, which was prepared by exchange with tritiated trifluoracetic acid, and which was of more than 96% radiopurity, Hebden et al. (1970) observed that circulating vinblastine was present mainly in blood platelets. The material transported by platelets consisted largely of unchanged drug, while the radioactivity present in the plasma was mainly in the form of vinblastine metabolites.

Little is presently known regarding the enzyme systems active in degrading vinblastine and the other Vinca alkaloids, or regarding the identity and possible pharmacological activity of the numerous metabolites.

## 5-Azacytidine

5-Azacytidine (Fig. 6) was prepared and shown to have significant antitumor activity by Czechoslovakian investigators (Šorm and Veselý, 1964; Hrodek and Veselý, 1971); considerable interest in this compound has recently developed because of its activity in acute myelogenous leukemia. The catabolism of 5-azacytidine appears to proceed nonenzymically. At neutral pH, the compound gives rise to 1-$\beta$-D-ribofuranosyl-3-guanylurea, $\alpha$-D-ribofuro-2-oxazolidone, guanidine, and D-ribose; under mild acidic conditions it yields 5-azacytosine, 5-azauracil, and D-ribose. None of the hydrolysis products shows biological activity comparable to that of the parent compound (Pıťhová et al., 1965).

Ehrlich ascites cells will convert 5-azacytidine to the mono-, di-, and triphosphate derivatives. No significant difference was found between the phosphorylating activity of normal and leukemic tissues. The compound is incorporated *in vivo* into RNA and the degree of incorporation appears to correlate well with its cytotoxic activity (Jurovčík et al., 1965). With L1210 cells in culture, the addition of cytidine greatly inhibited the phosphorylation of 5-azacytidine and its subsequent incorporation into polynucleotides (Li et al., 1970).

## Azaserine

Azaserine (Fig. 6) is a glutamine analog that acts by competing with glutamine to block amidination of $\alpha$-*N*-formylglycinamide ribonucleoside in the purine nucleotide biosynthetic pathway. Although little used clinically at the present time, azaserine is of potential interest because of its significant activity in a number of experimental tumor systems, when used in combination with thiopurines and other purine analogs (Sartorelli, 1965).

Azaserine is rapidly degraded to ammonia and pyruvate by an enzyme present in mouse liver (Reilly, 1954a, b). The enzyme appears to have a high degree of specificity, since under conditions which result in almost complete deamination of azaserine, no appreciable release of ammonia from any of 19 other amino acids tested was detectable. The azaserine analog of 6-diazo-5-oxo-L-norleucine was not a substrate. The structure-activity relationships for this enzyme are discussed more fully by Jacquez and Sherman (1962).

### References

Adamson, R. H.: Metabolism of anticancer agents in man. Ann. N. Y. Acad. Sci. **179**, 432—441 (1971).

Adamson, R. H., Loo, T. L., Morris, H. P.: Metabolism of $Cl^{36}$-Dichloromethotrexate by transplantable liver tumors. Proc. Soc. exp. Biol. (N. Y.) **111**, 566—568 (1962).

Adamson, R. H., Ague, S. L., Hess, S. M., Davidson, J. D.: The distribution, excretion and metabolism of hydroxyurea-$^{14}$C. J. pharmacol. exp. Ther. **150**, 322—334 (1965).

Allan, P. W., Schnebli, H. P., Bennett, L. L., Jr.: Conversion of 6-mercaptopurine and 6-mercaptopurine ribonucleoside to 6-methylmercaptopurine ribonucleotide in human epidermoid carcinoma no. 2 cells in culture. Biochim. biophys. Acta **114**, 647—650 (1966).

Baker, B. R., Wood, W. F., Kozma, J. A.: Irreversible enzyme inhibitors. CXXVI. Hydrocarbon interaction with xanthine oxidase by phenyl substitutents on purines and pyrazolo-(3,4-*d*)pyrimidines. J. med. Chem. **11**, 661—666 (1968).

Beer, C. T., Richards, J. F.: The metabolism of *Vinca* alkaloids. Part II. The fate of tritiated vinblastine in rats. Lloydia **27**, 352—360 (1964).

Bennett, L. L., Jr., Brockman, R. W., Schnebli, H. P., Chumley, S., Dixon, G. J., Schabel, F. M., Jr., Dulmadge, E. A., Skipper, H. E., Montgomery, J. A., Thomas, H. J.: Activity and mechanism of action of 6-methylthiopurine ribonucleoside in cancer cells resistant to 6-mercaptopurine. Nature (Lond.) **205**, 1276—1279 (1965).

Birnie, G. D., Kroeger, H., Heidelberger, C.: Studies of fluorinated pyrimidines. XVIII. The degradation of 5-fluoro-2′-deoxyuridine and related compounds by nucleoside phosphorylase. Biochemistry **2**, 566—572 (1963).

Bresnick, E.: The metabolism *in vitro* of antitumor imidazolyl derivatives of mercaptopurines. Fed. Proc. **18**, 371 (1959).

Brockman, R. W.: Biochemical aspects of mercaptopurine inhibition and resistance. Cancer Res. **23**, 1191—1201 (1963).

Buděšínský, Z., Jelínek, V., Přikryl, J.: 5-Halogenpyrimidine. I. Darstellung von 4-hydroxy-5-halogenpyrimidinen. Coll. Czech. Chem. Commun. **27**, 2550—2560 (1962).

Buděšínský, Z., Přikryl, J., Svátek, E.: 5-Halogenpyrimidine. II. Synthese des 2-hydroxy-5-fluoropyrimidins. Coll. Czech. Chem. Commun. **30**, 3895—3901 (1965).

Burchenal, J. H., Murphy, M. L., Ellison, R. R., Sykes, M. P., Tan, T. C., Leone, L. A., Karnofsky, D. A., Craver, L. F., Dargeon, H. W., Rhoads, C. P.: Clinical evaluation of a new antimetabolite, 6-mercaptopurine, in the treatment of leukemia and allied diseases. Blood **8**, 965—999 (1953).

Calabresi, P., Creasey, W. A., Prusoff, W. H., Welch, A. D.: Clinical and pharmacological studies with 5-iodo-2′-deoxycytidine. Cancer Res. **23**, 583—592 (1963).

Caldwell, I. C., Henderson, J. F., Paterson, A. R. P.: The enzymic formation of 6-(methylmercapto)purine ribonucleoside 5′-phosphate. Can. J. Biochem. **44**, 229—245 (1966).

Caldwell, I. C., Henderson, J. F., Paterson, A. R. P.: Resistance to purine ribonucleoside analogues in an ascites tumor. Can. J. Biochem. **45**, 735—744 (1967).

Caldwell, I. C., Henderson, J. F., Paterson, A. R. P.: The metabolism of formycin, an adenosine analogue. Can. J. Biochem. **47**, 901—908 (1969).

Camiener, G. W.: Studies of the enzymatic deamination of cytosine arabinoside. II. Properties of the deaminase of human liver. Biochem. Pharmacol. **16**, 1681—1690 (1967a).

Camiener, G. W.: Studies of the enzymatic deamination of cytosine arabinoside. III. Substrate requirements and inhibitors of the deaminase of human liver. Biochem. Pharmacol. **16**, 1691—1702 (1967b).

Camiener, G. W.: Studies of the enzymatic deamination of ara-cytidine. V. Inhibition *in vitro* and *in vivo* by tetrahydrouridine and other reduced pyrimidine nucleotides. Biochem. Pharmacol. **17**, 1981—1991 (1968).

Camiener, G. W., Smith, C. G.: Studies of the enzymatic deamination of cytosine arabinoside. I. Enzyme distribution and species specificity. Biochem. Pharmacol. **14**, 1405—1416 (1965).

Canellakis, E. S.: Pyrimidine metabolism. I. Enzymatic pathways of uracil and thymine degradation. J. biol. Chem. **221**, 315—322 (1956).

Canellakis, E. S.: Pyrimidine metabolism. III. The interaction of the catabolic and anabolic pathways of uracil metabolism. J. biol. Chem. **227**, 701—709 (1957).

Chalmers, A. H., Knight, P. R., Atkinson, M. R.: Conversion of azathioprine into mercaptopurine and mercaptoimidazole derivatives *in vitro* and during immunosuppressive therapy. Aust. J. exp. biol. Med. Sci. **45**, 681—691 (1967).

Chalmers, A. H., Knight, P. R., Atkinson, M. R.: 6-Thiopurines as substrates and inhibitors of purine oxidases: A pathway for conversion of azathioprine into 6-thiouric acid without release of 6-mercaptopurine. Aust. J. exp. biol. Med. Sci. **47**, 263—273 (1969).

Chaudhuri, N. K., Mukherjee, K. L., Heidelberger, C.: Studies on fluorinated pyrimidines. VII. The degradative pathway. Biochem. Pharmacol. **1**, 328—341 (1959).

Chu, M. Y.: Incorporation of arabinosyl cytosine into 2—7 S ribonucleic acid and cell death. Biochem. Pharmacol. **20**, 2057—2063 (1971).

Colvin, M., Bono, V. H., Jr.: The enzymatic reduction of hydroxyurea to urea by mouse liver. Cancer Res. **30**, 1516—1519 (1970).

Creasey, W. A.: Studies on the metabolism of 5-iodo-2′-deoxycytidine *in vitro*. Purification of nucleoside deaminase from mouse kidney. J. biol. Chem. **238**, 1772—1776 (1963).

Davidson, J. D., Oliverio, V. T.: The physiologic disposition of dichloromethotrexate-$Cl^{36}$ in man. Clin. Pharmacol. and Ther. **6**, 321—327 (1965).

Davidson, J. D., Winter, T. S.: Purine nucleotide pyrophosphorylases in 6-mercaptopurine-sensitive and -resistant human leukemias. Cancer Res. **24**, 261—267 (1964).

Durham, J. P., Ives, D. H.: Deoxycytidine kinase. I. Distribution in normal and neoplastic tissues and interrelationships of deoxycytidine and 1-β-D-arabinofuranosylcytosine phosphorylation. Mol. Pharmacol. **5**, 358—375 (1969).

DUSCHINSKY, R., PLEVEN, E., HEIDELBERGER, C.: The synthesis of 5-fluoropyrimidines. J. Amer. chem. Soc. **79**, 4559—4560 (1957).
EASTERN COOPERATIVE GROUP IN SOLID TUMOR CHEMOTHERAPY: Comparison of antimetabolites in the treatment of breast and colon cancer. J. Amer. Med. Assoc. **200**, 770—778 (1967).
ELFORD, H. L.: Effect of hydroxyurea on ribonucleotide reductase. Biochem. biophys. Res. Commun. **33**, 129—135 (1968).
ELION, G. B.: Biochemistry and pharmacology of purine analogues. Fed. Proc. **26**, 898—904 (1967).
ELION, G. B., BIEBER, S., HITCHINGS, G. H.: The fate of 6-mercaptopurine in mice. Ann. N. Y. Acad. Sci. **60**, 297—303 (1954).
ELION, G. B., MUELLER, S., HITCHINGS, G. H.: Studies on condensed pyrimidine systems. XXI. The isolation and synthesis of 6-mercapto-2,8-purinediol (6-thiouric acid). J. Amer. chem. Soc. **81**, 3042—3045 (1959).
ELION, G. B., CALLAHAN, S., BIEBER, S., HITCHINGS, G. H., RUNDLES, R. W.: A summary of investigations with 6-[(1-methyl-4-nitro-5-imidazolyl)thio]purine (B. W. 57—322). Cancer Chemother. Rep. **14**, 93—98 (1961).
ELION, G. B., CALLAHAN, S., NATHAN, H., BIEBER, S., RUNDLES, R. W., HITCHINGS, G. H.: Potentiation by inhibition of drug degradation: 6-Substituted purines and xanthine oxidase. Biochem. Pharmacol. **12**, 85—93 (1963a).
ELION, G. B., CALLAHAN, S., RUNDLES, R. W., HITCHINGS, G. H.: Relationship between metabolic fates and antitumor activities of thiopurines. Cancer Res. **23**, 1207—1217 (1963b).
ELION, G. B., BENEZRA, F. M., CARRINGTON, L. O., STRELITZ, R. A.: Metabolic fate of $^{14}$C-azathioprine. Fed. Proc. **29**, 607 (1970).
FARBER, S., DIAMOND, L. K., MERCER, R. D., SYLVESTER, R. F., Jr., WOLFF, J. A.: Temporary remissions in acute leukemia in children produced by folic acid antagonist, 4-aminopteroyl-glutamic acid (Aminopterin). New Eng. J. Med. **238**, 787—793 (1948).
FISHBEIN, W. N., CARBONE, P. P.: Hydroxyurea: mechanism of action. Science **142**, 1069—1070 (1963).
FÖLSCH, E., BERTINO, J. R.: Inactivation by mouse serum of a tightly bound inhibitor of dihydrofolate reductase. Molec. Pharmacol. **6**, 95—98 (1970).
GEDDES, E. W., FALKSON, G.: Malignant hepatoma in the Bantu. Cancer **25**, 1271—1278 (1970).
GENTRY, G. A., MORSE, P. A., Jr., DORSETT, M. T.: *In vivo* inhibition of pyrimidine catabolism by 5-cyanouracil. Cancer Res. **31**, 909—912 (1971).
GUARINO, A. M.: Metabolism of cancer chemotherapeutic agents *via* pathways utilized by xenobiotics. In: Handbook of Experimental Pharmacology, vol. XXXVIII, Part I, Antineoplastic and Immunosuppressive Agents, pp. 218—318 (A. C. SARTORELLI and D. G. JOHNS, Eds.). Berlin-Heidelberg-New York: Springer 1974.
HAKALA, M. T., LAW, L. W., WELCH, A. D.: Inhibitory activity of 6-azauracil, 6-uracil methyl sulfone and related compounds on the growth of mouse lymphomas and sarcoma 180. Proc. Amer. Assoc. Cancer Res. **2**, 113 (1956).
HAMILTON, L., ELION, G. B.: The fate of 6-mercaptopurine in man. Ann. N. Y. Acad. Sci. **60**, 304—314 (1954).
HEBDEN, H. F., HADFIELD, J. R., BEER, C. T.: The binding of vinblastine by platelets in the rat. Cancer Res. **30**, 1417—1424 (1970).
HEIDELBERGER, C.: Cancer chemotherapy with purine and pyrimidine analogues. Ann. Rev. Pharmacol. **7**, 101—124 (1967).
HEIDELBERGER, C., BOOHAR, J., KAMPSCHROER, B.: Fluorinated pyrimidines. XXIV. *In vivo* metabolism of 5-trifluoromethyluracil-2-$C^{14}$ and 5-trifluoromethyl-2'-deoxyuridine-2-$C^{14}$. Cancer Res. **25**, 377—381 (1965).
HRODEK, O., VESELÝ, J.: 5-Azacytidine in childhood leukemia. Neoplasma **18**, 493—503 (1971).
JACQUEZ, J. A., SHERMAN, J. H.: Enzymatic degradation of azaserine. Cancer Res. **22**, 56—61 (1962).
JOHNS, D. G., HOLLINGSWORTH, J. W., CASHMORE, A. R., PLENDERLEITH, I. H., BERTINO, J. R.: Methotrexate displacement in man. J. clin. Invest. **43**, 621—629 (1964).
JOHNS, D. G., IANNOTTI, A. T., SARTORELLI, A. C., BOOTH, B. A., BERTINO, J. R.: The identity of rabbit-liver methotrexate oxidase. Biochim. biophys. Acta (Amst.) **105**, 380—382 (1965).
JOHNS, D. G., IANNOTTI, A. T., SARTORELLI, A. C., BERTINO, J. R.: On the relative toxicities of methotrexate and aminopterin. Biochem. Pharmacol. **15**, 555—561 (1966a).
JOHNS, D. G., SARTORELLI, A. C., BERTINO, J. R., IANNOTTI, A. T., BOOTH, B. A., WELCH, A. D.: Enzymic hydroxylation of 5-fluoropyrimidines by aldehyde oxidase and xanthine oxidase. Biochem. Pharmacol. **15**, 400—403 (1966b).
JUROVČÍK, M., RAŠKA, K., ŠORMOVÁ, Z., ŠORM, F.: Anabolic transformation of a novel antimetabolite, 5-azacytidine, and evidence for its incorporation into ribonucleic acid. Coll. Czech. Chem. Commun. **30**, 3370—3376 (1965).

KAUFMAN, H. E., NESBURN, A. B., MALONEY, E. D.: IDU Therapy of herpes simplex. Arch. Ophthalmol. **67**, 583—591 (1962).
KNOX, W. E.: The quinine-oxidizing enzyme and liver aldehyde oxidase. J. biol. Chem. **163**, 699—711 (1946).
LEPAGE, G. A., WHITECAR, J. P., Jr.: Pharmacology of 6-thioguanine in man. Cancer Res. **31**, 1627—1631 (1971).
LI, L. H., OLIN, E. J., BUSKIRK, H. H., REINEKE, L. M.: Cytotoxicity and mode of action of 5-azacytidine on L1210 leukemia. Cancer Res. **30**, 2760—2769 (1970).
LOO, T. L., ADAMSON, R. H.: The enzymic oxidation of certain folic acid antagonists. Biochem. Pharmacol. **11**, 170—171 (1962).
LOO, T. L., ADAMSON, R. H.: The metabolite of 3′,5′-dichloro-4-amino-4-deoxy-$N^{10}$-methylpteroylglutamic acid (Dichloromethotrexate). J. med. Chem. **8**, 513—515 (1965).
LOO, T. L., LIM, C., JOHNS, D. G.: Enzymic hydroxylation of 6-methylthiopurine by hepatic aldehyde oxidase. Biochim. biophys. Acta (Amst.) **134**, 467—469 (1967).
LOO, T. L., LUCE, J. K., SULLIVAN, M. P., FREI, E., III: Clinical pharmacologic observations on 6-mercaptopurine and 6-methylthiopurine ribonucleoside. Clin. Pharmacol. Ther. **9**, 180—194 (1968).
LOO, T. L., MICHAEL, M. E., GARCEAU, A. J., REID, J. C.: 6-Thiouric acid — a metabolite of 6-mercaptopurine. J. Amer. chem. Soc. **81**, 3039—3041 (1959).
MANDEL, H. G.: The physiological disposition of some anticancer agents. Pharmacol. Rev. **11**, 743—838 (1959).
MANDEL, H. G.: The metabolism of analogs of endogenous substrates: Wider application of a limited concept. In: Handbook of experimental pharmacology, vol. 28, Concepts in Biochemical Pharmacology, part 2, pp. 654—683 (B. B. BRODIE and J. R. GILLETTE, Ed.). Berlin-Heidelberg-New York: Springer 1971.
MAZEL, P., HENDERSON, J. F., AXELROD, J.: S-Demethylation by microsomal enzymes. J. pharmacol. exp. Ther. **143**, 1—6 (1964).
MEAD, J. A. R., WOOD, H. B., Jr., GOLDIN, A.: Relationship of structure to antitumor activity in compounds related to folic acid. Cancer Chemother. Rep. (Part 2) **1**, 273—361 (1968).
MUKHERJEE, K. L., HEIDELBERGER, C.: Studies on fluorinated pyrimidines. IX. The degradation of 5-fluorouracil-6-$C^{14}$. J. biol. Chem. **235**, 433—437 (1960).
MIECH, R. P., PARKS, R. E., Jr., ANDERSON, J. H., Jr., SARTORELLI, A. C.: An hypothesis on the mechanism of action of 6-thioguanine. Biochem. Pharmacol. **16**, 2222—2227 (1967).
MIECH, R. P., YORK, R., PARKS, R. E., Jr.: ATP-GMP Phosphotransferase. II. Inhibition by 6-thioguanosine (6-thioGMP) of the enzyme isolated from hog brain and sarcoma 180 ascites cells. Molec. Pharmacol. **5**, 30—37 (1969).
MINNICH, V., MOORE, C. V., SMITH, D. E., ELLIOTT, G. V.: Studies on the acute toxic effects of 4-aminopteroyl-glutamic acid in dogs, guinea pigs, and rabbits. Arch. Path. **50**, 787—799 (1950).
MOORE, E. C., LEPAGE, G. A.: The metabolism of 6-thioguanine in normal and neoplastic tissues. Cancer Res. **18**, 1075—1083 (1958).
MULLIGAN, L. T., MELLETT, L. B.: Inhibition of arabinosyl cytosine deamination by tetrahydrouridine in the monkey. The Pharmacologist **12**, 221 (1970).
NAGYVARY, J.: Arabinonucleotides. II. The synthesis of $O^2$,2′-anhydrocytidine-3′-phosphate, a precursor of 1-$\beta$-D-arabinosylcytosine. J. Amer. chem. Soc. **91**, 5409—5410 (1969).
NEIL, G. L., WILEY, P. F., MANAK, R. C., MOXLEY, T. E.: Antitumor effect of 1-$\beta$-D-arabinofuranosylcytosine 5′-adamantoate (NSC 117614) in L1210 leukemic mice. Cancer Res. **30**, 1047—1054 (1970).
OLIVERIO, V. T., ZUBROD, C. G.: Clinical pharmacology of the effective antitumor drugs. Ann. Rev. Pharmacol. **5**, 335—356 (1965).
PIŤHOVÁ, P., PÍSKALA, A., PIŤHA, J., ŠORM, F.: Nucleic acid components and their analogues. LXVI. Hydrolysis of 5-azacytidine and its connection with biological activity. Coll. Czech. Chem. Commun. **30**, 2801—2811 (1965).
PRUSOFF, W. H., JAFFE, J. J., GÜNTHER, H., WELCH, A. D.: Studies of the pharmacology and antitumor activity of iododeoxyuridine, an analog of thymidine. Proc. Amer. Assoc. Cancer Res. **3**, 54 (1959).
PRUSOFF, W. H., JAFFE, J. J., GÜNTHER, H.: Studies in the mouse of the pharmacology of 5-iododeoxyuridine, an analogue of thymidine. Biochem. Pharmacol. **3**, 110—121 (1960).
RALL, D. P., PALLOTTA, A. J., ELSEA, J. R.: Comparative toxicity of amethopterin, 3′-monochloroamethopterin, and 3′,5′-dichloroamethopterin in rats and dogs. Proc. Amer. Assoc. Cancer Res. **3**, 54 (1959).
REDETZKI, H. M., REDETZKI, J. E., ELIAS, A. L.: Resistance of the rabbit to methotrexate: Isolation of a drug metabolite with decreased toxicity. Biochem. Pharmacol. **15**, 425—433 (1966).

REILLY, H. C.: Studies on the fate of azaserine in the animal body. Bact. Proc. **54**, 79 (1954a).
REILLY, H. C.: Inactivation of azaserine by a liver enzyme. Fed. Proc. **13**, 279 (1954b).
REMY, C. N.: Metabolism of thiopyrimidines and thiopurines. *S*-Methylation with *S*-adenosylmethionine transmethylase and catabolism in mammalian tissues. J. biol. Chem. **238**, 1078—1084 (1963).
REYES, P., HEIDELBERGER, C.: Fluorinated pyrimidines. XXV. The inhibition of thymidylate synthetase from Ehrlich ascites carcinoma cells by pyrimidine analogs. Biochim. biophys. Acta (Amst.) **103**, 177—179 (1965).
RUNDLES, R. W., LASZLO, J., ITOGA, T., HOBSON, J. B., GARRISON, F. E., Jr.: Clinical and hematologic study of 6-((1-methyl-4-nitro-5-imidazolyl)thio)purine (B. W. 57-322) and related compounds. Cancer Chemother. Rep. **14**, 99—115 (1961).
RUNDLES, R. W., WYNGAARDEN, J. B., HITCHINGS, G. H., ELION, G. B., SILBERMAN, H. R.: Effects of a xanthine oxidase inhibitor on thiopurine metabolism, hyperuricemia, and gout. Trans. Ass. Amer. Physicians **76**, 126—140 (1963).
RUTMAN, R. J., CANTAROW, A., PASCHKIS, K. E.: Studies in 2-acetylaminofluorene carcinogenesis. III. The utilization of uracil-2-$C^{14}$ by preneoplastic rat liver and rat hepatoma. Cancer Res. **14**, 119—123 (1954).
SARCIONE, E. J., STUTZMAN, L.: A comparison of the metabolism of 6-mercaptopurine and its 6-methyl analog in the rat. Cancer Res. **20**, 387—392 (1960).
SARTORELLI, A. C.: Approaches to the combination chemotherapy of transplantable neoplasms. Prog. Exp. Tumor Res. **6**, 228—288 (1965).
SARTORELLI, A. C., CREASEY, W. A.: The antineoplastic and biochemical effects of some 5-fluoropyrimidines. Cancer Res. **27**, 2201—2206 (1967).
SARTORELLI, A. C., CREASEY, W. A.: Cancer chemotherapy. Ann. Rev. Pharmacol. **9**, 51—72 (1969).
SCANNELL, J. P., HITCHINGS, G. H.: Thioguanine in deoxyribonucleic acid from tumors of 6-mercaptopurine-treated mice. Proc. Soc. exp. Biol. (N. Y.) **122**, 627—629 (1966).
SCHNEBLI, H. P., HILL, D. L., BENNETT, L. L., Jr.: Purification and properties of adenosine kinase from human tumor cells of type H. Ep. No. 2. J. biol. Chem. **242**, 1997—2004 (1967).
SHEEN, M. R., KIM, B. K., PARKS, R. E., Jr.: Purine nucleoside phosphorylase from human erythrocytes. III. Inhibition by the inosine analog formycin B of the isolated enzyme and of nucleoside metabolism in intact erythrocytes and sarcoma 180 cells. Molec. Pharmacol. **4**, 293—299 (1968).
SHEEN, M. R., MARTIN, H. F., PARKS, R. E., Jr.: The interaction of the nucleoside analogues, formycins A and B, with xanthine oxidase and hepatic aldehyde oxidase. Molec. Pharmacol. **6**, 255—265 (1970).
ŠORM, F., VESELÝ, J.: The activity of a new antimetabolite, 5-azacytidine, against lymphoid leukemia in AK mice. Neoplasma **11**, 123—130 (1964).
STANULOVIĆ, M., CHAYKIN, S.: Aldehyde oxidase: Catalysis of the oxidation of $N^1$-methylnicotinamide and pyridoxal. Arch. Biochem. Biophys. **145**, 27—34 (1971).
STOCK, J. A.: Other antitumor agents. In: Experimental chemotherapy, vol. 5, Chemotherapy of neoplastic diseases, Part II, pp. 333—416. (R. J. SCHNITZER and F. HAWKING, Eds.). New York-London: Academic Press 1967.
TOMCHICK, R., SASLAW, L. D., WARAVDEKAR, V. S.: Mouse kidney cytidine deaminase. Purification and properties. J. biol. Chem. **243**, 2534—2537 (1968).
UMEZAWA, H., SAWA, T., FUKUGAWA, Y., KOYAMA, G., MURASE, M., HAMADA, M., TAKEGUCHI, T.: Transformation of Formycin to Formycin B and their biological activities. J. Antibiot. (Tokyo) **18A**, 178—181 (1965).
VALERINO, D. M., JOHNS, D. G., ZAHARKO, D. S., OLIVERIO, V. T.: Studies of the metabolism of methotrexate by intestinal flora — I. Identification and study of biological properties of the metabolite 4-amino-4-deoxy-$N^{10}$-methylpteroic acid. Biochem. Pharmacol. **21**, 821—832 (1972).
VOGEL, C. L., ADAMSON, R. H., DEVITA, V. T., JOHNS, D. G., KYALWAZI, S. K.: Preliminary clinical trials of dichloromethotrexate in hepatocellular carcinoma. Cancer Chemother. Rep. **56** (1972).
WOLPERT, M. K., DAMLE, S. P., BROWN, J. E., SZNYCER, E., AGRAWAL, K. C., SARTORELLI, A. C.: The role of phosphohydrolases in the mechanism of resistance of neoplastic cells to 6-thiopurines. Cancer Res. **31**, 1620—1626 (1971).
WOLPERT, M. K., FARQUHAR, D., JOHNS, D. G.: Methotrexate esters as substrates for mammalian liver aldehyde oxidase. Abstr. Fifth International Congress on Pharmacology, 255 (1972).
YOUNG, C. W., BURCHENAL, J. H.: Cancer chemotherapy. Ann. Rev. Pharmacol. **11**, 369—386 (1971).
ZAHARKO, D. S., BRUCKNER, H., OLIVERIO, V. T.: Antibiotics alter methotrexate metabolism and excretion. Science **166**, 887—888 (1969).

Chapter 15

# Metabolism of Cancer Chemotherapeutic Agents via Pathways Utilized by Xenobiotics

A. M. Guarino and C. L. Litterst

With 3 Figures

## Introduction

The main factors which affect the duration and intensity of drug action are absorption, distribution, excretion, and metabolism; in this chapter attention will be focused on one important factor, the metabolism of antineoplastic agents. The metabolism of a drug can lead to an increase, a decrease, or no change in the pharmacologic or toxicologic activity of that drug. The catabolic reactions which are usually directed toward enhancing the elimination of a drug are emphasized in this and the preceding chapter. The anabolic processes by which conversion of drugs to more complex forms, and, in some cases, incorporation into body constituents occurs, have been discussed (Johns, Chapt. 14, this volume). In the latter case assimilation can occur only when the enzymes involved in intermediary anabolism cannot distinguish the antineoplastic compound from endogenous substrates because of a close resemblance in structural and/or physicochemical properties. Such a substitution of a drug for a natural metabolite is defined by the term "parametabolite" where substitution in a morphological, as well as a functional sense can occur. When the drug substitutes for the natural metabolite only in a morphological sense, with a resultant blockage in the normal biochemical process, the drug is called an antimetabolite.

Many antineoplastic agents undergo some sort of chemical transformation before they are eliminated into the air, bile, urine, or feces. The products of such biotransformations may be less active than the parent compound or inactive; they also can be equally active or more active. The usual, although not exclusive, goal of such biotransformations is in the direction of detoxication, where the metabolism of drugs represents some sort of advantage for the organism, since the products are less lipid soluble in character than the parent drug. This decrease in the lipid solubility of antineoplastic agents causes a change in the distribution of the products over the various compartments of the body: hydrophilic substances are more restricted to the extracellular phases of the body and hence are offered in higher concentrations to the excretory mechanisms. This hydrophilization may simultaneously cause a decrease in the extent and/or firmness with which the substances are bound to proteins or other body constituents. Hence, this reduction in tissue binding results in a substantial decrease in the volume of distribution, again favoring the excretory mechansims which are based on ultrafiltration processes. Another important factor is that the kidney is poorly equipped to excrete lipid-soluble substances and hence the lipid-soluble compounds would diffuse back into the plasma from the tubular compartment. Therefore, the reduction in lipophilic character of antineoplastic agents by metabolic action results in a reduction of the back absorption from the renal tubules and enhancement of urinary excretion of ultrafiltered substances.

While the catabolism of many antitumor agents via "endogenous" metabolic pathways has received considerable attention (see preceding chapter), the microsomal metabolism of a large number of antineoplastic agents is yet to be adequately studied. By necessity, therefore, much of this chapter will deal with metabolic pathways which are considered *possible* for such agents. Emphasis will be placed on the metabolism of substances which share structural moieties with antineoplastic agents. Specific examples are provided wherever possible.

The dominant types of biotransformations which can be expected to occur for anticancer drugs are the oxidative, reductive, and hydrolytic processes which lead to the introduction of groups into the drugs which render them suitable for conjugation with physiologically occurring substrates. These reactions are summarized in Fig. 1 where the width of the arrows suggests the relative dominance of the

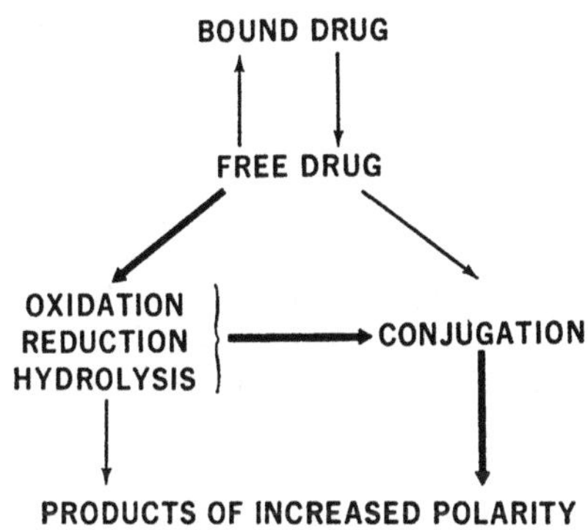


Fig. 1. Possible fate of drugs and other foreign compounds after administration to an animal

depicted pathway. The products of conjugative reactions are invariably less toxic and can be easily excreted via the bile or urine. The predominant pathways in the bioconversion of antineoplastic drugs are the oxidative reactions. They include aromatic hydroxylation, *O*-, *N*-, and *S*-dealkylation, oxidation of alkyl chains, *S*-oxidation, oxidative deamination, and epoxidation. For some agents the body makes use of reductive reactions such as the reduction of keto or nitro groups and the reductive cleavage of the azo bond. In the case of other agents, which are esters or amides, enzymatic hydrolysis occurs. The conjugation of antineoplastic drugs can occur by the synthesis of glucuronides, ethereal sulfates, mercapturic acids, amino acid conjugates, and acetylated aromatic amines. Other reactions involving the methylation of nitrogen in heterocyclic rings and of phenolic hydroxyl groups are also considered conjugation reactions.

In the metabolism of anticancer agents the liver plays the principal role. However, low levels of drug metabolizing enzymes also have been found in other tissues such as the kidney, lung, gastrointestinal tract, placenta, adrenal glands, heart, spleen, pancreas, brain, testis, thyroid, and muscle. The biotransformation of such agents in nonhepatic tissues cannot be neglected, since compounds that did not reach the liver, or that have escaped the metabolic conversion by this tiussue, can be altered near a possible site of action. For example, the drug metabolizing enzymes present in the gastrointestinal tract may be of particular importance with regard to the direct contact of people or animals with foreign chemicals in the environment. Such localized formation of metabolites in nonhepatic tissues may be of importance with regard to general and local toxicity, causation of specific organ lesions, allergy, and chemical carcinogenesis.

As far as the intracellular localization of drug-metabolizing enzyme systems is concerned, the most extensive studies which have been conducted have been carried out with liver tissue. A large class of drug-metabolizing enzymes appears to be bound to the membranes of the endoplasmic reticulum. When a tissue is homogenized, the disrupted membranes of the endoplasmic reticulum form small vesicles. These vesicles can be isolated by centrifugation of the 9000 × g supernatant of the homogenate at 105000 × g. The sediment thus obtained is generally called the "microsomal" fraction (CLAUDE, 1943), but really consists of several subcellular fractions. From a morphological point of view these fractions must be regarded as artifacts. Electron micrographs show that part of the membranes carries ribosomes; such membranes have been designated the rough endoplasmic reticulum and can be distinguished from the membranes without ribosomes, called the smooth endoplasmic reticulum. The enzymes which oxidize a number of antineoplastic agents undoubtedly are present in both subfractions. The enzyme systems designated NADPH-cytochrome c reductase and cytochrome P-450, involved in most of the drug-metabolizing reactions, are also localized in the microsomal subfraction. Solubilization of these systems has been attempted, but as might be expected a particular spatial organization of the various components involved is necessary, and such procedures have lead to such drastic changes in the microenvironment of the proteins that there have been dramatic changes in their activity. Detailed studies in this area must await the further development of gentler techniques of enzyme purification.

## Specificity of Drug-Metabolizing Enzymes

In the case of the synthetic antineoplastic agents, the question can arise as to how the body can handle a substance to which it has never been exposed. Obviously, if the drug is sufficiently like a natural metabolite it would fit into the normal metabolic systems. Enzymes of intermediary metabolism have a high affinity toward natural substrates, since they are geared to an effective organization of all cellular biochemical processes. In contrast, an attack on a xenobiotic compound apparently occurs via enzymes with low discrimination in their acceptance of substrates. Therefore, the metabolic attack on agents to which the body may not have been exposed previously depends largely on the recognition of the presence of a vulnerable site in the molecule. Other structural features in the drug molecule will regulate factors such as distribution in the body and affinity between the metabolizing enzyme and the drug substrate. Hence, because of the lipophilic nature of the endoplasmic reticulum, there can be little doubt that lipid-solubility is an important factor in controlling the rate of drug-metabolizing reactions. Other physical-chemical factors such as the steric structure and charge distribution over the molecule also are important. The metabolism of xenobiotic substances, such as the antineoplastic agents, is not a special function of the enzymes which have been designated "drug-metabolizing". It has been shown that many of the normal body constituents are metabolized by NADPH-dependent enzymes in liver microsomes. For example, the enzyme systems which metabolize steroidal hormones, such as estrogens, androgens, and glucocorticoids, also biotransform other xenobiotics (KUNTZMAN et al., 1964, 1968; CONNEY et al., 1965). According to WADA et al. (1968b), these microsomal enzymes are also involved with the ω-oxidation of fatty acids, in the formation of unsaturated fatty acids (MARSH and JAMES, 1962) and in the formation of bile acids (WADA et al., 1968a). The enzyme system which appears to be involved with the formation of glucuronides also seems to be involved in the normal formation of bilirubin glucuronide (SCHMID et al., 1957).

## Mechanism of Oxidation of Antineoplastic Agents

The microsomal enzyme systems for oxidative biotranformation of drugs were first extensively described by BRODIE et al. (1958) and AXELROD (1960). It has been shown by MASON (1957) that this type of enzymatic reaction has a requirement for both NADPH and free oxygen. He, therefore, introduced the term "mixed function oxidase" for this enzyme system. As far as the mechanism of reaction is concerned, at the present time most of the oxidative drug-metabolizing reactions are considered to belong to the general category of hydroxylations, wherein most reactions are regarded to have an −OH function as an intermediate and/or final product. The oxidative reactions require the mediation of an electron-transporting chain which consists of NADPH-cytochrome c reductase (an FAD-containing flavoprotein), a nonheme iron protein, and cytochrome P-450 (OMURA et al., 1965). In a scheme proposed by GILLETTE and GRAM (1969), the drug substrate first forms a complex with the oxidized form of a microsomal hemoprotein, cytochrome P-450. This complex is then reduced through other microsomal components by NADPH. The reduced cytochrome P-450-substrate complex quickly decomposes to form the oxidized substrate and the oxidized form of the cytochrome.

## Reductive Mechanisms

Many antineoplastic agents contain groups which can be biochemically reduced in the body. The enzyme systems involved in reduction appear to occur mainly in the liver, but low levels have been reported in other tissues, such as kidney and lung. Intracellularly, the enzyme systems are located mainly in the endoplasmic reticulum, but also have been found in the soluble fractions of the cell (FOUTS and BRODIE, 1957; UMAR and MITCHARD, 1968). These microsomal reductases are also NADPH-dependent, but reduction proceeds at a maximum rate under anaerobic conditions. The properties of the microsomal reduction mechanism resemble in some respects those of the oxidative reactions and appear to make use of the same system, wherein NADPH acts as a hydrogen donor and cytochrome P-450 or NADPH cytochrome c reductase participate.

Aromatic nitro compounds, such as chloramphenicol, *p*-nitrophenol, and *p*-nitrobenzoate, are reduced to the corresponding primary aromatic amines in mammalian tissues. Such reductions are attributed to enzymes present both in the endoplasmic reticulum (FOUTS and BRODIE, 1957) and in the supernatant fraction (KATO et al., 1969a). The early studies of OTSUKA (1961) are classic and worthy of consideration. He showed that the liver nitro-reducing system could be separated into two enzyme fractions: a nitro-reductase which catalyzed the reduction of a model substrate, such as *p*-nitrophenol to *p*-nitrosophenol, and a second fraction containing a nitroso-reductase which catalyzed the reduction of the nitroso derivative to *p*-hydroxylaminophenol. The conversion of this latter compound to the *p*-aminophenol is thought to proceed by a nonenzymatic reaction brought about by reduced pyridine nucleotides or by ferrous ions.

## Hydrolytic Enzyme Systems

In contrast to the oxidative and reductive drug-metabolizing enzymes which are located intracellularly, a considerable number of hydrolytic enzymes have been shown to be present both intracellularly and in blood plasma. LEE and LIVETT (1967) showed that various local anesthetics containing an ester link are hydrolyzed by esterases occurring in the liver. As examples of plasma esterases the following can be listed: aromatic esterases hydrolyzing phenol and *p*-nitrophenol esters, aliphatic esterases hydrolyzing aliphalic esters, and choline esterases preferentially hydrolyzing choline esters.

## Conjugation Reactions

Conjugation products suitable for excretion in urine or bile are synthesized by coupling the drug with a very polar, normal body substance. The molecule to be conjugated must possess one or more rather polar groups, and hence, if not already present, an earlier reaction such as hydroxylation must occur prior to the conjugation step (Fig. 1). Thus, conjugates are the end products of the metabolism of many natural and xenobiotic chemicals and often occur as the second step of other metabolic reactions involving oxidation, reduction, or hydrolysis. Although such reactions usually result in less toxic and more polar products, not all of the conjugation products are metabolically inert, since in some circumstances they may act as intermediates in transport processes where such relatively inactive forms of a compound are translocated from one location in the body to another. Yet, the general rule that such conjugation products are relatively nontoxic, water-soluble, excretory products seems to prevail in most cases.

Nearly all of the enzyme systems involved in the conjugation reactions have natural substrates, and all of the conjugating agents have roles in normal intermediary metabolism apart from those involving transformations of antineoplastic agents. The major conjugation reactions are few in number and the conjugating agents are derived mainly from the animal's carbohydrate and amino acid sources. For example, glycoside conjugations are limited mainly to glucose and its derivative glucuronic acid. Only a few of the 22 possible amino acids are used in conjugation reactions. These are glycine in hippuric acid formation, cysteine and glutamic acid in the formation of mercapturic acid conjugates, and methionine in methylation reactions. A few other amino acids are employed by particular species, and such variations occur more frequently with amino acid conjugations than with glycoside conjugations.

### A. Glucuronides

Glucuronide formation may occur with compounds bearing the OH-, COOH-, $NH_2$-, and SH-groups. Of all the conjugation reactions possible for antineoplastic agents, glucuronidation rather than sulfate, cysteine, and glycine conjugation, methylation, or acetylation, appears to be the most important, particularly because glucuronic acid reacts with a great number of different compounds. The enzymes required for conjugation reactions occur in many organs, but particularly in the liver, kidney, and intestine; furthermore, the major substrate for the conjugation reactions, glucuronic acid present as uridine diphosphate glucuronic acid (UDPGA), is easily generated from glucose via uridine diphosphate glucose (UDPG). This latter reaction, where glucose-1-phosphate combines with uridine triphosphate to give UDPG, is catalyzed by an enzyme called UDPG pyrophosphorylase. Work on the glucuronide conjugation of drugs has resulted in furthering the understanding of the biochemistry of bilirubin.

The question of the mechanism of the formation of glucuronides was not solved until DUTTON and STOREY (1952) discovered UDPGA in rabbit liver and elucidated its role as a cofactor in glucuronide formation. STROMINGER et al. (1954) were able to show that the glycoside UDPG was oxidized enzymatically to UDPGA, which then transferred its glucuronyl radical to the foreign compound by means of a glucuronyltransferase.

Since glucuronyltransferase is located within the microsomes, it is segregated by a lipid barrier which can be penetrated only by substances which possess the proper degree of lipid solubility (GAUDETTE and BRODIE, 1959). It must be emphasized that a number of endogenous compounds are also conjugated with glucuronic acid by these same enzyme systems which metabolize drugs, for example, steroidal hormones (JAYLE and PASQUALINI, 1966), bilirubin (SCHMID and LESTER, 1966), and vitamin A (LIPPEL and OLSON, 1968).

The observation by PARKE (1952) that administration of thiophenol increased the total glucuronide excretion in rabbit urine was one of the earliest observations of an *S*-glucuronide. KAMIL et al. (1953) detected extra amounts of glucuronic acid in the urine of rabbits receiving disulfiram, and KASLANDER (1963) extended these observations to man and found the *S*-glucuronide of this compound in urine.

*N*-Glucuronide synthesis is interesting, because under physiological conditions it can proceed enzymatically or nonenzymatically. BRIDGES and WILLIAMS (1962) mixed *in vitro* glucuronic acid with *p*-chloroaniline, aniline, or sulfanilamide. Interestingly, the $N^1$-glucuronide of sulfadimethoxine was synthesized enzymatically in monkey liver, while the $N^4$-glucuronide was formed spontaneously when the drug was added to human urine (BRIDGES et al., 1968).

There are four types of *N*-glucuronides: (1) those with aliphatic amino groups, (2) those with aromatic amino groups, (3) those with sulfonimido or a carbamoyl group, and (4) those with heterocyclic nitrogen (WILLIAMS, 1967). The former two glucuronides are extremely labile compounds in acid solution while those of the third group appear to be relatively stable. AXELROD et al. (1957) showed that several aromatic compounds formed *N*-glucuronides in the presence of guinea pig liver microsomes.

Inhibition of UDPGA transferases *in vitro* has been observed and one particular example of inhibition may be of significance in patients with neoplastic disease. FREZZA et al. (1968) found that bilirubin causes very strong inhibition of 4-methylumbelliferone glucuronide formation in human liver homogenates. Hence, in patients with hyperbilirubinemia this pathway of biotransformation may be inhibited.

Owing to the great amount of liver tissue in most animals and high glucuronyltransferase activity per unit weight, the liver is the main site of glucuronide production. However, hepatic glucuronidation capacity is dependent on glycogen content, because the latter substance is the initial precursor of UDPGA. Renal tissue is able to synthesize glucuronides, but the relative physiological significance of the process in the kidney must await further elucidation. On the other hand there are some studies which show that the kidney can, and in some cases does, compensate for the absence of the liver. Thus, in hepatectomized dogs, BOLLMAN and MENDEZ (1955) reported a slow conversion of bilirubin to the monoglucuronide, while in hepatectomized rats, BERAUD and VANNOTTI (1960) observed that the kidney could carry out glucuronidation of triiodothyronine. Glucuronyltransferase activity also is detectable throughout the gastrointestinal tract and appears to be localized in the mucosa, where most of the activity is contained in the microsomal fraction (STEVENSON and DUTTON, 1962). DAHM and BREUER (1966) found that human gastric mucosa contains both a soluble and a microsomal glucuronyltransferase. These observations suggest that patients with hepatic compromise from neoplastic disease and/or chemotherapy, may be able to use nonhepatic tissues to synthesize glucuronides. This transferase activity, like that of many other drug-metabolizing enzymes, seems to be connected with and dependent on the liver glycogen content in some unknown way (FOUTS, 1962). *In vitro* studies indicate that the largest specific activity is associated with the particulate glycogen fraction (HALAC and FRANK, 1960). In the rat liver depleted of glycogen by total fasting, this activity remains almost unchanged, while in the human liver, transferase activity appears to be reduced under these conditions (MIETTINEN and LESKINEN, 1963). Hence, the depleted glycogen stores associated with any chronic illness like neoplastic disease, would be expected to diminish this drug metabolism pathway. Studies concerned with the subcellular distribution of glucuronyltransferase activity utilizing various substrates seem to indicate that the transferases may be differentiated further on the basis of submicrosomal distribution (GRAM et al., 1968).

The rate at which glucose is metabolized via the glucuronic acid pathway is dependent not only on the activity of various enzymes, but also on the availability of glucose and other sugars, nucleotides, and the presence of other foreign compounds which may not have to be conjugated with glucuronic acid. Hence, under any circumstances where there are compromises in the dietary status of a patient, as would be expected in cases of neoplastic conditions, the activity of these enzymes may be profoundly altered.

Glucuronic acid conjugating enzymes have been reported to be inhibited *in vitro* by steroidal hormones, but the *in vivo* significance of such studies is currently unknown. It would seem, therefore, that patients with neoplastic diseases who are receiving large doses of hormones as part of their drug regimens should be tested for the possibility of having altered activities of these enzymes.

Studies of glucuronidation provide an interesting example of the role of relative organ sizes in the overall handling of a drug by this pathway. Since the activity of these enzymes *in vivo* is about the same magnitude per unit weight in the liver, kidney, and intestinal mucosa, the heaviest organ, usually the liver, will contribute the greatest rate of production of urinary glucuronides. Hence, under experimental conditions where there is an increase in the size of the liver or kidneys (e.g. where associated with phenobarbital induction), attempts to explain the capacity of the animal to excrete glucuronides should be expressed in terms of the enzyme activity of the whole organ rather than per unit weight of the tissue. For example, it has been reported that inducing agents such as phenobarbital, increase the biliary excretion of some drugs, even though there is no major change in the glucuronidation rate when expressed per unit weight of tissue (ROBERTS and PLAA, 1967). In these cases the change in excretion is attributable to the increased liver size. Another factor which limits the rate of glucuronidation is, of course, the rate of uptake of the parent drug. Hence, even if enzyme activities are increased several fold in the absence of a corresponding increase in the rate of uptake, no overall change in rate of formation of glucuronides will be observed.

One of the hallmarks of patients with neoplastic disease, especially as they approach the terminal phases of this disease, is a profound weight loss. Glucuronidation capacity, as judged from the results of anmial experiments, may be markedly reduced under these conditions. Studies by DIXON et al. (1960) suggest that oxidation, dealkylation, and hydroxylation reactions were limited for many drugs during fasting in mice. Accordingly, patients undergoing periods of different degrees of fasting may be especially sensitive to any drug (i.e. not only glucuronidation reactions may be compromised, but other mechanisms also may be slowed down). For example, sulfobromophthalein, which is removed in part via another conjugation mechanism (i.e. as its glutathione conjugate) is eliminated at a slower rate during fasting, than under usual dietary conditions (DUNCAN et al., 1964).

Since glucose metabolism is disturbed in diabetes mellitus, any of the drugs which have been reported to cause pancreatic changes [e.g. streptozotocin (RAKIETEN et al., 1963)], might be expected to alter not only glucuronic acid conjugation, but also other drug-metabolizing reactions.

## B. Sulfates

Sulfoconjugates are found in bacteria and higher plants, as well as throughout the animal kingdom, and constitute a very diverse group of compounds (DODGSON and ROSE, 1970). In the field of drug metabolism, the term sulfoconjugate is generally applied to the reactions in which sulfate is combined with steroids or phenols. Most of these conjugates can be classified as sulfuric acid esters in which the $C-O-SO_3^-$ linkage is present. Other conjugates exist in which sulfate is covalently attached by other linkages, such as $P-O-SO_3^-$, $N-SO_3^-$, $N-O-SO_3^-$ and $S-SO_3^-$.

Conjugates with $POSO_3^-$ linkages can be represented by two very important compounds, namely, adenylyl sulfate (APS) and 3′-phosphoadenylyl sulfate (PAPS). APS is the biosynthetic precursor of PAPS and both may be regarded as activated forms of sulfate analogous to activated forms of phosphate, such as ATP.

Arylsulfate esters are formed when a phenolic hydroxyl group is esterified with sulfuric acid. Such esters, for example those that occur by combination with estrogenic steroids, are found under normal circumstances in the urine. Other drugs and foreign compounds containing phenolic groups, or where phenolic groups are introduced by other enzymatic or nonenzymatic reactions in the body, also can be excreted in part as sulfate esters. These conjugates have the $COSO_3^-$ linkage.

With regard to APS and PAPS, it must be emphasized that enzymatic hydrolysis of both of these compounds occurs readily to yield a variety of products including adenosine, inosine, hypoxanthine, sulfate, and phosphate (FUJIWARA and SPENCER, 1962). Recent studies with rat liver showed that the activity of this enzyme is localized both in the lysosomal and supernatant fractions of the cell (KOIZUMI et al., 1969). A second and quite distinct sulfohydrolase which hydrolyzes APS to inorganic sulfate and AMP has recently been identified in rat liver by BAILEY-WOOD et al. (1969). These workers found that the enzymatic activity was localized in both the lysosomal and soluble fractions of the liver cell and after purification of the enzyme they were able to separate the APS sulfohydrolase from other APS-degrading enzymes.

Arylsulfate esters containing the $COSO_3^-$ linkage arise from simple phenols and phenolic acids, heterocyclic phenols such as indoxyl, and phenolic hormones such as estrone. However, the evidence for the occurrence of such sulfates is frequently indirect because these arylsulfates are relatively labile, are water-soluble and therefore difficult to separate from other components and are usually present only in small amounts.

In mammalian systems, apparently there are three kinds of sulfotransferases; namely, phenolsulfotransferase, estrogen sulfotransferase, and L-tyrosine methyl ester sulfotransferase. In mammals the phenolsulfotransferase activity is present in many tissues and, as far as the collective results can be interpreted, the bulk of this activity is localized in the soluble fraction of cell preparations.

Mammalian arylsulfohydrolase enzymes were originally reported to be present in the mitochondria, but the more recent work of VIALA and GIANETTO (1955) made it clear that these enzymes were lysosomal in origin. One of these enzymes has been designated arylsulfohydrolase "A"; two other types have been reported, "B" and "C", and according to MILSOM et al. (1968), this latter enzyme is localized in the smooth endoplasmic reticulum in the rat. Arylsulfoconjugation can be regarded as a protective mechanism whereby toxic phenols are rendered less toxic, while arylsulfohydrolases apparently can regenerate the parent phenol compound. It might then be asked why the mammalian organism should go to great lengths to protect itself by sulfoconjugating phenols and at the same time possess enzymes that are theoretically able to release the phenols from the conjugate. Apart from the probable decrease in toxicity arising from sulfoconjugation of phenols, the mechanism achieves a basic "detoxication" aim; namely, the production of a strongly acidic, water-soluble compound that can be excreted rapidly via the kidneys. Furthermore, the existence of the hydrolase enzymes raises the possibility that in some circumstances the controlled synthesis and degradation of arylsulfates in specific regions of the cell might be of some biological significance as yet unknown.

Steroid sulfohydrolases have been found in placental tissue and according to FRENCH and WARREN (1967) are localized in the microsomal fraction of this tissue. Simple alcohols, such as methanol, ethanol, and propanol, undergo sulfoconjugation by means of similar enzymes.

Conjugates which possess the $NSO_3^-$ linkage are called sulfamates and arise from substrates which are arylamines, such as aniline and 2-napthylamine. These compounds were reported to be excreted as the corresponding phenylsulfamate and napthyl 2-sulfamate by BOYLAND et al. (1957) and PARKE (1960).

## C. Amino Acid Conjugations

Any antineoplastic agent which contains an aromatic carboxylic acid can have this functional group combined with an amino acid through a secondary amide linkage. The most widespread of these reactions is with glycine. Hippuric acid was the first acid of this type reported to be so conjugated, and later studies showed that this reaction was a general one for most aromatic acids, since it also occurs for some substituted acetic and cinnamic acids. Another type of amino acid conjugation occurs with arylacetic acids via glutamine conjugation. The intracellular site of amino acid conjugations is of great interest, since in contrast to many of the other metabolic reactions of antineoplastic compounds, they occur in the mitochondria rather than in the microsomes. This may be related to the ability of the mitochondria to take up ionic forms of compounds, whereas in order for metabolism to occur in the microsomes lipid solubility seems to be more important.

## D. *N*-Hydroxy Conjugations

The *N*-hydroxylation of aromatic amines and their amide derivatives is carried out by enzymes located in the endoplasmic reticulum (KIESE and UEHLEKE, 1961; IRVING, 1964; BOOTH and BOYLAND, 1964). The enzyme system is NADPH-dependent, requires molecular oxygen and appears to be related to the other microsomal enzymes. These hydroxylases catalyze the incorporation of one atom of oxygen into the substrate, but unlike most other microsomal enzymes may not require the participation of cytochrome P-450, since no inhibition of this reaction by carbon monoxide was observed by KAMPFFMEYER and KIESE (1965).

LANGE (1967) offered evidence suggesting that there were different enzymes in the endoplasmic reticulum which catalyzed *N*- and *p*-hydroxylation of aromatic amines. There are very wide species differences in *N*- and *C*-hydroxylations (LOTLIKAR et al., 1967) which occur after treatment of animals with 3-methylcholanthrene. While this kind of study lends further credence to the hypothesis that there are separate enzymes involved with *N*- and *C*-hydroxylation, there are alternative explanations which might account for the species differences. For example, the lipid layer of the endoplasmic reticulum, which is in close contact with the hydroxylating enzyme, may concentrate the compound to be hydroxylated, permitting access to the enzyme. Consequently, differences in the lipid composition of various species or differences in the lipid composition caused by the administration of inducing agents might alter the metabolic rates. A variety of other factors such as administration of ACTH, partial hepatectomy, or administration of growth hormone, results in increased excretion of the glucuronide of a hydroxylated intermediate (MILLER et al., 1960). Like many other studies of this type, the increase was attributed to formation of increased amounts of *N*-hydroxylated metabolites in the animal; however, alterations in the amounts of urinary metabolites do not necessarily reflect differences in the activities of enzymes metabolizing these substrates. Measurement of urinary levels of metabolites is not a valid criterion for determining the extent of *N*-hydroxylation in the rat and probably not in any other species (IRVING et al., 1967).

Many of the *N*-hydroxylated compounds undergo further biotransformation via glucuronide formation. Other *N*-hydroxylations can similarly be followed by sulfate or methylation conjugation reactions. For example, *N*-acetyl-*N*-hydroxyurethan and *O*-acetyl-*N*-hydroxyurethan have been reported as urinary metabolites of urethan and *N*-hydroxyurethan, respectively (BOYLAND and NERY, 1965).

## E. Miscellaneous Conjugation Reactions

Methylation and mercapturic acid synthesis also require amino acids, but these conjugations do not result in the formation of a secondary amide link as in the case of most other conjugations. In methylation, for example, the amino acid methionine takes part in the reaction, but only its methyl group appears in the product. The tripeptide glutathione is involved in mercapturic acid synthesis, but only the cysteine moiety occurs in the final product. The first example of biological methylation was observed in dogs treated with pyridine acetate and consisted of the methylation of a tertiary nitrogen atom in an aromatic system (COHN, 1894). The relevance of the finding to cancer chemotherapy derives from the fact that the armamentarium of the chemotherapist contains many compounds with the pyridine nucleus. In addition to methylation of a tertiary nitrogen atom in an aromatic system, such reactions also occur with phenols, although rarely with monophenols. This type of *O*-methylation is usually characteristic of polyphenolic compounds containing two vicinal hydroxyl groups. SARCIONE and SOKAL (1958) reported a case of *S*-methylation when they observed that thiouracil was converted into 2-methylthiouracil in the rat. In addition, REMY (1963) has shown that 6-mercaptopurine is *S*-methylated to form 6-methylthiopurine.

The mechanism of methylation of foreign compounds has been worked out, largely due to the efforts of CANTONI (1953). It is now clear that methylation involving oxygen, nitrogen, or sulfur occurs when a methyl group is transferred from *S*-adenosylmethionine under the influence of methyl transferase enzymes.

Present day studies have shown that mercapturic acids arise mainly via glutathione conjugates and that the initial reaction in their formation is between the drug itself (or some form of the drug such as an epoxide) and glutathione, where the reactions are catalyzed by special transferase enzymes.

Acetylation is a potential reaction with any antineoplastic agent containing an amino group. Five types of amino groups (i.e. aliphatic $NH_2$, aromatic $NH_2$, α-amino acid $NH_2$, hydrazino group, and sulfonamide $NH_2$) can be distinguished and it appears probable that each one requires a different transacetylase for its acetylation.

## Factors Influencing the Metabolism of Anticancer Agents

The capacity of animals, and in all likelihood humans, to metabolize drugs varies with several endogenous factors, such as genetic background, hormonal changes, sex, and age, as well as with exogenous factors, such as certain environmental conditions, the nutritional status, and the ingestion of other xenobiotic chemicals. In this discussion, attention will be directed mainly toward agents which are associated with the stimulation or inhibition of drug biotransformation.

### A. Enzyme Induction

The enhanced metabolism of drugs evoked by pretreatment with drugs may lead to a tolerance or to an increased sensitivity of the organism to the action of the drug. The intentional introduction of substances into the body, or the accidental appearance in the body of substances previously encountered in the environment, can produce a wide variation in the ability of the body to metabolize drugs. Polycyclic hydrocarbons, barbiturates, insecticides, and a variety of other agents occurring in the environment can act as stimulators of drug metabolism. The increase in drug-metabolizing capacity appears to be mainly due to an increase in the concentration of enzyme proteins responsible for such reactions; this stimulation is referred to as enzyme induction. Recent studies have shown that induction of drug-metabolizing enzymes also can occur *in vitro* (Nebert and Gelboin, 1968). Some agents not only induce their own metabolism, but the levels of enzymatic activity are increased in a much more general manner. The inducers can be categorized into two groups: (1) drugs and insecticides that enhance the metabolism of a wide variety of drugs, and (2) a group mainly comprised of polycyclic hydrocarbons that stimulate the metabolism of only a few drugs. The prototype drug of the former group is phenobarbital, while 3-methylcholanthrene and 3,4-benzpyrene are often cited examples of the latter group. The different actions of the two groups of inducers not only reveal themselves in the variety of basic types of metabolic reactions that can occur, but also in the way in which the inducing agent may cause a particular substrate to be handled qualitatively or quantitatively in a different manner. Hence, the effects of a given substrate and a given inducing agent must remain speculative until the actual experiments are conducted using the agent and substrate in question. The central question is whether in a given type of reaction one or more enzymes are involved. There is evidence substantiating either of these views; for example, the extensive studies of Rubin et al. (1964) suggest that a single enzyme system is responsible for the metabolism of many drugs. Using the affinity of the enzyme for the substrates, Leibman and McAllister (1967) reported that there was no change in the $K_m$ after induction. On the other hand, Alvares et al. (1968) and Guarino et al. (1969) have shown that the apparent Michaelis constants in drug-metabolizing reactions are altered after induction. The inductions seen accompanying treatment with various agents can be caused by many mechanisms and four are indicated below:

1. Enhancement of enzyme synthesis
2. Synthesis of more active enzyme
3. Direct or indirect activation of existing enzyme
4. Stabilization of the enzyme against degradation.

At the present time, there is much evidence that the increased enzymatic activity is mainly due to a *de novo* synthesis of the enzyme (KATO et al., 1966; BARON and TEPHLY, 1969; LEVIN and KUNTZMAN, 1969). There is also some evidence that, as well as the *de novo* synthesis of microsomal enzymes, there is a decreased catabolism by means of stabilization of the components or by repression of catabolizing enzymes (HOLTZMAN and GILLETTE, 1968; GREIM and REMMER, 1969). LANG (1971) has also presented evidence of these changes occurring for steroids.

## B. Species Differences

As is the case with the development of new drugs in any field, in cancer chemotherapy extensive reliance is placed on the use of a variety of animal species in the early testing of potential antineoplastic agents. Depending on the species under test, a variety of different pharmacologic responses have been observed and in some cases these differences have been related to differences in the pathways or in the rates of drug metabolism (QUINN et al., 1958; KATO and GILLETTE, 1965). In attempting to elucidate the reasons for these species differences, *in vitro* studies have been much more productive than intact animal studies. It has been shown that species differences in drug-metabolizing reactions can be the result of variations in both the absolute amount and the kinetic properties of enzymes (GILLETTE, 1971). Several investigators have demonstrated, for example, that the rates of demethylation in the mouse, rat, rabbit, and guinea pig are due to differences both in the $K_m$ and $V_{max}$ of the enzyme system (CASTRO and GILLETTE, 1967; DAVIES et al., 1968; GILLETTE and GRAM, 1969). In spite of many extensive studies on drug metabolism in the past several years, comparative investigations in a wide range of species have rarely been performed (DEWAIDE, 1971). Most of the comparative studies published to date (DRING et al., 1966; ELLISON et al., 1966; BRIDGES et al., 1969a, b), have been based largely on *in vivo* experiments where measurements of the metabolites appearing in urine and feces are utilized. These data are always difficult to interpret because they often ignore the metabolism by gastrointestinal microorganisms and enterohepatic circulation of the drug and metabolites (SCHELINE, 1968; ZAHARKO et al., 1969).

## C. Presence of Neoplastic Disease

The possible effects that the presence of a tumor has on the ability of an organism to metabolize drugs in general, and specifically antineoplastic drugs reguire consideration. However, despite the importance of the liver in general metabolism, and particularly in the metabolism of drugs, relatively little work appears to have been done in connection with alterations in the ability of the liver to metabolize drugs in the presence of nonhepatic tumors. KATO et al. (1963) reported that the oxidation rate of drugs by liver microsomes was significantly lower than normal in rats bearing the Walker carcinosarcoma 256. MATTES et al. (1962) used the technique of measuring hexobarbital sleeping time as a measure of drug metabolism in mice with the ascites form of the Ehrlich tumor and found an increase in sleeping time in the tumor-bearing animals. These investigators, however, could not rule out altered drug distribution in the ascites fluid as a possible cause of the prolonged sleeping times. KANDASWAMY and HENDERSON (1963) offered preliminary evidence that ethidium bromide was not significantly metabolized by either normal mice or mice inoculated with Ehrlich ascites tumor cells. They did note, however, that tumor-bearing mice excreted only half as much of the drug as did normal mice 24 hours after treatment. This retention of the drug in tumor-bearing animals easily could have been mistaken for altered metabolism and certainly points to one of the pitfalls in using only urinary excretion data to reach a conclusion about the metabolism of antineoplastic agents. In some very elegant experiments, Brown et al. (1971) studied levels of a number of drug-metabolizing enzymes believed to be directly associated with the flow of electrons in the drug-oxidizing enzyme system in normal and tumor-bearing rats. They studied Morris hepatoma 7777 and dimethylaminobiphenyl-induced breast tumors. In comparing normal liver with liver from a hepatoma-bearing rat these changes were observed: NADPH oxidase and benzpyrene hydroxylase activities were not impressively different, while the levels of activities of NADPH-ferricyanide reductase and NADPH cytochrome c reductase, and the content of cytochrome P-450 were decreased from 30% to 50%. The levels of these components were all significantly decreased in the hepatoma tissue itself. In comparing normal rat liver and liver removed from animals with breast tumors it was found that NADPH oxidase activity, NADPH-ferricyanide reductase activity, P-450 content, and benzpyrene hydroxylase activity were significantly decreased from 38% to 46% of normal liver values. These studies rather definitively have established that the presence of tumors, even localized in tissues other than in the liver, can have significant effects on the metabolism of drugs including antineoplastic agents. Other workers, such as Rosso et al. (1968a, b) and Franchi and Rosso (1969), have also provided evidence suggesting that drug-metabolizing activity of liver microsomes in tumor-bearing animals is markedly reduced when compared with normal animals.

## D. Pretreatment with Antitumor Drugs

In a classic study addressed to the problem of alterations in drug-metabolizing activity following treatment with antineoplastic agents, Tardiff and Dubois (1969) employed three alkylating agents to ascertain the effects of such drugs on the synthesis of hepatic microsomal enzymes in the livers of weanling and adult male rats. None of the three drugs, cyclophosphamide, mechlorethamine ($HN_2$), or pipobroman, were effective inhibitors of the *N*-demethylase, *O*-demethylase, or phosphorothioate detoxication systems *in vitro*, indicating that they do not react directly with microsomal enzymes. However, these workers found that sublethal doses of the drugs given i.p. to 23-day-old male rats inhibited the increase in activity of the *N*-demethylase and phosphorothioate detoxifying systems which usually occurs in developing rats. Administration of the drugs to adult rats caused decreases in the activity of all enzymes studied. The time course of inhibition, as studied from one hour to 21 days after animals had received a single dose of the drug, produced a maximum inhibition of *O*-demethylation activity after 14 days for cyclophosphamide, after 7 days for $HN_2$, and after 5 days for pipobroman. This time course for maximum inhibition is noteworthy from the point of view that it was delayed and the effect was relatively persistent. From a clinical standpoint the inhibitory effect of alkylating agents on microsomal enzymes would be expected to alter the metabolism and consequently the toxicity of many other drugs. Especially in this era where combination chemotherapy is frequently employed (Rall, 1967), the possibility should be taken into consideration that levels of enzymes usually responsible for the detoxication of drugs may have been significantly depressed. Other workers have observed that a single administration of some antitumor drugs may impair the activity of liver-microsomal enzymes for several days (Donelli and Garattini, 1971). These workers employed *p*-nitroanisole as a substrate for *O*-demethylation, and aniline to measure parahydroxylation. They showed that the metabolism of both of these substrates is significantly decreased 3 or 6 days after treatment with either $HN_2$, chlorambucil, 5-fluorouracil, methotrexate, or daunomycin. Nine and 12 days after single administration of these agents there was an interesting "over compensation" in that the drug-metabolizing activity toward these two substrates was significantly elevated for chlorambucil, methotrexate, and cyclophosphamide, and the increase was particularly striking for 5-fluorouracil at 9 days after treatment. In general, measurement of the enhanced metabolism at later times showed increases of from 15% to 25% of control levels, whereas 5-fluorouracil treatment caused about an 80% to 120% increase over control levels after 9 days. Thus, these workers emphasize that drug-metabolizing activity of hepatic microsomes in animals after treatment with anti-tumor agents may be altered in either direction, depending on the schedule of treatment and the amount of time which has passed since the last treatment. LAVIN and KOSS (1971) conducted electron microscopic studies of the liver after single doses of cyclophosphamide and presented results apparently contrary to those presented by the two groups above. Although they did not directly assay the drug-metabolizing activity of their animals, they did note that 5 hours after injection of cyclophosphamide there was hypertrophy of the smooth endoplasmic reticulum and this is commonly assumed to be associated with increases in the activity of the microsomal enzymes. This whole area lacks a definitive study wherein simultaneous samples of liver are taken for electron microscopic measurement of the status of drug-metabolizing components, as well as for the measurement of drug-metabolizing enzymatic activity, utilizing a variety of substrates after several different times to establish the possible interrelationships between these events at the ultrastructural, biochemical, and enzymatic levels.

In an interesting study, DIXON (1968) was able to show that the antibiotic chloramphenicol reduced the lethality of cyclophosphamide and decreased the *in vivo* conversion of this drug to a metabolite capable of acting as an alkylating agent. Because of the rather well-established role of microsomes in the activation of this antineoplastic agent, it seems likely that chloramphenicol diminished the toxicity of cyclophosphamide by inhibiting its conversion to an active and presumably toxic metabolite.

THOMPSON and LARSON (1969) reported a prolongation in pentobarbital sleeping time in rats treated with single doses of BCNU [1,3-*bis*-(2-chloroethyl)-1-nitrosourea]. Following this suggestion of impaired drug metabolism, as measured by this preliminary criteria, LU and LARSON (1970) studied the metabolism of pentobarbital by 9000 × g supernatants from livers of BCNU-treated rats. Seven days after treatment with 20 mg/kg of BCNU, the rate of metabolism of pentobarbital was decreased to 72% of control, whereas after 21 days the rate of metabolism was decreased to 16% of control. This apparent continued decrease in drug-metabolizing function for three weeks after receiving a single dose of BCNU may be of profound clinical importance.

## Drug Latentiation as Affected by Drug Metabolism

Drug latentiation is the chemical modification of a biologically active compound to a derivative which can release the parent compound under *in vivo* conditions (HARPER, 1959). This concept has been evoked to explain the action of certain mustards and such a concept provided one of the early bases for a rational approach to the synthesis of potential antineoplastic agents. In one interesting early example, the oxidation of nitrogen mustard ($HN_2$) to its corresponding *N*-oxide was found by FARBER et al. (1956) to give a compound that had more activity in certain tumor systems than did $NH_2$. In this case the oxide is assumed to be a latent form of $HN_2$ that is activated *in vivo* by a reductive mechanism (IMAMURA, 1960). After it had been established that there are reductive cleavage enzymes which can operate on azo compounds to produce amines, a series of mustards was prepared which had the azo linkage; hence a relatively unreactive compound such as *N,N-bis*-(2-chloroethyl)-*p*-phenylazoaniline could serve as a precursor to the more active compound *N,N-bis*(2-chloroethyl)-*p*-phenylenediamine. ROSS and WARWICK (1956) provided evidence that the biological activity of a series of compounds containing the azo linkage could be related to the rate of reducibility of this linkage and the subsequent evolution of the corresponding amines.

The thinking behind preparation of another series of compounds reflected a further application of the concept of latentiation in formulating acyl derivatives which would require enzymatic hydrolysis for activation (EVERETT and ROSS, 1949). A number of amides derived from 2,2′-dichlorodiethylamine undergo *in vitro* hydrolysis and have good activity against Walker carcinosarcoma 256 (ROSS and WILSON, 1959).

A further outgrowth of the principle of latentiation came from the application of enzyme induction as a means of increasing the specificity of antitumor action of some alkylating agents. For example, an animal was pretreated with propylcarbanilate in an effort to induce in the tumor an enzyme capable of splitting the carbamoyl linkage of this compound. When the corresponding mustard, propyl-*p*-[*bis*(2-chloroethyl)amino]carbanilate, was then administered, it was much more effective than when the mustard derivative was used in the absence of the inducing treatment (DANIELLI et al., 1959).

## Identification of Antineoplastic Drugs in Body Tissues and Fluids

The complete description of the chemical structure of a compound isolated from patients or animals after treatment with an antineoplastic agent has ranged from difficult to impossible over the past few years. The identification of these drugs and metabolites in biological extracts has been made difficult in large part due to the following factors: (1) the brief half-lives of most of these antineoplastic agents, (2) the great toxicity and therefore usually low doses employed, (3) the rapid metabolism and/or spontaneous degradation of many of these agents and (4) the presence in tissues of chemically related compounds, especially in the case of antimetabolites.

The advent of an increasing variety of sensitive physical and chemical procedures has yet to receive adequate attention in the field of antineoplastic drug metabolism. No single procedure or observation is sufficient to identify a purified compound as a proposed metabolite and it may be impossible to isolate and purify enough material to accumulate evidence of the identity of a compound by means of infrared or mass spectra analysis. It is, therefore, often necessary to collect as much evidence as possible from several different sources. With unlabeled compounds, for example, chromatographic evidence of the identity of metabolites is most likely to be sought. Such methods as thin layer chromatography, counter current distribution, paper chromatography, and gas-liquid chromatography have been employed traditionally. In using any of the chromatographic systems, the material to be identified should appear at a reasonable $R_f$ value (i.e. it should not occur at either the origin or at the solvent front). In utilizing gas chromatographic procedures, reference compounds used as internal standards provide the best evidence.

Ultraviolet absorption spectra, as well as visible and fluorescent spectra, are easily measured, and can provide useful information on the presence of certain functional groups, but not on the identity of compounds. These techniques have the inherent advantage of being nondestructive.

Mass spectrometry is perhaps the most powerful method for the identification of antineoplastic agents. Spectra may be obtained with as little as 1 to 10 μg of a compound. This low requirement, as far as quantity is concerned, is much less than for most other physical methods. With equipment in which gas-liquid chromatography and mass spectrometry are combined, an excellent separation of compounds and an exceptionally reliable means for identification are obtained. This technique has been reviewed recently (GUARINO and FALES, 1971).

Infrared spectrometry is similar in scope to mass spectrometry, except that 10 to 100 times greater amounts of drug may be required. With infrared spectrometry the identity is based purely on a comparative basis, whereas with mass spectrometry structural elucidation sometimes can be achieved without a reference compound. Nuclear magnetic resonance spectrometry requires isolation of pure compounds, but can be a great aid in elucidating the structure of a metabolite.

## Spontaneous Reactions of Antineoplastic Agents

The possibility of spontaneous hydrolysis or tissue accelerated hydrolysis of anticancer agents has received only a moderate amount of attention. One of the best examples of spontaneous hydrolysis of drugs was reported by SCHUMACHER et al. (1965a) who studied the rapid conversion of thalidomide to a wide variety of carboxylic acids in buffer solutions of pH 7.4. It was expected, therefore, that most of an administered dose of thalidomide would be degraded nonenzymatically and thus show little species variation in the biologic half-life of the drug. In the monkey this half-life is about 2.7 hours, which is very similar to the half-life reported in rats and rabbits, and indeed was about the same as the half-life observed in the buffered solution at 37°. In comparing the distribution of this drug and its metabolites in plasma and various tissues, however, it was found that there were high levels of metabolites in the monkey liver suggesting that the drug was being degraded enzymatically, as well as nonenzymatically in this tissue. Hence, these workers (SCHUMACHER et al., 1965b) reported that ten minutes after an intravenous injection of 10 mg/kg of thalidomide, 90% of the radioactivity in muscle was present as unchanged thalidomide, while the liver at this time contained only 47% of the drug as parent drug. This interesting example of the possible occurrence of simultaneous degradation of a compound by both enzymatic and nonenzymatic means is important to consider in studies of antineoplastic agents.

WILLIAMSON et al. (1966) observed that there was an enzyme in serum that catalyzes the reaction between secondary nitrogen mustards and carbon dioxide to form substituted oxazolidinones. Although agents of the type nor-$HN_2$ are no longer of widespread interest, the results of these workers suggest an unusual pitfall encountered in studying the metabolism of these agents. The reaction they report causes the very rapid degradation of certain nitrogen mustards, such as nor-$HN_2$, because they are immediately transformed into products no longer capable of undergoing typical alkylation reactions. The substance in serum does not appear to react directly with nor-$HN_2$, but it does cause an accelerated loss of the compound in the presence of carbon dioxide. Apparently the substance is an enzyme, but is not carbonic anhydrase, is not inhibited by cyanide, and is nondialyzable. Hence, when mustards of this type are employed as chemotherapeutic agents, it must be recognized that the injected drugs can be immediately transformed into other compounds with the consequent unlikelihood of them behaving in the manner anticipated in their original design.

## Noncancer Uses of Anticancer Agents

In a recent excellent review dealing with the use of antineoplastic drugs in non-malignant diseases, STEINBERG et al. (1972) discuss some of the less common applications of these cytotoxic drugs. The use of cancer chemotherapeutic agents in the treatment of diseases of the connective tissue and skin, hematopoietic and nervous systems, and of the eye, liver, and kidney, as well as other systems and organs, is amply dealt with by these authors and will not be repeated here. Several more general applications, however, will be discussed briefly in the following paragraphs.

Agents such as methotrexate and 5-fluorouracil have been used in the treatment of refractory cases of psoriasis. Such uses of antineoplastic agents for relatively long periods of time provide an opportunity to study drug disposition in patients who have relatively normal host determinants; that is, such patients are usually free of hepatic and renal compromise and hence would be expected to remove the drug at normal rates. On the other hand, these chronic disease states may lead to therapy for periods longer than would be the case if the drugs were employed in the treatment of neoplastic disease. It would be of great interest to study rates of metabolism and rates of clearance of antineoplastic agents in such patients.

Another widespread use for drugs that were originally designed as antineoplastic agents is in the area of immunosuppression in patients receiving organ transplants. In cases where a diseased kidney is already present and a new kidney is being transplanted to the donor, one would expect severe limitations in the ability of such a patient to clear drugs normally excreted by the renal pathways. Likewise in the use of such agents in patients receiving other essential organs by transplantation, one might expect less than full capacity from such systems as the cardiovascular and hepatic. For example, it would be likely that a degree of anoxia could be associated with a failing heart, and hence replacement of this latter organ, with the consequent immunotherapy, could lead to exaggerated responses if the anoxia also affected the hepatocytes. Such diminished clearance and/or metabolism of these agents would therefore be dangerous in a patient hardly able to tolerate problems of drug toxicity after such major surgery.

## Metabolism of Specific Antineoplastic Agents

In this section emphasis will be placed on those metabolic pathways rather conclusively worked out for antineoplastic drugs, particularly where microsomal involvement is implicated. A summary of the agents and their pathways appears in Table 1.

### A. Alkylating Agents

#### I. Nitrogen Mustard (Mechlorethamine, $HN_2$, Mustargen)

The alkylating agents are usually very reactive compounds that combine most readily with nitrogen, sulfur, or oxygen atoms of biologically important molecules. The great chemical reactivity of the alkylating agents and the occurrence of a large number of nonselective reactions make it difficult to study the metabolism of these drugs. Although the properties of nitrogen mustards vary widely, $HN_2$ can

Table 1. *Summary of antineoplastic drugs known to be metabolized by microsomal enzymes*

| Drug | Species | Metabolic Pathway | Comments | Reference |
|---|---|---|---|---|
| *Alkylating agents* | | | | |
| Cyclophosphamide | rat | *N*-, *O*-Dealkylation | Requires NADPH and $O_2$; no metabolism detected in tumor homogenate | Brock and Hohorst (1967) |
| | rat | "Activation" | NADPH, $O_2$ required; phenobarbital inducible; carbon monoxide sensitive | Cohen and Jao (1970) |
| | rat, mouse | "Activation" | $K_m$ change following phenobarbital induction; *in vivo* and *in vitro* metabolism parallel | Sladek (1972) |
| | mouse | "Activation" | Duration of action increased following SKF-525A pretreatment | Field et al. (1972) |
| | mouse | "Activation" | NADPH required; inhibited by CO, SKF-525A | Hill et al. (1972) |
| OPSPA | rat, man | Hydrolysis | SKF-525A sensitive | Maller and Heidelberger (1957) |
| Mustargen | rat, rabbit | *N*-Dealkylation | Slight activity found in hepatoma homogenate | Trams and Nadkarni (1956) |
| Hydroxyurea | mouse | Reduction | Microsomes only 1/2 as active as mitochondria | Colvin and Bono (1970) |
| *Antimetabolites* | | | | |
| Butyl- and ethyl-mercaptopurine | man | *S*-glucuronidation | 50% to 70% of administered drug excreted as glucuronide | Hansen et al. (1963) |
| Methyl thiopurine | mouse | *S*-Demethylation | No activity in tumor tissue homogenate | Henderson and Mazel (1964) |
| *Antibiotics* | | | | |
| Puromycin | rodents | Demethylation | Phenobarbital inducible; SKF-525A sensitive | Mazel et al. (1966) |
| Mitomycins | rat | Reduction | Anaerobic; requires NADPH | Schwartz (1962) |
| *Miscellaneous* | | | | |
| Procarbazine | rat | *N*-Demethylation | Phenobarbital inducible; carbon monoxide sensitive | Wittkop et al. (1969) |
| | rat, swine | *N*-Demethylation | Phenobarbital induced enzyme is P-450 dependent | Prough et al. (1970) |
| Dialkyl triazenes | rat | Dealkylation | Requires NADPH and oxygen | Preussman et al. (1969) |
| Dialkyl triazeno-imidazoles | rat, man | Dealkylation | Metabolism *in vivo* (rat, man) and *in vitro* (rat); phenobarbital inducible | Skibba et al. (1970) |

be regarded as a prototype of this class of compounds. This compound is very toxic, a vesicant, and unstable. Even in buffer solutions at physiological pH, $HN_2$ is readily converted to the aziridinium ion, which in turn reacts with any available nucleophilic center.

SKIPPER et al. (1951) showed that about 15% of $^{14}$C-methyl labeled $HN_2$ was oxidized to carbon dioxide and exhaled by mice treated with 4 mg/kg of the drug. Using $^{14}$C-methyl $HN_2$, NADKARNI et al. (1959) found that the radioactivity was removed from the blood very rapidly with less than 10% being present 30 sec after injection. TRAMS and NADKARNI (1956) found that the *N*-methyl group was liberated and oxidized to formaldehyde, presumably by mediation of microsomal enzymes. Metabolism of the $\beta$-chloroethyl portion of the molecule was indicated by the finding that acetaldehyde could be detected in the incubation medium when $HN_2$ was added as the substrate. The physiological distribution of radioactive $^{14}$C-methyl-labeled $HN_2$ was similar to that of $^{14}$C-formate, and hence MANDEL (1959) suggested that the methyl group of $HN_2$ becomes detached and then incorporated into normal body constituents. The liver contains an enzyme that demethylates $HN_2$ to nor-$HN_2$ (SMITH et al., 1958) and a microsomal enzyme that can demethylate this agent was reported by TRAMS and NADKARNI (1956). WILLIAMSON et al. (1966) observed that an enzyme in the blood catalyzed the reaction between mustards such as nor-$HN_2$ and carbon dioxide to form substituted oxazolidinones which are incapable of undergoing typical alkylation reactions. Elucidation of all of the metabolites of radioactive $HN_2$ appearing in the urine is incomplete, but chromatographic analysis revealed the presence of at least eight labeled products, most of which were not further identified.

## II. Cyclophosphamide (Cytoxan, Endoxan, Procytoc, CTX)

Cyclophospamide (CTX) has particular importance in this chapter because it has no cytotoxic activity of its own, but rather requires conversion into alkylating substances in order to exert its pharmacologic effects. Once the antineoplastic activity of $HN_2$ had been established, a variety of potential antineoplastic agents was synthesized where the alkylating potential was either directly present, as in the case of $HN_2$, or was in a latent form such as occurs in CTX. In the case of this latter compound, a cyclic phosphamide was substituted for the *N*-methyl of $HN_2$. In this form the *bis*($\beta$-chloroethyl) portion of the molecule cannot be ionized until the cyclic group is cleaved at the phosphorus-nitrogen linkage. The parent compound is, therefore, inactive *in vitro*, but part of the rationale for the design of this compound was based on the observation that there were high phosphatase and phosphamidase activities in neoplastic tissues. The "activation" probably takes place primarily in the liver microsomes.

In a rather complete study of the *in vivo* activation of CTX, FIELD et al. (1972) were able to show by the use of a chemical assay that pretreatment with phenobarbital accelerated the production of alkylating metabolites of this agent, which was followed by a rapid depletion of the alkylating drug. Pretreatment with 2-diethylaminoethyl-2,2-diphenylvalerate (SKF-525A) retarded the activation process which resulted in the slow release of the drug over a longer period of time. In biological experiments these authors found that the duration of antileukemic activity was shortened by phenobarbital and lengthened by SKF-525A pretreatment. The similarity of the results of the biological and chemical studies relating to the effect of pretreatment on the metabolism of CTX suggests that the metabolites of this drug, as measured by chemical assay, are indeed responsible for the antileukemic activity. The chemical data show that pretreatment with SKF-525A increased, and pretreatment with phenobarbital decreased, the total amount of alkylating metabolites.

From a drug metabolism point of view, CTX perhaps provides one of the best examples of the problems in this area. The initial step in such studies was simply to set down all of the anticipated metabolites that would occur. This has been done in Fig. 2. Initially there are a variety of hydrolytic and oxidative reactions to consider.

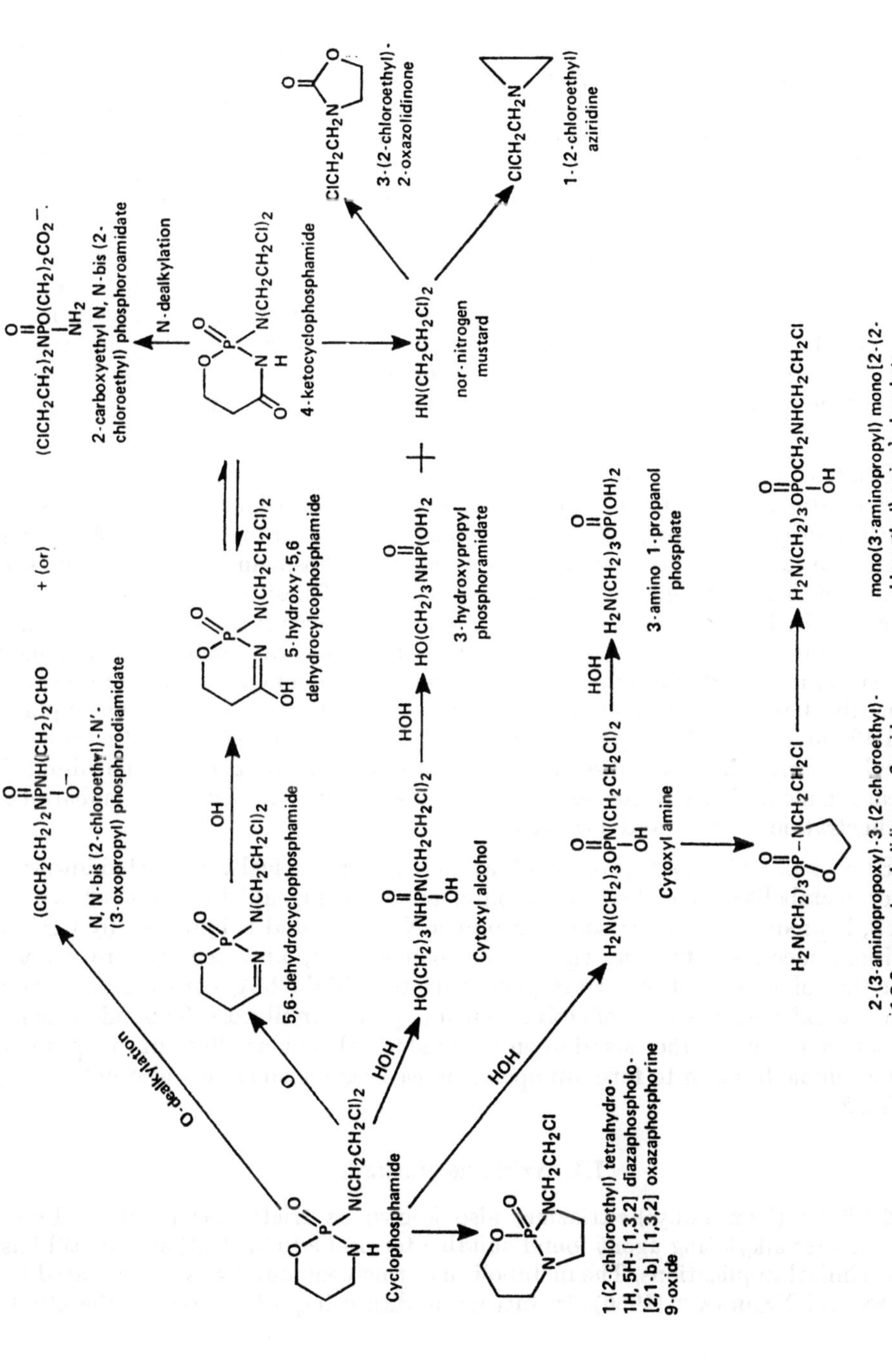


Fig. 2. Potential metabolites of cyclophosphamide

The secondary reactions may involve further hydrolysis and/or other degradative pathways. It is important to acknowledge that, despite several years of active research in this area and the testing of all possible metabolites considered to date, the active metabolite is yet to be isolated and identified. It seems likely that due to the instability of this "active metabolite" such a task may prove impossible.

The simple two-step hydrolysis of CTX to nor-$HN_2$, which was first proposed to account for the activation of this agent, cannot fully account for the observed biological effects. In further studies, evidence was proposed for the involvement of oxidation where 1-(2-chloroethyl)aziridine was formed via the oxidized and hydroxylated intermediates, 5,6-dehydrocyclophosphamide, and 5-hydroxy-5,6-dehydrocyclophosphamide. Further evidence was obtained from studies in rats which indicated that the specificity of action of CTX presumably occurs by an *O*-dealkylation reaction and/or an *N*-dealkylation reaction. Both cytoxylamine and cytoxyl alcohol are recognized as possible intermediates of this agent and the former did possess some *in vitro* antitumor activity (GRUNICKE et al., 1965). Cytoxyl alcohol and a structurally related phosphorodiamidic acid were also cytotoxic and comparable in activity to cyclophosphamide itself (FRIEDMAN et al., 1963; MADDOCK et al., 1966). It has been postulated further that a bicyclic intermediate (Fig. 2) may be the precursor of the major *in vitro* hydrolytic product (FRIEDMAN et al., 1963). Hence, it can be seen from this brief discussion that what was conceived as a simple latentiation of nor-$HN_2$ evolved into a very complex problem which remains to be solved.

STRUCK et al. (1971) have reported a number of urinary metabolites in dogs after treatment with CTX. The primary metabolite which they identified is 2-carboxyethyl *N,N-bis*(2-chloroethyl)phosphorodiamidate (Fig. 2). A minor metabolite found in these studies was 4-ketocyclophosphamide, the first known product of this drug which retains its ring structure. These workers also isolated a trace of $\beta$-hydroxypropionamide and proposed that this fragment was originally derived from the phosphorodiamidate moiety. The activation of cyclophosphamide by liver is mediated through mixed function oxidase enzymes which are located primarily, but not exclusively in liver microsomes. The enzyme system requires NADPH and molecular oxygen for full activity and is inhibited *in vitro* by compounds known to be metabolized by liver microsomes. The enzyme can be inhibited by carbon monoxide and the enzyme level is markedly increased by phenobarbital administration (COHEN and JAO, 1970).

HILL et al. (1972) have proposed that CTX is enzymatically converted into two major metabolites. The first metabolite, an open-ring aldehyde not shown in Fig. 2, is produced by microsomes, requires NADPH, and is inhibited by CO. In addition, nicotine, atropine, ephedrine, apomorphine, and cocaine are potent inhibitors of this reaction, while phenobarbital, SKF-525A, cytochrome c, and some steroid hormones are effective, but less potent inhibitors. This microsomal metabolite is then further acted upon by an aldehyde oxidase-like enzyme present in the soluble fraction to form an open-ring carboxyphosphamide also not shown in Fig. 2.

## III. Aziridine Mustards

2,4,6-*Tris*(1-aziridinyl)-*s*-triazine, also known as triethylmelamine or TEM, was the first alkylating agent found suitable for oral administration and still has some clinical applications. The metabolism of this compound was investigated by TRAMS and NADKARNI (1956). In further studies using a $^{14}C$ label on the ethyleneimino moiety of TEM, about 80% of TEM was recovered in mouse urine as cyanuric acid, urea, creatinine, and at least 14 other metabolites (GOLDENTHAL et al., 1958). Neither ethanolamine nor glycine appeared to be metabolites of this compound. The antineoplastic activity of TEM led to further studies wherein a series of phosphoramides were synthesized. The two most important ones in this group were *tris*(1-aziridinyl)phosphine oxide (triethylene phosphoramide or TEPA), and *tris*(1-aziridinyl)phosphine sulfide (thioTEPA). Unfortunately, most of the studies carried out with TEPA were done with the $^{32}P$ form of the compound, and therefore little is known about the fate and distribution of the rest of the molecule. In mice, 66% to 90% of the $^{32}P$-TEPA is recovered as inorganic phosphate, while in the rat most of the drug was reported to be excreted unchanged in the urine (CRAIG and JACKSON, 1955). MELLETT et al. (1962) studied $^{14}C$-thioTEPA and reported that less than 1% of the parent compound could be found in human or dog urine. ThioTEPA appears to be converted to the corresponding phosphoramide, TEPA, and hence further metabolism would follow the same pathways established for TEPA.

## IV. *N*-(3-Oxapentamethylene)-*N'N''*-diethylenethiophosphoramide (OPSPA)

OPSPA, another compound related to TEPA, is excreted in the urine largely as the corresponding phosphoramide, together with some morpholine and other unidentified metabolites (MALLER and HEIDELBERGER, 1957). The conversion of OPSPA to phosphoramide is inhibited by SKF-525A, suggesting that this reaction is catalyzed by microsomal enzymes.

## V. Methanesulfonate (Busulfan, Myleran, GT-41, 1,4-dimethanesulfonyloxybutane)

TRAMS et al. (1959) found that about 50% of labeled methanesulfonate (GT-41) appeared in the urine after two days. In man, 95% of GT-41 labeled with $^{35}S$ was recovered as methanesulfonic acid, whereas 75% of the administered dose of $^{14}C$ labeled GT-41 was reported by NADKARNI et al. (1959) to be excreted in the urine, and all of this radioactivity was associated with unidentifiable urinary metabolites. In several rodent species, methanesulfonic acid was also the predominant urinary metabolite after administration of $^{35}S$-GT-41, but as much as 25% of the parent compound along with two unidentified metabolites containing some inorganic sulfate were reported (TRAMS et al., 1959; FOX et al., 1960). In the rat, about 15% of $^{14}C$-GT-41 was converted to $CO_2$, while 6% of the radioactivity was recovered in the feces. Twenty urinary metabolites, including glucose, urea, oxylates, acetates, and 1,4-butanediol accounted for about 30% of the administered radioactivity. TRAMS et al. (1959) reported some unchanged compound was excreted, as well as propyl- and methyl-methanesulfonates which appeared to be excreted as cysteine conjugates. When $^{14}C$-ethyl methanesulfonate was administered, it was hydrolyzed to ethanol, metabolized to urinary serine, alanine, arginine, and *S*-ethylcysteine, and expired as $CO_2$ (ROBERTS and WARWICK, 1957, 1959).

## VI. Nitrosoureas

Studies of the fate and distribution of 1,3-*bis*(2-chloroethyl)-1-nitrosourea (BCNU) have been severely hampered by its rapid degradation. DEVITA et al. (1967) first investigated the stability of this compound in various aqueous systems and found that BCNU was relatively stable only at acidic pH. For example, at pH 3.5 about 90% of the drug remained intact after incubation for five hours. At pH 7.8, however, only 30% remained at five hours, while at pH 11 less than 3% was present at five hours. *In vivo* studies by these workers, using a combination of radioassays and thin layer chromatography, showed that as early as 15 min following drug dosage, none of the intact drug could be detected in urine or cerebrospinal fluid samples from monkeys. Their observation that the radioactivity from urine remained at the origin on thin-layer chromatography plates following development in chloroform suggests extensive conversion to very polar metabolites. It has been suggested (DEVITA et al., 1967) that BCNU may cleave at the bond between the nitrosated nitrogen and the carbonyl carbon leading to the immediate formation of chloroethylisocyanate, a very reactive compound. In aqueous solutions the identified decomposition products were 2-chloroethylamine hydrochloride, acetaldehyde, nitrogen, and carbon dioxide. Both BCNU and 1-(2-chloroethyl)-3-cyclohexyl-1-nitrosourea (CCNU) have been studied by *in vitro* decomposition techniques by MONTGOMERY et al. (1967), and CCNU has similarly been studied by BRAY et al. (1971) who published the following scheme (Fig. 3) for the decomposi-

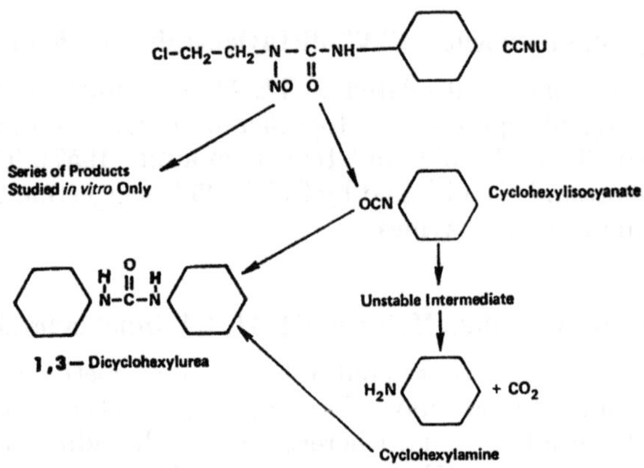


Fig. 3. Metabolites of the nitrosourea CCNU via pathways originally proposed by MONTGOMERY et al. (1967)

tion of CCNU. Accordingly, OLIVERIO et al. (1970) reported that the urine of mice treated with $^{14}$C-cyclohexyl labeled-CCNU contained about 4% of an administered dose as 1,3-dicyclohexylurea and about 16% as the cyclohexylamine metabolite. Such studies, however, have shed virtually no light on the fate of the chloroethyl group of CCNU, although a small amount of radioactive $CO_2$ does occur when the label is present in this position. Thus, approximately 75% of the $^{14}$C label in the cyclohexyl moiety of CCNU represents biotransformation products which are yet to be identified (OLIVERIO et al., 1970).

## B. Miscellaneous Compounds

### I. Procarbazine (Methylhydrazine, MIH, Natulan, Matulan)

Details of the metabolism of this interesting antineoplastic agent will be covered elsewhere in this book (REED, Chapt. 70, this volume), but a few points of interest will be made at this time. There have been several publications providing evidence of the *in vivo* lability of the *N*-methyl group of this compound. After labeling this methyl group with either $^3$H or $^{14}$C, radioactivity was found in the

*C*-1 pool, in purine bases, and in expired $CO_2$. Recently KREIS (1970) provided evidence for the *in vivo* transfer of the intact *N*-methyl group of procarbazine into cytoplasmic RNA. DOST and REED (1967) reported that methyl labeled procarbazine gave rise to not only radiolabeled carbon dioxide, but also radiolabeled methane. These workers further postulated that monomethylhydrazine may be an intermediate in the metabolism of procarbazine. In further studies attempting to characterize the nature of the microsomal metabolism of procarbazine and related alkylhydrazines, PROUGH et al. (1970) noted that there were two modes of metabolism: by alkylhydrazine oxidase, where conversion of alkylhydrazines results in formation of the corresponding alkenes, and also by *N*-methylhydrazine demethylase, where formation of formaldehyde results from the *N*-methyl group. Alkylhydrazine oxidase activity does not appear to be dependent upon cytochrome P-450 and the activity of this enzyme is not induced by prior treatment of rats with either phenobarbital or 3-methylcholanthrene. However, *N*-methylhydrazine demethylase activity in rats is inducible by these agents and the induced level of activity appears to be dependent upon the cytochrome P-450 content of the microsomes. The data are offered in support of the possibility of two enzyme systems being present in rat liver microsomes, both capable of demethylating *N*-methylhydrazines such as procarbazine. KATO et al. (1969b) studied the effects of a series of hydrazine derivatives on drug-metabolizing enzymes. Although procarbazine was not specifically studied, the findings suggest that these compounds inhibit drug-metabolizing enzymes and that the degree of inhibition is related to their lipid solubility. It would, therefore, be expected that procarbazine, because of its relatively great lipid solubility, would be a potent inhibitor of these enzymes. The possible clinical implicaton of these suggestions should be explored further.

## II. *o,p'*-DDD (*o,p'*-Dichlorodiphenyldichloroethane, Mitotane, Lysodren)

An astute histopathologic observation made by NELSON and WOODWARD (1949) led to the eventual use of this compound in adrenal cortical carcinoma. They observed that the insecticide DDD caused cytotoxic atrophy of the adrenal cortex and, although rare, tumors of the adrenal cortex have shown great sensitivity to the selective adrenolytic effect of *o,p'*-DDD. Some clues as to the possible metabolites of this compound are available from considerations of the metabolism of the insecticide DDD. In addition, MOY (1961) found that in humans about 60% of the administered dose of *o,p'*-DDD was eliminated by the feces as intact drug, 10% appeared in the urine as an unidentified metabolite, and 20% seemed to be retained and slowly released from the tissues and fat stores. The metabolism of this drug is treated in detail elsewhere in this book (STRAW and HART, Chapt. 74, this volume).

## III. Mitomycin

Mitomycin is generally nonreactive in the natural oxidized state, but after chemical or enzymatic reduction it behaves as a bifunctional alkylating agent. This activated form of mitomycin has been shown *in vitro* to interact with DNA by linking complementary strands. Although many of these activation studies have been conducted in bacterial lysates, there are several properties of these mitomycin-activating systems which are analogous to the mitomycin-reducing systems present in liver homogenates (SCHWARTZ and PHILIPS, 1961; SCHWARTZ, 1962; SCHWARTZ et al., 1963). It was concluded by IYER and SZYBALSKI (1964) that NADPH-dependent enzymatic reduction of mitomycin is a necessary prerequisite to DNA cross-linking, and they attributed this mechanism of action to the antibiotic.

## IV. Puromycin

The compound 6-dimethylaminopurine is demethylated by mouse liver microsomes, and this methylated purine analog has the same purine moiety found in the antibiotic puromycin. Furthermore, puromycin inhibits induction of the microsomal demethylase by either phenobarbital or 3-methylcholanthrene (CONNEY and GILMAN, 1963). The demethylation of puromycin and related compounds by rat liver microsomes has been demonstrated by MAZEL et al. (1966) who found that the enzyme catalyzing this reaction is localized in the liver and requires microsomes, oxygen, and NADPH. They further found that this demethylation of puromycin was inhibited by SKF-525A. These same workers substantiated this early evidence with further studies showing that pretreatment of rats with phenobarbital markedly stimulated the demethylation of puromycin and related compounds.

## V. 6-Methylthiopurine

Until the work of MAZEL et al. (1964) and HENDERSON and MAZEL (1964) *S*-demethylation by liver microsomes had not been described. These workers showed that rat liver microsomes can remove methyl groups from thioethers such as 6-methylthiopurine to yield formaldehyde and the free thioacids. They further showed that this *S*-demethylation required NADPH, glucose-6-phosphate, magnesium, oxygen and microsomes. These studies further emphasized the fact that the assumption that antimetabolites are metabolized only by enzymes which metabolize the natural products which they resemble was in serious error. Like cyclophosphamide, alkylthiopurines are themselves inactive as cancer chemotherapeutic agents and the dealkylation of these drugs must, therefore, be regarded as an activation step. Although this activation is pharmacologically the most important metabolic pathway, other pathways may be quantitatively more significant (see review by JOHNS, Chap. 14, this volume).

## References

ALVARES, A.P., SCHILLING, G.R., KUNTZMAN, R.: Differences in the kinetics of benzpyrene hydroxylation by hepatic drug-metabolizing enzymes from phenobarbital and 3-methylcholanthrene-treated rats. Biochem. biophys. Res. Commun. **30**, 588—593 (1968).

AXELROD, J.: Biochemical factors in the activation and inactivation of drugs. Naunyn-Schmiedebergs Arch. exp. Path. Pharmak. **238**, 24—35 (1960).

AXELROD, J., INSCOE, J.K., TOMKINS, G.M.: Enzymatic synthesis of *N*-glucuronic acid conjugates. Nature (Lond.) **179**, 538—539 (1957).

BAILEY-WOOD, R., DODGSON, K.S., ROSE, F.A.: A rat liver sulphohydrolase enzyme acting on adenylyl sulphate. Biochem. J. **112**, 257—258 (1969).

BARON, J., TEPHLY, T.R.: Effect of 3-amino-1,2,4-triazole on the stimulation of hepatic microsomal heme synthesis and induction of hepatic microsomal oxidases produced by phenobarbital. Molec. Pharmacol. **5**, 10—20 (1969).

BERAUD, T., VANNOTTI, A.: Comportement metabolique du rat hepatectomise. Acta Endocrinol. **35**, 324—333 (1960).

BOLLMAN, J.L., MENDEZ, F.L.: Separation of bile pigments by column chromatography. Fed. Proc. **14**, 399—400 (1955).

BOOTH, J., BOYLAND, E.: The biochemistry of aromatic amines. 10. Enzymic *N*-hydroxylation of arylamines and conversion of arylhydroxylamines into *o*-aminophenols. Biochem. J. **91**, 362—369 (1964).

BOYLAND, E., MANSON, D., ORR, S.F.D.: The biochemistry of aromatic amines. 2. The conversion of arylamines into arylsulfamic acids and arylamine-*N*-glucuronic acids. Biochem. J. **65**, 417—423 (1957).

BOYLAND, E., NERY, R.: The metabolism of urethane and related compounds. Biochem. J. **94**, 198—208 (1965).

BRAY, D.A., DEVITA, V.T., ADAMSON, R.H., OLIVERIO, V.T.: Effects of 1-(2-chloroethyl)-3-cyclohexyl-1-nitrosourea (CCNU; NSC-79037) and its degradation products on progression of L1210 cells through the cell cycle. Cancer Chemother. Rep. **55**, 215—220 (1971).

BRIDGES, J. W., WILLIAMS, R. T.: N-Glucuronide formation *in vivo* and *in vitro*. Biochem. J. **83**, 27P (1962).
BRIDGES, J. W., KIBBY, M. R., WALKER, S. R., WILLIAMS, R. T.: Species differences in the metabolism of sulphadimethoxine. Biochem. J. **109**, 851—856 (1968).
BRIDGES, J. W., KIBBY, M. R., WALKER, S. R., WILLIAMS, R. T.: Structure and species as factors affecting the metabolism of some methoxy-6-sulphanilamidopyrimidines. Biochem. J. **111**, 167—172 (1969a).
BRIDGES, J. W., WALKER, S. R., WILLIAMS, R. T.: Species differences in the metabolism and excretion of sulphasomidine and sulphamethomidine. Biochem. J. **111**, 173—179 (1969b).
BROCK, N., HOHORST, H. J.: Metabolism of cyclophosphamide. Cancer **20**, 900—904 (1967).
BRODIE, B. B., GILLETTE, J. R., LADU, B. N.: Enzymatic metabolism of drugs and other foreign compounds. Ann. Rev. Biochem. **27**, 427—454 (1958).
BROWN, H. D., CHATTOPADHYAY, S. K., PENNINGTON, S. N., SPRATT, J. S., MORRIS, H. P.: Mixed-function oxidation in tumors. Brit. J. Cancer **25**, 135—141 (1971).
CANTONI, G. L.: *S*-adenosylmethionine: a new intermediate formed enzymatically from *L*-methionine and adenosine triphosphate. J. biol. Chem. **204**, 403—416 (1953).
CASTRO, J. A., GILLETTE, J. R.: Species and sex differences in the kinetic constants for the *N*-demethylation of ethylmorphine by liver microsomes. Biochem. biophys. Res. Commun. **28**, 426—430 (1967).
CLAUDE, A.: The constitution of protoplasm. Science **97**, 451—456 (1943).
COHEN, J. L., JAO, J. Y.: Enzymatic basis of cyclophosphamide activation by hepatic microsomes of the rat. J. Pharmacol. exp. Ther. **174**, 206—210 (1970).
COHN, R.: Über das Verhalten einiger Pyridin- und Naphthalinderivate im thierischen Stoffwechsel. Hoppe-Seylers Z. physiol. Chem. **18**, 112—113 (1894).
COLVIN, M., BONO, V. H., JR.: The enzymatic reduction of hydroxyurea to urea by mouse liver. Cancer Res. **30**, 1516—1519 (1970).
CONNEY, A. H., GILMAN, A. G.: Puromycin inhibition of enzyme induction by 3-methylcholanthrene and phenobarbital. J. biol. Chem. **238**, 3682—3685 (1963).
CONNEY, A. H., SCHNEIDMAN, K., JACOBSON, M., KUNTZMAN, R.: Drug-induced changes in steroid metabolism. Ann. N. Y. Acad. Sci. **123**, 98—109 (1965).
CRAIG, A. W., JACKSON, H.: The mechanism of $^{32}$P-labelled triethylene-phosphoramide in relation to its anti-tumor activity. Brit. J. Pharmacol. **10**, 321—325 (1955).
DAHM, V. K., BREUER, H.: Enzymatische Untersuchungen über die Glucuronidierung von Östriol beim Menschen. Z. klin. Chem. **4**, 153—157 (1966).
DANIELLI, J. F., MONTAGU, K. A., BERNARD, P. J., PYE, A., PRICE, F. W., HAMERTON, J. L., COURTNEY, W. A. M.: A. R. Brit. Empire Cancer Campaign **37**, 575—576 (1959).
DAVIES, D. S., GIGON, P. L., GILLETTE, J. R.: Sex differences in the kinetic constants for the *N*-demethylation of ethylmorphine by rat liver microsomes. Biochem. Pharmacol. **17**, 1865—1872 (1968).
DEVITA, V. T., DENHAM, C., DAVIDSON, J. D., OLIVERIO, V. T.: Physiological disposition of the carcinostatic 1,3-*bis*(2-chloroethyl)-1-nitrosourea (BCNU) in man and animals. Clin. Pharmacol. Ther. **8**, 566—577 (1967).
DEWAIDE, J. H.: Metabolism of Xenobiotics. Ph. D. Thesis, Univ. of Nijmegen, Nijmegen, Netherlands (1971).
DIXON, R. L.: Effect of chloramphenicol on the metabolism and lethality of cyclophosphamide in rats. Proc. Soc. exp. Biol. (N. Y.) **127**, 1151—1155 (1968).
DIXON, R. L., SHULTICE, R. W., FOUTS, J. R.: Factors affecting drug metabolism by liver microsomes. IV. Starvation. Proc. Soc. exp. Biol. (N. Y.) **103**, 333—335 (1960).
DODGSON, K. S., ROSE, F. A.: Sulfoconjugation and sulfohydrolysis. In: Metabolic conjugation and metabolic hydrolysis (FISHMAN, W. H., Ed.) p. 240. New York: Academic Press 1970.
DONELLI, M. G., GARATTINI, S.: Drug metabolism after repeated treatments with cytotoxic agents. Europ. J. Cancer **7**, 361—364 (1971).
DOST, F. N., REED, D. J.: Methane formation *in vivo* from *N*-isopropyl α(2-methylhydrazino)-*p*-toluamide hydrochloride, a tumor-inhibiting methylhydrazine derivative. Biochem. Pharmacol. **16**, 1741—1746 (1967).
DRING, L. G., SMITH, R. L., WILLIAMS, R. T.: The fate of amphetamine in man and other mammals. J. pharm. Pharmacol. 18, 402—404 (1966).
DUNCAN, G. G., CRISTOFORI, F. C., YUE, J. K., MURTHY, M. S. J.: The control of obesity by intermittent fasts. Med. Clin. N. Amer. **48**, 1359—1372 (1964).
DUTTON, G. J., STOREY, I. D. E.: The isolation of a compound of uridine diphosphate and glucuronic acid from liver. Biochem. J. **53**, XXXVII (1953).
ELLISON, T. L., GUTZAIT, L., VAN LOON, E. J.: The comparative metabolism of *d*-amphetamine-$C^{14}$ in the rat, dog, and monkey. J. Pharmacol. exp. Ther. **152**, 383—387 (1966).
EVERETT. J. L., ROSS, W. C. J.: Aryl-2-halogenoalkylamines. Part II. J. chem. Soc. 1972—1983 (1949).

FARBER, S., TOCH, R., SEARS, E. M., PINKEL, D.: Advances in chemotherapy of cancer in man. Adv. Cancer Res. **4**, 1—71 (1956).
FIELD, R. B., GANG, M., KLINE, I., VENDITTI, J. M., WARAVDEKAR, V. S.: The effect of phenobarbital or 2-diethylaminoethyl-2,2-diphenyl-valerate on the activation of cyclophosphamide *in vivo*. J. Pharmacol. exp. Ther. **180**, 475—483 (1972).
FOUTS, J. R.: Interaction of drugs and hepatic microsomes. Fed. Proc. **21**, 1107—1111 (1962).
FOUTS, J. R., BRODIE, B. B.: The enzymatic reduction of chloramphenicol, *p*-nitrobenzoic acid and other aromatic nitro compounds in mammals. J. Pharmacol. exp. Ther. **119**, 197—207 (1957).
FOX, B. W., CRAIG, A. W., JACKSON, H.: The comparative metabolism of myleran-$^{35}$S in the rat, mouse, and rabbit. Biochem. Pharmacol. **5**, 27—29 (1960).
FRANCHI, G., ROSSO, R.: Metabolic fate of zoxazolamine in tumor bearing rats. Biochem. Pharmacol. 18, 236—238 (1969).
FRENCH, A. P., WARREN, J. C.: Properties of steroid sulphatase and aryl sulphatase activities of human placenta. Biochem. J. **105**, 233—241 (1967).
FREZZA, M., DESANDRE, G., PERONA, G., CORRICHER, R.: Bilirubin inhibition of 4-methylumbelliferone glucuro conjugation *in vitro* by the human liver. Clin. chim. Acta **21**, 509—512 (1968).
FRIEDMAN, O. M., PAPANASTASSIOU, Z. N., LEVI, R. S., TILL, H. R., JR., WHALEY, W. M.: Potential carcinolytic agents related to cyclophosphamide. J. med. Chem. **6**, 82—85 (1963).
FUJIWARA, T., SPENCER, B.: Adenyl deaminase of *Helix pomatia*. Biochem. J. **85**, 19P (1962).
GAUDETTE, L. E., BRODIE, B. B.: Relationship between the lipid solubility of drugs and their oxidation by liver microsomes. Biochem. Pharmacol. **2**, 89—96 (1959).
GILLETTE, J. R.: Factors affecting drug metabolism. Ann. N. Y. Acad. Sci. **179**, 43—66 (1971).
GILLETTE, J. R., GRAM, T. E.: Cytochrome P-450 reduction in liver microsomes and its relationship to drug metabolism. In: Microsomes and drug oxidations. (GILLETTE, J. R., CONNEY, A. H., COSMIDES, G. J., ESTABROOK, R. W., FOUTS, J. R., MANNERING, G. J., Eds., pp. 133—150. New York: Academic Press 1969.
GOLDENTHAL, E. I., NADKARNI, M. V., SMITH, P. K.: The excretion of radioactivity following administration of tri-C$^{14}$-ethylenimino-*s*-triazine in normal mice. J. Pharmacol. exp. Ther. **122**, 431—441 (1958).
GRAM, T. E., HANSEN, A. R., FOUTS, J. R.: The submicrosomal distribution of hepatic UDP-glucuronyl transferases in the rabbit. Biochem. J. **106**, 587—591 (1968).
GREIM, H., REMMER, H.: Abbauhemmung und Synthesesteigerung bei der Vermehrung mikrosomaler Cytochrome durch Phenobarbital. Naunyn-Schmiedebergs Arch. exp. Path. Pharmak. **264**, 238—239 (1969).
GRUNICKE, H., LIERSCH, M., HOLZER, H., ARNOLD, H.: Untersuchungen zum Wirkungsmechanismus von Endoxan. Biochem. Pharmacol. **14**, 1485—1490 (1965).
GUARINO, A. M., FALES, H. M.: Gas chromatography-mass spectrometry. Handbook exp. Pharmacol. XXVIII-2, 178—208 (1971).
GUARINO, A. M., GRAM, T. E., GIGON, P. L., GREENE, F. E., GILLETTE, J. R.: Changes in Michaelis and spectral constants for aniline in hepatic microsomes from phenobarbital-treated rats. Molec. Pharmacol. **5**, 131—136 (1969).
HALAC, E., JR., FRANK, S.: Glucuronyl transferase and glycogen deficiency in liver of Gunn rats. Biochem. biophys. Res. Commun. **2**, 379—383 (1960).
HANSEN, W. J., GILES, W. G., NADLER, S. B.: Metabolism of 9-ethyl-6-MP-S$^{35}$ and 9-butyl-6-MP-S$^{35}$ in humans. Proc. Soc. exp. Biol. (N. Y.) **113**, 163—165 (1963).
HARPER, N. J.: Drug latentiation. J. med. pharm. Chem. **1**, 467—500 (1959).
HENDERSON, J. F., MAZEL, P.: Demethylation of purine analogs by microsomal enzymes from mouse liver. Biochem. Pharmacol. **13**, 207—210 (1964).
HILL, D. L., LASTER, W. R., JR., STRUCK, R. F.: Enzymatic metabolism of cyclophosphamide and nicotine and production of a toxic cyclophosphamide metabolite. Cancer Res. **32**, 658—665 (1972).
HOLTZMAN, J. L., GILLETTE, J. R.: The effect of phenobarbital on the turnover of microsomal phospholipid in male and female rats. J. biol. Chem. **243**, 3020—3028 (1968).
IMAMURA, H.: Studies on carcinostatic substances. XXVIII. Activation of the derivatives of 2-chloroethylamine with latent activity. Chem. pharm. Bull. 8, 449—454 (1960).
IRVING, C. L.: Enzymatic *N*-hydroxylation of the carcinogen 2-acetylaminofluorene and the metabolism of *N*-hydroxy-2-acetylaminofluorene-9-$^{14}$C *in vitro*. J. biol. Chem. **239**, 1589—1596 (1964).
IRVING, C. L., WISEMAN, R., JR., HILL, J. T.: Biliary excretion of the *O*-glucuronide of *N*-hydroxy-2-acetylaminofluorene by the rat and rabbit. Cancer Res. **27**, 2309—2317 (1967).
IYER, V. N., SZYBALSKI, W.: Mitomycins and porfiromycin: chemical mechanism of activation and cross-linking of DNA. Science **145**, 55—58 (1964).

JAYLE, M. F., PASQUALINI, J. R.: In: Glucuronic acid: free and combined. Chemistry, biochemistry, pharmacology, and medicine, p. 507. (DUTTON, G. J., Ed.). New York: Academic Press 1966.

KAMIL, I. A., SMITH, J. N., WILLIAMS, R. T.: Studies in detoxication. 50. The isolation of methyl and ethyl glucuronides from the urine of rabbits receiving methanol and ethanol. Biochem. J. **54**, 390—392 (1953).

KAMPFFMEYER, H., KIESE, M.: The effect of carbon monoxide on the hydroxylation of aniline and *N*-ethylaniline by microsomal enzymes. Naunyn-Schmiedebergs Arch. exp. Path. Pharmak. **250**, 1—8 (1965).

KANDASWAMY, T. S., HENDERSON, J. F.: The metabolism of ethidium bromide in normal and neoplastic tissues. Cancer Res. **23**, 250—253 (1963).

KASLANDER, J.: Formation of an *S*-glucuronide from tetraethylthiuram disulfide (Antabuse®) in man. Biochem. biophys. Acta (Amst.) **71**, 730—732 (1963).

KATO, R., FRONTINO, G., VASSANELLI, P.: Decreased activities of liver microsomal drug-metabolizing enzymes in the rats bearing Walker carcinosarcoma. Experientia (Basel) **19**, 31—32 (1963).

KATO, R., GILLETTE, J. R.: Effect of starvation on NADPH-dependent enzymes in liver microsomes of male and female rats. J. Pharmacol. exp. Ther. **150**, 279—284 (1965).

KATO, R., JONDORF, W. R., LOEB, L. A., BEN, T., GELBOIN, H. V.: Studies on the mechanism of drug-induced microsomal enzyme activities. V. Phenobarbital stimulation of endogenous messenger RNA and polyuridylic acid-directed L-[$^{14}$C]-phenylalanine incorporation. Molec. Pharmacol. **2**, 171—186 (1966).

KATO, R., OSHIMA, T., TAKANAKA, A.: Studies on the mechanism of nitroreduction by rat liver. Molec. Pharmacol. **5**, 487—498 (1969a).

KATO, R., TAKANAKA, A., SHOJI, H.: Inhibition of drug-metabolizing enzymes of liver microsomes by hydrazine derivatives in relation to their lipid solubility. Jap. J. Pharmacol. **19**, 315—322 (1969b).

KIESE, M., UEHLEKE, H.: Der Ort der *N*-oxydation des Anilins im höheren Tier. Naunyn-Schmiedebergs Arch. exp. Phar. Pharmak. **242**, 117—129 (1961).

KOIZUMI, T., SUEMATSU, T., KAWASAKI, A., HIRAMATSU, K., IWABORI, N.: Synthesis and degradation of active sulfate in liver. Biochem. biophys. Acta (Amst.) **184**, 106—113 (1969).

KREIS, W.: Metabolism of an antineoplastic methylhydrazine derivative in a P815 mouse neoplasm. Cancer Res. **30**, 82—89 (1970).

KUNTZMAN, R., JACOBSON, M., SCHNEIDMAN, K., CONNEY, A. H.: Similarities between oxidative drug-metabolizing enzymes and steroid hydroxylases in liver microsomes. J. Pharmacol. exp. Ther. **146**, 280—285 (1964).

KUNTZMAN, R., LEVIN, W., JACOBSON, M., CONNEY, A. H.: Studies on microsomal hydroxylation and the demonstration of a new carbon monoxide binding pigment in liver microsomes. Life Sci. **7**, 215—224 (1968).

LANG, N.: Steroid hormones and enzyme induction. In: The biochemistry of steroid hormone action. (SMELLIE, R. M. S., Ed.) pp. 85—100. New York: Academic Press 1971.

LANGE, G.: Verschiedene Induktion der mikrosomalen N- und *p*-Hydroxylierung von Anilin und *N*-Äthylanilin bei Kaninchen. Naunyn-Schmiedebergs Arch. exp. Path. Pharmak. **257**, 230—256 (1967).

LAVIN, P., KOSS, L. G.: Effects of a single dose of cyclophosphamide on various organs in the rat. III. Electron microscopic study of the liver. Amer. J. Path. **62**, 159—168 (1971).

LEE, R. M., LIVETT, B. H.: A method for the colorimetric estimation of local anaesthetics containing an ester link, and its use in the determination of esterase activity. Biochem. Pharmacol. **16**, 1757—1765 (1967).

LEIBMAN, K. C., MCALLISTER, W. J., JR.: Metabolism of trichloroethylene in liver microsomes. III. Induction of the enzymic activities and its effect on excretion of metabolites. J. Pharmacol. exp. Ther. **157**, 574—580 (1967).

LEVIN, W., KUNTZMAN, R.: Biphasic decrease of radioactive hemoprotein from liver microsomal CO-binding particles. J. biol. Chem. **244**, 3671—3676 (1969).

LIPPEL, K., OLSON, J. A.: Biosynthesis of $\beta$-glucuronides of retinal and of retinoic acid *in vivo* and *in vitro*. J. Lipid Res. **9**, 168—175 (1968).

LOTLIKAR, P. D., ENOMOTO, M., MILLER, J. A., MILLER, E. C.: Species variation in the *N*- and ring-hydroxylation of 2-acetylaminofluorene and effects of 3-methylcholanthrene pretreatment. Proc. Soc. exp. Biol. (N. Y.) **125**, 341—346 (1967).

LU, I., LARSON, R. E.: Hepatic oxidative metabolism of pentobarbital following intoxication with 1,3-*bis*(2-chloroethyl)-1-nitrosourea (BCNU). Proc. Western Pharmacol. Soc. **13**, 78—82 (1970).

Maddock, C. L., Handler, A. H., Friedman, O. M., Foley, G. E., Farber, S.: Primary evaluation of alkylating agent cyclohexylamine salt of *N,N-bis*(2-chloroethyl)phosphorodiamidic acid (NSC-69945; OMF-59) in experimental antitumor assay systems. Cancer Chemother. Rep. **50**, 629—639 (1966).

Maller, R. K., Heidelberger, C.: Studies on OPSPA. II. Distribution and excretion of radioactivity following administration of OPSPA-$C^{14}$ and OPSPA-$P^{32}$ to the rat. Cancer Res. **17**, 284—290 (1957).

Mandel, H. G.: The physiological disposition of some anticancer agents. Pharmacol. Rev. **11**, 743—838 (1959).

Marsh, J. B., James, A. T.: The conversion of stearic to oleic acid by liver and yeast preparations. Biochim. biophys. Acta (Amst.) **60**, 320—328 (1962).

Mason, H. S.: In: Advances in enzymology. (Nord, F. F., Ed.), p. 1979. New York: Interscience 1957.

Mattes, L., Kruger, S., Schueler, F. W.: The effect of Ehrlich ascites tumor on the sleeping time of mice. Arch. int. Pharmacodyn. **87**, 166—172 (1962).

Mazel, P., Henderson, J. F., Axelrod, J.: *S*-demethylation by microsomal enzymes. J. Pharmacol. exp. Ther. **143**, 1—6 (1964).

Mazel, P., Kerza-Kwiatecki, A., Simanis, J.: Studies on the demethylation of puromycin and related compounds by liver microsomal enzymes. Biochim. biophys. Acta (Amst.) **114**, 72—82 (1966).

Mellett, L. B., Hodgson, P. E., Woods, L. A.: Absorption and fate of $C^{14}$ labeled *N, N′, N″*-triethylenethiophosphoramide (thio-TEPA) in humans and dogs. J. Lab. clin. Med. **60**, 818—825 (1962).

Miettinen, T. A., Leskinen, E.: Enzyme levels of glucuronic acid metabolism in the liver, kidney and intestine of normal and fasted rats. Biochem. Pharmacol. **12**, 565—575 (1963).

Miller, J. A., Cramer, J. W., Miller, E. C.: The *N*- and ring-hydroxylation of 2-acetylaminofluorene during carcinogenesis in the rat. Cancer Res. **20**, 950—962 (1960).

Milsom, S. W., Rose, F. A., Dodgson, K. S.: Assay of a microsomal marker enzyme: Rat liver aryl sulfatase. Biochem. J. **109**, 40P (1968).

Montgomery, J. A., James, R., McCaleb, G. S.: The modes of decomposition of 1,3-*bis*(2-chloroethyl)-1-nitrosourea and related compounds. J. med. Chem. **10**, 668—674 (1967).

Moy, R. H.: Studies of the pharmacology of *o,p′*-DDD in man. J. Lab. clin. Med. **58**, 296—304 (1961).

Nadkarni, M. V., Trams, E. G., Smith, P. K.: Preliminary studies on the distribution and fate of TEM, TEPA, and myleran in the human. Cancer Res. **19**, 713—718 (1959).

Nebert, D. W., Gelboin, H. V.: Substrate-inducible microsomal aryl hydroxylase in mammalian cell culture. I. Assay and properties of induced enzyme. J. biol. Chem. **243**, 6242—6249 (1968).

Nelson, A. A., Woodward, G.: Severe adrenal cortical atrophy (cytotoxic) and hepatic damage produced in dogs by feeding 2,2-*bis*(parachlorophenyl)-1,1-dichloroethane (DDD or TDE). Arch. Path. **48**, 387—394 (1949).

Oliverio, V. T., Vietzke, W. M., Williams, M. K., Adamson, R. H.: The absorption, distribution, excretion and biotransformation of the carcinostatic 1-(2-chloroethyl)-3-cyclohexyl-1-nitrosourea in animals. Cancer Res. **30**, 1330—1337 (1970).

Omura, T., Sato, R., Cooper, D. Y., Rosenthal, O., Estabrook, R. W.: Function of cytochrome P-450 of microsomes. Fed. Proc. **24**, 1181—1189 (1965).

Otsuka, S.: Studies on nitro-reducing enzymes of swine liver. Properties and cofactor requirements of nitro and nitroso reductases. J. Biochem. (Tokyo) **50**, 85—94 (1961).

Parke, D. V.: Studies in detoxication. 84. The metabolism of [$^{14}$C] aniline in the rabbit and other animals. Biochem. J. **77**, 493—503 (1960).

Parke, D. V.: Cited in: Detoxication mechanisms, 2nd ed. (Williams, R. T., Ed.) p. 492. Chapman and Hall 1952.

Preussmann, R., Vonhodenberg, A., Hengy, H.: Mechanism of carcinogenesis with 1-aryl-3,3-dialkyltriazenes. Enzymatic dealkylation by rat liver microsomal fraction *in vitro*. Biochem. Pharmacol. **18**, 1—13 (1969).

Prough, R. A., Wittkop, J. A., Reed, D. J.: Further evidence on the nature of microsomal metabolism of procarbazine and related alkylhydrazines. Arch. Biochem. Biophys. **140**, 450—458 (1970).

Quinn, G. P., Axelrod, J., Brodie, B. B.: Species, strain, and sex differences in metabolism of hexobarbitone, amidopyrine, antipyrine, and aniline. Biochem. Pharmacol. **1**, 152—159 (1958).

Rakieten, N., Rakieten, M. L., Nadkarni, M. V.: Studies on the diabetogenic action of Streptozotocin (NSC-37917). Cancer Chemother. Rep. **29**, 91—98 (1963).

RALL, D.P.: Pharmacologic aspects of selective chemotherapy of leukemia and Burkitt's tumor. Combination chemotherapy: advertent and inadvertent. Cancer Res. **27**, 2650—2655 (1967).

REMY, C.N.: Metabolism of thiopyrimidines and thiopurines. *S*-methylation with *S*-adenosylmethionine transmethylase and catabolism in mammalian tissues. J. biol. Chem. **238**, 1078—1084 (1963).

ROBERTS, R.J., WARWICK, G.P.: Mode of action of alkylating agents: formation of *S*-ethylcysteine from ethyl methanesulphonate *in vivo*. Nature (Lond.) **179**, 1181—1182 (1957).

ROBERTS, R.J., WARWICK, G.P.: Studies on the mode of action of alkylating agents. A. R. Brit. Empire Cancer Campaign. **37**, 40—43 (1959).

ROBERTS, R.J., PLAA, G.L.: Effect of phenobarbital on the excretion of an exogenous bilirubin load. Biochem. Pharmacol. **16**, 827—835 (1967).

ROSS, W.C.J., WARWICK, G.P.: Aryl-2-halogenoalkylamines. Part XVIII. The rates of reduction of substituted 4-di-(2-chloroethyl) aminoazobenzenes by stannous chloride, hydrazine, and the xanthine oxidase-xanthine system. J. chem. Soc. 1724—1732 (1956).

ROSS, W.C.J., WILSON, J.G.: Some *N*,*N*-di-2-chloroalkyl derivatives of carboxyamides and sulphonamides. J. chem. Soc., 3616—3622 (1959).

ROSSO, R., DOLFINI, L., DONELLI, M.G.: Prolonged effect of pontobarbital in tumor bearing rats. Europ. J. Cancer **4**, 133—135 (1968a).

ROSSO, R., DOLFINI, L., FRANCHI, G.: Metabolism of amphetamine in tumor bearing rats. Biochem. Pharmacol. **17**, 633—634 (1968b).

RUBIN, A., TEPHLY, T.R., MANNERING, G.J.: Kinetics of drug metabolism by hepatic microsomes. Biochem. Pharmacol. **13**, 1007—1016 (1964).

SARCIONE, E.J., SOKAL, J.E.: Detoxication of thiouracil by *S*-methylation. J. biol. Chem. **231**, 605—608 (1958).

SCHELINE, R.R.: Drug metabolism by intestinal microorganisms. J. pharm. Sci. **57**, 2021—2037 (1968).

SCHMID, R., HAMMAKER, L., AXELROD, J.: The enzymatic formation of bilirubin glucuronide. Arch. biochem. Biophys. **70**, 285—288 (1957).

SCHMID, R., LESTER, R.: In: Glucuronic acid: free and combined. Chemistry, biochemistry, pharmacology, and medicine, p. 493 (DUTTON, G.J., Ed.). New York: Academic Press 1966.

SCHUMACHER, H., SMITH, R.L., WILLIAMS, R.T.: The metabolism of thalidomide: the spontaneous hydrolysis of thalidomide in solution. Brit. J. Pharmacol. **25**, 324—337 (1965a).

SCHUMACHER, H., SMITH, R.L., WILLIAMS, R.T.: The metabolism of thalidomide: the fate of thalidomide and some of its hydrolysis products in various species. Brit. J. Pharmacol. **25**, 338—351 (1965b).

SCHWARTZ, H.S.: Pharmacology of mitomycin C. III. *In vitro* metabolism by rat liver. J. Pharmacol. exp. Ther. **136**, 250—258 (1962).

SCHWARTZ, H.S., PHILIPS, F.S.: Pharmacology of mitomycin C. II. Renal excretion and metabolism by tissue homogenates. J. Pharmacol. exp. Ther. **133**, 335—342 (1961).

SCHWARTZ, H.S., SODERGREN, J.E., PHILIPS, F.S.: Mitomycin C: chemical and biological studies on alkylation. Science **142**, 1181—1183 (1963).

SKIBBA, J.L., BEAL, D.D., RAMIREZ, G., BRYAN, G.T.: *N*-demethylation of the antineoplastic agent 4(5)-(3,3-dimethyl-1-triazeno)imidazole-5(4)-carboxamide in rats and man. Cancer Res. **30**, 147—150 (1970).

SKIPPER, H.E., BENNETT, L.L., JR., BRYAN, C.E., WHITE, L., JR., NEWTON, M.A., SIMPSON, L.: Carbamates in the chemotherapy of leukemia. VIII. Overall tracer studies on carbonyl-labeled urethane, methylene-labeled urethane and methylene-labeled ethyl alcohol. Cancer Res. **11**, 46—51 (1951).

SLADEK, N.E.: Therapeutic efficacy of cyclophosphamide as a function of its metabolism. Cancer Res. **32**, 535—542 (1972).

SMITH, P.K., NADKARNI, M.V., TRAMS, E.G., DAVISON, C.: Distribution and fate of alkylating agents. Ann. N. Y. Acad. Sci. **68**, 834—850 (1958).

STEINBERG, A.D., PLOTZ, P.H., WOLFF, S.M., WONG, V.G., AGUS, S.G., DECKER, J.L.: Cytotoxic drugs in treatment of nonmalignant diseases. Ann. intern. Med. **76**, 619—642 (1972).

STEVENSON, I.H., DUTTON, G.J.: Glucuronide synthesis in kidney and gastrointestinal tract. Biochem. J. **82**, 330—340 (1962).

STROMINGER, J.L., KALCKAR, H.M., AXELROD, J., MAXWELL, E.S.: Enzymatic oxidation of uridine diphosphate glucose to uridine diphosphate glucuronic acid. J. Amer. chem. Soc. **76**, 6411—6412 (1954).

STRUCK, R.F., KIRK, M.C., MELLETT, L.B., DAREER, S.E., HILL, D.L.: Urinary metabolites of the antitumor agent cyclophosphamide. Molec. Pharmacol. **7**, 519—529 (1971).

TARDIFF, R.G., DUBOIS, K.P.: Inhibition of hepatic microsomal enzymes by alkylating agents. Arch. int. Pharmacodyn. **177**, 445—456 (1969).

THOMPSON, G. R., LARSON, R. E.: The hepatotoxicity of 1,3-*bis*(2-chloroethyl)-1-nitrosourea (BCNU) in rats. J. Pharmacol. exp. Ther. **166**, 104—112 (1969).

TRAMS, E. G., NADKARNI, M. V.: Studies on the *N*-dealkylation of nitrogen mustard and triethylenemelamine by liver homogenates. Cancer Res. **16**, 1069—1075 (1956).

TRAMS, E. G., NADKARNI, M. V., DEQUATRO, V., MAENGWYN-DAVIES, G. C., SMITH, P. K.: Dimethane-sulphonoxybutane (myleran). Preliminary studies on distribution and metabolic fate in the rat. Biochem. Pharmacol. **2**, 7—16 (1959).

UMAR, M. T., MITCHARD, M.: The competitive inhibition of nitroreductase by some analogues of nitrofurantoin. Biochem. Pharmacol. **17**, 2057—2060 (1968).

VIALA, R., GIANETTO, R.: The binding of sulfatase by rat-liver particles as compared to that of acid phosphatase. Can. J. Biochem. Physiol. **33**, 839—844 (1955).

WADA, F., HIRATA, K., NAKAO, K., SAKAMOTO, Y.: Participation of P-450 in 7-$\alpha$ hydroxylation of cholesterol. J. Biochem. **64**, 415—417 (1968a).

WADA, F., SHIBATA, H., GOTTO, M., SAKAMOTO, Y.: Participation of the microsomal electron transport system involving cytochrome P-450 in $\omega$-oxidation of fatty acids. Biochim. biophys. Acta (Amst.) **162**, 518—524 (1968b).

WILLIAMS, R. T.: Patterns of excretion of drugs in man and other species. Ciba Found. Symp. drug Resp. in Man, 71—91 (1967).

WILLIAMSON, C. E., KIRBY, J. G., MILLER, J. I., SASS, S., KRAMER, S. P., SELIGMAN, A. M., WITTEN, B.: Enzyme-alterable alkylating agents. IX. The enzymatic transformation of some nitrogen mustards in the presence of carbon dioxide: implications in respiration. Cancer Res. **26**, 323—330 (1966).

WITTKOP, J. A., PROUGH, R. A., REED, D. J.: Oxidative demethylation of *N*-methylhydrazines by rat liver microsomes. Arch. Biochem. Biophys. **134**, 308—315 (1969).

ZAHARKO, D. S., BRUCKNER, H., OLIVERIO, V. T.: Antibiotics alter methotrexate metabolism and excretion. Science **166**, 887—888 (1969).

Chapter 16

# Theoretical Considerations in the Chemotherapy of Brain Tumors

ALAN L. COWLES and JOSEPH D. FENSTERMACHER

## Introduction

In the search for drugs with potential value for the treatment of brain tumors, one is confronted with an almost unlimited number of compounds. Because the screening of these agents is a time-consuming and expensive process, guidelines are required to predict which compounds should be subjected to screening and which should not. It is reasonable to make an initial selection of compounds on the basis of demonstrated antitumor activity in nonneural tumors; however, activity against nonneural tumors should not be the only criterion in choosing drugs for use against brain tumors. Some agents which are effective against tumors outside the central nervous system may not be able to enter brain tissue from the blood because of the blood-brain barrier. For this reason, not only demonstrated antitumor activity, but also a knowledge of the physical and chemical properties of the drug and the anatomical and physiological characteristics of blood-tissue exchange for brain and brain tumors helps to predict more precisely which compounds will be effective against brain tumors.

Drugs may be delivered to the central nervous system by way of the cerebrospinal fluid (CSF), as well as by the blood stream. When injected into the CSF, the depth of penetration of a drug and the extent of its accumulation in brain tissue are limited by its rates of diffusion, cellular uptake, and transcapillary exchange. Again, knowledge of the physical and chemical properties of drugs and the nature of CSF-brain exchange aids in predicting the effectiveness of antitumor drugs administered via this route.

In this chapter the theoretical considerations for selecting compounds and routes of administration for the treatment of brain tumors will be discussed.

## Administration of Drug Through the Vascular System

Most antineoplastic drugs are given by intravascular injection, with the expectation being that the drug will be carried in bulk by the blood stream to the brain capillaries and from there will diffuse rapidly across the brain capillary wall, through the brain extracellular space, and into the brain cells. The major factors that affect a drug's ability to get from the blood stream into the cell are the rate of perfusion of the tumor, the concentration of the drug in an unbound and therefore diffusible form in the plasma, and the ability of the drug to cross the brain capillary and brain cell membranes.

### A. Rate of Perfusion of the Tumor

Normal brain tissue is rapidly perfused by blood, each gram of brain tissue receiving approximately its own weight of blood every two minutes (WADE and

Bishop, 1962). Although some primary and metastatic brain tumors have higher rates of perfusion than normal brain, the swelling and pressure they produce may result in areas of local ischemia, both around and within the tumor (Cronqvist and Agee, 1968; Jaffe et al., 1970). Astrocytomas, acoustic neuromas, and metastatic tumors may outgrow their vascular supply and become necrotic. Any decrease in the rate of blood flow would be expected to shelter partially the tumor from any antineoplastic agent which is injected into the blood. On the other hand, part of the tumor may become ischemic and die if the decrease in perfusion is severe enough. The overall effect is unpredictable.

## B. Activity Gradients

For a drug to diffuse passively from the blood to the inside of a cell, a continuous activity gradient from the capillary lumen, through the extracellular fluid, and into the interior of the cell must exist. Thermodynamic activity is a measure of the concentration of the drug which is unbound and able to diffuse. Any degree of binding of the drug to components of the blood, such as to plasma proteins or to red blood cells, lowers the activity of the drug in the capillary, diminishes the capillary-cell activity gradient, and decreases the rate of diffusion of drug towards the cell. On the other hand, drugs which have a high affinity for the neoplastic cell or some component within it (high tumor: blood partition coefficient) will have a low thermodynamic activity within the cell, an increased activity gradient from the capillary to the cell, and a greater diffusion of drug from the capillary to the cell. It must be added that a continuous activity gradient is not necessary for drugs that are actively transported across either the capillary or cell membrane.

## C. The Blood-Brain Barrier

In the normal brain, the capillary wall consists of a single layer of capillary endothelial cells which have tight intercellular junctions, a relatively dense basement membrane, and an ensheathing pericapillary cuff of glial cells. The exchange of material across this complex membrane, the blood-brain barrier, is markedly different than across most other capillaries. Although lipid soluble, nonpolar compounds move readily across this membrane complex, there is very little exchange of most water soluble materials. Polar, lipid insoluble compounds enter the central nervous system slowly or not at all when given intravenously (Davson, 1955; Mayer et al., 1959; Schanker, 1964), and are generally ineffective within the brain when administered in this fashion. Less is known about the exchange of polar materials between blood and brain tumor. In electron microscopic studies of human brain tumors, Long (1970) has shown that the capillary ultrastructure is not constant throughout the tumor, but ranges from the apparently normal brain capillary membrane complex with tight endothelial intercellular junctions to markedly abnormal capillary endothelium with open intercellular junctions through which free diffusional exchange would be expected to occur. Torack (1961) has reported that the endothelial cells appear normal or slightly enlarged at the periphery of tumors but definitely abnormal (greatly proliferated) in the center.

Physiological differences also exist between normal brain and brain tumors. The ability of molecules that do not enter normal brain to penetrate into brain tumors has been used for the localization of brain tumors for many years (Moore, 1953; Shapiro and Ausman, 1969). Both inulin and para-aminohippurate, which do not penetrate normal brain, penetrate intracerebral ependymomas (Ausman and Levin, 1969). Although very little sucrose diffuses from blood into normal tissue, Bakay (1970b) found that a sizable amount of this polar compound is taken up by human brain tumors following intravenous infusion. In a companion study, which suggested an interesting relationship between anatomic and physiologic evidence, BAKAY (1970a) reported that the two cases (both glioblastomas) that gave the lowest tumor to normal brain ratio for chlormerodrin $^{203}Hg$, as determined by isotope scanning, had the most normal appearing capillaries.

In a study of the uptake of inulin and methotrexate by intracerebrally inoculated ependymoblastoma, rapid uptake occurred at the center of the tumor mass, whereas uptake at the periphery of the tumor was more like that of normal brain (LEVIN et al., 1972). This suggests that the area of the tumor which the drug must reach to be effective (i.e. the growing edge of the tumor) is the part with the closest to normal resistance to the entry of polar antineoplastic agents. Support for this suggestion comes from recent work on the chemotherapy of brain tumors. Methotrexate, a highly ionized, water-soluble compound, is excluded from normal brain by the blood-brain barrier (LEVIN et al., 1972). BCNU (1,3-*bis*(2-chloroethyl)-1-nitrosourea) and CCNU (1-(2-chloroethyl)-3-cyclohexyl-1-nitrosourea) are both highly lipid-soluble and cross the blood-brain barrier readily (LOO et al., 1966; OLIVERIO et al., 1970). As expected on the basis of their relative solubilities and the suggested "tightness" of the capillaries at the periphery of the tumor, methotrexate is not effective against brain tumors, whereas BCNU and CCNU are effective (BRODER and RALL, 1972; SHAPIRO et al., 1970).

## D. Diffusion Through Extracellular Fluid

Numerous physiological studies indicate that the size of the brain extracellular space (ECS) is about 20% of the total brain volume (PAPPIUS, 1969; LEVIN et al., 1970). For materials with tissue diffusion coefficients greater than $1 \times 10^{-6}$ cm²/sec, and tissue capillary beds with capillary radius to intracapillary distance ratios greater than 0.03, LEVITT (1971) has demonstrated mathematically that the ECS can be considered a well-stirred or uniformly mixed compartment. Since brain tissue diffusion coefficients for compounds smaller than inulin (MW = 5000) are larger than $1 \times 10^{-6}$ cm²/sec (LEVIN et al., 1970), and the ratio of capillary radius to intracapillary distance ranges from about 0.10 to 0.15 for the brain (KETY, 1951), diffusion from the capillary wall to cell surfaces (i.e. diffusion through the ECS) would be rapid and not rate limiting for the blood to brain exchange of most drugs.

## E. Cellular Uptake

Experimental and theoretical analysis of cellular membrane permeability has led to the development of a "mosaic" or lipid-filter theory to explain molecular transport into and out of cells (WILBRANDT, 1963; SCHANKER, 1964; DIAMOND and WRIGHT, 1969). This theory postulates that two parallel diffusion pathways, one for lipophilic and one for hydrophilic compounds, exist within the membrane. The lipid channels comprise the bulk of the membrane diffusion pathways (>99%). Molecular movement through this phase of the membrane is governed by the compound's lipid solubility (lipid: water partition coefficient) and diffusivity (a function of molecular size) in the lipid matrix of the membrane. The aqueous channels are small in size (approximately 8 Å in width) and occupy only a tiny fraction of the membrane surface. Permeation of hydrophilic materials through these channels is primarily limited by molecular size. Water-soluble compounds which are larger than the aqueous channels (MW > 150) do not enter cells to any appreciable extent, whereas smaller polar compounds such as water and urea enter cells rapidly. Diffusion of polar and nonpolar antineoplastic drugs into the cells would be expected to follow this general scheme.

In addition to entering cells by diffusion through aqueous channels, many water-soluble compounds such as glucose and leucine appear to be transported across cellular membranes by special carrier or pump systems (SCHANKER, 1964). Some of these systems require metabolic energy, are linked to inorganic ion transport, and lead to significant intracellular accumulation. Others are not energy or ion dependent and only lead to equilibration of material between extra and intracellular fluid compartments. Present evidence suggests that such transport systems also exist in brain cell membranes (LAJTHA and FORD, 1968).

### F. Timing of Injections

The antimetabolites (methotrexate, 5-fluorouracil, 5-fluoro-2′-deoxyuridine, cytosine arabinoside, 6-mercaptopurine, and 8-azaguanine) are only effective when the cell is actively synthesizing nucleic acids. For this reason, appropriate timing of injections of these drugs may enhance their effectiveness. For appropriate discussion, see Chapters 7 and 8 on Cell Cycle Kinetics or WILSON and HOSHINO, 1969).

### G. Local Infusion with Antidotes

Infusion of a tumor-inhibitory drug into the carotid artery with concurrent venous infusion of an antidote, in theory, should provide antitumor effectiveness while minimizing systemic toxicity. This has been attempted with methotrexate and its antidote, citrovorum factor (WATKINS and SULLIVAN, 1964), but the results have not been particularly good (WILSON and HOSHINO, 1969). If effective antidotes to drugs which cross the blood-brain barrier more readily than methotrexate are found, this method of administration may prove useful in the future.

## Models of Drug Uptake

The simultaneous uptake and distribution of a drug by the many organs and tissues of a patient as a whole is not easily visualized. Consideration of the many factors involved requires such complex computations that mathematical models implemented with digital or analog computers are required to make actual predictions of drug uptake and distribution. The primary value of such models is that they allow one to see the results of perfusion, binding, diffusion, and metabolism as they interact in the patient as a whole. A compartmental body model for the prediction of the uptake and distribution of antineoplastic drugs in a standard 70.0 kilogram man with assumed normal rates of tissue perfusion has been designed (COWLES et al., 1971). The standard man is divided into several compartments, each of which is either a single tissue or a group of tissues which have similar rates of perfusion and drug affinities. The compartments are as follows: (1) arterial blood, (2) lung tissue, (3) adrenals, thyroid, and kidneys, (4) heart, (5) brain, left half, (6) brain, right half, (7) red marrow, lymphoid tissue, and splanchnic tissue, (8) testes and spinal cord, (9) skin, subcutaneous tissue, and muscle, (10) yellow marrow and adipose tissue, (11) central venous blood, and (12) a capillary compartment associated with each solid tissue compartment.

Calculations are performed as follows: the entire course of drug uptake is divided into small time intervals (0.05 min) during which the concentration of drug in each compartment can be considered constant. Based on the concentration of drug, rates of blood flow, tissue volumes, partition coefficients, and rates of equilibration and metabolism for each compartment, the amounts of drug passing into and out of each compartment are calculated during each time interval. At the end of the time interval, the amounts of drug in each compartment are calculated and the whole process is repeated for each succeeding time interval. Time intervals of 0.05 min have been found to be sufficiently small, since division of the course of drug uptake into smaller intervals of 0.01 or 0.001 min does not significantly alter the results. The program was written in Fortran IV, and calculations were made using an IBM 370/165 computer.

For purposes of illustration, the simulated uptake and distribution of a drug with a tissue: blood partition coefficient of 1.0 for all tissues except fat (4.0) has been carried out, assuming 80% equilibration of the blood with the tissue with each passage of capillary blood through the tissue and assuming a metabolic half-life of 120 min. Right and left carotid blood were assumed to intermix to the extent of 10% at the Circle of Willis. Predictions were made for both intravenous and intracarotid routes of infusion since both are currently in use for brain tumor chemotherapy.

Table 1. *Peak drug concentrations (mg/l) predicted for a 70 kg man*

| Condition | Lung | Heart | Brain (L) | Brain (R) | Red marrow and splanchnic tissue | Muscle and skin | Fat | Brain (L)/Red marrow and splanchnic tissue |
|---|---|---|---|---|---|---|---|---|
| *Intravenous infusions* | | | | | | | | |
| Standard[a] | 7.64 | 5.94 | 5.18 | 5.18 | 4.61 | 1.24 | 1.72 | 1.12 |
| 20 min infusion | 3.84 | 3.66 | 3.56 | 3.56 | 3.45 | 1.23 | 1.71 | 1.03 |
| Increased brain partition coefficient (2.0) | 7.47 | 5.82 | 7.51 | 7.51 | 4.48 | 1.19 | 1.67 | 1.68 |
| Decreased rate of brain perfusion (1/2 normal) | 7.84 | 6.11 | 3.98 | 3.98 | 4.73 | 1.24 | 1.72 | 0.84 |
| 20% equilibration between brain and blood | 7.99 | 6.22 | 2.92 | 2.92 | 4.83 | 1.24 | 1.72 | 0.60 |
| 15 min half-life | 7.48 | 5.58 | 4.79 | 4.79 | 4.19 | 0.70 | 0.71 | 1.14 |
| *Left carotid infusions* | | | | | | | | |
| Standard[a] | 5.33 | 4.67 | 47.96 | 7.42 | 4.02 | 1.22 | 1.70 | 11.93 |
| 20 min infusion | 3.60 | 3.44 | 14.43 | 4.48 | 3.26 | 1.21 | 1.69 | 4.42 |
| Increased brain partition coefficient (2.0) | 3.91 | 3.63 | 65.97 | 9.25 | 3.30 | 1.16 | 1.63 | 19.97 |
| Decreased rate of brain perfusion (1/2 normal) | 4.11 | 3.85 | 64.92 | 8.20 | 3.50 | 1.20 | 1.68 | 18.54 |
| 20% equilibration between brain and blood | 6.76 | 5.27 | 20.29 | 3.79 | 4.14 | 1.20 | 1.70 | 4.90 |
| 15 min half-life | 5.04 | 4.11 | 45.27 | 6.98 | 3.34 | 0.63 | 0.65 | 13.56 |
| 25% L-R mixing | 5.33 | 4.67 | 40.36 | 15.02 | 4.02 | 1.22 | 1.70 | 10.03 |

[a] Standard conditions: infusion of 100 mg over 4 min; tissue: blood partition coefficients = 1.0 except fat (4.0); 80% equilibration of drug during each passage through the capillary; metabolic half-life = 120 min; rates of tissue perfusion are those of a normal adult male; each hemisphere assumed to be perfused by 90% blood from the ipsilateral carotid artery and 10% from the contralateral carotid artery.

Although examination of drug concentrations at various times is of interest, the model's predictions should be useful to suggest ways to improve drug effectiveness relative to toxicity. In order to do this, two aspects of the predicted tissue concentrations must be examined: (1) the predicted peak drug concentrations within the tissues (Table 1), a measure of the achievement of an effective drug concentration and (2) the integral of the concentrations of the drug in the tissues over time (Table 2), a measure of the maintenance of a drug concentration over a period of time. The integral of the concentration over time is called the *exposure* of the tissue to the drug. The effectiveness can be considered to be a function of target

Table 2. *Exposures of tissues (mg × min/l) to an antineoplastic drug predicted for a 70 kg man*

| Condition | Lung | Heart | Brain (L) | Brain (R) | Red marrow and splanchnic tissue | Muscle and skin | Fat | Brain (L)/ Red marrow and splanchnic tissue |
|---|---|---|---|---|---|---|---|---|
| *Intravenous infusions* | | | | | | | | |
| Standard[a] | 286 | 284 | 282 | 282 | 281 | 226 | 520 | 1.00 |
| 20 min infusion | 286 | 284 | 282 | 282 | 281 | 226 | 520 | 1.00 |
| Increased brain partition coefficient (2.0) | 280 | 277 | 544 | 544 | 275 | 221 | 507 | 1.98 |
| Decreased rate of brain perfusion (1/2 normal) | 286 | 284 | 279 | 279 | 281 | 226 | 520 | 0.99 |
| 20% equilibration between brain and blood | 287 | 284 | 271 | 271 | 281 | 226 | 520 | 0.96 |
| 15 min half-life | 86 | 81 | 78 | 78 | 75 | 27 | 32 | 1.03 |
| *Left carotid infusions* | | | | | | | | |
| Standard[a] | 283 | 281 | 503 | 304 | 278 | 223 | 514 | 1.81 |
| 20 min infusion | 283 | 281 | 503 | 304 | 278 | 223 | 514 | 1.81 |
| Increased brain partition coefficient (2.0) | 274 | 271 | 974 | 582 | 269 | 216 | 496 | 3.62 |
| Decreased rate of brain perfusion (1/2 normal) | 280 | 278 | 714 | 322 | 275 | 221 | 509 | 2.59 |
| 20% equilibration between brain and blood | 284 | 281 | 482 | 292 | 279 | 224 | 515 | 1.73 |
| 15 min half-life | 80 | 74 | 276 | 94 | 69 | 25 | 30 | 3.98 |
| 25% L-R mixing | 283 | 281 | 465 | 341 | 278 | 223 | 514 | 1.67 |

[a] Standard conditions: see Table 1.

organ (brain) peak concentrations and exposures, and toxicity can be considered to be a function of bone marrow and gastrointestinal tract peak concentrations and exposures (Mellett, 1973).

As measures of effectiveness relative to toxicity, the ratio of peak brain concentration to peak red marrow-splanchnic tissue compartment concentration, and the ratio of brain exposure to red marrow-splanchnic tissue compartment exposure have been calculated. The magnitudes of these ratios are not as important as the changes in the ratios induced by alterations in drug and tissue related variables. Factors which increase or decrease these ratios suggest ways of clinically increasing or decreasing effectiveness relative to systemic toxicity.

Examination of Tables 1 and 2 shows that infusion of the drug into the carotid artery produces both greater peak concentration ratios and exposure ratios and could be expected to improve effectiveness relative to toxicity[1]. When making a decision as to which route to use, complications such as arterial thrombosis, intoler-

1 This will not be true when the target organ capillaries are completely impermeable to the drug.

able local tissue toxicity, hematoma formation, catheter occlusion, and the difficulty and discomfort to the patient of placing a cannula in the carotid artery must be taken into account. Because of these problems, intracarotid infusion cannot be undertaken lightly.

Increasing the length of time of infusion has no effect on tissue exposures, but decreases the peak concentration ratio, particularly when the drug is given via the carotid artery. In a situation where effectiveness depends upon peak concentration, an increased duration of infusion can be expected to decrease effectiveness relative to toxicity, particularly if the drug is given by intra-arterial infusion. An increase in the affinity of the drug for the target organ (increased partition coefficient) increases both the peak concentration ratio and the exposure ratio for both routes of administration. Effectiveness is enhanced while systemic toxicity is decreased. A decreased rate of brain perfusion decreases the concentration and exposure ratios when the drug is given intravenously and can be expected to decrease effectiveness relative to toxicity. When the drug is given intra-arterially, both ratios are increased. This is because the lower rate of brain perfusion leads to less dilution of the infused drug in the cerebral circulation and slower washout of the drug from the tissue after the infusion is completed. However, if only the rate of perfusion of the tumor is decreased, the exposure of the drug to the tumor may not be enhanced with intra-arterial infusion because much of the drug may bypass the tumor via the normal brain circulation. Decreased equilibration between the capillary blood and the brain decreases both the concentration ratios and the exposure ratios, with the greatest effect being on the concentration ratios. It is to be expected that decreased equilibration will decrease effectiveness relative to toxicity.

An increase in the rate of metabolism has little effect on either ratio when the drug is given intravenously. With intracarotid infusion, the peak concentration ratio is increased significantly and the exposure ratio is more then doubled because much of the drug is metabolized before it has a chance to leave the brain. The effectiveness of BCNU and CCNU, both of which have short metabolic half-lives and are able to penetrate the blood-brain barrier (Loo et al., 1966; Oliverio et al. 1970), should be enhanced by intracarotid infusion.

An increased proportion of mixing of blood at the Circle of Willis decreases both the peak concentration ratio and the exposure ratio and can be expected to decrease effectiveness, relative to toxicity, with intracarotid infusion. With intravenous infusion there is no effect on the drug's distribution.

## Intrathecal Administration of Antineoplastic Drugs

Intrathecal infusions have been employed in brain tumor chemotherapy in attempts not only to bypass the blood-brain barrier and its restrictions to drug entry, but also to limit systemic toxicity. The brain and spinal cord distribution patterns obtained with various compounds administered in this manner are quite different than those found for the same compound following intravenous injection and are a function of the following factors: (1) the injection site, (2) the extent of bulk mixing within the CSF compartment, (3) the permeability of the ependymal and pia-glial borders to the drug, (4) the rate of transport of the compound through the extracellular fluid, (5) the diffusion distance from the nearest CSF-tissue interface, and (6) the permeability of the cellular and capillary membranes to the drug.

Of the several possible sites for intrathecal injection, the lumbar subarachnoid space is the most readily available and safest place of injection. This site, however, is quite remote from the brain and, thus, distribution of the drug to the brain surface may be poor. Injections into the cisterna magna may be performed but involve considerable risk, since vital centers in the medulla can be easily damaged by the incorrect placement of the needle. Some attempts to infuse drugs into the lateral or third ventricles have been made (Rubin et al., 1966). This approach requires special equipment and training and has proven to be time consuming and difficult (Korobkin et al., 1968).

The subsequent distribution of the infused drug throughout the CSF compartment is dependent upon bulk or convective flow, since the dimensions of the system (20 to 50 cm) are too great for diffusion to be an effective mechanism of mixing, except for regions within several millimeters of the injection site. The principle direction of CSF flow appears to be from the ventricular system, through the fourth ventricular foramina, and into the cisterna magna and the basal cisterns. From there the fluid spreads throughout the extensive, diffuse subarachnoid space of the brain and spinal cord (DiChiro, 1966). In work on anesthetized and unanesthetized cats, Korobkin et al. (1968) compared the distribution profiles of tracer sucrose and iodide in CSF, brain, and spinal cord six hours after injection or infusion at various intrathecal sites. Ventricular injections and infusions gave the highest levels of tracers in brain, spinal cord, and CSF. Somewhat lower tissue concentrations were obtained with intracisternal injections. The distribution of the materials from the lumbar sac was virtually limited to the lumbar CSF and spinal cord, indicating that this route of administration is the least effective. In an earlier study on the effects of the volume of solution injected, Rieselbach et al. (1962) found that injection into the lumbar sac of moderate sized volumes of fluid (10 to 20% of the CSF volume) yielded autoradiographically detectable amounts of the tracer in the basal cisterns one hour after administration. The injection of larger volumes (25 to 42% of the CSF volume) resulted in distribution of the labeled material throughout the cerebral subarachnoid space and the ventricular system. In addition, these authors noted that repeated injection and withdrawal did not enhance CSF mixing when either small, medium, or large volumes were used.

The ependymal and pia-glial borders appear to offer little or no restriction to CSF brain exchange of most molecules. Compounds with molecular weights of 5000 or less readily permeate these membranes (Rall, 1967; Levin et al., 1970). Significant movement of horseradish peroxidase (MW = 43000) (Brightman and Reese, 1969) and albumin (MW = 68000) (Curran et al., 1970) from ventricular CSF into brain parenchyma has been observed, indicating that even large compounds can exchange across the ependyma.

The effects of extracellular transport and capillary exchange on the tissue concentrations of drugs are different for intrathecal administration and intravascular administration. Although the rates of diffusion of various materials through the extracellular fluid of the brain would be the same in both cases, the distances from fluid interface to cell surfaces are markedly different. For CSF to brain diffusion, the distances range from microns to centimeters, whereas the distance from brain capillaries to the most remote cell is less than 40 μ (Kety, 1951). Table 3 lists the effective diffusion distance (defined in this instance as the point in the tissue where the concentration is 10% of the CSF concentration) for several different sized compounds at various times after beginning intrathecal infusion. As can be seen from the table, delivery of reasonable amounts of drug from CSF to brain tissue occurs for sites less than 2 cm from the surface. Only very small amounts of drug might be delivered to deeper tissue sites after long periods of time.

Once a drug has entered the extracellular fluid of the brain, significant loss from the tissue to the blood will occur if the capillaries are permeable to the drug, therefore, the intrathecal injection of drugs which can exchange across the blood-

Table 3. *Distance from the brain surface to the point in brain where the drug concentration in tissue fluid is 10% of the concentration in CSF*[a]

| Molecular weight (g/mole) | Tissue diffusion coefficient (cm²/sec) | Distance (cm) from surface to 10% point at time | | |
|---|---|---|---|---|
| | | 1 min | 1 hour | 1 day |
| 100 | $6 \times 10^{-6}$ | 0.044 | 0.34 | 1.68 |
| 1000 | $3 \times 10^{-6}$ | 0.031 | 0.24 | 1.18 |
| 10000 | $1.5 \times 10^{-6}$ | 0.022 | 0.17 | 0.84 |

[a] For these calculations it is assumed that: (1) the intrathecally infused drug immediately mixes throughout the CSF; (2) the concentration of drug in the CSF remains constant; (3) the tissue diffusion coefficient equals 50% of the water diffusion coefficient; and (4) no transcapillary exchange or tissue binding of drug occurs.

brain barrier leads to negligible tissue uptake throughout the brain. In contrast, intrathecally administered compounds which do not diffuse across the blood-brain interface will remain within the tissue unless special transport mechanisms mediate their transcapillary exchange. Experimental verification of this has been obtained in our laboratory with ventriculo-cisternal perfusion studies in monkeys. The lipid-soluble, capillary permeable antineoplastic agents such as triethylenethiophosphor-triamide (thio-TEPA) were found not to accumulate in periventricular brain tissue when delivered by ventricular perfusion; whereas, drugs with low brain capillary permeability, such as methotrexate and hydroxyurea, were found to accumulate in the tissue immediately adjacent to the CSF.

Attempts to treat both solid brain tumors and meningeal leukemia by intrathecal chemotherapy have been made over the last decade. As discussed by Shapiro and Ausman (1969), the solid tumor studies have been too recent, the number of cases too few, and the protocols too variable to adequately evaluate the efficacy of intrathecal drug infusion on this class of brain tumors. On the other hand, meningeal leukemia in both children and adults has been treated fairly extensively by intrathecal methotrexate and other antifolates (Shapiro and Ausman, 1969). The success achieved by the intrathecal treatment of meningeal leukemia with methotrexate supports our suggestion that effective delivery of drug to brain tissue would be expected in those cases where the malignant cells are at or near the CSF-tissue interface and the administered drug is not permeable to the capillaries.

## Comment

One of the most significant limitations to a consideration of the chemotherapy of brain tumors is the paucity of information about the fundamental pathophysiology of brain tumors. Without sound quantitative knowledge of the blood flow, capillary density, capillary permeability, cellular permeability, and the distribution of malignant cells within the tumor mass, any discussion of drug uptake and effectiveness by brain tumors remains speculative. It is for this reason that this chapter has attempted to give a broad general presentation of the basic parameters of *normal* blood-brain and CSF-brain exchange of materials and to suggest that the transport of drugs into brain tumors may be quite different than that in normal CNS tissue.

## Conclusions

Consideration of the chemical and physical properties of an antineoplastic drug and physiologic aspects of brain tumors enables one to suggest whether an antineoplastic drug will be effective against brain tumors. Tumor-inhibitory compounds of low molecular weight with an affinity for the tumor and which are lipid-soluble (and therefore able to pass the blood-brain barrier) should be effective against brain tumors when administered intravascularly. Compounds which do not cross the blood-brain barrier may be effective when administered intrathecally, but then only against tumors which are within a few millimeters of the brain surface. The rate of perfusion of the tumor, the timing of administration, the metabolic half-life of the drug and the use of antidotes against the drug may also influence effectiveness and toxicity. A mathematical model is used to demonstrate the effect of these factors on the uptake and distribution of the drug and to suggest ways of increasing effectiveness relative to toxicity.

## References


Ausman, J. I., Levin, V. A.: Intra- and extravascular distribution of standard drug molecules in brain tumor and brain, p. 41. Fourth International Congress of Neurological Surgery. (C. G. Drake and R. Duvoisin, Eds.) Amsterdam: Excerpta Medica Foundation 1970.

Bakay, L.: The extracellular space in brain tumours. I. Morphological considerations. Brain **93**, 693—698 (1970).

Bakay, L.: The extracellular space in brain tumours. II. The sucrose space. Brain **93**, 699—708 (1970).

Brightman, M. W., Reese, T. S.: Junctions between intimately apposed cell membranes in the vertebrate brain. J. Cell Biol. **40**, 648—677 (1969).

Broder, L. E., Rall, D. P.: Chemotherapy of brain tumors. In: Recent Advances in Brain Tumor Research. (W. G. Bingham, Jr., Ed.) in press.

Cowles, A. L., Borgstedt, H. H., Gillies, A. J.: Tissue weights and rates of blood flow in man for the prediction of anesthetic uptake and distribution. Anesthesiology **35**, 523—526 (1971).

Cronqvist, S., Agee, F.: Regional cerebral blood flow in intracranial tumours. Acta radiol. diag. **7**, 393—404 (1968).

Curran, R. E., Mosher, M. B., Owens, E. S., Fenstermacher, J. D.: Cerebrospinal fluid production rates determined by simultaneous albumin and inulin perfusion. Exp. Neurol. **29**, 546—553 (1970).

Davson, H.: A comparative study of the aqueous humor and cerebrospinal fluid in the rabbit. J. Physiol. **129**, 111—133 (1955).

Diamond, J. M., Wright, E. M.: Biological membranes: the physical basis of ion and non-electrolyte selectivity. Ann. Rev. Physiol. **31**, 581—646 (1969).

DiChiro, G.: Observations on the circulation of the cerebrospinal fluid. Acta radiol. diag. **5**, 988—1002 (1966).

Jaffe, M. E., McHenry, L. C., and Goldberg, H. I.: Regional cerebral flow measurement with small probes. II. Application of the method. Neurology **20**, 225—237 (1970).

Kety, S. S.: The theory and applications of the exchange of inert gas at the lungs and tissues Pharmacol. Rev. **3**, 1—40 (1951).

Korobkin, R. K., Lorenzo, A. V., Cutler, R. W. P.: Distribution of $C^{14}$-sucrose and $I^{125}$-iodide in the central nervous system of the cat after various routes of injection into the cerebrospinal fluid. J. Pharmacol. exp. Ther. **165**, 412—420 (1968).

Lajtha, A., Ford, D. H.: Brain barrier systems. In: Progress in brain research, Vol. 29, Amsterdam: Elsevier Publishing Co. 1968.

Levin, V. A., Clancy, T. P., Ausman, J. I., Rall, D. P.: Uptake and distribution of $^3$H-methotrexate by the murine ependymoblastoma. J. nat. Cancer Inst. **48**, 875—883 (1972).

Levin, V. A., Fenstermacher, J. D., Patlak, C. S.: Sucrose and inulin space measurements of cerebral cortex in four mammalian species. Amer. J. Physiol. **219**, 1528—1533 (1970).

Levitt, D. G.: Theoretical model of capillary exchange incorporating interactions between capillaries. Amer. J. Physiol. **220**, 250—255 (1971).

Long, D. M.: Capillary ultrastructure and the blood-brain barrier in human malignant brain tumors. J. Neurosurg. **32**, 127—144 (1970).

Loo, T. L., Dion, R. L., Dixon, R. L., Rall, D. P.: The antitumor agent, 1,3-*bis*(2-chloroethyl)-1-nitrosourea. J. pharm. Sci. **55**, 492—497 (1966).

Mayer, S., Maickel, R. P., Brodie, B. B.: Kinetics of penetration of drugs and other foreign compounds into cerebrospinal fluid and brain. J. Pharmacol. **127**, 205—211 (1959).

Mellett, L. B.: The constancy of the product of concentration and time. In: Antineoplastic and immunosuppresive agents. Handbook of experimental pharmacology, Vol. XXXVIII/Part I. (A. C. Sartorelli and D. G. Johns, Eds.) Berlin-Heidelberg-New York: Springer 1974.

MOORE, G. E.: Diagnosis and localization of brain tumors. Springfield, Ill. Charles C. Thomas, 1953.
OLIVERIO, V. T., VIETZKE, W. M., WILLIAMS, M. K., ADAMSON, R. H.: The absorption, distribution, excretion, and biotransformation of the carcinostatic 1-(2-chloroethyl)-3-cyclohexyl-1-nitrosourea in animals. Cancer Res. **30**, 1330—1337 (1970).
PAPPIUS, H. M.: Water spaces. In: Handbook of Neurochemistry, pp. 1—10, Vol. II, Structural Neurochemistry. (A. LAJTHA, Ed.) New York: Plenum Press 1969.
RALL, D. P.: Transport through the ependymal linings. Progr. Brain Res. **29**, 159—167 (1967).
RIESELBACH, R. E., DICHIRO, G., FREIREICH, E. J., RALL, D. P.: Subarachnoid distribution of drugs after lumbar injection. New Engl. J. Med. **267**, 1273—1278 (1962).
RUBIN, R. C., OMMAYA, A. K., HENDERSON, E. S., BERING, E. A., RALL, D. P.: Cerebrospinal fluid perfusion for central nervous system neoplasms. Neurology **16**, 680—692 (1966).
SCHANKER, L. S.: Physiological transport of drugs. In: Advances in Drug Research, pp. 71—106. (N. J. HARPER and A. B. SIMMONDS, Eds.) London: Academic Press 1964.
SHAPIRO, W. R., AUSMAN, J. I.: Chemotherapy of brain tumors: a clinical and experimental review. In: Recent Advances in Neurology, pp. 149—235. (F. PLUM, Ed.) F. Davis Co. 1969.
SHAPIRO, W. R., AUSMAN, J. I., RALL, D. P.: Studies on the chemotherapy of experimental brain tumors; evaluation of 1,3-*bis*(2-chloroethyl)-1-nitrosourea, cyclophosphamide, mithramycin, and methotrexate. Cancer Res. **30**, 2401—2413 (1970).
TORACK, R. M.: Ultrastructure of capillary reaction to brain tumors. Arch. Neurology **5**, 416—428 (1961).
WADE, O. L., BISHOP, J. M.: Cardiac output and regional blood flow. Oxford: Blackwell Scientific Publications 1962.
WATKINS, E., JR., SULLIVAN, R. D.: Cancer chemotherapy by prolonged arterial infusion. Surg. Gynec. Obstet. 118, 3—19 (1964).
WILBRANDT, W.: Transport through biological membranes. Ann. Rev. Physiol. **25**, 601—638 (1963).
WILSON, C. B., HOSHINO, T.: Current trends in the chemotherapy of brain tumors with special reference to glioblastomas. J. Neurosurg. **31**, 589—603 (1969).

Chapter 17

# The Constancy of the Product of Concentration and Time

L. B. MELLETT

With 5 Figures

## Introduction

The approach, that animal testing may predict pharmacological or toxicological responses in man, is undertaken with the conviction that there is a common plan for all living matter. The major biochemical discoveries of the last thirty years lend support to this conviction. It has been suggested that pharmacologic, toxic, and therapeutic effects of drugs can be directly related to the plasma or tissue concentration of the drug, i. e. the pharmacological responses of various species are similar for equal plasma or tissue levels of the drug. This suggestion is based on evidence that, in many instances, the receptors for a given type of drug are similar in various mammalian species. GILLETTE (1965), for example, showed that the paralytic effect of zoxazolamine lasted over sixty times longer in the rabbit than in the mouse, but found similar brain levels of the drug in both species at the time the righting reflex was restored. Similar observations with respect to brain levels were made in rats and guinea pigs, and in all four species serum levels were a reflection of brain drug levels. He also reported that carisoprodol had a 10-fold spread in duration of action in various animal species, but plasma levels on restoration of the righting reflex varied only about 30%. QUINN et al. (1958) observed a wide variation in the duration of the anesthetic action of hexobarbital among animal species, but found very little difference in plasma or brain levels of the drug when the animals recovered.

BRODIE and REID (1967) have noted that despite a 50-fold difference in the duration of action and rates of metabolism of barbiturates, various animal species and man recover from these drugs at similar plasma levels. They also noted the following comparisons. Compound ICI-33828

$$[CH_2 = CHCH(CH_3)NHCSNHNHCSNHCH_3]$$

inhibits pituitary gonadotrophic function at a plasma concentration of 3 μg/ml in animals and man despite a 200-fold difference in daily dosage requirements. Phenylbutazone exerts antirheumatic effects in man and anti-inflammatory effects in rabbits at similar drug plasma concentrations. Sodium retention produced in man and rats by phenylbutazone at doses of 5 to 10 mg/kg and 400 mg/kg, respectively, occurs in both species at the same drug plasma level. Similarly, the antipyretic effect of phenacetin in rats and man occurs at comparable plasma levels of the drug. The antidepressant effect of desipramine manifests itself in rats and man at comparable brain levels of the drug.

These observations, and others to be discussed subsequently, indicate that receptors for a given drug in various mammalian species exhibit similar sensitivities for a specified drug concentration. The observations also indicate that the doses required to produce these effects and the duration of effects in various species vary greatly. These species variations in dose and duration of effect are probably related to the persistence of the drug in a given species and thus are functions of the rate of metabolism and elimination of the drug in that species.

## Formulations of the Relationship of Concentration and Time and Biological Response

Many attempts have been made to formulate a relation between the quantity of a substance causing a physiological effect and the time necessary to produce this effect. CLARK (1933, 1937) published his remarkable monographs on the action of drugs on cells and general pharmacology approximately 35 years ago. In these works he reviewed the many attempts to establish a formulation for these relationships. In numerous instances the relation could be expressed by the formula $Ct=$ a constant. Stated in words, the formula indicated that to obtain a given biological effect when concentration ($C$) of the drug is changed, the time of exposure ($t$) must be suitably modified so that their product yields a constant value. This is obviously an oversimplification which does not account for either removal of drug from the system or changes in the rate of removal during exposure. CLARK was aware of the shortcomings of this formula and made suitable modifications.

SILVER (1945) made further modifications of CLARK's equations which allowed for graphical evaluation of the terms employed. The basic equation was expressed as follows:

$$Ct = K + at^{b+1},$$

where $C=$ concentration of the agent, $t=$ time of exposure, $K=$ a constant related to species susceptibility, $a=$ a constant related to the magnitude of the rate of drug removal, and $b=$ a constant related to the change in the rate of drug removal during exposure.

If the constants $K$, $a$, and $b$ are known, the relation between dosage ($C$) and time ($t$) to produce the biological effect may be calculated. A graphical evaluation of the terms may be made in the following manner. If $Ct$ is plotted against $t$, a line results which intercepts the $Ct$ axis at $K$ when $t$ is zero. This then defines $K$ as the dose producing the desired effect at zero time and is theoretically a measure of the susceptibility of the species for the agent. If $b=$ zero, the equation is first-order and the plot should produce a straight line, the slope of which is equal to $a$. The detoxication rate is then constant and equal to the slope of the line. If $b$ is not equal to zero, the plot results in a curved line and requires further manipulations for the estimation of $a$ and $b$.

If the original equation is rearranged to $(Ct - K) = at^{b+1}$ and the logarithms of both sides are taken, then

$$\log (Ct - K) = \log a + (b+1) \log t .$$

When log-log paper is employed for representation, all terms may be read directly without conversion to logarithms.

An example of this application when the detoxication rate is constant is shown in Fig. 1. In this instance, the median lethal concentrations of sulfur mustard, $S(CH_2CH_2Cl)_2$, for mice and rats exposed to an atmosphere containing the agent were determined. The slopes of the lines (a) are 0.009 and 0.002 mg/liter for mice and rats, respectively, indicating that the mouse eliminates the drug about four times faster than does the rat. The $Ct$ intercept, which is equivalent to $K$, is 840 and 835 mg · min/m³ for the mouse and rat, respectively, indicating that the two species are equally sensitive to the agent.

Similarly, in situations where the rate of drug elimination is not constant, the estimation of $b + 1$ and a may be made from an alternate plot as shown in Fig. 2. The slope of the lines for each species is equal to $b + 1$, and the $Ct - K$ intercept when $t = 1$ is equal to $a$.

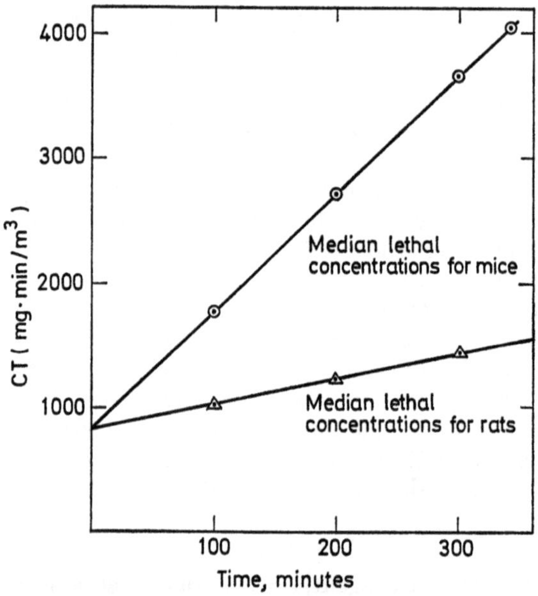


Fig. 1. Median lethal concentrations of sulfur mustard for mice and rats. $K$ (the $Ct$ intercept when $t = 0$) is equal to 840 mg · min/m³ for mice and 835 mg · min/m³ for rats. The slope of the line represents the detoxication rate and is 0.009 and 0.002 mg/liter for mice and rats, respectively. Adapted from SILVER (1945)

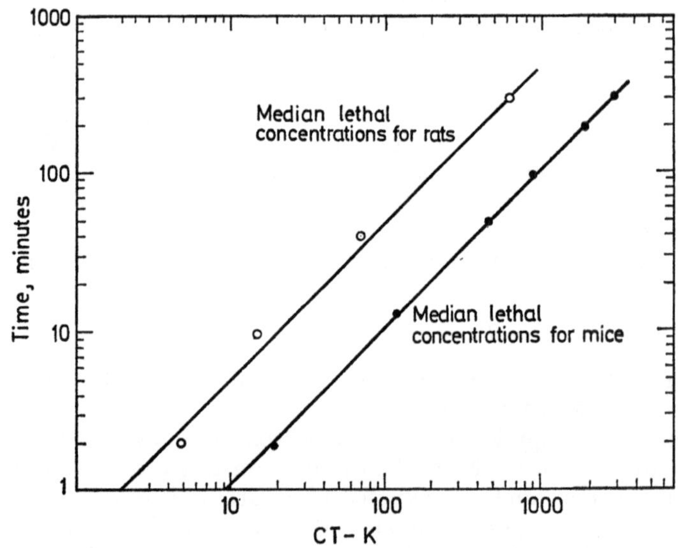


Fig. 2. Median lethal concentrations of sulfur mustard for mice and rats. $\text{Log}(Ct - K) = \log a + (b + 1) \log t$. Slope of the lines $= (b + 1)$ and $\log Ct - K = \log a$ when $t = 1$. The rate of detoxication or agent removal is read as the intercept of the $Ct - K$ axis and is 0.009 or 0.002 mg/liter for mice and rats, respectively. Adapted from SILVER (1945)

SKIPPER (1965) discussed the application of the $C \times t$ concept with respect to the killing of bacterial and leukemic cell populations and host toxicity. He demonstrated that for a given type of bacterium and a given drug, the $C \times t$ requirement for killing a given percentage of the population was constant within substantial variation of $C$ and $t$. Similarly, the $C \times t$ requirements for a 5-log kill of leukemic cells was constant. With respect to host toxicity, the $C \times t = K$ relationship can also be demonstrated. Maximum therapeutic advantage is achieved with a given agent when the exposure ($C \times t$) which produces maximum leukemic cell-kill has little or no effect on the host in terms of toxicity to normal cells. This simply indicates that the $C \times t$ value required to produce one biological effect may be greatly different than that required to produce a second biological effect.

## Relationships of Dose, Drug Metabolism Rates, Drug Plasma or Tissue Levels and Pharmacological Response in Various Species

In what practical way may a knowledge of dose, drug-metabolism rates, drug plasma or tissue levels, and pharmacological response be related in various species of animals? With regard to the quantitative consideration of rates of disappearance of drugs, BUTLER (1966) has made some pertinent observations. Even among closely related species (human and monkey) differences in drug metabolism rates may arise simply from differences in the size of the subjects. "A man could not be reduced to the size of a rhesus monkey without important physiological alterations that might be expected to affect the disposition of drugs. If the pattern of distribution of a drug in the tissues is the same in different species, the concentration of the drug at the site of action will be approximately proportional to the total amount of drug in the body divided by the body weight, regardless of the size of the animal or species. However, the processes removing the drug from the body are likely to be correlated not with the body weight itself, but with the body weight raised to a power less than unity." Many functions and physiological properties in different species of animals of diverse size are approximately proportional to powers of the body weight less than one. These are all functions and properties that in proportion to body weight are generally greater in small animals than in large. Aspects of these concepts have been discussed in detail by MELLETT (1969).

ADOLPH (1949) condensed an enormous amount of information about mammals for 34 biological characteristics and interrelations among all of them. The interrelations found imply quantitative orderliness among characteristics as diverse as urinary flow, renal clearances, duration of heartbeat, oxygen consumption, and biochemical composition in animals of widely varying sizes. The variation of these characteristics in different species was proportional to a power of the body weight less than one. To the extent that mammalian species are broadly similar and have corresponding organs and tissues, it is true that any body surface area will increase approximately with the two-thirds power of body weight. Thus the use of body surface area as a criterion for inter and intraspecies comparisons of function and composition receives support.

PINKEL (1958) first suggested the applicability of body surface area as a criterion for relating dosages of antitumor agents in laboratory and clinical studies. He reasoned that smaller animals had relatively larger surface areas, relative to body weight, than larger animals, and therefore, various functions and properties such as basal metabolic rate, blood volume, plasma volume, cardiac output, and renal function would be proportionately greater in smaller animals. He presented data which indicated that when doses were expressed in mg per square meter of body surface area, more meaningful correlations could be made between animal and human studies than when doses were expressed in mg per kg of body weight.

The most telling argument for the use of body surface area as a criterion for relating animal and human drug doses was presented by FREIREICH et al. (1966). They made a quantitative comparison of toxicity of 18 different anticancer agents in the mouse, rat, hamster, dog, monkey, and human. The compounds examined included antimetabolites and alkylating agents, as well as other types of antitumor drugs. Each animal species and all animal species combined were used to predict the toxic doses in man (based on dosage expressed as $mg/m^2$ of body surface area). The correlation of predicted toxic doses for humans derived from all animal systems for the 18 compounds studied is shown in Fig. 3. The authors concluded that relationships among various animal species and man are somewhat simpler and more direct when dosage is expressed on a $mg/m^2$ basis and that the experimental test systems used to evaluate the toxicities of potential anticancer drugs correlate remarkably closely with results in man. It is now considered standard practice in cancer chemotherapy to express doses in $mg/m^2$ of body surface area rather than mg/kg of body weight.

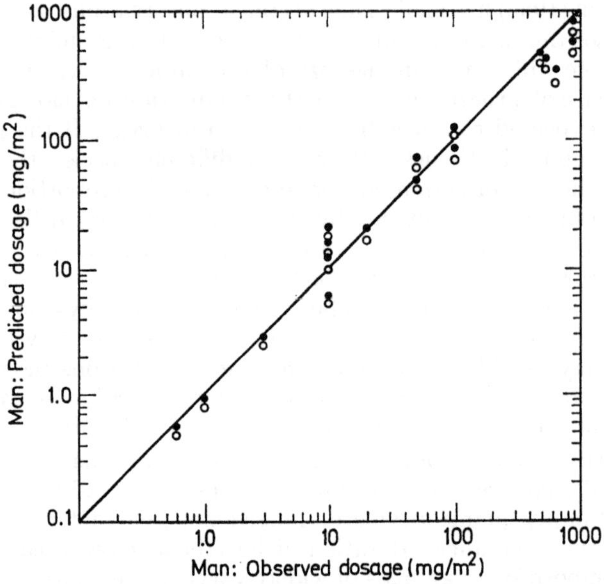


Fig. 3. Observed and predicted dosages ($mg/m^2$) in man using all animal systems. Model 1: ○; Model 2: ● weighted estimates. The reader is referred to the original publication for details of model descriptions and statistical treatment. Adapted from FREIREICH et al. (1966)

In an extension of these concepts, MELLETT (1969) examined the relationship between the dose (on a $mg/m^2$ basis) and serum levels of cyclophosphamide and methotrexate in animals and humans. The cyclophosphamide toxicologic data from animals (FREIREICH et al., 1966) indicated that the maximum tolerated dose for man should be 362 $mg/m^2$ on a 1 to 5 day schedule. The maximum tolerated dose determined from clinical data was 370 $mg/m^2$ for cyclophosphamide. In the case of methotrexate, the predicted toxic dose for man from animal studies was 15.7 $mg/m^2$ every day for 5 days, while the dose determined from clinical data was 15.0 $mg/m^2$ on the same schedule. Plasma levels per se are difficult to compare in various species because of differences in time relationships with respect to peak levels and rates of disappearance of the drug. Therefore, the area under the serum curve, represented by the product of drug concentration × time, $C \times t$ (μg/ml × min), was employed as an arithmetical measure of exposure for interspecies comparisons. The area under the serum curve at varying doses in various species was plotted against the dose expressed in mg/m² for both drugs. The results are shown in Figs. 4 and 5.

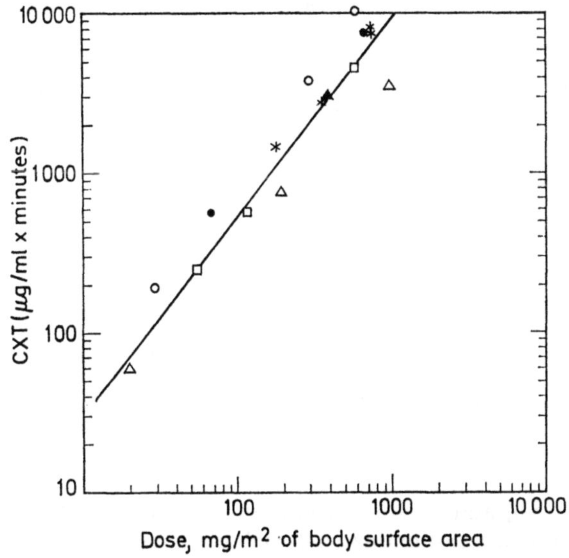


**Fig. 4.** Area under the serum curve vs dose of cyclophosphamide in mg/m² of body surface area. Mouse ○, hamster ▲, rat ●, dog □, monkey △, and man ✱. Adapted from MELLETT (1969)

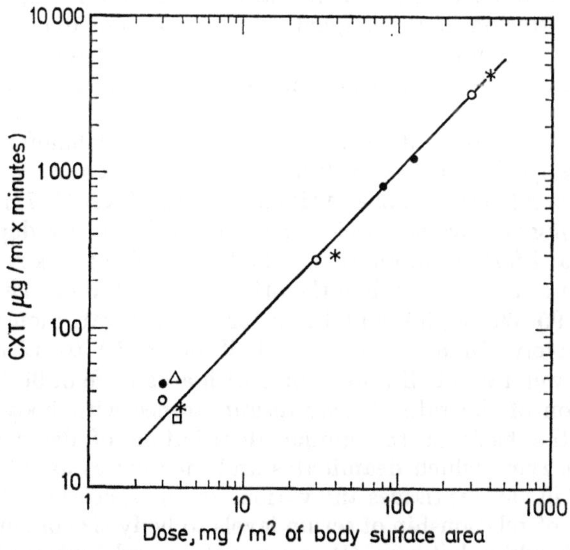


**Fig. 5.** Area under the serum curve vs dose of methotrexate in mg/m² of body surface area. Mouse ○, rat ●, dog □, monkey △, and man ✱. Adapted from MELLETT (1969); rat data provided by Dr. V. OLIVERIO (personal communication)

Several conclusions may be drawn from these data: (a) when doses are expressed on a mg/m² basis for various species, then equal doses give equivalent $Ct$ values in the different species, (b) equivalent $Ct$ values in various species give equivalent toxicological (or pharmacological) responses in the different species, and (c) the serum half-life of the drugs is shortest in small animals and longest in humans and is a prime determinant of the total $Ct$ value attained in the various species.

Similar though less extensive data have been obtained for $N,N',N''$-triethylenethiophosphoramide (thio-TEPA) in various species. These data are summarized in Table 1.

Table 1. *Comparison of the half-life and area under the serum curve for thio-TEPA in mice, rats, dogs, and man*[a]

| Species | Dose | | | Serum $t^{1/2}$ | Area under |
|---|---|---|---|---|---|
| | Route | mg/kg | mg/m² | (min) | serum curve (µg/ml × min) |
| Mouse[b] | i.p. | 2.0 | 6.0 | 10 | 24 |
| Rat | i.p. | 3.0 | 18.0 | 22 | 60 |
| Dog | i.v. | 3.0 | 60.0 | 40 | 200 |
| Man | i.v. | 0.3 | 11.1 | 60 | 35 |

[a] Data from MELLETT and WOODS (1960), MELLETT et al. (1962), RUDDON and MELLETT (1964).
[b] Data from CRAIG et al. (1959).

Loo et al. (1968b, and personal communication) have shown that parenteral doses of 5-(dimethyltriazeno)imidazole-4-carboxamide expressed on a mg/m² basis yield equivalent $Ct$ values in dogs and humans. They have also observed (Loo et al., 1968a) a similar relationship in children and adults treated parenterally with 6-mercaptopurine and 6-methylmercaptopurine ribonucleoside. Their data and data obtained in our laboratory indicate that these relationships do not hold after oral administration of these agents. In general, our experience with drugs which are slowly, incompletely, or erratically absorbed after oral administration indicates that these relationships do not hold as well as after parenteral administration.

The comparative rates of metabolism of 1-β-D-arabinofuranosyl cytosine (ara-C) in various species have been studied by CAMIENER and SMITH (1965), MULLIGAN and MELLETT (1968), MELLETT (1969), HO and FREI (1971). After administration of 50 mg/kg to various species, drug serum levels are depleted in an apparently haphazard fashion in relation to body size. The monkey and man metabolize the drug at a rate greater than the other species studied. The serum half-life of the drug was 95, 60, 30, 30, and 4 min for the dog, rat, mouse, hamster, and monkey, respectively. In man an initial half-life of 10 to 12 min was noted, followed by a slower rate of disappearance with a half-life of 90 to 150 min. This lack of correlation of the rate of drug disappearance with body surface area is explainable on the basis of the unique distribution of deoxycytidine aminohydrolase [the enzyme which deaminates and inactivates ara-C, MULLIGAN and MELLETT (1968)] in various tissues and various animal species (see MELLETT, 1969). Despite this lack of relationship of serum levels to body size or surface area, some interesting relationships between $Ct$ serum values and biological response were observed under a variety of conditions of drug administration. These relationships are summarized in Table 2.

Table 2. *Some relationships of area under the ara-C serum curve (Ct), dose, serum half-life, and toxicity in various species (data from the author's laboratory)*

| Species | Dose | | | Route | $t^{1/2}$ | $Ct$ | Toxicity comments |
|---|---|---|---|---|---|---|---|
| | ara-C | $H_4U$ | | | (min) | (μg/ml × min) | |
| | mg/kg | mg/kg | mg/m² | | | | |
| Mouse | 10 | | 30 | i.p. | 30 | 315 | no toxicity |
| | 30 | | 90 | i.p. | 30 | 900 | no toxicity |
| | 100 | | 300 | i.p. | 30 | 4800 | no toxicity |
| | 300 | | 900 | i.p. | 30 | 14400 | no toxicity |
| | 1000 | | 3000 | i.p. | 35 | 46000 | no toxicity |
| | 3000 | | 9000 | i.p. | 60 | 115000 | $LD_{10}$ |
| 24 hrs CI[a] | 250 | | 750 | i.p. | — | 8640 | no toxicity |
| 24 hrs CI | 3000 | | 9000 | i.p. | — | 144000 | $LD_{50}$ |
| Rat | 100 | | 600 | i.p. | 60 | 4200 | no toxicity |
| | 300 | | 1800 | i.p. | 60 | 13200 | no toxicity |
| | 2000 | | 12000 | i.p. | 70 | 125000 | $LD_{50}$ |
| Dog | 50 | | 1000 | i.v. | 88 | 6000 | nausea + vomiting without hematopoietic toxicity |
| | 50 | | 1000 | i.v. | 95 | 11700 | nausea + vomiting without hematopoietic toxicity |
| | 50 | | 1000 | i.v. | 95 | 9500 | nausea + vomiting without hematopoietic toxicity |
| | 100 | | 2000 | i.v. | 88 | 17800 | nausea + vomiting without hematopoietic toxicity |
| | 2000 | | 40000 | i.v. | 98 | 170000 | maximum tolerated dose re: hematopoietic toxicity |
| 24 hrs CI | 28 | | 550 | i.v. | — | 7200 | none |
| 24 hrs CI | 298 | | 5600 | i.v. | — | 105000 | maximum tolerated dose re: hematopoietic toxicity |
| Monkey | 50 | | 600 | i.v. | 4 | 210 | no toxicity |
| | 100 | | 1200 | i.v. | 4 | 600 | no toxicity |
| 24 hrs CI | 30 | | 360 | i.v. | — | 432 | no toxicity |
| 24 hrs CI | 300 | | 3600 | i.v. | — | 1680 | no toxicity |
| | 50 | 12.5 | | i.v. | 69 | 5000 | very slight hematopoietic effects |
| | 50 | 25.0 | | i.v. | 90 | 6000 | moderate hematopoietic effects |
| | 50 | 50.0 | | i.v. | 92 | 6300 | moderate hematopoietic effects |
| | 50 | 100.0 | | i.v. | 188 | 17000 | severe hematopoietic effects |
| | 50 | 1000.0 | | i.v. | 245 | 25000 | lethal hematopoietic effects |
| Man[b] | 1.4 | | 47 | i.v. | 10/100 | 20 | no toxicity |
| | 2.0 | | 67 | i.v. | 11/130 | 22 | no toxicity |
| | 5.7 | | 200 | i.v. | 12/150 | 200 | no toxicity |
| | 44.0 | | 1500 | i.v. | 10/90 | 1590 | no toxicity |
| | 88.0 | | 3000 | i.v. | 12/120 | 4380 | no toxicity |
| | 113.0 | | 4000 | i.v. | 12/100 | 5600 | no toxicity |

[a] CI, constant infusion; $H_4U$, tetrahydrouridine.
[b] Data from Ho and Frei (1971).

Some comments are in order regarding the data contained in Table 2. (a) Administration of the mouse single dose $LD_{10}$, the rat single dose $LD_{50}$, and the dog maximum tolerated single dose in the individual species produced essentially equivalent serum *Ct* values in each of the species. (b) Administration of an $LD_{50}$ dose by constant infusion (CI) for 24 h produced a *Ct* value in the mouse equivalent to that obtained in the dog when a maximum tolerated dose was infused for 24 h. The *Ct* values obtained for toxic doses administered by constant infusion were similar to those obtained with single toxic doses. (c) Administration of single doses of ara-C to monkeys and humans failed to produce toxicity because of rapid inactivation by metabolism of the drug which resulted in low *Ct* values for ara-C. (d) When the deaminase inhibitor, tetrahydrouridine ($H_4U$), was administered to monkeys prior to treatment with ara-C, graded degrees of toxicity to lethality were noted. It was possible to demonstrate toxicity in the monkey to a single dose of ara-C only through the use of the inhibitor. Similarly, constant infusion of 300 mg/kg of ara-C for 24 h resulted in relatively low *Ct* values and failed to produce toxicity in the monkey. (e) Since $H_4U$ by itself produces no toxicity in the monkey, the relatively low *Ct* value (25000 µg/ml · min) for the lethal combination of $H_4U$ and ara-C suggests that this species is more susceptible to ara-C toxicity than is the mouse, rat, or dog.

The techniques of tissue culture lend themselves effectively to demonstrating the relationships between biological response, concentration of a drug, and time required to produce the biological effect. In many instances the relationships are simplified because the drug is not metabolized to any significant degree in the tissue culture system. Thus, concentrations of the drug and time of exposure may be manipulated within wide ranges and related to the biological effect, e.g. total cell kill in the system.

HIMMELFARB et al. (1969) have devised an ingenious tissue culture apparatus which allows for the growth of murine leukemic cells to very high levels, and allows the investigator to manipulate drug exposures *in vitro* under conditions paralleling the situation *in vivo*. The unit incorporates a spinning filter which allows passage of large volumes of filtrate through the system without clogging by the retained cells. Regulation of flow rates and drug concentrations in the apparatus may be varied to yield drug half-times ($t^{1/2}$) observed *in vivo*. Subsequently, THAYER et al. (1970), from the same laboratory, demonstrated that continuous perfusion of methotrexate at varying rates to provide the same daily integrated concentration × time value resulted in equivalent cell killing effects over a two day period. The *Ct* value they obtained for equal cell killing effects was the same as that obtained by WILKOFF et al. (1967) where concentrations of methotrexate were held constant for 24 h.

SKIPPER et al. (1971) presented data obtained from tissue culture studies which indicated that the rate of cell kill for L1210 leukemic cells with ara-C was concentration dependent up to approximately 5 µg of drug per ml of medium. Above this level, the rate of cell kill was independent of drug concentration. THAYER (personal communication), utilizing the spin culture technique, pulsed doses of ara-C every three hours and controlled flow rates through the system to produce drug disappearance rates with a $t^{1/2}$ (20 to 30 min) equal to those observed *in vivo* in the mouse. The results of these studies were compared with results obtained in investigations where the concentration of drug was held constant. In both instances the cumulative *Ct* values were identical for equal cell killing effects. SKIPPER et al. (1971) further demonstrated that pulsed doses of ara-C every 3 h for 24 h in $BDF_1$ mice bearing L1210 leukemic cells were necessary to maintain continuous critical levels of the drug and to provide an *in vivo Ct* value to produce cures in the animals.

## Conclusions

It is the quantitative rate of drug disposition that is of practical importance in determining optimal dosage schedules. It is unlikely that we shall ever find a species of laboratory animal, primate or otherwise, that will consistently excrete and metabolize drugs at the same rate as man. We should, therefore, accept these rate differences and seek a means of relating them to drug effects in various species. The foregoing discussion has indicated some of the ways in which this may be approached.

(a) It can be demonstrated for many drugs that receptors for a given drug in various mammalian species exhibit similar sensitivities for a specified drug concentration.

b) The dose required to produce a given effect and the duration of the effect in various species vary greatly.

(c) The species variation in dose and duration of effect are related to the persistence of the drug in a given species and thus are functions of drug metabolism and elimination in the species.

d) The relation between the quantity of a drug causing a physiological effect and the time necessary to produce this effect may be related by the expression $Ct = K$, with suitable modifications to allow for drug removal from the system.

(e) The usefulness of body surface area rather than body weight as a criterion for relating drug dosages in laboratory and clinical studies can be demonstrated for many drugs on an empirical basis.

f) When doses of a drug are expressed on a mg per square meter of body surface area for various species, then equal doses give equivalent $Ct$ values in the different species.

(g) Equivalent $Ct$ values in various species give equivalent toxicological (or pharmacological) response in the different species.

(h) The serum or tissue half-life of a drug is shortest in small animals and longest in humans and is a prime determinant of the total $Ct$ value attained in the various species.

There are a number of phenomena which may invalidate these relationships.

(a) Distribution of the drug may increase at higher serum levels. This can be determined by establishing the linearity of the relation between serum curve areas for various doses and by estimating the volume of distribution at various doses.

(b) A unique sequestration in a particular tissue may occur. This may be determined by tissue distribution studies and methods of essential elimination of the drug.

(c) An enzyme system metabolizing the drug may become saturated at high serum levels, or a necessary cofactor or conjugating agent may fail to meet mobilization needs.

(d) The drug's metabolism may be stimulated by the drug itself or by another agent. This is likely to occur only with repeated administration or when we purposely introduce a second agent.

(e) The drug's metabolism may be inhibited by another agent. Again this is likely to occur only when we introduce a second agent.

(f) The plasma level of the drug may exceed the protein binding capacity. This can usually be tested by simple binding experiments at appropriate concentrations.

(g) If the drug is involved in active transport mechanisms in various tissues and the transport maximum is exceeded, these relationships may not prevail.

Such studies as suggested here may permit some reasonable extrapolations from experiments on lower animals to drug effects in the human species.

## References


ADOLPH, E. F.: Quantitative relations in the physiological constitutions of mammals. Science **109**, 579—585 (1949).

BRODIE, B. B., REID, W. D.: Some pharmacological consequences of species variation in rates of metabolism. Fed. Proc. **26**, 1062—1070 (1967).

BUTLER, T. C.: Conference on nonhuman primate toxicology. (C. O. MILLER, Ed.) Dept. Health, Education, and Welfare. Washington: 1966.

CAMIENER, G. W., SMITH, C. G.: Studies of the enzymatic deamination of cytosine arabinoside. I. Enzyme distribution and species specificity. Biochem. Pharmacol. **14**, 1405—1416 (1965).

CLARK, A. J.: The mode of action of drugs on cells, 1st ed. London: Arnold and Co. 1933.

CLARK, A. J.: General pharmacology, 1st ed. Berlin: Julius Springer 1937.

CRAIG, A. W., FOX, B. W., JACKSON, H.: Metabolic studies of $P^{32}$-labeled triethylenethiophosphoramide. Biochem. Pharmacol. **3**, 42—50 (1959).

FREIREICH, E. J., GEHAN, E. A., RALL, D. P., SCHMIDT, L. H., SKIPPER, H. E.: Quantitative comparison of toxicity of anticancer agents in mouse, rat, hamster, dog, monkey, and man. Cancer Chemother. Rep. **50**, 219—244 (1966).

GILLETTE, J. R.: Drug toxicity as a result of interference with physiological control mechanisms. Ann. N. Y. Acad. Sci. **123**, 42—54 (1965).

HIMMELFARB, P., THAYER, P. S., MARTIN, H. E.: Spin filter culture: The propagation of mammalian cells in suspension. Science **164**, 555—557 (1969).

HO, D. H., FREI, E. III: Clinical pharmacology of 1-β-D-arabinofuranosyl cytosine. Clin. Pharmacol. Ther. **12**, 944—954 (1971).

LOO, T. L., LUCE, J. K., SULLIVAN, M. P., FREI, E. III: Clinical pharmacologic observations on 6-mercaptopurine and 6-methylthiopurine ribonucleoside. Clin. Pharmacol. Ther. **9**, 180—190 (1968a).

LOO, T. L., TANNER, B. B., HOUSEHOLDER, G. E., SHEPARD, B. J.: Some pharmacokinetic aspects of 5-(dimethyltriazeno)imidazole-4-carboxamide in the dog. J. pharm. Sci. **57**, 2126—2129 (1968b).

MELLETT, L. B.: Comparative drug metabolism. In: Progress in drug research, Vol. 13, pp. 136—169. Basel and Stuttgart: Birkhäuser Verlag 1969.

MELLETT, L. B., HODGSON, P. E., WOODS, L. A.: Absorption and fate of $C^{14}$-labeled *N, N′, N″*-triethylenethiophosphoramide (thio-TEPA) in humans and dogs. J. Lab. clin. Med. **60**, 818—825 (1962).

MELLETT, L. B., WOODS, L. A.: The comparative physiological disposition of thio-TEPA and TEPA in the dog. Cancer Res. **20**, 524—532 (1960).

MULLIGAN, L. T., MELLETT, L. B.: Comparative metabolism of cytosine arabinoside and inhibition of deamination by tetrahydrouridine. Pharmacologist **10**, 167 (1968).

PINKEL, D.: The use of body surface area as a criterion of drug dosage in cancer chemotherapy. Cancer Res. **18**, 853—856 (1958).

QUINN, G. P., AXELROD, J., BRODIE, B. B.: Species, strain and sex differences in metabolism of hexobarbital, amidopyrine and aniline. Biochem. Pharmacol. **1**, 152—164 (1958).

RUDDON, R. W., MELLETT, L. B.: The distribution of $C^{14}$-labeled *N, N′, N″*-triethylenethiophosphoramide (thio-TEPA) and its metabolites in normal and tumor-bearing rats. Cancer Chemother. Rep. **39**, 7—13 (1964).

SILVER, S. D.: The relation of time to the dose required to produce a given physiological effect. Med. Div. Rep. No. 22, Edgewood Arsenal, Md.: Chemical Warfare Serv. 1945.

SKIPPER, H. E.: The effect of chemotherapy on the kinetics of leukemic cell behavior. Cancer Res. **25**, 1544—1550 (1965).

SKIPPER, H. E., SCHABEL, F. M., JR., MELLETT, L. B., MONTGOMERY, J. A., WILKOFF, L. J., LLOYD, H. H., BROCKMAN, R. W.: Implications of biochemical, cytokinetic, pharmacologic, and toxicologic relationships in design of optimal therapeutic schedules. Cancer Chemother. Rep. **54**, 431—450 (1971).

THAYER, P. S., HIMMELFARB, P., ROBERTS, D.: Effects of perfusion with amethopterin on L1210 leukemia cells in spin filter culture. Cancer Res. **30**, 1709—1714 (1970).

WILKOFF, L. J., WILCOX, W. S., BURDESHAW, J. A., DIXON, G. J., DULMADGE, E. A.: Effect of antimetabolites on kinetic behavior of proliferating L1210 leukemia cells. J. nat. Cancer Inst. **39**, 965—975 (1967).

Chapter 18

# Biochemical Aspects of Selective Toxicity

J. FRANK HENDERSON

## Introduction

Selective toxicity, i.e. differences in the biological consequences of drug action on normal and neoplastic cells, is the very basis of cancer chemotherapy, and the increasing effectiveness of drugs for the treatment of childhood leukemia, Burkitt's lymphoma, choriocarcinoma, and some other types of neoplastic disease, demonstrates that such selectivity can be achieved even in man. However, the large number of patients who still die of malignant disease testify that selectivity of drug action is not attained with sufficient frequency or reliability.

Despite numerous examples of the biological phenomenon of selective toxicity, very little is known about its biochemical basis. More than five years ago, reviewers of this subject reached conclusions, such as "there is at present no known metabolic basis for the design of drugs with specificity for cancer in general or for any particular cancer" (BENNETT and MONTGOMERY, 1967), and "even for ... agents. ... whose mechanism of action at a molecular level are reasonably well understood ... the reasons for their selective antineoplastic action remain largely obscure" (FREI, 1967). Although considerable progress has since been made in an understanding of the actions of cancer chemotherapeutic agents, we still do not know the biochemical bases of the selective toxicity of any drug. In part this deficiency is due to the difficulty of determining the primary biochemical effects of these drugs and the biological consequences of various biochemical effects; in particular, the biochemical causes of cell death following cessation of cell division are very little understood. In addition, the normal tissues most affected by antitumor drugs – bone marrow, intestinal mucosa, lymphatic tissue, and skin – have been particularly difficult subjects for biochemical investigation.

Because it is not possible to state definitively the biochemical basis of the selective toxicity of any cancer chemotherapeutic agent, this chapter will set out the many possible factors involved in this phenomenon and will provide examples of many of these. This can only be done by commingling the results of studies of many different drugs, and by including any type of selectivity of drug action. Thus, although selective toxicity in the strict sense refers to differences in the response to drug action of a tumor and the most sensitive normal tissue in a given host, selectivity is also observed when a drug has different effects on (a) two tumors in the same host or species, (including the phenomena of resistance, insensitivity, and pharmacological sanctuary), (b) tumors of the same origin in different species, (c) hosts of different species, (d) different normal tissues, and (e) tumors and their tissues of origin. Bases of differences in drug response between microorganisms and animal cells will in general not be discussed.

In the face of a very extensive but rather inconclusive literature on this subject, and the limitations of space, references have been chosen selectively to illustrate certain points, and no attempt has been made to be exhaustive. In general, more recent papers have been cited, from which older references can be found.

Selectivity of drug action in biochemical terms may be due to differences among cells of any of the factors required for drug action. In general these are the following: (a) the drug must be present in its biochemically active form at the site of action at a suitable concentration and for a suitable period; (b) it must interact with its target; (c) the target must be important for cell growth and/or function; (d) the cellular damage achieved must lead to damage to the tumor or the body as a whole. Each of these factors will now be further subdivided, and examples given where possible.

## Selectivity Due to Differences in the Concentration of Drug at the Biochemical Site of Action

Differences among cells which may affect the presence of the drug in its biochemically active form at the site of action at a suitable concentration and for a suitable period may exist (a) in the penetration of drug into cells, (b) in its conversion to active form(s) if this is required, (c) in the rates of catabolism of the drug or of its active form(s), and (d) in the loss of the drug or its active form(s) from the cell. The many important factors which affect the concentration of drug immediately outside normal and malignant cells are obviously relevant here, but are beyond the scope of this chapter.

### A. Entry into Cells

Drug concentrations in cells will depend first on the rate at which they traverse the cell membrane. This is affected not only by the extracellular concentration, but also by the mechanism by which the drug enters the cell. If a drug enters cells only by the process of passive diffusion, then relatively little variation from cell to cell would be expected in the rate of uptake at a given extracellular drug concentration. However, the rate of uptake of drugs which are partially ionized is known to depend on both intra and extracellular pH. Although the intracellular pH of tumor cells apparently is similar to that of normal cells (POOLE et al., 1964), the extracellular pH of solid tumors is relatively acidic (e.g. KAHLER and ROBERTSON, 1943; GUILLINO et al., 1965). In fact, however, this difference is not known to confer selectivity on any of the commonly used anticancer drugs.

The rate of entry into cells of drugs which require some carrier for their uptake may vary with the specificity, affinity, maximum velocity, and mechanism of the carrier-mediated process, and differences among cells in one or another of these factors have been shown to be related to different degrees of sensitivity to several drugs. Thus, FISCHER (1962) and others (e.g. WERKHEISER et al., 1963; SIROTNAK et al., 1968; NICHOL, 1968) have reported reduced rates of uptake in animal tumor lines selected for resistance to methotrexate, and KESSEL et al. (1965) found that there was a correlation between rates of uptake and sensitivity to this drug in ten transplanted mouse leukemias with a broad spectrum of response to methotrexate. JACQUEZ (1966) and KESSEL and HALL (1967) have also shown that the uptake of methotrexate was concentrative in Leukemia L1210 cells, whereas it was not so in Ehrlich ascites tumor cells; the former is much more sensitive to this drug than the latter. Some drug resistant human leukemia cells also demonstrated impaired uptake of methotrexate (HALL et al. 1966; KESSEL and HALL, 1965).

KESSEL et al. (1968) studied the nature and rate of methotrexate entry into normal and neoplastic leukocytes. Uptake into different types of normal cells varied widely in the following order: granulocytes > large lymphocytes > small lymphocytes; it was found that the mechanism and characteristics of the entry process were different in granulocytes and small lymphocytes. Studies with human leukemia cells showed that there was a much wider range of entry rates than in normal leukocytes, and that in general there was a correlation between rate of uptake and clinical sensitivity. Wide and overlapping ranges were encountered, however.

Nitrogen mustard is actively taken up by cells (GOLDENBERG et al., 1970), and several investigators (RUTMAN et al., 1968; CHUN et al., 1969; KLATT et al., 1969; WOLPERT and RUDDON, 1969; GOLDENBERG et al., 1970) have reported that Ehrlich ascites tumor lines selected for resistance to this drug are less permeable to it than drug sensitive cells. In most cases other factors apparently also contribute to the observed resistance. Recently, LYONS and GOLDENBERG (1972) have reported that the apparent Michaelis constant and maximum velocity of uptake were different in normal leukocytes and cells from patients with acute and chronic lymphoblastic leukemias. Both parameters were most favorable to high intracellular concentrations of nitrogen mustard in acute lymphoblastic leukemia cells.

Purine and pyrimidine nucleoside analogs and derivatives also enter cells by carrier mediated processes (e.g. OLIVER and PATERSON, 1971), and it may be expected that differences in rates of entry would be exhibited by different cells; however, concrete information on this point is not yet available.

## B. Conversion to Active Forms

Some drugs must be converted enzymatically to various derivatives in order to exert their cytotoxic effects, and variation in the rates of these activating reactions may be one basis for the selective toxicity of such compounds. Thus, animal tumor cells which lack adenine phosphoribosyltransferase, hypoxanthine-guanine phosphoribosyltransferase, or adenosine kinase, are resistant to the effects of those purine analogs and derivatives which are activated through the actions of these enzymes; numerous observations of such mechanisms of resistance have been reviewed by BROCKMAN (1963). Similarly, resistance to various pyrimidine analogs and derivatives may be caused by lack of uridine kinase, deoxycytidine kinase, or thymidine kinase.

Different rodent (MURRAY, 1966), monkey (KRENITSKY, 1969), and human (ROSENBLOOM et al., 1967) tissues vary widely in their purine phosphoribosyltransferase activities, and such differences are one basis for the observation that concentrations of thioguanine ribonucleotides are larger in bone marrow than in intestinal mucosa (MOORE and LEPAGE, 1958; MARCHESI and SARTORELLI, 1963); thioguanine is also more toxic in the former tissue. KESSEL and HALL (1969) measured the ability of bone marrow cells and normal and neoplastic leukocytes to convert 6-mercaptopurine to ribonucleotides, and found that normal bone marrow cells were most active in this respect. Cells from patients with chronic lymphocytic leukemia formed drug nucleotides at rather low rates, whereas those from other leukemia patients had very wide ranges of this activity.

Ho et al. (1968) studied a series of mouse tumors of different degrees of sensitivity to 6-methylmercaptopurine ribonucleoside, and found a good response between chemotherapeutic response and activity of adenosine kinase, the enzyme which converts this drug to its active form. However, no correlation between toxicity and adenosine kinase activity was noted in normal human and mouse tissues. In contrast, the inability of human bone marrow to phosphorylate α-deoxythioguanosine is believed by PEERY and LEPAGE (1969) to be the basis of its low toxicity to this tissue, whereas a number of human tumor specimens did phosphorylate it and would be expected to be sensitive to this antimetabolite.

The sensitivity of various animal tumors to cytosine arabinoside has been shown to be related to their relative abilities to phosphorylate this compound (e.g., KREIS et al., 1972); KESSEL et al. (1969) found wide differences in this regard among normal blood cells and different types of human leukemia cells. Greatest activity was found in small lymphocytes and cells from patients with chronic lymphocytic leukemia; as in most such studies of leukemic cells, great variation was exhibited in cells from individual patients. There was a general correlation between drug sensitivity and ability to phosphorylate cytosine arabinoside.

## C. Drug Catabolism

The ability of some tumors and normal tissues to catabolize drugs relatively rapidly appears to account for their insensitivity to several purine and pyrimidine analogs or derivatives. LEPAGE (1970), for example, has reviewed the extensive studies of his laboratory which showed that the sensitivity of both normal and neoplastic rodent cells to arabinofuranosyladenine and xylofuranosyladenine was inversely related to their adenosine deaminase activities, the deaminated derivatives being therapeutically inactive. Human solid tumor specimens also have a very wide range of deaminase activities, which would be expected to affect their chemotherapeutic response to these agents. Variation has also been observed in the ability of various human leukemia cell populations to deaminate cytosine arabinoside (KESSEL et al., 1969), although in this case deamination by liver seems to be a more important determinant of effectiveness.

Variations in guanine deaminase activity have also been related to the toxicity of some drugs. Thus, HIRSCHBERG et al. (1952) demonstrated several examples of the inverse relationship between the deaminating capacity of mouse tumors and their susceptibility to treatment with 8-azaguanine, and the toxicity of this compound to skin has been attributed to the low level of guanine deaminase activity in that tissue (GELLHORN, 1953). MARCHESI and SARTORELLI (1963) also have suggested that the rapid deamination of thioguanine by intestinal mucosa is one basis for its insensitivity to this drug, whereas the lack of guanine deaminase in bone marrow contributes to drug toxicity in the tissue.

The rates of degradation of azaserine by normal mouse tissues are in general correlated with their insensitivity to this drug. Liver, for example, is quite insensitive (MOORE and LEPAGE, 1958), and degrades this glutamine analog rapidly (JACQUEZ and SHERMAN, 1962), whereas intestinal mucosa is sensitive to azaserine and has a low rate of drug catabolism.

There are fewer reports of differences among cells in the catabolism of the active nucleotide derivatives of purine and pyrimidine analogs and derivatives. However, resistance of mouse tumors to 6-methylmercaptopurine ribonucleoside (HENDERSON et al., 1967) and thioguanine (WOLPERT et al., 1971) has been attributable to increased rates of dephosphorylation of drug nucleotides in a few cases.

## D. Loss of Drug from Cells

Among the factors which affect drug concentrations in cells is the rate at which drugs are lost from the cell. This depends not only on the metabolism and binding of the drug within the cell, but also on the rate and mechanism by which it crosses cell membranes from inside to outside. There appears to be no specific information relating this phenomenon to selective toxicity.

## Selectivity Due to Differences in the Interaction of Drugs with Their Biochemical Targets

Having attained a significant concentration of its active form within a normal or neoplastic cell, the drug must next interact in some way with its biochemical "target," which may be an enzyme or other protein, or one or another species of ribo- or deoxyribonucleic acid. The mode of interaction may be covalent (either by binding or incorporation) or non-covalent. Differences among cells with regard to the interaction of drug and target may arise with respect to (a) the effective concentration of the target, (b) the affinity of the drug for the target, (c) the mode of binding, and (d) the concentration of protecting metabolites.

### A. Effective Concentration of the Target

For antimetabolites that are incorporated into DNA (e.g., thioguanine, 6-mercaptopurine, iododeoxyuridine, bromodeoxyuridine), an effective concentration of target is available only when cells are synthesizing this polynucleotide. Hence, the target concentration is nil in permanently or temporarily nondividing cells, as well as in dividing cells outside of *S* phase. In a similar manner, vinblastine and other drugs that affect the mitotic apparatus, have an effective target with which to interact only during or immediately prior to mitosis. The importance of considering the availability of an effective concentration of target with respect to scheduling drug treatment has become increasingly apparent in recent years (e.g., SKIPPER, 1971).

### B. Affinity of the Target for the Drug

Several cases of apparent variation in the affinity of the target for the drug have been related to variation in chemotherapeutic sensitivity. Thus, HEIDELBERGER et al. (1960) studied a line of Ehrlich ascites tumor cells that was resistant to 5-fluorouracil, and concluded that its thymidylate synthetase did not bind 5-fluorodeoxyuridylate with the same affinity as did that of drug sensitive cells. In a similar manner, HENDERSON et al. (1967) concluded that the phosphoribosylpyrophosphate amidotransferase of a 6-methylmercaptopurine ribonucleoside-resistant tumor probably did not bind the nucleotide of this drug normally, or did not respond to the bound drug in the same way as did the enzyme of sensitive cells.

NICHOL (1968) has summarized differences among purified dihydrofolate reductases from Sarcoma 180, chicken liver, and Ehrlich ascites tumor cells with respect to effects of pH, urea and *p*-chloromercuribenzoate, enthalpy of activation and antigenic specificity.

### C. Mode of Binding

No cases are known in which differences in the mode of binding of the drug with the target lead to variation in drug toxicity in animal cells.

### D. Concentration of Protecting Metabolites

Although the effectiveness *in vitro* of inhibition by azaserine varies depending on the concentration of glutamine (e.g., FERNANDES et al., 1956), there is no evidence that variation of azaserine toxicity is inversely related to glutamine concentrations in tissues and tumors. Most other metabolites which prevent drug action do so by lowering the concentrations of the effective drug rather than by preventing its interaction with the target.

## Selectivity Due to Differences in the Effects of Drug-Target Interaction on Cell Growth

Effective interaction of a drug and its biochemical target does not necessarily lead to immediate and complete cessation of cell growth. Differences among cells with respect to the relatively immediate consequences of drug-target interaction may arise with respect to (a) the degree of completeness of inhibition, (b) the importance of the target for the cell, (c) amounts of metabolites or products accumulated "beyond" the block, and (d) the rates of repair or recovery from drug action.

### A. Completeness of Inhibition

Variation in effectiveness of a drug in different cells frequently is due to variation in the concentration of active form of the drug and its duration in cells. However, drug effectiveness may also be affected by the concentration of the biochemical target, inasmuch as a given amount of drug-target complex may be a large percentage of a small absolute amount of target or a small percentage of a large amount of target.

It is well known that treatment with methotrexate often leads to elevated cellular concentrations of dihydrofolate reductase, and that high levels of this enzyme are sometimes associated with resistance to this drug (e.g. NICHOL, 1968; BERTINO and HILLCOAT, 1968). HAKALA (1965) has concluded that even slight dissociation of the methotrexate-dihydrofolate reductase complex is a significant basis for drug resistance when the concentrations of this enzyme are elevated and when the permeability of cells to this drug is limited. This becomes particularly significant in view of the report of ROBERTS and HALL (1967) that uninhibited dihydrofolate reductase could be detected in extracts of leukemic leukocytes from patients who were receiving methotrexate and in which levels of this enzyme were elevated. It is also known that the concentrations of dihydrofolate reductase in various normal tissues vary widely (e.g. BERTINO, 1968).

### B. Importance of the Target

The importance of a particular biochemical target may vary in different cells depending on the needs of the cell and on the relative rates of alternative pathways or processes. Alternative pathways are most likely to be important factors in selective toxicity with respect to the relative rates of pathways of purine and pyrimidine ribo- and deoxyribonucleotide synthesis *de novo* and from preformed bases or nucleosides. The greater toxicity of azaserine to intestinal mucosa than to bone marrow, for example, has been attributed to the greater dependence of the former on purine nucleotide biosynthesis *de novo* and the greater dependence of the latter on preformed purines. Likewise, the lack of complete inhibition of tumor growth by azaserine under conditions of complete inhibition of purine nucleotide biosynthesis *de novo*, was attributed to the activity of alternative pathways of purine ribonucleotide metabolism (HENDERSON et al., 1957). Although the problem of alternative pathways continues to be of great potential significance as a basis for selective toxicity (e.g., SARTORELLI, 1969; SNEIDER and POTTER, 1969), its actual role is not yet clear.

Biochemical targets which are immediately involved in cell division are not usually important to permanently or temporarily nondividing cells, and are often most important to dividing cells only in specific phases of the cell cycle. Thus, inhibitors of ribonucleotide reductase (hydroxyurea, $\alpha$-($N$)-heterocyclic carboxaldehyde thiosemicarbazone derivatives), thymidylate synthetase (methotrexate, indirectly, 5-fluorodeoxyuridylate) and DNA polymerase (arabinosyl cytosine triphosphate, arabinosyl adenine triphosphate) are most effective on cells that are actively synthesizing DNA (although some have secondary effects as well).

### C. Amounts of Accumulated Products

The pharmacological result of inhibition of an enzyme will depend in part on the concentrations of products of the enzyme present in cells and the rate at which these are depleted. Hydroxyurea inhibits the synthesis of deoxyribonucleotides, and the concentrations of this compound which are equitoxic for different cell lines in tissue culture vary considerably from cell to cell (PFEIFFER and TOLMACH, 1967). YOUNG et al. (1967) have suggested that these differences may be due to variation in deoxyribonucleotide pools in these cells, and support this idea with observations that echinoderm ova, which are known to contain large concentrations of deoxyribonucleotides, are not affected by hydroxyurea for up to 3 to 4 divisions if drug is added at the time of fertilization. If added after the 5th division, hydroxyurea toxicity is expressed immediately, apparently because the large initial amounts of deoxyribonucleotides have been used up.

### D. Repair or Recovery

The effectiveness of interaction of drug and target also depends on the rate at which repair or recovery processes operate, and such events may take several different forms. Azaserine, for example, binds covalently to an enzyme of purine nucleotide biosynthesis *de novo*, and recovery depends on the synthesis of new enzymes. MOORE and LEPAGE (1957) and FERNANDES et al. (1956) have shown that the rates of recovery of purine biosynthesis from azaserine were different in liver, kidney, spleen, and Ehrlich ascites tumor cells, and SARTORELLI and LEPAGE (1958) have found that an azaserine-resistant mouse tumor recovered from inhibition more rapidly than did the sensitive parent line. The rate of repair of DNA damaged by treatment with alkylating agents also varies in different cells. Thus, BALL and ROBERTS (1970) observed that nitrogen mustard resistant Yoshida sarcoma cells removed the alkylating agent from the DNA more rapidly than did drug sensitive cells, and WALKER and REID (1971) similarly found that L-cells resistant to sulfur mustard removed alkylated products from DNA at 2 to 3 times the rate at which this occurred in sensitive cells. ROBERTS (1968) suggested that different normal tissues might vary in their rates of repair, but concrete data on this point are not yet available.

## Selectivity Due to Differences in the Effects of Inhibition of Cell Growth on Cell Viability and Cell Loss

Drug induced cessation of cell growth is not synonymous with cell death, but at the present time the biochemical events which lead from one event to the other are largely unknown. It is clear, however, that differences among tissues do exist in these factors, and this subject has recently been reviewed by FARBER (1971).

Studies using hydroxyurea provide a number of examples of variation in the effects of inhibition of cell division on cell viability. Chinese hamster cells in $S$ phase, for example, were killed after one hour's exposure to this drug (SINCLAIR, 1967), whereas HeLa cells were not killed after 18 h exposure under similar conditions (PFEIFFER and TOLMACH, 1967). In experiments *in vivo*, FARBER and BASERGA (1969) found that hydroxyurea inhibited DNA synthesis in continuously dividing cells and in quiescent tissues that were stimulated to divide. However, necrosis was observed only in the former (crypt cells of the small intestine, germinal centers of lymph follicles, and basal layers of the tongue epithelium), whereas no necrosis was observed in regenerating liver, folic acid-stimulated kidney and isoproterenol-stimulated salivary gland. Somewhat similar observations have been made by SCHWARZ et al. (1965), PHILIPS et al. (1967), and HENNINGS and DEVIK (1971).

Other examples need not be given, as the biochemical bases of such variability are not known. LIEBERMAN et al. (1970), however, have made the very important observation that inhibition of protein synthesis (by cycloheximide or tenuazonic acid) protects intestinal crypt epithelial cells from lethal damage by cytosine arabinoside, nitrogen mustard, and x-irradiation. The nature of the protein involved and the relationships between protein synthesis, inhibition of DNA metabolism and cell death remain to be clarified. FARBER (1971) has concluded "that the effect of an agent inducing rapid damage to some cells via a presumed action on DNA metabolism is as much a function of the metabolic organization of the cell as it is of the nature of the initial biochemical lesion."

## Conclusions

It may be concluded from the examples given above both that a large number of potential biochemical bases of selective toxicity of anticancer drugs exist, and at the same time that the biochemical basis of selective toxicity of no single drug is adequately understood. This is a defect which, it is hoped, will soon be remedied.

This chapter has adopted certain assumptions or hypotheses as a basic framework for discussion, and these should be made clear at this point. It has been assumed (a) that biochemical differences that affect drug action do exist between individual normal and malignant cells (understanding that each patient is unique), and (b) that these differences in the properties of individual cells are, in ways not presently understood, responsible for the selectivity of toxicity observed in tumor-bearing animals and patients. There is a fair amount of evidence to support the first assumption, but little to support the second, although both are more or less taken for granted by biochemists (e.g., HENDERSON, 1969).

These assumptions have recently come under both implicit and explicit attack. RALL (1968), for example, states that "minor quantitative differences may exist, but it is difficult to state that any agent possesses a selective toxicity because of any clear-cut biochemical mechanism." This school of thought assumes that there are no pharmacologically significant quantitative differences in drug effects between individual normal and malignant cells in the same state and phase of growth, but rather that differences do exist between normal and malignant cell populations, based on the relative proportions of cells in states and phases of growth with a greater or lesser degree of sensitivity to chemotherapeutic agents. Although the second part of this statement is certainly true, there is no experimental evidence in support of the first part. The recent recognition of biochemical differences at the level of cell populations is of great importance, but such differences also exist at the level of individual cells; investigations that concentrate exclusively on either approach seem equally shortsighted.

## References


BALL, C. R., ROBERTS, J.: DNA repair after mustard gas alkylation by sensitive and resistant Yoshida sarcoma cells *in vitro*. Chem. Biol. Interact. **2**, 321—329 (1970).

BERTINO, J. R., HILLCOAT, B. L.: Regulation of dihydrofolate reductase and other folate-requiring enzymes. Adv. Enzyme Regulat. **6**, 335—349 (1968).

BROCKMAN, R. W.: Resistance to purine antagonists in experimental leukemia systems. Cancer Res. **25**, 1596—1605 (1965).

CHUN, E. H. L., GONZALES, L., LEWIS, F. S., JONES, J., RUTMAN, R. J.: Differences in the *in vivo* alkylation and cross-linking of nitrogen mustard-sensitive and -resistant lines of Lettré-Ehrlich ascites tumors. Cancer Res. **29**, 1184—1194 (1969).

FARBER, E.: Biochemical pathology. Ann. Rev. Pharmacol. **11**, 71—96 (1971).

FARBER, E., BASERGA, R.: Differential effects of hydroxyurea on survival of proliferating cells *in vivo*. Cancer Res. **29**, 136—139 (1969).

FERNANDES, J. F., LEPAGE, G. A., LINDNER, A.: The influence of azaserine and 6-mercaptopurine on the *in vivo* metabolism of ascites tumor cells. Cancer Res. **16**, 154—161 (1956).

FISCHER, G. A.: Defective transport of amethopterin as a mechanism of resistance to the antimetabolite in L5178Y leukemic cells. Biochem. Pharmacol. **11**, 1233—1234 (1962).

GELLHORN, A.: Laboratory and clinical studies on 8-azaguanosine. Cancer **6**, 1030—1033 (1953).

GOLDENBERG, G. J., VANSTONE, C. L., ISRAELS, L. G., ILSE, D., BIHLER, I.: Evidence for a transport carrier of nitrogen mustard in nitrogen mustard-sensitive and -resistant L5178Y lymphoblasts. Cancer Res. **30**, 2285—2291 (1970).

GUILLINO, P. M., GRANTHAM, F. H., SMITH, S. H., HAGGERTY, A. C.: Modifications of the acid-base status of the internal milieu of tumors. J. nat. Cancer Inst. **34**, 857—869 (1965).

HAKALA, M. T.: On the role of drug penetration in amethopterin resistance of Sarcoma-180 cells *in vitro*. Biochim. biophys. Acta (Amst.) **102**, 198—209 (1965).

HALL, T. C., ROBERTS, D., KESSEL, D.: Methotrexate and folic reductase in human cancer. Europ. J. Cancer **2**, 135—142 (1966).

HEIDELBERGER, C., KALDOR, G., MUKHERJEE, K. L., DANNEBERG, P. B.: Studies on fluorinated pyrimidines. XI. *In vitro* studies on tumor resistance. Cancer Res. **20**, 903—909 (1960).

HENDERSON, J. F.: Variation in selective toxicity: Causes and consequences. Cancer Res. **29**, 2404—2406 (1969).

HENDERSON, J. F., CALDWELL, I. C., PATERSON, A. R. P.: Decreased feedback inhibition in a 6-(methylmercapto)purine ribonucleoside-resistant tumor. Cancer Res. **27**, 1773—1778 (1967).

HENDERSON, J. F., LEPAGE, G. A., MCIVER, F. A.: Observations on the action of azaserine in mammalian tissues. Cancer Res. **17**, 609—612 (1957).

HENNINGS, H., DEVIK, F.: Comparison of cytotoxicity of hydroxyurea in normal and rapidly proliferating epidermis and small intestine in mice. Cancer Res. **31**, 277—282 (1971).

HIRSCHBERG, E., KREAM, J., GELLHORN, A.: Enzymatic deamination of 8-azaguanine in normal and neoplastic tissues. Cancer Res. **12**, 524—528 (1952).

HO, D. H. W., LUCE, J. K., FREI, E.: Distribution of purine ribonucleoside kinase and selective toxicity of 6-methylthiopurine ribonucleoside. Biochem. Pharmacol. **17**, 1025—1035 (1968).

JACQUEZ, J. A.: Permeability of Ehrlich ascites tumor cells to folic acid, aminopterin and amethopterin. Cancer Res. **26**, 1616—1624 (1966).

JACQUEZ, J. A., SHERMAN, J. H.: Enzymatic degradation of azaserine. Cancer Res. **22**, 56—61 (1962).

KAHLER, H., ROBERTSON, W. B.: Hydrogen-ion concentration of normal liver and hepatic tumors. J. nat. Cancer Inst. **3**, 495—501 (1943).

KESSEL, D., HALL, T. C.: Uptake and efflux of tritiated methotrexate by leukocytes. Clin. Res. **13**, 338 (1965).

KESSEL, D., HALL, T. C.: Studies on drug transport by normal human leukocytes. Biochem. Pharmacol. **16**, 2395—2403 (1967).

KESSEL, D., HALL, T. C.: Retention of 6-mercaptopurine derivatives by intact cells as an index of drug response in human and murine leukemias. Cancer Res. **29**, 2116—2119 (1969).

KESSEL, D., HALL, T. C., ROBERTS, D.: Modes of uptake of methotrexate by normal and leukemic human leukocytes *in vitro* and their relation to drug response. Cancer Res. **28**, 564—570 (1968).

KESSEL, D., HALL, T. C., ROBERTS, D., WODINSKY, I.: Uptake as a determinant of methotrexate response in mouse leukemias. Science **150**, 752—754 (1965).

KESSEL, D., HALL, T. C., ROSENTHAL, D.: Uptake and phosphorylation of cytosine arabinoside by normal and leukemic human blood cells *in vitro*. Cancer Res. **29**, 459—463 (1969).

Klatt, O., Stehlin, J. S., Jr., McBride, C., Griffin, A. C.: The effect of nitrogen mustard treatment on the deoxyribonucleic acid of sensitive and resistant Ehrlich tumor cells. Cancer Res. **29**, 286—290 (1969).

Kreis, W., Drahovsky, D., Borberg, H.: Characterization of protein and DNA in P815 cells sensitive and resistant to 1-$\beta$-D-arabinofuranosylcytosine. Cancer Res. **32**, 696—701 (1972).

Krenitsky, T. A.: Tissue distribution of purine ribosyl- and phosphoribosyltransferases in the Rhesus monkey. Biochim. biophys. Acta (Amst.) **179**, 506—509 (1969).

LePage, G. A.: Alterations in enzyme activity in tumors and the implications for chemotherapy. Adv. Enzyme Regulat. **8**, 323—332 (1970).

Lieberman, M. W., Verbin, R. S., Landay, M., Liang, H., Farber, E., Lee, T. N., Starr, R.: A probable role for protein synthesis in intestinal epithelial cell damage induced *in vivo* by cytosine arabinoside, nitrogen mustard, or x-irradiation. Cancer Res. **30**, 942—951 (1970).

Lyons, R. M., Goldenberg, G. J.: Active transport of nitrogen mustard by normal and leukemic human lymphoid cells. Proc. Amer. Ass. Cancer Res. **13**, 15 (1972).

Marchesi, S. L., Sartorelli, A. C.: The biochemical basis for the differential sensitivity of intestinal mucosa and bone marrow to 6-thioguanine. Cancer Res. **23**, 1769—1773 (1963).

Moore, E. C., LePage, G. A.: *In vivo* sensitivity of normal and neoplastic mouse tissue to azaserine. Cancer Res. **17**, 804—808 (1957).

Moore, E. C., LePage, G. A.: The metabolism of 6-thioguanine in normal and neoplastic tissues. Cancer Res. **18**, 1075—1083 (1958).

Murray, A. W.: Purine-phosphoribosyltransferase activities in rat and mouse tissues and in Ehrlich ascites-tumor cells. Biochem. J. **100**, 664—670 (1966).

Nichol, C. A.: Studies on dihydrofolate reductase related to the drug sensitivity of microbial and neoplastic cells. Adv. Enzyme Regulat. **6**, 305—322 (1968).

Oliver, J. M., Paterson, A. R. P.: Nucleoside transport I. A mediated process in human erythrocytes. Canad. J. Biochem. **49**, 262—270 (1971).

Peery, A., LePage, G. A.: Nucleotide formation from $\alpha$ and $\beta$-2′-deoxythioguanosine in extracts of murine and human tissues. Cancer Res. **29**, 617—623 (1969).

Pfeiffer, S. E., Tolmach, L. J.: Inhibition of DNA synthesis in HeLa cells by hydroxyurea. Cancer Res. **27**, 124—129 (1967).

Philips, F. S., Sternberg, S. S., Schwartz, H. S., Cronin, A. P., Sodergren, J. E., Vidal, P. M.: Hydroxyurea. I. Acute cell death in proliferating tissues in rats. Cancer Res. **27**, 61—74 (1967).

Poole, D. T., Butler, T. C., Waddell, W. J.: Intracellular pH of the Ehrlich ascites tumor cell. J. nat. Cancer Inst. **32**, 939—946 (1964).

Rall, D. P.: Selective aspects of chemotherapy in acute leukemia and Burkitt's tumor. Cancer **21**, 575—579 (1968).

Roberts, D., Hall, T. C.: The reduction of folate and dihydrofolate by homogenates of leukocytes from patients with leukemia or with myeloid metaplasia. Cancer Res. **27**, 994—999 (1967).

Roberts, J. J., Crathorn, A. R., Brent, T. P.: Repair of alkylated DNA in mammalian cells. Nature (Lond.) **218**, 970—972 (1968).

Rosenbloom, F. M., Kelley, W. N., Miller, J., Henderson, J. F., Seegmiller, J. E.: Inherited disorder of purine metabolism. Correlation between central nervous system dysfunction and biochemical effects. J. Amer. med. Assoc. **202**, 175—177 (1967).

Rutman, R. J., Chun, E. H. L., Lewis, F. S.: Permeability difference as a source of resistance to alkylating agents in Ehrlich ascites tumor cells. Biochem. biophys. Res. Commun. **32**, 650—657 (1968).

Sartorelli, A. C.: Some approaches to the therapeutic exploitation of metabolic sites of vulnerability of neoplastic cells. Cancer Res. **29**, 2292—2299 (1969).

Sartorelli, A. C., LePage, G. A.: The development and biochemical characterization of resistance to azaserine in a TA3 ascites carcinoma. Cancer Res. **18**, 457—463 (1958).

Schwartz, H. S., Garofalo, M., Sternberg, S. S., Philips, F. S.: Hydroxyurea: Inhibition of deoxyribonucleic acid synthesis in regenerating liver of rats. Cancer Res. **25**, 1867—1870 (1965).

Sinclair, W. K.: Hydroxyurea: Effects on Chinese hamster cells grown in culture. Cancer Res. **27**, 297—308 (1967).

Sirotnak, F. M., Kurita, S., Hutchison, D. J.: On the nature of a transport alteration determining resistance to amethopterin in the L1210 leukemia. Cancer Res. **28**, 75—80 (1968).

Skipper, H. E.: The cell cycle and chemotherapy of cancer. In: The cell cycle and cancer. New York: Marcel Dekker 1971.

Sneider, T. W., Potter, V. R.: Alternative *de novo* and "salvage" pathways to thymidine triphosphate synthesis: Possible implications for cancer chemotherapy. Cancer Res. **29**, 2398—2403 (1969).

WALKER, I. G., REID, B. D.: Some properties of substrains of L-cells with a decreased sensitivity to *bis*(2-chloroethyl)sulfide. Cancer Res. **31**, 510—515 (1971).
WERKHEISER, W. C., LAW, L. W., ROOSA, R. A., NICHOL, C. A.: Further evidence that selective uptake modifies cellular response to 4-aminofolate antagonists. Proc. Amer. Ass. Cancer Res. **4**, 71 (1963).
WOLPERT, M. K., DAMLE, S. P., BROWN, J. E., SZNYCER, E., AGRAWAL, K. C., SARTORELLI, A. C.: The role of phosphohydrolases in the mechanism of resistance of neoplastic cells to 6-thiopurines. Cancer Res. **31**, 1620—1626 (1971).
WOLPERT, M. K., RUDDON, R. W.: A study on the mechanism of resistance to nitrogen mustard (HN2) in Ehrlich ascites tumor cells: Comparison of uptake of HN2-$^{14}$C into sensitive and resistant cells. Cancer Res. **29**, 873—879 (1969).
YOUNG, C. W., SCHOCHETMAN, G., KARNOFSKY, D. A.: Hydroxyurea-induced inhibition of deoxyribonucleotide synthesis: Studies in intact cells. Cancer Res. **27**, 526—534 (1967).

Chapter 19

# Mechanisms of Resistance

R. W. BROCKMAN

With 7 Figures

## Introduction

"The problem of resistance in neoplastic cells, as in microorganisms, will remain a most important perpetual threat to the successful use of therapeutic agents" (LAW, 1956). It also has been said, that as long as cancer cells are able to divide, Darwinian evolution is inevitable. The basis for these statements can be found by examining mechanisms by which a population of cells (microorganisms or neoplastic cells) adapt to the presence of a drug. *Physiologic adaptation*, in which the drug induces a change in the population, does not involve a genetic change and is not a stable characteristic. *Genetic adaptation*, in which mutants arising independently of the drug are selected in the presence of the drug, is characterized by stability of resistance. These mechanisms are not mutually exclusive, as pointed out by BRYSON and SZYBALSKI (1955), DEAN and HINSHELWOOD (1957), PETERS (1970), and others. Agents that are mutagenic, in some cases the anticancer drug itself, may increase the probability of the development of resistance by increasing the mutation frequency in a population of treated cells.

## Origins of Drug Resistance

There is ample evidence for the operation of random mutation and selection in the origin of stable resistance to drugs in bacteria (DEMEREC, 1945, 1948, 1957; LEDERBERG and LEDERBERG, 1952). Early experiments, to prove that mutational change was independent of drug, were based on adaptations of the fluctuation test of LURIA and DELBRÜCK (1943). This type of experiment, which originally was devised for the analysis of phage resistance, was adapted to a study of the origin of resistance to antibiotics in microorganisms (DEMEREC,1945, 1948) and of the origin of resistance to methotrexate in mouse leukemia L1210 (LAW, 1952). The fluctuation test is based on the assumption that mutations occurring at random would produce large variations in the frequency of occurrence of resistant cells, in samples taken from a series of independently maintained sublines, in contrast to much less variation in replicate samples from a single culture.

Modifications of the fluctuation test have been used to estimate mutation rates for resistance to growth inhibitors in nonneoplastic cells in culture. Table 1 summarizes findings of several investigators on the mutation rates for resistance to 8-azaguanine. The average value is about $5 \times 10^{-6}$, which is significantly lower than the average spontaneous mutation rate for ten different phenotypes in man (about $2 \times 10^{-5}$) and for eight loci in the mouse ($0.75 \times 10^{-5}$) (see NEEL, 1971). These average values for mutation rate must be considered only as gross estimates.

The mutation rate for resistance to puromycin, $4 \times 10^{-6}$, was similar to that for azaguanine, but that for resistance to arabinosylcytosine in mouse leukemia cells *in vitro* was much higher. The mutation rate, to intermediate levels of resistance to 8-azaguanine in bone marrow cells, of $5 \times 10^{-4}$ was comparable to that observed for resistance to arabinosylcytosine and for decreased thymidine transport (Table 1). These latter mutation rates are high compared with mutation rates of

Table 1. *Comparison of mutation rates in mammalian cells in culture*

| Resistance to | Cell line | Mutation rate[a] | Ref. |
|---|---|---|---|
| Puromycin | AMK-2 (mouse L cells)[b] | $4 \times 10^{-6}$<br>$1 \times 10^{-4}$ | LIEBERMAN and OVE (1959) |
| 8-Azaguanine | Human bone marrow[b] | $4.9 \times 10^{-4}$<br>$1 \times 10^{-6}$ | SZYBALSKI (1959) |
| | Chinese hamster cells (lung)[c] | $1.5 \times 10^{-8}$ | CHU et al. (1969) |
| | Mouse M-Mc cells[d] | $3 \times 10^{-6}$ | MORROW (1970) |
| | Human fibroblasts | $1 \times 10^{-6}$ | ALBERTINI and DEMARS (1970) |
| | Chinese hamster cells (lung) | $2.2 \times 10^{-5}$ | M. HARRIS (1971) |
| Arabinosyl-cytosine | Mouse leukemia cells *in vitro*[e] | $1 \times 10^{-4}$ | BACH (1969a) |
| Thymidine[f] | Chinese hamster fibroblasts (DON) | $2.6 \times 10^{-4}$ | BRESLOW and GOLDSBY (1969) |

[a] Spontaneous mutation rate per cell per generation.
[b] Mutation rate for the first and second step changes from sensitivity to resistance.
[c] A single high resistance level was detected.
[d] An intermediate level of resistance was detected; the mutation rate given is for the higher level of resistance. The cell line is similar to mouse L cells.
[e] No evidence for a mutagenic effect of arabinosylcytosine was found; however, the frequency of mutation to resistance was reduced significantly by treatment with quinacrine, an antimutagenic agent (BACH, 1969b).
[f] Cells were selected for loss of thymidine transport.

$10^{-9}$ to $10^{-6}$ in bacteria. Arabinosylcytosine-resistant populations of mouse leukemia and human leukemia appear to arise readily (F. M. SCHABEL, JR., personal communication; STEUART and BURKE, 1971).

M. HARRIS (1971) points out that fluctuation tests only establish the spontaneous or noninducible origin of a given change without distinguishing between (1) chromosomal mutations, (2) gene mutations, and (3) stable changes in phenotypic expression. Examples of mutational changes and of stable changes in phenotype accompanying resistance to anticancer agents are considered below.

## A. Chromosomal Changes

Evidence has been presented for an association between drug resistance in mouse leukemia and a specific chromosomal change (BIESELE et al., 1959; BIEDLER et al., 1963, 1965; SCHRECKER et al., 1963). The absence of the subtelocentric chromosome in a methotrexate-resistant subline of L1210 leukemia cells was correlated with elevated dihydrofolic acid reductase activity. Another methotrexate-resistant subline of L1210 leukemia exhibited normal dihydrofolic acid reductase activity (that is, activity comparable to that of the parent line) and decreased uptake of methotrexate, as a consequence of altered transport of the drug into the cell, but did not show karyotype alteration. Further passage of this cell line in the presence of methotrexate resulted in loss of the subtelocentric chromosome and a ten fold increase in dihydrofolate reductase activity (Sirotnak et al., 1968). Kit et al. (1963) observed loss of chromosomes in mouse fibroblasts accompanying resistance to 5-bromodeoxyuridine. However, it cannot be said that drastic alterations in karyotype necessarily accompany the development of resistance (Hakala and Ishihara, 1962; Hoshino et al., 1966; Hutchison, 1971; Biedler et al., 1972).

## B. Gene Mutations

Efforts have been made to demonstrate DNA mediated transformations with mammalian cells[1]. Szybalska and Szybalski (1962) described transformation of 8-azaguanine resistant bone marrow cells to sensitive cells by means of DNA isolated from sensitive cells; Ozer (1966) did not confirm this observation. Other reports of DNA mediated transformations to drug resistance include those of Podgajetskaya et al. (1964) who used DNA from sarcolysin resistant rat sarcoma cells in culture. Majumbar and Bose (1968) reported DNA transformation with 6-azathymine resistant human carcinoma cells, and Fox et al. (1969) observed DNA mediated transfer of resistance to 5-iodo-2′-deoxyuridine in mouse P388 plasma cells. Roosa and Bailey (1970) recently described the transformation of sensitive P388 cells to 8-azaguanine resistance by means of DNA prepared from resistant cells. Results of these experiments provide direct evidence for DNA mediated changes in sensitivity to anticancer agents in mammalian cells.

## C. Stable Changes in Phenotypic Expression

M. Harris (1971) found essentially no changes in mutation frequencies for heat resistance and 8-azaguanine resistance in diploid, tetraploid and octaploid Chinese hamster cells in culture. These results were difficult to interpret in terms of gene or chromosome changes and led Harris to suspect "that at least some variations may arise in somatic cells by stable shifts in phenotypic expression rather than by changes in genetic information". The end result still would be a stable heritable change resulting, in this case, in decreased sensitivity to a drug or to a physical change in the environment.

Mezger-Freed (1972) observed that exposure of haploid or pseudodiploid frog embryo cells to potent mutagens, ethylmethane sulfonate or N-methyl-N′-nitro-N-nitrosoguanidine, did not give consistent increased frequency of resistance to 5-bromodeoxyuridine. Resistance in this case was interpreted to be the result of decreased permeability as a consequence of a change in surface membrane in stable variant phenotypes of non mutational origin. Breslow and Goldsby (1969) have shown decreased permeability to thymidine in 5-bromodeoxyuridine resistant mutants rather than the loss of thymidine kinase observed by Kit et al. (1963).

Resistance to anticancer drugs frequently has been demonstrated to be a stable heritable characteristic of neoplastic cells *in vivo* and in cell culture by many investigators (see Law, 1956; Hutchison, 1963, 1965). In experimental studies of drug resistance, its origins are not always specified and may not be defined in the

1 Transformation to resistance to anticancer agents in microorganisms has been demonstrated clearly. For example, resistance to methotrexate in *Diplococcus pneumoniae* was induced by DNA from resistant cells (Drew, 1957). Sirotnak et al. (1960a) isolated 8-azaguanine resistant mutants of *D. pneumoniae* and demonstrated that the parent cells could be transformed to resistance by means of DNA isolated from the resistant organism.

terms considered above. Stability of the characteristic of drug resistance in the cell line under investigation is, of course, important in studies of biochemical mechanisms of drug resistance, and usually this is specified by the investigator. In clinical studies, the criterion for describing a neoplasm as resistant depends primarily on observation of response to the drug under study.

## D. Mechanisms for Transmission of Resistance

Drug resistance can be transferred between bacterial cells by means of DNA isolated from resistant cells, as mentioned earlier.[1] In addition, drug resistance can be transferred by means of bacteriophage, which introduces a portion of the genome of the resistant cell into the sensitive cell (transduction), and by mating, in which DNA of a donor cell is introduced into a recipient cell by direct contact between the cells (BRAUN, 1965).

The observations of SUBAK-SHARPE et al. (1969) on "metabolic cooperation" between mammalian cells in culture have significance with regard to circumvention of drug-resistance and possibly to transmission of resistance. In this study, natural mutant cells lacking hypoxanthine-guanine phosphoribosyltransferase (SUBAK-SHARPE, 1965) were grown in mixed culture with hamster fibroblast cells which possessed this enzyme activity and therefore had the capacity to incorporate hypoxanthine into polynucleotides. The enzyme deficient cells did not incorporate radioactive hypoxanthine into nucleic acid unless physical contact was established with the enzymically competent cells. Contact by means of a cytoplasmic connecting "bridge" was sufficient; VAN ZEELAND et al. (1972) showed that separation of cells by a fibrin layer prevented metabolic cooperation. It cannot be said with certainty that only labeled nucleotide or polynucleotide was transferred, and the possibility exists that enzyme, messenger RNA, or episomal DNA might have been transferred. COX et al. (1970) presented evidence for transfer of enzyme product, i.e. inosinic and guanylic acids, from normal cells to enzyme deficient cells by metabolic cooperation. FUJIMOTO and SEEGMILLER (1970) interpreted the presence of cells having enzyme activity intermediate between normal and deficient cells to be a consequence of transfer of enzyme or messenger RNA from normal to mutant cells in cultured skin fibroblasts from patients heterozygous for Lesch-Nyhan disease.

The transfer of resistance between microbial cells, particularly *Enterobacteriaceae*, by extrachromosomal elements, presumably by genes which are a part of such extrachromosomal elements, now is well established (for reviews see WATANABE, 1963; SHAW, 1971; MITSUHASHI, 1971; DAVIES and ROWND, 1972). The conventional view of the development of populations of drug-resistant bacteria by mutation-selection is being revised to include such extrachromosomal elements ("plasmids," "episomes," "R-factors"). Concern has been expressed that such transferable extrachromosomal elements might play a part in the spread of drug resistance in the malaria parasite (PETERS, 1970). As yet there is no evidence of a role of such factors in expression of resistance to anticancer agents in neoplastic cells.

Perhaps more cautious wording, such as "spontaneous intercellular variation followed by selection," should be used with reference to the development of resistance in neoplastic cells in order to make allowance for possible epigenetic changes in somatic cells, as well as for mutations at the genetic level. Stable changes in gene expression, as well as changes in the genes themselves, may account for variation in a tumor cell population.

## E. Drug-Resistant Cells as Tools in Genetic Research

Drug resistance in mammalian cells that is associated with specific enzyme deficiencies has provided valuable tools for the study of genetics of somatic cells and, in turn, such studies contribute to an understanding of genetic aspects of resistance. The technique of fusion of somatic cell lines to produce hybrid cells, first described by BARSKI et al. (1960), now is in use in several laboratories.[2] For example, LITTLEFIELD (1966) fused sublines of mouse L cells; one subline was resistant to 5-bromodeoxyuridine and lacked thymidine kinase (see KIT et al., 1963); the other subline was resistant to 8-azaguanine and lacked hypoxanthine-guanine phosphoribosyltransferase. Hybrid cells could be selected that possessed both enzyme activities and had regained sensitivity to 5-bromodeoxyuridine and 8-azaguanine. The method for selection of small numbers of hybrid cells in the presence of the parent cell lines depends on the enzyme deficiences associated with drug resistance. Parental sublines deficient in either thymidine kinase or hypoxanthine-guanine phosphoribosyltransferase cannot survive in medium containing methotrexate that is fortified with thymidine and hypoxanthine. Those hybrid cells that possess both enzyme activities utilize the exogenous substrates and survive exposure to methotrexate.

CHU et al. (1969) isolated genetic variants in a Chinese hamster cell line. One mutant line, incapable of utilizing L-glutamic acid, required L-glutamine for growth; another subline, selected for resistance to 8-azaguanine, was unable to utilize exogenous hypoxanthine. A hybrid cell line was derived by plating the glutamine-requiring and azaguanine-resistant cells together in an experimental medium in which neither of the parent cell lines could survive. The resultant hybrid, which underwent cell division, could utilize L-glutamic acid for growth and was sensitive to 8-azaguanine. The authors concluded that glutamine auxotrophy and azaguanine resistance behaved as recessive characters in the hybrid cell.

The hypoxanthine-guanine phosphoribosyltransferase deficiency associated with the Lesch-Nyhan syndrome (NYHAN, 1968) is known to involve mutation of a gene located on the X-chromosome (SEEGMILLER et al., 1967). By means of the hybridization technique and cell lines deficient in hypoxanthine-guanine phosphoribosyltransferase, the X-chromosomal linkage of this enzyme was confirmed in several laboratories (NABHOLZ et al., 1969; SILAGI et al., 1969; SINISCALCO et al., 1969; RUDDLE et al., 1971; GRZESCHIK et al., 1972). By means of specific techniques the latter group provided evidence for the localization of hypoxanthine-guanine phosphoribosyltransferase, glucose-6-phosphate dehydrogenase and phosphoglycerate kinase within the X-chromosome.

## F. The Problem of Drug Resistance

The studies cited in the previous section provide examples of the use of drug-resistant cell lines as tools for genetic studies in mammalian cells. Conversely, these studies provide strong evidence of a genetic basis for drug resistance in somatic cells. The development of drug resistance in large populations of neoplastic cells must be viewed as an inescapable biological fact by experimental and clinical

2 This interesting technique also has been used in producing hybrids from different types of cells, for example: (1) avian nucleated erythrocytes and mammalian cells (see HARRIS and WATKINS, 1965; SCHWARTZ et al., 1971); (2) human-mouse somatic hybrids (WEISS and GREEN, 1967; KUSANO et al., 1971); (3) human-Chinese hamster somatic cell hybrids (KAO and PUCK, 1970; WESTERVELD et al., 1971). Such hybrids are valuable in genetic analysis of somatic cells in culture (MATSUYA et al., 1968; H. HARRIS, 1971 a) and in analysis of malignancy (H. HARRIS, 1971 b).

chemotherapists (LAW, 1956; WELCH, 1959; KLEIN, 1961). This is not to say that the chemotherapist has no alternatives when faced with the spectre of resistance. As discussed elsewhere in this volume, judicious use of combination chemotherapy decreases the probability of the development of resistance in a population of neoplastic cells. A necessary condition for combination chemotherapy is that the drugs used in combination act by different mechanisms so that there is complete independence of possible mutational events leading to resistance to each drug. If the spontaneous mutation rate for resistance to each of the drugs is $10^{-6}$ and the conditions stated above are met, then the theoretical mutation rate for simultaneous resistance to both drugs would be $10^{-12}$. This was illustrated in bacteria by SZYBALSKI and BRYSON (1953) with a combination of *p*-aminosalicylic acid and isoniazid. The probability is small that a cell resistant to two drugs will arise in a population of cells.

## G. Other Aspects of the Problem of Drug Resistance

As used in the present context drug resistance refers to acquired resistance in cells initially sensitive to the drug. The ultimate criterion of sensitivity of a neoplasm to a drug is prolonged survival (cure) of the tumor-bearing host. In laboratory and clinical practice sensitivity of a neoplasm to a drug is measured in terms of increased life span, decreased tumor mass, decreased numbers of neoplastic cells, or other objective criteria that can be applied. With the advent of drugs active against some rapidly growing neoplasms came recognition that many neoplasms, particularly solid tumors, were unresponsive to chemotherapy. Such neoplasms are "naturally resistant" to a particular chemotherapeutic agent and resistance in these instances can be described as "innate," "intrinsic," or "inherent". A distinction must be made between *intrinsic* resistance in initially unresponsive neoplasms and *acquired* resistance, which develops in neoplasms that were initially responsive to chemotherapy and which will be the primary concern of this discussion.

## H. Cell Cycle Kinetics and Drug Resistance

Some comment should be made on intrinsic resistance, since this appellation may imply that no response to drug therapy is to be expected. Studies of the last two decades on the life cycle of cells and on the kinetics of cell proliferation provide a basis for understanding unresponsiveness in some tumors (BASERGA, 1971). Cells that are proliferating are recognized as undergoing mitosis; a prerequisite for mitosis is the replicative synthesis of DNA which occurs during a defined period of the cell cycle, the *S* phase. MENDELSOHN (1962, 1969) developed the concept of growth fraction; that is, that fraction of a given cell population that is "in cycle" and therefore progressing toward mitosis and cell division. STEEL (1967, 1968) has considered the factor of cell loss from neoplasms through cell death and lysis. Thus, the rate of growth of a population of tumor cells, the doubling time, is determined (1) by the cell cycle time, (2) by the fraction of the total population of cells that are in cycle, and (3) by the rate of cell death and subsequent loss of cells. For solid tumors other factors may be involved, such as anoxia or nutritional deficiencies, that may be a consequence of blood supply (TANNOCK, 1968, 1969). In simplest terms, the tissue that constitutes a population of tumor cells or normal cells consists of (1) continuously dividing cells, (2) nondividing cells, and (3) resting cells (SKIPPER, 1969). The latter cells may be brought into cycle by hormone stimulation, increased blood supply, and uncrowding of cells as a consequence of chemical, physical, or mechanical damage.

The concept has developed that cells in cycle are more vulnerable to attack by certain drugs; more specifically, cells may be vulnerable to certain drugs in only one phase of the cell cycle. Thus, agents, such as arabinosylcytosine that specifically interfere with DNA synthesis, are effective against those cells in the *S* phase of the cell life cycle. According to this concept, neoplasms with a large growth fraction probably would be more vulnerable to attack by inhibitors of DNA synthesis. The acute leukemias are particularly vulnerable to chemotherapeutic attack by inhibitors of DNA synthesis since most of the cells are in cycle. SKIPPER (1968, 1970, 1971a, b, c) has presented an extensive analysis of the proliferative state of neoplasms and response to chemotherapy based on consideration of cell cycle kinetics. In brief, it can be said that agents that specifically inhibit DNA synthesis are likely to be most effective when administered on schedules that take into account the cell cycle characteristics of the neoplasm so as to achieve effective levels of drug periodically in order to inhibit that portion of the cell population undergoing DNA replication (SKIPPER et al., 1967). The schedule should provide for recovery of damage done to proliferating host tissues that also would be sensitive to inhibitors of DNA synthesis, such as bone marrow and intestinal epithelium (SCHABEL, 1968; SKIPPER et al., 1970; DEVITA, 1971).

In contrast to the leukemias, many advanced solid tumors are unresponsive to chemotherapy with agents that are effective against rapidly growing neoplasms. One explanation is found in data which suggest that, as tumors increase in size, the growth fraction of the tumor decreases; that is, the number of tumor cells that are in cycle decreases (LASTER et al., 1969). Alkylating agents such as cyclophosphamide and BCNU damage cells that are in cycle, as well as resting cells. The optimal dose schedule for alkylating agents appears to be one in which relatively large single doses are given at intervals (see SKIPPER et al., 1970; SKIPPER, 1971a, b, c). SCHABEL (1969) suggests the use of sequential therapy in which treatment with agents that are not cell cycle specific (e.g. alkylating agents) is followed by treatment with agents that are specific for one phase of the cell cycle (e.g. cytosine arabinoside). The hypothesis is that the first agent kills both resting cells and cells in cycle; as a consequence of cell death and cell loss there results an increase in the growth fraction of the surviving tumor cells and an increased sensitivity to cell cycle specific agents. Also, the probability of resistant cells arising would be low, as discussed above.

This brief excursion into aspects of the cell cycle and its relationship to chemotherapy serves to indicate the significance of such kinetic studies and also serves to emphasize that one basis for intrinsic resistance of a neoplasm to chemotherapy may lie in this area rather than in some biochemical lesion in the neoplastic cells, such as failure to activate an inhibitor. Conversely, a neoplasm that lacks the capacity to metabolize an administered drug to its active form or that does not take up the drug cannot respond to therapy with that drug no matter what principles of cell cycle kinetics are applied. Although the emphasis in this presentation is on acquired mechanisms of resistance to agents initially effective against neoplastic cells, it is necessary to keep in mind other reasons for nonresponsiveness of neoplasms.

## Mechanisms of Resistance to Folic Acid Analogs

It is appropriate to begin the discussion of resistance mechanisms with folic acid analogs, since aminopterin, 4-amino-4-deoxyfolic acid (SEEGER et al., 1947, 1949), was the first antimetabolite used to advantage in the clinical treatment of leukemia (FARBER et al., 1948), and methotrexate, 4-amino-10-methyl-4-deoxyfolic acid (COSULICH and SMITH, 1948), continues to be a useful anticancer agent. Also, the study of acquired resistance to folic acid analogs, particularly resistance to methotrexate, provides several examples of resistance mechanisms: (1) increased level of the target enzyme, dihydrofolate reductase, (2) altered properties of the target enzyme, and (3) decreased uptake of the inhibitor by resistant cells. These and other mechanisms will be examined in some detail after brief consideration of the mode of action of folic acid antagonists.

Folic acid (F) is enzymically reduced to dihydrofolic acid (DHF) and tetrahydrofolic acid (THF) by NADPH and dihydrofolic acid reductase (EC 1.5.1.3):

$$\mathrm{F} + \mathrm{NADPH} + \mathrm{H}^+ \rightarrow \mathrm{DHF} + \mathrm{NADP}^+$$
$$\mathrm{DHF} + \mathrm{NADPH} + \mathrm{H}^+ \rightarrow \mathrm{THF} + \mathrm{NADP}^+.$$

The reduction of DHF to THF proceeds more rapidly than does the reduction of F to DHF. The enzyme is widely distributed and occurs in normal cells and in neoplastic cells (see HUENNEKENS, 1968; BLAKLEY, 1969). The interconversion of THF and various formyl and methyl derivatives, as well as the formation and subsequent utilization of these derivatives in the synthesis of thymidylic acid, purines, and amino acids is concisely summarized by BLAKLEY (1969) as shown in Fig. 1.

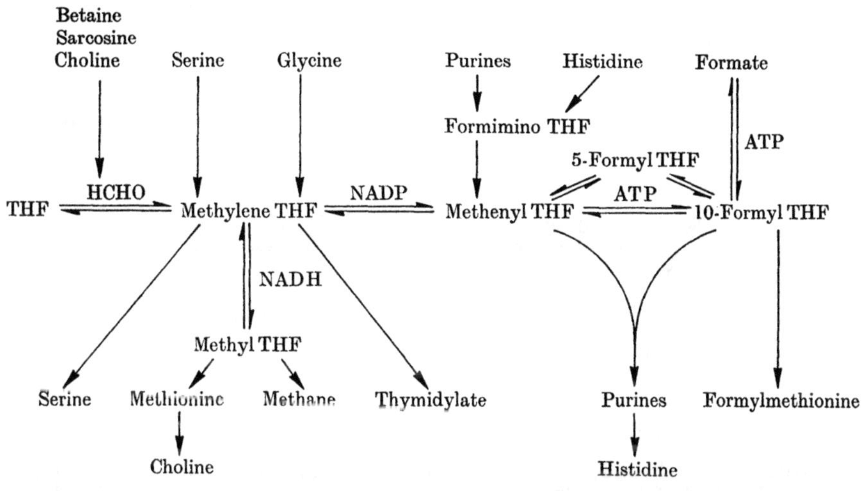


Fig. 1. Interconversion of tetrahydrofolate derivatives in relation to the generation and utilization of one-carbon units (from BLAKLEY, 1969, with permission of the author and Nord-Holland Publishing Company, Amsterdam)

The inhibition of dihydrofolate reductase is widely accepted as the primary effect of folic acid analogs (NICHOL and WELCH, 1950; FUTTERMAN, 1957; OSBORN et al., 1958; ZAKRZEWSKI and NICHOL, 1958, 1961). It is important to note that, except for the synthesis of thymidylic acid, there is no change in the oxidation state of the one-carbon unit transferred in the reactions depicted in Fig. 1. Also, the oxidation state of the pteridine ring is unaltered in the reactions mediated by folate coenzymes with the exception of thymidylic acid synthesis; that is, tetrahydrofolic acid is generated by transfer of the one-carbon unit with the exception of thymidylic acid synthesis, in which case dihydrofolic acid is formed.

Thymidylate synthetase catalyzes the synthesis of thymidylic acid by reaction of deoxyuridylic acid and 5, 10-methylene THF (HUMPHREYS and GREENBERG, 1958; FRIEDKIN, 1963; BLAKLEY, 1969). Dihydrofolic acid is generated in this reaction and THF is then regenerated by the action of dihydrofolate reductase; this sequence is represented by a cycle in Fig. 2 (HUENNEKENS et al., 1963; FRIEDKIN, 1963). Inhibition of dihydrofolate reductase results in a decrease in THF which in turn depletes the pool of 5, 10-methylene THF and also of other THF derivatives. The consequences of this are, first, inhibition of thymidylic acid synthesis and then inhibition of the synthesis of purine ribonucleotides and of serine, methionine, and histidine (see Fig. 1). Thus, the conversion of 5,10-methylene THF to DHF during thymidylate synthesis and the inhibition of DHF reductase are key factors in describing the metabolic effects of folic acid analogs.

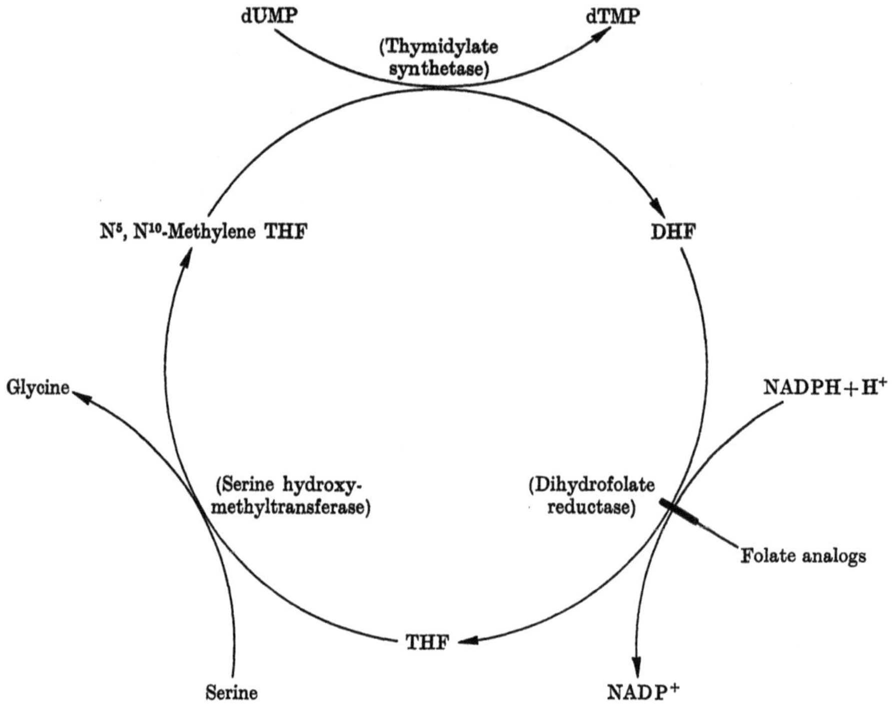


Fig. 2. Biosynthesis of thymidylic acid with accompanying formation of dihydrofolate. Folate analogs inhibit dihydrofolate reductase and thus prevent regeneration of THF and $N^5$, $N^{10}$-methylene THF, thereby blocking further synthesis of thymidylic acid

## A. Dihydrofolate Reductase Activity and Folate Analogs

The marked affinity of 4-amino-4-deoxyfolates for dihydrofolate reductase and the essential irreversibility of inhibition was noted by PETERS and GREENBERG (1959). Values for $K_i$ in the range of $10^{-10}$ to $10^{-11}$ have been estimated for rat liver reductase by WERKHEISER (1961) who was able to demonstrate a titration, or "stoichiometric inhibition," of this enzyme by aminopterin when folate was the substrate at pH 6.0. Analogous results were obtained under similar conditions, but with dihydrofolate reductase from different sources (ZAKRZEWSKI and NICHOL, 1961). In such cases it appears that essentially all inhibitor may be bound to enzyme when the concentration of inhibitor is less than the concentration of enzyme, and classical treatment of kinetic data cannot be used under these circumstances. It is important to note that the degree of dissociation of the methotrexate-dihydrofolate reductase complex varies with the source of the enzyme, the substrate (folate or dihydrofolate), and the pH at which the study is made (see BLAKLEY, 1969). BERTINO et al. (1964) demonstrated this clearly with dihydrofolate reductase of Ehrlich ascites tumor cells. With folate as substrate, methotrexate was a stoichiometric inhibitor at pH 5.3 to 6.2; with dihydrofolate as a substrate, methotrexate was not a stoichiometric inhibitor at pH 5.9; at pH 7.6 methotrexate acted as a competitive inhibitor by Michaelis-Menten kinetics. Similar results were obtained with dihydrofolate reductase from human leukemia cells (BERTINO, 1965).

## B. Resistance to Folate Analogs Accompanied by Increased Levels of Dihydrofolate Reductase

Three groups of investigators observed independently that the level of dihydrofolate reductase was greater in antifolate-resistant neoplasms than it was in the parent sensitive neoplasms (FISCHER, 1961; HAKALA et al., 1961; MISRA et al., 1961) and results of other studies have confirmed this observation (FRIEDKIN et al., 1962; HAKALA and ISHIHARA, 1962; BIEDLER et al., 1963, 1965, 1972; HAKALA, 1965a, b; HOSHINO et al., 1966; PERKINS et al., 1967; SCHRECKER et al., 1971). Experimental evidence indicates that these drug-resistant neoplasms consist of genetically stable mutant lines. From the preceding discussion of binding of antifolates to dihydrofolate reductase it follows that more drug would be required to inhibit mutant cells with an increased level of enzyme.

Consideration has been given to the idea of exploiting such an increased level of an enzyme to the detriment of the resistant cell. Friedkin and his associates examined homofolic acid and dihydrohomofolic acid with the idea that these analogs, as substrates for dihydrofolate reductase, would be converted to tetrahydrohomofolate, an inhibitor of thymidylate synthesis, more extensively in resistant cells than in sensitive cells or in normal tissue (GOODMAN et al., 1964; MEAD et al., 1966). Normal tissues *in vivo* do not appear to develop resistance to methotrexate (BERTINO, 1963). The idea is an attractive one since the "lethal synthesis" of tetrahydrohomofolate presumably would be more extensive in the resistant neoplasm than in normal tissues. Although hopes for such rational exploitation of a biochemical alteration accompanying resistance have not been realized (FRIEDKIN et al., 1971), this principle may yet be successfully applied in attacking resistant neoplastic cells.

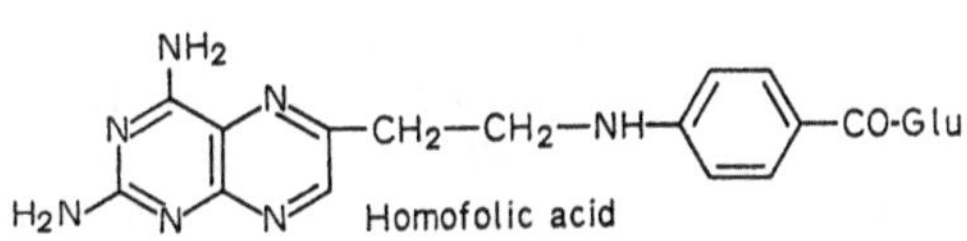

Homofolic acid

BERTINO et al. (1963) observed an apparent rapid rise in reductase activity in normal erythrocytes and leukocytes following methotrexate treatment of humans; this effect was pronounced in blood cells (HILLCOAT et al., 1967, 1971). The enzyme level in methotrexate-treated cells returned to normal levels after treatment was discontinued. Careful examination revealed that the level of enzyme activity observed was dependent on the pH at which the enzyme activity was determined *in vitro*. Thus, when measured at pH 8.5, a marked rise in leukocyte dihydrofolate reductase was apparent, a moderate increase in activity was seen at pH 7.0, and a decrease in activity was observed when the assay was carried out at pH 5.5. BERTINO (1965) concluded that methotrexate binding may protect the enzyme from normal inactivation. Tightly bound methotrexate inhibited enzyme activity when assays were done at low pH. However, at pH 8.5 in the presence of dihydrofolate, methotrexate was displaced from the enzyme, which then actively catalyzed reduction of dihydrofolate to tetrahydrofolate, revealing higher levels of enzyme in antifolate-treated cells.

Subsequent work has indicated that methotrexate does stabilize dihydrofolate reductase in cells in culture (HAKALA and SUOLINNA, 1966; HILLCOAT et al., 1967) and *in vivo* (HILLCOAT et al., 1971) by protecting the enzyme from degradation. The increased amount of enzyme present in methotrexate-treated human erythrocytes and leukocytes could not be distinguished from enzyme normally present in bone marrow cells or from enzyme isolated from methotrexate-resistant L1210 cells (BERTINO et al., 1970).

If studies of dihydrofolate activity *in vitro* are to be related to enzyme activity in the intact cell it is evident that care must be taken to perform the enzyme assays at near physiological pH values. The increased dihydrofolate reductase activity measured in blood cells following methotrexate treatment obviously is not a stable genetic change such as that observed in resistant microorganisms and neoplasms.

## C. Multiple Forms of Dihydrofolate Reductase in Cells Resistant to Folate Analogs

Dihydrofolate reductase of the parent strain of *S. faecium* has been purified and characterized (BLAKLEY and MCDOUGALL, 1961; ALBRECHT et al., 1966, 1969; HILLCOAT and BLAKLEY, 1966). The enzyme from the methotrexate-sensitive strain of *S. faecium*, SF/O, has been separated into two components; the major component is specific for reduction of dihydrofolate and the minor component catalyzes reduction of both folate and dihydrofolate (ALBRECHT et al., 1969). Methotrexate-resistant strains of *S. faecium* also possess the enzyme activity which utilizes both folate and dihydrofolate as substrates and which differs sufficiently in physical and chemical behavior to be distinctly separated from the enzyme that predominates in the sensitive strain (ALBRECHT et al., 1966; HILLCOAT and BLAKLEY, 1966; NIXON and BLAKLEY, 1968). The methotrexate-resistant mutant of *S. faecium*, designated SF/A, is about 300,000-fold resistant to methotrexate and the mutant designated SF/$A_k$ is about 30,000-fold resistant (HUTCHISON, 1958; JOHNSON and HUTCHISON, 1964). SF/$A_k$ and SF/A exhibit, respectively, about 6 times and 35 times the reductase activity of SF/O. The increased reductase activity of SF/A is due almost entirely to the presence of increased amounts of the enzyme which has the capacity to reduce both folic acid and dihydrofolic acid. ALBRECHT et al. (1969) concluded that the parent sensitive organism, SF/O, possessed two constitutive enzymes: a highly active, specific dihydrofolate reductase activity and, as a minor component, a folate reductase with extremely low activity. In fact, the latter enzyme was not detected in earlier work with this organism. In the methotrexate-resistant mutant, SF/$A_k$, there was only a doubling in the activity of the specific dihydrofolate reductase, whereas the nonspecific folate-dihydrofolate reductase activity increased several hundred-fold (ALBRECHT and HUTCHISON, personal communication). NIXON and BLAKLEY (1968) concluded from their analysis that the total concentration of the combined dihydrofolate reductases in methotrexate-resistant *S. faecium* was 87-fold increased over that of the sensitive strain. This increase seemed relatively insignificant compared to the high level of methotrexate resistance achieved; therefore, it seemed unlikely that the great degree of resistance was attributable solely to the amount of reductase available to bind methotrexate.

What is the significance of the presence of these two reductase enzymes? In the sensitive organism the nonspecific folate reductase, even at the low levels of activity present, provides the cell with a means of utilizing unreduced folate when it is available (ALBRECHT et al., 1969). The need for dihydrofolate reductase is essential for maintaining tetrahydrofolate for thymidylate biosynthesis (Fig. 2) and the cell maintains a constant level of this enzyme. In the sensitive organism methotrexate in small concentrations may inhibit first the folate-reducing enzyme present in small amounts and then, at larger concentrations, both enzyme activities are inhibited (see NIXON and BLAKLEY, 1968). In the resistant organism the decreased sensitivity to methotrexate appears to be a consequence of the greatly increased level of the folate-dihydrofolate reductase which permits the cell to utilize unreduced folate, thus increasing the concentration of dihydrofolate. It must then be assumed that sufficient amounts of tetrahydrofolate are formed in the resistant cells in the presence of methotrexate to maintain thymidylate synthesis.

## D. Altered Enzyme in Cells Resistant to Folate Analogs

Detailed analyses of genetic and biochemical aspects of resistance to folate analogs in *D. pneumoniae* have been presented by SIROTNAK and his colleagues; increased dihydrofolate reductase levels are present in the methotrexate-resistant mutants (SIROTNAK, 1969, 1970, 1971; SIROTNAK and HUTCHISON, 1966; SIROTNAK et al., 1964d, 1969). Resistant strains of *D. pneumoniae* have been isolated which synthesize an altered form of dihydrofolate reductase (SIROTNAK, 1969, 1970, 1972; SIROTNAK and HUTCHISON, 1965, 1966; SIROTNAK and HACHTEL, 1969; SIROTNAK and WILLIAMS, 1970; SIROTNAK et al., 1960b, 1964a–d, 1969). These mutants have been divided into two categories, A and B, on the basis of their interaction with dihydrofolic acid, folic acid, methotrexate and NADPH. Type A mutants exhibit a decrease in affinity for dihydrofolic acid and methotrexate and an increased affinity for NADPH. Also, reductase from Type A mutants is less stable than that from wild type (SIROTNAK, 1969, 1970; SIROTNAK and WILLIAMS, 1970), and the mutant enzyme is isolated in an associated form having molecular weights greater than the wild-type enzyme (SIROTNAK and HUTCHISON, 1965, 1966; SIROTNAK and WILLIAMS, 1970). Mutations of the A type also determine increases in the amount of the mutant enzyme (SIROTNAK, 1969, 1970, 1971; SIROTNAK et al., 1969).

Dihydrofolate reductase from Type B mutants shows a pronounced decrease in affinity for 4-amino-4-deoxyfolate analogs, but exhibits no differences from wild-type enzyme in binding of dihydrofolate, folate, or NADPH. The pH optimum of mutant enzyme of this type is shifted from pH 7.3 to 6.7, but no changes in physical properties, such as stability and molecular weight, were observed (SIROTNAK, 1972; SIROTNAK and HUTCHISON, 1966; SIROTNAK et al., 1964a, d). *D. pneumoniae* strains carrying both A and B mutations have been prepared by recombination (SIROTNAK and HACHTEL, 1969) and the dihydrofolate reductase characterized (SIROTNAK, 1972; SIROTNAK and HUTCHISON, 1966; SIROTNAK et al., 1964d).

The genetic and biochemical analysis of methotrexate-resistant mutants of *D. pneumoniae* provide eloquent testimony to the complexity and subtlety of the drug resistance problem. It is difficult to visualize such an extensive genetic analysis being made in mammalian cells; nevertheless, these studies clearly demonstrate some of the possibilities and consequences of enzyme alterations accompanying mutations to resistance to an inhibitor.

Results of several studies in drug-resistant mammalian cells indicated that dihydrofolate reductase was the same in sensitive and resistant cells although increased levels of enzyme activity were observed (KASHKET et al., 1964; RAUNIO and HAKALA, 1967; McCULLOUGH and BERTINO, 1971; NAKAMURA and LITTLEFIELD, 1972). On the other hand, BLUMENTHAL and GREENBERG (1970) presented evidence that methotrexate-resistant cells of leukemia L4946 produced a structurally altered enzyme. The resistant enzyme was immunologically distinguishable from the sensitive enzyme. Also, the $K_m$ of the resistant enzyme for dihydrofolic acid was lower than that for the sensitive enzyme by a factor of 10. The sensitive and resistant enzymes differed in chloride ion stimulation and in sensitivity to inhibition by *p*-chloromercuribenzoate. The resistant enzyme was functional in the presence of concentrations of methotrexate that completely inactivated the sensitive enzyme, a result similar to that obtained with mutant strains of *D. pneumoniae* (SIROTNAK, 1972; SIROTNAK et al., 1964a, c, d). ALBRECHT et al. (1972) also found a species of dihydrofolate reductase in methotrexate-resistant Chinese hamster cell lines that differed from the parent cell enzyme. The enzyme from resistant cells, the level of which was increased, exhibited decreased affinity for methotrexate. Whereas, methotrexate interacted stoichiometrically with the parent enzyme, it was a reversible inhibitor of the resistant enzyme.

It is also of interest that altered dihydrofolate reductase, as well as increased level of enzyme was observed in pyrimethamine resistant *Plasmodium berghei* (FERONE et al., 1969, 1970; FERONE, 1970; DIGGENS et al., 1970).

## E. Cofactor Binding to Dihydrofolate Reductases in Relation to Drug Resistance

HUENNEKENS et al. (1971) summarized characteristics of dihydrofolate reductases from different sources, including methotrexate sensitive and resistant microorganisms and neoplasms. In view of the observed variations in kinetic properties (e.g. $K_m$ values for substrates, turnover numbers, utilization of folate as substrate), no generalizations can be made. The existence of what appeared to be multiple forms of dihydrofolate reductase in chicken liver (MELL et al., 1968), leukemia L1210 (HARDING et al., 1970), and *L. casei* (DUNLAP et al., 1971a; GUNDERSEN et al., 1972) is a recently encountered variation of interest. Separation and characterization of multiple enzyme forms was accomplished by electrophoresis or by chromatography; form II of the enzyme had a greater net negative charge than form I. It now appears that these two separable forms of dihydrofolate reductase from *L. casei* can be distinguished by the presence or absence of NADPH: form I lacks bound NADPH, and form II has one equivalent of NADPH tightly, but not covalently bound. This also appears to be true of the chicken liver enzyme in which still a third form of the enzyme may exist (see HUENNEKENS et al., 1971). During the course of development of resistance to methotrexate in L1210 cells HARDING et al. (1970) observed a greater initial increase in enzyme II. Continued passage of L1210 cells in methotrexate treated animals resulted in cells completely resistant to drug; the resistant cells showed a further increase in the level of enzyme II. As suggested by HUENNEKENS et al. (1971), it is possible that NADPH binding to enzyme may be a factor governing the inhibition of dihydrofolate reductase by folate antagonists. This can be inferred from an earlier study by PERKINS and BERTINO (1966) who found that binding of 2,4,7-triamino-6-phenylpteridine (triamterene) to the dihydrofolate reductase isolated from methotrexate resistant L1210 cells was much tighter with an enzyme-NADPH complex than with enzyme alone.

## F. Decreased Uptake of Drug as a Mechanism of Resistance to Methotrexate

PINE (1960) observed that resistance to antifolates in *Bacillus subtilis* was accompanied by decreased capacity for transport. In the course of studying genetic aspects of the development of resistance to methotrexate in *D. pneumoniae*, SIROTNAK and his associates have described distinct classes of mutations. One class was a consequence of genetic modification both of structure and amount of enzyme, as discussed above, and the other class was shown to be a consequence of mutations which resulted in impairment in the transport of methotrexate (SIROTNAK et al., 1964b, 1967a, b). Dihydrofolate reductase was unaltered in these mutants but there was an increase in the $K_m$ of the transport system for methotrexate and a shift in pH optimum, suggesting an alteration in a permease.

FISCHER (1962) isolated a stable line of L5178Y leukemic cells from a methotrexate-resistant clone which took up the drug at a much slower rate than did the parent sensitive line. Sensitive cells concentrated the drug from the medium, whereas, at equilibrium, the drug concentration in resistant cells was significantly less than that in the medium. Dihydrofolate reductase activity in resistant cells was equal to that in sensitive cells and the enzyme was unaltered with respect to affinity for methotrexate. Subsequent work by WERKHEISER (1963) with P388 ascites tumor cells, by KESSEL et al. (1965) with resistant lines of L1210 and P288 leukemia, by BRAGANCA et al. (1967) with Yoshida sarcoma cells, by SIROTNAK et al. (1967c, 1968) with L1210 leukemia cells, and by HARRAP et al. (1971) with L5178Y leukemia have confirmed this mechanism of resistance to methotrexate.

SIROTNAK et al. (1968) and GOLDMAN et al. (1968) provided evidence that uptake of methotrexate in L1210 cells and in *D. pneumoniae* (SIROTNAK et al., 1967a) was mediated by an active transport system since uptake (1) occurred against a concentration gradient, (2) was temperature dependent, (3) required energy, (4) exhibited a pH optimum, and (5) followed Michaelis-Menten kinetics. A methotrexate-resistant subline, designated L1210/$XVI_4$, was impaired in uptake of methotrexate; an increased $K_m$ for the transport system with no appreciable change in maximum uptake velocity, $V_{max}$, was observed.

Continued transplantation of this subline in the presence of drug resulted in selection of a line with increased resistance, designated L1210/$XVI_{4a}$, which was characterized by an increased level of dihydrofolate reductase and by loss of the subtelocentric chromosome (SIROTNAK et al., 1967c, 1968). Thus, this line exhibited the kinetic properties of L1210/$XVI_4$ with respect to impaired transport of methotrexate in addition to an increased level of reductase. An interesting consequence of this dual change was that the rate of transport of methotrexate in L1210/$XVI_{4a}$ was like that of the parent methotrexate-sensitive line, L1210/V. The likely explanation for this finding is that the 10 fold increase in dihydrofolate reductase in L1210/$XVI_{4a}$ resulted in greater binding of methotrexate with consequent lowering of the intracellular concentration of free inhibitor. A steeper concentration gradient thus would be generated with resultant increased rate of transport despite the altered $K_m$ for methotrexate of the transport system in the resistant cells. This carefully documented study illustrates the complexity and the pitfalls that may be encountered in studies of drug resistance.

Evidence also has been presented for transport of methotrexate in Yoshida sarcoma cells (DIVEKAR et al., 1967) and in L1210 cells (KESSEL and HALL, 1967), but not in Ehrlich cells (KESSEL and HALL, 1967) or Sarcoma 180 (HAKALA, 1965a, b). The lack of concentrative uptake was offered as an explanation for the insensitivity of Ehrlich cells to methotrexate. An interesting feature of the studies with Sarcoma 180 cells was the demonstration that influx of methotrexate was slow, by diffusion, whereas efflux was a rapid, energy dependent process. HAKALA (1965a) pointed out that dissociation of the methotrexate-folate reductase complex then could result in loss of drug from the cell and it was considered that dissociation of the enzyme-inhibitor complex accounted for the lack of proportionality between the level of reductase in the cell and the degree of resistance.

## G. Intracellular Drug Alteration as a Mechanism of Resistance to Folate Antagonists

Studies of the metabolism of methotrexate in rodents and in man reveal that a large portion of administered drug is excreted unchanged (HENDERSON et al., 1965; JOHNS et al., 1966). Hepatic aldehyde oxidase from guinea pig and rabbit catalyzes the oxidation of methotrexate and of aminopterin to the 7-hydroxy derivative (JOHNS et al., 1966; REDETZKI et al., 1966; JOHNS and LOO, 1967); the rabbit enzyme was particularly active. ROTHENBERG (1969) obtained indirect evidence that methotrexate was altered in human leukemia cells, but no degradation product was identified. JACOBSEN and CATHIE (1960a, b) reported inactivation of aminopterin by chick embryo cells, chick fibroblasts, chick erythocytes, mouse liver, and mouse leukemia cells. The chemical nature of the inactivation was not defined; a cyclization of the glutamate moiety was postulated.

It can be seen from the preceding discussion that degradation of 4-amino-4-deoxyfolates does occur, but there is no evidence for increased degradation of folate analogs as a mechanism of acquired resistance to antifolates. Many of the studies on the uptake of methotrexate have been done with radioactive compound in order to measure accumulation. In cells where intracellular degradation is limited this may not be a problem, but it may introduce serious errors in studies with tissues, such as liver, that are known to oxidize folate analogs.

## H. Correlation of Changes in Biochemical Parameters with Response to Methotrexate

Acquired resistance to methotrexate in experimental neoplasms is mainly attributed to an increase in dihydrofolate reductase activity or to decreased uptake of the drug. Investigators seeking ways of predicting response to chemotherapy have compared the response of experimental neoplasms to methotrexate with levels of dihydrofolate reductase and with uptake of the drug.

In an examination of the response of transplantable rodent neoplasms to methotrexate, ROBERTS et al. (1965) found no correlation between dihydrofolate reductase levels and intrinsic resistance. Sublines of experimental neoplasms that had acquired resistance to methotrexate by prolonged passage *in vivo* did exhibit high levels of reductase. The same group of investigators observed a high degree of correlation between sensitivity to methotrexate and uptake of drug in ten transplantable rodent neoplasms (KESSEL et al., 1965). Two of these neoplasms, L1210/MTX and P288/MTX, had acquired resistance by exposure to methotrexate; they exhibited impaired uptake of drug as well as increased levels of dihydrofolate reductase. In subsequent studies, ROBERTS and WODINSKY (1968), ROBERTS and HALL (1969) and ROBERTS (1971) sought correlation between inhibition of reductase and incorporation of deoxyribonucleosides into DNA. Results of studies *in vivo* showed that doses of methotrexate that were therapeutic for the sensitive line completely inhibited dihydrofolic acid reductase prepared from washed cells for more than two hours both in sensitive and resistant lines. Inhibition of incorporation of deoxyuridine into DNA *in vivo* was more strongly inhibited in sensitive than in resistant cells. However, when methotrexate was administered to tumor bearing mice, which were then examined for deoxynucleoside incorporation *in vitro*, inhibition of incorporation of deoxyuridine into DNA was less pronounced than it was *in vivo* even though dihydrofolate reductase activity was strongly inhibited. Thus, correlation between dihydrofolate reductase activity and deoxyuridine incorporation was poor in these experiments. (See also HOFER, 1972, for related studies on $^{125}$I-iododeoxyuridine incorporation into DNA of L1210 cells.)

Increasing concentrations of methotrexate, when added to ascites tumor cells *in vitro*, inhibited deoxyuridine incorporation into DNA in a log-dose relationship in L1210 and P329 cells, but not in L1210/MTX cells. It was concluded that methotrexate levels in excess of the amount required to inhibit dihydrofolate reductase were necessary to inhibit deoxyuridine incorporation into DNA. This interpretation finds support in earlier work of WAHBA and FRIEDKIN (1961) and in more recent studies by BORSA and WHITMORE (1969a, b), which emphasized the inhibition of thymidylate synthetase by larger concentrations of methotrexate. Interest has been focused on the relationship between dihydrofolate reductase and thymidylate synthetase (DUNLAP et al., 1971b).

The generalization that methotrexate kills proliferating cells, but not non-proliferating cells, has been linked with the concept of thymineless death, in which DNA synthesis is selectively inhibited (RUECKERT and MUELLER, 1960; COHEN, 1971); RNA synthesis, protein synthesis and other cellular metabolic processes continue for a period of time. Intracellular concentrations of methotrexate in excess of that required to inhibit dihydrofolate reductase may directly affect other metabolic areas, but the depletion of intracellular tetrahydrofolate levels, a consequence of inhibition of dihydrofolate reductase, and the resultant secondary effects on synthesis of purine nucleotides, protein, and lipids (Fig. 1) provides an attractive basis for understanding the effectiveness of antifolates in rapidly proliferating tissues. But neither this knowledge, nor an understanding of mechanisms of resistance to antifolates, has enabled investigators to define criteria for clearly predicting the response of proliferating neoplasms, experimental or human, to methotrexate.

## Mechanisms of Resistance to Purine and Pyrimidine Analogs

It is generally accepted that nucleotides are biologically active forms of natural purines and pyrimidines as well as analogs (see BALIS, 1968; KIT, 1970; ROY-BURMAN, 1970, for recent reviews). KIDDER and DEWEY (1949) were among the first to recognize this from their study of 8-azaguanine. Examples of exceptions to this generalization are nucleosides such as psicofuranine (MAGEE and EBERTS, 1961; FUKUYAMA and MOYED, 1964), 9-$\beta$-D-arabinosyl-6-mercaptopurine (LEPAGE et al., 1969), and perhaps arabinosyladenine (TONO and COHEN, 1962); these nucleosides appear to be active without phosphorylation in some biological systems. Also, certain 9-alkylpurines are known to have growth-inhibitory effects (KELLEY et al., 1962; KIMBALL and LEPAGE, 1963); these derivatives cannot be phosphorylated and are active as such.

The major pathway for utilization of bases was not clearly recognized until KORNBERG et al. (1955a) identified 5-phosphoribosyl-1-pyrophosphate (PRPP). It was found that PRPP plays a key role in the synthesis of orotidylic acid (LIEBERMAN et al., 1955; HURLBERT and REICHARD, 1955) and in the utilization of natural purine bases (KORNBERG et al., 1955b; KORN et al., 1955), as well as of analogs of purine bases (LUKENS and HERRINGTON, 1957; WAY and PARKS, 1958).

The reactions of bases with PRPP are catalyzed by phosphoribosyltransferases (nucleotide pyrophosphorylases) in the presence of $Mg^{++}$.

$$\text{Base} + \text{PRPP} \xrightleftharpoons{Mg^{++}} \text{Ribonucleotide} + \text{PPi}$$

The synthesis of orotidylic acid by reaction of orotate and PRPP is readily reversible, in contrast to uracil and purine phosphoribosyltransferase activities, which favor nucleotide synthesis (KORNBERG, 1957). The Enzyme Commission recognizes four such enzymes (Table 2). Xanthine phosphoribosyltransferase activity appeared to be a distinct enzyme in *Streptococcus faecalis* mutants (BROCKMAN et al., 1961) and in *Salmonella typhimurium* (KALLÉ and GOTS, 1961), but this activity was weak in most mammalian cells studied (BROCKMAN et al., 1959b, c; POMALES et al., 1965; KELLEY et al., 1967). Guanine is a substrate for hypoxanthine-guanine phosphoribosyltransferase, which now is considered as a single enzyme (KRENITSKY et al., 1969; HENDERSON, 1969). However, it should be noted that KALLÉ and GOTS (1961) were led to consider the possibility that hypoxanthine and guanine phosphoribosyltransferases might exist as isozymes in *Salmonella typhimurium* (see GOTS, 1971).

Table 2. *Purine and pyrimidine phosphoribosyltransferase activities*[a]

| EC No. | Systematic name | Trivial name | Substrates |
|---|---|---|---|
| 2.4.2.7 | AMP: pyrophosphate phosphoribosyl-transferase | Adenine phosphoribosyltransferase<br>AMP pyrophosphorylase | Adenine, 4-amino-5-imidazolecarboxamide, 2,6-diaminopurine, 4-aminopyrazolo(3,4-d)pyrimidine, 2-fluoroadenine |
| 2.4.2.8 | IMP: pyrophosphate phosphoribosyltransferase | Hypoxanthine phosphoribosyltransferase<br>IMP pyrophosphorylase | 6-Mercaptopurine, hypoxanthine, 4-hydroxypyrazolo (3,4-d)-pyrimidine, guanine, 8-azaguanine, 6-thioguanine |
| 2.4.2.9 | UMP: pyrophosphate phosphoribosyl-transferase | Uracil phosphoribosyltransferase<br>UMP pyrophosphorylase | Uracil, 5-fluorouracil |
| 2.4.2.10 | Orotidine-5′-phosphate: pyrophosphate phosphoribosyltransferase | Orotate phosphoribosyltransferase<br>OMP pyrophosphorylase | Orotic acid, 5-fluoroorotic acid |
| | | Pyrimidine phosphoribosyltransferase[b] | Orotic acid, uracil, 5-fluorouracil, xanthine, uric acid |

[a] These enzymes originally were designated pyrophosphorylases by analogy with phosphorylases. Because their primary function is in the formation of nucleotides they are better regarded as synthetases (KORNBERG, 1962); therefore, the trivial name phosphoribosyltransferase is preferable to pyrophosphorylase.

[b] This enzyme appears to be distinct from orotate phosphoribosyltransferase of mammalian cells.

Pyrimidine phosphoribosyltransferases require special attention since there appear to be distinctive differences between the enzymes of microorganisms and of mammalian cells. A specific UMP pyrophosphorylase has been purified from bacterial cells that require uracil for growth (CANELLAKIS, 1957; CRAWFORD et al., 1957). In an *E. coli* strain, which contained both orotate and uracil phosphoribosyltransferase activities, it was observed that a fluorouracil resistant mutant had lost activity for both uracil and 5-fluorouracil; orotate phosphoribosyltransferase activity was unaltered in the resistant mutant (BROCKMAN et al., 1960). The presence of uracil phosphoribosyltransferase activity in mammalian cells has been open to question and the major pathway for utilization of uracil was considered to be by the sequential action of uridine phosphorylase and uridine kinase (REICHARD, 1959). SKÖLD (1958, 1960) demonstrated that 5-fluorouracil serves as a substrate for these enzymes with the formation of 5-fluorouridine and 5-fluorouridylic acid. Unexpectedly, 5-fluorouracil was found to be a substrate for a pyrimidine phosphoribosyltransferase of calf thymus; a similar enzyme was described in lymphosarcoma cells (KASBEKAR and GREENBERG, 1963; KASBEKAR et al., 1964) and in beef erythrocytes (HATFIELD and WYNGAARDEN, 1964). These interesting observations have been extended by REYES (1969) and by REYES and HALL (1969) who examined mouse neoplasms for 5-fluorouracil phosphoribosyltransferase activity. It appears that this enzyme is distinct from orotate phosphoribosyltransferase.

Enzymatic reactions may be directly inhibited by nucleotide analogs such as 6-mercaptopurine ribonucleotide, 6-methylthiopurine ribonucleotide, 6-azauridylic acid, 5-fluorodeoxyuridylic acid, and arabinosylcytosine triphosphate; other nucleotide analogs can be incorporated into nucleic acids in place of natural bases. For example, nucleotides of 8-azaguanine, 6-thioguanine, and arabinosylcytosine may be incorporated into both RNA and DNA; 5-fluorouridylic acid and 5-azacytidylic acid are incorporated into RNA; 5-azadeoxycytidylic acid is incorporated into DNA. Cells that have undergone deletion or loss of activity of those enzymes (phosphorylases, kinases, phosphoribosyltransferases) that "activate" analogs by converting them to nucleotides then would be insensitive to analogs of bases and nucleosides. Thus, the concept has grown that enzymatic syntheses of nucleotides from base analogs can be considered as examples of "lethal syntheses," to use the terminology of PETERS (1952).

While it is clear that failure to form the analog nucleotide results in loss of sensitivity to the analog base or nucleoside, it is also evident that mechanisms other than deletion of nucleotide-forming enzymes may result in acquired resistance to analogs of interest in cancer chemotherapy. Resistance mechanisms that contribute to failure of purine and pyrimidine analogs and that will be discussed are: (A) decreased activity of purine and pyrimidine nucleotide-forming enzymes; (B) failure of resistant cells to metabolize an initially formed nucleotide to a more inhibitory form or failure to incorporate the analog nucleotide into polynucleotides; (C) alteration of the target enzyme in resistant cells in such a way that it becomes less sensitive to the analog nucleotide; (D) increased degradation of the analog itself or of the analog nucleotide by the resistant cells; (E) failure of the analog to gain entry into resistant cells (or failure of the analog to gain access to the site of its activation within the cell); and (F) increased production of metabolites capable of overcoming the inhibitory effects of the analog.

## A. Decreased Activity of Purine and Pyrimidine Nucleotide-Forming Enzymes

### I. 6-Mercaptopurine

Recognition that the phosphoribosyltransferases provided a major pathway by which nucleotide derivatives of purines and analogs could be formed was followed by observations that bacteria and leukemia cells resistant to purine analogs, such as 6-mercaptopurine, 8-azaguanine, and 6-thioguanine, lacked the capacity to form ribonucleotides and were deficient in hypoxanthine-guanine phosphoribosyltransferase activities (Table 3, see BROCKMAN, 1963). Earlier studies on the failure of 8-azaguanine-resistant L1210 cells to incorporate the analog into nucleic acids

(Bennett et al., 1953) and on the inability of 6-mercaptopurine-resistant microorganisms to utilize hypoxanthine for growth (Elion et al., 1953, 1954a; Hutchison, 1954; Balis et al., 1957, 1958a) were interpretable in terms of decrease or loss of capacity to form nucleotides of these bases. Many such examples of resistance to purine analogs have been encountered in microorganisms, in mammalian cells in culture and in neoplasms *in vivo* (Brockman et al., 1957, 1959a, b, c, 1961, 1962; Brockman, 1960, 1963).

Table 3. *Examples of enzyme deficiencies accompanying resistance to purine and pyrimidine analogs*

| Resistance to analog | Decrease or loss of enzyme activity |
|---|---|
| 2,6-Diaminopurine<br>8-Azaadenine<br>2-Fluoroadenine | Adenine phosphoribosyltransferase; EC 2.4.2.7 |
| 6-Mercaptopurine<br>8-Azaguanine<br>8-Azahypoxanthine<br>6-Thioguanine | Hypoxanthine-guanine phosphoribosyltransferase; EC 2.4.2.8 |
| 8-Azaxanthine (microorganisms) | Xanthine phosphoribosyltransferase |
| 5-Fluorouracil (microorganisms) | Uracil phosphoribosyltransferase; EC 2.4.2.9 |
| 5-Fluorouracil (mammalian cells) | Pyrimidine phosphoribosyltransferase |
| 6-Methylthiopurine ribonucleoside<br>Formycin B<br>2-Fluoroadenosine | Adenosine kinase; EC 2.7.1.20 |
| 5-Fluorodeoxyuridine<br>5-Bromo- and 5-iododeoxyuridine | Thymidine (deoxyuridine) kinase; EC 2.7.1.21 |
| 5-Fluorouridine<br>6-Azauridine<br>5-Azacytidine | Uridine (cytidine) kinase; EC 2.7.1.48 |
| Arabinosylcytosine<br>5-Azacytidine<br>5-Azadeoxycytidine | Deoxycytidine kinase |
| 5-Fluorouracil | Uridine phosphorylase; EC 2.4.2.3 |

A significant study by Davidson and Winter (1964) of hypoxanthine phosphoribosyltransferase activity in human leukemia cells that had acquired clinical resistance to 6-mercaptopurine, as judged by lack of therapeutic response, revealed that decreased enzyme activity occurred only in one of fifteen resistant leukemias. Thus, although decreased enzymic capacity for formation of IMP, GMP, and 6-mercaptopurine ribonucleotide did occur in human leukemia, this mechanism did not account for most cases of resistance in this study. Kessel and Hall (1969) were able to correlate response of rodent leukemias to 6-mercaptopurine with capacity to convert the analog into nondiffusible cellular metabolites, predominantly nucleotides. This study was extended to include human leukemias with the indication that those leukemias sensitive to 6-mercaptopurine possessed relatively high capacities for conversion of drug to nondiffusible products *in vitro*; drug resistance was associated with low conversion of drug. In these experiments low conversion of drug to nucleotide might be a consequence not only of decreased hypoxanthine phosphoribosyltransferase activity, but also of increased degradation of drug or decreased uptake of drug. The mechanism of resistance to 6-mercaptopurine so readily encountered in experimental systems (Table 3) may be encountered less frequently in human leukemia, perhaps because the selective pressure exerted on the leukemic cell population in the clinical situation is not as great.

### II. 6-Thioguanine

It is known that 6-thioguanine is converted by hypoxanthine-guanine phosphoribosyltransferase of tumor cells to 6-thioguanylic acid (MOORE and LEPAGE, 1958) and that this nucleotide analog accumulates in susceptible tumor cells (SARTORELLI et al., 1964; BIEBER and SARTORELLI, 1964). Three sites of action of 6-thioguanine have been explored and all three require nucleotide formation. They are (1) incorporation of the analog into DNA (LEPAGE, 1960, 1963), (2) feedback inhibition of purine nucleotide biosynthesis (LEPAGE and JONES, 1961; MCCOLLISTER et al., 1964), and (3) inhibition of GMP kinase (MIECH et al., 1967, 1969). Mechanisms that operate to decrease nucleotide formation, whether by decreased uptake of drug, by decreased phosphoribosyltransferase activity, by increased degradation of the base analog, or by increased degradation of the analog nucleotide result in diminished effectiveness of the analog as a growth inhibitor. In the case of agents that are incorporated into DNA, such as 6-thioguanine, impairment of further metabolism of the analog to the deoxyribonucleotide or impairment of subsequent phosphorylation to the analog deoxyribonucleoside triphosphate offers additional opportunities for biochemical alterations that could lead to resistance (LEPAGE, 1971).

Examples of resistance to 6-thioguanine as a consequence of decrease or loss of hypoxanthine-guanine phosphoribosyltransferase activity were found in Ehrlich cells and in L1210 cells by ELLIS and LEPAGE (1963) and in L1210 cells by STUTTS and BROCKMAN (1963). The former investigators found thioguanine-resistance in Adenocarcinoma 755 cells, in Sarcoma 180 cells, and in one subline of Ehrlich cells not to be accompanied by decreased phosphoribosyltransferase activity. Nevertheless, incorporation of labeled 6-thioguanine into acid-soluble nucleotides and into nucleic acids was significantly diminished in these resistant sublines (see Section B, below).

### III. 6-Methylmercaptopurine Ribonucleoside

HENDERSON (1963), HENDERSON and KHOO (1965), and BENNETT et al. (1965) recognized that 6-methylmercaptopurine ribonucleoside was an active inhibitor of purine nucleotide biosynthesis. This nucleoside acted as a feedback inhibitor and was inhibitory to the growth of 6-mercaptopurine-resistant neoplasms that lacked hypoxanthine-guanine phosphoribosyltransferase, suggesting that it might be phosphorylated by action of a kinase (BENNETT et al., 1965). Subsequently and independently, BENNETT et al. (1966a) and CALDWELL et al. (1966) found this postulate to be correct. Adenosine kinase, purified 175-fold from human epidermoid carcinoma cells grown in culture, utilized as substrates adenosine, deoxyadenosine, 6-methylmercaptopurine ribonucleoside, 2-fluoroadenosine and other adenosine analogs; inosine, guanosine, 6-mercaptopurine ribonucleoside, and a number of other nucleosides were not phosphorylated by this enzyme (SCHNEBLI et al., 1967; LINDBERG et al., 1967). 6-Methylmercaptopurine ribonucleoside was not a substrate for purine nucleoside phosphorylase and so was not cleaved to 6-methylmercaptopurine, which was inactive (PATERSON and SUTHERLAND, 1964). 6-Methylmercaptopurine ribonucleoside 5′-phosphate was dephosphorylated prior to or during entry into Ehrlich ascites tumor cells, that is, the ionized nucleotide as such did not gain entry into cells (HO, 1971). The ribonucleoside was readily taken up by human erythrocytes *in vitro*, phosphorylated, and thereby retained (LOO et al., 1969).

Tumor cells selected for resistance to 6-methylmercaptopurine ribonucleoside were deficient in purine nucleoside kinase (BENNETT et al., 1966a; CALDWELL et al., 1967; LOMAX and HENDERSON, 1972). Tumor cell lines selected for resistance to 2-fluoroadenine were deficient in adenine phosphoribosyltransferase but retained purine nucleoside kinase activities (BENNETT et al., 1966b). Mutants have been selected that are resistant to both 2-fluoroadenine and 2-fluoroadenosine; this subline was deficient in both enzyme activities. Strains of *E. coli* resistant to 2-fluoroadenine and to 2-fluoroadenosine showed a specific decrease in adenine phosphoribosyltransferase (PITTILLO et al., 1965); 2-fluoroadenosine probably was converted to the nucleotide after it was cleaved to 2-fluoroadenine.

HILL and BENNETT (1969) and TAY et al. (1969) showed 6-methylmercaptopurine ribonucleotide to be a potent inhibitor of 5-phosphoribosyl-1-pyrophosphate amidotransferase (EC 2.4.2.14), the site of feedback inhibition by natural purine nucleotides (CASKEY et al., 1964). The methylated derivative was effective at less than one-tenth the effective concentration of 6-mercaptopurine ribonucleotide. Therefore, it is significant that 6-mercaptopurine is metabolized in neoplastic cells not only to 6-mercaptopurine ribonucleotide but also to 6-methylmercaptopurine ribonucleotide (BENNETT and ALLEN, 1971), as outlined in Fig. 3. REMY (1967) found that 6-mercaptopurine ribonucleotide was an acceptor of the methyl group from *S*-adenosylmethionine in the presence of a thiopurine methyltransferase from mammalian cells, thus offering a metabolic route for formation of the methylated nucleotide. The effectiveness of 6-methylmercaptopurine ribonucleotide as a feedback inhibitor makes attractive the hypothesis that this derivative is responsible for inhibition of purine nucleotide synthesis *de novo* as observed in Ehrlich ascites tumor cells (HENDERSON, 1963, 1965; SHANTZ et al., 1972), in human epidermoid carcinoma cells in culture and in leukemia L1210 cells (BENNETT et al., 1965), in Adenocarcinoma 755 cells in culture (BENNETT and ADAMSON, 1970), and in normal human fibroblasts (HENDERSON and MERCER, 1966; ROSENBLOOM et al., 1968a, b). As depicted in Fig. 3, 6-mercaptopurine ribonucleotide may exert inhibitory effects on the interconversion of ribonucleotides (see ELION, 1967; BALIS, 1968) or, after its metabolic conversion to 6-thioguanine nucleotides, on GMP kinase (MIECH et al., 1967) and on DNA as a consequence of its incorporation in place of guanine (SCANNELL and HITCHINGS, 1966). The significance of inhibition of purine nucleotide synthesis *de novo* is evident in the observation that 4-aminoimidazole-5-carboxamide and hypoxanthine completely reversed the inhibition of growth of Adenocarcinoma 755 cells in culture produced by relatively small concentrations (3.5 μM) of 6-methylmercaptopurine ribonucleoside (BENNETT and ADAMSON, 1970). SHANTZ et al. (1972) made similar observations in Ehrlich ascites tumor cells. These results were analagous to those of TOMIZAWA and ARONOW (1960) and HAKALA and NICHOL (1964), who found that 4-aminoimidazole-5-carboxamide and hypoxanthine effectively reversed the growth-inhibitory action of 6-mercaptopurine in Earle's L cells and in Sarcoma 180 cells in culture. The study of SHANTZ et al. (1972) adds support to the view that the observed inhibition of purine nucleotide synthesis *de novo* contributes significantly to the antitumor effect of 6-methylmercaptopurine ribonucleoside.

## IV. 6-Azauracil

Studies of the pyrimidine analog 6-azauracil and its ribonucleoside, 6-azauridine, revealed that the nucleotide, 6-azauridylic acid, was the active inhibitor of orotidylic acid decarboxylase (Fig. 4) (see HANDSCHUMACHER and WELCH, 1960; HANDSCHUMACHER et al., 1962; ŠKODA, 1963). A mutant of *S. faecalis* was unable to

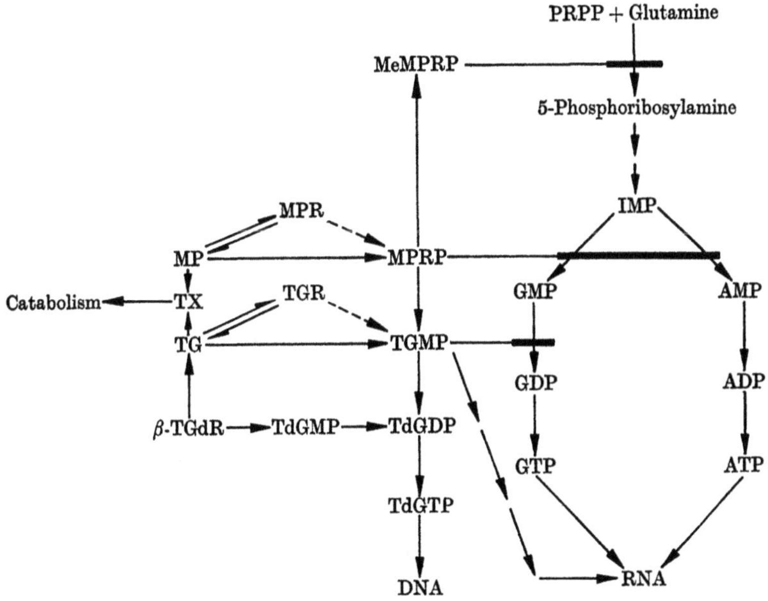


Fig. 3. Outline of biosynthesis and interconversion of purine nucleotides and loci of inhibition by 6-thiopurines. Abbreviations: MP, 6-mercaptopurine; MPR, 6-mercaptopurine ribonucleoside; MPRP, 6-mercaptopurine ribonucleotide; MeMPRP, 6-methylmercaptopurine ribonucleotide; TG, 6-thioguanine; TGR, 6-thioguanine ribonucleoside; TGMP, 6-thioguanylic acid; β-TGdR, 6-thiodeoxyguanosine; TX, 6-thioxanthine. MP and TG also compete with hypoxanthine and guanine for phosphoribosyltransferase and thus inhibit utilization of these purine bases. 6-Methylmercaptopurine ribonucleoside is phosphorylated directly to MeMPRP by the action of adenosine kinase

convert uracil or 6-azauracil to nucleotide derivatives, but could anabolize uridine and was not cross-resistant to 6-azauridine, suggesting a deficiency in uridine phosphorylase activity with retention of uridine kinase activity (HANDSCHUMACHER, 1957). An azauridine-resistant subline of L5178Y leukemia in culture was unable to form significant amounts of 6-azauridine 5′-monophosphate from 6-azauridine and was unable to phosphorylate uridine as a consequence of a uridine kinase deficiency (PASTERNAK et al., 1961). Uridine kinase, like other nucleoside kinases, probably is the rate-limiting enzyme of this pathway; uridine kinase is known to be subject to feedback inhibition by UTP, CTP, and by analog nucleoside triphosphates (ANDERSON and BROCKMAN, 1964; ORENGO, 1969; VESELÝ et al., 1971a, b).

## V. 5-Fluorouracil

An excellent summary of the metabolism and inhibitory effects of fluorinated pyrimidines has been presented by HEIDELBERGER (1965). Resistance to 5-fluorouracil also has been associated with decreased activity of anabolic enzymes. REICHARD et al. (1959, 1962) found resistance to 5-fluorouracil in Ehrlich ascites tumor cells and in L1210 leukemia to be accompanied by decreased activities of uridine phosphorylase and uridine kinase (Fig. 5). Sköld et al. (1962) demonstrated the selective advantage conferred by uridine kinase deficiency in a mixed population of sensitive and resistant cells exposed to 5-fluorouracil. Goldberg et al. (1966) found

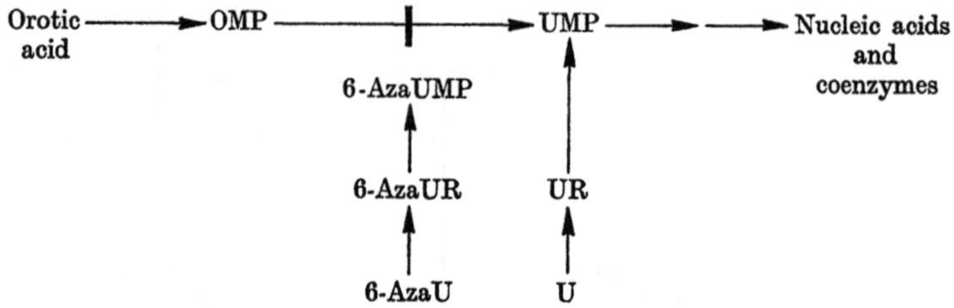


Fig. 4. Locus of action of 6-azauridylic acid (after Handschumacher et al., 1962)

resistance in L1210 cells accompanied by decreased uridine phosphorylase while uridine kinase activity remained unchanged. Brockman et al. (1960) observed loss of uracil phosphoribosyltransferase activity in *E. coli* highly resistant to 5-fluorouracil. Kasbekar and Greenberg (1963) made the interesting observation that a 5-fluorouracil resistant line of the Gardner lymphosarcoma exhibited a significant decrease in orotidylate decarboxylase activity. The partially purified orotidylate decarboxylase preparation possessed orotate and 5-fluorouracil phosphoribosyltransferase activities; these activities were separable by starch gel electrophoresis (Kasbekar et al., 1964; see also Appel, 1968). Orotidylate decarboxylase preparations from the fluorouracil-resistant neoplasm lacked the capacity to catalyze the formation of 5-fluorouridylic acid by reaction of 5-fluorouracil with 5-phosphoribosyl-1-pyrophosphate.

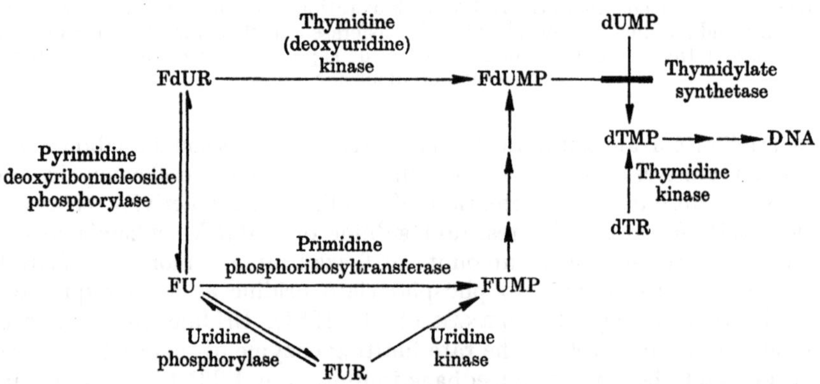


Fig. 5. Pathways for formation of nucleotides of 5-fluorouracil (see Heidelberger, 1965)

Wolberg (1964) examined the capacity of human tumors to incorporate pyrimidine precursors, uridine-$^3$H and thymidine-$^3$H, into RNA and DNA and evaluated the effect of fluoropyrimidines on their incorporation in an effort to correlate biochemical effects and response to chemotherapy. In some cases, tumor resistance was attributed to a deficiency in nucleotide-forming capacity. Kessel et al. (1966) extended this approach and showed that the capacity of tumor cells to convert 5-fluorouracil to nucleotides could be correlated with response to chemotherapy with fluorouracil. Subsequently, REYES and HALL (1969) correlated increase in survival of fluorouracil-treated mouse neoplasms with the specific activity of fluorouracil phosphoribosyltransferase in cell-free extracts from these neoplasms.

It is recognized that 5-fluorodeoxyuridylic acid is the most potent inhibitory derivative of fluorouracil (HEIDELBERGER, 1963, 1965, 1967). The formation of this nucleotide, which represents only a small portion of the total fluorouracil nucleotides formed, may be the determining factor in responsiveness of a given neoplasm. KESSEL et al. (1969a) noted that a subline of the plasma cell neoplasm P388 that was resistant to a terephthalanilide had a lowered capacity for formation of fluorouracil nucleotides and yet was responsive to fluorouracil therapy. The formation of fluorodeoxyuridylic acid from fluorouracil in this neoplasm was not examined. It is possible that the intracellular concentration of 5-fluoro-2′-deoxyuridylic acid was maintained at a level inhibitory to thymidylate synthetase, even though the formation of 5-fluorouridine-5′-mono-, di-, and triphosphates was diminished. WOLBERG (1972) assessed the effect of 5-fluorouracil on the incorporation of formate-$^{14}C$ into DNA; in this manner, a measure of inhibition of thymidylate synthetase was obtained and, therefore, an indirect assessment of levels of fluorodeoxyuridylic acid.

## VI. 5-Fluoro-2′-Deoxyuridine

Fluorodeoxyuridine is phosphorylated directly by thymidine (deoxyuridine) kinase to yield 5-fluoro-2′-deoxyuridylic acid. As might be anticipated, cells that have diminished thymidine kinase activity are less sensitive to fluorodeoxyuridine; examples of this resistance mechanism are known (DUBBS and KIT, 1964; MORSE and POTTER, 1965; HEIDELBERGER, 1965; WOLBERG, 1970). Cell lines selected for resistance to fluorodeoxyuridine may retain pathways for metabolism of 5-fluorouracil and therefore are not completely resistant to fluorodeoxyuridine, which is degraded to fluorouracil by the action of pyrimidine deoxyribonucleoside phosphorylase (Fig. 5).

On the other hand, KESSEL and WODINSKY (1970) observed higher levels of thymidine kinase in transplantable mouse leukemias that were insensitive to fluorodeoxyuridine. A basis for understanding this result may also be found in the fact that fluorodeoxyuridine is not only a substrate for thymidine (deoxyuridine) kinase, but also for pyrimidine deoxyribonucleoside phosphorylase. The latter enzyme rapidly degrades fluorodeoxyuridine to fluorouracil (BIRNIE et al., 1963) which must then be metabolized through multiple biochemical steps to fluorodeoxyuridylic acid, the active inhibitor (Fig. 5). Although some fluorodeoxyuridine is phosphorylated directly, a significant portion of administered drug is converted to fluorouracil. Inhibition of thymidylate synthetase by fluorodeoxyuridylic acid decreases the pool of thymine deoxynucleotides; one consequence of this is a compensatory rise in the thymidine kinase level as the inhibited cell attempts to maintain DNA synthesis (IVES et al., 1963; WOLBERG, 1972). When such a situation exists, those cells having the greater thymidine kinase capacity may escape fluorodeoxyuridylate inhibition, assuming that an exogenous source of thymidine is available.

## VII. Arabinosylcytosine

Arabinosylcytosine (1-β-D-arabinofuranosylcytosine) has proven to be inhibitory to the multiplication of many experimental tumors and DNA viruses

(COHEN, 1966) and it is clinically interesting as an antileukemic agent (see LIVINGSTON and CARTER, 1970). As shown in Fig. 6, arabinosylcytosine is converted to phosphorylated derivatives by the action of appropriate nucleoside and nucleotide phosphotransferases (CARDEILHAC and COHEN, 1964; CHU and FISCHER, 1965) and is an inhibitor of DNA synthesis (CHU and FISCHER, 1962; KIM and EIDINOFF, 1965). Subsequent work has shown that arabinosylcytosine is phosphorylated by deoxycytidine kinase of mammalian cells (CHU and FISCHER, 1965; MOMPARLER and FISCHER, 1968; KESSEL, 1968a, b; DURHAM and IVES, 1970). The substrate specificity of this enzyme may vary depending on the source and purification of the enzyme, but it is clear that deoxycytidine and arabinosylcytosine are phosphorylated by the same enzyme. The 5′-triphosphate of arabinosylcytosine (AraCTP) is the predominant form of this analog in mammalian cells (SCHRECKER and URSHEL, 1968; MOMPARLER et al., 1968). This nucleotide inhibited DNA polymerase from Ehrlich ascites tumor cells (KIMBALL and WILSON, 1968), calf thymus and bovine lymphosarcoma (FURTH and COHEN, 1968), human leukemic leukocytes (INAGAKI et al., 1969), and L cells (GRAHAM and WHITMORE, 1970b). AraCTP did not replace deoxycytidine 5′-triphosphate as a substrate for DNA polymerase in the study of FURTH and COHEN (1968), but was competitive with the natural substrate. These investigators, as well as GRAHAM and WHITMORE (1970a), considered the inhibition of DNA synthesis to be a consequence of inhibition of DNA polymerase.

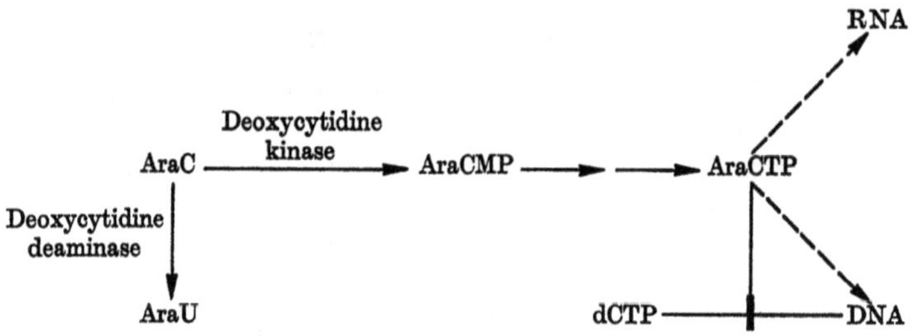


Fig. 6. Pathways of metabolism of arabinosylcytosine

In an earlier study (CARDEILHAC and COHEN, 1964) it was found that AraCTP did not inhibit the *E. coli* DNA polymerase of KORNBERG, now designated *E. coli* DNA polymerase I. More recently, REDDY et al. (1971) and STAUB et al. (1972) found that AraCTP inhibited *E. coli* DNA polymerase II, which is considered to be a candidate for the role of a replicative DNA polymerase. DNA polymerase III, which may function in replication, was inhibited to a lesser extent; DNA polymerase I was not inhibited, in agreement with CARDEILHAC and COHEN (1964). The studies of STAUB et al. (1972) were performed in toluene-treated *E. coli* which lacked DNA polymerase I, but which carried out replicative DNA synthesis. More than one DNA-dependent DNA polymerase activity now has been described in mammalian cells (see for examples BARIL and LASZLO, 1971; WEISSBACH et al., 1971; CRISS, 1971) and it is not yet clear in mammalian cells which of these polymerases is responsible for DNA replication and which is responsible for DNA repair. A number of investigators have found that arabinosylcytosine inhibition of tumor cells results in unbalanced growth as a consequence of *S*-phase specific inhibition of DNA synthesis (for example SILAGI, 1965; KIM and EIDINOFF, 1965; DOERING et al., 1966; YOUNG and FISHER, 1968; KARON and SHIRAKAWA, 1969; BREMERSKOV et al., 1970; GRAHAM and WHITMORE, 1970a) and there can be little doubt that replicative DNA synthesis is inhibited by this agent.

Other investigators have reported incorporation of arabinosylcytosine into DNA (CHU and FISCHER, 1965; SILAGI, 1965; CREASEY et al., 1966). MOMPARLER (1969) and WAQAR et al. (1971) considered arabinosylcytosine to be a DNA chain terminator; however, GRAHAM and WHITMORE (1970b) and FURLONG and GRESHAM (1971) presented evidence supporting the view that arabinosylcytosine was incorporated into internucleotide linkages. CHU and FISCHER (1965, 1968) reported the incorporation of arabinosylcytosine into RNA; more recently CHU (1971) described the incorporation of the analog into a low molecular weight RNA. It was suggested that incorporation of the analog into nucleic acids contributes to the lethal effect to the cell (SILAGI, 1965; CHU and FISCHER, 1968).

The earlier postulate of CHU and FISCHER (1962) that arabinosylcytosine inhibited the reduction of ribonucleotides to deoxyribonucleotides was not supported by a direct examination of the effect of nucleotides of arabinosylcytosine on ribonucleotide reductase from Novikoff hepatoma (MOORE and COHEN, 1967); these results were confirmed *in vivo* by KAPLAN et al. (1968) and by GRAHAM and WHITMORE (1970a).

At this time it remains uncertain whether arabinofuranosylcytosine 5'-triphosphate always inhibits DNA polymerase directly or whether, in some systems, it may alter the template by incorporation either in internucleotide or terminal positions. However, in these and the other mechanisms considered above it is quite clear that arabinosylcytosine must first be phosphorylated in order to become inhibitory.

Several groups of investigators have found that resistance to arabinosylcytosine in neoplastic cells was accompanied by a decreased capacity for phosphorylation of the analog (CHU and FISCHER, 1965; SCHRECKER and URSHEL, 1968; KESSEL et al., 1967; UCHIDA and KREIS, 1969; KESSEL et al., 1969b). More specifically, resistant cells were found to be deficient in deoxycytidine kinase activity (CHU and FISCHER, 1965; SCHRECKER, 1970; DRAHOVSHY and KREIS, 1970). The findings of KREIS et al. (1972) are particularly interesting in this regard; evidence was obtained by immunological techniques for the presence of enzymatically inactive protein in arabinosylcytosine resistant cells which behaved electrophoretically like deoxycytidine kinase.

$$\text{dCyR or AraC} \xrightarrow[\text{Deoxycytidine kinase}]{\text{ATP,Mg}^{++}} \text{dCMP or AraCMP}$$

KESSEL and his associates obtained positive correlation of capacity for nucleotide formation with response to arabinosylcytosine therapy in experimental mouse leukemias (1967) and in human leukemias (1969b). As KESSEL (1971) has pointed out, the prospect of measuring levels of a particular enzyme, such as deoxycytidine kinase, as a means of predicting clinical response to a drug, arabinosylcytosine, is attractive as a means of designing relevant chemotherapeutic regimens.

## VIII. 5-Azacytidine

PÍSKALA and ŠORM (1964) synthesized 5-azacytidine and the Czechoslovak group has done most of the biological and biochemical work with this compound and with the related drug, 5-aza-2'-deoxycytidine. As has occurred before in chemotherapy research, a compound prepared initially by the organic chemist, later was subsequently isolated as an antibiotic[3]. HANKA et al. (1967) isolated an antibiotic from the fermentation beer of *Streptoverticillium ladakanus* and identified it as 5-azacytidine. This compound was found to possess significant anticancer activity against AKR leukemia (ŠORM and VESELÝ, 1964) and against L1210 leukemia (HANKA et al., 1967). Azacytidine was found to be highly mutagenic in *E. coli* (FUČIK et al., 1965) and was shown to be incorporated into *E. coli* DNA (PAČES et al., 1968). The chemical instability of 5-azacytidine, which undergoes ring opening at neutral or basic pH, raised the possibility that the compound might undergo decomposition after incorporation into polynucleotide and that this might account for mutagenic effects observed in microorganisms (PÍTHOVÁ et al., 1965). However, subsequent work has shown that azacytidine can be recovered intact from *E. coli* RNA (PAČES et al., 1968). Azacytidine was phosphorylated to the corresponding mono-, di-, and triphosphate levels (Fig. 7) and was incorporated into the RNA of mouse liver (ČIHÁK et al., 1965) and of Ehrlich ascites tumor cells *in vivo* (JUROVČÍK et al., 1965). Inhibitory effects of azacytidine on protein synthesis in mammalian cells appear to be related to its incorporation into newly synthesized RNA and to changes in polyribosome patterns, namely, loss of heavy polyribosomes in regenerating rat liver (ČIHÁK et al., 1968; LEVITAN and WEBB, 1969). Also, 5-azacytidine inhibited the increase in thymidine kinase levels in regenerating liver (ČIHÁK and VESELÝ, 1969) and inhibited substrate induction of tryptophan pyrrolase in rat liver (ČIHÁK et al., 1969). Another effect of azacytidine was found to be an inhibition of the utilization of orotic acid for pyrimidine synthesis *in vivo;* this was related to an inhibition of orotidylic acid decarboxylase activity (VESELÝ et al., 1968a), probably by 5-azacytidine 5′-phosphate. In this respect the actions of 5-azacytidine and 6-azauridine were similar.

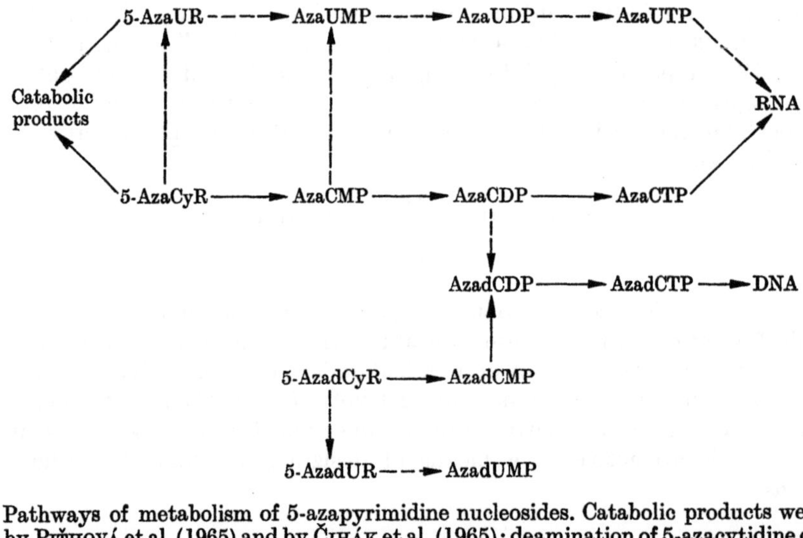


Fig. 7. Pathways of metabolism of 5-azapyrimidine nucleosides. Catabolic products were described by PÍTHOVÁ et al. (1965) and by ČIHÁK et al. (1965); deamination of 5-azacytidine occurs in microorganisms (ČIHÁK and ŠORM, 1965) and to some extent in mammalian cells

3 Other examples are afforded by 8-azaguanine and 6-thioguanine. Azaguanine was originally synthesized by ROBLIN et al. (1945) and was subsequently isolated from fermentation broths (ANZAI and SUZUKI, 1961). 6-Thioguanine was synthesized as a candidate anticancer agent (ELION and HITCHINGS, 1955) and has recently been isolated from the fermentation broth of a *Pseudomonas* specie (SCANNELL et al., 1971).

Li et al. (1970a) also found that azacytidine was phosphorylated in intact leukemic cells to yield primarily the triphosphate. These investigators confirmed the incorporation of azacytidine into RNA and, in addition, reported the formation of nucleotides of 5-azadeoxycytidine and their incorporation into the DNA of L1210 cells in culture. 5-Azacytidine inhibition of DNA synthesis was more pronounced than was inhibition of RNA synthesis in rhesus monkey kidney cells in culture (Šorm et al., 1966) and in L1210 cells in culture (Li et al., 1970a). The observations that azacytidine inhibited mitosis and that it was most toxic to mammalian cells in culture when they were in *S*-phase (Li et al., 1970b) are in agreement with the view that one effect of azacytidine is on DNA synthesis (Li et al., 1970a).

In an examination of the effect of 5-azacytidine on cell-free enzymes it was noted that the analog did not interfere with the phosphorylation of uridine (Li et al., 1970a), an unexpected finding since azacytidine is a substrate for uridine (cytidine) kinase (Veselý et al., 1970). The latter group of investigators observed that 5-azacytidine did not inhibit uridine phosphorylation even when the concentration of analog was 10 times that of the natural substrate, thus indicating that azacytidine is a relatively poor substrate. Azacytidine did not inhibit ribonucleoside diphosphate reductase or DNA polymerase activities from L1210 cells (Li et al., 1970a), but such inhibition would not be expected unless the analog was first phosphorylated in the enzyme reaction mixture. It was assumed that the inhibition of DNA in intact cells by azacytidine might be a consequence of its incorporation into DNA after first being phosphorylated and reduced to the deoxyribonucleotide. Another possibility for inhibition of DNA synthesis is by competition between 5-aza-2′-deoxycytidine 5′-triphosphate and dCTP for DNA polymerase, as has been shown to occur with arabinosylcytosine 5′-triphosphate. However, if this were a major effect of azacytidine then one might expect deoxycytidine to alleviate azacytidine inhibition of DNA synthesis, which was not observed (Li et al., 1970a).

The development of resistance to 5-azacytidine in AKR leukemia was accompanied by cross-resistance to 5-fluorouracil and by decreased activity of uridine phosphorylase and uridine kinase (Veselý et al., 1966). Also, resistance was accompanied by decreased incorporation of uridine, cytidine, and 5-azacytidine into ribonucleic acids and by a concurrent decrease in uridine kinase activity (Veselý et al., 1967, 1968b, 1970). Decreased deoxycytidine kinase activity also was observed to accompany resistance to 5-azacytidine and, as a consequence, this subline was cross-resistant to 5-aza-2′-deoxycytidine. An unexpected observation in this connection was the finding that deoxycytidine-2-$^{14}$C incorporation into nucleic acids of this azacytidine resistant line was comparable to that in the sensitive line. Although the deoxycytidine kinase activity of the resistant line was decreased, it was sufficient to supply dCMP-2-$^{14}$C for subsequent phosphorylation and incorporation into DNA. Veselý et al. (1970) observed that 5-aza-2′-deoxycytidine was a poor substrate for deoxycytidine kinase relative to the natural substrate. Thus, decreased enzyme activity evidently resulted in diminished phosphorylation of the analog in intact cells to levels that were not inhibitory. It is interesting that the partially purified uridine kinase from azacytidine-resistant leukemia was found to be more stable to heat and to *p*-chloromercuribenzoate than was the enzyme from sensitive cells, suggesting structural or conformational changes in the enzyme (Veselý et al., 1971a, b). Enzymes from both sensitive and resistant cells retained sensitivity to feedback inhibition by cytidine 5′-triphosphate, even after treatment with *p*-chloromercuribenzoate and heat (Veselý et al., 1971b). It would be of interest also to examine the effect of 5-azacytidine 5′-triphosphate on uridine kinase from sensitive and resistant cells.

Another intriguing aspect of the metabolic alterations accompanying resistance to 5-azacytidine was the observation that the activities of DNA-dependent DNA polymerase and DNA-dependent RNA polymerase from resistant cells were increased relative to the activities of these enzymes in the parent sensitive AKR leukemia (VESELÝ et al., 1970). The enhancement of these polymerase activities does not appear to be directly related to the development of resistance, and VESELÝ (1971) has suggested that perhaps this may be a compensatory response to impairment of salvage pathways for pyrimidine nucleosides.

### IX. 5-Aza-2′-Deoxycytidine

This deoxycytidine analog was synthesized by PLIML and ŠORM (1964) and found to be active against AKR mouse leukemia (ŠORM and VESELÝ, 1968). As might be anticipated, the analog inhibited the incorporation of deoxycytidine into DNA of mouse leukemia cells (VESELÝ et al., 1969) and the natural substrate partially reversed the antileukemic effect of the analog (ŠORM and VESELÝ, 1968). The incorporation of deoxyuridine into nucleic acids of mouse leukemia also was inhibited by azadeoxycytidine, which suggests that the analog may be deaminated to some extent in mammalian cells as it is in *E. coli* (DOSKOČIL and ŠORM, 1970) or, perhaps, that 5-azadeoxyuridylic acid, formed either by phosphorylation of azadeoxyuridine or by deamination of 5-azadeoxycytidylic acid, inhibited thymidylate synthetase (see Fig. 7). There is no direct evidence for such inhibition; furthermore, thymidine did not reverse the antileukemic effect of azadeoxycytidine (ŠORM and VESELÝ, 1968). In contrast to azacytidine, azadeoxycytidine did not affect RNA or protein synthesis and had no effect on inducible enzymes in rat liver (ČIHÁK et al., 1968; VESELÝ et al., 1968b; VESELÝ, 1971).

Resistance to 5-aza-2′-deoxycytidine in mouse leukemia cells is accompanied by partial loss of deoxycytidine kinase activity and cross-resistance to arabinosylcytosine; uridine-cytidine kinase activity was unaltered and cells resistant to azadeoxycytidine retained sensitivity to 5-azacytidine (VESELÝ et al., 1970).

## B. Failure of Resistant Cells to Metabolize an Initially Formed Nucleotide to a More Inhibitory Form or Failure to Incorporate an Analog Nucleotide into Polynucleotides

The possibilities for such a mechanism can be briefly illustrated by examples. LEPAGE et al. (1964) made the observation that Mecca lymphosarcoma ascites tumor cells *in vivo* readily metabolized 6-thioguanine-8-$^{14}$C to acid-soluble nucleotides and incorporated radioactivity into RNA, but not into DNA. In contrast, radioactivity from 2′-deoxy-6-thioguanosine-8-$^{14}$C was incorporated into acid-soluble nucleotides and also into DNA (Fig. 3). This neoplasm was not responsive to 6-thioguanine, but did respond somewhat to the deoxyribonucleoside. LEPAGE et al. (1964) made the interesting suggestion that the Mecca lymphosarcoma might be limited in its capacity for conversion of ribonucleotides to deoxyribonucleotides or, more specifically, it might be deficient in the capacity to reduce 6-thioguanosine 5′-diphosphate to the corresponding deoxyribonucleotide. The major biosynthetic pathway for formation of deoxyribonucleotides is by the action of ribonucleoside diphosphate reductase on purine and pyrimidine ribonucleoside 5′-diphosphates (REICHARD, 1968). Cells probably would not survive loss of capacity for reduction of natural purine and pyrimidine ribonucleotides but it is conceivable that an enzyme might be formed which had altered substrate specificity such that natural purine ribonucleotides, but not 6-thioguanosine 5′-diphosphate, were reduced. This explanation for the failure of this thioguanine insensitive neoplasm to incorporate thioguanylic acid into DNA is plausible but no enzymatic evidence has been presented in its support. One also can speculate that alterations in DNA polymerase could occur and, as a consequence, that 6-thiodeoxyguanylic acid might be excluded from incorporation into DNA.

A similar situation is offered in the case of 5-fluorouracil. If 5-fluoro-2′-deoxyuridine 5′-diphosphate were not formed from 5-fluorouridine 5′-diphosphate by the action of ribonucleoside diphosphate reductase in a given neoplasm, then that neoplasm would be unresponsive to 5-fluorouracil, even though ribonucleotide derivatives of 5-fluorouracil were formed (see Fig. 5). This type of resistance mechanism was mentioned by HEIDELBERGER et al. (1960b) as a possible basis for understanding resistance to 5-fluorouracil in an Ehrlich ascites tumor; however, this did not prove to be the basis for resistance (see Sec. C below).

A third example is offered by the observation, discussed earlier, that 6-mercaptopurine ribonucleotide is methylated to 6-methylmercaptopurine ribonucleotide, which is a more potent inhibitor of purine nucleotide biosynthesis *de novo* than is 6-mercaptopurine ribonucleotide (Fig. 3). In some neoplasms sensitivity to 6-mercaptopurine may be related to the capacity of cells to accomplish this methylation. Conversely, resistance to 6-mercaptopurine might be attributed in part to decreased formation of 6-methylmercaptopurine ribonucleotide. DIXON et al. (1970) observed that Adenocarcinoma 755 cells in culture were more sensitive to feedback inhibition by 6-mercaptopurine than were Sarcoma 180 cells, which correlates with the relative sensitivity of these neoplasms to 6-mercaptopurine. Both cell lines possessed 6-mercaptopurine phosphoribosyltransferase activity. It is an interesting speculation that decreased sensitivity of Sarcoma 180 cells might be related to the extent of methylation of 6-mercaptopurine ribonucleotide or, as discussed below, to altered sensitivity of the target enzyme.

## C. Alteration of the Target Enzyme in Resistant Cells in Such a Way that it Becomes Less Sensitive to the Analog Nucleotide

HEIDELBERGER et al. (1960a, b) studied a fluorouracil resistant line of Ehrlich ascites tumor in which chemotherapeutic doses of 5-fluorouracil did not inhibit significantly the incorporation of formate-$^{14}$C or uracil-2-$^{14}$C into DNA thymine. In the parent sensitive line, under comparable experimental conditions, fluorouracil inhibition of incorporation of these same precursors was marked, and persisted for as long as 18 hours after fluorouracil treatment. Both the sensitive and the resistant line converted 5-fluorouracil to its ribo- and deoxyribonucleotides; there was approximately equal conversion of 5-fluorouracil to 5-fluorodeoxyuridylic acid in these tumor lines. Thus, in this resistant cell line there was no evidence for decreased activities of uridine phosphorylase or uridine kinase and no evidence of failure to form 5-fluorodeoxyuridylic acid. HEIDELBERGER et al. (1960b) concluded that there might be an alteration in thymidylate synthetase such that 5-fluorodeoxyuridylic acid was less inhibitory to the enzyme of the resistant mutant. This was shown to be the case by direct experiment; thymidylate synthetase preparations were made from sensitive and resistant cells and the effect of 5-fluorodeoxyuridylic acid was determined. At a concentration of $10^{-4}$ M, 5-fluorodeoxyuridylic acid strongly inhibited the enzyme from sensitive cells, but was without significant effect on the enzyme from resistant cells. The sensitive enzyme was significantly inhibited even at a concentration of $10^{-6}$ M fluorodeoxyuridylic acid.

In studies of resistance to 5-fluorouracil in four other resistant lines of Ehrlich ascites tumor cells, the sensitivity of thymidylate synthetase to 5-fluorodeoxyuridylic acid was comparable in sensitive and resistant lines (Häggmark, 1962). Resistance in these neoplasms was accompanied by decreased uridine kinase activity, as discussed earlier.

Henderson et al. (1967) observed decreased sensitivity of 5-phosphoribosylpyrophosphate amidotransferase to 6-methylmercaptopurine ribonucleotide in a drug resistant neoplasm. Their experimental results suggest the interesting possibility that resistant cells possessed an altered enzyme such that the enzyme affinity for 6-methylmercaptopurine ribonucleoside 5′-monophosphate was lower or that the altered enzyme was less inhibited by the analog. Feedback inhibition by adenine was equally effective in sensitive and resistant lines, but guanine was less effective in the resistant cells. Caskey et al. (1964) presented evidence that the allosteric binding site of 5-phosphoribosylpyrophosphate amidotransferase has separate but interrelated binding sites for 6-aminopurine ribonucleotides and 6-hydroxypurine ribonucleotides. Perhaps the 6-hydroxypurine ribonucleotide binding site was altered and this was the binding site for the 6-methylthiopurine; the results of Hill and Bennett (1969) offer support for this view.

## D. Increased Degradation of the Analog Itself or of the Analog Nucleotide

A mechanism by which tumor cells might become resistant to purine analogs is the logical one of increased degradation of the analog. Roush and Norris (1950) made observations which indicated that 8-azaguanine could be deaminated to 8-azaxanthine by guanine deaminase of bacterial and mammalian cells. Hirschberg et al. (1952, 1953) suggested that resistance to 8-azaguanine in neoplastic cells might be a consequence of deaminase activity, since 8-azaxanthine was devoid of carcinostatic activity. However, subsequent investigation failed to reveal any consistent relationship between 8-azaguanine deaminase activity and lack of response to 8-azaguanine (Shacter and Law, 1957; Mandel, 1959). No significant differences in xanthine oxidase and uricase levels were found in 8-azaguanine sensitive and resistant L1210 cells (Feigelson et al., 1959) and so cross-resistance to 6-mercaptopurine in the 8-azaguanine resistant L1210 cannot be accounted for by this mechanism.

Elion (1967) concisely summarized catabolic pathways of metabolism of 6-mercaptopurine, which include enzymic oxidation to 6-thioxanthine as well as methylation to 6-methylthiopurine; the latter compound serves as a substrate for hepatic aldehyde oxidase (Loo et al., 1967). Thioguanine can be deaminated to yield thioxanthine or it may first be methylated to 6-methylthioguanine, which also can be deaminated and oxidized.

Sartorelli et al. (1958) selected a subline of Ehrlich ascites carcinoma that was resistant to 6-thioguanine and cross-resistant to 6-mercaptopurine. Less analog nucleotide was present in the resistant line compared to the sensitive line following a standard dose of 6-thioguanine; however, pretreatment with azaserine eliminated this difference, indicating that the resistant cell line possessed the capacity to metabolize 6-thioguanine to 6-thioguanine nucleotides. In the absence of azaserine pretreatment, less 6-thioguanine was converted to 6-thioguanylic acid in the resistant cell line and therefore more 6-thioguanine was available as substrate for deaminase and xanthine oxidase activities. Under these circumstances resistant cells appeared to be somewhat more active than the sensitive line in the degradation of 6-thioguanine to 6-thioxanthine and to 6-thiouric acid; this was considered to be a basis for resistance in this cell line (SARTORELLI et al., 1958).

Another possible degradative route for 6-thiopurines is their conversion to 6-hydroxypurines by desulfuration. This has been observed in microorganisms (BALIS et al., 1958b; CAREY and MANDEL, 1960; COGGIN et al., 1966), in mammalian tissue, including neoplasms (ELION et al., 1954b; SARTORELLI et al., 1958), and in human leukemia cells (MARTIN et al., 1972). Increased conversion of thiopurines to purines occurred in 6-mercaptopurine resistant *E. coli*, presumably at the nucleotide level (COGGIN et al., 1966). The recent report by MARTIN et al. (1972) that 6-mercaptopurine ribonucleotide was converted to inosine is of interest as a potential resistance mechanism in leukemia cells.

Attention has been directed to yet another degradative mechanism in experimental neoplasms. BIEBER and SARTORELLI (1964) suggested that increased catabolism of 6-thioguanylic acid was a factor in resistance to 6-thioguanine in Sarcoma 180 cells. BENNETT et al. (1969) concluded that resistance to 4-aminopyrazolo-(3,4-*d*)pyrimidine in neoplastic cells in culture was associated with a higher rate of degradation of the analog ribonucleotides in resistant cells. WOLPERT et al. (1971) found that cell-free extracts of a 6-thioguanine-resistant subline of Sarcoma 180 possessed increased alkaline phosphatase activity. This enzyme activity was localized primarily in particulate fractions of the neoplasm. It was noted that phosphatase activities of sensitive and resistant neoplasms were similar at pH 6.4 and 8.4; phosphatase activity dropped sharply in the sensitive cell line at pH 9.2, whereas enzyme activity increased at that pH in the resistant cell line, resulting in an 8 fold difference in activity. One might question the significance of such a difference observed only at a pH value far removed from physiological pH. Relevant to this question is the work of NELSON and PARKS (1972), who showed that the half-life of 6-thioguanine nucleotides was only about 3 hours in the resistant cell compared to a half-life of about 7 hours in the sensitive tumor. It cannot be said that alkaline phosphatase activity was solely responsible for this difference, but this observation fits well with the observed increase in phosphatase activity. No differences were noted, between the sensitive and 6-thioguanine-resistant neoplasms, in uptake or catabolism of 6-thioguanine or in the capacity to form thioguanylic acid (WOLPERT et al., 1971). Presumably, natural purine nucleotides might be protected from degradation by this phosphatase activity, since they are present predominantly as triphosphate derivatives. The intracellular pool of 6-thioguanine nucleotides consists predominantly of 6-thioguanosine 5'-monophosphate (MOORE and LEPAGE, 1958; NELSON and PARKS, 1972), which is known to be a substrate for the alkaline phosphatase; however, data on the activity of nucleoside 5'-triphosphates as substrates for this enzyme were not presented (WOLPERT et al., 1971).

Arabinosylcytosine is deaminated in experimental animals (CAMIENER and SMITH, 1965) and in man (CREASEY et al., 1966) to arabinosyluracil, which has no chemotherapeutic activity. Efforts have been made to find inhibitors of deamination as a means of enhancing the chemotherapeutic effectiveness of the drug (CAMIENER, 1968). Tetrahydrouridine was found to be a good inhibitor of the enzymatic deamination of arabinosylcytosine (CAMIENER, 1968; MULLIGAN and MELLETT, 1970) and this agent enhanced the activity of arabinosylcytosine in the treatment of L1210 leukemic mice (NEIL et al., 1970). Thus, the level of deaminase activity of the host animal and of the neoplastic cell are factors in the effectiveness of this agent. STEUART and BURKE (1971) noted that initial therapeutic responses to arabinosylcytosine in human leukemia were correlated with lower deaminase activities. Furthermore, during the course of therapy of human leukemias with arabinosylcytosine the deaminase level increased and the duration of remission decreased. It is not known whether this increased deaminase activity was a consequence of selection of a specific population of cells or whether enzyme activity was induced. This same mechanism of resistance obviously could occur with 5-azacytidine since it also can be inactivated by deamination. MALEY and MALEY (1971) reported that tetrahydrodeoxyuridine and the corresponding nucleotide also inhibited deoxycytidine deaminase.

## E. Failure of the Analog to Gain Entry into Resistant Cells (or Failure of the Analog to Gain Access to the Site of its Activation within the Cell)

PATERSON (1959) isolated and identified 6-mercaptopurine ribonucleotide from Ehrlich ascites carcinoma cells and showed that the di- and triphosphates were not formed in detectable amounts. A 6-mercaptopurine-resistant subline of the Ehrlich carcinoma was developed and characterized as cross-resistant to 6-mercaptopurine ribonucleoside and 6-thioguanine. In intact cells of this resistant line almost no nucleotide was formed from 6-mercaptopurine, 6-mercaptopurine ribonucleoside, or 6-thioguanine (PATERSON, 1960a, b). A study then was made of purine nucleotide metabolism in the intact cells of the sensitive and 6-mercaptopurine-resistant lines *in vitro* and no differences were revealed; the rates at which adenine-8-$^{14}$C, guanine-8-$^{14}$C and hypoxanthine-8-$^{14}$C were metabolized to purine nucleotides were similar in both lines (PATERSON and HORI, 1962). However, as was the case *in vivo*, the resistant subline failed to form 6-mercaptopurine ribonucleotide in intact cells *in vitro*. PATERSON (1962) evaluated the capacity of cell-free extracts to catalyze the reaction of 6-mercaptopurine with 5-phosphoribosylpyrophosphate and found that the sensitive and mercaptopurine-resistant Ehrlich ascites carcinoma possessed similar capacities for synthesis of 6-mercaptopurine ribonucleotide. The formation of the nucleotide was strictly dependent on the presence of 5-phosphoribosylpyrophosphate in the enzyme incubation mixture. The conclusion drawn from this thorough series of investigations was that 6-mercaptopurine fails to gain access to the site of nucleotide synthesis in the intact resistant cell (PATERSON, 1963). The simplest postulate is that resistance was acquired through loss of transport of 6-mercaptopurine through the cell membrane, perhaps by a highly specific alteration of a permease. However, studies of permeability to adenine and to pyrimidine bases in Ehrlich ascites cells lead to the conclusion that these bases gained entry into the cells by diffusion (JACQUEZ and GINSBERG, 1960; JACQUEZ, 1962); unfortunately for the present discussion, hypoxanthine and 6-mercaptopurine were not included in this study. Whether or not a permease is involved, PATERSON's studies provide a clear example of what may be termed an intact cell effect. It may be that the synthesis of purine nucleotides from exogenous bases takes place within a compartment of the cell and that 6-mercaptopurine was selectively excluded from that compartment. But this is only a more elaborate way of describing the observation.

In *E. coli* the uptake of purines has been related to the activity of purine phosphoribosyltransferase activities associated with cell membrane structures (HOCHSTADT-OZER and STADTMAN, 1971a, b). There is no evidence for a similar relationship in mammalian cells, but it is known that greater uptake of exogenous bases takes place in mammalian cells that possess phosphoribosyltransferase activity than occurs in mutant cells that lack the appropriate enzyme. This is a consequence of metabolism of base to nucleotide within the enzymically competent cell, which results in a decreased intracellular concentration of free base and, therefore, a favorable concentration gradient for continued diffusion of base from the medium into the cell.

## F. Increased Production of Metabolites Capable of Overcoming the Inhibitory Effects of the Analog

In an examination of mechanisms of resistance to 6-mercaptopurine in mutants of *Streptococcus faecalis* (HUTCHISON, 1958), BALIS et al. (1958b) considered one mutant, SF/MPcc, to be resistant as a consequence of an increased capacity for purine nucleotide synthesis *de novo*. It was considered that the increased formation of purine nucleotides *de novo* accounted for the growth of SF/MPcc in the presence of 6-mercaptopurine. This mutant had not lost hypoxanthine-guanine phosphoribosyltransferase activity and therefore formed 6-mercaptopurine ribonucleotide from the base. Another mutant, SF/MP, was found to be resistant as a consequence of decreased phosphoribosyltransferase activity.

A mutant of L5178Y lymphoma partially resistant to arabinosylcytosine was not deficient in deoxycytidine kinase activity; neither was there evidence for increased catabolism or decreased incorporation of deoxycytidine, arabinosylcytosine, or thymidine into nucleotides (MOMPARLER et al., 1968). There was an increased incorporation of uridine and cytidine into nucleotides and a decreased incorporation of deoxycytidine into DNA of this resistant subline, an observation that suggested an increased pool of deoxycytidine nucleotides. The pool size of deoxycytidine nucleotides was measured and found to be elevated about 4 fold in the resistant line. An increased concentration of deoxycytidine nucleotides, particularly dCTP, could have several modifying effects. Deoxycytidine triphosphate, an inhibitor of deoxycytidine kinase (MALEY and MALEY, 1962), could inhibit phosphorylation of arabinosylcytosine, but this effect was not observed by MOMPARLER et al. (1968). An increased level of deoxycytidine triphosphate also could overcome inhibition of DNA synthesis by arabinosylcytosine 5'-triphosphate and, by competition, decrease the incorporation of arabinosylcytosine into nucleic acids. Increased ribonucleoside diphosphate reductase activity could be a means by which cells generate an increased pool of deoxycytidine nucleotides; this mechanism of resistance has not yet been established, but it offers interesting possibilities.

## G. Other Mechanisms of Resistance to Purine and Pyrimidine Analogs

It would be unwise not to leave this discussion open-ended for there are, or will be, other mechanisms of resistance to be considered. For example, BIEBER et al. (1961) made the intriguing observation that a 6-mercaptopurine-resistant subline of Adenocarcinoma 755 incorporated radioactivity from 6-mercaptopurine-$^{35}S$ into nucleic acids more extensively than did the parent sensitive line. SCANNELL and HITCHINGS (1966) demonstrated that 6-mercaptopurine-8-$^{14}C$ was metabolized and incorporated into the DNA of this resistant subline as 6-thiodeoxyguanylic acid. Obviously there was no impairment in the resistant line of nucleotide formation, of metabolism of 6-mercaptopurine ribonucleotide to 6-thioguanylic acid and 6-thiodeoxyguanylic acid, or incorporation of 6-thiodeoxyguanylic acid into DNA.

LEPAGE (1963) correlated inhibitory effects of 6-thioguanine with extent of incorporation of analog into DNA, and SCANNELL and HITCHINGS (1966) found that the level of incorporation of 6-mercaptopurine into DNA, as thioguanine, was comparable to the incorporation of 6-thioguanine into DNA. What, then, is the mechanism by which this cell line achieved resistance to 6-mercaptopurine? The answer to this question probably will provide a new resistance mechanism.

## Resistance to Alkylating Agents

From the standpoint of cancer chemotherapy an alkylating agent may be broadly defined as a compound that generates a reactive alkyl group which reacts with a nucleophilic receptor in a biological system under physiological conditions. The reactive group may be an ethylenimmonium ion, an aziridino group, an epoxide, or a carbonium ion. The source of these reactive moieties may be a 2-chloroethylamine (nitrogen mustard), an aziridine (triethylene melamine, mitomycin C), an epoxy compound or a compound that can generate an epoxide (1,2,3,4-diepoxybutane, dibromomannitol), or molecules that can generate carbonium ions (myleran, *N*-alkyl-*N*-nitrosoureas, triazenes). Representatives from each of these groups are well-known chemotherapeutic agents, (for reviews see MONTGOMERY et al., 1970; OCHOA and HIRSCHBERG, 1967; ROSS, 1962). The biological receptor groups for an alkylating moiety may be organic anions, amines, nitrogen atoms of heterocyclic molecules, or sulfides. It is generally agreed that nucleic acids are targets for alkylation (WHEELER, 1962, 1967; WARWICK, 1963; LAWLEY, 1966; ALEXANDER, 1969), that the purine and pyrimidine moieties of RNA and DNA are prime sites of alkylation, and that the most extensively alkylated site is the 7-position of guanine (LAWLEY, 1966).

WHEELER (1963), in reviewing mechanisms of resistance to biological alkylating agents, concluded, at that time, that two mechanisms appeared most plausible: (A) altered cell permeability and (B) increased cellular concentration of protective agents, such as sulfhydryl compounds; more recently another mechanism has attracted interest: (C) increased capacity of resistant neoplasms for repair of DNA damaged by alkylation.

### A. Altered Cell Permeability

Decreased uptake of labeled nitrogen mustard by mammalian cells resistant to this agent was reported by several groups of investigators (RUTMAN et al., 1968; WOLPERT and RUDDON, 1969; CHUN et al., 1969; GOLDENBERG et al., 1970). Less binding of nitrogen mustard to macromolecules was observed in resistant cells than in sensitive cells. REID and WALKER (1966) showed reduced binding of sulfur mustard to DNA of resistant L cells. However, decreased permeability was considered by most of these investigators to be but one factor that contributed to resistance in tumor cells. WOLPERT and RUDDON (1969) and GOLDENBERG et al. (1970) provided good evidence that, in neoplastic cells *in vitro*, the uptake of nitrogen mustard was mediated by an active transport system. This conclusion was based on observations that uptake was temperature dependent, that it proceeded against a concentration gradient, and that it was partially inhibited by agents which affect membrane function, such as ouabain. GOLDENBERG et al. (1971) extended these investigations and obtained results indicating that the transport of nitrogen mustard and its hydrolysis product, which is not an alkylating agent, was mediated by the same carrier that acts in the transport of choline; structural similarities between these agents can be seen:

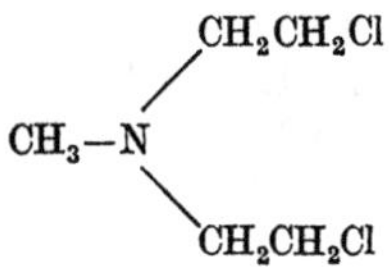

Nitrogen mustard

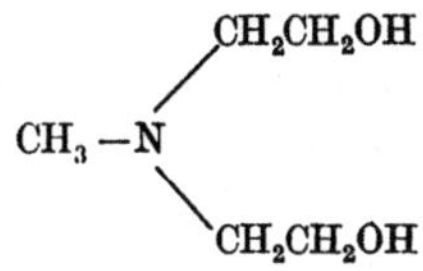

Hydrolysis product
of nitrogen mustard

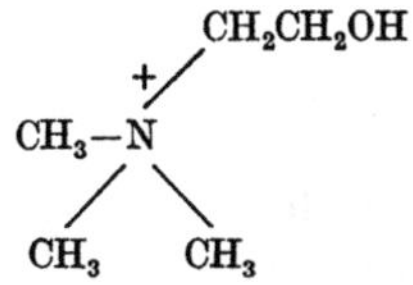

Choline

Competition between these compounds for transport into L5178Y lymphoma cells was observed. In this connection it is interesting that structural analogs of nitrogen mustard, such as chlorambucil, phenylalanine mustard, and cyclophosphamide, did not inhibit the uptake of nitrogen mustard, suggesting chemical specificity for the transport mechanism (GOLDENBERG et al., 1970).

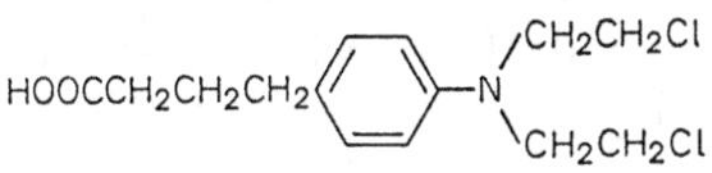

Chlorambucil

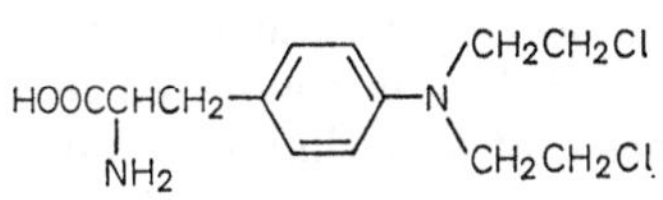

Phenylalanine mustard (Sarcolysin, melphalan)

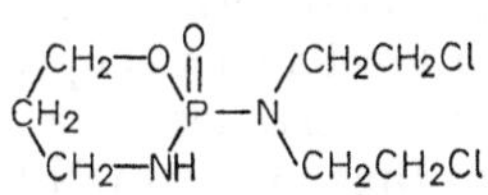

Cyclophosphamide (Cytoxan, Endoxan)

Other investigators have not observed decreased uptake of alkylating agent in resistant cells. For example, WHEELER and ALEXANDER (1964) found no difference in binding of $^{14}$C-labeled nitrogen mustard to subcellular fractions of sensitive and resistant hamster plasmacytomas *in vivo*. Similarly, CRATHORN and ROBERTS (1965) observed no difference in binding of sulfur mustard-$^{35}$S to macromolecules of sensitive and resistant L5178Y lymphoma cells growing in culture. The extent of gross alkylation of nucleic acids in sensitive and resistant cells was similar and it appears that mechanisms other than altered cell permeability must account for resistance in the neoplasms studied by WHEELER and ALEXANDER and by CRATHORN and ROBERTS.

## B. Increased Cellular Concentration of Protective Agents, Such as Sulfhydryl Compounds

HIRONO (1960, 1961) found elevated nonprotein sulfhydryl levels in nitromin-resistant Yoshida sarcoma cells, and CALCUTT and CONNORS (1963), BALL et al. (1966), UJHÁZY and WINKLER (1965), and GOLDENBERG (1969) provided support for this observation. An increased intracellular concentration of a nonessential thiol could protect cells against the toxicity of an alkylating agent by reacting with it, thereby protecting more vital targets within the cell. However, such a relationship has been shown to exist for only a small number of transplanted tumors. Contrary to these findings was the observation of REID and WALKER (1966) that L cells resistant to sulfur mustard generally had a lower acid-soluble sulfhydryl content than did the sensitive line. (For further discussion of aspects of this mechanism of resistance to alkylating agents see CONNORS, 1966.)

## C. Increased Capacity of Resistant Neoplasms for Repair of DNA Damaged by Alkylation[4]

The process of repair of DNA damaged by alkylation is considered to be similar to the repair of damage produced in the DNA of bacteria and mammalian cells by ultraviolet light. The process consists of a series of steps outlined as follows: (1) deletion of alkylated bases (chemical or enzymatic hydrolysis) and cleavage of the damaged strand of DNA; (2) excision of deoxyribonucleotides by exonuclease activity to produce a gap in the DNA strand; (3) addition of deoxynucleotides by the action of DNA polymerase; the undamaged DNA strand serves as template to rebuild the damaged strand; (4) joining of the reconstructed DNA to the rest of the strand by the action of a ligase.

CRATHORN and ROBERTS (1966) found that alkylated products were excised from the DNA of mustard-treated HeLa cells; these were thought to consist of oligonucleotides containing alkylguanine residues. Alkylated purines can be lost hydrolytically from alkylated DNA (LAWLEY, 1966) without the necessity for enzyme action. ROBERTS et al. (1968) made the significant observation that nonsemiconservative DNA synthesis (repair) occurred in HeLa cells following alkylation with a variety of agents; this was confirmed in P388 cells by AYAD et al. (1969). Thus, there is evidence that a mechanism analogous to the repair of lesions induced by ultraviolet irradiation exists for the removal of alkylation damage from the DNA of mammalian cells (ROBERTS et al., 1971a, b; ROBERTS, 1972). The extent to which such a repair mechanism is operative could be a significant factor in determining sensitivity or resistance to cytotoxic alkylating agents. Also, inhibition of repair by agents that bind to DNA (CLEAVER, 1969) should enhance the cytotoxicity of alkylating agents and x-rays.

GAUDIN and YIELDING (1969) proposed that the response of cytoxan-resistant hamster plasmacytomas to cytoxan, nitrogen mustard, and x-rays might be increased by treating tumor-bearing animals with known inhibitors of repair, such as caffeine and chloroquine. The effects of such combinations on malignant melanomas grown in the hamster also were examined by GAUDIN et al. (1971). These investigators reported that such combination therapy did limit growth of the resistant plasmacytoma and the refractory melanoma. They were careful to point out that these results do not provide direct evidence that repair capacity was implicated in tumor resistance but, by whatever mechanism, the inhibition of growth is of interest for further study.

RAUTH et al. (1970) examined the effect of caffeine on mitomycin-treated mouse L cells in culture and showed that caffeine enhanced the lethal effect of mitomycin C. Cells exposed to mitomycin C in the $G_1$ phase of a synchronized culture escaped the effect of caffeine, provided they were not exposed to it until after the cells had gone through S phase; cells exposed to mitomycin C in $G_2$ were vulnerable to caffeine for much longer periods. The ability of mitomycin C-treated

4 The subject of repair mechanisms is beyond the scope of this discussion; the reader is referred to a recent symposium on molecular and cellular repair processes (BEERS et al., 1972).

cells to escape from caffeine toxicity as a function of the time of incubation after treatment was seen to be analogous to results of a previous study in which L cells were irradiated with UV light (DOMON and RUATH, 1969). If mitomycin C or other alkylating agents produces damage in tumor cells that is repairable, then agents that block repair should increase the effectiveness of the alkylating agent. The hazard, of course, is that the toxicity to vulnerable normal tissues also would be enhanced.

## Resistance to other Agents

Brief reference will be made to studies of resistance to other important chemotherapeutic agents: tumor-inhibitory enzymes, e.g. L-asparaginase; steroid hormones; anticancer agents of complex structure that bind to cellular components, e.g. actinomycin, daunomycin, mitomycin, vincristine, vinblastine, colchicine, phthalanilides.

### A. L-Asparaginase

KIDD (1953a, b) observed that guinea pig serum had a lethal effect on transplanted mouse lymphomas in the absence of toxicity for the host. BROOME (1961, 1963a, b) identified the active component of guinea pig serum as L-asparaginase and MASHBURN and WRISTON (1964) showed that the L-asparaginase of *E. coli* also was inhibitory for mouse lymphoma 6C3HED. It was known from the work of MCCOY et al. (1956, 1959a, b) that a number of experimental neoplasms require an exogenous source of asparagine for growth. Such neoplasms lack the capacity for intracellular synthesis of asparagine and thus must be supplied with asparagine from blood. Asparaginase, which cleaves asparagine to aspartic acid, acts to deprive the tumor cell of this metabolite and thus inhibits its growth. In experimental animal work, the presence of asparagine synthetase (PATTERSON and ORR, 1967, 1968) has been correlated with resistance to tumor growth inhibition by L-asparaginase (BROOM and SCHWARTZ, 1967; PRAGER and BACHYNSKY, 1968; HOROWITZ et al., 1968). Resistant tumors respond to L-asparaginase by relatively large increases in the level of asparagine synthetase, whereas normal tissues and sensitive neoplasms, including human leukemia (HASKELL and CANELLOS, 1969), showed a low level, or a transient increase, of asparagine synthetase activity.

The use of an enzyme in cancer chemotherapy is not without its difficulties since, as might be anticipated, the host responds to the enzyme as a foreign protein; also, as seen above, neoplasms may become resistant. The use of this enzyme does represent a new approach in the treatment of cancer and it is possible that other metabolites will be recognized for which tumor cells have a greater requirement than normal cells, thus providing additional possibilities for enzyme therapy. (For more comprehensive coverage of literature on L-asparaginase see COONEY and HANDSCHUMACHER, 1970; CAPIZZI et al., 1970; PRAGER, 1971; CROWTHER, 1971).

### B. Steroid Hormones

The hormone-dependent variety of the carcinogen-induced mammary carcinoma of the rat (HUGGINS et al., 1961) was shown to have an affinity for estrogen *in vivo* and *in vitro* (KING et al., 1965; MOBBS, 1966; JENSEN et al., 1967; SANDER and ATTRAMADAL, 1968; TERENIUS, 1968). Recently, it was found that the dimethylbenzanthracene-induced mammary carcinomas that regress after ovariectomy contain a specific cytoplasmic 17$\beta$-estradiol-binding protein whereas autonomous mammary tumors lack this protein (MCGUIRE and JULIAN, 1971). Similarly, a transplantable rat mammary carcinoma (R3230AC), one that did not regress after ovariectomy and that did not bind estradiol-$^3$H to chromatin, was shown to be deficient in estradiol-binding protein. It was demonstrated that failure to bind estradiol to chromatin was a consequence of the deficiency in estradiol-binding protein (McGuire et al., 1972).

The autonomous mammary carcinoma, which is unresponsive to hormone, may be viewed as a resistant neoplasm; resistance in this case is a consequence of the loss of capacity of the tumor cell to produce a specific protein which binds estradiol. Analogy can be drawn between this deficiency and the deficiency of certain drug-resistant neoplasms to form an enzyme that is essential for activation of the drug.

## C. Anticancer Agents of Complex Structure that Bind to Cellular Components

Anticancer agents that bind to DNA include actinomycin D, daunomycin, mithramycin, and mitomycin C (see Newton, 1970). The vinca alkaloids (vincristine and vinblastine) and colchicine and its derivatives, although structurally unrelated, are considered together, since these agents are known to arrest mitosis during metaphase, although this may not be their only effect (for reviews see Dustin, 1963; Johnson et al., 1963). The phthalanilides, from a chemical standpoint, are aromatic diamidines (Bennett, 1965) and are of interest as experimental antileukemic agents. Resistance to phthalanilides is known to be accompanied in some neoplasms by cross-resistance to several of the structurally complex agents named above.

This reviewer was led to group these agents together in this discussion of resistance because of recent work on cellular resistance by Bosmann (1971), Bosmann and Kessel (1970), and Kessel and Bosmann (1970). Results of these studies, in agreement with earlier work in bacteria (Slotnick and Sells, 1964), in HeLa cells (Goldstein et al., 1966), and in murine leukemias (Kessel and Wodinsky, 1968), demonstrated that resistance to actinomycin D was related to membrane permeability, which appears to be related to altered membranes and to altered membrane synthesis. Biedler and Riehm (1970) developed resistance to actinomycin D over a wide range of concentrations; 2500 fold resistance was attained in Chinese hamster cells in culture. The extent of labeling of the nucleus by $^3$H-actinomycin decreased as resistance to actinomycin increased; actinomycin inhibition of RNA synthesis also decreased as resistance increased. Results obtained in this study revealed that the actinomycin D cells were cross-resistant to mithramycin, vinblastine, vincristine, puromycin, daunomycin, demecolcine (colcemid), and mitomycin C. Such cross-resistance was related, in a general way, to the molecular weight of the agent; that is, the greater the molecular weight the greater the degree of cross-resistance. Also, graded increases in resistance to actinomycin D were accompanied by similar resistance to vincristine and daunomycin and resistance to daunomycin was accompanied by cross-resistance to actinomycin D. Riehm and Biedler (1972) observed that the nonionic detergent Tween 80 potentiated the effect of actinomycin and daunomycin on the resistant neoplasm and increased the uptake of the tritium-labeled antibiotics. These results support the view that acquired resistance to these antibiotics was related to changes in the capacity of the cell to admit these structures, perhaps as a consequence of changes in the cellular membrane.

Bosmann and Kessel (1970) isolated sublines of P388 that were resistant to vincristine and to a phthalanilide (NSC38280; see Bennett, 1965). Both of these sublines were resistant to vincristine, actinomycin D, and daunomycin. Such mutual cross-resistance between these structurally unrelated compounds had been observed earlier by Kessel et al. (1968) and by Burchenal et al. (1962, 1963). Hakala (1971) also has observed cross-resistance between Sarcoma 180 cell lines resistant to vincristine and to a phthalanilide. Sarcoma 180 cells resistant to an aromatic *bis*-guanylhydrazone also were cross-resistant to a phthalanilide; these cells took up the inhibitor at a reduced rate (HAKALA, 1971).

Reduced levels of a spectrum of glycosidases were associated with the development of resistance to this heterogeneous group of drugs, an observation which suggested possible alterations in the biosynthesis and degradation of membrane constituents. BOSMANN (1971) has developed the hypothesis that acquired resistance to actinomycin D occurs through selection of cells with altered surface membranes, possibly as a consequence of altered membrane synthetic apparatus, and that such cells are less permeable to actinomycin D. Cross-resistance to other large, structurally complex molecules logically could be accounted for by the same mechanism.

SIMARD and CASSINGENA (1969) derived an actinomycin D-resistant subline of a hamster neoplasm in cell culture and found it to be cross-resistant to nogalamycin and to chromomycin (see NEWTON, 1970). There was somewhat less $^{3}$H-actinomycin D bound to chromatin of resistant cells than to that of sensitive cells and these investigators suggested that mechanisms other than altered cell permeability might be involved; enzymatic inactivation of actinomycin within the cell was suggested but supporting data was not presented. DANØ et al. (1972) also concluded that a resistance mechanism other than decreased permeability was involved in resistance to daunorubicin in Ehrlich ascites tumor cells.

## Conclusions

Studies of mechanisms of resistance to anticancer agents in neoplastic cells provide evidence of the variety of ways by which such cells may adapt to an adverse environment. In the course of such studies much has been learned about cell metabolism and about mechanisms of action of anticancer agents. The selection of a resistant population of cells from one initially sensitive to a drug is not necessarily disastrous; the resistant cell may be more vulnerable to attack by a different agent. Also, the resistant cell may be less oncogenic or more immunogenic than the parent cell, changes that probably are interrelated.

Drug-resistant cell lines have proven to be useful tools in exploring mechanisms of action of new drugs. They have also proven to be valuable tools for genetic studies in mammalian cells; such studies now are contributing to an understanding of malignancy.

## References


ALBERTINI, R. J., DEMARS, R.: Diploid azaguanine-resistant mutants of cultured human fibroblasts. Science **169**, 482—485 (1970).

ALBRECHT, A. M., BIEDLER, J. L., HUTCHISON, D. J.: Two different species of dihydrofolate reductase in mammalian cells differentially resistant to amethopterin and methasquin. Cancer Res. **32**, 1539—1546 (1972).

ALBRECHT, A. M., PALMER, J. L., HUTCHISON, D. J.: Differentiating properties of the dihydrofolate reductases of amethopterin-resistant *Streptococcus faecalis*/$A_k$ and the sensitive parent strain. J. biol. Chem. **241**, 1043—1048 (1966).

ALBRECHT, A. M., PEARCE, F. K., SULING, W. J., HUTCHISON, D. J.: Folate reductase and specific dihydrofolate reductase of the amethopterin-sensitive *Streptococcus faecium* var. *durans*. Biochemistry **8**, 960—967 (1969).

ALEXANDER, P.: Comparison of the mode of action by which some alkylating agents and ionizing radiations kill mammalian cells. Ann. N. Y. Acad. Sci. **163**, 652—674 (1969).

ANDERSON, E. P., BROCKMAN, R. W.: Feedback inhibition of uridine kinase by cytidine triphosphate and uridine triphosphate. Biochim. biophys. Acta (Amst.) **91**, 380—386 (1964).

Anzai, K., Suzuki, S.: Chemical structure of pathocidin. J. Antibiot. (Japan) **14** A, 253 (1961).

Appel, S. H.: Purification and kinetic properties of brain orotidine 5′-phosphate decarboxylase. J. biol. Chem. **243**, 3924—3929 (1968).

Ayad, S. R., Fox, M., Fox, B. W.: Non-semiconservative incorporation of labelled 5-bromo-2′-deoxyuridine in lymphoma cells treated with low doses of methyl methanesulphonate. Mutat. Res. **8**, 639—645 (1969).

Bach, M. K.: Biochemical and genetic studies of a mutant strain of mouse leukemia L1210 resistant to 1-β-D-arabinofuranosylcytosine (cytarabine) hydrochloride. Cancer Res. **29**, 1036—1044 (1969a).

Bach, M. K.: Reduction in the frequency of mutation to resistance to cytarabine in L1210 murine leukemic cells by treatment with quinacrine hydrochloride. Cancer Res. **29**, 1881—1885 (1969b).:

Balis, M. E.: Antagonists and nucleic acids. In: Neuberger, A., Tatum, E. L. (Eds.): Frontiers of biology, Vol. 10. Amsterdam: North-Holland Publishing Co. 1968.

Balis, M. E., Hylin, V., Coultas, M. K., Hutchison, D. J.: Metabolism of resistant mutants of *Streptococcus faecalis*. II. Incorporation of exogenous purines. Cancer Res. **18**, 220—225 (1958a).

Balis, M. E., Hylin, V., Coultas, M. K., Hutchison, D. J.: Metabolism of resistant mutants of *Streptococcus faecalis*. III. The action of 6-mercaptopurine. Cancer Res. **18**, 440—444 (1958b).

Balis, M. E., Levin, D. H., Brown, G. B., Elion, G. B., Nathan, H. C., Hitchings, G. H.: The effects of 6-mercaptopurine on *Lactobacillus casei*. Arch. Biochem. Biophys. **71**, 358—366 (1957).

Ball, C. R., Connors, T. A., Double, J. A., Ujhazy, V., Whisson, M. E.: Comparison of nitrogen mustard-sensitive and-resistant Yoshida sarcoma. Int. J. Cancer **1**, 319—327 (1966).

Baril, E., Laszlo, J.: Sub-cellular localization and characterization of DNA polymerases from rat liver and hepatomas. In: Weber, G., (Ed.): Advances in enzyme regulation, Vol. 9, pp. 183—204. Oxford: Pergamon Press 1971.

Barski, G., Sorieul, S., Cornefert, C. A. F.: Production dans des cultures *in vitro* de deux souches cellulaires en association, de cellules de caratére hybridge. C. R. Acad. Sci. (Paris) **251**, 1825—1827 (1960).

Baserga, R. (Ed.): The cell cycle and cancer. New York: Marcel Dekker, Inc. 1971.

Beers, R. F., Jr., Herriott, R. M., Tilghman, R. C.: Molecular and cellular repair processes. In: Fifth international symposium on molecular biology. Baltimore: Johns Hopkins University Press, 1972.

Bennett, L. L., Jr.: Phthalanilides and some related dibasic and polybasic compounds: A review of biological activities and modes of action. In: Homburger, F. (Ed.): Progress in experimental tumor research, Vol. 7, pp. 259—325. Basel: S. Karger 1965.

Bennett, L. L., Jr., Adamson, D.: Reversal of the growth inhibitory effects of 6-methylthiopurine ribonucleoside. Biochem. Pharmacol. **19**, 2172—2176 (1970).

Bennett, L., L., Jr., Allan, P. W.: Formation and significance of 6-methylthiopurine ribonucleotide as a metabolite of 6-mercaptopurine. Cancer Res. **31**, 152—158 (1971).

Bennett, L. L., Jr., Allan, P. W., Smithers, D., Vail, M. H.: Resistance to 4-aminopyrazolo-(3,4-d)pyrimidine. Biochem. Pharmacol. **18**, 725—740 (1969).

Bennett, L. L., Jr., Brockman, R. W., Schnebli, H. P., Chumley, S., Dixon, G., Schabel, F. M., Jr., Dulmadge, E. A., Skipper, H. E., Montgomery, J. A., Thomas, H. J.: Activity and mechanism of action of 6-methylthiopurine ribonucleoside in cancer cells resistant to 6-mercaptopurine. Nature (Lond.) **205**, 1276—1279 (1965).

Bennett, L. L., Jr., Schnebli, H. P., Vail, M. H., Allan, P. W., Montgomery, J. A.: Purine ribonucleoside kinase activity and resistance to some analogs of adenosine. Molec. Pharmacol. **2**, 432—443 (1966a).

Bennett, L. L., Jr., Skipper, H. E., Law, L. W.: Incorporation of 8-azaguanine-2-$C^{14}$ into 8-azaguanine-susceptible and 8-azaguanine-dependent leukemic tumors. Fed. Proc. **12**, 300—301 (1953).

Bennett, L. L., Jr., Vail, M. H., Chumley, S., Montgomery, J. A.: Activity of adenosine analogs against a cell culture line resistant to 2-fluoroadenine. Biochem. Pharmacol. **15**, 1719—1728 (1966b).

Bertino, J. R.: The mechanism of action of the folate antagonists in man. Cancer Res. **23**, 1286—1306 (1963).

Bertino, J. R.: Current studies of the folate antagonists in patients with acute leukemia. Cancer Res. **25**, 1614—1619 (1965).

Bertino, J. R., Booth, B. A., Bieber, A. L., Cashmore, A., Sartorelli, A. C.: Studies of the inhibition of dihydrofolate reductase by the folate antagonists. J. biol. Chem. **239**, 479—485 (1964).

BERTINO, J. R., CASHMORE, A. R., HILLCOAT, B. L.: "Induction" of dihydrofolate reductase: purification and properties of the induced human erythrocyte and leukocyte enzyme and normal bone marrow enzyme. Cancer Res. **30**, 2372—2378 (1970).

BERTINO, J. R., DONOHUE, D. M., SIMMONS, B., GABRIO, B. W., SILBER, R., HUENNEKENS, F. M.: The "induction" of dihydrofolic reductase activity in leukocytes and erythrocytes of patients treated with amethopterin. J. clin. Invest. **42**, 466—475 (1963).

BIEBER, S., DIETRICH, L. S., ELION, G. B., HITCHINGS, G. H., MARTIN, D. S.: The incorporation of 6-mercaptopurine-$S^{35}$ into the nucleic acids of sensitive and nonsensitive transplantable mouse tumors. Cancer Res. **21**, 228—231 (1961).

BIEBER, A. L., SARTORELLI, A. C.: The metabolism of 6-thioguanine in purine analog-resistant cells. Cancer Res. **24**, 1210—1215 (1964).

BIEDLER, J. L., ALBRECHT, A. M., HUTCHISON, D. J.: Cytogenetics of mouse leukemia L1210. I. Association of a specific chromosome with dihydrofolate reductase activity in amethopterin-treated sublines. Cancer Res. **25**, 246—257 (1965).

BIEDLER, J. L., ALBRECHT, A. M., HUTCHISON, D. J.: Drug response, dihydrofolate reductase, and cytogenetics of amethopterin-resistant Chinese hamster cells *in vitro*. Cancer Res. **32**, 153—161 (1972).

BIEDLER, J. L., RIEHM, H.: Cellular resistance to actinomycin D in Chinese hamster cells *in vitro:* cross-resistance, radioautographic, and cytogenetic studies. Cancer Res. **30**, 1174—1184 (1970).

BIEDLER, J. L., SCHRECKER, A. W., HUTCHISON, D. J.: Selection of chromosomal variants in amethopterin-resistant sublines of leukemia L1210 with increased levels of dihydrofolate reductase. J. nat. Cancer Inst. **31**, 575—601 (1963).

BIESELE, J. J., BIEDLER, J. L., HUTCHISON, D. J.: The chromosomal status of drug-resistant sublines of mouse leukemia L1210. In: Genetics and cancer, pp. 295—307. Austin: University of Texas Press 1959.

BIRNIE, G. D., KROEGER, H., HEIDELBERGER, C.: Studies of fluorinated pyrimidines. XVIII. The degradation of 5-fluoro-2'-deoxyuridine and related compounds by nucleoside phosphorylase. Biochemistry **2**, 566—572 (1963).

BLAKLEY, R. L.: The biochemistry of folic acid and related pteridines. In: Frontiers of biology, Vol. 13. Amsterdam-London: North-Holland Publishing Co. 1969.

BLAKLEY, R. L., MCDOUGALL, B. M.: Dihydrofolic reductase from *Streptococcus faecalis* R. J. biol. Chem. **236**, 1163—1167 (1961).

BLUMENTHAL, G., GREENBERG, D. M.: Evidence for two molecular species of dihydrofolate reductase in amethopterin resistant and sensitive cells of the mouse leukemia L4946. Oncology **24**, 223—229 (1970).

BORSA, J., WHITMORE, G. F.: Studies relating to the mode of action of methotrexate. II. Studies on sites of action in L-cells *in vitro*. Molec. Pharmacol. **5**, 303—317 (1969a).

BORSA, J., WHITMORE, G. F.: Studies relating to the mode of action of methotrexate. III. Inhibition of thymidylate synthetase in tissue culture cells and in cell-free systems. Molec. Pharmacol. **5**, 318—332 (1969b).

BOSMANN, H. B.: Mechanisms of cellular drug resistance. Nature (Lond.) **233**, 566—569 (1971).

BOSMANN, H. B., KESSEL, D.: Altered glycosidase levels in drug-resistant mouse leukemias. Molec. Pharmacol. **6**, 345—349 (1970).

BRAGANCA, B. M., DIVEKAR, A. Y., VAIDYA, N. R.: Defective transport of aminopterin in relation to development of resistance in Yoshida sarcoma cells. Biochim. biophys. Acta (Amst.) **135**, 937—946 (1967).

BRAUN, W.: Bacterial genetics, 2nd ed. Philadelphia: W. B. Saunders 1965.

BREMERSKOV, V., KADEN, P., MITTERMAYER, C.: DNA synthesis during the life cycle of L cells: Morphological, histochemical and biochemical investigations with arabinosylcytosine and thioarabinosylcytosine. Europ. J. Cancer **6**, 379—392 (1970).

BRESLOW, R. E., GOLDSBY, R. A.: Isolation and characterization of the thymidine transport mutant of Chinese hamster cells. Exp. Cell Res. **55**, 339—346 (1969).

BROCKMAN, R. W.: A mechanism of resistance to 6-mercaptopurine: Metabolism of hypoxanthine and 6-mercaptopurine by sensitive and resistant neoplasms. Cancer Res. **20**, 643—653 (1960).

BROCKMAN, R. W.: Mechanisms of resistance to anticancer agents. In: HADDOW, A., WEINHOUSE, S., (Eds.): Advances in Cancer Research, Vol. 7., pp. 129—234. New York: Academic Press 1963.

BROCKMAN, R. W., BENNETT, L. L., JR., SIMPSON, M. S., WILSON, A. R., THOMSON, J. R., SKIPPER, H. E.: A mechanism of resistance to 8-azaguanine. II. Studies with experimental neoplasms. Cancer Res. **19**, 856—869 (1959b).

BROCKMAN, R. W., DAVIS, J. M., STUTTS, P.: Metabolism of uracil and 5-fluorouracil by drug-sensitive and by drug-resistant bacteria. Biochim. biophys. Acta (Amst.) **40**, 22—32 (1960).

Brockman, R. W., Kelley, G. G., Stutts, P., Copeland, V.: Biochemical aspects of resistance to 6-mercaptopurine in human epidermoid carcinoma cells in culture. Nature (Lond.) **191**, 469—471 (1961).

Brockman, R. W., Roosa, R. A., Law, L. W., Stutts, P.: Purine ribonucleotide pyrophosphorylase activity and resistance to purine analogs in P388 murine lymphocytic leukemia J. cell. comp. Physiol. **60**, 65—84 (1962).

Brockman, R. W., Sparks, M. C., Hutchison, D. J., Skipper, H. E.: A mechanism of resistance to 8-azaguanine. I. Microbiological studies on the metabolism of purines and 8-azapurines. Cancer Res. **19**, 177—188 (1959a).

Brockman, R. W., Sparks, M. C., Simpson, M. S.: A comparison of the metabolism of purines and purine analogs by susceptible and drug-resistant bacterial and neoplastic cells. Biochim. biophys. Acta (Amst.) **26**, 671—672 (1957).

Brockman, R. W., Sparks, M. C., Simpson, M. S., Skipper, H. E.: Decreased ribonucleotide pyrophosphorylase activity of *Streptococcus faecalis* and L1210 leukemia resistant to purine antagonists. Biochem. Pharmacol. **2**, 77—79 (1959c).

Broome, J. D.: Evidence that the L-asparaginase activity of guinea pig serum is responsible for its antilymphoma effects. Nature (Lond.) **191**, 1141—1115 (1961).

Broome, J. D.: Evidence that the L-asparaginase of guenea pig serum is responsible for its antilymphoma effects. I. Properties of the L-asparaginase of guinea pig serum in relation to those of the antilymphoma substance. J. exp. Med. **118**, 99—120 (1963a).

Broome, J. D.: Evidence that the L-asparaginase of guinea pig serum is responsible for its antilymphoma effects. II. Lymphoma 6C3HED cells cultured in a medium devoid of L-asparaginase lose their susceptibility to the effects of guinea pig serum *in vivo*. J. exp. Med. **118**, 121—148 (1963b).

Broome, J. D., Schwartz, J. H.: Differences in the production of L-asparagine in asparaginase-sensitive and resistant lymphoma cells. Biochim. biophys. Acta (Amst.) **138**, 637—639 (1967).

Bryson, V., Szybalski, W.: Microbial drug resistance. In: Advances in genetics, vol. 7, pp. 1—46. New York: Academic Press 1955.

Burchenal, J. H., Coley, V., Purple, J. R., Bucholz, E., Lyman, M. S., Kreis, W.: Studies on the mechanisms of action of various phthalanilide derivatives by cross resistance and tissue culture. Cancer Res. **23**, 1364—1374 (1963).

Burchenal, J. H., Lyman, M. S., Purple, J. R., Coley, V., Smith, S., Bucholz, E.: Therapeutic, combination and resistance studies on certain imidazolin phthalanilide derivatives in mouse leukemia. Cancer Chemother. Rep. **19**, 19—29 (1962).

Calcutt, G., Connors, T. A.: Tumor sulphydryl levels and sensitivity to the nitrogen mustard meraphan. Biochem. Pharmacol. **12**, 839—845 (1963).

Caldwell, I. C., Henderson, J. F., Paterson, A. R. P.: The enzymic formation of 6-(methylmercapto)purine ribonucleoside 5′-phosphate. Canad. J. Biochem. **44**, 229—245 (1966).

Caldwell, I. C., Henderson, J. F., Paterson, A. R. P.: Resistance to purine ribonucleoside analogues in an ascites tumor. Canad. J. Biochem. **45**, 735—744 (1967).

Camiener, G. W.: Studies of the enzymatic deamination of aracytidine. V. Inhibition *in vitro* and *in vivo* by tetrahydrouridine and other reduced pyrimidine nucleosides. Biochem. Pharmacol. **17**, 1981—1991 (1968).

Camiener, G. W., Smith, C. G.: Studies on the enzymatic deamination of cytosine arabinoside. I. Enzyme distribution and species specificity. Biochem. Pharmacol. **14**, 1405—1416 (1965).

Canellakis, E. S.: Pyrimidine metabolism. II. Enzymatic pathways of uracil anabolism. J. biol. Chem. **227**, 329—338 (1957).

Capizzi, R. L., Bertino, J. R., Handschumacher, R. E.: L-Asparaginase. Ann. Rev. Med. **21**, 433—444 (1970).

Cardeilhac, P. T., Cohen, S. S.: Some metabolic properties of nucleosides of 1-β-D-arabinofuranosylcytosine. Cancer Res. **24**, 1595—1603 (1964).

Carey, N. H., Mandel, H. G.: The metabolism of 6-mercaptopurine by *Bacillus cereus*. Biochem. Pharmacol. **5**, 64—78 (1960).

Caskey, C. T., Mashton, D., Wyngaarden, G. B.: The enzymology of feedback inhibition of glutamine phosphoribosylpyrophosphate amidotransferase by purine ribonucleotides. J. biol. Chem. **239**, 2570—2579 (1964).

Chu, E. H. Y., Brimer, P., Jacobsen, K. B., Merriam, E. V.: Mammalian cell genetics. I. Selection and characterization of mutants auxotrophic for L-glutamine or resistant to 8-azaguanine in Chinese hamster cells *in vitro*. Genetics **62**, 359—377 (1969).

Chu, M. Y.: Incorporation of arabinosyl cytosine into 2—7 S ribonucleic acid and cell death. Biochem. Pharmacol. **20**, 2057—2063 (1971).

Chu, M. Y., Fischer, G. A.: A proposed mechanism of action of 1-β-D-arabinofuranosylcytosine as an inhibitor of the growth of leukemic cells. Biochem. Pharmacol. **11**, 423—430 (1962).

CHU, M. Y., FISCHER, G. A.: Comparative studies of leukemic cells sensitive and resistant to cytosine arabinoside. Biochem. Pharmacol. **14**, 333—341 (1965).
CHU, M. Y., FISCHER, G. A.: The incorporation of $^3$H-cytosine arabinoside and its effect on murine leukemic cells (L5178Y). Biochem. Pharmacol. **17**, 753—767 (1968).
CHUN, E. L., GONZALES, L., LEWIS, F. S., JONES, J., RUTMAN, R. J.: Differences in the in vivo alkylation and cross-linking of nitrogen mustard-sensitive and -resistant lines of Lettré Ehrlich ascites tumors. Cancer Res. **29**, 1184—1194 (1969).
ČIHÁK, A., ŠORM, F.: Biochemical effects and metabolic transformations of 5-azacytidine in *Escherichia coli*. Collect. Czech. Chem. Commun. **30**, 2091—2102 (1965).
ČIHÁK, A., VESELÁ, H., ŠORM, F.: Thymidine kinase and polyribosome distribution in regenerating rat liver following 5-azacytidine. Biochim. biophys. Acta (Amst.) **166**, 277—279 (1968).
ČIHÁK, A., VESELÝ, J.: Altered liver regeneration in partially hepatectomized rats following 5-azacytidine treatment. Collect. Czech. Chem. Commun. **34**, 910—918 (1969).
ČIHÁK, A., VESELÝ, J., ŠORM, F.: Incorporation of 5-azacytidine into liver ribonucleic acids of leukemia mice sensitive and resistant to 5-azacytidine. Biochim. biophys. Acta (Amst.) **108**, 516—518 (1965).
ČIHÁK, A., VESELÝ, J., ŠORM, F.: Substrate-induced tryptophan pyrrolase in rat liver after 5-azacytidine administration. Collect. Czech. Chem. Commun. **34**, 1060—1066 (1969).
CLEAVER, J. E.: Repair replication of mammalian cell DNA: Effects of compounds that inhibit DNA synthesis or dark repair. Radiat. Res. **37**, 334—348 (1969).
COGGIN, J. H., LOOSEMORE, M., MARTIN, W. R.: Metabolism of 6-mercaptopurine by resistant *Escherichia coli* cells. J. Bact. **92**, 446—454 (1966).
COHEN, S. S.: Introduction to the biochemistry of D-arabinosyl nucleosides. In: DAVIDSON, J. N., COHN, W. E. (Eds.): Progress in nucleic acid research and molecular biology, Vol. 5, pp. 1—88 New York: Academic Press 1966.
COHEN, S. S.: On the nature of thymineless death. Ann. N. Y. Acad. Sci. **186**, 292—301 (1971).
CONNORS, T. A.: Protection against the toxicity of alkylating agents by thiols: The mechanism of protection and its relevance to cancer chemotherapy. A review. Europ. J. Cancer **2**, 293—305 (1966).
COONEY, D. A., HANDSCHUMACHER, R. E.: L-Asparaginase and L-asparagine metabolism. Ann. Rev. Pharmacol. **10**, 421—440 (1970).
COUSLICH, D. B., SMITH, J. M., JR.: Analogs of pteroylglutamic acid. I. $N^{10}$-Alkylpteroic acid and derivatives. J. Amer. chem. Soc. **70**, 1922—1926 (1948).
COX, R. P., KRAUSS, M. R., BALIS, M. E., DANCIS, J.: Evidence for transfer of enzyme product as the basis of metabolic cooperation between tissue culture fibroblasts of Lesch-Nyhan disease and normal cells. Proc. nat. Acad. Sci. (Wash.) **67**, 1573—1579 (1970).
CRATHORN, A. R., ROBERTS, J. J.: Reactions of cultured mammalian cells of varying radiosensitivity with the radiomimetic alkylating agent, mustard gas. Progr. Biochem. Pharmacol. **1**, 320—326 (1965).
CRATHORN, A. R., ROBERTS, J. J.: Mechanism of the cytotoxic action of alkylating agents in mammalian cells and evidence for the removal of alkylated groups from deoxyribonucleic acid. Nature (Lond.) **211**, 150—153 (1966).
CRAWFORD, I., KORNBERG, A., SIMMS, E. S.: Conversion of uracil and orotate to uridine 5'-phosphate by enzymes in Lactobacilli. J. biol. Chem. **226**, 1093—1101 (1957).
CREASEY, W. A., PAPAC, R. J., MARKIW, M. E., CALABRESI, P., WELCH, A. D.: Biochemical and pharmacological studies with 1-β-D-arabinofuranosylcytosine in man. Biochem. Pharmacol. **15**, 1417—1428 (1966).
CRISS, W. E.: A review of isozymes in cancer. Cancer Res. **31**, 1523—1542 (1971).
CROWTHER, D.: L-Asparaginase and human malignant disease. Nature (Lond.) **229**, 168—171 (1971).
DANØ, K., FREDERIKSEN, S., HELLUNG-LARSEN, P.: Inhibition of DNA and RNA synthesis by daunorubicin in sensitive and resistant Ehrlich ascites tumor cells *in vitro*. Cancer Res. **32**, 1307—1314 (1972).
DAVIDSON, J. D., WINTER, T. S.: Purine nucleotide pyrophosphorylases in 6-mercaptopurine-sensitive and -resistant human leukemias. Cancer Res. **24**, 261—267 (1964).
DAVIES, J. E., ROWND, R.: Transmissible multiple drug resistance in Enterobacteriaceae. Science **176**, 758—768 (1972).
DEAN, A. C. R., HINSHELWOOD, C.: Aspects of the problem of drug resistance in bacteria. In: WOLSTENHOLME, G. E. W., O'CONNOR, C. M. (Eds.): Drug resistance in microorganisms. CIBA foundation symposium, pp. 4—29. London: Churchill, 1957.
DEMEREC, M.: Production of *Staphylococcus* strains resistant to various concentrations of penicillin. Proc. nat. Acad. Sci. (Wash.) **31**, 16—24 (1945).
DEMEREC, M.: Origin of bacterial resistance to antibiotics. J. Bact. **56**, 63—74 (1948).

Demerec, M.: Genetic aspects of drug resistance. In: Wolstenholme, G.E.W., O'Connor, C.M. (Eds.): Drug resistance in microorganisms. CIBA foundation symposium, pp. 47—58. London: Churchill, 1957.
DeVita, V.T.: Cell kinetics and the chemotherapy of cancer. Cancer Chemother. Rep. 2, 23—33 (1971).
Doering, A., Keller, J., Cohen, S.S.: Some effects of D-arabinosyl nucleosides on polymer synthesis in mouse fibroblasts. Cancer Res. 26, 2444—2450 (1966).
Domon, M., Rauth, A.M.: Ultraviolet-light irradiation of mouse L cells: Effects on cells in the DNA synthetic phase. Radiat. Res. 40, 414—429 (1969).
Doskočil, J., Šorm, F.: The mode of action of 5-aza-2′-deoxycytidine in *Escherichia coli*. Europ. J. Biochem. 13, 180—187 (1970).
Diggens, S.M., Gutteridge, W.E., Trigg, P.I.: Altered dihydrofolate reductase associated with a pyrimethamine-resistant *Plasmodium berghei* produced in a single step. Nature (Lond.) 228, 579—580 (1970).
Divekar, A.Y., Vaidya, N.R., Braganca, B.M.: Active transport of aminopterin in Yoshida sarcoma cells. Biochim. biophys. Acta (Amst.) 135, 927—936 (1967).
Dixon, G.J., Dulmadge, E.A., Brockman, R.W.: Feedback inhibition of purine biosynthesis in Adenocarcinoma 755 and Sarcoma 180 cells in culture. J. nat. Cancer Inst. 45, 681—685 (1970).
Drahovsky, D., Kreis, W.: Studies on drug resistance. II. Kinase patterns in P815 neoplasms sensitive and resistant to 1-β-D-arabinofuranosylcytosine. Biochem. Pharmacol. 19, 940—944 (1970).
Drew, R.M.: Induction of resistance to A-methopterin in *Diplococcus pneumoniae* by deoxyribonucleic acid. Nature (Lond.) 179, 1251—1252 (1957).
Dubbs, D.R., Kit, S.: Effect of halogenated pyrimidines and thymidine on growth of L-cells and a subline lacking thymidine kinase. Exp. Cell Res. 33, 19—28 (1964).
Dunlap, R.B., Gundersen, L.E., Huennekens, F.M.: Interconversion of the multiple forms of dihydrofolate reductase from amethopterin-resistant *Lactobacillus casei*. Biochem. biophys. Res. Commun. 42, 772—777 (1971a).
Dunlap, R.B., Harding, N.G.L., Huennekens, F.M.: Thymidylate synthetase and its relationship to dihydrofolate reductase. Ann. N. Y. Acad. Sci. 186, 153—165 (1971b).
Durham, J.P., Ives, D.H.: Deoxycytidine kinase. J. biol. Chem. 245, 2276—2284 (1970).
Dustin, P., Jr.: New aspects of the pharmacology of antimitotic agents. Pharmacol. Revs. 15, 449—480 (1963).
Elion, G.B.: Biochemistry and pharmacology of purine analogues. Fed. Proc. 26, 898—903 (1967).
Elion, G.B., Bieber, S., Hitchings, G.H.: The fate of 6-mercaptopurine in mice. Ann. N.Y. Acad. Sci. 60, 297—303 (1954b).
Elion, G.B., Hitchings, G.H.: The synthesis of 6-thioguanine. J. Amer. chem. Soc. 77, 1676 (1955).
Elion, G.B., Singer, S., Hitchings, G.H.: The purine metabolism of a 6-mercaptopurine-resistant *Lactobacillus casei*. J. biol. Chem. 204, 35—41 (1953).
Elion, G.B., Singer, S., Hitchings, G.H.: Microbiological effects of 6-mercaptopurine. Ann. N. Y. Acad. Sci. 60, 200—206 (1954a).
Ellis, D.B., LePage, G.A.: Biochemical studies of resistance to 6-thioguanine. Cancer Res. 23, 436—443 (1963).
Farber, S., Diamond, L.K., Mercer, R.D., Sylvester, R.F., Jr., Wolff, S.A.: Temporary remissions in acute leukemia in children produced by folic acid antagonists, 4-aminopteroyl glutamic acid (Aminopterin). New Engl. J. Med. 238, 787—793 (1948).
Feigelson, P., Ultmann, J.E., Harris, S., Dashman, T.: Cellular xanthine oxidase and uricase levels in leukemic and normal mouse leukocytes. Cancer Res. 19, 1230—1233 (1959).
Ferone, R.: Dihydrofolate reductase from pyrimethamine-resistant *Plasmodium berghei*. J. biol. Chem. 245, 850—854 (1970).
Ferone, R., Burchall, J.J., Hitchings, G.H.: *Plasmodium berghei* dihydrofolate reductase: Isolation, properties, and inhibition by antifolates. Molec. Pharmacol. 5, 49—59 (1969).
Ferone, R., O'Shea, M., Yoeli, M.: Altered dihydrofolate reductase associated with drug-resistance transfer between rodent plasmodia. Science 167, 1263—1264 (1970).
Fischer, G.A.: Increased levels of folic acid reductase as a mechanism of resistance to amethopterin in leukemic cells. Biochem. Pharmacol. 7, 75—77 (1961).
Fischer, G.A.: Defective transport of amethopterin (methotrexate) as a mechanism of resistance to the antimetabolite in L5178Y leukemic cells. Biochem. Pharmacol. 11, 1233—1234 (1962).
Fox, M., Fox, B.W., Ayad, S.R.: Evidence for genetic expression of integrated DNA in lymphoma cells. Nature (Lond.) 222, 1086—1087 (1969).
Friedkin, M.: Enzymatic aspects of folic acid. Ann. Rev. Biochem. 32, 185—214 (1963).

Friedkin, M., Crawford, E. J., Humphreys, S. R., Goldin, A.: The association of increased dihydrofolate reductase with amethopterin resistance in mouse leukemia. Cancer Res. **22**, 600—606 (1962).
Friedkin, M., Crawford, E. J., Plante, L. T.: Empirical vs. rational approaches in cancer chemotherapy. Ann. N. Y. Acad. Sci. **186**, 209—213 (1971).
Fučík, V., Zadražil, S., Šormová, Z., Šorm, F.: Mutagenic effects of 5-azacytidine in bacteria. Collect. Czech. Chem. Commun. **30**, 2883—2886 (1965).
Fujimoto, W. Y., Seegmiller, J. E.: Hypoxanthine-guanine phosphoribosyltransferase deficiency: Activity in normal, mutant and heterozygote-cultured human skin fibroblasts. Proc. nat. Acad. Sci. (Wash.) **65**, 577—584 (1970).
Fukuyama, T. T., Moyed, H. S.: A separate antibiotic-binding site in xanthosine-5'-phosphate aminase: Inhibitor- and substrate-binding studies. Biochemistry **3**, 1488—1492 (1964).
Furlong, N. B., Gresham, C.: Inhibition of DNA synthesis but not of poly-dAT synthesis by the arabinose analogue of cytidine *in vitro*. Nature (Lond.) **233**, 212—213 (1971).
Furth, J., Cohen, S. S.: Inhibition of mammalian DNA polymerase by the 5'-triphosphate of 1-β-D-arabinofuranosylcytosine and the 5'-triphosphate of 9-β-D-arabinofuranosyladenine. Cancer Res. **28**, 2061—2067 (1968).
Futterman, S.: Enzymatic reduction of folic acid and dihydrofolic acid. J. biol. Chem. **228**, 1031—1038 (1957).
Gaudin, D., Yielding, K. L.: Response of a "resistant" plasmacytoma to alkylating agents and x-ray in combination with the excision repair inhibitors caffeine and chloroquine. Proc. Soc. exp. Biol. (N. Y.) **131**, 1413—1416 (1969).
Gaudin, D., Yielding, K. L., Stabler, A., Brown, J.: The effect of DNA repair inhibitors on the response of tumors treated with x-ray and alkylating agents. Proc. Soc. exp. Biol. (N.Y.) **137**, 202—206 (1971).
Goldberg, A. R., Mechledt, J. H., Pardee, A. R.: On the action of 5-fluorouracil on leukemia cells. Cancer Res. **26**, 1611—1615 (1966).
Goldenberg, G. J.: Properties of L5178Y lymphoblasts highly resistant to nitrogen mustard. In: Biological effects of alkylating agents. Ann. N. Y. Acad. Sci. **163**, 936—953 (1969).
Goldenberg, G. J., Vanstone, C. L., Bihler, I.: Transport of nitrogen mustard on the transport-carrier for choline in L5178Y lymphoblasts. Science **172**, 1148—1149 (1971).
Goldenberg, G. J., Vanstone, C. L., Israels, L. G., Ilse, D., Bihler, I.: Evidence for a transport carrier of nitrogen mustard in nitrogen mustard-sensitive and -resistant L5178Y lymphoblasts. Cancer Res. **30**, 2285—2291 (1970).
Goldman, I. D., Lichtenstein, N. S., Oliverio, V. T.: Carrier mediated transport of the folic acid analogue, methotrexate, in the L1210 leukemia cell. J. biol. Chem. **243**, 5007—5017 (1968).
Goldstein, M. N., Hamm, K., Amrod, E.: Incorporation of tritiated actinomycin D into drug-sensitive and drug-resistant HeLa cells. Science **151**, 1555—1556 (1966).
Goodman, L., DeGraw, J., Kisliuk, R. L., Friedkin, M., Pastore, E. M., Crawford, E. J., Plante, L. T., Alnahas, A., Morningstar, J. F., Jr., Kwok, G., Wilson, L., Donovan, E. F., Ratzan, J.: Tetrahydrohomofolate, a specific inhibitor of thymidylate synthetase. J. Amer. chem. Soc. **86**, 308—309 (1964).
Gots, J. S.: Regulation of purine and pyrimidine metabolism. In: Vogel, H. J. (Ed.): Metabolic pathways. 3rd ed., Vol. V., pp. 225—255. New York: Academic Press 1971.
Graham, F. L., Whitmore, G. F.: The effect of 1-β-D-arabinofuranosylcytosine on gowth, viability, and DNA synthesis of mouse L-cells. Cancer Res. **30**, 2627—2635 (1970a).
Graham, F. L., Whitmore, G. F.: Studies in mouse L-cells on the incorporation of 1-β-D-arabinofuranosylcytosine into DNA and on inhibition of DNA polymerase by 1-β-D-arabinofuranosylcytosine 5'-triphosphate. Cancer Res. **30**, 2636—2644 (1970b).
Grzeschik, K. H., Allerdice, P. W., Grzeschik, A., Optiz, J. M., Miller, O. J., Siniscalco, M.: Cytological mapping of human x-linked genes by use of somatic cell hybrids involving an x-autosome translocation. Proc. nat. Acad. Sci. (Wash.) **69**, 69—73 (1972).
Gundersen, L. E., Dunlap, R. B., Harding, N. G. L., Freisheim, J. H., Otting, F., Huennekens, F. M.: Dihydrofolate reductase from amethopterin-resistant *Lactobacillus casei*. Biochemistry **11**, 1018—1023 (1972).
Häggmark, A.: Studies on resistance against 5-fluorouracil. II. Thymidylate synthetase from drug-resistant tumor lines. Cancer Res. **22**, 568—572 (1962).
Hakala, M. T.: On the role of drug penetration in amethopterin resistance of Sarcoma-180 cells *in vitro*. Biochim. biophys. Acta (Amst.) **102**, 198—209 (1965a).
Hakala, M. T.: On the nature of permeability of Sarcoma 180 cells to amethopterin *in vivo*. Biochim. biophys. Acta (Amst.) **102**, 210—225 (1965b).
Hakala, M.: Uptake and distribution of 4,4'-diacetyl-diphenyl-urea-*bis*-guanylhydrazone in sensitive and resistant Sarcoma 180 cells *in vitro*. Biochem. Pharmacol. **20**, 81—95 (1971).

Hakala, M. T., Ishihara, T.: Chromosomal constitution and amethopterin resistance in cultured mouse cells. Cancer Res. **22**, 987—992 (1962).

Hakala, M. T., Nichol, C. A.: Prevention of the growth-inhibitory effect of 6-mercaptopurine by 4-aminoimidazole-5-carboxamide. Biochim. biophys. Acta (Amst.) **80**, 665—668 (1964).

Hakala, M. T., Suolinna, E. M.: Specific protection of folate reductase against chemical and proteolytic inactivation. Molec. Pharmacol. **2**, 465—480 (1966).

Hakala, M. T., Zakrzewski, S. F., Nichol, C. A.: Relation of folic acid reductase to amethopterin resistance in cultured mammalian cells. J. biol. Chem. **236**, 952—958 (1961).

Handschumacher, R. E.: Studies of bacterial resistance to 6-azauracil and its riboside. Biochim. biophys. Acta (Amst.) **23**, 428—430 (1957).

Handschumacher, R. E., Calabresi, P., Welch, A. D., Bono, V., Fallon, H., Frei, E.: Summary of current information on 6-azauridine. Cancer Chemother. Rep. **21**, 1—18 (1962).

Handschumacher, R. E., Welch, A. D.: Agents which influence nucleic acid metabolism. In: Chargaff, E., Davidson, J. N. (Eds.): The nucleic acids, Vol. III, pp. 453—526. New York: Academic Press, 1960.

Hanka, L. J., Evans, J. S., Mason, D. J., Dietz, A.: Microbiological production of 5-azacytidine. I. Production and biological activity, pp. 619—624. In: Antimicrobial agents and chemotherapy — 1966. Ann Arbor: American Society of Microbiologists 1967.

Harding, N. G. L., Martelli, M. F., Huennekens, F. M.: Amethopterin-induced changes in the multiple forms of dihydrofolate reductase from L1210 cells. Arch. Biochem. Biophys. **137**, 295—296 (1970).

Harrap, K. R., Hill, B. T., Furness, M. E., Hart, L. I.: Sites of action of amethopterin: intrinsic and acquired drug resistance. Ann. N. Y. Acad. Sci. **186**, 312—324 (1971).

Harris, H.: The expression of genetic information: A study with hybrid animal cells, pp. 1—32. In: The Harvey lectures, Series 65. New York: Academic Press, 1971a.

Harris, H.: Cell fusion and the analysis of malignancy. Proc. Royal Soc. (Lond.) **B179**, 1—20 (1971b).

Harris, H., Watkins, J. F.: Hybrid cells derived from mouse and man: Artificial heterokaryons of mammalian cells from different species. Nature (Lond.) **205**, 640—646 (1965).

Harris, M.: Mutation rates in cells at different ploidy levels. J. Cell. Physiol. **78**, 177—184 (1971).

Haskell, C. M., Canellos, G. P.: L-Asparaginase resistance in human leukemia-asparagine synthetase. Biochem. Pharmacol. **18**, 2578—2580 (1969).

Hatfield, D., Wyngaarden, J. B.: I. Synthesis of (3-ribosyluric acid) 5′-phosphate and (3-ribosylxanthine) 5′-phosphate by a pyrimidine ribonucleotide pyrophosphorylase of beef erythrocytes. J. biol. Chem. **239**, 2580—2586 (1964).

Heidelberger, C.: Biochemical mechanisms of action of fluorinated pyrimidines. Exp. Cell Res. **9**, 462—471 (1963).

Heidelberger, C.: Fluorinated pyrimidines. In: Davidson, J. N., Cohn, W. E. (Eds.): Progress in nucleic acid research and molecular biology, Vol. 4, pp. 2—50. New York: Academic Press 1965.

Heidelberger, C.: Cancer chemotherapy with purine and pyrimidine analogues. Ann. Rev. Pharmacol. **7**, 101—124 (1967).

Heidelberger, C., Ghobar, A., Baker, R. K., Mukherjee, K. L.: Studies on fluorinated pyrimidines. X. In vivo studies on tumor resistance. Cancer Res. **20**, 897—902 (1960a).

Heidelberger, C., Kaldor, G., Mukherjee, K. L., Danneberg, P. B.: Studies on fluorinated pyrimidines. XI. In vitro studies on tumor resistance. Cancer Res. **20**, 903—909 (1960b).

Henderson, E. S., Adamson, R. H., Oliverio, V. T.: The metabolic fate of tritiated methotrexate. III. Absorption and excretion in man. Cancer Res. **25**, 1018—1024 (1965).

Henderson, J. F.: Feedback inhibition of purine biosynthesis in ascites tumor cells by purine analogues. Biochem. Pharmacol. **12**, 551—556 (1963).

Henderson, J. F.: Hypoxanthine-guanine phosphoribosyltransferase: further evidence for the identity of the binding sites for hypoxanthine and guanine. Canad. J. Biochem. **47**, 69—71 (1969).

Henderson, J. F., Caldwell, I. C., Paterson, A. R. P.: Decreased feedback inhibition in a 6-(methylmercapto)purine ribonucleotide-resistant tumor. Cancer Res. **27**, 1773—1778 (1967).

Henderson, J. F., Khoo, M. K. Y.: On the mechanism of feedback inhibition of purine biosynthesis *de novo* in Ehrlich ascites tumor cells *in vitro*. J. biol. Chem. **240**, 3104—3109 (1965).

Henderson, J. F., Mercer, N. J. H.: Feedback inhibition of purine biosynthesis de novo in mouse tissues in vivo. Nature (Lond.) **212**, 507—508 (1966).

Hill, D. L., Bennett, L. L., Jr.: Purification and properties of 5-phosphoribosyl pyrophosphate amidotransferase from Adenocarcinoma 755 cells. Biochemistry **8**, 122—130 (1969).

HILLCOAT, B. L., BLAKLEY, R. L.: Dihydrofolate reductase of *Streptococcus faecalis*. I. Purification and some properties of reductase from the wild strain and from strain A. J. biol. Chem. **241**, 2995—3001 (1966).
HILLCOAT, B. L., MARSHALL, L., GAULDIE, J., HIEBERT, M.: Stabilization of dihydrofolate reductase by inhibitors *in vivo* and *in vitro*. Ann. N. Y. Acad. Sci. **186**, 187—205 (1971).
HILLCOAT, B. L., SWETT, V., BERTINO, J. R.: Increase of dihydrofolate reductase activity in cultured mammalian cells after exposure to methotrexate. Proc. nat. Acad. Sci. (Wash.) **58**, 1632—1637 (1967).
HIRONO, I.: Non-protein sulphydryl group in the original strain and subline of the ascites tumor resistant to alkylating reagents. Nature (Lond.) **186**, 1059—1060 (1960).
HIRONO, I.: Mechanism of natural and acquired resistance to methyl-*bis*($\beta$-chloroethyl)amine *N*-oxide in ascites tumors. Gann **52**, 39—48 (1961).
HIRSCHBERG, E., KREAM, J., GELLHORN, A.: Enzymatic deamination of 8-azaguanine in normal and neoplastic tissues. Cancer Res. **12**, 524—528 (1952).
HIRSCHBERG, E., MURRAY, M. R., PETERSON, E. R., KREAM, J., SCHAFRANEK, R., POOL, J. L.: Enzymatic deamination of 8-azaguanine in normal human brain and in glioblastoma multiforme. Cancer Res. **13**, 153—157 (1953).
HO, D. H. W.: Metabolism of 6-methylthiopurine ribonucleoside 5′-phosphate. Biochem. Pharmacol. **20**, 3538—3539 (1971).
HOCHSTADT-OZER, J., STADTMAN, E. R.: The regulation of purine utilization in bacteria. II. Adenine phosphoribosyltransferase in isolated membrane preparations and its role in transport of adenine across the membrane. J. biol. Chem. **246**, 5304—5311 (1971a).
HOCHSTADT-OZER, J., STADTMAN, E. R.: The regulation of purine utilization in bacteria. III. The involvement of purine phosphoribosyltransferases in the uptake of adenine and other nucleic acid precursors by intact resting cells. J. biol. Chem. **246**, 5312—5320 (1971b).
HOFER, K. G.: *In vivo* effects of methotrexate inhibition of DNA synthesis and cell death in sensitive and resistant L1210 ascites populations. Chemotherapy **17**, 59—70 (1972).
HOROWITZ, B., MADRAS, B. K., MEISTER, A., OLD, L. J., BOYSE, E. A., STOCKERT, E.: Asparagine synthetase activity of mouse leukemias. Science **160**, 533—535 (1968).
HOSHINO, A., ALBRECHT, A. M., BIEDLER, J. L., HUTCHISON, D. J.: Amethopterin resistance in clonal lines of L1210 mouse leukemia: some associated biologic and biochemical alterations. Cancer Res. **26**, 1397—1407 (1966).
HUENNEKENS, F. M.: Folate and $B_{12}$ coenzymes. In: SINGER, T. P. (Ed.): Biological oxidations. New York: Interscience Publishers 1968.
HUENNEKENS, F. M., BERTINO, J. R., SILBER, R., GABRIO, B. W.: Antimetabolites in the chemotherapy of leukemia. Exp. Cell Res. **9**, 441—461 (1963).
HUENNEKENS, F. M., DUNLAP, R. B., FREISHEIM, J. H., GUNDERSEN, L. E., HARDING, N. G. L., LEVISON, S. A., MELL, G. P.: Dihydrofolate reductases: structural and mechanistic aspects. Ann. N. Y. Acad. Sci. **186**, 85—99 (1971).
HUGGINS, C., GRAND, L. C., BRILLANTES, F. P.: Mammary cancer induced by a single feeding of polynuclear hydrocarbons and its suppression. Nature (Lond.) **189**, 204—207 (1961).
HUMPHREYS, G. K., GREENBERG, D. M.: Studies on the conversion of deoxyuridylic acid to thymidylic acid by a soluble extract from rat thymus. Arch. Biochem. Biophys. **78**, 275—287 (1958).
HUTCHISON, D. J.: Biological activities of 6-mercaptopurine: Effects on *Streptococcus faecalis*. Ann. N. Y. Acad. Sci. **60**, 212—219 (1954).
HUTCHISON, D. J.: Metabolism of resistant mutants of *Streptococcus faecalis*. I. Isolation and characterization. Cancer Res. **18**, 214—219 (1958).
HUTCHISON, D. J.: Cross resistance and collateral sensitivity studies in cancer chemotherapy. In: Advances in Cancer Research, Vol. 7, pp. 235—350. New York: Academic Press 1963.
HUTCHISON, D. J.: Studies on cross-resistance and collateral sensitivity (1962—1964). Cancer Res. **25**, 1581—1595 (1965).
HUTCHISON, D. J.: Antifolate resistance and the genetic control of dihydrofolate reductase activity. Ann. N. Y. Acad. Sci. **186**, 172—181 (1971).
HURLBERT, R. B., REICHARD, P.: The conversion of orotic acid to uridine nucleotides *in vitro*. Acta chem. scand. **9**, 251—262 (1955).
INAGAKI, A., NAKAMURA, T., WAKISAKA, G.: Studies on the mechanism of action of 1-$\beta$-D-arabinofuranosylcytosine as an inhibitor of DNA synthesis in human leukocytes. Cancer Res. **29**, 2169—2176 (1969).
IVES, D. H., MORSE, P. A., JR., POTTER, V. R.: Feedback inhibition of thymidine kinase by thymidine triphosphate. J. biol. Chem. **238**, 1467—1474 (1963).
JACOBSEN, W., CATHIE, I. A. B.: The inactivation of folic acid antagonists by normal and leukemic cells. Biochem. Pharmacol. **5**, 130—142 (1960a).
JACOBSEN, W., CATHIE, I. A. B.: The nature of aminopterin inactivated by normal and leukemic tissues. Biochem. Pharmacol. **5**, 143—156 (1960b).

Jacquez, J. A.: Permeability of Ehrlich cells to uracil, thymine and fluorouracil. Proc. Soc. exp. Biol. (N. Y.) **109**, 132—135 (1962).

Jacquez, J. A., Ginsberg, F.: Permeability of Ehrlich ascites cells to adenine. Proc. Soc. exp. Biol. (N. Y.) **105**, 478—480 (1960).

Jensen, E. V., DeSombre, E. R., Jungblut, P. W.: Estrogen receptors in hormone responsive tissues and tumors. In: Wissler, R. W., Dao, T. L., Wood, S., Jr. (Eds.): Endogenous factors influencing host-tumor balance, pp. 15—30. Chicago: Chicago University Press 1967.

Johns, D. G., Iannotti, A. T., Sartorelli, A. C., Bertino, J. R.: The relative toxicities of methotrexate and aminopterin. Biochem. Pharmacol. **15**, 555—561 (1966).

Johns, D. G., Loo, T. L.: Metabolite of 4-amino-4-deoxy-$N^{10}$-methylpteroylglutamic acid (methotrexate). J. pharm. Sci. **56**, 356—359 (1967).

Johnson, A. H., Hutchison, D. J.: Folic acid metabolism in antifolic-resistant mutants of *Streptococcus faecalis*. J. Bact. **87**, 786—791 (1964).

Johnson, I. S., Armstrong, J. G., Gorman, M., Burnett, J. P., Jr.: The vinca alkaloids: A new class of oncolytic agents. Cancer Res. **23**, 1390—1427 (1963).

Jurovčík, M., Raška, K., Šormová, Z., Šorm, F.: Anabolic transformation of a novel antimetabolite, 5-azacytidine, and evidence for its incorporation into ribonucleic acid. Collect. Czech. Chem. Commun. **30**, 3370—3376 (1965).

Kallé, G. P., Gots, J. S.: Alterations in purine nucleotide pyrophosphorylases and resistance to purine analogues. Biochim. biophys. Acta (Amst.) **53**, 166—173 (1961).

Kao, F. T., Puck, T. T.: Genetics of somatic mammalian cells. VII. Induction and isolation of nutritional mutants in Chinese hamster cells. Nature (Lond.) **228**, 329—332 (1970).

Kaplan, A. S., Brown, M., Ben-Porat, T.: Effect of 1-$\beta$-D-arabinofuranosylcytosine on DNA synthesis. I. In normal rabbit kidney cell cultures. Molec. Pharmacol. **4**, 131—138 (1968).

Karon, M., Shirakawa, S.: The locus of action of 1-$\beta$-D-arabinofuranosylcytosine in the cell cycle. Cancer Res. **29**, 687—696 (1969).

Kasbekar, D. K., Greenberg, D. M.: Studies on tumor resistance to 5-fluorouracil. Cancer Res. **23**, 818—824 (1963).

Kasbekar, D. K., Nagabhushanam, A., Greenberg, D. M.: Purification and properties of orotic acid-decarboxylating enzymes from calf thymus. J. biol. Chem. **239**, 4245—4249 (1964).

Kashket, E. R., Crawford, E. J., Friedkin, M., Humphreys, S. R., Goldin, A.: On the similarity of dihydrofolate reductases from amethopterin-sensitive and amethopterin-resistant mouse leukemia (L1210) cells. Biochemistry **3**, 1928—1931 (1964).

Kelley, G. G., Wheeler, G. P., Montgomery, J. A.: The effects of a series of 9-alkylpurines on the growth of sensitive and 6-MP-resistant H. Ep.-2 cells. Cancer Res. **22**, 329—333 (1962).

Kelley, W. N., Rosenbloom, F. M., Henderson, J. F., Seegmiller, J. E.: Xanthine phosphoribosyltransferase in man: relationship to hypoxanthine-guanine phosphoribosyltransferase. Biochem. biophys. Res. Commun. **28**, 340—345 (1967).

Kessel, D.: Properties of deoxycytidine kinase partially purified from L1210 cells. J. biol. Chem. **243**, 4739—4744 (1968a).

Kessel, D.: Some observations on the phosphorylation of cytosine arabinoside. Molec. Pharmacol. **4**, 402—410 (1968b).

Kessel, D.: Relevance in *in vitro* tests for predicting responsiveness to antitumor agents. In: Hall, T. C. (Ed.): Prediction of response in cancer therapy. Nat. Cancer Inst. Monograph 34, pp. 138—143. Bethesda: Nat. Cancer Inst. 1971.

Kessel, D., Bosmann, H. B.: On the characteristics of actinomycin D resistance in L5178Y cells. Cancer Res. **30**, 2695—2701 (1970).

Kessel, D., Botterill, V., Wodinsky, I.: Uptake and retention of daunomycin by mouse leukemic cells as factors in drug response. Cancer Res. **28**, 938—941 (1968).

Kessel, D., Hall, T. C.: Amethopterin transport in Ehrlich ascites carcinoma and L1210 cells. Cancer Res. **27**, 1539—1543 (1967).

Kessel, D., Hall, T. C.: Retention of 6-mercaptopurine derivatives by intact cells as an index of drug response in human and murine leukemias. Cancer Res. **29**, 2116—2119 (1969).

Kessel, D., Hall, T. C., Reyes, P.: Metabolism of uracil and 5-fluorouracil in P388 murine leukemia cells. Molec. Pharmacol. **5**, 481—486 (1969a).

Kessel, D., Hall, T. C., Roberts, D., Wodinsky, I.: Uptake as a determinant of methotrexate response in mouse leukemias. Science **150**, 752—754 (1965).

Kessel, D., Hall, T. C., Rosenthal, D.: Uptake and phosphorylation of cytosine arabinoside by normal and leukemic human blood cells *in vitro*. Cancer Res. **29**, 459—463 (1969b).

Kessel, D., Hall, T. C., Wodinsky, I.: Nucleotide formation as a determinant of 5-fluorouracil response in mouse leukemias. Science **154**, 911—913 (1966).

Kessel, D., Hall, T. C., Wodinsky, I.: Transport and phosphorylation as factors in the antitumor action of cytosine arabinoside. Science **156**, 1240—1241 (1967).

KESSEL,D., WODINSKY,I.: Uptake *in vivo* and *in vitro* of actinomycin D by mouse leukemias as factors in survival. Biochem. Pharmacol. **17**, 161—164 (1968).

KESSEL,D., WODINSKY,I.: Thymidine kinase as an index of fluorodeoxyuridine response in mouse leukemias. Molec. Pharmacol. **6**, 251—254 (1970).

KIDD,J.G.: Regression of transplanted lymphomas induced *in vivo* by means of normal guinea pig serum. I. Course of transplanted cancers of various kinds in mice and rats given guinea pig serum, horse serum, or rabbit serum. J. exp. Med. **98**, 565—582 (1953a).

KIDD,J.G.: Regression of transplanted lymphomas induced *in vivo* by means of normal guinea pig serum. II. Studies on the nature of the active serum constituent: Histological mechanism of the regression: Tests for effects of guinea pig serum on lymphoma cells *in vitro:* Discussion. J. exp. Med. **98**, 583—606 (1953b).

KIDDER,G.W., DEWEY,V.C.: The biological activity of substituted purines. J. biol. Chem. **179**, 181—187 (1949).

KIM,J.H., EIDINOFF,M.L.: Action of 1-$\beta$-D-arabinofuranosylcytosine on the nucleic acid metabolism and viability of HeLa cells. Cancer Res. **25**, 698—702 (1965).

KIMBALL,A.P., LEPAGE,G.A.: Metabolic effects of 9-butyl-6-thioguanine *in vivo*. Cancer Res. **23**, 1792—1799 (1963).

KIMBALL,A.P., WILSON,M.J.: Inhibition of DNA polymerase by $\beta$-D-arabinosylcytosine and reversal of inhibition by deoxycytidine-5'-triphosphate. Proc. Soc. exp. Biol. (N. Y.) **127**, 429—432 (1968).

KING,R.J.B., COWAN,D.M., INMAN,D.R.: The uptake of 6,7-$^3$H oestradiol by dimethylbenzanthracene-induced rat mammary tumors. J. Endocrinol. **32**, 83—90 (1965).

KIT,S.: Nucleotides and nucleic acids. In: GREENBERG,D.M. (Ed.): Metabolic pathways. 3rd ed., Vol. IV, pp. 69—275. New York: Academic Press 1970.

KIT,S., DUBBS,D.R., PIEKARSKI,L.J., HSU,T.C.: Deletion of thymidine kinase activity from L cells resistant to bromodeoxyuridine. Exp. Cell Res. **31**, 297—312 (1963).

KLEIN,G.: Population changes and drug resistance in tumors. In: HARRIS,R.J.C. (Ed.): Biological approaches to cancer chemotherapy, pp. 201—217. New York: Academic Press 1961.

KORN,E.D., REMY,C.N., WASILEJKO,H.C., BUCHANAN,J.M.: Biosynthesis of the purines. VII. Synthesis of nucleotides from bases by partially purified enzymes. J. biol. Chem. **217**, 875—883 (1955).

KORNBERG,A.: Pyrophosphorylases and phosphorylases in biosynthetic reactions. Adv. Enzymol. **18**, 191—240 (1957).

KORNBERG,A.: On the metabolic significance of phosphorolytic and pyrophosphorolytic reactions. In: KASHA,M., PULLMAN,B. (Eds.): Horizons in biochemistry, pp. 251—264. New York: Academic Press 1962.

KORNBERG,A., LIEBERMAN,I., SIMMS,E.S.: Enzymatic synthesis and properties of 5-phosphoribosylpyrophosphate. J. biol. Chem. **215**, 389—402 (1955a).

KORNBERG,A., LIEBERMAN,I., SIMMS,E.S.: Enzymatic synthesis of purine nucleotides. J. biol. Chem. **215**, 417—427 (1955b).

KREIS,W., DRAHOVSKY,D., BORBERG,H.: Characterization of protein and DNA in P815 cells sensitive and resistant to 1-$\beta$-D-arabinofuranosylcytosine. Cancer Res. **32**, 696—701 (1972).

KRENITSKY,T.A., PAPAIOANNOU,R., ELION,G.B.: Human hypoxanthine phosphoribosyltransferase. J. biol. Chem. **244**, 1263—1270 (1969).

KUSANO,T., LONG,C., GREEN,H.: A new reduced human-mouse somatic cell hybrid containing the human gene for adenine phosphoribosyltransferase. Proc. nat. Acad. Sci. (Wash.) **68**, 82—86 (1971).

LASTER,W.R.,JR., MAYO,J.G., SIMPSON-HERREN,L., GRISWOLD,D.P.,JR., LLOYD,H.H., SCHABEL,F.M.,JR., SKIPPER,H.E.: Success and failure of the treatment of solid tumors. II. Kinetic parameters and "cell cure" of moderately advanced carcinoma 755. Cancer Chemother. Rep. **53**, 169—188 (1969).

LAW,L.W.: Origin of the resistance of leukemic cells to folic acid antagonists. Nature (Lond.) **169**, 628—629 (1952).

LAW,L.W.: Differences between cancers in terms of evolution of drug resistance. Cancer Res. **16**, 698—716 (1956).

LAWLEY,P.D.: Effects of some chemical mutagens and carcinogens on nucleic acids. Progr. nucl. Acid Res. Molec. Biol. **5**, 89—131 (1966).

LEDERBERG,J., LEDERBERG,E.M.: Replica plating and indirect selection of bacterial mutants. J. Bact. **63**, 399—406 (1952).

LEPAGE,G.A.: Incorporation of 6-thioguanine into nucleic acids. Cancer Res. **20**, 403—408 (1960).

LEPAGE,G.A.: Basic biochemical effects and mechanism of action of 6-thioguanine. Cancer Res. **23**, 1202—1206 (1963).

LePage, G. A.: Resistance to purine analogs. In: Clark, R. L., Cumley, R. W., McCay, J. E., Copeland, M. M. (Eds.): Experimental cancer therapy, Vol. II, pp. 275—278. Chicago: Yearbook Medical Publishers 1971.
LePage, G. A., Bell, J. P., Wilson, M. J.: Arabinosyl-6-mercaptopurine and arabinosyl-6-mercaptopurine-5′-phosphate: Comparison of their metabolic effects. Proc. Soc. exp. Biol. (N. Y.) **131**, 1038—1041 (1969).
LePage, G. A., Jones, M.: Further studies on the mechanism of action of 6-thioguanine. Cancer Res. **21**, 1590—1594 (1961).
LePage, G. A., Junga, I. G., Bowman, B.: Biochemical and carcinostatic effects of 2′-deoxythioguanosine. Cancer Res. **24**, 835—840 (1964).
Levitan, I. B., Webb, T. E.: Effects of 5-azacytidine on polyribosomes and on the control of tyrosine transaminase activity in rat liver. Biochim. biophys. Acta (Amst.) **182**, 491—500 (1969).
Li, L. H., Olin, E. J., Buskirk, H. H., Reineke, L. M.: Cytotoxicity and mode of action of 5-azacytidine on L1210 leukemia. Cancer Res. **30**, 2760—2769 (1970a).
Li, L. H., Olin, E. J., Fraser, T. J., Bhuyan, B. K.: Phase specificity of 5-azacytidine against mammalian cells in tissue culture. Cancer Res. **30**, 2770—2775 (1970b).
Lieberman, I., Kornberg, A., Simms, E. S.: Enzymatic synthesis of pyrimidine nucleotides. Orotidine-5′-phosphate and uridine-5′-phosphate. J. biol. Chem. **215**, 403—415 (1955).
Lieberman, I., Ove, P.: Estimation of mutation rates with mammalian cells in culture. Proc. nat. Acad. Sci. (Wash.) **45**, 872—877 (1959).
Lindberg, B., Klenow, H., Hansen, K.: Some properties of partially purified mammalian adenosine kinase. J. biol. Chem. **242**, 350—356 (1967).
Littlefield, J. W.: The use of drug-resistant markers to study the hybridization of mouse fibroblasts. Exp. Cell Res. **41**, 190—196 (1966).
Livingston, R. B., Carter, S. K.: Single agents in cancer chemotherapy. New York: Plenum Publishing Corp. 1970.
Lomax, C. A., Henderson, J. F.: Phosphorylation of adenosine and deoxyadenosine in Ehrlich ascites carcinoma cells resistant to 6-(methylmercapto)purine ribonucleoside. Can. J. Biochem. **50**, 423—427 (1972).
Loo, T. L., Ho, D. H. W., Blossom, D. R., Shepard, B. J., Frei, E., III: Cellular uptake of purine antimetabolites *in vitro*. II. Uptake of 6-methylthiopurine ribonucleoside by human erythrocytes. Biochem. Pharmacol. **18**, 1711—1725 (1969).
Loo, T. L., Lim, C., Johns, D. G.: Enzymic hydroxylation of 6-methylthiopurine by hepatic aldehyde oxidase. Biochim. biophys. Acta (Amst.) **134**, 467—469 (1967).
Lukens, L. N., Herrington, K. A.: Enzymic formation of 6-mercaptopurine ribotide. Biochim. biophys. Acta (Amst.) **24**, 432—433 (1957).
Luria, S. E., Delbrück, M.: Mutations in bacteria from virus sensitivity to virus resistance. Genetics **28**, 491—511 (1943).
Magee, W. E., Eberts, F. S., Jr.: Studies with psicofuranine in the tumor-bearing rat. Cancer Res. **21**, 611—619 (1961).
Majumbar, A., Bose, S. K.: DNA-mediated genetic transformation of a human cancerous cell line cultured *in vitro*. Brit. J. Cancer **22**, 603—613 (1968).
Maley, F., Maley, G. F.: On the nature of a sparing effect by thymidine on the utilization of deoxycytidine. Biochemistry **1**, 847—851 (1962).
Maley, F., Maley, G. F.: Tetrahydrodeoxyuridylate: A potent inhibitor of deoxycytidylate deaminase. Arch. Biochem. Biophys. **144**, 723—729 (1971).
Mandel, H. G.: The physiological disposition of some anticancer agents. Pharmacol. Revs. **11**, 743—838 (1959).
Martin, W. R., Crichton, I. K., Yang, R. C., Evans, A. E.: The metabolism of thioinosinic acid by 6-mercaptopurine sensitive and resistant leukemic leukocytes. Proc. Soc. exp. Biol. (N. Y.) **140**, 423—428 (1972).
Mashburn, L. T., Wriston, J. C., Jr.: Tumor inhibitory effect of L-asparaginase from *Escherichia coli*. Arch. Biochem. Biophys. **105**, 450—452 (1964).
Matsuya, Y., Green, H., Basilico, C.: Properties and uses of human-mouse hybrid cell lines. Nature (Lond.) **220**, 1199—1202 (1968).
McCollister, R. J., Gilbert, W. R., Ashton, D. M., Wyngaarden, J. B.: Pseudofeedback inhibition of purine synthesis by 6-mercaptopurine ribonucleotide and other purine analogues. J. biol. Chem. **239**, 1560—1563 (1964).
McCoy, T. A., Maxwell, M.: Some nutritional aspects of a 3′-methyl-4-dimethylaminoazobenzene-induced hepatoma *in vitro*. J. nat. Cancer Inst. **23**, 385—393 (1959b).
McCoy, T. A., Maxwell, M., Neuman, R. E.: The amino acid requirements of the Walker carcinosarcoma 265 *in vitro*. Cancer Res. **16**, 979—984 (1956).
McCoy, T. A., Maxwell, M., Kruse, P. F., Jr.: The amino acid requirements of the Jensen sarcoma *in vitro*. Cancer Res. **19**, 591—595 (1959a).

McCullough, J.L., Bertino, J.R.: Dihydrofolate reductase from mouse liver and spleen: Purification, properties and inhibition by substituted 2,4-diaminopyrimidines and 4,6-diaminotriazines. Biochem. Pharmacol. **20**, 561—574 (1971).

McGuire, W.L., Julian, J.A.: Comparison of macromolecular binding of estradiol in hormone-dependent and hormone-independent rat mammary carcinoma. Cancer Res. **31**, 1440—1445 (1971).

McGuire, W.L., Huff, K., Jennings, A., Chamness, G.C.: Mammary carcinoma: A specific biochemical defect in autonomous tumors. Science **175**, 335—336 (1972).

Mead, J.A.R., Goldin, A., Kisliuk, R.L., Friedkin, M., Plante, L., Crawford, E.J., Kwok, G.: Pharmacologic aspects of homofolate derivatives in relation to amethopterin-resistant murine leukemia. Cancer Res. **26**, 2374—2379 (1966).

Mell, G.P., Martelli, M., Kirchner, J., Huennekens, F.M.: Multiple forms of dihydrofolate reductase. Biochem. biophys. Res. Commun. **33**, 74—79 (1968).

Mendelsohn, M.L.: Autoradiographic analysis of cell proliferation in spontaneous breast cancer of $C_3H$ mouse. III. Growth fraction. J. nat. Cancer Inst. **28**, 1015—1029 (1962).

Mendelsohn, M.L.: Cell cycle kinetics and mitotically linked chemotherapy. Cancer Res. **29**, 2390—2393 (1969).

Mezger-Freed, L.: Effect of ploidy and mutagens on bromodeoxyuridine resistance in haploid and diploid frog cells. Nature (Lond.) **235**, 245—246 (1972).

Miech, R.P., Parks, R.E., Jr., Anderson, J.H., Jr., Sartorelli, A.C.: An hypothesis on the mechanism of action of 6-thioguanine. Biochem. Pharmacol. **16**, 2222—2227 (1967).

Miech, R.P., York, R., Parks, R.E., Jr.: Adenosine triphosphate-guanosine-5′-phosphate phosphotransferase. II. Inhibition by 6-thioguanosine-5′-phosphate of the enzyme isolated from hog brain and Sarcoma 180 ascites cells. Molec. Pharmacol. **5**, 30—37 (1969).

Misra, D.K., Humphreys, S.R., Friedkin, M., Goldin, A., Crawford, E.J.: Increased dihydrofolate reductase activity as a possible basis of drug resistance in leukemia. Nature (Lond.) **189**, 39—42 (1961).

Mitsuhashi, S.: Transferable drug resistance factor R. Baltimore-London-Tokyo: University Park Press 1971.

Mobbs, B.G.: The uptake of tritiated oestradiol by dimethylbenzanthracene-induced mammary tumors of the rat. J. Endocrinol. **36**, 409—414 (1966).

Momparler, R.L.: Effect of cytosine arabinoside 5′-triphosphate on mammalian DNA polymerase. Biochem. biophys. Res. Commun. **34**, 465—471 (1969).

Momparler, R.L., Chu, M.Y., Fischer, G.A.: Studies on a new mechanism of resistance to L5178Y murine leukemia cells to cytosine arabinoside. Biochim. biophys. Acta (Amst.) **161**, 481—492 (1968).

Momparler, R.L., Fischer, G.A.: Mammalian deoxynucleoside kinase. I. Deoxycytidine kinase: purification, properties, and kinetic studies with cytosine arabinoside. J. biol. Chem. **243**, 4298—4304 (1968).

Montgomery, J.A., Johnston, T.P., Shealy, Y.F.: Drugs for neoplastic diseases. In: Burger, A. (Ed.): Medicinal chemistry. 3rd ed. Part I, pp. 680—783. New York: Wiley Interscience 1970.

Moore, E.C., Cohen, S.S.: Effects of arabinonucleotides on ribonucleotide reduction by an enzyme system from rat tumor. J. biol. Chem. **242**, 2116—2118 (1967).

Moore, E.C., LePage, G.A.: The metabolism of 6-thioguanine in normal and neoplastic tissues. Cancer Res. 18, 1075—1083 (1958).

Morrow, J.: Genetic analysis of azaguanine resistance in an established mouse cell line. Genetics **65**, 279—287 (1970).

Morse, P.A., Jr., Potter, V.R.: Pyrimidine metabolism in tissue culture cells derived from rat hepatomas. I. Suspension cell cultures derived from the Novikoff hepatoma. Cancer Res. **25**, 499—508 (1965).

Mulligan, L.T., Mellett, L.B.: Inhibition of arabinosylcytosine deamination by tetrahydrouridine. Pharmacologist **12**, 221 (1970).

Nabholz, M., Miggiano, V., Bodmer, W.: Genetic analysis with human-mouse somatic cell hybrids. Nature (Lond.) **223**, 358—363 (1969).

Nakamura, H., Littlefield, J.W.: Purification, properties and synthesis of dihydrofolate reductase from wild type and methotrexate-resistant hamster cells. J. biol. Chem. **247**, 179—187 (1972).

Neel, J.V.: The detection of increased mutation rates in human populations. Perspect. Biol. Med. **14**, 522—537 (1971).

Neil, G.L., Moxley, T.E., Manak, R.C.: Enhancement by tetrahydrouridine of 1-$\beta$-D-arabinofuranosylcytosine (Cytarabine) oral activity in L1210 leukemic mice. Cancer Res. **30**, 2166—2172 (1970).

Nelson, J. A., Parks, R. E., Jr.: Biochemical mechanisms for the synergism between 6-thioguanine and 6-(methylmercapto)purine ribonucleoside in Sarcoma 180 cells. Cancer Res. **32**, 2034—2041 (1972).

Newton, B. A.: Chemotherapeutic compounds affecting DNA structure and function. In: Garattini, S., Goldin, A., Hawking, F., Kopin, I. J. (Eds.): Advances in pharmacology and chemotherapy, Vol. 8, pp. 149—184. New York: Academic Press 1970.

Nichol, C. A., Welch, A. D.: On the mechanism of action of aminopterin. Proc. Soc. exp. Biol. (N. Y.) **74**, 403—411 (1950).

Nixon, P. F., Blakley, R. L.: Dihydrofolate reductase of *Streptococcus faecium*. II. Purification and some properties of two dihydrofolate reductases from the amethopterin-resistant mutant, *Streptococcus faecium* var. *Durans* Strain A. J. biol. Chem. **243**, 4722—4731 (1968).

Nyhan, W. L.: Clinical features of the Lesch-Nyhan syndrome. Introduction — clinical and genetic features. Fed. Proc. **27**, 1027—1033 (1968).

Ochoa, M., Jr., Hirschberg, E.: Alkylating agents. In: Schnitzer, R. J., Hawking, F. (Eds.): Experimental chemotherapy, Vol. 5, pp. 1—132. New York: Academic Press 1967.

Orengo, A.: Regulation of enzymic activity by metabolites. I. Uridine-cytidine kinase of Novikoff ascites rat tumors. J. biol. Chem. **244**, 2204—2209 (1969).

Osborn, M. J., Freeman, M., Huennekens, F. M.: Inhibition of dihydrofolate reductase by aminopterin and amethopterin. Proc. Soc. exp. Biol. (N. Y.) **97**, 429 (1958).

Ozer, H. L.: Purine pyrophosphorylase as a selective genetic marker in a mouse lymphoma, P388, in cell culture. J. cell Physiol. **68**, 61—68 (1966).

Pačes, V., Doskočil, J., Šorm, F.: Incorporation of 5-azacytidine into nucleic acids of *Escherichia coli*. Biochim. biophys. Acta (Amst.) **161**, 352—360 (1968).

Pasternak, C. A., Fischer, G. A., Handschumacher, R. E.: Alterations in pyrimidine metabolism in L5178Y leukemia cells resistant to 6-azauridine. Cancer Res. **21**, 110—117 (1961).

Paterson, A. R. P.: The formation of 6-mercaptopurine riboside phosphate in ascites tumor cells. Canad. J. Biochem. Physiol. **37**, 1011—1023 (1959).

Paterson, A. R. P.: The development of resistance to 6-mercaptopurine in a subline of the Ehrlich ascites carcinoma. Canad. J. Biochem. Physiol. **38**, 1117—1127 (1960a).

Paterson, A. R. P.: Thiopurine nucleotide synthesis in a 6-MP-resistant subline of the Ehrlich ascites carcinoma and growth inhibition by certain antimetabolites. Canad. J. Biochem. **38**, 1129—1136 (1960b).

Paterson, A. R. P.: Resistance to 6-mercaptopurine. II. The synthesis of thioinosinate in a 6-mercaptopurine-resistant subline of the Ehrlich ascites carcinoma. Canad. J. Biochem. Physiol. **40**, 195—206 (1962).

Paterson, A. R. P.: Biochemical mechanisms of resistance to antimetabolites, pp. 417—438. In: Canadian Cancer Conference, Vol. 5. New York: Academic Press 1963.

Paterson, A. R. P., Hori, A.: Resistance to 6-mercaptopurine. I. Biochemical differences between the Ehrlich ascites carcinoma and a 6-mercaptopurine-resistant subline. Canad. J. Biochem. Physiol. **40**, 181—194 (1962).

Paterson, A. R. P., Sutherland, A.: Metabolism of 6-mercaptopurine ribonucleoside by Ehrlich ascites carcinoma cells. Canad. J. Biochem. **42**, 1415—1423 (1964).

Patterson, M. K., Jr., Orr, G.: L-Asparagine biosynthesis by nutritional variants of the Jensen Sarcoma. Biochem. biophys. Res. Commun. **26**, 228—233 (1967).

Patterson, M. K., Jr., Orr, G.: Asparagine biosynthesis by the Novikoff hepatoma. J. biol. Chem. **243**, 376—380 (1968).

Perkins, J. P., Bertino, J. R.: Dihydrofolate reductase from L1210R murine lymphoma. Fluorimetric measurements of the interaction of the enzyme with coenzymes, substrates and inhibitors. Biochemistry **5**, 1005—1012 (1966).

Perkins, J. P., Hillcoat, B. L., Bertino, J. R.: Dihydrofolate reductase from a resistant subline of the L1210 lymphoma. J. biol. Chem. **242**, 4771—4776 (1967).

Peters, R. A.: Lethal synthesis. Proc. Royal Soc. (Lond.) **139B**, 143—170 (1952).

Peters, W.: Chemotherapy and drug resistance in malaria. London-New York: Academic Press 1970.

Peters, J. M., Greenberg, D. M.: Studies of folic acid reduction. Biochim. biophys. Acta (Amst.) **32**, 273—274 (1959).

Pine, M. J.: Uptake of aminopterin in *Bacillus subtilis*. J. Bact. **79**, 827—834 (1960).

Pískala, A., Šorm, F.: Synthesis of 1-glycosyl derivatives of 5-azauracil and 5-azacytosine. Coll. Czech. Chem. Commun. **29**, 2060—2076 (1964).

Pithová, P., Pískala, A., Pitha, J., Šorm, F.: Nucleic acid components and their analogues. LXVI. Hydrolysis of 5-azacytidine and its connection with biological activity. Coll. Czech. Chem. Commun. **30**, 2801—2811 (1965).

Pittillo, R. F., Moncrief, C., Brockman, R. W., Chambers, P.: Antimicrobial activity of 2-fluoroadenosine and 2-fluoroadenine, pp. 474—484. In: Antimicrobial Agents and Chemotherapy — 1964, 1965.

PLIML, J., ŠORM, F.: Synthesis of a 2-deoxy-D-ribofuranosyl-5-azacytosine. Coll. Czech. Chem. Commun. **29**, 2576—2578 (1964).

PODGAJETSKAYA, D.J., BRESLER, V.M., SURIKOV, I.M., IGNATOVA, T.N., OLENOV, J.M.: The transforming action of deoxyribonucleic acid isolated from sarcolysine-resistant tumors or sarcolysine-sensitive tumors. Biochim. biophys. Acta (Amst.) **80**, 110—115 (1964).

POMALES, R., ELION, G.B., HITCHINGS, G.H.: Xanthine as a precursor of nucleic acid purines in the mouse. Biochim. biophys. Acta (Amst.) **95**, 505—506 (1965).

PRAGER, M.D.: Tumor inhibitory enzymes. In: CLARK, R.L., CUMLEY, R.W., MCCAY, J.E., COPELAND, M.M. (Eds.): Oncology 1970. Experimental Cancer Chemotherapy, Vol. II, pp. 237—253. Chicago: Yearbook Medical Publishers 1971.

PRAGER, M.D., BACHYNSKY, N.: Asparagine synthetase in normal and malignant tissues: Correlation with tumor sensitivity to asparaginase. Arch. Biochem. Biophys. **127**, 645—654 (1968).

RAUNIO, R.P., HAKALA, M.T.: Comparison of folate reductases of Sarcoma 180 cells, sensitive and resistant to amethopterin. Molec. Pharmacol. **3**, 279—283 (1967).

RAUTH, A.M., BARTON, B., LEE, C.P.Y.: Effects of caffeine on L-cells exposed to mitomycin C. Cancer Res. **30**, 2724—2729 (1970).

REDDY, G.V.R., GOULIAN, M., HENDLER, S.S.: Inhibition of *E. coli* DNA polymerase II by ara-CTP. Nature (Lond.) **234**, 286—288 (1971).

REDETZKI, H.M., REDETZKI, J.E., ELIAS, A.L.: Resistance of the rabbit to methotrexate: Isolation of a drug metabolite with decreased cytotoxicity. Biochem. Pharmacol. **15**, 425—433 (1966).

REICHARD, P.: The enzymic synthesis of pyrimidines. Advances in enzymology, Vol. 21, pp. 263—294. New York: Academic Press 1959.

REICHARD, P.: The biosynthesis of deoxyribose. CIBA lectures in biochemistry, New York: John Wiley and Sons 1968.

REICHARD, P., SKÖLD, O., KLEIN, G.: Possible enzymic mechanism for the development of resistance against fluorouracil in ascites tumors. Nature (Lond.) **183**, 939—941 (1959).

REICHARD, P., SKÖLD, O., KLEIN, G., RÉVÉSZ, L., MAGNUSSON, P-H.: Studies on resistance against 5-fluorouracil. I. Enzymes of the uracil pathway during development of resistance. Cancer Res. **22**, 235—243 (1962).

REID, B.D., WALKER, I.G.: Resistance to sulfur mustard: A comparison of some properties of strain L cells and a resistant subline. Cancer Res. **26**, 1801—1805 (1966).

REMY, C.N.: Ribonucleotides and ribonucleosides as methyl acceptors for 5-adenosylmethionine: (amino- and thio-)purine methyltransferases. Incorporation of 6-amino-2-methylaminopurine into ribonucleic acids. Biochim. biophys. Acta (Amst.) **138**, 258—275 (1967).

REYES, P.: The synthesis of 5-fluorouridine 5'-phosphate by a pyrimidine phosphoribosyltransferase of mammalian origin. I. Some properties of the enzyme from P1534J mouse leukemic cells. Biochemistry **8**, 2057—2062 (1969).

REYES, P., HALL, T.C.: Synthesis of 5-fluorouridine 5'-phosphate by a pyrimidine phosphoribosyltransferase of mammalian origin. II. Correlation between the tumor levels of the enzyme and the 5-fluorouracil-promoted increase in survival of tumor-bearing mice. Biochem. Pharmacol. **18**, 2587—2590 (1969).

RIEHM, H., BIEDLER, J.L.: Potentiation of drug effect by Tween 80 in Chinese hamster cells resistant to actinomycin D and daunomycin. Cancer Res. **32**, 1195—1200 (1972).

ROBERTS, D.: In search of a key. In: Prediction of response in cancer therapy. Nat. Cancer Inst. Monograph 34. Bethesda: National Cancer Institute 1971.

ROBERTS, D., HALL, T.C.: Enzyme activities and deoxynucleoside utilization of leukemic leukocytes in relation to drug therapy and resistance. Cancer Res. **29**, 166—173 (1969).

ROBERTS, D., WODINSKY, I.: On the poor correlation between the inhibition by methotrexate of dihydrofolate reductase and of deoxynucleoside incorporation into DNA. Cancer Res. **28**, 1955—1962 (1968).

ROBERTS, D., WODINSKY, I., HALL, T.C.: Studies on folic reductase. III. The level of enzyme activity and response to methotrexate of transplantable mouse tumors. Cancer Res. **25**, 1899—1903 (1965).

ROBERTS, J.J.: Repair of alkylated DNA in mammalian cells. In: BEERS, R.F., JR., HERRIOTT, R.M., TILGHMAN, R.C. (Eds.): Molecular and cellular repair processes. Baltimore: Johns Hopkins University Press 1972.

ROBERTS, J.J., CRATHORN, A.R., BRENT, T.P.: Repair of alkylated DNA in mammalian cells. Nature (Lond.) **218**, 970—972 (1968).

ROBERTS, J.J., PASCOE, J.M., PLANT, J.E., STURROCK, J.E., CRATHORN, A.R.: Quantitative aspects of the repair of alkylated DNA in cultured mammalian cells. I. The effect on HeLa and Chinese hamster cell survival of alkylation of cellular macromolecules. Chem. Biol. Interact. **3**, 29—47 (1971a).

Roberts, J. J., Pascoe, J. M., Smith, B. A., Crathorn, A. R.: Quantitative aspects of the repair of alkylated DNA in cultured mammalian cells. II. Non-semi-conservative DNA synthesis ("repair synthesis") in HeLa and Chinese hamster cells following treatment with alkylating agents. Chem. Biol. Interact. **3**, 49—68 (1971b).

Roblin, R. O., Jr., Lampen, J. O., English, J. P., Cole, Q. P., Vaughan, J. R., Jr.: Studies in chemotherapy. VIII. Methionine and purine antagonists and their relation to the sulfonamides. J. Amer. chem. Soc. **67**, 290—294 (1945).

Roosa, R. A., Bailey, E.: DNA-mediated transformation of mammalian cells in culture. Increased transforming efficiency following sonication. J. Cell. Physiol. **75**, 137—150 (1970).

Rosenbloom, F. M., Henderson, J. F., Caldwell, I. C., Kelley, W. N., Seegmiller, J. E.: Biochemical bases of accelerated purine biosynthesis de novo in human fibroblasts lacking hypoxanthine-guanine phosphoribosyltransferase. J. biol. Chem. **243**, 1166—1173 (1968a).

Rosenbloom, F. M., Henderson, J. F., Kelley, W. N., Seegmiller, J. E.: Accelerated purine biosynthesis de novo in skin fibroblasts deficient in hypoxanthine-guanine phosphoribosyltransferase activity. Biochim. biophys. Acta (Amst.) **166**, 258—260 (1968b).

Ross, W. C. J.: Biological alkylating agents. London: Butterworths 1962.

Rothenberg, S. P.: Alteration of methotrexate by leukemic cells: Loss of affinity for an anion exchange resin. Cancer Res. **29**, 2047—2055 (1969).

Roush, A., Norris, E. R.: Deamination of 8-azaguanine by guanase. Arch. Biochem. **29**, 124—129 (1950).

Roy-Burman, P.: Analogues of nucleic acid components. In: Rentchnick, P. (Ed.): Recent Results in Cancer Research, Vol. 25. Berlin-Heidelberg-New York: Springer 1970.

Ruddle, F. H., Chapman, V. M., Ricciuti, F., Klebe, R., Murnane, M., Meera-Khan, P.: Linkage relationships of seventeen human gene loci as determined by man-mouse somatic cell hybrids. Nature (Lond.) **232**, 69—73 (1971).

Rueckert, R. R., Mueller, G. C.: Studies on unbalanced growth in tissue culture. I. Induction and consequences of thymidine deficiency. Cancer Res. **20**, 1584—1591 (1960).

Rutman, R. J., Chun, E. H. L., Lewis, F. S.: Permeability difference as a source of resistance to alkylating agents in Ehrlich tumor cells. Biochem. biophys. Res. Commun. **32**, 650—657 (1968).

Sander, S., Attramadal, A.: The *in vivo* uptake of oestradiol-17$\beta$ by hormone responsive and unresponsive breast tumors of the rat. Acta pathol. microbiol. scand. **74**, 169—178 (1968).

Sartorelli, A. C., LePage, G. A., Moore, E. C.: Metabolic effects of 6-thioguanine. I. Studies on thioguanine-resistant and -sensitive Ehrlich ascites cells. Cancer Res. **18**, 1232—1239 (1958).

Sartorelli, A. C., Upchurch, H. F., Bieber, A. L., Booth, B. A.: Some metabolic effects exerted by azaserine and purine analogs *in vivo*. Cancer Res. **24**, 1202—1209 (1964).

Scannell, J. P., Hitchings, G. H.: Thioguanine in deoxyribonucleic acid from tumors of 6-mercaptopurine-treated mice. Proc. Soc. exp. Biol. (N. Y.) **122**, 627—629 (1966).

Scannell, J. P., Pruess, D. L., Kellett, M., Demny, T. C., Stempel, A.: Antimetabolites produced by microorganisms. III. 2-Aminopurine-6-thiol (thioguanine). J. Antibiot. (Japan) **24**, 328—329 (1971).

Schabel, F. M., Jr.: *In vivo* leukemia cell kill kinetics and "curability" in experimental systems, pp. 379—408. In: The Proliferation and Spread of Neoplastic Cells (M. D. Anderson Symposium). Baltimore: Williams and Wilkins Co. 1968.

Schabel, F. M., Jr.: The use of tumor growth kinetics in planning "curative" chemotherapy of advanced solid tumors. Cancer Res. **29**, 2384—2389 (1969).

Schnebli, H. P., Hill, D. L., Bennett, L. L., Jr.: Purification and properties of adenosine kinase from human tumor cells of type H. Ep. No. 2. J. biol. Chem. **242**, 1997—2004 (1967).

Schrecker, A. W.: Metabolism of 1-$\beta$-D-arabinofuranosylcytosine in leukemia L1210: Nucleoside and nucleotide kinases in cell-free extracts. Cancer Res. **30**, 632—641 (1970).

Schrecker, A. W., Mead, J. A. R., Greenberg, N. H., Goldin, A.: Dihydrofolate reductase activity of leukemia L1210 during development of methotrexate resistance. Biochem. Pharmacol. **20**, 716—718 (1971).

Schrecker, A. W., Urshel, M. J.: Metabolism of 1-$\beta$-D-arabinofuranosylcytosine in leukemia L1210: studies with intact cells. Cancer Res. **28**, 793—801 (1968).

Schrecker, A. W., Venditti, J. M., Greenberg, N. H., Biedler, J. L., Robinson, D. L., Hutchison, D. J.: Association of increased dihydrofolate reductase levels and chromosome alteration in amethopterin-resistant sublines of leukemia L1210. J. nat. Cancer Inst. **31**, 557—574 (1963).

Schwartz, A. G., Cook, P. R., Harris, H.: Correction of a genetic defect in a mammalian cell. Nature (Lond.) **230**, 5—8 (1971).

Seeger, D. R., CousLich, D. B., Smith, J. M., Jr., Hultquist, M. E.: Analogs of pteroylglutamic acid. III. 4-Amino derivatives. J. Amer. chem. Soc. **71**, 1753—1758 (1949).

SEEGER, D. R., SMITH, J. M., JR., HULTQUIST, M. E.: Antagonist of pteroylglutamic acid. J. Amer. chem. Soc. **69**, 2567 (1947).
SEEGMILLER, J. E., ROSENBLOOM, F. M., KELLEY, W. N.: Enzyme defect associated with sex-linked human neurological disorder and excessive purine synthesis. Science **155**, 1682—1684 (1967).
SHACTER, B., LAW, L. W.: Azaguanine-deaminase activity of several lymphocytic leukemias of mice. J. nat. Cancer Inst. **18**, 77—81 (1957).
SHANTZ, G. D., FONTENELLE, L. J., HENDERSON, J. F.: Inhibition of purine biosynthesis *de novo* and of Ehrlich ascites tumor cell growth by 6-methylmercaptopurine ribonucleoside. Biochem. Pharmacol. **21**, 1203—1206 (1972).
SHAW, W. V.: Biochemical mechanisms of transferable drug resistance, Vol. 9. (GARATTINI, S., GOLDIN, A., HAWKING, F., KOPIN, L. J., Eds.) New York: Academic Press 1971.
SILAGI, A.: Metabolism of 1-$\beta$-D-arabinofuranosylcytosine in L cells. Cancer Res. **25**, 1446—1453 (1965).
SILAGI, S., DARLINGTON, G., BRUCE, S. A.: Hybridization of two biochemically marked human cell lines. Proc. nat. Acad. Sci. (Wash.) **62**, 1085—1092 (1969).
SIMARD, R., CASSINGENA, R.: Actinomycin resistance in cultured hamster cells. Cancer Res. **29**, 1590—1597 (1969).
SINISCALCO, M., KILNGER, H. P., EAGLE, H., KOPROWSKI, H., FUJIMOTO, W. Y., SEEGMILLER, J. E.: Evidence for intergenic complementation in hybrid cells derived from two human diploid strains each carrying an x-linked mutation. Proc. nat. Acad. Sci. (Wash.) **62**, 793—799 (1969).
SIROTNAK, F. M.: Dual consequences of mutation in the dihydrofolate reductase gene of *Diplococcus pneumoniae*. Biochem. biophys. Res. Commun. **36**, 603—607 (1969).
SIROTNAK, F. M.: Increased dihydrofolate reductase synthesis in *Diplococcus pneumoniae* following translatable alteration of the structural gene. III. Further evidence on the extent of genomic involvement. Genetics **65**, 391—406 (1970).
SIROTNAK, F. M.: High dihydrofolate reductase levels in *Diplococcus pneumoniae* after mutation in the structural gene: biochemical and immunological evidence for increased synthesis. J. Bact. **106**, 318—324 (1971).
SIROTNAK, F. M.: On the mode of binding of folate antagonists to dihydrofolate reductase. An analysis of genetic effects in a microbial system. (in press).
SIROTNAK, F. M., DONATI, G. J., HUTCHISON, D. J.: Evidence for a genetic alteration of dihydrofolate reductase associated with amethopterin resistance in *Diplococcus pneumoniae*. Biochem. biophys. Res. Commun. **14**, 292—295 (1964a).
SIROTNAK, F. M., DONATI, G. J., HUTCHISON, D. J.: Dihydrofolate reductase in genotypically distinguishable amethopterin-resistant *Diplococcus pneumoniae*. J. biol. Chem. **239**, 2677—2682 (1964c).
SIROTNAK, F. M., DONATI, G. J., HUTCHISON, D. J.: Genetic modification of the structure and amount of dihydrofolate reductase in amethopterin-resistant *Diplococcus pneumoniae*. J. biol. Chem. **239**, 4298—4302 (1964d).
SIROTNAK, F. M., HACHTEL, S. L.: Increased dihydrofolate reductase synthesis in *Diplococcus pneumoniae* following translatable alteration of the structural gene. I. Genotype derivation and recombinational analyses. Genetics **61**, 293—312 (1969).
SIROTNAK, F. M., HACHTEL, S. L., WILLIAMS, W. A.: Increased dihydrofolate reductase synthesis in *Diplococcus pneumoniae* following translatable alteration of the structural gene. II. Individual and dual effects on the properties and rate of synthesis of the enzyme. Genetics **61**, 313—326 (1969).
SIROTNAK, F. M., HUTCHISON, D. J.: Gel filtration properties of mutant and wild-type dihydrofolate reductase from *Diplococcus pneumoniae*. Biochem. biophys. Res. Commun. **19**, 734—738 (1965).
SIROTNAK, F. M., HUTCHISON, D. J.: Purification and properties of mutant and wild-type dihydrofolate reductase from *Diplococcus pneumoniae*. J. biol. Chem. **241**, 2900—2906 (1966).
SIROTNAK, F. M., KURITA, S., HUTCHISON, D. J.: On the nature of a transport alteration determining resistance to amethopterin in the L1210 leukemia. Cancer Res. **28**, 75—80 (1968).
SIROTNAK, F. M., KURITA, S., SARGENT, M. G., ROBINSON, D. L., HUTCHISON, D. J.: Sequential biochemical alteration to antifolate resistance in L1210 leukemia. Nature (Lond.) **216**, 1236—1237 (1967c).
SIROTNAK, F. M., LUNT, R. B., HUTCHISON, D. J.: Transformation of resistance to 8-azaguanine in *Diplococcus pneumoniae*. Nature (Lond.) **187**, 800—801 (1960a).
SIROTNAK, F. M., LUNT, R. B., HUTCHISON, D. J.: Genetic studies on amethopterin resistance in *Diplococcus pneumoniae*. J. Bact. **80**, 648—653 (1960b).
SIROTNAK, F. M., LUNT, R. B., HUTCHISON, D. J.: The distribution of mutational sites affecting resistance to amethopterin in *Diplococcus pneumoniae*. Genetics **49**, 439—452 (1964b).

Sirotnak, F.M., Sargent, M.G., Hutchison, D.J.: Genetically alterable transport of amethopterin in *Diplococcus pneumoniae*. I. Physiological properties and kinetics of the wild-type system. J. Bact. **93**, 309—314 (1967a).
Sirotnak, F.M., Sargent, M.G., Hutchison, D.J.: Genetically alterable transport of amethopterin in *Diplococcus pneumoniae*. II. Impairment of the system associated with various mutant genotypes. J. Bact. **93**, 315—319 (1967b).
Sirotnak, F.M., Williams, W.A.: A dissociable mutant form of dihydrofolate reductase from *Diplococcus pneumoniae*. Arch. Biochem. Biophys. **136**, 580—582 (1970).
Skipper, H.E.: Cellular kinetics associated with "curability" of experimental leukemias. In: Dameshek, W., Dutcher, R.M. (Eds.): Perspectives in leukemia, pp. 187—216. New York: Grune and Stratton 1968.
Skipper, H.E.: Improvement of the model systems. Cancer Res. **29**, 2329—2333 (1969).
Skipper, H.E.: The cell cycle and chemotherapy of cancer. In: The cell cycle and cancer. New York: Marcel Dekker 1971a.
Skipper, H.E.: Cancer chemotherapy is many things: G. H. A. Clowes Memorial Lecture. Cancer Res. **31**, 1173—1180 (1971b).
Skipper, H.E.: Kinetic behavior versus response to chemotherapy. In: Prediction of response in cancer therapy. Nat. Cancer Inst. Monograph 34. Bethesda: Nat. Cancer Inst. 1971c.
Skipper, H.E., Schabel, F.M., Jr., Mellett, L.B., Montgomery, J.A., Wilkoff, L.J., Lloyd, H.H., Brockman, R.W.: Implications of biochemical, cytokinetic, pharmacologic and toxicologic relationships in the design of optimal therapeutic schedules. Cancer Chemother. Rep. **54**, 431—450 (1970).
Skipper, H.E., Schabel, F.M., Jr., Wilcox, W.S.: Experimental evaluation of antitumor agents. XXI. Scheduling of arabinosylcytosine to take advantage of its *S*-phase specificity against leukemia cells. Cancer Chemother. Rep. **51**, 125—165 (1967).
Škoda, J.: Mechanism of action and application of azapyrimidines. In: Davidson, S.N., Cohn, W.E. (Eds.): Progress in nucleic acid research, Vol. 2, pp. 197—219. New York: Academic Press 1963.
Sköld, O.: Enzymic arbosidation and ribotidation of 5-fluorouracil by extracts of the Ehrlich-ascites tumor. Biochim. biophys. Acta (Amst.) **29**, 651 (1958).
Sköld, O.: Nucleoside and nucleotide derivatives of 5-fluorouracil. Arkiv für Kemi **17**, 59—71 (1960).
Sköld, O., Magnusson, P-H., Revesz, L.: Studies on resistance against 5-fluorouracil. III. Selective value of resistant, uridine kinase-deficient tumor cells. Cancer Res. **22**, 1226—1229 (1962).
Slotnick, I.J., Sells, B.H.: Actinomycin resistance in *Bacillus subtilis*. Science **146**, 407—408 (1964).
Šorm, F., Šormová, Z., Raška, K., Jr., Durovčik, M.: Comparison of the metabolism and inhibitory effect of 5-azacytidine and 5-aza-2′-deoxycytidine in mammalian tissues. Rev. Roumaine Biochim. **3**, 139—147 (1966).
Šorm, F., Veselý, J.: Effect of 5-aza-2′-deoxycytidine against leukemic and hemopoietic tissues in AKR mice. Neoplasma **15**, 339—343 (1968).
Šorm, F., Veselý, J.: The activity of a new antimetabolite, 5-azacytidine, against lymphoid leukemia in AK mice. Neoplasma **11**, 123—130 (1964).
Staub, M., Warner, H.R., Reichard, P.: Selective inhibition of DNA replication in *Escherichia coli* by 1-β-D-arabinosylcytosine triphosphate. Biochem. biophys. Res. Commun. **46**, 1824—1829 (1972).
Steel, G.G.: Cell loss as a factor in the growth rate of human tumors. Europ. J. Cancer **3**, 381—387 (1967).
Steel, G.G.: Cell loss from experimental tumors. Cell Tissue Kinet. **1**, 193—207 (1968).
Struart, C.D., Burke, P.J.: Cytidine deaminase and the development of resistance to arabinosylcytosine. Nature (Lond.) **233**, 109—110 (1971).
Stutts, P., Brockman, R.W.: A biochemical basis for resistance of L1210 mouse leukemia to 6-thioguanine. Biochem. Pharmacol. **12**, 97—104 (1963).
Subak-Sharpe, H.: Biochemically marked variants of the Syrian hamster fibroblast cell line BHK 21 and its derivatives. Exp. Cell Res. **38**, 106—119 (1965).
Subak-Sharpe, H., Bürk, R.R., Pitts, J.D.: Metabolic co-operation between biochemically marked mammalian cells in tissue culture. J. Cell Sci. **4**, 353—367 (1969).
Szybalska, E.H., Szybalski, W.: Genetics of human cell lines. IV. DNA mediated heritable transformation of a biochemical trait. Proc. nat. Acad. Sci. (Wash.) **48**, 2026—2034 (1962).
Szybalski, W.: Genetics of human cell lines. II. Method for determination of mutation rates to drug resistance. Exp. Cell Res. **18**, 588—590 (1959).
Szybalski, W., Bryson, V.: One step resistance development to isoniazid and sodium *p*-aminosalicylate. J. Bact. **66**, 468—469 (1953).

TANNOCK, I. F. A.: The relation between cell proliferation and the vascular system in a transplanted mouse mammary tumor. Brit. J. Cancer **22**, 258—273 (1968).
TANNOCK, I. F. A.: Comparison of cell proliferation parameters in solid and ascites Ehrlich tumors. Cancer Res. **29**, 1527—1534 (1969).
TAY, B. S., LILLEY, M. R., MURRAY, A. W., ATKINSON, M. R.: Inhibition of phosphoribosyl pyrophosphate amidotransferase from Ehrlich ascites-tumour cells by thiopurine nucleotides. Biochem. Pharmacol. **18**, 936—938 (1969).
TERENIUS, L.: Selective retention of estrogen isomers in estrogen-dependent breast tumors of rat demonstrated by *in vitro* methods. Cancer Res. **28**, 328—337 (1968).
TOMIZAWA, S., ARONOW, L.: Studies on drug resistance in mammalian cells. II. 6-Mercaptopurine resistance in mouse fibroblasts. J. Pharmacol. exp. Ther. **128**, 107—114 (1960).
TONO, H., COHEN, S. S.: The activity of nucleoside phosphorylase on 1-β-D-arabinosyluracil within *Escherichia coli*. J. biol. Chem. **237**, 1271—1282 (1962).
UCHIDA, K., KREIS, W.: Studies on drug resistance. I. Distribution of 1-β-D-arabinofuranosylcytosine, cytidine and deoxycytidine in mice bearing Ara-C-sensitive and -resistant P815 neoplasms. Biochem. Pharmacol. **18**, 1115—1128 (1969).
UJHÁZY, V., WINKLER, A.: Nitrogen mustard-resistant Yoshida sarcoma and cross-resistance studies. Neoplasma **12**, 11—14 (1965).
VAN ZEELAND, A. A., VAN DIGGELEN, M. C. E., SIMONS, J. W. I. M.: The role of metabolic cooperation in selection of hypoxanthine-guanine-phosphoribosyl-transferase-(HG-PRT)-deficient mutants from diploid mammalian cell strains. Mutat. Res. **14**, 355—363 (1972).
VESELÝ, J.: Resistance to pyrimidine analogs. In: CLARK, R. L., CUMLEY, R. W., MCCAY, J. E., COPELAND, M. M., (Eds.): Oncology 1970, Vol. II, Experimental Cancer Therapy, pp. 265—274. Chicago: Yearbook Medical Publishers 1971.
VESELÝ, J., ČIHÁK, A., ŠORM, F.: Biochemical mechanisms of drug resistance. IV. Development of resistance to 5-azacytidine and simultaneous depression of pyrimidine metabolism in leukemic mice. Int. J. Cancer **2**, 639—646 (1967).
VESELÝ, J., ČIHÁK, A., ŠORM, F.: Biochemical mechanisms of drug resistance. VII. Inhibition of orotic acid metabolism by 5-azacytidine in leukemic mice sensitive and resistant to 5-azacytidine. Biochem. Pharmacol. **17**, 519—524 (1968a).
VESELÝ, J., ČIHÁK, A., ŠORM, F.: Characteristics of mouse leukemic cells resistant to 5-azacytidine and 5-aza-2′-deoxycytidine. Cancer Res. **28**, 1995—2000 (1968b).
VESELÝ, J., ČIHÁK, A., ŠORM, F.: Biochemical mechanisms of drug resistance. IX. Metabolic alterations in leukemic cells following 5-aza-2′-deoxycytidine. Collect. Czech. Chem. Commun. **34**, 901—909 (1969).
VESELÝ, J., ČIHÁK, A., ŠORM, F.: Association of decreased uridine and deoxycytidine kinase with enhanced RNA and DNA polymerase in mouse leukemic cells resistant to 5-azacytidine and 5-aza-2′-deoxycytidine. Cancer Res. **30**, 2180—2186 (1970).
VESELÝ, J., ČIHÁK, A., ŠORM, F.: Enhanced stability of uridine kinase from mouse leukemic cells resistant to 5-azacytidine. Europ. J. Biochem. **22**, 551—556 (1971b).
VESELÝ, J., DVOŘÁK, M., ČIHÁK, A., ŠORM, F.: Biochemical mechanisms of drug resistance. XII. Uridine kinases from mouse leukemic cells sensitive and resistant to 5-azacytidine. Int. J. Cancer 8, 310—319 (1971a).
VESELÝ, J., SEIFERT, J., ČIHÁK, A., ŠORM, F.: Biochemical changes associated with the development of resistance to 5-azacytidine in AKR leukemic mice. Int. J. Cancer **1**, 31—40 (1966).
WAHBA, A. J., FRIEDKIN, M.: Direct spectrophotometric evidence for the oxidation of tetrahydrofolate during the enzymatic synthesis of thymidylate. J. biol. Chem. **236**, PC 11—12 (1961).
WAQAR, M. A., BURGOYNE, L. A., ATKINSON, M. R.: Deoxyribonucleic acid synthesis in mammalian nuclei. Incorporation of deoxyribonucleotides and chain-terminating nucleotide analogues. Biochem. J. **121**, 803—809 (1971).
WARWICK, G. P.: The mechanism of action of alkylating agents. Cancer Res. **23**, 1315—1333 (1963).
WATANABE, T.: Infective heredity of multiple drug resistance in bacteria. Bact. Rev. **27**, 87—115 (1963).
WAY, J. L., PARKS, R. E., JR.: Enzymatic synthesis of 5′-phosphate nucleotides of purine analogues. J. biol. Chem. **231**, 467—480 (1958).
WEISS, M. C., GREEN, H.: Human-mouse hybrid cell lines containing partial complements of human chromosomes and functioning human genes. Proc. nat. Acad. Sci. (Wash.) **58**, 1104—1111 (1967).
WEISSBACH, A., SCHLABACH, A., FRIDLENDER, B., BOLDEN, A.: DNA polymerases from human cells. Nature (Lond.) **231**, 167—170 (1971).
WELCH, A. D.: The problem of drug resistance in cancer chemotherapy. Cancer Res. **19**, 359—371 (1959).

Werkheiser, W. C.: Specific binding of 4-amino folic acid analogues by folic acid reductase. J. biol. Chem. **236**, 888—893 (1961).
Werkheiser, W. C.: The biochemical, cellular and pharmacological action and effects of the folic acid antagonists. Cancer Res. **23**, 1277—1285 (1963).
Westerveld, A., Visser, R. P. L. S., Khan, P. M., Bootsma, D.: Loss of human genetic markers in man-Chinese hamster somatic cell hybrids. Nature (Lond.) **234**, 20—24 (1971).
Wheeler, G. P.: Studies related to the mechanisms of action of cytotoxic alkylating agents: a review. Cancer Res. **22**, 651—688 (1962).
Wheeler, G. P.: Studies related to mechanisms of resistance to biological alkylating agents. Cancer Res. **23**, 1334—1349 (1963).
Wheeler, G. P.: Some biochemical effects of alkylating agents. Fed. Proc. **26**, 885—890 (1967).
Wheeler, G. P., Alexander, J. A.: Studies with mustards. V. *In vivo* fixation of $C^{14}$ of labeled alkylating agents by bilaterally grown sensitive and resistant tumors. Cancer Res. **24**, 1331—1337 (1964).
Wolberg, W. H.: Studies on the mechanism of human tumor resistance to the fluorinated pyrimidines. Cancer Res. **24**, 1437—1447 (1964).
Wolberg, W. H.: Development of resistance of Novikoff hepatoma to 5-fluoro-2′-deoxyuridine. Int. J. Cancer **6**, 261—269 (1970).
Wolberg, W. H.: Response of DNA thymidine synthesis in human tumor and normal tissue to 5-fluorouracil. Cancer Res. **32**, 130—132 (1972).
Wolpert, M. K., Damle, S. P., Brown, J. E., Sznycer, E., Agrawal, K. C., Sartorelli, A. C.: The role of phosphohydrolases in the mechanism of resistance of neoplastic cells to 6-thiopurines. Cancer Res. **31**, 1620—1626 (1971).
Wolpert, M. K., Ruddon, R. W.: A study of the mechanism of resistance to nitrogen mustard (HN2) in Ehrlich ascites tumor cells: Comparison of uptake of $HN2\text{-}^{14}C$ into sensitive and resistant cells. Cancer Res. **29**, 873—879 (1969).
Young, R. S. K., Fischer, G. A.: The action of arabinosylcytosine on synchronously growing populations of mammalian cells. Biochem. biophys. Res. Commun. **32**, 23—29 (1968).
Zakrzewski, S. F., Nichol, C. A.: On the enzymic reduction of folic acid by a purified hydrogenase. Biochim. biophys. Acta (Amst.) **27**, 425—426 (1958).
Zakrzewski, S. F., Nichol, C. A.: Evidence for a single enzyme reducing folate and dihydrofolate. J. biol. Chem. **235**, 2984—2988 (1961).

Chapter 20

# Combination Chemotherapy: Basic Considerations

ABRAHAM GOLDIN, JOHN M. VENDITTI, and NATHAN MANTEL

With 6 Figures

## Introduction

Recent progress in the chemotherapy of human malignancy, and especially in the treatment of leukemias and lymphomas, has resulted from the discovery of more effective antitumor drugs, the optimization of treatment schedules, the increased effectiveness of supportive care, and the application of concomitant and sequential combination chemotherapy. It is beyond the scope of this chapter to review clinical results in support of this conclusion. However, much has been written with respect to the clinical efficacy of combination therapy and the reader is referred to the recent reviews of BRODSKY et al. (1972), EVANS (1972), FAUST et al. (1972), FREI (1972), GOLD and BAIG (1972), GONICK (1972), HALL (1972), KRAKOFF (1972), LACHER (1972), MASTRANGELO and WEISS (1972), REGELSON (1972 a, b), and SHNIDER (1972); to the earlier papers of BURCHENAL (1969), DEVITA et al. (1969), FREIREICH et al. (1968), HART et al. (1969), MANDEL and RALL (1969), and HENDERSON and SAMAHA (1969) and the references cited therein. In outlining the historical progression toward improved clinical therapy, HOLLAND (1968) and FREI (1972) emphasized the increasingly effective interaction of clinical scientists with laboratory scientists. In the present chapter, an attempt is made to cite experimental studies that relate to current concepts of combination therapy. Experimental data[1], both old and new, are presented when they exemplify principles of applied combination therapy.

## Some Principles of Combination Drug Evaluation

In Chapter 2 emphasis was placed on finding progressively more effective therapies through the use of an experimental research program. These same considerations can simplify the problem of studying drug combinations, while at the same time bringing out the true points of complexity.

In previous reviews of the combination chemotherapy of neoplasia (GOLDIN and MANTEL, 1957; VENDITTI and GOLDIN, 1964a), the point was made that different investigators used varying definitions of what constituted drug synergism and that, in a number of instances, synergism could be demonstrated in accordance with the investigator's definition. In general, there was little concern with whether any demonstrated synergisms had any carryover in terms of improved therapy. Our

1 Experimental data are included from published and unpublished experiments conducted by I. KLINE et al. at Microbiological Associates, Inc., Bethesda, Maryland; F. M. SCHABEL and H. E. SKIPPER and their colleagues at the Southern Research Institute, Birmingham, Alabama; and I. WODINSKY et al. at Arthur D. Little, Inc., Cambridge, Massachusetts under contract to the National Cancer Institute.

own view, cited from yet earlier publications (GOLDIN et al., 1955b; VENDITTI et al., 1956) was that if synergism indicated the cooperative action of agents to produce some effect, then we should be free to define the desired effect as improved therapy, hence the term "therapeutic synergism".

A principal competitive definition of synergism relates to whether drug requirements, when they are used in combination, are lower than when they are used separately (i.e. the drugs in combination show greater than dose-wise additivity). In nonmedical situations, as for example, with insecticidal combinations, this may be a reasonable definition, for when such synergism exists it can result in financial savings. But in medical situations this is inappropriate where many drugs are or can be made abundant. Perhaps one may instinctively feel that if drug dosage can be reduced by employing combinations which are synergistic under this definition, then there will be an advantageous reduction in toxicity for the patient. But if two drugs are synergistic in their effects on the disease process they may also be equally synergistic in their toxic effects for the patient so that no net gain results. In fact, it should be possible for two drugs with antagonistic effects to provide an improved therapy if their antagonism relative to patient toxicity outweighs their antagonism relative to the disease process. The illustration of delayed citrovorum factor enhancing the efficacy of antifolics can be considered an example of antagonistic agents providing therapeutic synergism (GOLDIN et al., 1955b, c).

Essentially, under this competitive definition of synergism we are postulating a model by which the two agents are equivalent except for a factor of relative potency. A contradiction of this model under which drug requirements are decreased is taken as synergism, while an increase in drug requirements would indicate antagonism. But the model can be completely wrong, with neither synergism nor antagonism occurring; further, any demonstration of such synergism may have no relationship to improved therapeutic efficacy. This view point can be enlarged to cover other null models for combined drug effects. Suppose that we postulate a model of effect-wise additivity (the effect of 1 unit of $A$ + 1 unit $B$ should equal the effect of 1 unit of $A$ + the effect of 1 unit of $B$). If the data are inconsistent with this model, it could be interpreted as a demonstration of synergism or antagonism, depending on the data. Alternatively, it may only mean that too simple a null model is being postulated, and in any case there is again no carryover of any such demonstrated synergism to improved efficacy.

A notion which attends the concepts of some investigators regarding synergism is that of inexplicability. In the examples above, the demonstrations of synergism were related to the failure of particular simple models to explain the data. Suppose, however, that sometime after a demonstration of synergism, a simple explanation for the observed result is forthcoming; should a claim of synergism be allowed to stand? Under the definition of therapeutic synergism, the answer would be yes, just so long as an improved therapy resulted from the use of agents in combination. One might wish to differentiate between explained and unexplained therapeutic synergism, according to whether or not the rationale is known for the improved result. Thus, one rationale for an improved result could be that neither agent $A$ nor agent $B$ alone could kill more than 99.9% of tumor cells at nontoxic levels, the resistant 0.1% of cells ultimately killing the host. If resistance mechanisms to the drug are independent, the agents in combination at the same levels could kill 99.9999% of the tumor cells and so could extinguish a finite cell population, with cure resulting. Note that in this example the drugs are acting independently and the improved results can be explained; yet the end result is a desired one unattainable with either drug alone so that our requirement for therapeutic synergism is met. The notion of inexplicability did not attend earlier workers' concepts for using drugs in combination; thus, a practitioner might recommend the simultaneous use of two agents, one for obtaining an immediate effect, the other for a sustained effect; each agent is acting just as expected, but the practitioner recognizes the value of the combined regimen.

A pervading problem in combination drug testing is that there is no simple identification of the combination of two agents, say agents $A$ and $B$. If $A$ and $B$ are to be administered simultaneously, should they be administered in about equal proportions, or in equal adjusted proportions with allowance made for any difference in the doses at which they are individually effective? Suppose one of the agents in the combination is individually ineffective. Or perhaps in some way agent $A$ synergizes with agent $B$ so that it takes only a small amount of $A$ to heighten the efficacy of $B$, or vice versa. Our approach here has been to consider the $A + B$ combination as defining an infinity of drugs with different ratios of $A$ to $B$, varying from $0\% A + 100\% B$ to $100\% A + 0\% B$. A spectrum of the possible ratios is then tested, for instance employing $5\% A + 95\% B$, $10\% A + 90\% B$, $25\% A + 75\% B$, $50\% A + 50\% B$, $75\% A + 25\% B$, $90\% A + 10\% B$, $95\% A + 5\% B$, as well as $A$ by itself and $B$ by itself. This spectrum approach becomes more complicated for combinations of more than two drugs, and previously a systematic spectrum approach for combinations of three drugs was described (GOLDIN et al., 1968).

In employing the spectrum approach, each relative $A + B$ combination is considered as a drug in its own right, that is as a pseudo-drug. Each such pseudo-drug is tested over a range of dosage levels, using the approaches described in Chapter 2. If some $A + B$ pseudo-drug is more efficacious than the better of the separate drugs, this would be indicative of therapeutic synergism. This approach is taken whether we are using limited treatment as in GOLDIN et al. (1955a, c), where the superior agent was defined as the one giving greater antitumor effect for given toxicity for the host, or whether continued treatment was used so that the superior agent is taken as the one yielding the greater increase in survival time at its optimal dose (VENDITTI et al., 1956). Experimental designs have been described for applying this latter approach (MANTEL, 1958).

When drugs are used in combination they may or may not be administered simultaneously, adding another complication to the evaluation of the combination. Suppose $A$ and $B$ given on alternate days prove efficacious; this could be in part due to the efficacy of the combination of drugs and in part due to the fact that some treatment is given every day rather than only every other day. To determine whether the efficacy of $A + B$ indicates therapeutic synergism, it is necessary to employ each individual drug daily and on alternate days. Indeed, there may be almost endless ways of using drugs $A$ and $B$ in combination. When therapeutic synergism is not observed, it is still possible that some untried way of combining the drugs (e.g. alternative proportions of $A$ to $B$ or alternative schedules of concomitant, alternating, or sequential treatment) may yet be more effective. Conversely, there may be some particularly efficacious, but untried way of using one of the drugs. The latter eventuality is the less likely because the optimal conditions for individual drug usage are more easily determined than the optimal conditions for drug combinations (VENDITTI, 1971). However, neither possibility need constitute a problem if we take the developmental approach viewpoint that we are seeking treatment methods that are particularly effective. If we eventually find that some way of using $A$ alone is superior to what had previously appeared to be a synergistic $A + B$ combination, we have nevertheless made a therapeutic advance. Having two drugs to work with gives us more possibilities to explore, and a still better way of using $A + B$ may yet arise.

One rationale for combination chemotherapy could be that treatment with a single drug may fail because of selective or developing resistance; by using two drugs, successful therapy might be achieved because resistance to both drugs may not develop as rapidly (VENDITTI and GOLDIN, 1964a). However, even this rationale may not apply if adaptation of the tumor cells is to an environment and not to just a single drug. If we use two agents simultaneously or closely proximate in time, we may create just a single new environment to which the cells need adapt. With this alternative rationale we should alternate intervals or courses of treatment with two or more agents, shifting to the next agent before resistance to the current one has developed and reintroducing a previously used agent at some later time. Of course, the efficacy of varied durations of treatment with each agent alone would have to be investigated. Our intended point here is not so much to emphasize any particular way of using drugs in combination, but rather to bring out that there can be imaginative scope for using combinations. The goal remains to attain progressively improved results against progressively more serious challenges, and the use of combination therapy provides an additional device.

Current concepts relative to the evaluation of alternative antitumor therapies are a logical development of the emphasis by MARSHALL (1952) on the host-parasite-drug relationship and of the concept of "selective toxicity" (ALBERT, 1960). Essentially, where therapeutic synergism has occurred there has been an increase in selective toxicity against the tumor relative to the host. This may result from a decrease in toxicity for the host without a concomitant decrease in effectiveness against the tumor or from an increase in effectiveness against the tumor without a corresponding increase in toxicity for the host. Combination treatment may be said to exhibit therapeutic synergism when it has elicited a therapeutic response which exceeds that observed for each of the individual therapies when used separately.

## Therapeutic Synergism Resulting from Decreased Host Toxicity without Concomitant Decrease in Effectiveness against the Tumor

### A. Differential Protection of the Host by a Metabolite Employed in Conjunction with an Antimetabolite

One procedure that may be employed in an attempt to improve therapeutic efficacy is to treat with a combination of a metabolite plus a corresponding antimetabolite. For example, it had been observed that treatment with folic acid (FA) given one hour prior to treatment with the antifolate, aminopterin, reversed the toxicity of aminopterin for mice (GOLDIN et al., 1953). However, when FA was administered simultaneously with or after aminopterin, there was no protection against lethal toxicity. On the other hand, citrovorum factor (leucovorin, CF) protected against the lethal toxicity of aminopterin or methotrexate (MTX) when the CF was given as late as 12 to 24 h after the antagonist. In mice with leukemia L1210, simultaneous administration of CF and aminopterin resulted in a diminution of the therapeutic efficacy of the aminopterin. However, when CF was delayed for 12 to 24 h following the administration of aminopterin there was an increase in therapeutic efficacy (GOLDIN et al., 1955c). These studies were extended to the combination of MTX plus CF (GOLDIN et al., 1955b). Again, simultaneous administration of CF plus MTX failed to provide a therapeutic advantage over treatment with MTX alone. With MTX plus delayed CF, however, it was possible to obtain greater increases in survival time and a larger percentage of animals in which the disease had been eradicated, as compared with treatment with MTX alone. The advantage of the combinations was attributed to the ability of delayed CF to still protect the host against the toxicity of aminopterin or methotrexate, whereas during the same period, the action of the antimetabolite against the tumor cells appeared to be complete. This in turn permitted a larger dose of antimetabolite to be given and resulted in enhanced therapeutic efficacy. Thus, therapeutic synergism was achieved by virtue of a reduction in drug toxicity for the host without an equivalent reduction in toxicity for the tumor cells.

Deoxycytidine has been shown to block cytosine arabinoside (ara-C) cytotoxicity *in vitro* (RENIS and JOHNSON, 1962; CHU and FISCHER, 1962) and to inhibit both marrow suppression (PAPAC et al., 1965) and antitumor activity (EVANS and MENGEL, 1964) of a single ara-C treatment *in vivo*. Studies using daily ara-C treatment over a wide range of dosage levels and varying time intervals following administration of daily deoxycytidine illustrate the competitive nature of the metabolite-antimetabolite relationship *in vivo* (Table 1, I. KLINE et al., unpublished data). In mice with early leukemia L 1210, daily deoxycytidine increased the daily dose of ara-C required to attain maximum antitumor efficacy. However, the combination did not provide a greater therapeutic effect than ara-C alone. One possible explanation of the failure to "cure" mice with combinations of deoxycytidine given 30 min prior to or simultaneously with ara-C might be the failure to give the antimetabolite at a dosage level sufficiently high to compensate for the protective action of deoxycytidine for the tumor. Thus, in these instances the maximum ara-C dosage was not determined. From the data available in Table 1 it is concluded that the combination of deoxycytidine and ara-C resulted in a decrease in toxicity to the host that was offset by an essentially equivalent decrease in toxicity to the tumor. Therefore, therapeutic synergism was not obtained.

Table 1. *Effect of the Temporal relationship between deoxycytidine and cytosine arabinoside (ara-C) on the optimal antileukemic (L1210) dose of ara-C*[a,b]

| Ara-C daily dose | Ara-C alone | Time (min) of administration of 320 mg/kg/day deoxycytidine relative to ara-C —120 | —60 | —30 | 0 | +30 | +60 |
|---|---|---|---|---|---|---|---|
| Mg/kg | | Median day of death (number of 70-day survivors/8 mice) | | | | | |
| 65 | 12.0(0) | 23.0(0) | >97.0(5) | 42.5(0) | 29.0(0) | 72.0(2) | 18.0(0) |
| 39 | 41.0(2) | >97.0(5) | 33.0(0) | 31.0(0) | 25.0(0) | >87.5(4) | 78.5(2) |
| 23 | >97.0(5) | 80.0(2) | 29.0(0) | 27.0(0) | 23.5(0) | 49.5(3) | >97.0(6) |
| 14 | 79.5(3) | 44.0(0) | 28.5(0) | 23.0(0) | 14.0(0) | 32.0(0) | 54.0(2) |
| 0 | — | Deoxycytidine alone, median survival time — 10 days (no survivors). | | | | | |
| | | Untreated controls, median survival time — 11 days (no survivors). | | | | | |

[a] I. KLINE et al. (unpublished data).

[b] Subcutaneous (SC) treatment was begun on day 3 after SC tumor implantation and continued daily to death or day 70. Long-term survivors from daily ara-C treatment is unusual. Typically, ara-C treatment is "curative" against early L1210 leukemia when it is given $q3$ h/24 h/$q4$ days or on a similar intensive intermittent schedule (SKIPPER et al., 1970). It is possible that in this experiment the number of viable tumor cells in the inoculum was low although 100% of untreated mice succumbed. Nevertheless, the ability of deoxycytidine to block ara-C toxicity to the host and to the tumor is evident by the progressive increase in the ara-C optimal dose with decreasing interval between administration of the agents.

## B. Differential Protection of the Host Against Toxicity of an Antitumor Agent by a Therapeutically Inactive Drug

CONNORS and ELSON (1962) reported that a number of thiols including cysteine reduced the toxicity of the more chemically reactive nitrogen mustards. In extending these studies, CONNORS and his coworkers (see CONNORS, 1966) showed a positive correlation between the degree of protection by cysteine and the associated increase in the level of protein-free *SH*-groups in spleen, liver, and thymus. BRINKER (1964) reported that mice were protected from cyclophosphamide toxicity by pre or post administration of cysteine hydrochloride, and PRIMACK (1971) reported that irrigation of bladders of monkeys and dogs with acetylcysteine protected against cyclophosphamide-induced cystitis. These findings prompted investigation of the effects of *N*-acetylcysteine (NAC) on the toxicity and antileukemic (L1210) effectiveness of cyclophosphamide and the cyclophosphamide derivative, isophosphamide (Table 2) (KLINE et al., 1972; VENDITTI et al., unpublished data). When normal mice were treated with a single injection of 833 or 500 mg/kg of isophosphamide, lethal toxicity was generally observed. However, when 750 to 1500 mg/kg of NAC was administered ten minutes prior to isophosphamide, some animals survived 833 mg/kg isophosphamide and most of the animals survived 500 mg/kg. When the combination of NAC plus isophosphamide was employed in the treatment of leukemia L1210 a marked therapeutic advantage over treatment with isophosphamide alone was achieved. In the experiment summarized in Table 2, the optimal dose of isophosphamide alone (300 mg/kg) increased the median survival time of the mice from 9 days (untreated controls) to 23.5 days. At 500 mg/kg, isophosphamide alone was frankly lethal as evidenced by the median survival time of 3.5 days. When NAC was given at 1000 or 1500 mg/kg from 60 minutes prior to ten minutes after isophosphamide there was no reduction in the efficacy of 300 mg/kg isophosphamide and an actual increase in efficacy in some instances. It is particularly noteworthy, however, that the combination of NAC plus 500 mg/kg isophosphamide provided a therapy that was superior to that achievable with isophosphamide alone at any dosage level. With the combination of 1500 mg/kg NAC given simultaneously with 500 mg/kg isophosphamide, 100% of the mice survived for 90 days (Table 2). Similarly, enhancement of cyclophosphamide antileukemic activity was observed on prior administration of NAC, but the therapeutic advantage obtained with this combination was less than that observed with NAC plus isophosphamide. The degree to which bladder cystitis might contribute to lethality of isophosphamide in mice, or the mechanism whereby NAC protected against isophosphamide toxicity in the present experiments, is unknown. However, it is clear that NAC did protect the host against the toxicity of isophosphamide with little or no reversal of antitumor effectiveness. Consequently, an increase in antitumor specificity was achievable because a larger dose of the active drug could be employed.

## C. Differential Protection of the Host Against an Antitumor Agent by a Second Therapeutically Active Drug

The therapeutic synergism exhibited by combinations of antifolics plus delayed citrovorum factor or NAC plus isophosphamide resulted from the ability of an agent devoid of antitumor activity to selectively protect the host from the toxicity of the active antitumor drug. However, therapeutic synergism has also been achieved with two active antitumor agents because one was capable of diminishing the host toxicity of the other. Such an example is provided by the combination of ICRF-159 [1,2-*bis*(3,5-dioxopiperazin-1-yl)propane] (Fig. 1) plus daunomycin or adriamycin. The anti-L1210 activity of each of these drugs has been reported

Table 2. *Influence of N-acetylcysteine on isophosphamide lethal toxicity and anti-leukemic (L1210) activity*[a]

| N-Acetylcysteine[b] IP-day 1 only | | Isophosphamide-IP-day 1 only[c] | | | | | | | | |
|---|---|---|---|---|---|---|---|---|---|---|
| | | 300 mg/kg | | | 500 mg/kg | | | 833 mg/kg | | |
| | | Leukemic | | Normal | Leukemic | | Normal | Leukemic | | Normal |
| Dose (mg/kg) | Time relative to isophosphamide (min) | MST[d] (days) | Day 90 (S/T)[e] | Day 90 (S/T)[e] | MST[d] (days) | Day 90 (S/T)[e] | Day 90 (S/T)[e] | MST[d] (days) | Day 90 (S/T)[e] | Day 90 (S/T)[e] |
| 0 | — | 23.5 | 3/8 | 5/6 | 3.5 | 1/8 | 1/6 | 2.0 | 0/8 | 0/6 |
| 1500 | —60 | 23.5 | 2/8 | 6/6 | 83.5 | 3/8 | 1/6 | 6.5 | 2/8 | 2/6 |
| 1500 | —30 | 22.5 | 3/8 | 6/6 | 68.5 | 0/8 | 6/6 | 2.0 | 0/8 | 0/6 |
| 1500 | —10 | 22.5 | 1/8 | 5/6 | >90.0 | 5/8 | 5/6 | 22.0 | 0/8 | 2/6 |
| 1500 | 0 | 24.5 | 0/8 | 6/6 | >90.0 | 8/8 | 4/6 | 7.0 | 0/8 | 0/6 |
| 1500 | +10 | 23.0 | 1/8 | 6/6 | >83.5 | 4/8 | 5/6 | 9.0 | 0/8 | 0/6 |
| 1000 | —60 | 26.0 | 2/8 | 6/6 | >88.0 | 4/8 | 2/6 | 4.0 | 1/8 | 0/6 |
| 1000 | —30 | 19.0 | 0/8 | 6/6 | >90.0 | 6/8 | 0/6 | 5.0 | 1/8 | 1/6 |
| 1000 | —10 | >63.5 | 4/8 | 2/6 | 59.0 | 3/8 | 0/6 | 6.0 | 1/8 | 3/6 |
| 1000 | 0 | 21.0 | 1/8 | 6/6 | >73.0 | 4/8 | 3/6 | 13.0 | 0/8 | 2/6 |
| 1000 | +10 | >72.0 | 4/8 | 3/6 | >90.0 | 7/8 | 4/6 | 10.0 | 0/8 | 0/6 |
| 750 | —60 | 23.0 | 0/8 | 5/6 | 5.0 | 1/8 | 4/6 | 3.0 | 0/8 | 1/6 |
| 750 | —30 | 30.5 | 3/8 | 5/6 | >87.0 | 4/8 | 5/6 | >48.5 | 4/8 | 0/6 |
| 750 | —10 | 18.5 | 0/8 | 6/6 | >90.0 | 5/8 | 4/6 | 3.0 | 0/8 | 0/6 |
| 750 | 0 | 17.0 | 2/8 | 0/6 | 82.5 | 2/8 | 2/6 | 4.0 | 2/8 | 0/6 |
| 750 | +10 | 25.0 | 3/8 | 6/6 | >90.0 | 6/8 | 3/6 | 4.5 | 0/8 | 0/6 |

[a] Data of VENDITTI et al. (see KLINE et al. 1972).

[b] N-Acetylcysteine alone at 1500, 1000, or 750 mg/kg or no treatment resulted in a median survival time of 9.0 days, no survivors among leukemic mice, and no deaths among normal mice.

[c] 180 mg/kg isophosphamide alone elicited a median survival time of 15.5 days, no leukemic survivors, and no deaths among normal mice. Thus, for isophosphamide alone treatment, the 300 mg/kg dose was optimal.

[d] MST = Median survival time.

[e] S/T = No. of survivors/total no. of mice in each group.

previously (CREIGHTON et al., 1969; SANDBERG et al., 1970; VENDITTI, 1971; VENDITTI et al., 1966). Cardiac toxicity or electrocardiogram abnormalities have been described in clinical studies of daunomycin and adriamycin (BONADONNA et al., 1969; CORTES et al., 1972; LIVINGSTON and CARTER, 1970). In attempting to elucidate the mechanisms of their cardiac effects, HERMAN et al. (1972) found that the

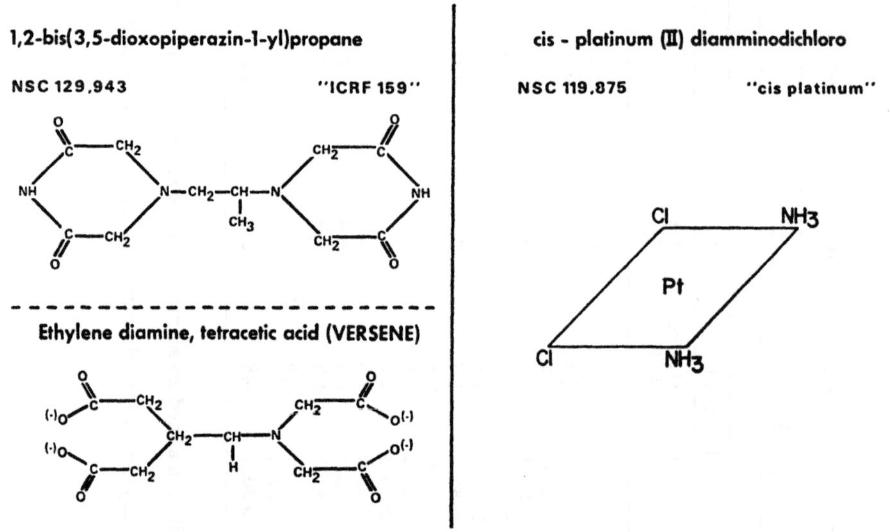


Fig. 1. Structures of ICRF-159, versene (EDTA), and *cis*-platinum (II) diamminodichloro

toxic effects of daunomycin or adriamycin on the isolated dog heart could be partially reversed by pre-perfusion of the tissue with the chelating agent versene (EDTA, Fig.1) or the structurally related compound ICRF-159. It seemed appropriate to investigate the extent to which EDTA or ICRF-159 might protect against daunomycin or adriamycin toxicity *in vivo*, and , if so, whether such protection might lead to enhanced antitumor effectiveness for the combination (WOODMAN et al., 1972). Table 3 summarizes an experiment in which normal mice were given one injection of daunomycin alone or in conjunction with EDTA or ICRF-159. The results indicate that the single treatment $LD_{50}$ for daunomycin alone (<5.0 mg/kg)

Table 3. *Protection against lethal toxicity of daunomycin in mice by EDTA or ICRF-159*[a,b]

| Daunomycin | EDTA (mg/kg) | | | | | ICRF-159 (mg/kg) | | | | |
|---|---|---|---|---|---|---|---|---|---|---|
| | 0 | 50 | 100 | 200 | 400 | 50 | 100 | 200 | 400 | 800 |
| (mg/kg) | (Number of 60-day survivors/ten mice per group) | | | | | | | | | |
| 20 | 0 | 0 | 0 | 0 | — | 0 | 0 | 2 | 1 | — |
| 10 | 0 | 0 | 0 | 0 | — | 1 | 8 | 9 | 9 | — |
| 5 | 0 | 0 | 4 | 6 | — | 10 | 10 | 10 | 10 | — |
| 0 | 10 | 10 | 10 | 10 | 10 | 10 | 10 | 10 | 10 | 8 |

[a] Data of WOODMAN et al. (1972).
[b] A single IP injection of EDTA or ICRF-159 was given 10 min prior to a single IP injection of daunomycin.

was approximately doubled by the concomitant administration of 200 mg/kg EDTA. Significantly, only one of ten mice that had received 200 or 400 mg/kg ICRF-159 plus 10 mg/kg daunomycin succumbed. The antileukemic (L1210) effectiveness of ICRF-159 and daunomycin, separately and combined, is summarized in Tables 4 and 5. With therapy limited to one treatment on the day following tumor implantation (Table 4), daunomycin alone was relatively ineffective in increasing the survival time of the leukemic mice and, at doses as low as 5.0 mg/kg, killed all of the normal mice treated in parallel. The optimal dose of ICRF-159

Table 4. *Effectiveness of ICRF-159 and daunomycin, separately and combined, against early leukemia L1210; treatment on day 1 only*[a]

| ICRF-159 (mg/kg — IP-Day 1 only) | Daunomycin | Leukemic mice MST[b] (Days) | ILS[c] (%) | Normal mice S/T[d] (Day 60) |
|---|---|---|---|---|
| 800 | — | 6.5 | 0 | 1/6 |
| 400 | — | 15.0 | 67 | 5/6 |
| 200 | — | 13.0 | 44 | 6/6 |
| 100 | — | 10.0 | 11 | 6/6 |
| — | 20 | 6.5 | 0 | 0/6 |
| — | 10 | 9.0 | 0 | 0/6 |
| — | 5.0 | 10.5 | 17 | 0/6 |
| — | 2.5 | 11.0 | 22 | 6/6 |
| 400 | 20 | 7.0 | 0 | 0/6 |
| 400 | 10 | 16.0 | 78 | 4/6 |
| 400 | 5.0 | 15.0 | 67 | 6/6 |
| 400 | 2.5 | 14.5 | 61 | 5/6 |
| 200 | 20 | 8.0 | 0 | 3/6 |
| 200 | 10 | 14.5 | 61 | 6/6 |
| 200 | 5.0 | 15.0 | 67 | 6/6 |
| 200 | 2.5 | 14.0 | 55 | 6/6 |
| 100 | 10 | 13.0 | 44 | 0/6 |
| 100 | 5.0 | 13.5 | 50 | 6/6 |
| 100 | 2.5 | 13.0 | 44 | 6/6 |
| Untreated controls | | 9.0 | — | 6/6 |

[a] Data of WOODMAN et al. (1972).
[b] Median survival time.
[c] Increase in lifespan (MST) over controls.
[d] Survivors/total.

Table 5. *Therapeutic synergism against early leukemia L1210 of ICRF-159 plus daunomycin given daily or every fourth day*[a]

| Treatment | IP Treatment schedule | Optimal dose (mg/kg) S[b] | C[c] | Increase in lifespan over controls (%) S[b] | C[c] | Survivors/total S[b] | C[c] |
|---|---|---|---|---|---|---|---|
| Daunomycin | qd; Days 1—9 | 1.0 | 2.0 | 33 | 111 | 0/8 | 0/8 |
| + ICRF-159 | qd; Days 1—9 | 50 | + 50 | 61 | | 0/8 | |
| Daunomycin | q4d; Days 1,5,9 | 2.0 | 4.0 | 22 | >500 | 0/8 | 4/8 |
| + ICRF-159 | q4d; Days 1,5,9 | 400 | +400 | 155 | | 0/8 | |

[a] Data of WOODMAN et al. (1972).
[b] S = Individual drug treatment.
[c] C = Combination treatment.

alone (400 mg/kg) elicited a 67% increase in the lifespan of leukemic mice and was lethal to one of six normal mice. The maximally effective combination (400 mg/kg ICRF-159 plus 10 mg/kg daunomycin) increased the lifespan of leukemic mice by 78% and was lethal to two of six normal mice. Thus, with the treatment schedule used, the combination failed to provide an antileukemic effect that was superior to treatment with ICRF-159 alone, but the protection by ICRF-159 against daunomycin toxicity was evident (Table 4). SANDBERG et al. (1970) did not find daunomycin markedly schedule dependent against the L1210 leukemia although a single treatment was inferior to a number of alternative treatment schedules. Studies of the schedule dependency of ICRF-159 against the L1210 tumor indicated the inferiority of a single treatment and the superiority of intermittent therapy (e.g., once every fourth day or *q* 3 h/24 h/*q* 4 day) (VENDITTI, 1971, Fig. 2). When ICRF-159 plus

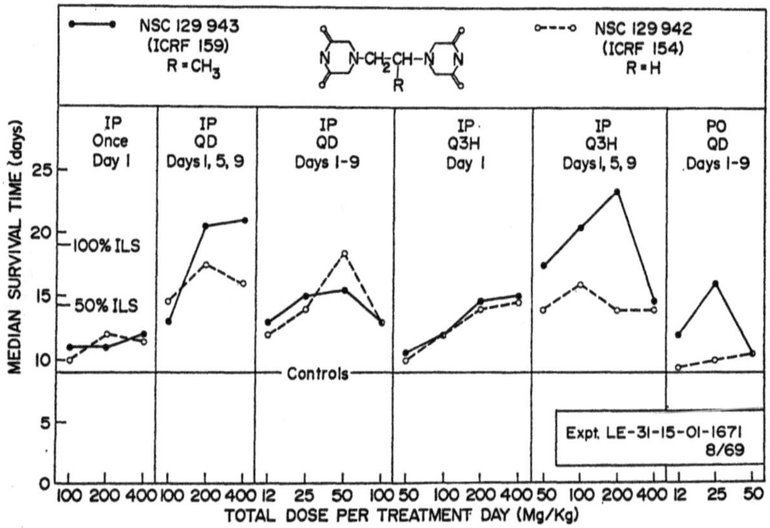


Fig. 2. Influence of treatment schedule on activity of bisdiketopiperazines against IP implanted leukemia L1210 (VENDITTI, 1971)

daunomycin were combined against the L1210 leukemia using daily or intermittent treatment, the therapeutically synergistic qualities of the combination became evident (Table 5). When treatment was given daily, optimal combination dosage was approximately twice as effective as optimal treatment with ICRF-159 alone and three times more effective than optimal treatment with daunomycin alone. The synergistic effect of the combination was more pronounced when treatment was given every fourth day; 50% of the combination treated mice showing long-term survival, as compared with none of the individual drug-treated mice. With each of the multiple treatment schedules (Table 5), as well as with day 1 only treatment (Table 4), the optimal combination dosage included ICRF-159 at its optimal dose when used alone, plus daunomycin at a dosage level which was greater than the optimal dose for daunomycin alone treatment. The study of the ICRF-159 plus daunomycin combination was important for a number of reasons. A new therapeutically synergistic drug combination was identified, which provided an example of therapeutic synergism with two antitumor drugs arising from the ability of one to diminish the host toxicity of the other, thereby permitting the administration of more total antitumor drug. It further emphasized the importance of the treatment schedule as a factor influencing the effectiveness of combination therapy.

In preliminary experiments employing a limited number of treatment schedules, ICRF-159 failed to protect normal mice against the toxicity of adriamycin. Nevertheless, under appropriate conditions, the combination of ICRF-159 plus adriamycin did provide therapeutic synergism against leukemia L1210 (WOODMAN et al., personal communication, Table 6). SANDBERG et al. (1970) reported that, in

Table 6. *Effectiveness of ICRF-159 plus adriamycin against early mouse leukemia L1210*[a]

| Treatment (IP-q3 h/24 h on day 1 only) | Optimal dose (mg/kg/injection) | ILS[b] (%) | S/T[c] |
|---|---|---|---|
| ICRF-159 alone | 50 | 60 | 0/8 |
| Adriamycin alone | 2.0 | 60 | 0/8 |
| ICRF-159+Adriamycin | 25+2.0 | >500 | 6/8 |

[a] Unpublished data of I. KLINE, R. WOODMAN, and J. M. VENDITTI.
[b] Increase in lifespan over controls.
[c] Survivors/total.

contrast to daunomycin, the anti-L1210 effectiveness of adriamycin was treatment schedule dependent and that eight treatments given at three-hour intervals on day 1 after tumor implantation was more effective than a single treatment or any mode of continued treatment beyond day 1. The *q* 3 h/24 h/day 1 only schedule was not particularly effective for ICRF-159 alone (VENDITTI, 1971, Fig. 2). Nevertheless, combination of ICRF-159 plus adriamycin on the *q* 3 h/24 h/day 1 only schedule yielded six of eight survivors (Table 6). It should be emphasized that neither ICRF-159 alone, nor adriamycin alone, has produced long-term survivors among mice with L1210 leukemia, although each drug has been examined in detail using a number of diverse treatment schedules (VENDITTI, 1971). The precise mechanisms responsible for the synergistic action of ICRF-159 plus daunomycin or adriamycin are not known. MHATRE and HERMAN (1972) reported that ICRF-159 modified the uptake and metabolism of daunomycin and adriamycin in hamsters and suggested this as a possible mechanism for influencing both cardiac toxicity and antitumor activity.

Favorable reports of the effectiveness of the combination of ara-C and 6-thioguanine (6-TG) in the treatment of human adult acute leukemia (GEE et al. 1968, 1969) prompted intensive laboratory investigations leading to the observations that, under appropriate conditions of treatment scheduling, ara-C protected mice against the lethal toxicity of 6-TG and that the combination was therapeutically synergistic against leukemia L1210 (SCHMIDT et al., 1970; SCHABEL et al., personal communication). Interest in combinations of ara-C and purine analogs stemmed from observations that daily treatment with ara-C plus 6-mercaptopurine (6-MP) was more effective than daily treatment with the individual drugs alone against the L1210 leukemia (BURCHENAL and DOLLINGER, 1967). In the latter study, maximum efficacy was obtained with one-half of the optimal ara-C dose alone plus twice the optimal 6-MP dose alone (Table 7). Moreover, the combination of the drugs at the full optimal dose for each agent alone was more effective than either of the individual drugs. The results indicated a minimum degree of additive toxicity for the host and suggested that a moderately effective level of ara-C may have actu-

Table 7. *Effectiveness of cytosine arabinoside (ara-C) plus 6-Mercaptopurine (6-MP) against early leukemia L1210; treatment IP, daily, days 1 to 10*[a]

| 6-MP (mg/kg/Day) | Ara-C (mg/kg/Day) 0 | 5 | 10 | 20 |
|---|---|---|---|---|
| | Pct. ILS[b] (50-day survivors/10) | | | |
| 0 | 0 (0) | 51 (0) | 85 (0) | 98 (0) |
| 5 | 37 (0) | — | — | 149 (0) |
| 10 | 68 (0) | 104 (0) | >201 (1) | 164 (0) |
| 20 | 50 (0) | 141 (0) | >293 (4) | 158 (0) |

[a] From BURCHENAL and DOLLINGER (1967).
[b] Percentage increase in life span.

ally protected the host against the toxicity of 6-MP. It was not clear that daily treatment with the combination would have been more effective than ara-C alone if given on its optimal treatment schedule, $q$ 3 h/24 h/$q$ 4 days (BURCHENAL and DOLLINGER, 1967; SCHABEL, 1968a; SKIPPER et al., 1967). SCHABEL et al. (unpublished data) confirmed the therapeutic advantage of daily ara-C plus daily 6-MP over daily treatment with either drug alone and also demonstrated the marked advantage of the combination against the L1210 leukemia using the $q$ 3 h/24 h/$q$ 4 day schedule (Table 8). However, in the latter experiment, there was no suggestion that ara-C protected against 6-MP toxicity to the host. VENDITTI and GOLDIN (1964a), in discussing mechanisms of action and resistance relative to the use of drug combinations, pointed out the importance of the observation that 6-TG was incorporated into DNA in significant amounts (LEPAGE, 1963), while 6-MP was not. GOLDIN et al. (1960) reported that although 6-MP and 6-TG exhibited approximately the same degree of therapeutic efficacy against advanced L1210 leukemia, the optimal daily dose of 6-MP was approximately 50-times greater than the optimal daily dose of 6-TG. The experiments of SARTORELLI and LEPAGE (1957) and LEPAGE (1963) clearly implicated the incorporation of 6-TG into DNA as a major factor contributing to its marked toxicity. LEPAGE and KANEKO (1969) proposed that ara-C, by inhibiting DNA polymerase (FURTH and COHEN, 1968) blocked the incorporation of 6-TG into DNA and found this to be the case, but only under specific conditions of timing of the treatments. The same investigators found

Table 8. *Effectiveness of cytosine arabinoside (ara-C) plus 6-mercaptopurine (6-MP) against early leukemia L1210; treatment IP q3 h/24 h on days 1,5,9,13*[a]

| Treatment | Optimal dose (mg/kg/injection) | ILS[b] (%) | Day 45 S/T[c] |
|---|---|---|---|
| Ara-C alone | 15 | 366 | 1/10 |
| 6-MP alone | 10 | 83 | 0/10 |
| Ara-C + 6-MP | 11 + 7.5 | >400 | 5/10 |

[a] Unpublished data of F. M. SCHABEL, Jr. et al. Tumor inoculum —$10^7$ cells, IP.
[b] Increase in life span.
[c] Survivors per number of mice treated.

that daily treatment with ara-C plus 6-TG was no more effective than daily ara-C treatment alone against the L1210 leukemia, but emphasized the limitation of their studies with respect to combination dosages and treatment schedule (LePage and Kaneko, 1969). Schabel et al. (unpublished data) found that daily ara-C plus daily 6-TG was moderately more effective against the L1210 tumor than daily treatment with either drug alone when the approximate optimal doses for the drugs used individually were combined (Table 9). Also, using the $q$ 3 h/24 h/$q$ 4 day

Table 9. *Efficacy of daily treatment with cytosine arabinoside (ara-C) plus 6-thioguanine (6-TG) against early leukemia L1210*[a]

| Treatment IP daily (Days 1 to 15) | Optimal dose (mg/kg/Day) | ILS[b] (%) | Survivors |
|---|---|---|---|
| Ara-C alone | 32 | 171 | 0 |
| 6-TG-alone | 0.67 | 71 | 0 |
| Ara-C + 6-TG | 36 + 0.5 | 278 | 0 |

[a] F. M. Schabel, Jr. et al. unpublished data. Tumor inoculum —$10^6$ cells, IP.
[b] Increase in life span.

schedule for both drugs, Schmidt and Schabel and their colleagues (Schmidt et al., 1970) found the combination of ara-C plus 6-TG to be markedly synergistic against leukemia L1210 (Table 10). Moreover, the superiority of the combination over individual drug therapy was clearly associated with a reduction in the host toxicity of 6-TG, permitting the advantageous use of a larger dose of 6-TG when combined with ara-C (Tables 10 and 11). The importance of the treatment schedule to the manifestation of syn-

Table 10. *Effectiveness of divided-intermittent treatment with cytosine arabinoside (ara-C) plus 6-thioguanine (6-TG) against leukemia L1210*[a]

| IP dose (mg/kg) $q$3 h/24 h days 1,5,9,13 | | Mice with tumor | | | Normal mice | |
|---|---|---|---|---|---|---|
| Ara-C | 6-TG | ILS[b] (%) | S/T[c] | Pct. Surv. | S/T | Pct. Surv. |
| 22 | 0 | 345 | 1/27 | 4 | 28/49 | 57 |
| 15 | 0 | 480 | 0/30 | 0 | 47/48 | 98 |
| 10 | 0 | 422 | 0/29 | 0 | 46/49 | 94 |
| 6.7 | 0 | 327 | 0/29 | 0 | 48/48 | 100 |
| 0 | 1.0 | 125 | 0/20 | 0 | 1/30 | 3 |
| 0 | 0.67 | 105 | 0/30 | 0 | 29/50 | 58 |
| 0 | 0.45 | 60 | 0/30 | 0 | 47/49 | 96 |
| 15 | 1.0 | 604 | 9/18 | 50 | 12/20 | 60 |
| 10 | 1.0 | 625 | 6/19 | 32 | 11/17 | 65 |
| 15 | 0.67 | 606 | 7/20 | 35 | 15/18 | 83 |
| 10 | 0.67 | 558 | 9/29 | 31 | 27/29 | 93 |
| 6.7 | 0.67 | 550 | 1/10 | 10 | 10/10 | 100 |

[a] Data of L. H. Schmidt and F. M. Schabel, Jr. (see Schmidt et al., 1970). Tumor inoculum —$10^6$ cells, IV.
[b] Increase in life span.
[c] Survivors per number of mice treated.

Table 11. *Protection by 6-thioguanine (6-TG) against lethality of cytosine arabinoside (ara-C) in normal mice*[a]

| 6-TG mg/kg/ injection[b] | Ara-C (mg/kg/injection)[b] 0 | 0.47 | 0.94 | 1.88 | 3.75 | 7.5 | 15 |
|---|---|---|---|---|---|---|---|
| | Number of survivors/total | | | | | | |
| 0 | 39/40 | 10/10 | 10/10 | 10/10 | 10/10 | 10/10 | 10/10 |
| 0.45 | 7/7 | 10/10 | 10/10 | 10/10 | 9/9 | 10/10 | 9/10 |
| 0.90 | 0/10 | 9/10 | 9/10 | 10/10 | 10/10 | 10/10 | 10/10 |
| 1.35 | 1/10 | 1/10 | 9/10 | 9/9 | 10/10 | 8/10 | 9/10 |
| 1.80 | 0/10 | 0/10 | 0/10 | 3/10 | 3/10 | 4/10 | 0/10 |

[a] Data of L. H. SCHMIDT and F. M. SCHABEL, JR. (see SCHMIDT et al., 1970).
[b] Treatment q3 h/24 h/days 1,5,9,13.

ergism between ara-C and 6-TG was emphasized further by the preliminary results of SCHABEL et al. (personal communication) that alternating intermittent therapy consisting of ara-C given *q* 3 h/24 h/days 2,5 and 8 plus 6-TG *q* 3 h/24 h/days 4,7 and 10 enhanced toxicity with little evidence of a therapeutic advantage over individual drug treatment.

## Therapeutic Synergism Resulting from Selective Increase in Antitumor Toxicity Using Combinations of Individually Active Agents

Combinations of antitumor agents have generally been employed in attempts to obtain therapeutic synergism. In the most extensively employed procedure in such testing for therapeutic synergism, dose-survival time response curves are generally established for the drugs employed individually (preferably on optimal schedules) and for the drugs in combination. Comparisons are then made of the maximum increases in survival time obtained at optimal dosage, and when the increase in survival time for the combination of drugs is more extensive than that observed with the drugs employed individually, therapeutic synergism is considered to have occurred. Where such therapeutic synergism is observed for combination therapy, it is generally the result of a selective increase in antitumor toxicity in which the increase in antitumor effectiveness is proportionately greater than the increase in toxicity for the host.

A number of combinations of drugs administered on concomitant treatment schedules have demonstrated therapeutic synergism in the leukemia L1210 system and a partial listing of such combinations is given in Table 12. For these combinations therapeutic synergism is manifested by increased survival time and in a number of instances by an increase in percentage "cures". The wide range of chemical structures for which combination chemotherapy in experimental systems has been advantageous is notable and many such combinations have not as yet received clinical attention.

## Attempts to Improve Therapy by Altering the Concentration ($C$) and Duration of Effectiveness ($T$) of an Antitumor Agent

SKIPPER et al. (1970), in discussing cytokinetic, biochemical, toxicologic and pharmacologic factors that may influence antitumor efficacy, emphasized the importance of the product $C \times T$ at the target site. In most cases, alterations in $C \times T$ leading to improved therapy have been effected by modifications of the treatment schedule. An alternative method of altering the $C \times T$ of an antitumor

Table 12. *Examples of therapeutic synergism employing combinations of antitumor agents*

| Drug[a] | Tumor site inoculum level (cells/mouse) | Treatment (route and schedule) | Activity at optimal or greatest non-lethal dose: ILS (%) S[b] | ILS (%) C[c] | Surv. (%) S[b] | Surv. (%) C[c] | Ref.[d] |
|---|---|---|---|---|---|---|---|
| Methotrexate | IP-$10^5$ | IP-daily, days 1—9 | 111 | 178 | 0 | 37 | [5] |
| Guanazole | | IP-$q$3 h/24h/days 1,5,9 | 100 | | 0 | | |
| Methotrexate | SC-$10^6$ | SC-daily, day 5-death | 137 | 237 | 0 | 0 | [1] |
| Actinomycin D | | SC-weekly, day 5-death | 37 | | 0 | | |
| Methotrexate | SC-$10^6$ | SC-daily, days 5—19 | 83 | 161 | 0 | 0 | [5] |
| Camptothecin, Na | | SC-weekly, days 5—19 | 44 | | 0 | | |
| 6-Thioguanine | IP-$10^5$ | IP-daily, days 1—15 | 100 | 225 | 0 | 20 | [2] |
| 6-Me-MP-R | | IP-daily, days 1—15 | 100 | | 0 | | |
| 6-Thioguanine | IP-$10^6$ | IP-once, day 2 | 71 | 443 | 0 | 40 | [6] |
| Ara-C-5′-palmitate | | IP-once, day 2 | 221 | | 10 | | |
| 6-Mercaptopurine | IP-$10^5$ | IP-daily, days 1—15 | 68 | 162 | 0 | 0 | [3] |
| 6-Me-MP-R | | IP-daily, days 1—15 | 75 | | 0 | | |
| 6-Mercaptopurine | IP-$10^5$ | IP-daily, days 1—15 | 75 | 175 | 0 | 0 | [2] |
| Daunomycin | | IP-daily, days 1—15 | 62 | | 0 | | |
| 6-Mercaptopurine | SC-$10^6$ | SC-$q$2D, day 7-death | 67 | 483 | 0 | 4 | [5] |
| BCNU | | SC-once, day 7 | 289 | | 0 | | |
| 5-Fluorouracil | IP-$10^5$ | IP-once, day 3 | 80 | 120 | 0 | 0 | [4] |
| *cis*-Pt-II | | IP-once, day 3 | 45 | | 0 | | |
| Cyclophosphamide | IV-$10^7$ | IP-once, day 2 | 313 | >900 | 10 | 30 | [6] |
| DIC | | IP-once, day 2 | 112 | | 0 | | |
| Cyclophosphamide | IV-$10^7$ | IP-once, day 2 | 400 | >900 | 0 | 50 | [6] |
| BIC | | IP-once, day 2 | 250 | | 0 | | |
| Cyclophosphamide | IV-$10^7$ | IP-once, day 2 | 225 | 387 | 0 | 40 | [3] |
| BCNU | | IP-once, day 2 | 250 | | 0 | | |
| Cyclophosphamide | IV-$10^7$ | IP-once, day 2 | 300 | 331 | 0 | 20 | [6] |
| CCNU | | IP-once, day 2 | 306 | | 12 | | |
| Cyclophosphamide | IV-$10^7$ | IP-once, day 2 | 225 | 487 | 0 | 50 | [6] |
| Methyl-CCNU | | IP-once, day 2 | 350 | | 40 | | |
| Cyclophosphamide | SC-$10^6$ | SC-once, day 6 | 85 | 290 | 0 | 0 | [5] |
| Ara-C | | SC-$q$2D, days 2—34 | 110 | | 0 | | |
| Cyclophosphamide | IP-$10^5$ | IP-once, day 3 | 135 | >500 | 37 | 75 | [4] |
| cis-Pt-II | | IP-once, day 3 | 45 | | 0 | | |
| BIC | IV-$10^7$ | IP-once, day 2 | 212 | >700 | 0 | 90 | [6] |
| CCNU | | IP-once, day 2 | 512 | | 0 | | |
| DIC | IP-$10^5$ | IP-daily, days 3—17 | 55 | 139 | 0 | 0 | [5] |
| Adriamycin | | IP-$q$3 h/24 h/Day 1 | 61 | | 0 | | |
| Ara-C | SC-$10^6$ | SC-$q$3 h/24 h/days 5, 9,13 | 122 | 211 | 0 | 0 | [5] |
| Procarbazine | | SC-daily, days 5—13 | 78 | | 0 | | |
| Ara-C | SC-$10^6$ | SC-$q$3 h/24 h/days 5,9,13,17 | 100 | 235 | 0 | 20 | [5] |
| BIC | | SC-weekly, days 5—19 | 95 | | 0 | | |
| BIC | IP-$10^5$ | IP-once, day 3 | 78 | 117 | 12 | 37 | [4] |
| *cis*-Pt-II | | IP-once, day 3 | 55 | | 0 | | |
| Isophosphamide | IP-$10^5$ | IP-once, day 3 | 100 | >469 | 0 | 50 | [4] |
| *cis*-Pt-II | | IP-once, day 3 | 55 | | 0 | | |

[a] 6-Me-MP-R = 6-methylmercaptopurine ribonucleoside, BCNU = 1,3-*bis*(2-chloroethyl)-1-nitrosourea, CCNU = 1-(2-chloroethyl)-3-cyclohexyl-1-nitrosourea, Methyl-CCNU = 1-(2-chloroethyl)-3-(4-methylcyclohexyl)-1-nitrosourea, *cis*-Pt-II = *cis*-Platinum (II) diammino-dichloride, DIC = 5-(3,3-dimethyl-1-triazeno)imidazole-4-carboxamide, BIC = 5-[3,3-*bis*-(2-chloroethyl)-1-triazeno]imidazole-4-carboxamide.

[b] S = Results of individual drug treatment.

[c] C = Results of combination treatment.

[d] [1] VENDITTI and GOLDIN (1970). [2] SCHABEL et al. (1968). [3] SCHABEL (1968b). [4] WOODMAN et al. (in press, Chemotherapy). [5] Unpublished data, I. KLINE et al. [6] Unpublished data, F. M. SCHABEL, JR. et al.

drug is to utilize another drug to modify its rate of metabolic biotransformation. For example, the cytotoxicity of cyclophosphamide (Cy) depends on its biotransformation to an active metabolite by the action of microsomal enzymes, mainly those of the liver (Foley et al., 1961; Brock and Hohorst, 1963, 1967; Cohen and Jao, 1970; Connors et al., 1970). Liver microsomal enzyme activity can be stimulated by phenobarbital (Remmer and Merker, 1963; Shuster and Jick, 1966) and inhibited by 2-diethylaminoethyl-2,2-diphenylvalerate hydrochloride (SKF-525A) (Fouts, 1965; Mannering, 1968). Pretreatment with either phenobarbital or SKF-525A has been shown to increase and retard, respectively, the conversion of Cy to its active metabolite (Rauen and Kramer, 1964; Remmer, 1965; Mellett et al., 1969a, b). Recently, Field et al. (1972) studied the influence of phenobarbital and SKF-525A on the activation of Cy in leukemic (L1210) mice. The mice, having been pretreated with phenobarbital or SKF-525A, were given Cy at various times prior to tumor implantation. Chemical determinations of the alkylating metabolites of Cy in plasma at varying times after Cy administration showed that pretreatment with phenobarbital accelerated the production and subsequent depletion of the metabolites, whereas pretreatment with SKF-525A retarded the activation of the drug (Field et al., 1972). Survival times of parallel groups of tumor-bearing mice showed that the duration of time following Cy administration during which the drug was active was shortened by phenobarbital treatment and lengthened by SKF-525A (Field et al., 1972, Table 13). On concomitant administration, phenobarbital plus Cy or SKF-525A plus Cy appeared more effective than Cy in increasing survival time. However, by comparison over a series of time intervals, neither phenobarbital nor SKF-525A plus Cy appeared to provide a therapeutic advantage

Table 13. *Influence of pretreatment with phenobarbital or SKF-525A on the duration of effective levels of cyclphosphamide activity against leukemia L1210*[a]

| Cyclophosphamide IP-180 mg/kg | Cyclphosphamide Alone | | Phenobarbital[b] + Cyclophosphamide | | SKF-525A[c] + Cyclophosphamide | |
|---|---|---|---|---|---|---|
| Time prior to tumor inoculation (min) | Exp. 1 | Exp. 2 | Exp. 1 | Exp. 2 | Exp. 1 | Exp. 2 |
| | Mean survival time in days (no. of 60-day survivors/total)[d] | | | | | |
| 0 | 29.4 (3/10) | 27.5 (2/10) | 41.3 (5/10) | 53.4 (8/10) | 50.2 (8/10) | 37.2 (5/10) |
| 20 | 43.4 (5/8) | 32.5 (3/8) | 22.1 (0/8) | 18.4 (1/8) | 43.3 (4/6) | 42.9 (5/8) |
| 40 | 11.6 (0/8) | 11.9 (0/8) | 8.6 (0/8) | 10.1 (0/8) | 40.5 (4/7) | 32.1 (3/8) |
| 60 | 8.7 (0/8) | 10.4 (0/8) | 8.4 (0/8) | 8.7 (0/8) | 25.0 (2/8) | 26.5 (1/4) |
| 90 | — | — | — | — | — | 13.4 (0/7) |
| 180 | — | — | — | — | — | 11.5 (0/8) |
| Untreated controls | 9.1 (0/16) | 8.9 (0/16) | | | | |
| Phenobarbital alone | 9.2 (0/8) | 8.3 (0/7) | | | | |
| SKF-525A alone | 10.5 (0/8) | 10.3 (0/8) | | | | |

[a] Field et al. (1972). Tumor inoculum —$10^5$ cells, IP.

[b] Phenobarbital (35 mg/kg) was given IP every 12 h × 5; last injection 6 h prior to cyclophosphamide.

[c] SKF-525A (35 mg/kg) was given IP one hour prior to cyclophosphamide.

[d] 60-Day survivors were assigned day 60 as the day of death for calculation of mean survival time.

over Cy alone; nor was it clear that the toxicity of Cy had been modified. Hoshi et al. (1969) reported the failure of phenobarbital to potentiate Cy activity against mouse Sarcoma 180. In the same study, imipramine was reported to enhance Cy activity against Sarcoma 180, but did not influence Cy activating enzyme systems.

Preliminary studies (Field and Kline, personal communication) have indicated that iproniazid, an inhibitor of monamine oxidase and demethylation (Koechlin and Iliev, 1959; Anders and Mannering, 1966), was capable of protecting mice against Cy toxicity. The net effect of iproniazid plus Cy in leukemic (L 1210) mice was to shift the optimal dose of Cy to a greater level with no enhancement of therapeutic efficacy. Iproniazid alone was ineffective.

The antibiotic chloramphenicol has been reported to inhibit microsomal enzymes responsible for the activation of Cy (Dixon, 1968). In recent studies by Kline et al. (personal communication) prior treatment with chloramphenicol reduced the toxicity of Cy in normal mice and in mice with leukemia L 1210. However, no marked therapeutic improvement over treatment with Cy alone was observed with the combination. Chloramphenicol alone was ineffective.

None of the aforementioned attempts to improve the therapeutic efficacy of Cy by altering the rate at which its active metabolite is produced or depleted was successful. However, the experimental conditions over which the combinations were tested were quite limited (with the exception of the phenobarbital or SKF-525A plus Cy studies). In view of the recognized importance of the time interval between injections in maintaining optimally effective levels of many antitumor drugs (Venditti, 1971), the potential for manipulating effective drug levels by altering rates of biotransformation should not be overlooked.

## Schedule Dependency in Combination Chemotherapy

In discussing the problem of interpretation of results of combination treatment, the point was made earlier that failure to demonstrate therapeutic synergism for a drug pair using any particular treatment schedule does not remove the possibility that the potential for synergism exists and might be expressed using a yet untried schedule. Conversely, the demonstration of a therapeutic advantage for a combination should be interpreted with caution if there is a reasonable possibility of finding a more efficacious way of using one of the individual drugs. The elucidation of the therapeutically synergistic combination of ara-C plus 6-TG described earlier in this chapter resulted from a number of significant successive observations (i.e. the advantage of the daily combination treatment over daily individual drug treatment, the finding that one of the drugs (ara-C) was remarkably effective when used alone on an alternative schedule (*q* 3 h/24 h/*q* 4 days) and finally that the combination given *q* 3 h/24 h/*q* 4 days cured a high percentage of tumor-bearing mice). The demonstration of the therapeutic synergism of ICRF-159 plus daunomycin, described earlier in this chapter, also depended on finding the right treatment schedule for maximum combination efficacy.

In a previous review (Venditti and Goldin, 1964a), the influence of treatment schedule on the activity against advanced L 1210 of combinations of azaserine plus 6-MP, MTX plus Cy, and MTX plus 6-MP was discussed. For example, azaserine alone and 6-MP alone displayed approximately the same effectiveness when given twice daily, daily, or every second day. The combination given twice daily provided no therapeutic advantage. When given every second day, however, the combination was approximately twice as effective as individual drug treatments. Daily combination treatment was superior to individual drug treatment, but inferior to every second day combination treatment (Goldin et al., 1960). More recently, the activity of azaserine alone against early L1210 leukemia was found to be remarkably enhanced using the *q* 3 h/24 h/*q* 4 day schedule (VENDITTI, 1971). This raises obvious questions. Does the schedule dependency of azaserine against the early tumor carry over to treatment of advanced leukemia L1210 and, if so, would the combination of azaserine plus 6-MP on this intermittent schedule be more effective than azaserine alone? The combination of MTX plus 6-MP given every three days to mice with advanced leukemia L1210 was more effective than either of the individual drugs given every three days (VENDITTI et al., 1956). However, when the drugs were given separately and combined using a daily treatment schedule, the combination was less effective than daily MTX alone. Moreover, the combination given every three days was inferior to daily MTX alone, the latter being the optimal schedule for MTX against very advanced L1210 leukemia (GOLDIN et al., 1956).

A further example of the schedule dependency of combination chemotherapy against the L1210 tumor is provided by the synergistic combination of ICRF-159 and *cis*-platinum (II) diammino-dichloride (*cis*-Pt-II) (Fig. 1) (WOODMAN et al., 1971). In the experiment summarized in Fig. 3, *cis*-Pt-II was given every fourth day because experience has shown this drug to be maximally effective when given once only, or at widely-spaced intervals (WOODMAN et al., unpublished observations.) In this experiment, ICRF-159 was used on two treatment schedules. When used alone, ICRF-159 was more effective given *q* 3h/24h/*q* 4 days than when given once every 4 days, and with either schedule, ICRF-159 alone was superior to *cis*-Pt-II alone. When ICRF-159 and *cis*-Pt-II were combined on the *q* 3 h/24 h/*q* 4 day schedule, over the dose range employed the combination was not more effective than ICRF-159 alone. However, *q* 4 day treatment with the combination provided a therapeutic effect superior to that achieved with optimal treatment with ICRF-159 alone.

The combination of *cis*-Pt-II plus Cy has shown a remarkable degree of therapeutic synergism against early or advanced L1210 leukemia (WOODMAN et al., unpublished observations). Although the therapeutic advantage of the combination over each of the individual drugs was evident using a number of treatment schedules, the most effective consisted of a single treatment with each drug.

The influence of the temporal relationship in the administration of two drugs on the demonstration of therapeutic synergism was illustrated by studies of VADLAMUDI et al. (1972) in which a survey was made of various schedules of methotrexate plus L-asparaginase in the treatment of mouse leukemia L5178 Y. A therapeutic advantage for the combination was observed over a wide range of treatment schedules. In this study therapeutic synergism was observed when methotrexate was administered on days 3 to 7 following leukemic inoculation and L-asparaginase on days 10 to 14. However, the survival time of mice treated with L-asparaginase on days 3 to 7 followed by methotrexate on days 10 to 14 was less than that observed with either of the drugs alone.

In the examples cited above, modifications in treatment schedule involved variations in the interval between successive treatments. Another scheduling factor that may influence combination chemotherapy efficacy relates to the state of advancement of the disease at the time of treatment initiation. For example, daily treatment with 5-(3,3-dimethyl-l-triazeno)imidazole-4-carboxamide (DIC) plus 5-fluorouracil (5-FU) was considerably more effective than daily treatment with either drug alone against leukemia L1210 if therapy was begun on the first day after tumor implantation. When treatment was delayed until day 5, however, the advantage of the combination was diminished considerably (KLINE et al., 1971b, Table 14). 5-FU alone displayed about the same efficacy against early or advanced disease. In contrast, DIC alone, effective against early disease, was relatively ineffective against advanced disease. For the data summarized in Table 14, one might question the validity of the conclusion that the day of treatment initiation was the only factor influencing the relative success of combination therapy inasmuch as

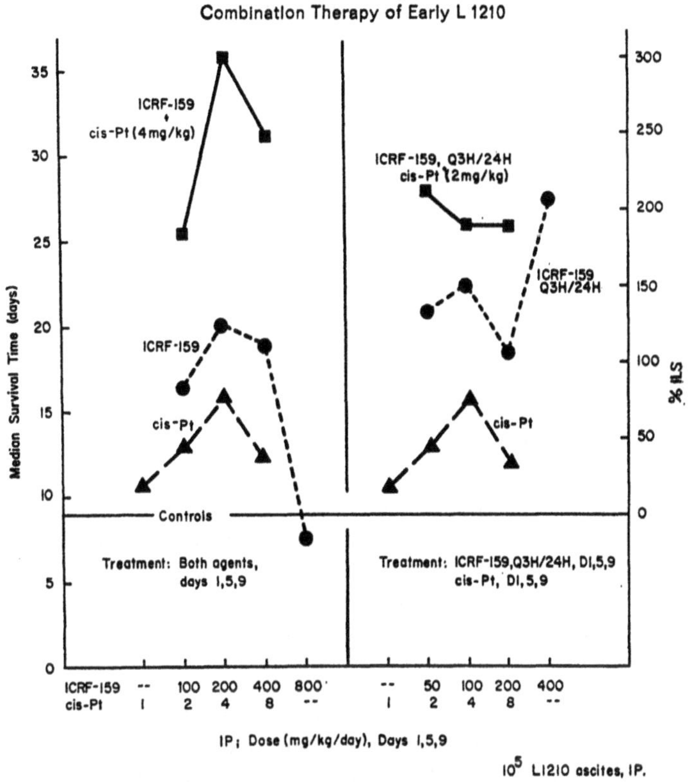


Fig. 3. Influence of treatment schedule on the effectiveness of *cis*-Pt-II plus ICRF-159 against early IP implanted leukemia L1210 (see WOODMAN et al., 1971)

Table 14. *Influence of the day of treatment initiation on response of leukemic (L1210) mice to 5-(3,3-dimethyl-1-triazeno)imidazole-4-carboxamide (DIC) and 5-fluorouracil (5-FU), separately or in combination*[a]

| Treatment | Optimal dose (mg/kg/day) | Increase in lifespan over controls (%) |
|---|---|---|
| | (Treatment daily from days 1—18) | |
| FU alone | 14 | 95 |
| DIC alone | 300 | 67 |
| FU + DIC | 23 + 65 | 250 |
| | (Treatment daily from days 5—18) | |
| FU alone | 14 | 100 |
| DIC alone | 300 | 20 |
| FU + DIC | 8.4 + 23 | 144 |

[a] KLINE et al. (1971b).

the total number of days of treatment was also altered (i.e. 18 days for mice with early leukemia L1210 and 14 days for mice with advanced leukemia L1210, Table 14). Whether continuation of combination treatment would have benefited mice with advanced disease is questionable, but the experiment does exemplify an additional complication in studies of schedule dependency of combinations and individual drugs as well. As has been pointed out many times in the past (VENDITTI et al., 1956, 1957; GOLDIN et al., 1960), the treatment schedule for individual drugs may be modified in a number of demonstrably important ways including the time when treatment is begun, the total duration of treatment and the interval between treatments. This same principle applies to combination therapy (GOLDIN and MANTEL, 1957; VENDITTI and GOLDIN, 1964a).

## Sequential Combination Chemotherapy

An additional way of modifying the treatment schedules in combination chemotherapy is to employ the drugs in some sequential or alternating fashion rather than simultaneously. In view of the generally observed inverse relationship between the size of the tumor cell population and treatment efficacy (GOLDIN et al., 1955d), studies have been conducted on the ability of a priming dose of drug A to selectively reduce the tumor cell population and thereby increase the susceptibility of the disease to subsequent treatment with drug *B*. In general, drug *A* is selected on the basis of schedule dependency studies indicating at least moderate effectiveness when given as a single treatment or treatment for some very limited duration. For example, following the demonstration that 2-chloro-4′,4″-di-2-imidazolin-2-ylterephthalanilide (Chloro-TIC) or Cy produced substantial increases in the survival of mice with advanced leukemia L1210 when given as a single treatment (VENDITTI et al., 1959, 1962), studies were conducted to determine what influence a single priming treatment with Chloro-TIC or Cy might have on the efficacy and schedule dependency of subsequent MTX therapy of advanced disease. It had been shown (GOLDIN et al., 1956) that against early L1210 leukemia, MTX was more effective when given intermittently every fourth day than when given daily. In contrast, against advanced leukemia L1210, there was a sharp diminution in the efficacy of the intermittent schedule and daily MTX was more effective. The loss of intermittent MTX effectiveness against advanced disease was attributed to the relative ineffectiveness of a single treatment with MTX, with the result that the short remaining lifetime of the mice after the initiation of therapy abrogated the opportunity for effective intermittent MTX therapy. An initial single treatment with either Chloro-TIC or Cy followed by MTX either daily or intermittently was considerably more effective than any of the individual drug therapies. Moreover, the priming treatment with Chloro-TIC or Cy resulted in a 3- to 4-fold increase in the efficacy of subsequent intermittent MTX therapy (VENDITTI and GOLDIN, 1964a, b).

A number of subsequent studies have demonstrated the value of a single treatment with 1,3-*bis*(2-chloroethyl)-1-nitrosourea (BCNU), 5-FU, or 6-MP plus continuous treatment with MTX (VENDITTI et al., 1965; KLINE et al., 1966a; GOLDIN and VENDITTI, 1970). Although in some instances the "priming" drug was given on the same day that MTX treatment was begun, the effectiveness of intermittent MTX against the advanced L1210 tumor was enhanced. Other studies have shown the advantage of sequential combination therapy of advanced leukemia L1210 using BCNU followed by ara-C (GOLDIN and VENDITTI, 1970), 5-FU followed by ara-C (HOFFMAN et al., 1969) and ara-C followed by 1-(2-chloroethyl)-3-cyclohexyl-1-nitrosourea (CCNU) (SCHABEL, personal communication).

Schabel (1968a, b) demonstrated the superiority of ara-C plus CCNU over ara-C alone or CCNU alone when both drugs were given concomitantly *q*3 h/24 h/ *q*4 days beginning on day 2 or 3. In Schabel's study of sequential treatment with ara-C and CCNU (Table 15) mice were implanted intravenously with $10^7$ L1210 cells and, under these conditions, 29/30 succumbed four days later, the

Table 15. *Sequential treatment of advanced leukemia L1210 with CCNU followed by ara-C and ara-C followed by CCNU*[a]

| IP treatment | Treatment schedule[b] | Dose per injection (mg/kg) | Leukemic mice: Median survival[c] (days) | Leukemic mice: Day 45 survivors/ total | Normal mice: Day 45 survivors/ total |
|---|---|---|---|---|---|
| Controls | — | — | 4.0 | 0/30 | 9/10 |
| Ara-C alone | *q*3 h/24 h, days 2, 6, 10, 14 | 15 | 20 | 0/10 | 8/10 |
| CCNU alone | Once, day 2 | 50 | 15 | 0/10 | 4/10 |
| | | 37.5 | 14 | 0/10 | 8/10 |
| | | 25 | 9.5 | 0/10 | 10/10 |
| Ara-C → CCNU | *q*3 h/24h/day 2 once, day 5 | 15 37.5 | 39 | 4/10 | 10/10 |
| CCNU → Ara-C | Once, day 2 *q*3 h/24 h/day 5 | 37.5 15 | 10 | 0/10 | 0/10 |
| CCNU → Ara-C | Once, day 2 *q*3 h/24 h/day 5 | 25 15 | 16 | 0/10 | 6/10 |

[a] Selected unpublished data of F. M. Schabel, Jr. Tumor inoculum — $10^7$ cells, IV.

[b] The *q*3 h/24 h/*q*4 day schedule for ara-C alone represented an appropriate control in this experiment since it was known to be superior to divided or single treatment on days 1 or 2 only against early or advanced L1210 leukemia (Skipper et al. 1970; Venditti, 1971). Against SC-implanted advanced leukemia L1210, treatment with ara-C alone has generally not elicited long-term survivors (Venditti, 1971). Thus, there was no evidence from this or other studies that an alternative schedule for ara-C alone would have been more effective than the one used in this experiment. The single treatment schedule was optimal for CCNU treatment of early L1210 leukemia (Skipper et al. 1970). In other studies, a single treatment of CCNU on day 2 has provided long-term survivors in the IV-L1210 leukemia assay used here (Schabel, 1968a, b). The $LD_{10}$ dose for ara-C given *q*3h/24 h/*q*4 days × 4 was reported to be 16 mg/kg/ injection and the $LD_{10}$ single dose of CCNU was reported to be 57 mg/kg (Skipper et al., 1970).

[c] Surviving mice were included in the determination of median survival times.

remaining control animal dying on day 5. When ara-C was given *q*3 h/24 h on day 2 only and followed by CCNU given once on day 5 there was a marked enhancement in therapeutic efficacy over treatment with either ara-C alone or CCNU alone (on day 2). In contrast, when CCNU was given on day 2 followed by ara-C on day 5, the sequential therapy provided no therapeutic advantage. Moreover, survival among normal mice treated in parallel suggested that ara-C followed by CCNU did not result in additive toxicity, whereas there was considerable additive toxicity when CCNU was followed by ara-C (Table 15). The study is important for several reasons. First, it emphasizes further the advantage that can be realized using sequential chemotherapy, although it was not clear that sequential use of this particular combination was superior to its use concomitantly (Schabel, 1968a, b). Secondly, the study showed that the order in which two drugs are used in sequence may have a profound influence on efficacy and toxicity. Additionally, in view of the cell cycle stage specific (CCSS) action of ara-C and the non-CCSS action of nitrosoureas (SKIPPER et al., 1970), the advantage of ara-C followed by CCNU against leukemia L1210 may, at least in part, be a reflection of the presence of a very high proliferative fraction of viable L1210 cells even in the advanced disease state (SIMPSON-HERREN and LLOYD, 1970).

In contrast, SCHABEL (1969) and GRISWOLD et al. (1970) have provided evidence that advanced solid tumors, which exhibit a smaller proliferative fraction and are generally insensitive to CCSS drugs, might be treated effectively by sequential therapy employing a non-CCSS drug followed by a CCSS drug. Improved therapy could be a consequence of the capacity of the non-CCSS drug to reduce the total viable tumor cell population and increase the proliferative fraction of the surviving viable cells. Thus, Cy followed by ara-C was more effective than Cy alone against advanced plasmacytoma no. 1 in hamsters, while ara-C alone was ineffective (GRISWOLD et al., 1970). Tumors of Cy treated animals exhibited thymidine indices that were 2- to 5-times greater than those of untreated animals, the difference increasing progressively with time after treatment (GRISWOLD et al., 1970). Against advanced mouse carcinoma 755, Cy followed by 6-MP was considerably more effective than Cy alone or 6-MP alone (SCHABEL, 1969). SCHABEL (1969) considered that a rational approach to the chemotherapy of advanced solid tumors would involve sequential therapy with a non-CCSS drug followed by a CCSS drug; and existing experimental data appear to support this proposition.

An additional example of the cytokinetic approach to combination chemotherapy was provided by VADLAMUDI and GOLDIN (1971) who demonstrated the ability to obtain therapeutic synergism against leukemia L1210 by synchronizing the tumor cell population with a mitotic inhibitor and following at an appropriate interval with ara-C; thus, specifically inhibiting DNA synthesis with ara-C when a maximum number of tumor cells are in the *S*-phase of the cell cycle. Colcemid treatment arrested the leukemic cells in metaphase, but colcemid alone, at the dose employed did not increase the lifespan of the mice. Therapeutic synergism was observed when colcemid was followed by ara-C treatment at a time when the leukemic cells were estimated to be in *S*-phase, i.e. 15 h after colcemid or 9 h after metaphase arrest. When the time interval between the colcemid and ara-C treatments was less or more than 15 h, the effectiveness of the combination was reduced. Under the conditions of the experiment, colcemid plus ara-C, at the optimal interval between treatments, was approximately 3-times more effective than ara-C alone. Similarly, vinblastine a mitotic inhibitor with moderate anti-L1210 leukemia activity, followed by ara-C, 15 to 24 hours later, was more effective than either vinblastine alone or ara-C alone. SKIPPER et al. (1967) suggested that a more effective therapy with a specific *S*-phase inhibitor such as ara-C could be achieved if the number of cells in *S*-phase could be controlled. The studies of GRISWOLD et al. (1970), SCHABEL (1969) and VADLAMUDI and GOLDIN (1971) discussed above demonstrated the feasibility of exerting such control.

## The Dosage Ratio in Drug Combinations

The influence of the dosage levels and in particular the ratio of the dose of drug *A* to the dose of drug *B* on the therapeutic efficacy of the combination has been discussed previously (VENDITTI and GOLDIN, 1964a). With the combination of methylglyoxal bis-guanylhydrazone (Me-GAG) and 6-MP, over a series of daily dosage levels, for each of five Me-GAG/6-MP dosage ratios ranging from 80% Me-GAG plus 20% 6-MP to 20% Me-GAG plus 80% 6-MP on a mg/kg basis, each dosage ratio exhibited an optimal dosage level, and comparison of these optimal dosages defined the optimal ratio for the combination in the treatment of leukemia L1210. For Me-GAG plus 6-MP, maximum therapeutic synergism was observed when the drugs were combined in the mg/kg ratio of 33% Me-GAG plus 67% 6-MP, and the optimal combination dosage in that ratio consisted of one-half the optimal dose of each drug when used alone (VENDITTI and GOLDIN, 1964a). Table 16 summarizes a recent study of the anti-L1210 leukemia efficacy of the synergistic

Table 16. *Effectiveness of ICRF-159 and camptothecin, sodium salt, separately and combined, against early leukemia L1210*[a]

| ICRF-159 IP-days 1, 5, 9 (mg/kg/day) | Camptothecin IP-days 1, 5, 9 (mg/kg/day) | Mg/kg dosage ratio ICRF-159/ camptothecin | Fraction of individual drug optimal dose | | Increase in lifespan (%) | Number 60-day survivors/ total |
|---|---|---|---|---|---|---|
| | | | ICRF-159 | Camptothecin | | |
| 800 | 0 | — | 2.0 | — | 0 | 0/8 |
| **400** | 0 | — | **1.0** | — | **155** | **1/8** |
| 200 | 0 | — | 0.50 | — | 111 | 0/8 |
| 100 | 0 | — | 0.25 | — | 83 | 0/8 |
| 50 | 0 | — | 0.125 | — | 67 | 0/8 |
| 0 | 80 | — | — | 2.0 | 78 | 0/8 |
| 0 | **40** | — | — | **1.0** | **122** | **0/8** |
| 0 | 20 | — | — | 0.50 | 83 | 0/8 |
| 0 | 10 | — | — | 0.25 | 55 | 0/8 |
| 0 | 5 | — | — | 0.125 | 22 | 0/8 |
| 400 | 20 | 20/1 | 1.0 | 0.50 | 44 | 2/8 |
| **200** | **10** | **20/1** | **0.50** | **0.25** | **133** | **0/8** |
| 100 | 5 | 20/1 | 0.25 | 0.125 | 111 | 0/8 |
| 400 | 40 | 10/1 | 1.0 | 1.0 | 28 | 1/8 |
| **200** | **20** | **10/1** | **0.50** | **0.50** | **411** | **2/8** |
| 100 | 10 | 10/1 | 0.25 | 0.25 | 144 | 0/8 |
| 50 | 5 | 10/1 | 0.125 | 0.125 | 88 | 0/8 |
| **200** | **40** | **5/1** | **0.50** | **1.0** | **>560** | **5/8** |
| 100 | 20 | 5/1 | 0.25 | 0.50 | 172 | 1/8 |
| 50 | 10 | 5/1 | 0.125 | 0.25 | 100 | 0/8 |
| **100** | **40** | **2.5/1** | **0.25** | **1.0** | **189** | **1/8** |
| 50 | 20 | 2.5/1 | 0.125 | 0.5 | 133 | 0/8 |

[a] Unpublished data of I. KLINE et al. Tumor inoculum —$10^5$ cells, IP. The optimal treatment level for each of the alternative therapies is shown in boldface.

combination of ICRF-159 plus camptothecin sodium. In this case, maximum efficacy was observed when one-half the optimal dose of ICRF-159 was combined with the full optimal dose of camptothecin alone.

The importance of examining drug combinations over a wide range of dosage levels and dosage ratios is illustrated by the studies of KLINE et al. (1966a) on the anti-L1210 leukemia effectiveness of the combination of MTX and 5-FU. When mice with advanced leukemia L1210 were treated daily, a moderate degree of therapeutic synergism was observed, but only at combination doses consisting of the full optimal dose of MTX alone plus a low dose of 5-FU, which was ineffective when used alone (Table 17). As might be expected, considering the lethality of 5-FU in parallel groups of normal mice, combinations of therapeutically effective doses of 5-FU and small ineffective doses of MTX were no better than optimal treatment with MTX alone (I. KLINE, personal communication). In the experi-

Table 17. *Effectiveness of daily treatment with methotrexate (MTX) and 5-fluorouracil (5-FU), separately and combined against advanced leukemia L1210*[a,b]

| Daily dose (mg/kg/day) | | Leukemic mice | | Normal mice |
|---|---|---|---|---|
| MTX | 5-FU | ILS[c] (%) | 70-Day survivors/ total | 70-Day survivors/ total |
| 1.6 | — | 67 | 0/10 | 1/10 |
| **0.8** | **—** | **144** | **0/10** | **10/10** |
| 0.4 | — | 11 | 0/10 | 10/10 |
| — | 205 | 50 | 0/10 | 0/10 |
| **—** | **102** | **56** | **0/10** | **0/10** |
| — | 51 | 50 | 0/10 | 0/10 |
| — | 26 | 11 | 0/10 | 0/10 |
| — | 13 | 0 | 0/10 | 7/10 |
| 1.6 | 26 | 83 | 0/10 | 0/10 |
| **0.8** | **13** | **189** | **0/10** | **6/10** |
| 0.4 | 6.4 | 11 | 0/10 | 10/10 |

[a] Kline et al. (1966a).
[b] SC treatment beginning 6 days after SC tumor implantation. The optimal treatment level for each of the alternative therapies is boldface.
[c] Increase in life span.

ment summarized in Table 17, the undesirable toxicity of 5-FU was avoided by the use of a very small daily dosage level which nevertheless was capable of contributing to therapeutic efficacy. An alternative way of attempting to diminish the adverse effects of a drug with an apparent narrow margin of safety is to limit the duration of treatment. In the experiment summarized in Table 18, mice with

Table 18. *Effectiveness of a single treatment with 5-fluorouracil (5-FU) plus daily treatment with methotrexate (MTX) against leukemia L1210*[a]

| SC-treatment | Optimal dose (mg/kg) | ILS[b] (%) |
|---|---|---|
| 5-FU, day 6 only | 108 | 88 |
| MTX, daily from day 6 | 1.1 | 112 |
| 5-FU, day 6 only + MTX, daily from day 6 | 23.0+1.1 | 200 |

[a] Kline et al. (1966a).
[b] Increase in life span.

advanced leukemia L1210 were given one 5-FU treatment and this was combined with daily MTX treatment (Kline et al., 1966a). In similarity to the situation when both drugs were given daily, therapeutic synergism was observed when the full optimal daily dose of MTX was combined with a small relatively ineffective single dose of 5-FU.

## Biochemical Rationale in the Choice of Drug Combinations

With increasing knowledge of the specific biochemical sites of action of antitumor drugs, it may be possible to select a greater number of drug combinations for studies of therapeutic synergism on this basis (Sartorelli, 1965, 1969).

In discussing the biochemical basis for antitumor synergism, VENDITTI and GOLDIN (1964a) reviewed studies relating the synergistic action of combinations such as MTX plus fluorinated pyrimidines, 6-MP plus azaserine and 6-MP plus MTX to the concurrent or sequential blockade of critical steps in the pathways of nucleic acid biosynthesis. The possible biochemical basis for the protection by ara-C against host toxicity by 6-TG and the resultant therapeutic advantage of the combination were discussed earlier in this chapter.

## A. Combinations of Cytosine Arabinoside (ara-C) and Inhibitors of Ribonucleoside Diphosphate Reductase

Ara-C, an inhibitor of DNA polymerase (FURTH and COHEN, 1968), and the ribonucleoside diphosphate reductase inhibitors, guanazole, hydroxyurea, picolinaldehyde thiosemicarbazone (PT) and 5-hydroxypicolinaldehyde thiosemicarbazone (5-HP) (KRAKOFF et al., 1968; SARTORELLI et al., 1969; BROCKMAN et al., 1970a, b) (Fig 4.) have been shown to be maximally effective against early leukemia

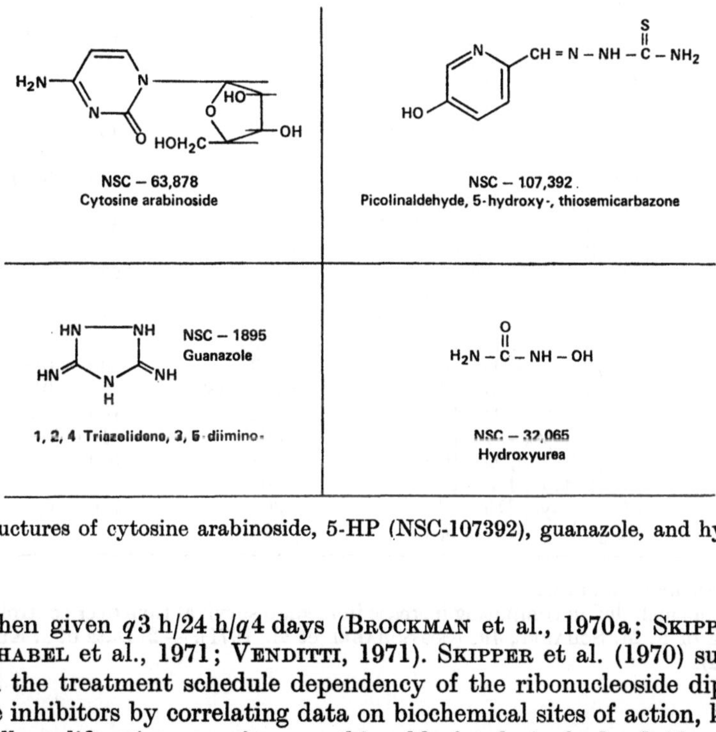


Fig. 4. Structures of cytosine arabinoside, 5-HP (NSC-107392), guanazole, and hydroxyurea

L1210 when given $q$3 h/24 h/$q$4 days (BROCKMAN et al., 1970a; SKIPPER et al., 1970; SCHABEL et al., 1971; VENDITTI, 1971). SKIPPER et al. (1970) successfully predicted the treatment schedule dependency of the ribonucleoside diphosphate reductase inhibitors by correlating data on biochemical sites of action, kinetics of tumor cell proliferation, maximum achievable levels in body fluids, minimum levels required for effective tumor cell destruction, and the effect of drug concentration and time at the target cell on the rate of tumor cell kill. In relating biochemical sites of inhibition to patterns of resistance and cross-resistance among specific inhibitors of DNA synthesis, SCHABEL et al. (1971) found that a variant of the L1210 leukemia developed for resistance to ara-C retained sensitivity to the ribonucleoside diphosphate reductase inhibitors and that L1210 tumor variants selected for resistance to hydroxyurea or PT retained sensitivity to ara-C, but were resistant to hydroxyurea, guanazole, and the picolinaldehyde thiosemicarbazones.

These observations prompted studies showing that combinations of ara-C plus hydroxyurea, guanazole, or picolinaldehyde thiosemicarbazones were more effective than the individual drugs against the parent line of leukemia L1210 (Table 19). The sites of biochemical inhibition implicated in the synergistic action of ara-C plus ribonucleoside diphosphate reductase inhibitors are illustrated in Fig. 5.

Table 19. *Combination therapy of leukemia L1210 with cytosine arabinoside (ara-C) plus guanazole (Guan), hydroxyurea (Hydrox), picolinaldehyde thiosemicarbazone (PT), or 5-hydroxypicolinaldehyde thiosemicarbazone (5-HP)*

| Treatment | Route and schedule | GNLD[a] (mg/kg per injection) | ILS[b] (%) | 60-Day S/T | Ref.[c] |
|---|---|---|---|---|---|
| Ara-C alone | IP-$q$3 h × 8, D2, 6, 10, 14 | 15 | 271 | 0/10 | [1] |
| | IP-$q$3 h × 8, D2, 6 | 15 | 228 | 1/10 | |
| Hydroxy alone | IP-$q$3 h × 8, D2, 6, 10, 14 | 60 | 42 | 0/10 | [1] |
| | IP-$q$3 h × 8, D2, 6 | 60 | 42 | 0/10 | |
| PT alone | IP-$q$3 h × 8, D2, 6, 10, 14 | 6.0 | 243 | 2/10 | [1] |
| | IP-$q$3 h × 8, D2, 6 | 6.0 | 143 | 1/10 | |
| Guan alone | IP-$q$3 h × 8, D2, 6, 10, 14 | 600 | 157 | 0/10 | [1] |
| | IP-$q$3 h × 8 D2, 6 | 600 | 92 | 0/10 | |
| Ara-C | IP-$q$3 h × 8, D2, 6 | 10 | 271 | 2/10 | [1] |
| + Hydrox | IP-$q$3 h × 8, D10, 14 | + 40 | | | |
| Ara-C | IP-$q$3 h × 8, D2, 6, 10, 14 | 10 | >750 | 6/10 | [1] |
| + Hydrox | IP-$q$3 h × 8, D2, 6, 10, 14 | + 40 | | | |
| Ara-C | IP-$q$3 h × 8, D2, 6 | 10 | 464 | 3/10 | [1] |
| + PT | IP-$q$3 h × 8, D10, 14 | + 4.0 | | | |
| Ara-C | IP-$q$3 h × 8, D2, 6, 10, 14 | 10 | 586 | 3/10 | [1] |
| + PT | IP-$q$3 h × 8, D2, 6, 10, 14 | + 4.0 | | | |
| Ara-C | IP-$q$3 h × 8, D2, 6 | 10 | 257 | 3/10 | [1] |
| + Guan | IP-$q$3 h × 8, D10, 14 | +450 | | | |
| Ara-C | IP-$q$3 h × 8, D2, 6, 10, 14 | 10 | 214 | 2/10 | [1] |
| + Guan | IP-$q$3 h × 8, D2, 6, 10, 14 | +450 | | | |
| 5-HP alone | SC-$q$3 h × 8, D5, 9, 13 | 23 | 90 | 0/8 | [2] |
| | SC-$q$2 days, D5—13 | (180—1388) | < 25 | 0/8 | |
| Ara-C alone | SC-$q$3 h × 8, D5, 9, 13 | 14 | 100 | 0/8 | [2] |
| | SC-$q$2 days, D5—13 | 500 | 115 | 0/8 | |
| Ara-C | SC-$q$3 h × 8, D5, 9, 13 | 14 | 140 | 0/8 | [2] |
| + 5-HP | SC-$q$2 days, D5—13 | +108 | | | |
| Ara-C | SC-$q$2 days, D5—13 | 300 | 180 | 0/8 | [2] |
| + 5-HP | SC-$q$3 h × 8, D5, 9, 13 | + 14 | | | |

[a] Greatest nonlethal dose.
[b] Survivors included in computing increase in median survival time over controls (ILS, %).
[c] 1. Data of F. M. SCHABEL, JR. (See SCHABEL et al., 1971). — 2. Data of I. KLINE et al., unpublished).

## B. Combination Chemotherapy of Mouse Leukemias Using Glutamine Analogs and L-Asparaginase

The role of glutamine analogs (e. g. azaserine, azotomycin, duazomycin A and 6-diazo-5-oxo-L-norleucine) as inhibitors of glutamine utilization has been reviewed by LIVINGSTON et al. (1970). Historically, antitumor activity of agents such as azaserine had been related to their ability to inhibit glutamine utilization in nucleic acid biosynthesis (see VENDITTI and GOLDIN, 1964a, and references cited therein). However, LIVINGSTON et al. (1970) in discussing the role of L-glutamine as a precursor of L-asparagine biosynthesis cited a number of previous studies showing that tumors with low levels of intracellular asparagine synthetase activity (e. g. leukemia L5178Y) generally require an extracellular source of L-asparagine and are sensitive to L-asparaginase treatment. In contrast, tumors with relatively high levels of asparagine synthetase activity (e. g. leukemia L1210)

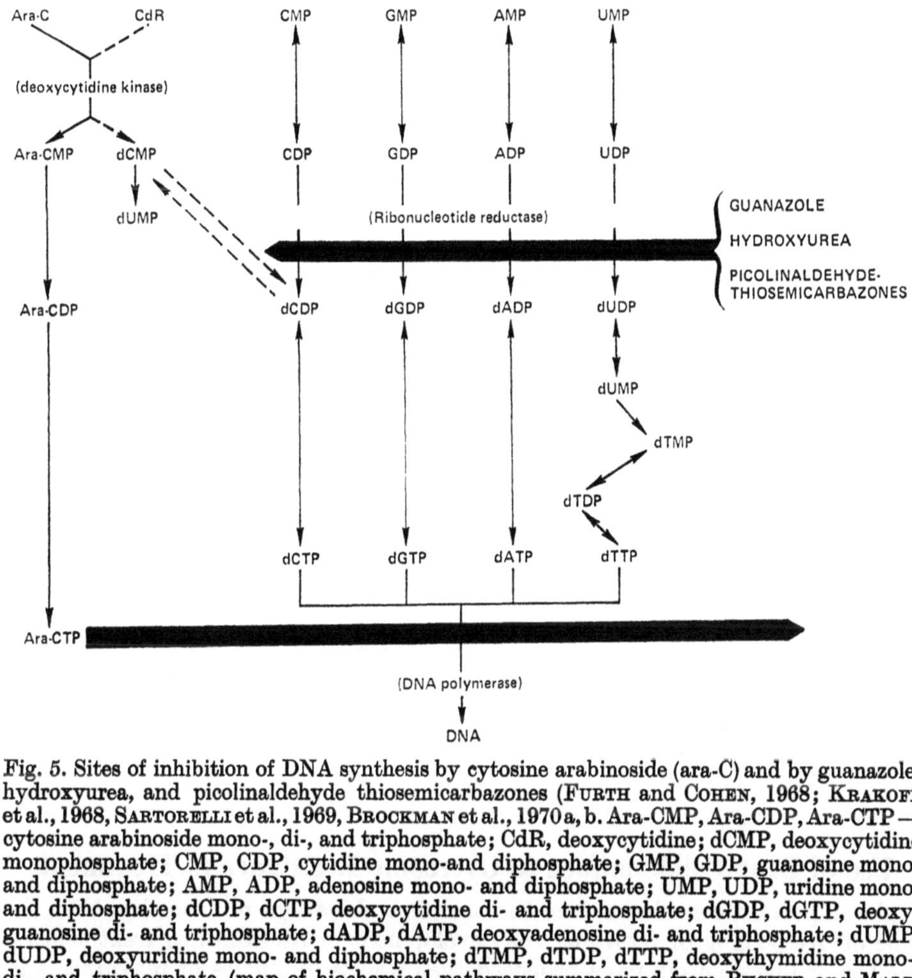


Fig. 5. Sites of inhibition of DNA synthesis by cytosine arabinoside (ara-C) and by guanazole, hydroxyurea, and picolinaldehyde thiosemicarbazones (FURTH and COHEN, 1968; KRAKOFF et al., 1968, SARTORELLI et al., 1969, BROCKMAN et al., 1970a, b. Ara-CMP, Ara-CDP, Ara-CTP — cytosine arabinoside mono-, di-, and triphosphate; CdR, deoxycytidine; dCMP, deoxycytidine monophosphate; CMP, CDP, cytidine mono-and diphosphate; GMP, GDP, guanosine mono- and diphosphate; AMP, ADP, adenosine mono- and diphosphate; UMP, UDP, uridine mono- and diphosphate; dCDP, dCTP, deoxycytidine di- and triphosphate; dGDP, dGTP, deoxyguanosine di- and triphosphate; dADP, dATP, deoxyadenosine di- and triphosphate; dUMP, dUDP, deoxyuridine mono- and diphosphate; dTMP, dTDP, dTTP, deoxythymidine mono-, di-, and triphosphate (map of biochemical pathways summarized from BUCHER and MALT, 1971)

are generally not dependent on circulating L-asparagine and are insensitive to L-asparaginase. JACOBS et al. (1970) conducted extensive studies of combinations of L-asparaginase plus other antitumor agents, including a number of glutamine antagonists. *L*-Asparaginase treatment alone was effective against leukemia L5178Y, but ineffective against leukemia L1210. Azaserine or azotomycin was effective against both L5178Y and L1210 leukemias. Combinations of L-asparaginase plus azaserine or azotomycin provided a high degree of therapeutic synergism against leukemia L5178Y, but were no more effective than azaserine or azotomycin alone against the L1210 tumor. Livingston et al. (1970) suggested two possible mechanisms for the observed synergism against leukemia L5178Y i.e. that depletion of circulating L-asparagine was maximized as a result of deamidation by L-asparaginase and inhibition by glutamine antagonists of the precursor for its biosynthesis in the host and/or that synergism may have resulted from L-asparagine depletion and concurrent block of *de novo* purine nucleotide biosynthesis. The failure of L-asparaginase to provide a therapeutic advantage when combined with azaserine or azotomycin against leukemia L1210 suggested that any inhibition of glutamine utilization for L-asparagine biosynthesis was insufficient to create dependence of the tumor on circulating L-asparagine (Livingston et al., 1970). Jacobs et al. (1970) also reported therapeutic synergism against the L5178Y tumor for combinations of L-asparaginase plus actinomycin D or 6-MP. Wodinsky et al. (personal communication) reported a marked synergistic effect against leukemia L5178Y by L-asparaginase plus 5-azacytidine (Table 20).

Table 20. *Effectiveness of L-asparaginase and 5-azacytidine, separately and combined, against mouse leukemia L5178 Y*[a]

| L-Asparaginase (IU/mouse/day)[b] | 5-Azacytidine (mg/kg/Day)[b] | ILS[c] (%) | 60-Day survivors/ total |
|---|---|---|---|
| 16 | 0 | 100 | 1/10 |
| 8 | 0 | 95 | 0/10 |
| 4 | 0 | 79 | 0/10 |
| 0 | 6.0 | 141 | 0/10 |
| 0 | 3.0 | 58 | 0/10 |
| 0 | 1.5 | 35 | 0/10 |
| 0 | 0.75 | 16 | 0/10 |
| 16 | 6.0 | >341 | 5/10 |
| 16 | 3.0 | >399 | 7/10 |
| 16 | 1.5 | 233 | 4/10 |
| 16 | 0.75 | 108 | 4/10 |

[a] Unpublished data of I. Wodinsky et al.
[b] IP treatment, daily, days 1—5.
[c] Increase in life span.

## Use of Drug Combinations to Overcome Resistance to Treatment

An important consideration in the use of combinations of drugs has been the hope of overcoming or retarding the development of resistance to treatment. A number of investigators have proposed that results of studies of resistance and cross-resistance can be used to select appropriate drugs for combination chemotherapy studies. Although some therapeutically synergistic drug pairs have been selected on this basis, the demonstration that enhanced efficacy resulted from retardation of resistance to treatment requires a more complex experimental model. One such model was provided by Venditti and Goldin (1964a) who demonstrated that the synergistic combination of MTX plus Chloro-TIC actually delayed the onset of resistance in the treatment of leukemia L1210. In this study the L1210 tumor was treated *in vivo* over successive transplant generations with optimal levels of MTX alone, Chloro-TIC alone, or the combination. The rate at which resistance developed in each of the tumor variants was measured with respect to (a) the number of successive transplant generations required, (b) the total number of treatments required and (c) the elapsed time from the initial treatment of the first treated transplant generation to the development of resistance in a subsequent transplant generation. Chloro-TIC treatment alone resulted in the rapid development of a variant tumor resistant to Chloro-TIC in the first post-parental transplant generation. The leukemic subline which was developed by treating with MTX alone over successive transplant generations displayed a high degree of resistance to MTX in the third generation. The leukemic subline developed by treatment with the combination was still very sensitive to MTX alone and to the combination in the third transplant generation, and displayed resistance to either therapy in the fourth transplant generation. Significantly, the latter subline remained partially sensitive to Chloro-TIC throughout five transplant generations. The study was important because it described an experimental model that permitted the measurement of the degree to which a synergistic drug combination delayed the onset of resistance *in vivo*.

Recently, KLINE et al. (1971a) reported that in the treatment of advanced L1210 leukemia, the combination of 5-(3,3-dimethyl-1-triazeno)imidazole-4-carboxamide (DIC) plus ara-C was superior to either of the individual drugs. Bioassay studies showed that surviving tumor cells taken from mice that were effectively treated with ara-C and implanted into recipient mice were resistant to ara-C therapy, suggesting the possibility that the development of resistance to ara-C may have also finally limited the effectiveness of the DIC plus ara-C combination. Ara-C, DIC, or MTX therapy administered sequentially after termination of DIC plus ara-C treatment provided additional increases in lifespan over the DIC plus ara-C combination of 0 to 17%, 28%, and 58%, respectively. The results indicated that, during the course of DIC plus ara-C treatment, the disease had become resistant to ara-C, retained some degree of sensitivity to DIC or ara-C plus DIC, but was most effectively treated by discontinuing the initial combination treatment and initiating a sequential treatment with a third drug (MTX) (KLINE et al., 1971a). Extension of these studies (KLINE et al., personal communication) has shown that treatment with DIC plus ara-C followed sequentially by BCNU or the combination of MTX plus BCNU was more effective than continuation of DIC plus ara-C therapy (Table 21). The combination of MTX plus BCNU displayed a marked degree of therapeutic synergism against advanced L1210 leukemia when used concomitantly or sequentially (VENDITTI et al., 1965).

Table 21. *Effectiveness of sequential treatment following therapy of leukemia L1210 with the synergistic combination of ara-C plus DIC*[a]

| Treatment following initial course of ara-C + DIC[b] | Additional ILS after discontinuance of ara-C + DIC (%) |
|---|---|
| Ara-C + DIC (continuation of treatment) | 30 |
| Ara-C | 0—17 |
| DIC | 28 |
| MTX | 58 |
| BCNU | 90—105 |
| MTX + BCNU | 110 |

[a] KLINE et al. (1971a) and unpublished data.

[b] Ara-C, DIC, MTX, 4—5 days following ara-C + DIC; BCNU, MTX + BCNU, 3—5 days following ara-C + DIC.

## Combination Chemotherapy of Meningeal Leukemia

A serious complication in the therapy of human leukemia is the development of meningeal disease. Similarly, meningeal leukemia has been observed to limit the therapy of advanced mouse leukemia L1210 (THOMAS et al., 1962). Nitrosourea derivatives such as BCNU are capable of crossing the "blood-brain barrier" and exerting an effect against L1210 cells in the brain (SCHABEL et al., 1963). Ara-C has also been shown to be effective against intracranially (IC) inoculated L1210 leukemia (KLINE et al., 1966b). The marked synergism against SC implanted advanced leukemia L1210 upon treatment with BCNU followed sequentially by ara-C has been demonstrated (TYRER et al., 1967). The effectiveness of both drugs against IC leukemia suggests that such activity may have contributed at least in part to the therapeutic improvement observed on sequential therapy of advanced SC implanted L1210 tumor, for which penetration of L1210 cells into the brain may pose a serious problem in therapy.

Figure 6 illustrates a recent study which demonstrates the therapeutic synergism of ICRF-159 plus ara-C against IC implanted L1210 leukemia. While ICRF-159 was only minimally effective when used alone, the combination was considerably more effective than therapy with ara-C alone.

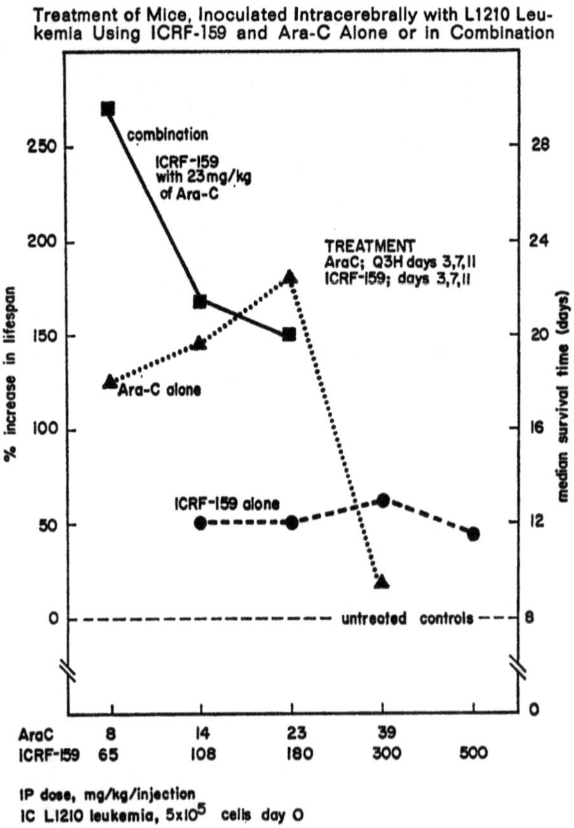


Fig. 6. Effectiveness of ara-C plus ICRF-159, separately and in combination, against intracranially (IC) implanted leukemia L1210. Ara-C was given IP alone or in combination q 3h/24 h on days 3, 7 and 11. ICRF-159 was given IP alone or in combination once each day on days 3, 7 and 11. For combination treatment one dosage level of ara-C (23 mg/kg) was combined with each of three ICRF-159 doses (8,14, or 23 mg/kg)

## Combination Chemotherapy of Spontaneous AKR Lymphoma

SCHABEL et al. (1969, 1970), SKIPPER et al. (1969) and GOLDBERG et al. (1972) described the growth characteristics of spontaneous lymphoma in AKR mice and the ability of the combination of vincristine (VCR) and prednisone to induce remission of the disease. The development of this model assay was inportant for at least two reasons. The combination of VCR and prednisone is one of the most effective treatments for inducing remission in acute lymphocytic leukemia (MATHÉ et al., 1967; HENDERSON, 1969). Moreover, since the VCR plus prednisone combination is capable of inducing remission in approximately 60% of treated mice (GOLDBERG et al., 1972), the model provides an opportunity to study subsequent therapy for its ability to maintain remissions. GOLDBERG et al. (1972) examined ten drugs for their relative efficacy in maintaining VCR plus prednisone induced remissions of spontaneous AKR lymphoma. Of these, Cy was the most effective. While VCR plus prednisone followed by Cy increased survival time 250% over VCR plus prednisone followed by placebo, the sequential treatment did not appear to be more effective than Cy used alone from the initiation of treatment. Nevertheless, the assay system does present an experimental model for evaluating the remission maintenance potential of a drug, and further emphasizes the complications in evaluation of results for multiple drug assays.

## Chemotherapy Plus Immunotherapy

Attempts have been made to improve chemotherapeutic effectiveness by the utilization of immune enhancing agents (HENDERSON and LEVENTHAL, 1972; REGELSON, 1972a) and by employing immunological programs such as those involving adoptive immunity (GLYNN et al., 1968, 1969; MIHICH, 1969; FEFER, 1971a; GLYNN and KENDE, 1971; GOLDBERG and GLYNN, 1972; HENDERSON and LEVENTHAL, 1972). GLYNN et al. (1969) showed that allogeneic spleen cells specifically sensitized to the Moloney virus-induced transplantation antigens in conjunction with Cy can be used to successfully eradicate the virus-induced lymphoma, while neither Cy treatment alone nor treatment with sensitized allogeneic cells alone could achieve this effect. Cy alone, however, was effective in increasing the survival time of the mice. BONMASSAR et al. (1970) investigated precisely defined genetic systems to determine whether a difference in a minor histocompatibility gene could result in immunological potentiation of a chemotherapeutic effect. It was found that host immune responses directed against tumor antigens, specified by only a single minor histocompatibility gene, were capable of producing a significant increase in the antileukemic effect of BCNU. These authors (BONMASSAR et al., 1970) cited a number of studies in which additive or synergistic effects between drugs and transplantation immunity were reported in animals and in man. The studies demonstrate that immune allograft reactions directed against transplantation antigens of tumors may increase the antitumor activity of drugs.

FEFER (1971b) and STOLFI et al. (1971) have reviewed the current status of the combination of chemotherapy and immunotherapy and emphasized that antitumor drugs, in addition to their beneficial cytotoxicity against tumor cells, may suppress or enhance the host's immune response. Moreover, the immune suppressive or enhancing properties of drugs, as well as their cytotoxic action may be dependent on dosage and treatment schedule. Thus, it would seem important to determine, for any active antitumor drug, the conditions for maximal immunosuppressive activity so that such regimens can be avoided when it is used alone or when combined with immunotherapy.

## Surgery and Chemotherapy (Surgical-Adjuvant Therapy)

Earlier in this chapter, in discussing sequential combination chemotherapy, a number of studies were cited in which a "priming" treatment with drug *A* reduced the total tumor cell population and rendered the remaining viable cells more susceptible to subsequent treatment with drug *B*. Alternatively, a number of investigators have indicated that the appropriate use of surgery in combination with chemotherapy may be more effective than surgery alone, radiation alone, or chemotherapy alone (Venditti and Goldin, 1964a; Karrer and Humphreys, 1967; Humphreys and Karrer, 1970; Laster et al., 1971; Stolfi et al., 1971). Karrer and Humphreys (1967) and Humphreys and Karrer (1970) demonstrated that, although established primary or metastatic Lewis lung carcinoma in mice is not curable either by treatment with Cy alone or surgery alone, surgical removal of the primary tumor followed by Cy treatment resulted in cures. Laster et al. (1971) observed that 1-(2-chloroethyl)-3-(4-methylcyclohexyl)-1-nitrosourea (MeCCNU) was unusually effective against subcutaneous implanted Lewis lung carcinoma and that surgical removal of the primary tumor followed by MeCCNU treatment significantly increased the number of long-term survivors over that achieved by MeCCNU treatment alone or surgery alone.

The possible effect of a reduction in viable tumor cell population in increasing the growth fraction of surviving viable cells and consequentially increasing their susceptibility to therapy with antimetabolites (see "Sequential Chemotherapy" above) is also applicable to surgery followed by chemotherapy.

Stolfi et al. (1971) have reviewed the rational for using surgical treatment to potentiate chemotherapy and the current status of multiple combined therapy (chemotherapy, immunotherapy, and surgery) in the treatment of a spontaneous mammary carcinoma in mice.

## Conclusions

The choice of drugs for experimental studies of combination chemotherapy can be made entirely empirically; that is, combinations have been selected because of demonstrated antitumor activity of the individual drugs or because the individual drugs displayed different qualitative toxicities. However, we have cited some examples in which specific combinations were examined in rationally based attempts to enhance antitumor specificity: (a) by selectively decreasing toxicity to the host without decreasing cytotoxicity to tumor cells, (b) by selectively increasing the toxicity for the tumor without a proportionate increase in toxicity for the host, (c) influencing the concentration and duration of effect of an active drug at the target site, (d) by reducing the tumor cell population or modifying the growth characteristics of the tumor and thereby altering its sensitivity to subsequent therapy, and (e) by retarding the development of resistance to treatment. With increasing knowledge, it may be possible in the above to take increasing advantage of knowledge of specific biochemical sites of action. The potential for enhancing antitumor efficacy with combinations of surgery plus drugs as well as immunotherapy plus drugs was reviewed briefly. As knowledge of the actions of new agents increases at the cytokinetic, biochemical, toxicologic, and pharmacologic levels, as we learn to maximize the efficacy of individual drugs, as we learn how to better utilize drugs as adjuvants to surgery or irradiation, and as we learn how to take better advantage of host defense mechanisms to enhance the response to drugs or how to use drugs to enhance immune responses, we may look forward to the emergence of still more effective means of controlling human cancers.

## References

ALBERT, A.: Selective toxicity. London: Methuen & Co. 1960.

ANDERS, M. W., MANNERING, G. J.: Inhibition of drug metabolism. I. Kinetics of the inhibition of the *N*-demethylation of ethylmorphine by 2-diethylaminoethyl-2,2-diphenylvalerate HCl (SKF-525 A) and related compounds. Molec. Pharmacol. **2**, 319—327 (1966).

BONADONNA, G., MONFARDINI, S., DELENA, M., FOSSATI-BELLANI, F., BERETTA, G.: Phase I and preliminary phase II evaluation of adriamycin (NSC-123127). Cancer Res. **30**, 2572—2582 (1970).

BONMASSAR, E., CUDKOWITZ, G., VADLAMUDI, S., GOLDIN, A.: Influence of tumor-host differences at a single histocompatibility locus (H-1) on the antileukemic effect of 1,3-*bis* (2-chloroethyl)-1-nitrosourea (NSC-409962). Cancer Res. **30**, 2538—2542 (1970).

BRINKER, H.: Protection of C3H-mice against toxic effects of endoxan by means of cysteine HCl. Acta path. microbiol. Scand. 61, 321—332 (1964).

BROCK, N., HOHORST, H. J.: Über die Activierung von Cyclophosphamid in vivo und in vitro. Arzneimittel-Forschung **13**, 1021—1031 (1963).

BROCK, N., HOHORST, H. J.: Metabolism of cyclophosphamide. Cancer **20**, 900—904 (1967).

BROCKMAN, R. W., SHADDIX, S., LASTER, W. R., JR., SCHABEL, F. M., JR.: Inhibition of ribonucleotide reductase, DNA synthesis, and L-1210 leukemia by guanazole. Cancer Res. **30**, 2358—2368 (1970a).

BROCKMAN, R. W., SIDWELL, R. W., ARNETT, G., SHADDIX, S.: Heterocyclic thiosemicarbazones: correlation between structure, inhibition of ribonucleotide reductase, and inhibition of DNA viruses. Proc. Soc. exp. Biol. (N. Y.) **133**, 609—614 (1970b).

BRODSKY, I., KAHN, S. B., CONROY, J. F.: The effects of androgens on cancer chemotherapy. In: BRODSKY, I., KAHN, S. B., MOYER, J. H. (Eds): Cancer chemotherapy II (The Twenty-second Hahnemann Symposium), pp. 303—314. New York: Grune & Stratton 1972.

BUCHER, N. L. R., MALT, R. A.: Regeneration of Liver and Kidney, Chapter 4, DNA synthesis (replication), pp. 55—77. Boston: Little, Brown & Co. 1971.

BURCHENAL, J. H.: Success and failure in present chemotherapy and the implications of asparaginase. Cancer Res. **29**, 2262—2269 (1969).

BURCHENAL, J. H., DOLLINGER, M. R.: Cytosine arabinoside (NSC-63878) in combination with 6-mercaptopurine (NSC-755), methotrexate (NSC-740), or 5-fluorouracil (NSC-19893) in L1210 mouse leukemia. Cancer. Chemother. Rep. **51**, 435—438 (1967).

CHU, M. Y., FISCHER, G. A.: A proposed mechanism of action of 1-$\beta$-D-arabinofuranosylcytosine as an inhibitor of the growth of leukemic cells. Biochem. Pharmacol. **11**, 423—430 (1962).

COHEN, J. L., JAO, J. Y.: Enzymatic basis of cyclophosphamide activation by hepatic microsomes of the rat. J. Pharmacol. exp. Ther. **174**, 206—210 (1970).

CONNORS, T. A.: Protection against the toxicity of alkylating agents by thiols: the mechanism of protection and its relevance to cancer chemotherapy. A review. Europ. J. Cancer **2**, 293—305 (1966).

CONNORS, T. A., ELSON, L. A.: Reduction of the toxicity of "radiomimetic" alkylating agents in rats by thiol pretreatment. Biochem. Pharmacol. **11**, 1221—1232 (1962).

CONNORS, T. A., GROVER, P. L., MCLOUGHLIN, A. M.: Microsomal activation of cyclophosphamide in vivo. Biochem. Pharmacol. **19**, 1533—1535 (1970).

CORTES, E. P., ELLISON, R. R., YATES, J. W.: Adriamycin (NSC-123127) in the treatment of acute myelocytic leukemia. Cancer Chemother. Rep. **56**, 237—243 (1972).

CREIGHTON, A. M., HELLMAN, K., WHITECROSS, S.: Antileukemic activity in a series of bis diketopiperazines. Nature (Lond). **222**, 384—385 (1969).

DEVITA, V. T., SERPICK, A., CARBONE, P. P.: Combination chemotherapy of advanced Hodgkins disease: the NCI program, a progress report. Proc. Am. Ass. Cancer Res. **10**, 19 (1969).

DIXON, R. L.: Effect of chloramphenicol on the metabolism and lethality of cyclophosphamide in rats. Proc. Soc. exp. Biol. (N. Y.) **127**, 1151—1155 (1968).

EVANS, A. E.: Refinements in the treatment of children with solid tumors. In: BRODSKY, I., KAHN, S. B., MOYER, J. H. (Eds.): Cancer chemotherapy II, pp. 181—187. New York: Grune & Stratton 1972.

EVANS, J. S., MENGEL, G. D.: The reversal of cytosine arabinoside activity in vivo by deoxycytidine. Biochem. Pharmacol. **13**, 989—994 (1964).

FAUST, D. S., BRADY, L. W., ANTONIADES, J.: Hyberbaric oxygen with chemotherapy and radiation therapy in cancer. In: BRODSKY, I., KAHN, S. B., MOYER, J. H. (Eds.): Cancer chemotherapy II, pp. 459—464. New York: Grune & Stratton 1972.

FEFER, A.: Adoptive chemoimmunotherapy of a Moloney lymphoma. Int. J. Cancer **8**, 364—373 (1971a).

FEFER, A.: Experimental approaches to immunotherapy of cancer. In: Current concepts in the management of leukemias and lymphomas. Recent results in cancer research, pp. 182—192. New York: Springer 1971b.

Field, R. B., Gang, M., Kline, I., Venditti, J. M., Waravdekar, V. S.: The effect of phenobarbital or 2-diethylaminoethyl-2,2-diphenylvalerate on the activation of cyclophosphamide in vivo. J. Pharmacol. exp. Ther. **180**, 475—483 (1972).
Foley, G. E., Friedman, O. M., Drolet, B. P.: Studies on the mechanism of action of cytoxan. Evidence of activation in vivo and in vitro. Cancer Res. **21**, 57—63 (1961).
Fouts, J. R.: Impairment of drug metabolism in drug toxicity. In: Brodie, B. B., Gillette, J. R. (Eds.): Drugs and enzymes, pp. 261—276. New York: The Macmillan Co. 1965.
Frei, E., III: Chemotherapy of acute leukemia. In: Brodsky, I., Kahn, S. B., Moyer, J. H. (Eds.): Cancer chemotherapy II, pp. 315—325. New York: Grune & Stratton 1972.
Freireich, E. J., Henderson, E. S., Karon, M. R., Frei, E., III: The treatment of acute leukemia considered with respect to cell population kinetics. In: The proliferation and spread of neoplastic cells. pp. 441—452. Baltimore: Williams and Wilkins Co. 1968.
Furth, J. J., Cohen, S. S.: Inhibition of mammalian DNA polymerase by the 5′-triphosphate of 1-$\beta$-D-arabinofuranosylcytosine and the 5′-triphosphate of 9-$\beta$-D-arabinofuranosyladenine. Cancer Res. **28**, 2061—2067 (1968).
Gee, T. S., Yu, K. P., Augustin, B. T., Krakoff, I. H., Clarkson, B. D.: Combination chemotherapy of adult leukemia with thioguanine (TG) and 1-$\beta$-D-arabinofuranosylcytosine (CA). Proc. Amer. Ass. Cancer Res. **9**, 23 (1968).
Gee, T. S., Yu, K. P., Clarkson, B. D.: Treatment of adult acute leukemia with arabinosylcytosine and thioguanine. Cancer **23**, 1019—1032 (1969).
Glynn, J. P., Fefer, A., Halpern, B. L.: Cyclophosphamide-induced chimerism. Cancer Res. **28**, 41—43 (1968).
Glynn, J. P., Halpern, B. L., Fefer, A.: An immunochemotherapeutic system for the treatment of a transplanted Moloney virus-induced lymphoma in mice. Cancer Res. **29**, 515—520 (1969).
Glynn, J. P., Kende, M.: Treatment of Moloney virus-induced leukemia with cyclophosphamide and specifically sensitized allogeneic cells. Cancer Res. **31**, 1383—1388 (1971).
Gold, G. L., Baig, M.: Chemotherapy and hormonal therapy in neoplasms of the ovary and uterus. In: Brodsky, I., Kahn, S. B., Moyer, J. H. (Eds.): Cancer chemotherapy II, pp. 125—130. New York: Grune & Stratton 1972.
Goldberg, A. I., Glynn, J. P.: Adoptive immunotherapy following chemotherapy against AKR lymphoma. Proc. Amer. Ass. Cancer Res. **13**, 56 (1972).
Goldberg, A. I., Glynn, J. P., Kende, M., Mantel, N., Goldin, A.: A two-stage therapeutic design in the spontaneous AKR lymphoma system. Cancer Res. **32**, 1321—1328 (1972).
Goldin, A., Mantel, N.: The employment of combinations of drugs in the chemotherapy of neoplasia. A review. Cancer Res. **17**, 635—645 (1957).
Goldin, A., Mantel, N., Greenhouse, S. W., Venditti, J. M., Humphreys, S. R.: Estimation of antileukemic potency of the antimetabolite aminopterin, administered alone and in combination with citrovorum factor or folic acid. Cancer Res. **13**, 843—850 (1953).
Goldin, A., Venditti, J. M.: In vivo testing of anti-tumor agents. In: Progress in antimicrobial and anticancer therapy. Proc. 6th Internat. Cong. Chemother. (Tokyo) Vol. II, pp. 864—877 (1970).
Goldin, A., Venditti, J. M., Humphreys, S. R., Dennis, D., Mantel, N., Greenhouse, S. W.: An investigation into the synergistic antileukemic action of amethopterin and 6-mercaptopurine in mice. J. nat. Cancer Inst. **16**, 129—138 (1955a).
Goldin, A., Venditti, J. M., Humphreys, S. R., Dennis, D., Mantel, N.: Studies on the management of mouse leukemia (L1210) with antagonists of folic acid. Cancer Res. **15**, 724—747 (1955b).
Goldin, A., Venditti, J. M., Humphreys, S. R., Dennis, D., Mantel, N., Greenhouse, S. W.: Factors influencing the specificity of action of an antileukemic agent (aminopterin). Multiple treatment schedules plus delayed administration of citrovorum factor. Cancer Res. **15**, 57—61 (1955c).
Goldin, A., Venditti, J. M., Humphreys, S. R., Mantel, N.: The influence of concentration of leukemic inoculum on the effectiveness of treatment. Science **123**, 840 (1955d).
Goldin, A., Venditti, J. M., Humphreys, S. R., Mantel, N.: Modification of treatment schedules in the management of advanced mouse leukemia with amethopterin. J. Nat. Cancer Inst. **17**, 203—212 (1956).
Goldin, A., Venditti, J. M., Humphreys, S. R., Shuster, L., Darrow, R. A., Mantel, N.: Advanced leukemia as a tool for chemotherapy studies. Acta Un. int. le Cancer **16**, 642—650 (1960).
Goldin, A., Venditti, J. M., Mantel, N., Kline, I., Gang, M.: Evaluation of combination chemotherapy with three drugs. Cancer Res. **28**, 950—960 (1968).
Gonick, P.: Chemotherapy of genitourinary neoplasms. In: Brodsky, I., Kahn, S. B., Moyer, J. H. (Eds.): Cancer chemotherapy II, pp. 189—194. New York: Grune & Stratton 1972.

GRISWOLD, D. P., JR., SIMPSON-HERREN, L., SCHABEL, F. M., JR.: Altered sensitivity of a hamster plasmacytoma to cytosine arabinoside (NSC-63878). Cancer Chemother. Rep. **54**, 337—346 (1970).

HALL, T. C.: Biochemical factors predicting response to chemotherapeutic agents. In: BRODSKY, I., KAHN, S. B., MOYER, J. H. (Eds.): Cancer chemotherapy II, pp. 93—101. New York: Grune & Stratton 1972.

HART, J. S., SHIRAKAWA, S., TRUJILLO, J., FREI, E., III: The mechanism of induction of complete remission in acute myeloblastic leukemia in man. Cancer Res. **29**, 2300—2307 (1969).

HENDERSON, E. S.: The treatment of acute leukemia. Semin. Hematol. **6**, 271—319 (1969).

HENDERSON, E. S., LEVENTHAL, B. G.: Immunotherapy of leukemia. In: BRODSKY, I., KAHN, S. B., MOYER, J. H. (Eds.): Cancer chemotherapy II, pp, 327—345. New York: Grune & Stratton 1972.

HENDERSON, E. S., SAMAHA, R. J.: Evidence that drugs in multiple combinations have materially advanced the treatment of human malignancies. Cancer Res. **29**, 2272—2280 (1969).

HERMAN, E. H., MHATRE, R. H., LEE, I. P., WARAVDEKAR, V. S.: Prevention of the cardiac effects of adriamycin and daunomycin in the isolated dog heart. Proc. Soc. exp. Biol. (N. Y.) **140**, 234—239 (1972).

HOFFMAN, G. S., KLINE, I., GANG, M., TYRER, D. D., GOLDIN, A., MANTEL, N., VENDITTI, J. M.: Sequential chemotherapy with cyclophosphamide (NSC-26271) and cytosine arabinoside (NSC-63878) in mice with advanced leukemia L1210. Cancer Chemother. Rep. **53**, 265—271 (1969).

HOLLAND, J. F.: Methods in cancer chemotherapy research in man. In: BUSCH, H. (Ed.): Methods in cancer research, vol. 4, pp. 255—283. New York: Academic Press 1968.

HOSHI, A., KANZAWA, F., KURETANI, K.: Enhancement of antitumor activity of cyclophosphamide with imipramine. Chem. pharm. Bull. **17**, 1694—1697 (1969).

HUMPHREYS, S. R., KARRER, K.: Relationship of dose schedules to the effectiveness of adjuvant chemotherapy. Cancer Chemother. Rep. **54**, 379—392 (1970).

JACOBS, S. P., WODINSKY, I., KENSLER, C. J., VENDITTI, J. M.: Combination therapy studies with L-asparaginase (NSC-109229) and other antitumor agents. Cancer Chemother. Rep. **54**, 329—335 (1970).

KARRER, K., HUMPHREYS, S. R.: Continuous and limited courses of cyclophosphamide (NSC-26271) in mice with pulmonary metastasis after surgery. Cancer Chemother. Rep. **51**, 439—449 (1967).

KLINE, I., GANG, M., VENDITTI, J. M.: Therapeutic value of combination therapy with cytosine arabinoside (ara-C, NSC-63878) plus 5-(3,3-dimethyl-1-triazeno)imidazole-4-carboxamide (DIC, NSC-45388) and enhancement of the combination with sequential methotrexate (MTX, NSC-740) in advanced murine leukemia L1210. Proc. Amer. Ass. Cancer Res. **12**, 21 (1971a).

KLINE, I., VENDITTI, J. M., MEAD, J. A. R., TYRER, D. D., GOLDIN, A.: The antileukemic effectiveness of 5-fluorouracil and methotrexate in the combination chemotherapy of advanced leukemia L1210 in mice. Cancer Res. **26**, 848—852 (1966a).

KLINE, I., VENDITTI, J. M., TYRER, D. D., MANTEL, N., GOLDIN, A.: Chemotherapy of leukemia L1210 in mice with 1-β-D-arabinofuranosylcytosine hydrochloride II. Effectiveness against intracerebrally and subcutaneously inoculated L1210 cells. Cancer Res. **26**, 1930—1937 (1966b).

KLINE, I., WOODMAN, R. J., GANG, M., WARAVDEKAR, V. S., GOLDIN, A., and VENDITTI, J. M.: Enhanced response of leukemic (L1210) mice to combination chemotherapy with 5-(3,3-dimethyl-1-triazeno)imidazole-4-carboxamide (NSC-45388) and 5-fluorouracil (NSC-19893). Cancer **27**, 1363—1368 (1971b).

KLINE, I., WOODMAN, R. J., VENDITTI, J. M.: Protection with N-acetylcysteine (NAC) against isophosphamide (Isoph, NSC-109724) host toxicity and enhancement of therapy in early murine leukemia L1210, Proc. Am. Ass. Cancer Res. **13**, 29 (1972).

KOECHLIN, B., ILIEV, V.: The metabolism of iproniazid. Ann. N. Y. Acad. Sci. **80**, 864—872 (1959).

KRAKOFF, I. H.: Chemotherapy and hormonal therapy of carcinoma of the breast. In: BRODSKY, I., KAHN, S. B., MOYER, J. H. (Eds.): Cancer chemotherapy II, pp. 109—116. New York: Grune & Stratton 1972.

KRAKOFF, I. H., BROWN, N. C., REICHARD, P.: Inhibition of ribonucleoside diphosphate reductase by hydroxyurea. Cancer Res. **28**, 1559—1565 (1968).

LACHER, M. J.: Chemotherapy of Hodgkin's disease. In: BRODSKY, I., KAHN, S. B., MOYER, J. H. (Eds.): Cancer chemotherapy II, pp. 417—430. New York: Grune & Stratton (1972).

LASTER, W. R., JR., MAYO, J. G., ANDREWS, C. M., SCHABEL, F. M., JR.: Lewis lung carcinoma as an experimental model for studies with anticancer drugs as surgical adjuvants. Proc. Amer. Ass. Cancer Res. **12**, 7 (1971).

LEPAGE, G. A.: Basic biochemical effects and mechanism of action of 6-thioguanine. Cancer Res. **23**, 1202—1206 (1963).

LEPAGE, G. A., KANEKO, T.: Effective means of reducing toxicity without concomitant sacrifice of efficacy of carcinostatic therapy. Cancer Res. **29**, 2314—2318 (1969).

LIVINGSTON, R. B., CARTER, S. K.: Single agents in cancer chemotherapy, p. 367. New York: IFI/Plenum 1970.

LIVINGSTON, R. B., VENDITTI, J. M., COONEY, D. A., CARTER, S. K.: Glutamine antagonists in chemotherapy. In: GARATTINI, S., GOLDIN, A., HAWKING, F., KOPIN, I. J. (Eds.): Advances in pharmacology and chemotherapy, Vol. 8, pp. 57—120. New York: Academic Press 1970.

MANDEL, H. G., RALL, D. P.: The present status of cancer chemotherapy. A summary of papers delivered at the Cherry Hill Conference on "A Critical Evaluation of Cancer Chemotherapy". Cancer Res. **29**, 2478—2485 (1969).

MANNERING, G. J.: Significance of stimulation and inhibition of drug metabolism in pharmacological testing. In: BURGER, A. (Ed.): Selective pharmacological testing methods, pp. 51—119. New York: Marcel Dekker 1968.

MANTEL, N.: An experimental design in combination chemotherapy. Ann. N. Y. Acad. Sci. **76**, 909—914 (1958).

MARSHALL, E. K., JR.: The dosage schedule of chemotherapeutic agents. Pharmacol. Rev. **4**, 85—105 (1952).

MASTRANGELO, M. J., WEISS, A. J.: Chemotherapy of neoplasms of the respiratory tract. In: BRODSKY, I., KAHN, S. B., MOYER, J. H. (Eds.): Cancer Chemotherapy II, pp. 195—208. New York: Grune & Stratton 1972.

MATHÉ, G., SCHWARZENBERG, L., SCHNEIDER, M., SCHLUMBERGER, J. R., HAYAT, M., AMIEL, J. L., CATTAN, A., JASMIN, C.: Acute lymphoblastic leukemia treated with a combination of prednisone, vincristine, and rubidomycin. Value of pathogen-free rooms. Lancet II, 380—382 (1967).

MELLETT, L. B., EL DAREER, S. M., LUCE, J. K., FREI, E., III: Activation of cyclophosphamide metabolism in various species. Pharmacologist **11**, 273 (1969a).

MELLETT, L. B., EL DAREER, S. M., RALL, D. P., ADAMSON, R. H.: Metabolism of cyclophosphamide —$C^{14}$ by various marine species. Arch. int. Pharmacodyn. **177**, 60—70 (1969b).

MHATRE, R. M., HERMAN, E. H.: Effect of ICRF-159 (NSC-129943) on the metabolic breakdown of daunomycin (NSC-82151) and adriamycin (NSC-123127) in the Syrian golden hamster. Proc. Amer. Ass. Cancer Res. **13**, 100 (1972).

MIHICH, E.: Modification of tumor regression by immunologic means. Cancer Res. **29**, 2345—2350 (1969).

PAPAC, R. J., CALABRESI, P., HOLLINGSWORTH, J. W., WELCH, A. D.: Effects of 1-β-D-arabinofuranosylcytosine hydrochloride on regenerating bone marrow. Cancer Res. **25**, 1459—1462 (1965).

PRIMACK, A.: Amelioration of cyclophosphamide induced cystitis. J. nat. Cancer Inst. **47**, 223—228 (1971).

RAUEN, H. M., KRAMER, K. P.: Der Gesamtalkylation-Blutspiegel von Ratten nach Verabreichung von Cyclophosphamid und Acyclophosphamid. Arzneimittel-Forsch. **14**, 1066—1067 (1964).

REGELSON, W.: Immunologic factors and chemotherapy. In: BRODSKY, I., KAHN, S. B., MOYER, J. H. (Eds.): Cancer chemotherapy II, pp. 69—83. New York: Grune & Stratton (1972a).

REGELSON, W.: Chemotherapy of gastrointestinal neoplasms. In: BRODSKY, I., KAHN S. B., MOYER, J. H. (Eds.): Cancer chemotherapy II, pp. 117—124. New York: Grune & Stratton 1972b.

REMMER, H.: The fate of drugs in the organism. Ann. Rev. Pharmacol. **5**, 405—428 (1965).

REMMER, H., MERKER, H. J.: Drug-induced changes in the liver and endoplasmic reticulum: association with drug metabolizing enzymes. Science **142**, 1657—1658 (1963).

RENIS, H. E., JOHNSON, H. G.: Inhibition of plaque formation of Vaccinia virus by cytosine arabinoside hydrochloride. Bact. Proc. **45**, 140 (1962).

SANDBERG, J. S., HOWSDEN, F. L., DIMARCO, A., GOLDIN, A.: Comparison of the antileukemic effect in mice of adriamycin (NSC-123127) with daunomycin (NSC-82151). Cancer Chemother. Rep. **54**, 1—7 (1970).

SARTORELLI, A. C.: Approaches to the combination chemotherapy of transplantable neoplasms. Prog. exp. Tumor Res. **6**, 228—288 (1965).

SARTORELLI, A. C.: Some approaches to the therapeutic exploitation of metabolic sites of vulnerability of neoplastic cells. Cancer Res. **29**, 2292—2299 (1969).

SARTORELLI, A. C., BOOTH, B. A., MOORE, E. C.: Studies on the site of action of pyrimidine aldehyde thiosemicarbazones. Proc. Am. Ass. Cancer Res. **10**, 76 (1969).

SARTORELLI, A. C., LEPAGE, G. A.: Modification of thioguanine toxicity in tumor bearing mice with bone marrow transplants. Proc. Amer Ass. Cancer Res. **2**, 246 (1957).

SCHABEL, F. M., JR.: In vivo leukemic cell kill kinetics and "curability" in experimental systems. In: The proliferation and spread of neoplastic cells, pp. 379—408. Baltimore: The Williams and Wilkins Co. 1968a.

SCHABEL, F. M., JR.: Improvement of therapeutic activity of antileukemic agents in experimental systems by varying dose schedules and by combination chemotherapy. In: HALL, T. C., KARRER, K. (Eds.): Pharmacological principles in antitumor chemotherapy, pp. 65—82. Vienna: Verlag der Wiener Medizinischen Akademie 1968b.

SCHABEL, F. M., JR.: The use of tumor growth kinetics in planning "curative" chemotherapy of advanced solid tumors. Cancer Res. **29**, 2384—2389 (1969).

SCHABEL, F. M., JR., JOHNSTON, T. P., MCCALEB, G. S., MONTGOMERY, J. A., LASTER, W. R., JR., SKIPPER, H. E.: Experimental evaluation of anticancer agents VIII. Effects of certain nitrosoureas on intracerebral L1210 leukemia. Cancer Res. **23**, 725—733 (1963).

SCHABEL, F. M., JR., LASTER, W. R., JR., TRADER, M. W.: Therapeutic potentiation of antileukemic drugs. Proc. Amer Ass. Cancer Res. **9**, 62 (1968).

SCHABEL, F. M., JR., LASTER, W. R., JR., TRADER, M. W.: Specific DNA inhibitors vs. leukemia L1210. Development of resistance to ara-C and ribonucleotide reductase inhibitors. Proc. Amer. Ass. Cancer Res. **12**, 67 (1971).

SCHABEL, F. M., JR., SKIPPER, H. E., TRADER, M. W., LASTER, W. R., JR., SIMPSON-HERREN, L.: Spontaneous AKR leukemia (lymphoma) as a model system. Cancer Chemother. Rep. **53**, 329—344 (1969).

SCHABEL, F. M., JR., SKIPPER, H. E., LASTER, W. R., JR., TRADER, M. W., WELLS, J. R.: Remission induction of spontaneous lymphoma in AKR mice with prednisone and vincristine. Proc. Amer. Ass. Cancer Res. **11**, 69 (1970).

SCHMIDT, L. H., MONTGOMERY, J. A., LASTER, W. R., JR., SCHABEL, F. M., JR.: Combination therapy with arabinosylcytosine and thioguanine. Proc. Amer. Ass. Cancer Res. **11**, 70 (1970).

SHNIDER, B. I.: Soft-tissue sarcomas. In: BRODSKY, I., KAHN, S. B., MOYER, J. H. (Eds.): Cancer Chemotherapy II, pp. 209—220. New York: Grune & Stratton 1972.

SHUSTER, L., JICK, H.: Turnover of microsomal protein in the livers of phenobarbital-treated mice. J. biol. Chem. **241**, 5361—5365 (1966).

SIMPSON-HERREN, L., LLOYD, H. H.: Kinetic parameters and growth curves for experimental tumor systems. Cancer Chemother. Rep. **54**, 143—174 (1970).

SKIPPER, H. E., SCHABEL, F. M., JR., WILCOX, W. S.: Experimental evaluation of potential anticancer agents XXI. Scheduling of arabinosylcytosine to take advantage of its S-phase specificity against leukemic cells. Cancer Chemother. Rep. **51**, 125—165 (1967).

SKIPPER, H. E., SCHABEL, F. M., JR., MELLETT, L. B., MONTGOMERY, J. A., WILKOFF, L. J., LLOYD, H. H., BROCKMAN, R. W.: Implications of biochemical, cytokinetic, pharmacologic, and toxicologic relationships in the design of optimal therapeutic schedules. Cancer Chemother. Rep. **54**, 431—450 (1970).

SKIPPER, H. E., SCHABEL, F. M., JR., TRADER, M. W., LASTER, W. R., JR.: Response to therapy of spontaneous, first passage, and long passage lines of AKR leukemia. Cancer Chemother. Rep. **53**, 345—366 (1969).

STOLFI, R. L., MARTIN, D. S., FUGMANN, R. A.: Spontaneous murine mammary adenocarcinoma: model system for evaluation of combined methods of therapy. Cancer Chemother. Rep. **55**, 239—251 (1971).

THOMAS, L. B., CHIRIGOS, M. A., HUMPHREYS, S. R., GOLDIN, A.: Pathology of the spread of L1210 leukemia in the central nervous system of mice and effect of treatment with cytoxan. J. nat. Cancer Inst. **28**, 1355—1389 (1962).

TYRER, D. D., KLINE, I., VENDITTI, J. M., GOLDIN, A.: Separate and sequential chemotherapy of mouse leukemia L1210 with 1-$\beta$-D-arabinofuranosylcytosine hydrochloride and 1,3-bis-(2-chloroethyl)-1-nitrosourea. Cancer Res. **27**, 873—879 (1967).

VADLAMUDI, S., GOLDIN, A.: Influence of mitotic cycle inhibitors on the antileukemic activity of cytosine arabinoside (NSC-63878) in mice bearing leukemia L1210. Cancer Chemother. Rep. **55**, 547—555 (1971).

VADLAMUDI, S., SUBBA REDDY, V. V., GOLDIN, A.: Schedule dependent therapeutic synergism for L-asparaginase and methotrexate in leukemic mice. Proc. Amer. Ass. Cancer Res. **13**, 31 (1972).

VENDITTI, J. M.: Treatment schedule dependency of experimentally active antileukemic (L1210) drugs. Cancer Chemother. Rep. (part 3) **2**, 35—59 (1971).

VENDITTI, J. M., ABBOTT, B. J., DIMARCO, A., GOLDIN, A.: Effectiveness of daunomycin (NSC-82151) against experimental tumors. Cancer Chemother. Rep. **50**, 659—665 (1966).

VENDITTI, J. M., GOLDIN, A.: Drug synergism in antineoplastic chemotherapy. In: GOLDIN, A., HAWKING, F. (Eds.): Advances in chemotherapy, Vol. 1, pp. 397—498. New York: Academic Press 1964a.
VENDITTI, J. M., GOLDIN, A.: Chemotherapy of advanced mouse leukemia L1210. Comparison of methotrexate alone and in sequential therapy. Cancer Res. **24**, 1457—1460 (1964b).
VENDITTI, J. M., GOLDIN, A., KLINE, I.: Studies on the effectiveness of 4',4''-di-2-imidazolin-2-ylterephthalanilides against mouse leukemia L1210 and resistant variants. Cancer Chemother. Rep. **19**, 5—11 (1962).
VENDITTI, J. M., HUMPHREYS, S. R., GOLDIN, A.: Investigation of the activity of Cytoxan against leukemia L1210 in mice. Cancer Res. **19**, 986—995 (1959).
VENDITTI, J. M., HUMPHREYS, S. R., MANTEL, N., GOLDIN, A.: Combined treatment of advanced leukemia (L1210) in mice with amethopterin and 6-mercaptopurine. J. nat. Cancer Inst. **17**, 631—638 (1956).
VENDITTI, J. M., HUMPHREYS, S. R., MANTEL, N., GOLDIN, A.: Influence of duration of treatment with a-methopterin on the survival time of mice with advanced leukemia L1210. Cancer Res. **17**, 917—922 (1957).
VENDITTI, J. M., KLINE, I., TYRER, D. D., GOLDIN, A.: 1,3-*Bis*(2-chloroethyl)-1-nitrosourea (NSC-409962) and methotrexate (NSC-740) as combination therapy for advanced mouse leukemia L1210. Cancer Chemother. Rep. **48**, 35—39 (1965).
WODINSKY, I., KENSLER, C. J.: Activity of selected compounds in a subline of leukemia L1210 resistant to cytosine arabinoside (NSC-63878). Cancer Chemother. Rep. **43**, 1—3 (1964).
WOODMAN, R. J., KLINE, I., VENDITTI, J. M.: Protection by (1,2-*bis*(3,5-dioxopiperazin-1-yl)-propane) (ICRF-159) against daunomycin (DAU) toxicity and enhanced antileukemic (L1210) efficacy of the combination. Proc. Amer. Ass. Cancer Res. **13**, 31 (1972).
WOODMAN, R. J., VENDITTI, J. M., SCHEPARTZ, S. A., KLINE, I.: ICRF-159 (1,2-*bis* (3,5-dioxopiperazin-1-yl)propane) (NSC-129943). Activity against intracerebrally inoculated L1210; therapeutic superiority against IP L1210 in combination with *cis*-platinum (II) diamminodichloride (*cis*-Pt-II: NSC-119875). Proc. Amer. Ass. Cancer Res. **12**, 24 (1971).

Chapter 21

# Combination Chemotherapy: Clinical Considerations

EMIL FREI, III and JEFFREY A. GOTTLIEB

## Introduction

The experimental design for the evaluation of a single agent in cancer can be complex, and the results from different centers vary considerably. The variables involved in the evaluation of combinations of agents, as compared to single agents, increase substantially. Thus, in the construction of clinical trials involving combination chemotherapy, major emphasis should be given to the problem of experimental design.

Over the past 20 years, cancer chemotherapy has moved from a largely empirical science to one involving sophisticated clinical investigation and interaction with the basic and bridging sciences. The construction of clinical trials involving combination chemotherapy is increasingly based on experimental therapeutics, molecular biological studies, pharmacologic and cytokinetic investigations, studies of drug resistance, and biologic and toxicologic evaluations. Investigations based on sound rational hypotheses with rigid experimental designs may provide important leads to the correlation of clinical and experimental toxicology and therapeutics, as well as provide information on some of the above mentioned scientific disciplines. Even if clinically negative, such studies may solve an important objective. On the other hand, empirical combinations chosen with little concern for experimental design, if negative or even if marginally positive, do not provide the building blocks for a step-wise approach to improved treatment. Accordingly, the organization of this chapter will follow the scientific lines described above.

The different effects that may occur when drugs are given in combination may be defined as follows: An *antagonistic* combination is one in which the combined effect of several drugs is less than that produced by the individual agents used alone. *Subadditive* refers to a combination in which the effect is greater than that seen for the individual agents used alone, but less than the sum of the actions of the component drugs. *Additive* indicates that the combination has activity equivalent to the sum of the agents involved, while *synergism* implies that the efficacy of the combination exceeds the sum of activity of the individual agents used alone.

## Molecular Biology

In contrast to tissue culture systems involving established cell lines and to many of the transplanted tumor systems in rodents, there is evidence for substantial biological and biochemical heterogeneity within a given human tumor. This is particularly true with solid tumors. With melanoma, for example, cytogenetic studies indicate substantial vaıying hyperdiploidy which suggests a major cytogenetic instability in the tumor with the resultant rapid development of new clones (WHANG-PENG and KNUTSEN, 1970). Similarly, the biochemical and cytokinetic variations and the degrees of drug responsiveness seen in individual clones of cells from a given solid tumor indicate substantial heterogeneity. These observations indicate that it is unlikely that a single agent would be effective against all of the neoplastic cells within such a tumor, and strongly support a multifaceted approach. While these observations are at present empirical, increasing research and information in the area of predictive systems, together with improved cloning techniques may allow for a more rational approach to combination chemotherapy. Treatment individualized for a given patient may be possible in the not too distant future.

Biochemical approaches to combination chemotherapy have classically been divided as follows (Sartorelli and Creasey, 1973):

## A. Sequential Biochemical Blockade

This approach involves the use of compounds which block enzymes on the multienzyme sequence of a biosynthetic pathway. An example of this approach is the use of a glutamine analog which interrupts glutamine-dependent purine nucleotide biosynthesis and thiopurines which inhibit biosynthesis of this pathway at the initial step and at the level of purine nucleotide interconversions. Such combinations involving, for example, azaserine and 6-mercaptopurine, are highly synergistic in experimental systems (Livingston et al., 1970). While uncontrolled clinical trials indicate promising results with this combination in several solid tumor systems, definitive controlled studies in patients with acute leukemia have failed to demonstrate a therapeutic advantage (Livingston et al., 1970).

## B. Concurrent Biochemical Blockade

This is defined as inhibition of separate biochemical pathways leading to a common and essential metabolite. Examples might include combinations of cytosine arabinoside (ara-C) or methotrexate, which primarily inhibit pyrimidine nucleotide biosynthesis, with substances which interfere with purine nucleotide biosynthesis, such as the purine analogs. Examples of such combinations include methotrexate and 6-mercaptopurine which are synergistic in experimental systems (Venditti et al., 1956), but not in man, and ara-C and 6-mercaptopurine or thioguanine which are synergistic in experimental systems (Burchenal and Dollinger, 1967). Ara-C and thioguanine are synergistic in the treatment of acute myelogenous leukemia in man (Gee et al., 1969), but it is questionable as to whether the thioguanine is acting as an inhibitor of purine nucleotide biosynthesis in this combination.

## C. Complementary Blockade

This involves combination of an agent which inhibits the biosynthetic pathway to a macromolecule with an agent that directly damages the macromolecular product of the synthetic pathway. An example would be the combination of an antimetabolite which inhibits purine or pyrimidine nucleotide biosynthesis with an alkylating agent which directly damages DNA. Since substances which interfere with DNA function are often non-cell-cycle specific, this rationale, which generally combines cell-cycle-specific and non-cell-cycle-specific substances, overlaps substantially with that of a cytokinetic approach (see below). Combinations of ara-C and alkylating agents, such as mitomycin C, the nitrosoureas, or cyclophosphamide, are highly synergistic in experimental systems (Preisler and Henderson, 1971) and there is evidence that this is true for man (see below).

There are an increasing number of approaches to combination chemotherapy based on biochemical factors. Thus, DNA repair mechanisms may determine the responsiveness of a given tissue to alkylating agents or to substrate analogs which are incorporated into DNA, such as thioguanine. Recent evidence concerning inhibition of DNA repair mechanisms by several agents (GAUDIN et al., 1971) offers an approach to combination chemotherapy and to chemotherapy combined with radiotherapy. Another aspect of this approach would be the use of drugs which produce point mutations, thus leading to error amplification (SARTORELLI and CREASEY, 1973).

## Pharmacology

This section includes the modification of the pharmacological or biological action of an active drug by another agent. An example is the use of regional methotrexate with systemic protection by citrovorum factor. Thus, in the treatment of meningeal leukemia, the tolerated single dose of methotrexate given intrathecally is 12 to 15 mg/m². However, when citrovorum factor is given concurrently by the intramuscular or intravenous route, in excess of 60 mg/m² of methotrexate can be delivered intrathecally. It has been demonstrated that this provides substantially greater concentrations of methotrexate within the spinal fluid. However, the distribution of methotrexate within the spinal fluid is not uniform, and whether methotrexate followed by citrovorum factor is superior clinically to methotrexate alone in the treatment of meningeal leukemia remains to be determined.

However, it has been demonstrated in experimental tumor systems that methotrexate, followed after a short time interval by citrovorum factor "rescue", improves the therapeutic index. This rationale is based primarily on cytokinetic factors. Studies of this combination, particularly in patients with head and neck cancer and to a lesser extent in other diseases, are being actively pursued (MITCHELL et al., 1968). At present, there is suggestive evidence that this combination is superior to methotrexate alone in patients with metastatic head and neck cancer, particularly in the avoidance of dose limiting toxicity (LEFKOWITZ et al., 1967). As with the regional approach, there is other clinical evidence that much larger doses of systemic methotrexate can be delivered if followed by citrovorum factor, as compared to methotrexate given alone (GOTTLIEB and SERPICK, 1970).

A recent ingenious variation of this approach has been applied to low growth fraction tumors, e.g. lung cancer (DJERASSI et al., 1970). Methotrexate is given in large doses over a 4 to 6 h period. This is followed by citrovorum factor rescue which is continued for 12 to 24 h. The methotrexate damage to rapidly proliferating normal cells (i.e. gastrointestinal tract and bone marrow stem cells) is largely ameliorated by providing the product of the inhibited enzyme dihydrofolate reductase, and thus the cells divide and "dilute" the methotrexate-bound dihydrofolate reductase. On the other hand, it is hypothesized that resting cells have methotrexate bound pseudoirreversably to dihydrofolate reductase, which persists until the cells enter mitosis, at which time the cells "self-destruct" because of inhibition of their folic acid system.

The pharmacology of antitumor agents can be modified in a number of ways. For example, allopurinol will decrease the degradation of 6-mercaptopurine by xanthine oxidase and thus permit utilization of smaller doses of this thiopurine (ELION et al., 1963). Substances, such as phenobarbital, which stimulate hepatic microsomal enzymes, will significantly increase the activation of cyclophosphamide (MELLETT et al., 1969). Organic acids, which displace methotrexate from protein binding sites, thereby alter the pharmacology of this agent (LIEGLER et al., 1969). While the approaches considered in this paragraph result in substantial and quantitative modification of the toxicology of these antitumor agents, there is no evidence to date that they provide a therapeutic advantage.

Another pharmacologic approach involves drug distribution. Most of the currently effective antileukemic agents do not enter the central nervous system. Accordingly, the combination of these agents with antitumor drugs that will enter this pharmacologic sanctuary provides a further pharmacologic approach to combination chemotherapy.

## Cytokinetics

Experimental and clinical cytokinetic studies are providing an increasing number of rational approaches to therapeutics. Many antitumor agents, such as ara-C, hydroxyurea, and the vinca alkaloids, affect DNA synthesis or the process of mitosis and thus affect dividing cells exclusively; that is, they are cell-cycle specific. Other drugs capable of producing cell death in resting cells are considered non-cell-cycle-specific agents, and identification of compounds of this type has recently received increasing emphasis. Important examples of non-cell-cycle-specific agents include the nitrosoureas, bleomycin, and the anthracycline derivatives daunorubicin and adriamycin. Cell-cycle- and non-cell-cycle-specific agents are frequently combined. Thus, combinations of ara-C with nitrosoureas are highly synergistic in experimental systems (Preisler and Henderson, 1971) and are probably so in man (see below). Similarly, the use of cyclophosphamide to decrease tumor size and thus increase the proportion of cells in cycle (i.e. "recruitment") followed by ara-C is a combination based on this rationale, which is highly effective in rodent tumors (Skipper et al., 1967). In experimental *in vitro* systems, and to a limited extent in *in vivo* systems, some degree of synchrony of tumor cells and of normal host cells (i.e. bone marrow and gastrointestinal tract) can be achieved by chemotherapeutic manipulations. Clinically, such approaches remain complex because of our inability to date to effectively synchronize neoplastic cells, as compared to normal rapidly proliferating host tissues.

There is evidence that the regular circadian rhythm of cytokinetic activity is less evident in tumor tissue, as compared to normal host tissues such as the bone marrow. This offers an approach which has yet to be exploited to therapeutic advantage. There is increasing emphasis on humoral cytokinetic and differentiation control mechanisms. In solid tumors particularly, substances that might selectively stimulate $G_0$-cells into cycle and thus make them sensitive to cell-cycle-specific agents have substantial potential. One approach might involve the use of a hormone for hormone-dependent tumors; such an approach has been shown in experimental systems to substantially increase the labeling index. In estrogen-dependent breast cancer for example, this rationale would presumably increase the growth fraction and thus increase responsiveness to certain antitumor agents. Clinical trials based on this rationale have not been reported.

## Drug Resistance

While many tumors show initial and very substantial responsiveness to a given agent, relapse eventually occurs in the majority of cases and is associated with drug resistance. The mechanisms for drug resistance are complex and will not be discussed here. The heterogeneity of human tumors, both cytogenetically and with respect to drug responsiveness of different clones from the same tumor, is consistent with the probability that drug resistant lines may be readily selected (Whang-Peng and Knutsen, 1970). The use of combinations of agents aimed at several critical targets should substantially reduce the rate at which resistant cells or clones develop or are selected. Such an approach might involve the concurrent administration of antitumor agents or their cyclic administration. The latter is based on the evidence that the development of drug resistance takes a minimum period of drug exposure and that alternating therapy at intervals shorter than this minimum period should not permit development of resistance to the individual agents. Since drug resistance may develop very rapidly, the superiority of combination chemotherapy in a number of diseases may relate to the decreasing development of drug resistance. Cyclic chemotherapy, particularly in acute leukemia, has been substantially studied. The experimental and theoretical basis for this approach is compelling and numerous clinical trials are based on this rationale (ZUELZER, 1964).

## Biologic Approaches

Many biologic approaches interrelate with some of the above cytokinetic approaches. In experimental systems such as the AKR lymphoma, there is evidence that viral reinduction of the tumor following cellular eradication is responsible for relapse (SKIPPER et al., 1972). This has served as a basis for combination antitumor and antiviral chemotherapy. Many of the antitumor agents are immunosuppressive, and there is increasing evidence that the schedule of drug administration may modify substantially the degree of this immunosuppression (HERSH et al., 1971). Since immunosuppression may be associated with an increased incidence of newly developing malignancies (SCHNECK and PENN, 1971), as well as infectious complications, a shortening of the period of immunosuppression is clearly of practical advantage. Finally, the combination of immunosuppressive agents with immune stimulants such as BCG (Bacillus Calmette-Guerin) has demonstrated in experimental systems that immunosuppression can, in substantial degree, be attenuated (PIESSENS et al., 1971).

## Toxicologic Approaches

The major clinical basis for combination chemotherapy has been the demonstration that agents which are active when given alone against a given disease and which have qualitatively different toxicities and mechanisms of action will result in increased activity when used in combination. This results from the fact that such agents can be used in combination at the same doses as when given alone if

Table 1. *A basis for combination chemotherapy*

| Antileukemic agent | Major toxicity |
|---|---|
| Methotrexate (MTX) | Marrow depression |
| Prednisone (Pred) | Cushing's syndrome |
| Vincristine (VCR) | Peripheral nervous system |
| 6-Mercaptopurine (6-MP) | Marrow depression |
| Cyclophosphamide (Cyclo) | Marrow depression |
| **Combinations** | **Tolerated dose in man % of a single dose** |
| MTX and 6-MP | 60 + 60 |
| Pred and 6-MP | 100 + 100 |
| VCR and Pred | 100 + 100 |
| Pred and Cyclo | 100 + 100 |
| Pred, 6-MP, MTX and VCR | 100 + 60 + 60 + 100 |

From FREI et al. (1966).

their spectrum of toxicity does not overlap. A variation in this approach may involve the use of two agents in combination, both of which affect the same normal organ but at different times. For example, ara-C produces myelosuppression with maximum depression occurring at approximately 2 to 3 weeks, whereas the nitrosoureas take 4 to 6 weeks to produce myelosuppression. Thus, these agents may be given together in combination at nearly full doses. This will result in a more prolonged myelosuppression, but not in an increase in the degree of myelosuppression at any one time. Table 1 gives examples of various drugs that have different major toxicities and thus permit combinations without overlapping toxicity. Vincristine and prednisone have little if any myelosuppressive toxicity. Thus, the dose of these two agents need not be altered when a drug with myelosuppressive dose-limiting toxicity is added. Methotrexate and 6-mercaptopurine, on the other hand, both have a pronounced effect on the bone marrow, and when used in combination require a reduction in the dosage of both agents.

## Clinical Combination Chemotherapy

The effects of various combination chemotherapeutic regimens as compared to single agent chemotherapy will be considered by disease category. An exhaustive review of all the combinations that have been studied will not be undertaken; these are given in more comprehensive reviews (Henderson, 1969; Henderson and Samaha, 1969; Nathanson et al., 1969; Carter, 1971). Our analysis will involve those studies which illustrate certain principles and progressive inprovement in combination chemotherapy programs. In order to consider combination chemotherapy, particularly of the leukemias, a definition of terms is essential.

### A. Remission Induction

This involves the treatment of a patient with clinically evident disease. During this time, bone marrow failure is also present which may complicate therapy and require substantial supportive care. The essential goal of remission induction therapy is to produce a complete remission. This involves the reduction of the number of neoplastic cells from $10^{12}$ (an order of magnitude estimate) to less than $10^{10}$ (i.e. at least a two log reduction) (Frei and Freireich, 1965).

### B. Maintained Remission

Once a patient enters complete remission his bone marrow returns to normal. The number of neoplastic cells present is usually less than $10^9$ and in general cannot be detected and quantified. It has been clearly demonstrated that treatment with agents active in remission maintenance may prolong the duration of remission.

### C. Duration of Unmaintained Remission

This is defined as the duration of remission from the end of treatment to relapse. Studies of the duration of unmaintained remission have primarily been employed to estimate the number of persisting neoplastic cells at the end of treatment. In experimental systems and probably in man, there is an inverse correlation between the number of cells persisting at the end of treatment and the duration of unmaintained remission (Frei and Freireich, 1965).

### D. Maintenance Therapy

This consists of the continued use of drug therapy during remission in an attempt to prolong the duration of remission.

### E. Reinduction during Maintenance

This refers to the use of effective short-term induction therapy such as vincristine and prednisone treatment at intervals during maintenance treatment with other agents.

## Acute Lymphocytic Leukemia of Children

The effects of active single agents used alone and in combination chemotherapy regimens for remission induction in acute lymphocytic leukemia of childhood are presented in Table 2. Single agents used alone produced remission rates varying

Table 2. *Remission induction in acute lymphocytic leukemia of childhood*

| Agent | Number of patients | Percent achieving complete remission | Ref. |
|---|---|---|---|
| MTX | 48 | 22 | FREI et al. (1961) |
| 6-MP | 43 | 27 | FREI et al. (1961) |
| Daunorubicin (DNR) | 32 | 33 | BERNARD et al. (1968) |
| VCR | 103 | 57 | KARON et al. (1966) |
| Pred | 337 | 63 | WOLFF et al. (1967) |
| MTX and 6-MP | 39 | 45 | FREI and FREIREICH (1965) |
| Pred and 6-MP | 154 | 82 | FREI et al. (1965) |
| Pred and VCR | 287 | 85 | HOLLAND and GLIDEWELL (1968) |
| POMP[a] | 35 | 94 | HENDERSON (1967) |
| Pred, VCR and DNR | 33 | 97 | BERNARD et al. (1968) |

[a] Pred, Oncovin (VCR), MTX, and Purinethol (6-MP).

from 22% for methotrexate up to 63% for prednisone. The combination of vincristine and prednisone has been most widely employed for complete remission induction in childhood acute lymphocytic leukemia. Complete remission rates in excess of 85% are regularly reported. Attempts to improve this by larger doses of prednisone, have to date not been successful (LEIKIN et al., 1968). Other combinations, including the four drug combination POMP [an acronym derived from the first letters of the four drugs in the regimen [i.e. prednisone, Oncovin (vincristine), methotrexate, and Purinethol (6-mercaptopurine)] have also produced complete remission in excess of 85% (HENDERSON, 1968). The comparative effects of different regimens when the standard is in the neighborhood of 85% is difficult to assess, since it would take a very large number of patients in a comparative study to demonstrate superiority for different combinations. The remission rates for combinations of drugs are significantly superior to those for individual agents, and in the case of vincristine and prednisone, for example, are superior to the effects of the individual agents, assuming independent drug action. Thus, for this combination, there is evidence for synergism. In the combinations indicated in Table 2, with the exception of POMP and the combination of methotrexate and 6-mercaptopurine, the agents were used at full doses. This is possible because their toxicities are independent. Thus, the rationale for combination chemotherapy in these instances is based on independent toxicology, as discussed above. It may be concluded that combination chemotherapy for children with acute lymphocytic leukemia significantly increases the complete remission rate.

## Unmaintained Remission for Acute Lymphocytic Leukemia of Childhood

As already discussed, the duration of unmaintained remission after treatment has been employed in experimental systems to measure the number of residual cells persisting at the end of treatment. Thus, particularly for combination chemotherapy, the duration of unmaintained remission measures, with many assumptions, the degree of destruction of leukemic cells produced by treatment. The duration of unmaintained remission following remission induction with vincristine or prednisone, or combinations of these two agents, is approximately 1.5 to 2 months (Table 3). Assuming a 4-day doubling time, this finding is consistant with a three-log reduction in the number of leukemic cells (i.e. $10^{12}$ to $10^{9}$). The initial combination employing more than two agents was the VAMP program (vincristine, methotrexate, mercaptopurine, and prednisone) (Freireich et al., 1968). In this instance, ten day courses of the combination were given at four to six week intervals for a total of five courses. Thus, both the intensity and the duration of chemotherapy were increased. That both factors are important in the duration of unmaintained remission is evident when the program is compared to the POMP regimen. This involves the same agents with slightly different doses and schedules (Henderson, 1968). The major difference is that POMP treatment was continued for a total of 16 months and the VAMP for a total of 7 months. The duration of subsequent unmaintained remission was 8 and 5 months, respectively. Again assuming a 4-day doubling time, one cell would have to undergo 40 doublings (i.e. approximately 5 months) for the appearance of clinically evident disease ($10^{12}$ cells). Thus, unmaintained remission durations in excess of 5 months, which have occurred for the POMP program, are consistant with experimental evidence indicating that the obstacles to cellular eradication and cure, when one approaches cellular cure, probably involve highly selected cells in term of cytokinetics, biochemistry, and perhaps anatomical sites (i.e. "pharmacological sanctuaries"). The possibility of reinduction of disease also remains. In any event, appropriate exploitation of combination chemotherapy with an increase in the length of treatment can substantially prolong the duration of unmaintained remission.

Table 3. *Unmaintained remissions in acute lymphoblastic leukemia of childhood*

| Treatment | | Median of treatment duration | Median duration of unmaintained remission | Ref. |
|---|---|---|---|---|
| Remission induction | Early remission | (months) | (months) | |
| Pred | None | 1.5 | 1.5 | Frei and Freireich (1965) |
| VCR | None | 1.5 | 2 | Frei and Freireich (1965) |
| Pred and VCR | None | 1.5 | 2 | Frei and Freireich (1965) |
| Pred and VCR | MTX → 6MP → Cyclo | 3.5 | 4 | Holland (1968) |
| Pred and VCR | MTX → 6MP → Cyclo → BCNU | 4 | 5 | Holland (1968) |
| VAMP[a] | None | 7 | 5 | Freireich et al. (1968) |
| BIKE | (MTX → 6MP → Cyclo) × 2 | 7 | 5 | Freireich et al. (1968) |
| POMP[b] | None | 16 | 8 | Henderson (1967) |
| Pred and VCR | (MTX ⇆ Pred and VCR) | 10 | 10.5 | Holland (1968) and Henderson (1968) |

[a] VCR, methotrexate, mercaptopurine (6-MP), pred.
[b] See Table 2.

Durations of maintained remissions are presented in Table 4. With vincristine and prednisone induction, methotrexate induces a median duration of maintained remission of 3 months. In experimental systems and in man the schedule of methotrexate administration markedly influences the therapeutic index. This is demonstrated in Table 4 where twice weekly methotrexate was significantly superior to daily methotrexate, and 5 day courses of methotrexate followed by twice

Table 4. *Durations of maintained remissions in acute lymphoblastic leukemia of childhood*

| Remission induction therapy | Maintenance regimen | Numbers of patients | Median duration of remission | Ref. |
|---|---|---|---|---|
| | | | (months) | |
| VCR and Pred | MTX, daily orally | 17 | 3 | SELAWRY (1965) |
| | MTX, twice weekly, orally | 22 | 10.4 | ALGB (1969) |
| | MTX, (5 day courses) × 3; then twice weekly, orally | 57 | 18.5 | HOLLAND and GLIDEWELL (1968) |
| Pred | 6-MP | 33 | 8 | FREIREICH et al. (1963) |
| 6-MP and Pred | 6-MP and MTX | 154 | 8 | FREI et al. (1963) |
| VCR and Pred | 6-MP + MTX + Cyclo + Intrathecal MTX + brain irradiation | 21 | 33 | PINKEL et al. (1971) |

weekly methotrexate produced an even greater effect, a median duration of remission of 18.5 months (HOLLAND and GLIDEWELL, 1968). This illustrates the complexities of combination chemotherapy and shows the importance of utilizing both the optimal schedule of drug administration, as well as the optimal ratio of doses in the various combinations. It is generally assumed that the optimal schedule of the agent used alone will also apply to the combination. This is a guarded assumption, however, which is under study in experimental systems. For 6-mercaptopurine maintenance, the median duration of remission is 8 months, and in contrast to methotrexate, differing dose schedules of 6-mercaptopurine have not improved the duration of remission. When methotrexate and 6-mercaptopurine were both given daily following vincristine and prednisone induction, the doses of each were of necessity lower, since they have similar myelosuppressive toxicity, and the duration of remission was not prolonged. Recently, a combination of vincristine and prednisone followed by cyclic methotrexate, 6-mercaptopurine, cyclophosphamide and prophylactic brain irradiation has been used in an intensive maintenance regimen. This combination has resulted in a median duration of remission in excess of two years with an extrapolated duration of 3 to 4 years (PINKEL et al., 1971).

## Survival and Cure

Studies involving improved remission induction and improved remission maintenance have resulted in increasing median and 5 year survivals. Some of the current studies are producing direct or extrapolated 5 year survival rates of 10% to 35% (PINKEL et al., 1971). In a retrospective study, it has been observed that patients who survived beyond 5 years have a 25 to 50% chance of remaining disease free (BURCHENAL, 1968).

## Acute Myelogenous Leukemia of Adults

The results of single agent and combination therapy in terms of complete remission induction and duration of complete remissions in acute myelogenous leukemia of adults are presented in Table 5. It should be emphasized that in all of these studies, where the duration of response is given, the patients were maintained with the same treatment program employed to induce complete remission. Comparison of the figures presented in Table 5 must be guarded, since with few exceptions these do not involve comparative studies, and certain prognostic factors, such as age, may vary among the series. It is important to note, however, that all of the agents effective in adult myelogenous leukemia are myelosuppressive.

Table 5. *Acute myelocytic leukemia of adults*

| Agent | Percent achieving complete remission | Median duration of response (months) | Ref. |
|---|---|---|---|
| Cyclo | <10 | — | Hoogstraten (1962) |
| 6-MP | 10 | 6 | Frei et al. (1961) |
| DNR | 20—50 | — | Bernard (1967); Bernard et al. (1968) |
| Cytosine arabinoside (ara-C) | 21—44 | 3-10 | Ellison et al. (1968); Henderson et al. (1968) |
| Ara-C and Cyclo | 40 | — | Bodey et al. (1968) |
| Ara-C and 6-thioguanine | 36 | 4 | Gee et al. (1969) |
| COAP[a] | 50 | 14 | Whitecar et al. (1970) |
| POMP[b] | 30—50 | 10 | Henderson and Serpick (1967); Henderson (1968) |
| Ara-C and DNR | 62 | — | Crowther et al. (1970) |

[a] Cyclo, Oncovin (VCR), ara-C, pred.
[b] See Table 2.

Vincristine and prednisone are marginally effective in adults with acute myelogenous leukemia, although they are effective in acute myelogenous leukemia in children. Thus, the rationale of most of the chemotherapy combinations in adults with acute myelogenous leukemia, in contrast to those employed in acute lymphocytic leukemia, do not involve independent toxicity. The response rate for single agents varies from less than 10% for cyclophosphamide to as much as 50% for daunorubicin. Ranges are given for certain other drugs, since drug schedule manipulation and certain tactical maneuvers, as well as the intensity of supportive care, may influence the complete remission rate achieved. There is evidence both in experimental systems and in man, that cytosine arabinoside given in courses of twice the generation time of the leukemic cells, with interruption between courses to allow for host recovery, is superior to daily or other schedules of administration of this drug (Skipper et al., 1967). This finding is evident in man in that 5-day courses of cytosine arabinoside given every 2 to 3 weeks produce a 30 to 40% complete remission rate, as compared to a 15 to 25% complete remission rate for cytosine arabinoside given daily (Bodey et al., 1970).

The rationale for the combination of cytosine arabinoside with an alkylating agent has already been presented. In summary, this regimen constitutes complementary biochemical blockade (i.e., interruption of DNA synthesis and direct damage to DNA, respectively) along with cytokinetic rationale involving the use of a cell-cycle-specific drug plus a non-cell-cycle-specific agent. The combination of cytosine arabinoside and cyclophosphamide produced a 40% complete remission rate in a small number of patients (Bodey et al., 1970). When vincristine and prednisone were added to this combination (i.e. the COAP program – cyclophosphamide, Oncovin[R], arabinosyl cytosine, and prednisone), a 50% complete remission rate was achieved (Whitecar et al., 1970). In a direct comparison of 5 day courses of cytosine arabinoside versus the COAP program, the latter was superior in terms of both the complete remission rate and the duration of maintained remission (Bodey and Freireich, 1972).

In experimental systems, it has been demonstrated that ara-C and thiopurines are synergistic (Burchenal and Dollinger, 1967). Ara-C and thioguanine have been shown to produce complete remission in 36% of adults with acute myelogenous leukemia (Gee et al., 1969). The remissions tend to be of relatively short duration. The basis for the superiority of this combination over other treatment regimens remains to be determined. The antitumor effect of thioguanine may be dependent upon its incorporation into DNA (LePage and Jones, 1961). In comparative studies the mixture of ara-C and thioguanine has proven to be superior to ara-C plus 6-mercaptopurine in remission induction in adults with acute myelogenous leukemia (acute leukemia group B, 1970). In experimental toxicological studies, ara-C, by inhibiting DNA synthesis, allows the tolerance of larger doses of thioguanine by the host, as compared to thioguanine given alone (LePage, 1972). This appears to be consistent with an ara-C induced inhibition of DNA synthesis, which produces a decreased uptake of thioguanine into the DNA of susceptible host tissues. How this applies to the antileukemic effects remains to be determined. It is postulated that ara-C decreases thioguanine uptake into DNA to a greater extent in normal stem cells, as compared to leukemic cells.

A generality that pertains to most combination chemotherapy in man is that the best combinations are likely to involve drugs which have potent activity when used alone. The best agents used alone for adults with acute myelogenous leukemia are ara-C and daunorubicin (Table 5). The combination of these two agents has produced a 62% complete remission rate (Crowther et al., 1970). In contrast to acute lymphocytic leukemia, where drug combinations are often additive and perhaps synergistic, the combination of cytosine arabinoside and daunorubicin would appear to be subadditive. This is again probably because the agents were not used at full doses, since dose limiting toxicity for each involves myelosuppression. Daunorubicin is effective against nonproliferating cells and damages the formation of DNA, as well as DNA-dependent RNA biosynthesis (Calendi et al., 1965). Thus, on a biochemical basis, the above combination may well produce complementary blockade.

## Hodgkin's Disease

As in acute leukemia of children, there are now some 8 agents capable of producing complete remissions in patients with Hodgkin's disease (Ultmann and Nixon, 1969). For several of these (e.g. prednisone, vincristine, and bleomycin), myelosuppression is not dose limiting. Thus, this disease presents a major opportunity for combination chemotherapy based on independent toxicity. The complete response rate for single agents used alone varies from 10 to 30% (Table 6). For the 3-drug combination of cyclophosphamide, Oncovin[R], and prednisone (COP), a 36% complete remission rate was achieved (Luce et al., 1971), and with the 4-drug combination, [the MOPP program – Mustargen (nitrogen mustard), Oncovin[R], procarbazine, and prednisone] complete remission rates of 70 to 80% have been attained (DeVita et al., 1970; Frei, 1972). All of the data given in Table 6

Table 6. *Combination chemotherapy of Hodgkin's disease*

| Agent | Percent achieving complete remission | Median duration of response (months) maintained | unmaintained | Ref. |
|---|---|---|---|---|
| Pred | <10 | <6 | — | Ezdinli et al. (1969) |
| Nitrogen mustard | <10 | 8 | 3 | Jacobs et al. (1968)<br>Scott (1963)<br>Spear and Patno (1962) |
| Cyclo | 11 | 4.5 | 3 | Livingston and Carter (1972) |
| VCR | 13 | — | — | Bohannon et al. (1963) |
| Procarbazine | 18 | 3 | — | DeConti (1971) · |
| Cyclo, VCR, pred | 36 | 11 | 5 | Luce et al. (1971) |
| MOPP[a] | 81 | — | 48 | DeVita et al. (1970) |
| MOPP | 72 | 60[b] | 23 | Frei (1972) |

[a] Mustargen (nitrogen mustard), Oncovin (VCR), procarbazine, pred.
[b] Extrapolated figure.

relates to patients with Stages III B and IV Hodgkin's disease. Thus, within a short span of time (i.e. 5 years), a major saltation in the complete remission rate has been achieved. Single agent remission induction with cyclophosphamide or vinblastine results in short durations of unmaintained remission (median: 2 to 3 months) (Ezdinli and Stutzman, 1968). In contrast, combination chemotherapy, and particularly the MOPP program, has produced median durations of unmaintained remission in a multi-institute study of 2 years (Frei, 1972), and in the study of the National Cancer Institute of 4 years (DeVita et al., 1970). Following radiotherapy, it is considered that patients who remain relapse-free for 3 to 4 years have an 80 to 90% chance of being cured (Kaplan, 1966). The 2 to 4 year median duration of unmaintained remission for patients with advanced Hodgkin's disease achieved with chemotherapy is therefore most impressive. Again, for continued treatment during remission (i.e. maintained remission), the duration of remission is longer. This pertains to single agents and is also true for the MOPP program. Thus, in a multi-institute study, with patients in which remission was induced by MOPP, a random half were maintained with courses of MOPP every 2 months for a total of 24 months of treatment, and the other half were unmaintained following the 6 month induction course. The duration of complete remission was significantly longer in the maintained group with an extrapolated median duration of 5 years (Frei, 1972).

## Non-Hodgkin's Lymphoma

As in Hodgkin's disease, single agents have produced complete remission rates in the range of 10 to 20% (Ultmann and Nixon, 1969; Livingston and Carter, 1970). Combinations of vincristine, prednisone, and cyclophosphamide have produced complete remission rates in the range of 40 to 50% and have improved to some extent the duration of unmaintained and maintained remissions (Luce et al., 1971). The improvement with combination chemotherapy has been significant, but the saltatory step seen in Hodgkin's disease has not yet been achieved.

## Multiple Myeloma

In contrast to most of the hematologic malignancies, multiple myeloma in relapse is a "slow growing," so called low growth fraction tumor. It has generally been felt that since most cancer chemotherapeutic approaches probably exploit qualitative differences between tumor cells and normal host organs, faster growing tumors would be more susceptible to chemotherapy. Multiple myeloma is a notable exception to this generality. The first agent clearly effective in multiple myeloma was phenylalanine mustard (melphalan). As with other systems it was demonstrated that the schedule of drug administration significantly influenced response. Thus, the objective response for melphalan given in 4 day courses every 6 weeks is 35% as compared to 19% with melphalan given daily (ALEXANIAN et al., 1969). While corticosteroids are marginally active when used alone in the treatment of multiple myeloma (MASS, 1962), it has been observed that corticosteroids added to melphalan significantly increase the initial response rates to approximately 70 % (ALEXANIAN et al., 1969). Recent cytokinetic studies indicate that this combination produces approximately a 3-log reduction in the number of myeloma cells (i.e. $10^{12}$ down to $10^{9}$), and no further reduction occurs in spite of the continuing melphalan therapy (SALMON and SMITH, 1970). Nevertheless, melphalan produces subjective and objective improvement, particularly when employed in the proper schedule and combined with prednisone, in the majority of patients and has increased median survival from 9 months to approximately 2 years (ALEXANIAN et al., 1969). Recent evidence suggests that during remission the cytokinetic behavior of the myeloma cells changes substantially. This evidence is primarily in the form of a substantially increased labeling index suggesting a larger growth fraction (SALMON, 1972). Thus, the use of cell-cycle-specific agents such as ara-C and vincristine and others which have been notably ineffective in the treatment of overt myeloma (i.e. $10^{12}$) may prove effective in treatment during remission. Such studies are underway (ALEXANIAN, 1972).

## Solid Tumors

### A. Introduction

Chemotherapy, including combination chemotherapy, has not been as effective in the treatment of solid tumors as it has been in the hematologic malignancies. There are a number of reasons for the relative lack of efficacy of drug combinations. First, there are relatively few solid tumors in which complete remissions with single agents occur with any frequency. In the hematologic malignancies, on the other hand, where complete remissions are not so rare, it has only been through the combination of agents capable of producing complete remissions individually that an additive or synergistic effect has been demonstrated. Secondly, there are relatively few solid tumors in which more than one or 2 agents have significant efficacy. It has generally been true that the addition of an inactive agent to an active agent has not increased the effect of the latter. The third problem in solid tumor combination chemotherapy studies is the relative lack of ability to quantitate the amount of disease as compared to the leukemias. Differences and difficulties in establishing criteria for response and a relative lack of control of dosing and scheduling in the different studies are further problems in this field. Most of the above features are involved in explaining the variation in response of a given disease reported for single agent treatment from different centers. An example of this is shown in Table 7 with respect to the effect of 5-fluorouracil in colorectal cancer. Again, it must be emphasized that these tumors are often difficult to measure, that complete responses rarely occur, and that the extent of disease, the duration of disease, and prior treatment are variables that differ substantially among the different studies.

Table 7. *Response rate in colorectal carcinoma with 5-fluorouracil*

| Ref. | Number of patients | Percent achieving objective response |
|---|---|---|
| Sharp and Benefiel (1962) | 13 | 85 |
| Rochlin et al. (1962) | 47 | 55 |
| Allaire et al. (1961) | 17 | 47 |
| Field (1963) | 37 | 41 |
| Weiss and Jackson (1961) | 37 | 35 |
| Hurley (1964) | 150 | 31 |
| Eastern Coop. Group (1967) | 48 | 27 |
| Brennan et al. (1964) | 183 | 23 |
| Ansfield (1963) | 141 | 17 |
| Moertel et al. (1969) | 144 | 15 |
| Ellison (1962) | 87 | 12 |
| Kennedy (1964) | 22 | 9 |

As in acute leukemia, some definitions are again obligatory. An *objective response* is usually defined as a 50% or greater decrease in the total area of measurable disease. A *complete response* denotes the complete disappearance of all disease, as well as symptoms referrable to the tumor.

## B. Breast Cancer

The tumor which has received major attention with respect to combination chemotherapy in recent years has been metastatic breast cancer. This disease shares with the hematologic malignancies the fact that there are a number of agents capable of producing tumor regression. However, unlike the hematologic malignancies, such regressions are relatively infrequent and rarely complete.

5-Fluorouracil has been effective in producing an objective response rate of approximately 30% in metastatic breast carcinoma. For cyclophosphamide, a similar rate has been reported, while for methotrexate the rate is approximately 20%; for vincristine and vinblastine it is also approximately 20% (Livingston and Carter, 1970). New agents such as adriamycin and the nitrosoureas also have activity in breast cancer (Middleman et al., 1970; Bonnet and Brownlee, 1971). In addition, hormonal agents such as the androgens, estrogens and corticosteroids have effectiveness varying up to 30% depending upon the age of the patient and other variables (Kennedy, 1970). Because of these factors, various combinations have been employed in patients with breast cancer. A 5-drug regimen involving vincristine, methotrexate, 5-fluorouracil, cyclophosphamide, and prednisone was initially introduced by Cooper (1969). This regimen and modifications thereof have subsequently been studied by a number of groups. This combination involves 2 agents which are nonmyelosuppressive (i.e. vincristine and prednisone), 2 cell-cycle-specific agents (i.e. 5-fluorouracil and methotrexate), as well as a non-cell-cycle specific agent (i.e. cyclophosphamide); all of the agents, as indicated above, have some effectiveness when used alone in breast cancer. In several studies, partial response rates of 50 to 70% have been reported with complete responses in the range of 10 to 20% (Ansfield et al., 1971). The duration of response has also varied substantially. In the initial study, a median duration of complete response was reported to be 12 months (COOPER, 1969), while in subsequent studies, with possibly a different patient population, complete remission durations ranging from 4 to 12 months with the median in the range of 6 months have been reported (ANSFIELD et al., 1971). Ongoing studies are currently comparing the use of intermittent combinations with continuous chemotherapy; some investigations employ androgens and estrogens as well. As with other combination chemotherapy studies, the possibility remains that the initial higher objective response rate may be offset by more effective sequential use of the same agents.

### C. Other Solid Tumors

Other solid tumors in which combination chemotherapy has been suggestively superior to single agent treatment include neuroblastoma and testicular tumors. In neuroblastoma, there is suggestive but not conclusive evidence that vincristine and cyclophosphamide given either concurrently or sequentially are superior to either agent alone (PINKEL et al., 1968). In testicular neoplasms, actinomycin D has demonstrated some degree of activity (MACKENZIE, 1966). Combinations employing actinomycin D together with other drugs, particularly an alkylating agent and methotrexate have also been studied (LI et al.,1960). It remains questionable as to whether this combination is more effective than actinomycin D alone (MACKENZIE, 1966).

There have been a number of studies of combination chemotherapy in a broad spectrum of solid tumors. One such regimen is the COMF program, which includes cyclophosphamide, Oncovin, methotrexate and 5-fluorouracil. In several large studies, response rates approaching 30% (mainly partial responses) have been achieved (COSTANZI and COLTMAN, 1969; COLTMAN et al., 1971). While this would appear promising, the range of response rates for the single agents, such as 5-fluorouracil varies up to and beyond 30% (see Table 7), so that the question of whether the combination is superior remains unanswered.

## Conclusions

It may be concluded that combination chemotherapy has resulted in marked improvement in the therapy of some of the hematologic malignancies. Drug mixtures are producing long-term, tumor-free survival rates in childhood acute lymphocytic leukemia and disseminated Hodgkin's disease. For most of the hematologic malignancies, there are a number of agents that are individually active, some of which have independent toxicity and thus can be combined at full doses. These two assets do not apply to most of the solid tumors. This difference is, at least in part, the reason for the much less impressive effects of combination chemotherapy in solid tumors. As indicated in the above discussion of the rationale for the approach to combination chemotherapy, the heterogeneity of tumor cells within a given tumor in a given patient is such as to make a very strong theoretical case for combination chemotherapy. The same is true for the problem of the development of resistance. The ever increasing extension of molecular, pharmacologic, cytokinetic, drug-resistance, and biologic data, along with the discovery of new agents, will supply an increasing number of hypotheses and approaches for combination chemotherapy. With this background and with the increasing application of better experimental designs and techniques for the evaluation of therapeutic effects, a number of studies with increasing efficacy may be anticipated for the combination chemotherapy of cancer.

## References


Acute Leukemia Group B: Acute lymphocytic leukemia in children. Maintenance therapy with methotrexate administered intermittently. J. Amer. med. Ass. 207, 923—928 (1969).

Acute Leukemia Group B: Unpublished data (1970).

Alexanian, R.: Unpublished data of the Southwest Cancer Chemotherapy Study Group (1972).

Alexanian, R., Hart, A., Khan, A. U., Lane, M., McKelvey, E. M., Migliore, P. J., Stuckey, W. J. Jr., Wilson, H. E.: Treatment for multiple myeloma; combination chemotherapy with different melphalan dose regimens. J. Amer. med. Ass. 208, 1680—1685 (1969).

Allaire, F. J., Thieme, E. T., Korst, D. R.: Cancer chemotherapy with 5-fluorouracil alone and in combination with X-ray therapy. Cancer Chemother. Rep. 14, 59—75 (1961).

Ansfield, F. J.: Further clinical comparison between 5-fluoro-2'-deoxyuridine (5-FUDR) and 5-fluorouracil (5-FU). Proc. Amer. Ass. Cancer Res. 4, 2 (1963).

Ansfield, F. J., Ramirez, G., Korbitz, B. C., Daus, H. L., Jr.: Five drug therapy for advanced cancer: a phase I study. Cancer Chemother. Rep. 55, 183—188 (1971).

Bernard, J.: Acute leukemia treatment. Cancer Res. 27, 2565—2569 (1967).

Bernard, J., Boiron, M., Jacquillat, E., Weill, M.: Rubidomycin: 400 patients with leukemia and other malignancies. Abstracts of the XII Congress of the Int. Society of Hemat., p. 5 (1968).

Bodey, G. P., Freireich, E. J.: Unpublished data of Southwestern Cancer Chemotherapy Study Group (1972).

Bodey, G. P., Luce, J. K., Harris, J. E., Frei, E., III: The effect of cytosine arabinoside on metastatic cancer and acute leukemia, p. 6. Abstracts of XII Congress, Inst. Soc. Hemat. (1968).

Bodey, G. P., Rodriguez, V., Whitecar, J. P., Hart, J., Freireich, E. J.: The treatment of acute leukemia in adults. In: Leukemia-Lymphoma, a collection of papers presented at the 14th annual clinical conference at M. D. Anderson Hospital and Tumor Institute pp. 333—346. Chicago: Yearbook Medical Publishers, Inc. 1970.

Bohannon, R. A., Miller, D. G., Diamond, H.: Vincristine in the treatment of lymphomas and leukemias. Cancer Res. 23, 613—621 (1963).

Bonnet, J. D., Brownlee, R. W.: Unpublished data of the Southwest Cancer Chemotherapy Study Group (1971).

Brennan, M. J., Talley, R. W., Sandiego, E. L., Burrows, J. H., O'Brien, R. M., Vaitkevicius, V. M., Horeyland, S.: Critical analysis of 594 cancer patients treated with 5-fluorouracil. In: Plattner, P. A. (Ed.): Proceedings of the international symposium of chemotherapy of cancer, pp. 148—150. New York: American Elsevier 1964.

Burchenal, J. H.: Long term survivors in acute leukemia. In: Zarafonetis, C. J. D. (Ed.): Proceedings of the international conference on leukemia-lymphoma, pp. 469—474. Philadelphia: Lea Febiger 1968.

Burchenal, J. H., Dollinger, M. R.: Cytosine arabinoside (NSC-63878) in combination with 6-mercaptopurine (NSC-755), methotrexate (NSC-740) or fluorouracil (NSC-19893) in L1210 mouse leukemia. Cancer Chemother. Rep. 51, 435—438 (1967).

Calendi, E., DiMarco, A., Reggiani, M., Scarpinato, B., Valentini, L.: On physico-chemical interactions between daunomycin and nucleic acids. Biochim. biophys. Acta (Amst.) 103, 25—49 (1965).

Carter, S.: Clinical trials and combination chemotherapy. Cancer Chemother. Rep. 2, 81—97 (1971).

Coltman, C. A., Costanzi, J. J., Dudley, G. M., III., Haut, A., Lane, M., Gehan, E. A.: Further clinical studies of combination chemotherapy using cyclophosphamide, vincristine, methotrexate, and 5-fluorouracil. Amer. J. med. Sci. 261, 73—78 (1971).

Cooper, R. G.: Combination chemotherapy in hormone resistant breast cancer. Proc. Amer. Ass. Cancer Res. 10, 15 (1969).

Costanzi, J. J., Coltman, C. A.: Combination chemotherapy using cyclophosphamide, vincristine, methotrexate, and 5-fluorouracil. Cancer 23, 589—596 (1969).

Crowther, D., Bateman, C. J. T., Vartan, C. P., Whitehouse, J. M. A., Malpas, J. S., Fairley, G. H., Scott, R. B.: Combination chemotherapy using L-asparaginase, daunorubicin, and cytosine arabinoside in adults with acute myelogenous leukemia. Brit. med. J. 4, 513—517 (1970).

DeConti, R. C.: Procarbazine in the management of late Hodgkin's disease. J. Amer. med. Ass. 215, 927—930 (1971).

DeVita, V. T., Serpick, A. A., Carbone, P. P.: Combination chemotherapy in the treatment of advanced Hodgkin's disease. Ann. intern. Med. 73, 881—895 (1970).

Djerassi, I., Rominger, C. J., Kim, J., Turcui, J., Meyer, E.: Methotrexate — citrovorum in patients with lung cancer. Proc. Amer. Ass. Cancer Res. 11, 21 (1970).

Eastern Cooperative Group in Solid Tumor Chemotherapy: Comparison of antimetabolites in the treatment of breast and colon cancer. J. Amer. med. Ass. **200**, 770—778 (1967).

ELION, G. B., CALLAHAN, S. N., NATHAN, H., BIEBER, S., RUNDLES, R. W., HITCHINGS, G. M.: Potentiation of inhibition of drug degradation: 6-substituted purines and xanthine oxidase. Biochem. Pharmacol. **12**, 85—93 (1963).

ELLISON, R. R.: Experience with fluorinated pyrimidines in adenocarcinoma of the lower intestinal tract. N. Y. J. Med. **62**, 2364—2369 (1962).

ELLISON, R. R., HOLLAND, J. F., WEIL, M., JACQUILLAT, C., BOIRON, M., BERNARD, J., SAWITSKY, A., ROSNER, F., GUSSOTT, B., SILVER, R. T., KARAMAS, A., CUTTNER, J., SPURR, C. L., HAYES, D. M., BLOM, J., LEONE, L. A., MAURANI, F., KYLE, R., HUTCHISON, J. L., FORCIER, R. J., MOON, J. N.: Arabinosyl cytosine: a useful agent in the treatment of acute leukemia in adults. Blood **32**, 507—523 (1968).

EZDINLI, E. Z., STUTZMAN, L.: Vinblastine vs. nitrogen mustard therapy of Hodgkin's disease. Cancer **22**, 473—479 (1968).

EZDINLI, E. Z., STUTZMAN, L., AUNGST, C. W., FIRAT, D.: Corticosteroid therapy for lymphomas and chronic lymphocytic leukemia. Cancer **23**, 900—909 (1969).

FIELD, J. B.: 5-Fluorouracil (NCS 9803) treatment of advanced cancer in ambulatory patients. Cancer Chemother. Rep. **33**, 45—49 (1963).

FREI, E., III.: Southwestern Chemotherapy Study Group data; manuscript in preparation, 1972.

FREI, E., III., DEVITA, V. T., MOXLEY, J. N., CARBONE, P. P.: Approaches to improving the chemotherapy of Hodgkin's disease. Cancer Res. **26**, 1284—1289 (1966).

FREI, E., III., FREIREICH, E. J.: Progress and perspectives in the chemotherapy of acute leukemias. Advanc. Chemother. **2**, 269—298 (1965).

FREI, E., III., FREIREICH, E. J., GEHAN, E., PINLEY, D., HOLLAND, J. F., SELAWRY, O., HAURAMI, F., SPURR, C. L., HAYES, D. M., JONES, G. W., ROTHBERG, H., SODEE, D. B., RUNTLES, R. W., SHROEDER, L. R., KOOGSTRATEN, B., WOLMAN, I. J., TRAGGIS, D. G., COOPER, T., GERDEL, B. R., EBAUGH, F., TAYLOR, R.: Studies of sequential and combination antimetabolite therapy in acute leukemia: 6-mercaptopurine and methotrexate, from the acute leukemia Group B. Blood **18**, 431—454 (1961).

FREI, E., III., KARON, M., LEVIN, R. M., FREIREICH, E. J., TAYLOR, R. J., MANANIAN, J., SELAWRY, O., HOLLAND, J. F., NOOGSTRATEN, B., WOLMAN, I. J., ABIR, E., SAWITSKY, A., LEE, S., MILLS, S. D., BURGERT, E. O., JR., SPURR, C. L., PATTERSON, R. B., EBAUGH, F. G., JAMES, G. W., III., MOON, J. N.: The effectiveness of combinations of antileukemic agents in inducing and maintaining remission in children with acute leukemia. Blood **26**, 642—656 (1965).

FREIREICH, E. J., GEHAN, E., FREI, E., III., SCHROEDER, L. R., WOLMAN, I. J., ANBORI, R., BURGERT, E. O., MILLS, S. D., PINKEL, D., SELAWRY, O. S., MOON, J. N., GENDEL, B. R., SPURR, G. L., STORRS, R., MAURANI, F., NOOGSTRATEN, B., LEE, S.: The effect of 6-mercaptopurine on the duration of steroid-induced remission in acute leukemia: A model for evaluation of other potentially useful therapy. Blood **21**, 699—716 (1963).

FREIREICH, E. J., HENDERSON, E. S., KARON, M. R., FREI, E., III.: The treatment of acute leukemia considered with respect to cell population kinetics. In: The proliferation and spread of neoplastic cells, pp. 441—452. Baltimore: Williams and Wilkins 1968.

GAUDIN, D., YIELDING, K. L., STABLER, A., BROWN, J.: The effect of DNA repair inhibitors on the response of tumors treated with x-ray and alkylating agents. Proc. Soc. exp. Biol. (N. Y.) **137**, 202—206 (1971).

GEE, T. S., YU, K. P., CLARKSON, B. D.: Treatment of adult acute leukemia with arabinosyl cytosine and thioguanine. Cancer **23**, 1019—1032 (1969).

GOTTLIEB, J. A., SERPICK, A. A.: Prolonged intravenous methotrexate therapy in the treatment of acute leukemia and solid tumors. Cancer Res. **30**, 2132—2138 (1970).

HENDERSON, E. S.: Combination chemotherapy of acute lymphocytic leukemia of childhood. Cancer Res. **27**, 2570—2572 (1967).

HENDERSON, E. S.: Treatment of acute leukemia. Ann. intern. Med. **69**, 628—629 (1968).

HENDERSON, E. S.: Treatment of acute leukemia. Semin. Hemat. **6**, 271—319 (1969).

HENDERSON, E. S., SAMAHA, R. J.: Evidence that drugs in multiple combinations have materially advanced the treatment of human malignancies. Cancer Res. **29**, 2272—2280 (1969).

HENDERSON, E. S., SERPICK, A. A.: The effect of combination drug therapy and prophylactic oral antibiotic treatment in adult acute leukemia. Clin. Res. **15**, 336 (1967).

HENDERSON, E. S., SERPICK, A. A., LEVENTHAL, B. G., HENRY, P.: Cytosine arabinoside infusions in adult and childhood acute myelocytic leukemia. Proc. Amer. Ass. Cancer Res. **9**, 29 (1968).

HERSH, E. M., WHITECAR, J. P., JR., MCCREDIE, K. B., BODEY, G. P., FREIREICH, E. J.: Chemotherapy, immunocompetence, immunosuppression and prognosis in acute leukemia. N. Engl. J. Med. **285**, 1211—1216 (1971).

Holland, J. F.: Clinical studies of unmaintained remission in acute lymphocytic leukemia. In: The proliferation and spread of neoplastic cells, pp. 453—462. Baltimore: Williams & Wilkins 1968.

Holland, J. F., Glidewell, O.: Induction, consolidation, intensification, reinduction and maintenance chemotherapy of acute lymphocytic leukemia. Abstracts of the XII Congress, Int. Soc. Hemat., p. 9. 1968.

Hoogstraten, B.: Cyclophosphamide in acute leukemia. Cancer chemother. Rep. 16, 167—171 (1962).

Hurley, J. D.: Treatment of advanced cancer with 5-fluorouracil. Acta Un. int. Cancer. 20, 363—365 (1964).

Jacobs, E. M., Peters, F. C., Luce, J. K., Zippin, C., Wood, D. A.: Mechlorethamine HCl and cyclophosphamide in the treatment of Hodgkin's disease and the lymphomas. J. Amer. med. Ass. 203, 392—398 (1968).

Kaplan, H. S.: Long-term results of palliative and radical radiotherapy of Hodgkin's disease. Cancer Res. 26, 1250—1252 (1966).

Karon, M., Freireich, E. J., Frei, E., III., Taylor, R., Wolman, I. J., Djerassi, I., Lee, S. L., Sawitsky, A., Hananian, J., Selawry, O., James, D., Jr., George, P., Patterson, R. B., Burgert, I., Haurani, F. I., Oberfield, R. A., Macy, C. T., Hoogstraten, B., Blom, T.: The role of vincristine in the treatment of childhood acute leukemia. Clin. Pharmacol. Ther. 7, 332—339 (1966).

Kennedy, B. J.: Chemotherapy of colon cancer. Lancet 84, 131—133 (1964).

Kennedy, B. J.: Hormonal therapies in breast cancer: Androgens versus estrogens. In: Breast cancer early and late, pp. 381—386. Chicago: Yearbook Medical Publishers 1970.

Lefkowitz, E., Papac, R. J., Bertino, J. R.: Head and neck cancer. III. Toxicity of 24-hour infusions of methotrexate (NSC 740) and protection by leucovorin (NSC 3590) in patients with epidermoid carcinomas. Cancer Chemother. Rep. 51, 305—311 (1967).

Leikin, J. L., Brubaker, C., Hartmann, J. R., Murphy, M. L., Wolff, J. A., Perrin, E.: Varying prednisone dosage in remission induction of previously untreated childhood leukemia. Cancer 21, 346—351 (1968).

LePage, G. A.: Unpublished data (1972).

LePage, G. A., Jones, M.: Further studies on mechanism of action of 6-thioguanine. Cancer Res. 21, 1590—1594 (1961).

Li, M. D., Whitmore, W. F., Jr., Golbey, R., Gragstald, M.: Effects of combined drug therapy on metastatic cancer of the testis. J. Amer. med. Ass. 174, 1291—1301 (1960).

Liegler, D. G., Henderson, E. S., Hahn, M. A., Oliverio, V. T.: The effect of organic acids on renal clearance of methotrexate in man. Clin. Pharmacol. Ther. 10, 849—857 (1969).

Livingston, R., Carter, S.: Single agents in cancer chemotherapy. New York: Plenum 1970.

Livingston, R. B., Venditti, J. M., Cooney, D. A., Carter, S. K.: Glutamine antagonists in chemotherapy. Advanc. Pharmacol. Chemother. 8, 57—120 (1970).

Luce, J. K., Gamble, J. F., Wilson, N. E., Monto, R. W., Isaacs, B. L., Palmer, R. L., Coltman, C. A., Jr., Hewlett, J. S., Gehan, E. A., Frei, E., III.: Combined cyclophosphamide, vincristine and prednisone therapy of malignant lymphoma. Cancer 28, 306—317 (1971).

MacKenzie, A. R.: Chemotherapy of metastatic testis cancer. Results in 154 patients. Cancer 19, 1369—1376 (1966).

Mass, R. E.: A comparison of the effect of prednisone and a placebo in the treatment of multiple myeloma. Cancer Chemother. Rep. 16, 257—259 (1962).

Mellett, L. B., El Da Reer, S. M., Luce, J. K., Frei, E., III.: Activation of cyclophosphamide in various species. Pharmacologist 11, 273 (1969).

Middleman, E., Luce, J. K., Frei, E., III.: Clinical trials with adriamycin. Cancer 28, 844—850 (1971).

Mitchell, M. S., Wawro, N. W., DeConti, R. C., Kaplan, S. R., Papac, R., Bertino, J. R.: Effectiveness of high dose infusions of methotrexate followed by leucovorin in carcinoma of the head and neck. Cancer Res. 28, 1088—1094 (1968).

Moertel, C. G., Reitemeier, R. J., Kahn, R. G.: Therapy with the fluorinated pyrimidines. In: Moertel, C. G., Reitemeier, R. J. (Eds.): Advanced gastrointestinal cancer. Clinical management and chemotherapy, pp. 86—107. New York: Harper & Row 1969.

Nathanson, L., Hall, T. C., Schilling, A., Miller, S.: Concurrent combination chemotherapy of human solid tumors: experience with a three-drug regimen and review of the literature. Cancer Res. 29, 419—425 (1969).

Piessens, W. F., Keimann, R., Legrus, N., Keuson, J. C.: Effect of BCG on mammary tumor formulation and cellular immunity in DMBA-treated rats. Cancer Res. 31, 1061—1065 (1971).

Pinkel, D., Hernandez, K., Borella, L., Holton, C., Aur, R., Samoy, G., Pratt, C.: Drug dosage and remission duration in childhood lymphocytic leukemia. Cancer 27, 247—256 (1971).

PINKEL, D., PRATT, C., HOLTON, C., JAMES, D., JR., WRENN, E., JR., HUSTU, H. O.: Survival of children with neuroblastoma treated with combination chemotherapy. J. Pediat. **73**, 928—931 (1968).

PREISLER, H. D., HENDERSON, E. S.: Effect of cytosine arabinoside and 1,3-bis-2-chloroethyl-1-nitrosourea on hematopoietic precursors in the mouse. J. nat. Cancer Inst. **47**, 971—977 (1971).

ROCHLIN, D. B., SHINER, J., LANGDON, E., OTTOMAN, R.: Use of 5-fluorouracil in disseminated solid neoplasms. Ann. Surg. **156**, 105—113 (1962).

SALMON, S. E.: Personal communication (1972).

SALMON, S. E., SMITH, B. A.: Immunoglobulin synthesis and total body tumor cell number in IgG multiple myeloma. J. clin. Invest. **49**, 1114—1121 (1970).

SARTORELLI, A. C., CREASEY, W. A.: Combination chemotherapy. In: HOLLAND, J. F., FREI, E., III. (Eds.): Cancer medicine. Philadelphia: Lea & Febiger 1973.

SCHNECK, S. A., PENN, J.: De Novo brain tumours in renal transplant recipients. Lancet **1**, 983—986 (1971).

SCOTT, J. L.: The effect of nitrogen mustard and maintenance chlorambucil in the treatment of advanced Hodgkin's disease. Cancer Chemother. Rep. **27**, 27—32 (1963).

SELAWRY, O. S.: New treatment schedule with improved survival in childhood leukemia: Intermittent parenteral daily oral administration of methotrexate for maintenance of induced remission. J. Amer. med. Ass. **194**, 75—81 (1965).

SHARP, G. S., BENEFIEL, W. W.: 5-Fluorouracil in the treatment of inoperable carcinoma of the colon and rectum. Cancer Chemother. Rep. **20**, 97—101 (1962).

SKIPPER, H. E., SCHABEL, F. M., TRADER, M. W., LASTER, W. R., SIMPSON, L., LLOYD, M. M.: Basic and therapeutic trial results obtained in the spontaneous AKR leukemia (lymphoma) model. Cancer Chemother. Rep. (in press).

SKIPPER, H. E., SCHABEL, F. M., JR., WILCOX, W. S.: Experimental evaluation of potential anticancer agents. XXI. Scheduling of arabinosyl cytosine to take advantage of its 5-phase specificity against leukemia cells. Cancer Chemother. Rep. **51**, 125—141 (1967).

SPEAR, P., PATNO, M.: A comparative study of the effectiveness of $HN_2$ and cyclophosphamide in bronchogenic carcinoma, Hodgkin's disease and lymphosarcoma. Cancer Chemother. Rep. **16**, 413—415 (1962).

ULTMANN, J. E., NIXON, D. D.: The therapy of lymphoma. Semin. hemat. **6**, 376—403 (1969).

VENDITTI, J. M., HUMPHREYS, S. R., MANTEL, N., GOLDIN, A.: Combined treatment of advanced leukemia (L1210) in mice with amethopterin and 6-mercaptopurine. J. nat. Cancer. Inst. **17**, 631—638 (1956).

WEISS. A. J., JACKSON, L.: The effect of 5-fluorouracil upon carcinomas of the gastrointestinal tract and related organs. Amer. J. Gastroent. **35**, 138—146 (1961).

WHANG-PENG, C. P., KNUTSEN, T.: Polyploidy in malignant melanoma. Cancer **25**, 1216—1223 (1970).

WHITECAR, J. P., JR., BODEY, G. P., FREIREICH, E. J.: Combination chemotherapy (COAP) of adult acute leukemia. Proc. Amer. Ass. Cancer Res. **11**, 83 (1970).

WOLFF, J. A., BRUBAKER, C. A., MURPHY, M. L., PIERCE, M. I., SEVERO, N.: Prednisone therapy of acute childhood leukemia: Prognosis and duration of response in 330 treated patients. J. Pediat. **70**, 626—631 (1967).

ZUELZER, W. W.: Implications of long-term survival in acute stem cell leukemia of childhood treated with composite cyclic therapy. Blood **24**, 477—494 (1964).

Chapter 22

# Tests Predictive of Cytotoxic Activity

THOMAS C. HALL

## Introduction

Tests predictive of cytotoxicity are of three general types; those that select agents for antitumor cytotoxicity, those that predict host cytotoxicity, and those applied to predict the toxicity/benefit ratio of a drug of generally accepted potency in a particular patient with a specific tumor. The first type is fundamental to the other two, since the agent involved must be able to inhibit cell growth in order to deserve any consideration, and agents that show such activity will then be studied in more detail for their effects upon the tumor-bearing host. The latter two types of tests are basic, therefore, respectively, to screening of potential new drugs in subhuman systems and to initial human trials. Screening for tumor cytotoxicity has been discussed in Chapter 2 of this volume, and many of the considerations in regard to host toxicity of known effective agents have been discussed in Chapter 18. The present chapter will, therefore, deal primarily with tests predictive of antitumor toxicity of a specific drug in a specific patient.

## Sensitivity Testing

The use of antibiotic sensitivity testing in infectious diseases has made it possible to increase the effectiveness of first therapy, to reduce the number of drugs used to combat an infection to the one or ones having most cytotoxicity to the invading microorganism, and to reduce unwanted side effects and drug interactions. In addition to these desiderata, in the tumor patient, predictions of marked antitumor toxicity may permit justifiable increases in the doses of the effective agents, and achieve more rapid and complete responses, by inducing greater decreases in the body burden of tumor.

The first methods used were akin to those used for microbiologic testing: drugs were added to cultures of tumor cells from the patient, and the alterations in specific aspects of the metabolism of these cultured cells were studied. Correlations were sought between drug-induced *in vitro* derangements and the clinical effects of the drug upon the tumor in the patient. Among the culture methods used were short-term outgrowths from solid explants (LAZARUS et al., 1966), short-term growth of separated cells from biopsies (BICKIS et al., 1966), short-term monolayers (DENDY et al., 1970) and organ cultures (YARNELL et al., 1964). Since most of such cells were not demonstrated to grow after explantation, cytotoxic inhibition of dividing tumor cells could not easily be shown. The effect of the test drugs was, therefore, commonly studied by means of changes in $G_1$ metabolism as reflected in loss of capacity of treated cells to reduce methylene blue (DIPAOLA and DOWD, 1961), or the activity of succinic dehydrogenase (KONDO et al., 1966). These tests have had a variable utility in spite of their simplicity, and most workers do not now feel that there are good correlations between the effects seen *in vitro* and later clinical responses to the drug. This is hardly surprising since most antitumor agents are designed to inhibit growing cell populations. In addition, the complex *in vitro* problems of drug activation, catabolism, excretion, and plasma protein binding can not easily be reproduced in cell culture.

Establishment of stable human tumor lines has been attempted, but the success rate of these maneuvers is very low; only a few human tumors have been established in long-term culture. Even then there is doubt as to whether the cells which propagate are tumor cells or fibroblasts, or if they are tumor cells, whether they are truly representative of the cells that made up the bulk of the tumor in the host. Attempts to study short-range drug effects *in vitro* upon the replication of cancer cells in pieces of tumor removed at operation were undertaken by WOLBERG (1971) by adding the fresh tissue to incubation mixtures containing drug and DNA precursors such as $^{3}$H-thymidine and $^{3}$H-deoxyuridine. The correlations with later response to the drug were less than satisfactory for a clinical predictive test, but were more often correlated with the effect of drugs in man than were the older tests. In addition, such assays are primarily done upon tissues obtained at the time of initial surgery, and the data may not be relevant to the metastatic lesions appearing later.

For a number of drugs to be effective, critical pathways of drug transport, metabolic activation, and critical amounts of target enzyme are needed. In the case of methotrexate, for example, an increased amount of the target enzyme dihydrofolate reductase is found in mouse ascites tumors made resistant to the drug (FISCHER, 1961). However, this is not found to be a factor in "natural" or innate resistance to methotrexate in a spectrum of mouse ascites tumors (ROBERTS et al., 1965). In most mouse ascites tumors, transmembrane transport of the drug into the cell is critical (KESSEL et al., 1965). This finding, first suggested by studies of methotrexate transport in cell cultures (FISCHER, 1962), appears to be the determinant of cytotoxicity in human leukemias (KESSEL et al., 1968). So it is now possible to predict possible cytotoxicity of methotrexate in man by removing leukemic cells and incubating them with labeled drug. A negative prediction is always apt to be more accurate, because there may be other factors blocking the action of a drug even after it gains access to the cell. There are also major differences between degrees of innate drug resistance, which is commonly based upon one parameter such as drug uptake or phosphorylation, and induced or acquired resistance, which is commonly accompanied by the development of several pathways of resistance. For example, in induced methotrexate resistance, there may be the simultaneous appearance of high levels of dihydrofolic reductase, decreased transport of methotrexate, and a shift toward the use of relatively more thymidine as a DNA precursor. This suggests that tests useful in predicting cytotoxicity in previously untreated human patients may have to be applied with great caution to those who have relapsed after an initial response to chemotherapy.

Most antipurine and antipyrimidine drugs require phosphorylation in order to be activated. The final drug product may be the result of a number of reactions, deletion of any of which may interfere with the cytotoxicity. Assays for those enzymes can be used to predict cytotoxicity. A simple approach is to examine the ability of the tumor cell to metabolize the drug to a phosphorylated derivative which, being charged, will not diffuse out readily. Such measurements are relatively feasible for the isolated cells of leukemia and malignant effusions, but can not readily be applied to solid tumors from which it is difficult to separate intact single cells in large numbers and feel confident that they represent the whole tumor mass. In the latter case, homogenates of tumor can be analyzed for their enzymatic capacity. The ability to reconstitute a truly representative biochemical environment may be difficult in a broken cell system, since the physical separation of enzymatic functions within the cell is disrupted, and the pool sizes of substrates are apt to be unphysiological. In the case of the antimetabolite, 5-fluorouracil (FU), its effectiveness against murine (Kessel et al., 1966) and human leukemia (Hall et al., 1968) is well correlated with cellular conversion to nucleotides. In the case of solid tumors, the development of FU resistance seems most likely correlated with their content of orotidine 5′-phosphoribosyltransferase (Kasbekar and Greenberg, 1963). This also appears to be the resistance-determining enzyme in certain mouse solid tumors (Reyes and Hall, 1969). However, the existence of an adequate amount of 5-fluorodeoxyuridine 5′-monophosphate may be rendered noncytotoxic, if the cell can use another method for getting the thymidine needed for DNA synthesis. The "salvage" pathway for utilization of preformed thymidine requires thymidine kinase, and in mouse leukemias, there is a tendency for resistance to be correlated with high levels of this enzyme (Kessel et al., 1970). A completely accurate prediction system for FU cytotoxicity for solid tumors could, therefore, depend upon the measurement of the enzymes involved in several possible pathways for FU phosphorylation, as well as the activity of the "salvage" pathway(Everson et al., 1970).

Drug catabolism has been suggested as a possible factor in constructing a predicting equation for cytotoxicity. Wolpert et al. (1971) have shown that intracellular hydrolysis of 6-thiopurine nucleotides may contribute to neoplastic cell resistance. In other instances, for example cytosine arabinoside, the host liver may be of more importance as a source of degradation by deamination (Camiener and Smith, 1965). This host destruction before the drug reaches the tumor cell appears to be more of a problem than the content of deaminase in the leukemic cell itself (Hall and Levine, 1967). The capacity of target tumor cells to metabolize steroids by conjugation with sulfuric acid has been reported by Dao and Libby (1971) to predict for the cytotoxicity of estradiol to mammary tumor tissue and for the beneficial effect of adrenalectomy. Bulbrook (1970) has spent a great deal of effort to relate the patterns of steroid excretion in urine to responsiveness to hormone manipulation. This can be considered a measurement of net steroid metabolism involving host and tumor. The correlations have not been sufficient, however, to justify the use of urinary steroids as a predictive test.

The host can contribute other factors that are involved in prediction of cytotoxicity. Plasma protein binding is one such factor. The folic acid analogs are bound to different degrees by the plasma protein of different species, and this may predict the possibility for free drug cytotoxicity to the hosts or tumor tissue. There is little evidence to date of differential binding by different human patients' plasma proteins of methotrexate or of other antitumor drugs; hense, this factor can probably be ignored as a test predictive of drug cytotoxicity in a specific patient.

Other cellular factors in the tumor which are predictive of cytotoxicity include the presence or absence of steroid hormone receptors (Jensen et al., 1966). These have been described for almost all steroids and can be analyzed in the cell sap of disrupted tumor tissue. Jensen et al. (1971) have found a suggestive relation between the content of estrogen-binding protein and response to adrenalectomy. In the animal (Terenius, 1968) and in breast cancer patients (Braunsberg et al., 1971) uptake of radiolabeled steroid by the tumor has been found to correlate with estrogen responsiveness.

There may be intrinsic limitations in any *in vitro* analysis for factors predictive of *in vivo* cytotoxicity. The multiple metabolic factors, both intrinsic to tumor and to host, heterogeneity of the tumor mass, instability of the tumor genome, and differences between the genetic composition of different hosts, all make the pharmacologic interaction of drug, tumor, and host highly individual. Hence, analyses based more intimately upon the reactivity of a specific patient and his tumor to treatment by a specific drug or combination of drugs may require examination of that particular interaction. Most cytotoxic drugs create specific lesions in the cell replication system of the tumor which occur soon after the administration of the drug; however, it is not until repeated doses have been administered and time has passed to permit removal of the dead cell population that clinical shrinkage of tumor can be seen. There must be monitorable drug-induced changes at the single ($10^0$) to thousands ($10^3$) of cells level, observable during relatively short cell cycles (e.g. 8 to 48 h) which precede the changes in cell numbers observed weeks later at the 100 g (i.e. $10^{11}$ cell) level of the clinical "mass" lesion. In a general way, one could predict that neoplasms with slow growth rates and low fractions of their cell populations in the mitotic cycle, such as chronic lymphocytic leukemia and lung cancer, would be relatively unresponsive to $S$-phase active drugs, such as the antimetabolites inhibiting the synthesis of DNA, and more responsive to alkylating agents and corticosteroids which also affect cells in the $G_1$ phase of the cell cycle. However, these are very general concepts which may aid in the selection of classes of drugs, but do not permit prediction of cytotoxicity in a given patient. A number of attempts have been made to monitor the early effects of therapy in a patient and relate these to the ultimate outcome of the clinical use of the drug, and in this way simplify and integrate the multiple variables mentioned above.

One of the earliest of such an *in vivo* predictive system was that of SKY-PECK et al. (1960), in which $^{14}C$-formate incorporation into breast cancer nodules was monitored during the first hours after steroid administration. However, this test required repeated biopsy of accessible lesions, and attempts were made thereafter to use as a cytotoxicity-predictive test, incorporation of a radioactive precursor that was related to new DNA synthesis and could be monitored externally. $^{32}P$ uptake by tumor nodules seemed to correlate well with response to treatment with steroids, alkylating agents, antimetabolites, and radiation therapy (NEVINNY and HALL, 1961). However, because of the short range of the $\beta$ emission of $^{32}P$, a more energetic isotope has been sought. Initial studies with $^{131}I$-5-iodo-2′-deoxyuridine have shown some promise and should be pursued further (NATHANSON and HALL, 1968). Quite recently, sequential study of cesium-131 uptake by tumors has shown a predictive correlation between changes in early uptake of the isotope and the clinical results of drug (FERGUSON and HARPER, 1967).

Patients with "liquid" tumors such as leukemia or malignant effusions, commonly provide an easily accessible supply of neoplastic cells whose short-range response to therapy can commonly be studied by repeated sampling. Using single doses of drug given in the usual therapeutic amounts, it has been possible to measure the inhibition of the incorporation of precursors into nucleic acids. CLINE et al. (1968) used $^3H$-uridine into RNA, but as might be expected, correlations with cytotoxicity were poor. Correlations between inhibition of DNA synthesis from $^3H$-thymidine were quite good (HALL, 1971), and these results have been confirmed by others (WILMANNS, 1971).

## Conclusions

Substantial progress has been made toward developing an understanding of the components of a predictive equation for patient response to a possibly effective drug. These include host factors, drug factors, and tumor target characteristics. The interaction ultimately is designed to result in selective inhibition of DNA synthesis in the target tumor. Analyses can be made of the individual components in tumor homogenates, or of the early net change in macromolecular synthesis by the target cell in tumors yielding whole tumor cells and susceptible to repeat biopsies. Indirect estimates may be possible for deep-seated tumor DNA synthesis by external monitoring of $^{32}P$, $^{131}I$-5-iodo-2′-deoxyuridine, cesium-131 and other tumor-seeking isotopes. Assays for succinic dehydrogenase or RNA synthesis have not been helpful. We are not at the point of a predictive system for cytotoxicity comparable to that now available for antibacterials, but substantial progress has been made and there are exploitable leads of promise, so that one can anticipate with confidence that helpful predictive systems will be developed.

## References


Bickis, I. J., Henderson, I. W., Quastel, J. H.: Biochemical studies of human tumors. II. *In vitro* studies of individual tumor sensitivity to anticancer agents. Cancer **19**, 103—113 (1966).

Braunsberg, H., Carter, A. E., Irvine, W. T., James, F., James, V. H. T.: Estrogens in breast cancer. In: Hall, T. C. (Ed.): NCI Monograph 34. Prediction of response in cancer therapy pp. 71—75. Washington: U.S. Govt. Printing Office 1971.

Bulbrook, R. D.: Techniques for predicting response to treatment and survival. Oncology **3**, 367—370 (1970).

Camiener, G. W., Smith, C. C.: Studies of the enzymatic deamination of cytosine arabinoside I. Enzyme distribution and species specificity. Biochem. Pharmacol. **14**, 1405—1416 (1965).

Cline, M. J., Rosenbaum, E.: Prediction of in vivo cytotoxicity of chemotherapeutic agents by their in vitro effect on leukocytes from patients with acute leukemia. Cancer Res. **28**, 2516—2521, (1968).

Dao, T. L., Libby, P. R.: Enzymatic synthesis of steroid sulfate by mammary cancer and its clinical implications. In: Hall, T. C. (Ed.): NCI Monograph 34. Prediction of response in cancer therapy, Washington: U.S. Govt. Printing Office 1971.

Dendy, P. P., Bozman, E., Wheeler, T. K.: *In vitro* screening test for human malignant tumours before chemotherapy. Lancet **2**, 68 (1970).

DiPaolo, J. A., Dowd, J. E.: Evaluations of inhibition of human tumor tissue by cancer chemotherapeutic drugs with an *in vitro* test. J. nat. Cancer Inst. **27**, 807—815 (1961).

Everson, R., Kessel, D., Hall, T. C.: Enzymatic determinants of responsiveness of LPC-1 plasma cell tumors to fluorouracil and fluorodeoxyuridine. Biochem. Pharmacol. **19**, 2932—2934 (1970).

Ferguson, D. J., Harper, P. V.: Early effects of cancer therapy on uptake of Cesium-131 by tumor: Correlation with clinical result. Surg. Clin. N. Amer. **47**, 1507—1515 (1967).

Fischer, G. A.: Increased levels of folic acid reductase as a mechanism of resistance to amethopterin in leukemic cells. Biochem. Pharmacol **7**, 75 (1961).

Fischer, G. A.: Defective transport of amethopterin (methotrexate) as a mechanism of resistance to the antimetabolite. Biochem. Pharmacol. **11**, 1233 (1962).

Hall, T. C.: Selecting drug regimens in human leukemia. In: Hall, T. C. (Ed.): NCI Monograph 34. Prediction of response in cancer therapy, pp. 140—146. Washington: U.S. Govt. Printing Office 1971.

Hall, T. C., Kessel, D., Roberts, D.: Cellular pharmacology of effective anticancer drugs in man. Nebraska State med. J. **53**, 592 (1968).

Hall, T. C., Levine, R.: Deamination of cytosine arabinoside by normal and malignant tissues. Proc. Amer. Assoc. Cancer Res. **8**, 57 (1967).

Jensen, E. V., Block, G. E., Smith, S., Kyser, K., and DeSombre, E. R.: Estrogen receptors and breast cancer response to adrenalectomy. In: Hall, T. C. (Ed.): NCI Monograph 34. Prediction of response in cancer therapy, pp. 55—79. Washington: U.S. Govt. Printing Office 1971.

Jensen, E. V., Jacobson, H. I., Fisher, J. W., Saha, N. N., Gupta, G. N., Smith, S., Colucci, V., Shiplacoff, D., Neumann, H. G., DeSombre, E. R., Jungblut, P. W.: Estrogen receptors in target tissues. In: Nakao, T., Pincus, G., Tait, J. (Eds.): Steroid dynamics, pp. 133—157. New York: Academic Press 1966.

Kasbekar, D. K., Greenberg, D. M.: Studies on tumor resistance to 5-fluorouracil. Cancer Res. **23**, 818—825 (1963).

Kessel, D., Hall, T. C., Roberts, D: Modes of uptake of methotrexate by normal and leukemic leukocytes *in vitro* and their relation to drug response. Cancer. Res. **28**, 564—570 (1968).

Kessel, D., Hall, T. C., Roberts, D., Wodinsky, I.: Uptake as a determinant of methotrexate response in mouse leukemias. Science **150**, 752—754 (1965).

KESSEL, D., HALL, T.C., WODINSKY, I.: Nucleotide formation as a determinant of 5-fluorouracil response in mouse leukemias. Science 145, 911—913 (1966).
KESSEL, D., REYES, P., HALL, T.C.: Thymidine kinase as a determinant of 5-fluoro-2'-deoxyuridine resistance in transplantable murine leukemias. J. molec. Pharmacol. 6, 251—254 (1970).
KONDO, T., IMAMURA, T., ICHIHASHI, H.: *In vitro* test for sensitivity of tumor to carcinostatic agents. Gann 57, 113—121 (1966).
LAZARUS, H., TEGELER, W., MAZZONE, H.M., LEROY, J.G., BONNE, B.A., FOLEY, G.E.: Determinants of sensitivity of individual biopsy specimens to potential inhibitory agents: Evaluation of some explant culture methods of assay systems. Cancer Chemother. Rep. 50, 543—555 (1966).
NATHANSON, L., HALL, T.C.: External monitoring of cancer seeking isotopes. Clin. Res. 16, 360 (1968).
NEVINNY, H.B., HALL, T.C.: *In situ* determination of the antitumor effect of chemotherapeutic compounds. Proc. 2nd int. Symp. Chemother. (Naples) 3, 219—225 (1961).
REYES, P., HALL, T.C.: Synthesis of 5-fluorouridine 5'-phosphate by a pyrimidine phosphoribosyltransferase of mammalian origin. 11. Correlation between the tumor levels of the enzyme and the 5-fluorouracil promoted increase in survival of tumor-bearing mice. Biochem. Pharmacol. 18, 2587—2590 (1969).
ROBERTS, D., WODINSKY, I., HALL, T.C.: Studies on folic reductase, III. The level of enzyme activity and response to methotrexate of transplantable mouse tumors. Cancer Res. 25, 1899—1903 (1965).
SKY-PECK, H.H., KOFMAN, S., TAYLOR, S.G., WINZLER, R.J.: The incorporation of formate-$C^{14}$ into human breast cancer *in vitro*. Cancer Res. 20, 125—132 (1960).
TERENIUS, L.: Selective retention of estrogen isomers in estrogen dependent breast tumors of rats demonstrated by *in vitro* methods. Cancer Res. 28, 328—337 (1968).
WILMANNS, W.: DNA Synthesis in leukemic cells under the action of cytotoxic agents *in vitro* and *in vivo*. In: HALL, T.C. (Ed.): NCI Monograph 34. Prediction of response in cancer therapy, pp. 147—153. Washington: U.S. Govt. Printing Office 1971.
WOLBERG, W.H.: Biochemical approaches to prediction of responses in solid tumors. In: HALL, T.C. (Ed.): NCI Monograph 34. Prediction of response in cancer therapy. Washington: U.S. Govt. Printing Office 1971.
WOLPERT, M.K., DAMLE, S.P., BROWN, J.E., SZNYCER, E., AGRAWAL, K.C., SARTORELLI, A.C.: The role of phosphohydrolases in the mechanism of resistance of neoplastic cells to 6-thiopurines. Cancer Res. 31, 1620 (1971).
YARNELL, M., AMBROSE, E.J., SHEPLEY, K., TCHAO, R.: Drug assays on organ cultures of biopsies from human tumours. Brit. med. J. 2, 490 (1964).

Chapter 23

# Metabolic Changes Induced by Ionizing Radiations

PAUL TODD

With 2 Figures

## Introduction

Metabolic changes induced by ionizing radiations fall into two categories: those that follow the primary radiation events and lead to subcellular damage and cell lethality and those that are consequences of cell lethality and tissue damage. The former are observable shortly after irradiation and can be found in isolated cellular systems. The latter cannot be observed in isolated cell systems and are limited to whole organisms, usually with considerable lag after radiation exposure.

Historical examples of each are very pertinent to treatment in man. MITCHELL (1942) pointed out that radiation doses similar in magnitude to those used therapeutically disturb nucleic acid metabolism, and he correctly concluded that DNA ("thymonucleic acid") synthesis was inhibited. The sudden onset of nausea and vomiting that occurred in irradiated patients was considered indicative of metabolic disturbance to the extent that the phenomenon was termed *Strahlenkater* (radiation hangover) by GROEDEL and LOSSEN (1922).

## Effects of Ionizing Radiations on Biological Molecules

Most simply (and perhaps over-generally) stated, the chemistry of irradiated biological molecules is the chemistry of free radicals. This chemical statement has several predictable consequences: irradiated water will affect solute molecules; radiation-produced free radicals will be reactive toward oxygen and sulfur; and the 5 and 6 carbons of pyrimidines, the thiol groups of proteins, the hydroxyl groups of sugars and unsaturated carbon atoms in fats will be affected by radiation. Specific examples follow, so that the underlying causes of subcellular damage may be better understood.

### A. Nucleic Acids and Their Substituents

The first noticeable modification in irradiated pyrimidines is the appearance of an unpaired electron on the 5 carbon (PRUDEN et al., 1965), rendering the 5-6 double-bonded structure susceptible to reaction with nearby molecules (SCHOLES and WEISS, 1953). In pyrimidine nucleosides, unpaired electrons may occur on the carbon atoms of the furanose ring (SNIPES and HENRIKSEN, 1970), and the free-radical yield in irradiated nucleotides is greater than that in nucleosides, which is, in turn, greater than that for the bases, so that in the dry state the free-radical yield increases with molecular dimensions. Pyrimidines irradiated in aqueous solution react with radicals produced in water to form hydroxyl adducts, which may in turn react with oxygen if it is present, producing a hydroperoxide. The yield of the hydroperoxide in the presence of oxygen is approximately twice that of the hydroxyl adduct that occurs in the absence of oxygen. These chemical processes are summarized in Fig. 1.

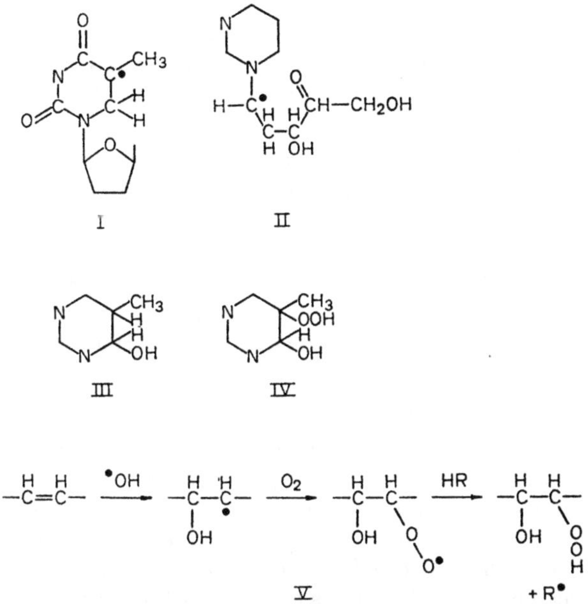

Fig. 1. Effects of ionizing radiation on the pyrimidine molecule. I. Unpaired electron on the 5 carbon of irradiated crystallized thymidine (PRUDEN et al., 1965). II. One of four possible furanose radicals in irradiated crystallized thymidine (SNIPES and HENRIKSEN, 1970). III. Hydroxyl adduct of thymine. IV. Hydroperoxide of thymine formed in irradiated aerated aqueous solution (SCHOLES and WEISS, 1959). V. Proposed general mechanism of hydroperoxide formation

Strand scission occurs in DNA irradiated in aqueous solutions (PEACOCKE and PRESTON, 1958), and this process accounts for a large fraction of the loss of biological activity of virus DNA (TAYLOR and GINOZA, 1967). Strand scission is also observed in DNA removed from irradiated bacteria (MCGRATH and WILLIAMS, 1966) and mammalian cells (LETT et al., 1967). In all cases where reasonably careful experiments and calculations have been done, it has been found that about 60 eV of energy produces one single-strand break (ELKIND and KAMPER, 1970). The term "single-strand" break arises from the technique of DNA analysis after irradiation involving molecular weight estimations by sedimentation velocity in the ultracentrifuge (STUDIER, 1965); cells are lysed and strands are separated at high pH, possibly leading to further chemical damage so the radiation effects are perhaps more accurately termed "alkali-labile lesions" (HEWITT and MARBURGER, 1971). That strand breaks may not be the immediate consequence of irradiation of DNA in cells is also evidenced by the observation that free "ends" (as evaluated enzymatically) appear several seconds after irradiation (MOSS et al., 1971). It is unlikely that this delay is due to the "after effects" observed in heavily-irradiated pure DNA (SCHOLES and WEISS, 1953). Alkali-labile lesions and free ends are sealed by living cells in about 10 min at 37° (LETT et al., 1967; DALRYMPLE et al., 1969).

## B. Proteins

Irradiation of dry proteins leads to unpaired electrons on their sulfur atoms (GORDY et al., 1955). Enzymes that depend upon free sulfhydryl groups for their activity are inhibited by ionizing radiation exposure (BARRON and DICKMAN, 1949). Irradiation of aqueous solutions of reduced cysteine or glutathione with moderate (ca. 10000 rads) doses liberates $H_2S$ in readily detectable amounts; the yield is concentration dependent and is optimum at pH 6, clearly indicating the involvement of the indirect effect (participation of radiolysis products of water) and the specificity of the indirect effect (DALE and DAVIES, 1951).

The behavior of irradiated histones in a monomolecular layer on a Langmuir trough indicates that ca. 100000 rads fragments the molecules, as the irradiated monolayer is compressible into a larger area. It is suggested that sulfhydryl groups are liberated and that the residual charge per molecule is reduced (KARGAONKAR and DESAI, 1959; TKACH and SIDYAKIN, 1961).

It has been claimed that the effects of doses as low as 400 rads can be detected in human serum albumin in aqueous solution when the end-point is the ability of the protein to bind methionine (PAVLOVSKAYA et al., 1955).

## C. Lipids and Carbohydrates

Unsaturated fats, in the presence of water and oxygen, are very susceptible to forming peroxides and hydroperoxides (Fig. 1). The same is true for sterols having ring double bonds (SCHOLES and WEISS, 1959). It is not uncommon to find that peroxide yields in the presence of oxygen are 10 times those in its absence (BECKER et al., 1956). An "after effect" due to autooxidation occurs in irradiated fats, and it has been claimed that doses as low as a thousand rads yield significant radiation products of linoleic acid in aqueous solution; the after effect leads to a paradoxical (inverse) dose-rate dependence of yield in this material (MEAD, 1952). The radiation-induced oxidations of fats and carbohydrates are of paramount interest in the food irradiation industry, as both are important in nutrition, taste, and palatability.

Carbohydrates are important nutritional and structural components of cells; among other important roles, they occur in glycoproteins and mucopolysaccharides in the outer surfaces of cells. These substances provide the cells' immediate microenvironment in such exposed places as the intestinal villi, and they confer immunological and tissue-specific individuality on the cell.

High-dose irradiation of dry monosaccharides leads to decomposition of the carbon chain. In aqueous solution the decomposition is preceded by oxidation of a terminal hydroxyl to a keto group (WOLFROM et al., 1959). Decomposition products include formaldehyde, glyoxal and dihydroxyacetone. When simple polysaccharides (starch and inulin) are irradiated in solution with high doses, the same decomposition products result, along with monosaccharides; the molecules are depolymerized and decomposed.

Doses below 1000 rads have been claimed to decrease significantly the viscosity of hyaluronic acid irradiated in aqueous solutions, and a slight "after effect" is reported (SCHOENBERG et al., 1951).

## D. Macromolecular Complexes

Much interest has centered around the radiation response of mixtures and aggregates of DNA with other macromolecules. Under some conditions, the presence of protein may "sensitize" the DNA by donating its free radical from sulfur to DNA thymine (LENHERR et al., 1967). Solutions of freshly-extracted nucleohistone (DNA with its native histone associated) are extremely viscous (BUTLER, 1956). SPARROW and ROSENFELD (1946) were the first to notice that the viscosity of irradiated extracted nucleohistone decreases exponentially with dose. Sensitive chemical techniques reveal significant radiation effects on nucleohistone fibers at very low doses. For example, viscosity changes in native nucleohistone have been claimed following doses as low as 10 rads (FISHER et al., 1959), and the solubilization of radioactive phosphorus from prelabeled DNA of nucleohistone after 100 rads has been reported (BUDILOVA and KUZIN, 1957). Following 800 rads or more, enhanced release of DNA from nucleohistone by tryptic digestion is noted (COLE and ELLIS, 1956).

It is more pertinent to examine the effects of radiation on nucleohistone in intact cells or nuclei. The observation that irradiated (1000 rads) nuclei lose their capacity to swell in water led to the interpretation that the deoxyribonucleoprotein of the nucleus is dissociated into DNA and protein (BERNSTEIN, 1954; KAUFMAN et al., 1955). To these observations should be added, first, that the radiation "target sizes" for these phenomena are enormous, as evidenced by their sensitivity, implying strong dependence on indirect effects and the involvement of large macromolecular aggregates; second, that dense deoxyribonucleoprotein aggregates are found associated with the nuclear membrane in multiplying cells and that the extent of aggregation depends upon ion concentration (ROBBINS and PEDERSON, 1971); and finally, the radiation sensitivity of lipids and its oxygen dependence suggest that the effects of radiation on the physical properties of nuclei may not be limited to modifications of DNA and protein molecules.

Large-target macromolecular complexes from the nuclei of irradiated cultured mammalian cells have been analysed on the basis of sedimentation velocity in the ultracentrifuge. Disruption of complexes has been interpreted in two different ways: DNA subunits of $5.5 \times 10^9$ molecular weight are held together by "linkers" that are easily broken by 400 to 800 rads (LETT, 1971) or large pieces of DNA are bound in a complex structure to nuclear membrane subunits, and this complex structure is dissociated by 300 to 700 rads (ELKIND, 1971).

## E. Summary of Molecular Effects

The effects of ionizing radiations on each of the classes of biological molecules discussed above is summarized in Table 1. Each effect can be characterized by its significant primary radical, the chemical product in aqueous solution and doses involved in producing the most sensitive effect.

Table 1. *Summary of effects of ionizing radiation on biological molecules*

| Type of molecule | Position of radical | Product in aqueous solution | Approximate minimum dose |
|---|---|---|---|
| DNA | Pyrimidine ring | Strand scission | 300 rads (in cells) |
| Protein | Sulfur | Enzyme inhibition, $H_2S$ | 400 rads (in solution, for methionine binding) |
| Lipid | Unsaturated carbons | Peroxides, hydroperoxides | 1000 rads (in solution) |
| Carbohydrate | | Carbon-chain decomposition, OH oxidation | 1000 rads (in solution, hyaluronic acid) |
| DNA-Histone | | Partial dissociation | 10 rads (viscosity change) |

## Subcellular and Early Metabolic Changes

The metabolism, and particularly the synthesis, of each of the classes of macromolecules discussed above is affected by exposure to ionizing radiation of the cells in which the syntheses occur.

### A. The Synthesis of DNA and Its Precursors

The use of ionizing radiation as an antineoplastic agent led to Mitchell's (1942) discovery that cells in the tumors of irradiated patients experienced a reduction in rate of DNA increase. This finding, made by quantitative cytological techniques, was rapidly confirmed in Jensen's rat sarcoma (Euler and Hevesy, 1944), in which a reduced incorporation of $P^{32}$ phosphate into DNA was noted.

Radiation also inhibits DNA synthesis in normal tissue (Ahlström et al., 1945). The inhibition of DNA synthesis occurs immediately after radiation exposure, and it is very effective, with 1000 rads being sufficient to reduce incorporation of precursors by 50% within 0.5 hours (Gronow and Todd, 1969), as shown in Fig.2.

In addition to the inhibition of ongoing DNA synthesis in normal and malignant mammalian cells, it appears that the initiation of DNA synthesis is also very effectively inhibited by radiation (Holmes, 1956; Stocken, 1968; Little, 1970). A few hundred rads can delay the initiation of DNA synthesis several hours. The extreme radiosensitivity of this process may be related to the sensitivity of nuclear phosphorylation, which is discussed in greater detail below.

The vital role of thymidylic acid as a precursor to DNA (Rueckert and Mueller, 1960) has led to the suspicion that radiation effects upon its synthesis may influence DNA synthesis rates (Soška et al., 1961). Indeed, it has been found, for example, that small (less than 1000 rads) doses of radiation reduce the activities of deoxycytidylate deaminase (Sugino and Potter, 1960), methyl transferase (Winchell et al., 1968), and thymidine kinase (Gelbard et al., 1970). A clear-cut causal relationship between radiation-inhibited precursor synthesis and DNA synthesis inhibition remains to be firmly established, although the protective effect of exogenously supplied deoxyribonucleotides is very suggestive (Soška et al., 1960; Petrovič et al., 1964).

### B. RNA Synthesis

Radiation doses that inhibit DNA synthesis in multiplying cells also inhibit RNA synthesis (Holmes, 1949). The process whereby radiation leads to inhibition of RNA synthesis appears to be closely related to the process that leads to reproductive death of the cell, as radiation and actinomycin D have very similar effects on reproductive viability of cultured mammalian cells (Elkind et al., 1969).

The sensitivity to radiation of the process of RNA synthesis varies widely among cell types, but RNA synthesis in isolated thymocyte nuclei is noticeably reduced after 50 rads (Logan et al., 1959). It should be noted that all biochemical processes so far studied in the nuclei of cells from lymphatic tissues are very radiation sensitive.

### C. Protein Synthesis

Soon after the availability of radioisotopes for biological studies, it was noted that incorporation of radioactive precursors into substances other than nucleic acids was not particularly inhibited (Hevesy, 1949). Doses in excess of 100000 rads lead to detectable inhibition of protein synthesis in microorganisms, and the sensitive target within the cell appears to be the ribosome (Pollard, 1961). On the other hand, the synthesis of specific inducible enzymes during induction is quite sensitive, and responds significantly to less than 10000 rads in microorganisms. The sensitive process is not considered to be protein synthesis per se, but the transcription of new messenger RNA which must precede protein synthesis (POLLARD and DAVIS, 1970). The reentry of cultured mammalian cells into DNA synthesis appears to require first RNA then protein synthesis (BECKER and LEVITT, 1968). This raises the question of a possible relationship between the radiosensitivity of transcription and the radiosensitivity of the initiation of DNA synthesis.

## D. Histones

Although protein synthesis in general is hardly affected by radiation doses that severely affect nucleic acid synthesis, the synthesis of histones deserves special consideration, as their synthesis is considered closely coupled to that of DNA (ROBBINS and BORUN, 1967). It is apparent that meaningful studies of radiation effects on histone synthesis must be done on cell populations in which active DNA synthesis occurs. The immediate inhibition of DNA synthesis following 1000 rads in ascites tumor cells (Fig 2) is not accompanied by an immediate inhibition of histone synthesis (GRONOW and TODD, 1969). Radiation appears to be the only pharmacological agent thus far studied that has this uncoupling effect. Further studies of multiplying cell populations indicate that a delayed inhibition of histone synthesis occurs several hours after irradiation (BASES and MENDEZ, 1971) and that

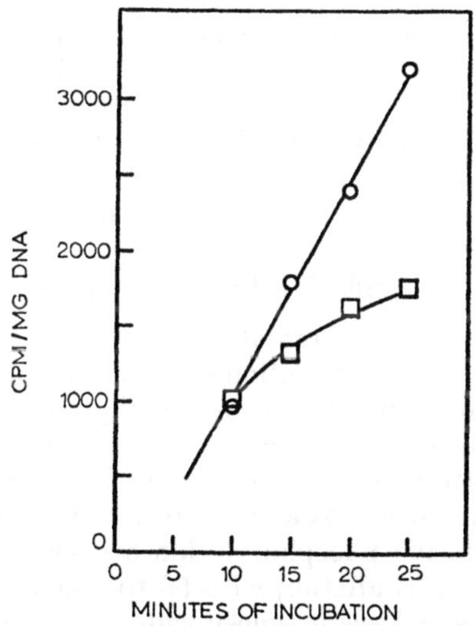


Fig. 2. Incorporation of labeled precursors into DNA in rat hepatoma cells after 1000 rads of $^{60}Co$ gamma irradiated (squares) compared with unirradiated control cells (circles). Irradiation was *in vivo*, and incorporation occurred in cells after removal from the peritoneum (GRONOW and TODD, 1969). Copyright by Academic Press, Inc.

there is a gradual accumulation of histone (EVANS et al., 1970), presumably the $f_3$ component in the nuclei of irradiated cells, and this accumulation may be responsible for the well-known radiation-induced $G_2$ block (GURLEY et al., 1970). Possible relationships between this uncoordinated synthesis and cell lethality are suggested by the rescuing effect of the deliberate inhibition of protein synthesis in irradiated DNA-synthesizing cultured human cells (PHILLIPS and TOLMACH, 1966).

Apart from effects on the synthesis of histones, structural or chemical modifications have been reported; for example, some DNA-bound histone is thought to become unbound in irradiated thymocytes (WHITFIELD et al., 1964), and 1000 rads is reported to diminish histone phosphorylation (see next section) and lead to oxidation of fraction $f_3$ sulfhydryl groups (ORD and STOCKEN, 1968).

## E. Nuclear Phosphorylation

Isolated thymus nuclei are capable of synthesizing ATP from AMP under aerobic conditions (OSAWA et al., 1957), as are nuclei isolated from other lymphatic tissues and lymphatic tumors, with the possible exception of those from lymph nodes (KLOUWEN, 1965). The nuclear synthesis of ATP appears to be a very radiation sensitive process (CREASEY and STOCKEN, 1959). In thymocyte nuclei isolated from whole-body irradiated rats, nuclear ATP synthesis is abolished 2 h after 500 rads, 8 h after 150 rads, and noticeably reduced 1 h after as little as 25 rads (DEAKIN et al., 1963). Although lymphosarcoma cell nuclei do synthesize ATP, the process is not inhibited by radiation, and is only reduced as the cells undergo mitotic death (KLOUWEN, 1965).

In addition to the nuclear synthesis of ATP in lymphatic cells, it has been reported that phosphorylation of histones precedes DNA replication and transcription in various tissues of rats (STEVELY and STOCKEN, 1968), that this process is stimulated by adenosine-3′,5′-monophosphate (LANGAN, 1968) and that it is inhibited to a noticeable degree by 1000 rads of gamma rays (ORD and STOCKEN, 1966, 1968).

A role for phosphate in the interphase death of thymocytes has been proposed by WHITFIELD (1965), who postulates that the reduced ATP synthesis results in an increased phosphate ion concentration, which in turn dissociates histone from DNA, which in turn leads to thymocyte death. In summary, the immunosuppressive effects of radiation must be considered with due regard for the radiation inhibition of nuclear phosphorylation, which occurs mainly in lymphatic tissues.

## F. Oxidative Phosphorylation

Aside from the early effects of radiation on the synthesis of macromolecules, immediate biochemical effects of radiation are seldom found after moderate (50 to 2000 rads) doses except in lymphatic tissues (i.e., thymus, spleen and tonsils). These cells characteristically have very little cytoplasm, consisting almost entirely of nucleus, and have a small number of mitochondria. Evidently the phosphate metabolism of such cells is in delicate balance, and it is in cells of these tissues where radiation effects on oxidative phosphorylation are seen (POTTER and BETHELL, 1952, VAN BEKKUM, 1957). Irradiation with 50 to 100 rads *in vivo* leads to detectable depression of ATP synthesis in spleen cells. No such inhibition of oxidative phosphorylation is found in irradiated liver, ascites tumor, or HeLa cells except after very large doses (SCAIFE and HILL, 1962).

There exist reports of increased oxygen consumption (10 to 40%) after 50 to 600 rads in isolated erythrocytes (LESSLER, 1958).

Inhibition studies with dinitrophenol indicate that some aspects of DNA repair in irradiated cultured mammalian cells require ATP produced by oxidative phosphorylation (DALRYMPLE et al., 1969).

## G. Sulfhydryl Compounds

Despite the well-known protective effects of reduced sulfhydryl compounds in irradiated cells (PATT et al., 1949), there is very little evidence that favors *in vivo* oxidation by ionizing radiation of intracellular sulfhydryl groups when cells are exposed to doses of therapeutic magnitude. It is worth noting in this regard that 1000 rads corresponds to about $10^{15}$ primary ionizations per gram of tissue; if reduced sulfhydryls are present in the cell in a concentration of $10^{-4}$M, then there are $10^{19}$ sulfhydryls to be oxidized in each gram. If every primary ionization oxidized one sulfhydryl group, less than 0.01% of them would be oxidized, and this would be undetectable. Nevertheless, in the nucleus of the thymocyte, where biochemical radiation effects are magnified, DEAKIN et al. (1963) noted a decrease in sulfhydryl content after 1000 rads, *provided* nuclear glutathione reductase was inhibited by zinc ions (ORD and STOCKEN, 1963). In a study of a number of nuclear functions in irradiated cells of rat liver and thymus, ORD and STOCKEN (1968) reported evidence for the oxidation of thiol groups of histone fraction $f_3$, which appear to play a role in the transcription-inhibiting effect of this histone fraction (i.e. oxidized histone $f_3$ inhibits transcription more effectively than $f_3$-SH) (HILTON and STOCKEN, 1966).

### H. Transport Phenomena

Although radiation inhibition of membrane transport phenomena, such as active sodium transport, is found to occur only after large (several thousand rads) doses in mammalian systems, a few radiosensitive transport phenomena have been discovered. Notable is the work of BRINKMAN and LAMBERTS (1958, 1960) who built up a subcutaneous pressure of 100 to 500 mm mercury by saline injection and irradiated overlying skin with less than 200 rads of 35 kVp x-rays; the subcutaneous pressure dropped during the irradiation, and the radiation effect was protected against by cysteamine. Also, evidence has been found that membrane structure in isolated mitochondria is altered by low doses of x-rays (FRITZ-NIGGLI, 1956) on the basis of reduced citrate oxidation. Changes in membrane permeability may be attributed to radiation effects on either active or passive transport; the apparently active transport of glycine by ascites tumor cells is inhibited by moderate doses (HAGEMANN and EVANS, 1968). The rapidity of the BRINKMAN-LAMBERTS (1958) effect and the knowledge that the cell maintains lytic enzymes surrounded by membranes that prevent their action (lysosomes) has lead to a theory of radiation action on cells known as the "Enzyme Release Hypothesis" (BACQ and ALEXANDER, 1961).

## Whole-Body Metabolic Changes

Although changes in metabolism at the cellular level are expected to be reflected in the metabolic behavior of the irradiated organism, the changes observed are not simply a scaled-up version of the cellular changes. Most whole-body metabolic changes are subsequent to the loss of cells of specific types, and the metabolism of the whole body reflects the loss of these cells rather than reflecting the metabolic changes that occur in these cells.

### A. Pertinent Tissue Pathology

The reproductive lethality of multiplying cells appears to be the most important effect of ionizing radiation as far as the acutely-irradiated organism is concerned. This is especially evident in organs that depend upon the continous replacement of cells. The fastest is almost certainly the intestinal epithelium. About 1.5 days after 400 rads or more, the typical mammal is without intestinal villi, as they have not been replaced by the multiplying cells that normally exist in the intestinal crypts.

The preceding discussion clearly points out that lymphatic tissues are very radiosensitive. Pathology bears this out in the irradiated animal; thus one day after 200 rads the circulating lymphocyte count is below 10% of its normal value in rats (SUTER, 1947). Much abnormal cell division and mitotic death is observed in the bone marrow, the consequence of which can be seen about 8 days later, when the circulating erythrocyte and platelet counts fall to dangerous levels after exposure to 500 rads or more (BOND et al., 1965). Skin also depends upon multiplying cells for its replacement; doses in the range 1000 to 4000 rads lead to progressively more severe effects, usually classified as detectable erythema, severe erythema, dry desquamation, and skin loss. Although it is not clear whether multiplying cells are involved, it is evident that doses in excess of 500 rads lead to capillary fragility, the consequence of which is usually hemorrhage if the radiation exposure has also caused thrombopenia. Finally, the widespread destruction of cells throughout the body often leads to the release of large quantities of potassium into the blood, especially after large doses, thereby creating problems of electrolyte balance and neuron function (JACKSON et al., 1958).

## B. Metabolic Changes Due to Intestinal Effects

Nutrient, water, and electrolyte intake occur through the intestine. The exposure of the upper abdomen to 150 rads leads to nausea and vomiting known as the prodromal response, and it occurs within a few hours after exposure (GROEDEL and LOSSEN, 1922; LUSHBAUGH et al., 1966). The metabolic changes responsible for this physiological reaction remain poorly understood, but their effects are counteracted by antihistamines, narcotics, and tranquilizers, implying that tissue destruction and the autonomic nervous system play important roles.

Water and electrolyte content of the serum is modified to a clinically observable extent after a few hundred rads (JACKSON et al., 1958), and serum protein and lipid concentrations are elevated, mainly due to dehydration. The destruction of the intestinal barrier has numerous, almost predictable, metabolic sequelae: the denuded lining is a good culture medium for uncontrolled bacterial growth, especially in an organism with impaired immunological response; water is lost freely into the intestines, and a reduction of over 50% in plasma volume may occur (SWIFT and TAKETA, 1958); along with water, sodium is lost, and up to 20% of the total body sodium can be lost from rats following 1500 rads (JACKSON et al., 1958); bile salts cease to be absorbed in the distal ileum and gain entrance to the small intestine and colon, where they cause diarrhea (SULLIVAN, 1962); and transaminase activity is reduced by more than 95% (BRIN and MCKEE, 1964), presumably as a result of cell depletion of a similar magnitude. In summary, the metabolic changes associated with the intestinal effects of radiation are mainly consequences of cell loss.

## C. Metabolic Changes Associated with Effects on Lymphatic Tissues

At the cellular level, as was pointed out above, biochemical changes are most readily detectable in lymphatic cells, including small lymphocytes. Circulating lymphocytes have a mean lethal dose of less than 50 rads (SUTER, 1947). The expected metabolic consequences include reduced resistance of the organism to infection, when considered along with the effects of radiation on the bone marrow. Indeed, small (i.e. less than 200 rads) doses suppress antibody formation (BENJAMIN and SLUKA, 1908; KOHN, 1951). Oddly enough, however, the changes in serum globulins after whole body irradiation appear to be associated with irradiation of the intestine (PALMER and SULLIVAN, 1958); in this regard it should be pointed out that circulating albumin is more severely affected than are the globulins.

Although lymphocytes and the lymphatic organs play an important role in the immune response, it is fairly evident that the critical cell is the granulocyte. Mortality with infection among a variety of mammalian species correlates well with granulocytopenia, but not with the lymphocyte count. Additionally, spleen transplants in irradiated mice did not change this picture (BOND et al., 1965).

## D. Metabolic Changes Associated with Bone-Marrow Effects

Protection against infection plays an important role in the survival of the irradiated animal. Radiation is a well-known immunosuppressive agent, and the importance of granulocytes has been previously mentioned. The effects of radiation (650 rads) on mature neutrophils is negligible, but 3 days after exposure, neutropenia is apparent, and microorganisms are free to multiply in the blood of deliberately infected animals (SMITH et al., 1963). Thus, the metabolism of the bone marrow depleted organism is that of one with a severe infection, and rectal temperatures of 105° F have been recorded in moribund dogs. In man, treatment of the symptoms of infection (i.e. fever, etc.) is recommended. It should be pointed out that acute bacteremia in the midlethally irradiated rodent is common, but that the infections seldom spread to the blood of man and primates. The infecting organism is usually indigenous to the intestine (WARREN and WHIPPLE, 1923). It is quite possible to avoid the lethal effects of neutrophil depletion with modern pharmacological techniques.

The bone marrow also supplies erythrocytes, the depletion of which also has serious consequences. During the postirradiation period, when no new erythrocytes are contributed to the circulation, mature erythrocytes are lost at the rate of 1% per day, as the mean life of circulating erythrocytes is 100 days. The oxygen carrying capacity of the blood is therefore impaired and the metabolism of iron in the spleen and bone marrow is altered. Specifically, marrow suspensions from irradiated (800 rads) rabbits immediately after exposure, consume oxygen and synthesize heme at about twice the normal rate, after which the rate of incorporation of $^{14}C$ into heme falls to 10% of normal over the next few days. One week after exposure, the synthesis of globin has fallen to $^1/_3$ normal, due to the depletion of functional reticulocytes, but heme synthesis at the same time is returning to normal. The picture in the spleen is slightly different. Heme synthesis remains high, and globin synthesis passes through a maximum on the first day and declines thereafter. It is important to point out that the studies were done on lethally irradiated rabbits (RICHMOND et al., 1951).

There are practically no reticulocytes in the marrow of the lethally irradiated and near-lethally irradiated human between the 3rd and 14th day after exposure (FLIEDNER, 1960), and a corresponding reduction in iron metabolism is observed in $LD_{50}$-irradiated animals. In addition to this obviously depressed rate of red-cell formation, there is also an increased rate of red cell loss, as evidenced by the increased rate of disappearance of prelabeled ($^{59}Fe$) red cells in monkeys about 8 days after an $LD_{50}$ exposure (GILBERT et al., 1962). The increased rate of loss is almost certainly due to hemorrhage.

The bone marrow is also the source of blood platelets, essential for clotting. The platelet depression (thrombocytopenia) that follows the bone marrow syndrome leads, possibly along with other metabolic changes, to increased clotting time. Controversial findings have been presented concerning the possible existence of a radiation induced heparin-like anticoagulating factor (JACKSON et al., 1952). Radiation-induced clotting defects appear to be almost entirely due to thrombocytopenia, which might cause, but certainly aggravates, the hemorrhagic syndrome (Sire et al., 1961).

The metabolic changes accompanying the bone-marrow syndrome are those associated with pancytopenia; the irradiated individual is deprived of oxygen transport, phagocytosis, antibody synthesis, clotting, and a certain amount of reticuloendothelial function. The indicated treatment is transfusion of platelets, whole blood, and marrow, if possible. It is generally considered that such treatment in the human situation is useful, but the success with which it actually prevents lethality in man remains unknown (Mathé et al., 1959).

### E. Some General Metabolic Effects

Although the most pertinent metabolic changes in the irradiated organism are associated with the major syndromes discussed above, other modifications are observed, and some of these are of more than passing interest. Immediately after irradiation of mammals in the mean lethal dose range or below, there is either no change or a slight increase in the rate of oxygen consumption or the basal metabolic rate. Metabolic changes of this sort are more apparent in starving or anesthetized animals. Transient accumulations of glycogen are observed in livers (Kay and Entenman, 1956) and brains (Miquel et al., 1963) of moderately irradiated rats. Cortisone is known to have this effect, so it may be a consequence of the general adaptation syndrome (Selye, 1950). Indeed, this phenomenon does not occur in the livers of adrenalectomized rats (McKee and Brin, 1956), but it does occur in locally irradiated brains, only in the irradiated area.

Additional metabolic changes, too numerous to mention, also occur; some of these are at some distance from the irradiated area and are considered a secondary consequence of the radiation "stress" to the whole body.

## Conclusions

Radiation induces radicals in water or critical biological molecules, and the latter then undergo functional impairment. This damage is expressed in the metabolism of the irradiated cells. In particular, cells which normally multiply are reproductively impaired, due to critical molecular effects. Which molecular effects are critical is one of the central issues of modern radiation biology. The death of reproductively incapacitated cells leads to functional impairment of the organs they supply. In the case of the intestine, metabolism is severely altered, and fluid and electrolyte balance consequently changed. In the case of the bone marrow, the cells it supplies to the rest of the body are reduced in number, and oxygen transport, clotting, and the immune response are all subsequently impaired. Extensive cell loss (tissue destruction) releases histamine and serotonin to the system, leading to a stress response, and, at extremely large doses, not discussed here, tissue destruction may also release sufficient potassium to affect neurological function.

## References

Ahlström, L., von Euler, H., von Hevesy, G.: Die Wirkung der Röntgenstrahlen auf den Nucleinsäureumsatz in den Organen der Ratte. Arkiv Kemi Mineral. Geol. 19 A, 1—16 (1944).

Bacq, Z. M., Alexander, P.: Fundamentals of radiobiology, 2nd ed. Oxford: Pergamon Press 1961.

Barron, E. S. G., Dickman, S. R.: Studies on the mechanism of ionizing radiations. II. Inhibition of sulfhydryl enzymes by alpha, beta, and gamma rays. J. gen. Physiol. 32, 595—607 (1949).

BASES, R., MENDEZ, F.: Delayed inhibition of histone synthesis despite prompt inhibition of DNA synthesis in x-irradiated HeLa cells. Radiat. Res. **47**, 258 (1971).

BECKER, R. R., KUNG, H-C., BARR, N. F., PEARSON, C. S., KING, C. G.: Nutritional and biochemical effects of irradiation. Food Technol. **10**, 61—64 (1956).

BECKER, Y., LEVITT, J.: Stimulation of macromolecular processes in $BSC_1$ cells due to medium replenishment. Exp. Cell Res. **51**, 1—11 (1968).

BENJAMIN, E., SLUKA, E.: Antikörperbildung nach Experimenteller Schädigung des Hematopoetischen Systems durch Röntgenstrahlen. Wien. Klin. Wochenschr. **21**, 311—313 (1908).

BERNSTEIN, M. H.: Deoxyribonucleoprotein of cell nuclei: sensitivity to x-rays. Nature (Lond.) **174**, 463 (1954).

BOND, V. P., FLIEDNER, T. M., ARCHAMBEAU, J. O.: Mammalian radiation lethality. New York: Academic Press 1965.

BRIN, M., MCKEE, R. W.: Effects of x-irradiation, nitrogen mustard, fasting, cortisone, and adrenalectomy on transaminase activity in the rat. Arch. Biochem. Biophys. **61**, 384—389 (1964).

BRINKMAN, R., LAMBERTS, H. B.: Direct registration of an instantaneous x-ray effect in rats and man. Nature (Lond.) **181**, 774—775 (1958).

BRINKMAN, R., LAMBERTS, H. B.: Examples of immediate low-level x-ray effects: their significance for the study of chemical protection. Int. J. Radiat. Biol. Suppl. **1**, 167 (1960).

BUDILOVA, E. V., KUZIN, A. M.: Disaggregation by ionizing radiation in deoxyribose nucleoprotein filaments. Biofizika **2**, 476—479; Biophysics **2**, 467—470 (1957).

BUTLER, J. A. V.: The action of ionizing radiation on biological materials. Radiat. Res. **4**, 20—32 (1956).

COLE, L. J., ELLIS, M. E.: Physicochemical alterations in spleen deoxyribonucleoprotein after *in vitro* x-irradiation with 850 R. Radiat. Res. **5**, 252—266 (1956).

CREASEY, W. A., STOCKEN, L. A.: The effect of ionizing radiation on nuclear phosphorylation in the radiosensitive tissues of the rat. Biochem. J. **72**, 519—523 (1959).

DALE, W. M., DAVIES, J. V.: The liberation of sulphide hydrogen by x-radiation from cysteine and glutathione. Biochem. J. **48**, 129—132 (1951).

DALRYMPLE, G. V., SANDERS, J. L., MOSS, A. J., JR., BAKER, M. L., WILKINSON, K. P.: Energy dependent nucleolytic processes are responsible for the production of many post-irradiation breaks in L-cell DNA. Biochem. biophys. Res. Comm. **36**, 284—288 (1969).

DEAKIN, H., ORD, M. G., STOCKEN, L. A.: Glucose-6-phosphate dehydrogenase activity and thiol content of thymus nuclei from control and x-irradiated rats. Biochem. J. **89**, 296—304 (1963).

ELKIND, M. M.: DNA: a principal target (or a target of principle) in the radiation lethality o mammalian cells? Radiat. Res. **47**, 315 (1971).

ELKIND, M. M., KAMPER, C.: Two forms of repair in mammalian cells following irradiation. Biophys. J. **10**, 237—245 (1970).

ELKIND, M. M., SAKAMOTO, K., KAMPER, C.: Age dependent toxic properties of actinomycin D and x-rays in cultured Chinese hamster cells. Cell Tissue Kinet. **1**, 209—224 (1969).

EULER, H. V., HEVESY, G. V.: Wirkung der Röntgenstrahlen auf den Umsatz der Nukleinsäure in Jensen-Sarkom. Akiv. Kemi Mineral. Geol. **17A**, 1—60 (1944).

EVANS, T. C., LEEPER, D. B., SCHENKEN, L. L.: Further analysis of the effects of fractionation of x-irradiation on DNA synthesis and mitosis in ascites tumor cells. Radiat. Res. **43**, 217—218 (1970).

FISHER, W. D., ANDERSON, N. G., WILBUR, K. M.: Studies on nuclei. II. Effects of x-rays on deoxyribonucleoprotein from rat thymus. Exp. Cell Res. **18**, 481—493 (1959).

FLIEDNER, T. M.: Zur Hämatologie des Akuten Strahlensyndroms. Strahlentherapie **112**, 543—560 (1960).

FRITZ-NIGGLI, H.: Enzymatische Strahlenschädigung von Lebermitochondrien durch die minimale Röntgendosis von 0,1 r. Naturwiss. **43**, 225—226 (1956).

GELBARD, A. S., PEREZ, A. H., KIM, J. H.: The effect of irradiation on thymidine kinase activity in synchronous populations of HeLa cells. Radiat. Res. **43**, 219 (1970).

GILBERT, C. W., PATERSON, E., HAIGH, M. V., SCHOFIELD, R.: Red-cell and plasma-volume changes in the Rhesus monkey after whole-body irradiation by x-rays. Int. J. Radiat. Biol. **5**, 9—23 (1962).

GORDY, W., ARD, W. B., SHIELDS, H.: Microwave spectroscopy of biological substances. I. Paramagnetic resonance in x-irradiated amino acids and proteins. Proc. nat. Acad. Sci. (Wash.) **41**, 983—996 (1955).

GROEDEL, F., LOSSEN, H.: Über den Röntgenkater. Strahlentherapie **13**, 756—757 (1922).

GRONOW, M., TODD, P.: The synthesis of deoxyribonucleic acid and nuclear proteins by rat hepatoma cells immediately after gamma irradiation. Radiat. Res. **39**, 705—715 (1969).

GURLEY, L. R., HARDIN, J. M., WALTERS, R. A.: The response of histone fractions to x-irradiation in cultured Chinese hamster cells. Biochem. biophys. Res. Commun. **38**, 290—297 (1970).
HAGEMANN, R., EVANS, T. C.: The effect of x-irradiation on glycine transport in Ehrlich Ascites tumor cells. Radiat. Res. **33**, 371—380 (1968).
HEVESY, G. V.: Effect of x-rays on the incorporation of carbon-14 into animal tissue. Nature (Lond.) **164**, 269 (1949).
HEWITT, R., MARBURGER, K.: UV sensitivity of DNA containing 5-bromouracil. Biophys. Soc. Abstr. **11**, 279 (1971).
HILTON, J., STOCKEN, L. A.: The role of thiol groups in the modification of the template activity of histone-deoxyribonucleic acid complexes. Biochem. J. **100**, 21 C (1966).
HOLMES, B. E.: The indirect effect of x-rays on the synthesis of nucleic acids *in vivo*. Brit. J. Radiol. **22**, 487 (1949).
HOLMES, B. E.: Influence of radiation on metabolism of regenerating rat liver. Ionizing radiation and cell metabolism, (WOLSTENHOLME, G. E. W. and O'CONNOR, C. M., Eds.). pp. 225—283. London: Ciba 1956.
JACKSON, D. P., CRONKITE, E. P., LEROY, G. V., HALPERN, B.: Further studies on the nature of the hemorrhagic state in radiation injury. J. Lab. clin. Med. **39**, 449—461 (1952).
JACKSON, K. L., RHODES, R., ENTENMAN, C.: Electrolyte excretion in the rat after severe intestinal damage by x-irradiation. Radiat. Res. **8**, 361—373 (1958).
KARGAONKAR, K. S., DESAI, A. M.: Monolayer technique to study effects of ionizing radiations on histone. Radiat. Res. **11**, 625—635 (1959).
KAUFMAN, B. P., MCDONALD, M. R., BERNSTEIN, M. H.: Cytochemical studies of changes induced in cellular materials by ionizing rudiations. Ann. N. Y. Acad. Sci. **59**, 553—566 (1955).
KAY, R. E., ENTENMAN, C.: Hyperglycemia and increased liver glycogen in rats after x-irradiation. Proc. Soc. exp. Biol. (N. Y.) **91**, 143—146 (1956).
KLOUWEN, H. M.: Radiosensitivity of nuclear ATP synthesis and its relation to inhibition of mitosis, pp. 142—166. In: Cellular radiation biology. Baltimore: Williams and Wilkins 1965.
KOHN, H. I.: Effect of x-rays upon hemolysin production in the rat. J. Immunol. **66**, 525—533 (1951).
LANGAN, T. A.: Histone phosphorylation: stimulation by adenosine 3',5'-monophosphate. Science **162**, 579—580 (1968).
LENHERR, A. D., CHARLESBY, A., SINGH, B. B.: Energy transfer in nucleoproteins. Int. J. Rad. Biol. **12**, 51—60 (1967).
LESSLER, M. A.: Modification of human erythrocyte respiration by x-rays. Radiat. Res. **9**, 144 (1958).
LETT, J. T.: The restoration of chromosomal DNA structure in x-irradiated cells. Radiat. Res. **47**, 313—314 (1971).
LETT, J. T., CALDWELL, I., DEAN, C. J., ALEXANDER, P.: Rejoining of x-ray induced breaks in the DNA of leukaemia cells. Nature (Lond.) **214**, 790—792 (1967).
LITTLE, J. B.: Differential response of cultured human cells to irradiation in the exponential and plateau phases of growth. Radiat. Res. **39**, 504—505 (1970).
LOGAN, R., ERRERA, M., FICQ, A.: The effect of x-rays and ultraviolet light on the uptake *in vitro* of (8-$^{14}$C)-adenine and (2-$^{14}$C)-phenylalanine by isolated nuclei. Biochim. biophys. Acta (Amst.) **32**, 147—155 (1959).
LUSHBAUGH, C. C., COMAS, F., SAENGER, E. L., JACOBS, M., HOFSTRA, R., ANDREWS, G. A.: Radiosensitivity of man by extrapolation from studies of total body irradiation of patients. Radiat. Res. **27**, 487—488 (1966).
MATHÉ, G., JAMMET, H. P., PENDIC, B., SCHWARZENBERG, L., DUPLAN, J. F., MAUPIN, B., LATARJET, R., LAURIEN, M. J., KALIC, D., DJUKIC, L.: Transfusions et grefes de moelle osseusl homologue chez de humains irradiés à haute dose accidentellement. Rev. Franc. Etudes Clin. Biol. **4**, 226—238 (1959).
MCGRATH, R. A., WILLIAMS, R. W.: Reconstruction *in vivo* of irradiated *Escherichia coli* DNA and the rejoining of broken pieces. Nature (Lond.) **212**, 534—535 (1966).
MCKEE, R. W., BRIN, M.: Effects of x-irradiation on glyconeogenesis, glycogenesis and gluconeogenesis in the rat. Arch. Biochem. Biophys. **61**, 390—396 (1956).
MEAD, J. F.: The irradiation-induced autoxidation of linoleic acid. Science **115**, 470—472 (1952).
MIQUEL, J., KLATZO, I., MENZEL, D. B., HAYMAKER, W.: Glycogen changes in x-irradiated rat brain. Acta neuropath. **2**, 482—493 (1963).
MITCHELL, J. S.: Disturbance of nucleic acid metabolism produced by therapeutic doses of x- and $\gamma$-radiation. III. Inhibition of synthesis of thymonucleic acid by radiation. Brit. J. exp. Path. **23**, 309—315 (1942).
MOSS, A. J., JR, DALRYMPLE, G. V., SANDERS, J. L., WILKINSON, K. P., NASH, J. C.: Dinitrophenol inhibits the rejoining of radiation induced DNA breaks by L cells. Biophys. Soc. Abstr. **11**, 30a (1971).

ORD, M. G., STOCKEN, L. A.: Biochemical effects of x-irradiation and the sulfhydryl hypothesis: a re-appraisal. Nature (Lond.) **200**, 136—138 (1963).
ORD, M. G., STOCKEN, L. A.: Phosphorylation of histones from natural and $\gamma$-irradiated rats. Biochem. J. **101**, 34 P (1966).
ORD, M. G., STOCKEN, L. A.: The biochemical effects of ionizing radiation on nuclear function in animal cells. Proc. Roy. Soc. Edinburgh **70** B, 117—124 (1968).
OSAWA, S., ALLFREY, V., MIRSKY, A. E.: Mononucleotides of the cell nucleus. J. gen. Physiol. **40**, 491—513 (1957).
PALMER, R. F., SULLIVAN, M. F.: Hanford Atomic Prod. Operation Report HW-56414 (17. June 1958).
PATT, H. M., TYREE, E. B., STRAUBE, H. L., SMITH, D. E.: Cysteine protection against x-irradiation. Science **110**, 213—214 (1949).
PAVLOVSKAYA, T. E., VULKOVA, M. S., PASYNSKII, A. G.: Izmenenie svyazyvaniya metionina $S^{35}$ syvorotkoi krovi pri detanuratsii oblucheniem i nagrevaniem. Dokl. A. N. USSR **101**, 723—726 (1955).
PEACOCKE, A. R., PRESTON, B. N.: The action of $\gamma$-rays on sodium deoxyribonucleate in solution. II. Degradation. Proc. Roy. Soc. Lond. Ser. **B**, **153**, 90—102 (1960).
PETROVIĆ, D., MILETIĆ, B., BRDAR, B.: Restoration of viability of x-irradiated L-strain cells by isologous subcelluar fractions. Int. J. Radiat. Biol. **7**, 131—139 (1964).
PHILLIPS, R. A., TOLMACH, L. J.: Repair of potentially lethal damage in x-irradiated HeLa cells. Radiat. Res. **29**, 413—432 (1966).
POLLARD, E. C.: The action of ionizing radiation on the cellular synthesis of protein. In: HARRIS, R. J. C. (Ed.): The initial effects of ionizing radiations on cells, (HARRIS, R. J. C., Ed.). pp. 68—89 New York: Academic Press 1961.
POLLARD, E. C., DAVIS, S. A.: The action of ionizing radiation on transcription (and translation) in several strains of *E. coli*. Radiat. Res. **41**, 375—399 (1970).
POTTER, R. L., BETHELL, F. H.: Oxidative phosphorylation in spleen mitochondria. Fed. Proc. **2**, 270 (1952).
PRUDEN, H., SNIPES, W., GORDY, W.: Electron spin resonance of an irradiated single crystal of thymidine. Proc. nat. Acad. Sci. (Wash.) **53**, 917—924 (1965).
RICHMOND, J. E., ALTMAN, K. I., SOLOMON, K.: The effect of x-radiation on the biosynthesis of hemoglobin. J. biol. Chem. **190**, 817—825 (1951).
ROBBINS, E., BORUN, T. W.: The cytoplasmic synthesis of histones in HeLa cells and its temporal relation to DNA replication. Proc. Nat. Acad. Sci. (Wash.) **57**, 409—416 (1967).
ROBBINS, E., PEDERSON, T.: On the role of ions in mitosis. In Vitro **6**, 323—334 (1971).
RUECKERT, R. R., MUELLER, G. C.: Studies on the unbalanced growth in tissue culture. I. Induction and consequences of thymidine deficiency. Cancer Res. **20**, 1584 (1960).
SCAIFE, J. F., HILL, B.: The uncoupling of oxidative phosphorylation by ionizing radiation. Canad. J. Biochem. Physiol. **40**, 1025—1042 (1962).
SCHOENBERG, M., BROOKS, R., HALL, I., SCHNEIDERMAN, M.: Effect of irradiation on the hyaluronidase-hyaluronic acid system. Arch. Biochem. **30**, 333—340 (1951).
SCHOLES, G., WEISS, J.: Oxygen effect and formation of peroxides in aqueous solutions. Radiat. Res. Suppl. **1**, 177—189 (1959).
SELYE, H.: The physiology and pathology of exposure to stress. Montreal: Acta, Inc. 1950.
SIRE, H. S., GAUTHIER, J., BECKER, R., BOLGER, J.: Blood coagulation factors in total body irradiation. Blood **18**, 702—709 (1961).
SMITH, M. R., FLEMING, D. U., WOOD, W. B., JR.: The effect of acute radiation on phagocytic mechanisms of antibacterial defense. J. Immunol. **90**, 914—924 (1963).
SNIPES, W., HENRIKSEN, T.: Radiation-induced radicals in thymidine single crystals at 77° K. Int. J. Radiat. Biol. **17**, 367—373 (1970).
SOŠKA, J., BENEŠ, L., DRÁŠIL, V., KARPFEL, Z., PALEČEK, E., SKALKA, M.: The significance of free deoxyribonucleotides in radiation damage. In: The initial effects of ionizing radiations on cells, HARRIS, R. J. C. (Ed.): pp. 153—163. New York: Academic Press 1961.
SPARROW, A. H., ROSENFELD, F. M.: X-ray-induced depolymerization of thymonucleohistone and of sodium thymonucleate. Science **104**, 245—248 (1946).
STEVELY, W. S., STOCKEN, L. A.: Phosphorylation of rat thymus histone. Biochem. J. **100**, 20 C (1966).
STEVELY, W. S., STOCKEN, L. A.: Histone phosphorylation and cell division. Biochem. J. **109**, 24 P—25 P (1968).
STOCKEN, L. A.: Some observations on the effects of ionizing radiation on the metabolism of DNA in animal tissues. Advanc. Biol. med. Phys. **12**, 239—243 (1968).
STUDIER, F. W.: Sedimentation studies of the size and shape of DNA. J. molec. Biol. **11**, 373—390 (1965).
SUGINO, Y., POTTER, R. L.: Deoxycytidylic acid deaminase in regenerating rat thymus. Radiat. Res. **12**, 477 (1960).

Sullivan, M. F.: Dependence of radiation diarrhea on the presence of bile in the intestine. Nature (Lond.) **195**, 1217—1218 (1962).
Suter, G. M.: Response of hematopoietic system to x-rays. U.S. Atomic Energy Commission Document MDDC-824 (1947).
Swift, M. N., Taketa, S. T.: Effect on circulating blood volume of partial shielding of rat intestine during x-irradiation. Radiat. Res. **8**, 516—525 (1958).
Taylor, W. D., Ginoza, W.: Correlation of $\gamma$-ray inactivation and strand scission in the replicative form of ∅X174 bacteriophage DNA. Proc. Natl. Acad. Sci. U.S. **58**, 1753—1757 (1967).
van Bekkum, D. W.: The effects of x-rays on phosphorylations *in vivo*. Biochim. biophys. Acta (Amst.) **25**, 487—493 (1957).
Warren, S. L., Whipple, G. H.: Roentgen ray intoxication. I. Bacterial invasion of the blood stream as influenced by x-ray destruction of the mucosal epithelium of the small intestine. J. exp. Med. **38**, 713—723 (1923).
Whitfield, J. F.: How radiation causes cell death. Euratom Bull. **4**, 116—121 (1965).
Whitfield, J. F., Brohee, H., Youdale, T.: Changes in nuclear histone of irradiated rat thymocytes. Exp. Cell Res. **36**, 417—421 (1964).
Winchell, H. S., Vimoksant, S. L., Raley, R. B.: Relative effects of radiation on *de novo* DNA base synthesis and thymidine incorporation into DNA. University of California Radiation Laboratory Report UCRL-18347, 149—154 (1968).
Wolfrom, M. L., Binkley, W. W., McCabe, L. I., Shenhan, T. M., Michelakis, A. M.: The effect of ionizing radiations on carbohydrates. Radiat. Res. **10**, 37—47 (1959).

Chapter 24

# Radiation Research: Survival Kinetics

L. J. Tolmach and L. E. Hopwood

With 7 Figures

## Introduction

The lethal action of ionizing radiations on mammalian cells has been observed for almost as long as the existence of these radiations has been known, but even today, with a large body of experimental observations at our disposal, understanding of the mechanisms by which the initial deposition of energy and breakage of chemical bonds lead to cell death is far from complete. Nevertheless, significant progress has been made in recent years, largely through the application of kinetic analysis. This discussion will be restricted mainly to kinetic aspects of cell killing by x- and $\gamma$-rays; only cursory consideration will be given to the molecular bases of the phenomena and the cellular organelles involved. It will be apparent that many of the concepts and experimental approaches mentioned apply also to the lethal action of cytotoxic drugs.

## A. Cell Killing

Because of the profound differences that exist among mammalian cells, and the complexity of the lethal process(es), the term cell killing must be clearly defined. For differentiated cells that do not proliferate, such as nerve, muscle, or secretory cells, death can be defined as the loss of specific function. For proliferating cells such as hematopoietic stem cells or cells growing in culture, the microbiological definition, loss of the capacity for sustained proliferation ("reproductive death"), is appropriate. Not only can this function be assessed quite accurately by measuring the colony-forming ability of the cells, or their capacity to initiate tumor growth, but proliferation is a particularly meaningful end-point in the treatment of neoplasia because the use of radiation, like cytotoxic drugs, in cancer therapy is based on its ability to prevent proliferation of the cancer cells. In general, destruction of differentiated cell function in nonproliferating systems requires much higher radiation doses (of the order of 20 krads) than does inactivation of proliferative capacity: mean lethal doses are usually less than 200 rads. It is evident, however, that a cell, or the progeny of a cell, which has been irradiated and has lost its capacity for sustained proliferation will sooner or later lose both morphological and physiological integrity, and cell death can be examined in terms of these changes as well, even for proliferating cells exposed to moderate doses of radiation. Hence, the particular criterion of cell death that is under consideration in any discussion must be clearly specified. Here we will be concerned with both loss of proliferative capacity and subsequent cellular disintegration.

### B. Loss of Proliferative Capacity

The ability of a cell to grow into a macroscopic colony is a convenient measure of its capacity for sustained proliferation. The loss of this ability as a function of the dose of radiation is described by the dose-survival curve. Such curves provide a useful way of correlating data pertaining to various types of cells growing or treated under different conditions; their study constitutes an important area of cellular radiation biology.

Radiation survival data for many different lines of mammalian cells, malignant and normal, growing *in vivo* and *in vitro*, have been reported, analyzed, and reviewed in depth. The treatise by Elkind and Whitmore (1967) presents the pertinent theoretical background and a thorough discussion of the experimental techniques and data, as well as their inadequacies. The volume of Okada (1970) provides a more recent compilation of relevant data. Because of the great similarity in the response of different types of cells to irradiation, as attested to by the data summarized in these and other publications (e. g. Whitmore and Till, 1964), the present discussion will adopt the point of view that despite measurable variations among cells in their radiation response, all dose-survival curves are qualitatively and quantitatively similar, and that the dose-response of most types of cells depends in a predictable fashion on the conditions under which the radiation is applied.

### C. Postirradiation Growth and Cell Disintegration

Mammalian cells subjected to moderate, though lethal, doses of x-rays do not lose their proliferative, metabolic, or morphological integrity immediately, but continue to metabolize for some time, and will usually undergo several rounds of growth and division during which a variety of abnormalities may be manifested. Study of postirradiation growth can provide information important for elucidating the mechanisms by which the initial molecular lesions develop and ultimately cause cell destruction. Furthermore, in the case of human tumors, postirradiation change in tumor mass is the most immediate, albeit unreliable, information the therapist obtains about the response to treatment. In addition, optimization of treatment with respect to such factors as dose fractionation or the application of combined therapeutic agents requires knowledge of the growth kinetics of the cells that are being treated. Hence, the kinetics of cell proliferation following insult by radiation constitutes another important area of cellular radiation biology.

Information about postirradiation growth kinetics, as derived especially from time-lapse cinemicrographic studies, is more recent and less abundant than are data concerning loss of proliferative capacity; accordingly, it will be discussed in some detail. We will not be concerned, however, with the radiation responses of lymphoid cells whose postirradiation behavior is not typical of most cell types [i.e. cells which undergo disintegration within a few hours even after treatment with only moderate x-ray doses (Okada, 1970, Chapter VII)].

## Loss of Proliferative Capacity

### A. Theoretical Considerations

X-radiation consists of packets of electromagnetic energy called photons, which behave as particles that travel with the speed of light and have no rest mass. Their energy is often in the range 1 to 300 KeV (wave length 0.004 to 1 nm). $\gamma$-Rays are identical except for their origin; they arise in nuclear reactions. The average amount of energy deposited in each interaction of such a photon with matter, 60 eV, is enough to break any chemical bond in a cell (RAUTH and SIMPSON, 1964), and is independent of the cell's molecular composition, since all cellular constituents have approximately the same atomic composition. Thus, the interaction of x-rays with the cell results in a number of random and independent primary ionizations; the larger the dose, the more ionizations occur. This characteristic led to the development of the target theory (LEA, 1955) which, in its simplest form, is based on the idea that one crucial primary ionization (hit) per cell is lethal. In a population of cells irradiated with a very small dose, a certain number of cells will be hit. As the dose is increased, this numbei increases, but because the probability that some of the hits will occur in cells that have already been hit increases also, the dependence is not linear with dose, but rather approaches 100% asymptotically. Poisson statistics apply; at an average of one hit per cell, for example, 37% ($1/e$) of the cells will not have received any hits, 37% will have sustained one hit, and the remainder will have received two or more hits. Thus, if the fraction of surviving cells (i. e. cells receiving no hits) is plotted against the dose, a curve with a continuously decreasing slope (exponential) is obtained. The number of cells inactivated by a given increment of dose is less at large doses than at smaller doses, but the fraction of the remaining viable cells inactivated is identical for each equal increment of dose. This is expressed mathematically by the relation

$$\frac{-dN}{N} = kdD,$$

where $N$ is the number of viable cells, $dN$ is the increment killed when the incremental dose $dD$ is applied, and $k$ is a proportionality constant. On integration, this yields the relation

$$\log_e (N/N_0) = -kD,$$

or

$$N/N_0 = S = \exp(-kD),$$

where $N_0$ is the number of viable cells before the dose $D$ is applied, and $S$ is the surviving fraction of cells. Thus, the fraction of cells surviving decreases exponentially with dose, and a plot of the logarithm of the surviving fraction against dose gives a straight line.

Dose survival curves for viruses exposed to x-rays were indeed found to be exponential (LEA, 1955). The target size can be calculated from the survival curve and radiation parameters; in several instances it was found to correspond to the size of the virus (LEA, 1955), or to its nucleic acid content (EPSTEIN, 1953), as determined by other methods. In these cases, therefore, one hit occurring anywhere in the "cell", or in its genome, is lethal. While much of the damage sustained by a cell is presumably the result of ionizations occurring directly in critical structures, chemically reactive free radicals are also produced in the surrounding volume, and these can diffuse to the critical sites and there produce similar damage ("indirect effect"). The distance over which such free radicals can diffuse before reacting is of the order of 3 nm (HUTCHINSON, 1961). Hence, this phenomenon effetively increases the size of the target.

With bacteria that exhibit simple exponential survival curves, the calculated target size is considerably smaller than the cell or its genome (KAPLAN and MOSES, 1964; SPARROW et al., 1967). This discrepancy can reflect differential effectiveness of ionizations that occur in a restricted portion of the cell (i. e. the target); it might also arise from the intervention of repair processes subsequent to irradiation. Under certain conditions, bacteria and mammalian cells generally have been found to respond less to low doses of x-rays than predicted from simple target theory: there is a "shoulder" region on the survival curve where an increment of dose has little effect on the surviving fraction (Fig. 1). Curves of this type

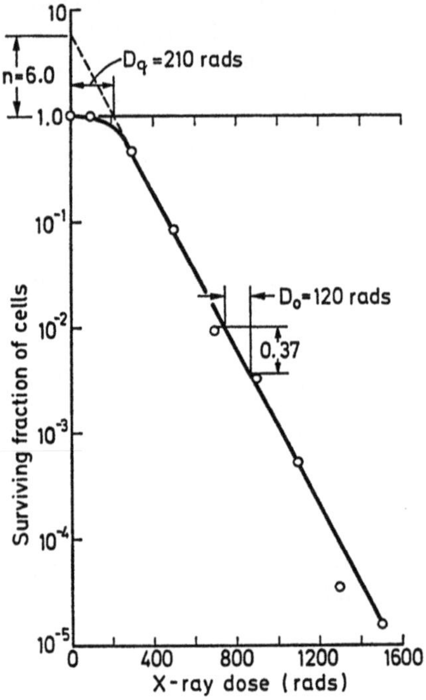


Fig. 1. Dose-survival curve for Chinese hamster CHO cells. Samples of (synchronous) cells, plated in growth medium, were irradiated (in mid-$G_1$) with graded doses of 220 kV x-rays, and incubated for 8 days. The number of colonies was then scored and the surviving fraction calculated. The method of estimating the survival curve parameters, assuming the curve to be exponential after the initial shoulder, is shown. The value 0.37 indicates the surviving fraction at the lower arrow if that at the upper arrow is taken as 1.0

are generally characterized by two parameters: the slope ($-k$) of the exponential region ($1/k$ is denoted $D_0$) and the extrapolation of this line on the ordinate (denoted $n$). The extrapolation number provides a measure of the width of the "shoulder." A related and sometimes more useful measure is the quasi-threshold dose, $D_q$, which is the intercept of the extrapolated exponential line on the abscissa at 100% survival (Alper et al., 1962). The relation between the three parameters is given by:

$$D_q = D_0 \log_e n.$$

None of them specify the shape of the curve in the shoulder region.

The existence of a region of smaller response at low doses implies that radiation damage must accumulate before it is lethal. This type of dose-response can be accommodated into target theory by postulating a multiplicity of identical targets, all of which must be inactivated before the cell is killed, yielding the multitarget, single-hit relation:

$$S = 1\text{-}[1\text{-}\exp(\text{-}kD)]^n.$$

Other elaborations of target theory provide for a number of discrete hits being required to inactivate a single target (the single-target, multi-hit model) and for both a multi-target and multi-hit condition. While the multi-hit relation does not yield a strict exponential response even at high doses, the deviation would generally be difficult to demonstrate, so that distinction between the models cannot be made on experimental grounds (BENDER and GOOCH, 1962).

These theoretical formulations can provide a useful basis for comparing data, but the target model on which they are based is generally a vast oversimplification, and they have not provided a great deal of insight into the fundamental cellular processes that occur as a consequence of irradiation. For example, their utility in estimating target sizes is severely compromised by the intervention of repair processes. Nevertheless, there is considerable evidence that irradiation of all the regions of a eukaryotic cell is not equally effective in producing cellular damage, i. e., that targets do exist even if target theory is generally inadequate for quantitative prediction. In particular, the nucleus is a much more effective target than is the cytoplasm (MUNRO, 1959; MARIN and BENDER, 1963). Furthermore, allowing for inefficiencies (e. g. energy degradation to heat, without bond breakage), the breakage of a few thousand bonds distributed throughout the entire nucleus is sufficient to bring about cell death. This indicates that the initial damage is greatly amplified, and suggests that the cell's genetic apparatus, in which amplification of information is of course a normal function, is the target likely to sustain the primary lethal damage. There are a number of additional indications of intimate genetic involvement in cellular response to irradiation: chromosome aberrations are produced (e. g. DEWEY and HUMPHREY, 1964), DNA synthesis is affected, mutations arise, and physiological death is delayed several generations (i. e. the damage is inherited but its expression is delayed) (PUCK, 1959). However, other potential targets are not excluded.

## B. *In Vitro* Determination of Dose-Survival Curves

The first dose-survival curve for a mammalian cell was obtained by PUCK and MARCUS (1956), using their *in vitro* single-cell plating technique (PUCK and MARCUS, 1955; PUCK et al., 1956). This technique, which exploits the capacity of cells to proliferate into colonies after disaggregation of an *in vitro* culture, or even, in some cases, of intact tissue, provided the means whereby the sensitivity of cells to radiation could be examined in terms of loss of the capacity for sustained proliferation. Employing the HeLa S3 strain (the clonal isolation of which had also been carried out by means of single-cell plating), they found that the dose-survival curve was apparently exponential with a shoulder region at low doses, $D_0$ and $n$ having the values 130 rads and 2, respectively.

The dose-survival curves subsequently obtained for different cultured cell lines have shown essentially the same characteristics as those for HeLa S3 cells: a region of increasing response followed by an exponential curve. In addition, virtually all subsequent measurements have yielded values of $D_0$ remarkably similar to that for HeLa cells, reported values being between about 50 and 300 rads (WHITMORE and TILL, 1964). Extrapolation numbers are generally found to fall in the region 1 to 10, though higher values have sometimes been reported. There is almost as much variation found within one cell line, as measured by different investigators, as among different cell lines. The property of malignancy does not influence the value of $D_0$; for example, an extended series of benzpyrene-induced rat fibrosarcomas yielded $D_0$ values ranging from 81 to 737 rads (though most of the values were below 300 rads), and $n$ values from 1 to 5, when their x-ray response was measured *in vitro* 1 to 120 days after explantation (MADOC-JONES et al., 1968).

Neither does the chromosomal content appear to play an important role at least among closely related cell lines; for example, various sublines of mouse L cells with mean chromosome numbers, and probably chromatin content, differing more than two-fold, yielded identical survival curves (TILL, 1961). [There is, however, an inverse relation between DNA content and $D_0$ among cells of different species (SPARROW et al., 1967). Indeed, among the viruses, monera, and protista, as well as cells of higher organisms, several groups of species (sometimes phylogenetically related) can be distinguished on the basis of the proportionality factor. Mammalian cells, together with certain yeasts and bacteria, appear to constitute one such group.]

It should be noted that some published survival curves do not show any exponential region, but instead have a continuously increasing slope (BARENDSEN et al., 1960). In this case it is impossible to obtain the previously described parameters. It is not certain that measurements yielding such curves are entirely free from experimental artifacts, but if they do accurately represent the response of a cell population, they might arise from the occurrence of more than one kind of lethal damage, each having a different dose-response. Another type of deviation from the usual shape of the dose-survival curve involves a decrease in slope at some point in the exponential region. Such a curve can arise from heterogeneity in the population's sensitivity, (e. g. POWERS and TOLMACH, 1963).

## C. *In Vivo* Determinations of Dose-Survival Curves

A single general method is not applicable for the generation of cell survival curves *in vivo*, though in several instances, techniques conceptually identical to the *in vitro* colony-forming method are available. For example, survival curves for bone marrow stem cells (MCCULLOCH and TILL, 1962) and for lymphoma cells as well (BRUCE and VAN DER GAAG, 1963), irradiated either *in situ* or *in vitro*, can be determined by scoring the number of colonies that develop in the spleens of lethally irradiated recipient mice. (For the bone marrow cell assay, the recipients must be pre-irradiated with a dose of about 1000 rads.) A small fraction of the cells infiltrate and colonize the spleen; the colonies appear as nodules which can be counted easily after proper fixation. $D_0$ and $n$ values of about 100 rads and 2.0, respectively, have been reported.

An alternative method of measurement has yielded similar results. When mammals are irradiated with whole-body doses of the order of 1000 rads, they normally die within 9 to 14 days from infection and hemorrhage resulting from the depletion of leukocytes with rapid turn-over times. By injecting isologous bone marrow cells, an animal can be "rescued," and the loss of the ability of the transplanted cells to effect such rescue, as a function of x-ray dose delivered to the marrow, can be determined. $D_0$ values ranging from 71 to 115 rads and values of $n$ from 1 to 2.5 have been found (MCCULLOCH and TILL, 1960).

Measurements of the radiation response of skin epithelial cells and of stem cells in the crypts of the jejunum have been carried out, again using colony formation, this time *in situ*, as the end-point. A ring of skin is irradiated with a large dose (e. g. 3000 rads) to define an area, initially shielded, that is subsequently irradiated with a specific smaller dose. Cells surviving in the test area form nodules (i. e. colonies), the heavily irradiated ring providing a barrier against migrating cells from the surrounding untreated region. The dose of radiation and the size of the test field are adjusted to yield a number of nodules small enough to ensure that each arises from a single cell. Survival can be measured over only a limited dose range, and since no value can be determined for zero or low doses, the extrapolation number cannot be determined, but the value of $D_0$ reported for the mouse is again close to that for other mammalian cells, 135 rads (WITHERS, 1967). A similar procedure, involving exteriorization of the jejunum, has been described for studying the radiation response of intestinal epithelial cells (WITHERS and ELKIND, 1969). A segment, terminated at both ends by heavily irradiated regions, is given the test dose, and the number of viable crypts is scored several days after the laparotomy and irradiation were performed. A $D_0$ value of about 100 rads, and an estimated value of *n* of about 40, have been reported for the mouse (WITHERS and ELKIND, 1969).

For malignant cells that are maintained by serial transplantation in isologous animals, the induction of a tumor, or death of the animal from proliferation of the malignant cells, provide useful criteria of cell death, often in conjunction with an end-point dilution procedure (HEWITT, 1958). Indeed, shortly after the dose-survival curve for HeLa cells was described, the radiation response of mouse leukemia cells was measured by such a method (HEWITT and WILSON, 1959). As in *in vitro* experiments, the fraction of cancer cells surviving irradiation is based on non-irradiated controls, but the change in the number of cells required to produce the adopted end-point, rather than in the number of proliferating cells, is determined; the latter is then inferred from the former. It is convenient to use as an end-point the number of cells needed to induce tumors in one-half of a group of test animals ($TD_{50}$), or to kill one-half of a group ($LD_{50}$). For example, the 6C3HED mouse lymphosarcoma requires about 3 cells to produce a tumor and kill the animal (POWERS et al., 1967); for a solid CBA mouse sarcoma, the $TD_{50}$ is 85 cells (HEWITT and WILSON, 1961); while for Ehrlich ascites cells the $TD_{50}$ depends on the age of the recipient, 1.4 cells being required for 1 to 2 day old mice and 6000 cells for 50 day old animals (SILINI and HORNSEY, 1961). Immediately following irradiation of the tumor cells, the $TD_{50}$ (or $LD_{50}$) will of course be increased, as some or most of the cells will not be viable; measurement of this increase permits construction of a dose-survival curve. For the three types of cells mentioned, the survival curves are amazingly similar: $D_0$ ranges from 110 to 165 rads, and *n* from about 1 to 2.4 (except for the hypotetraploid Ehrlich ascites cells) (SILINI and HORNSEY, 1962).

From these examples, it is clear that the sensitivities of mammalian cells irradiated *in vivo* are closely similar to sensitivities measured *in vitro*, and when the same cell system is irradiated *in situ* or *in vitro*, nearly identical results are obtained (McCULLOCH and TILL, 1962; PHILPOTT et al., 1962). Hence, the environment would not appear to play any large role in the radiation response of a cell's proliferative ability. That it does play a measurable role, however, and very likely a crucial role with respect to cancer therapy, will become clear in the subsequent discussion.

## D. Modulation of the Dose-Survival Response

A number of factors, physical, chemical, and biological, affect the responses of cells to ionizing radiations. One such factor is the submicroscopic distribution of energy deposition in the irradiated material. This is conveniently and approximately measured by the average linear energy transfer (LET) of the radiation (i. e. the rate of energy loss along the path traveled by the particle). The LET increases with increasing mass and charge of the ionizing particle, and decreases with increasing energy. The relative biological effectiveness (RBE), as compared with that of 200 kV x-rays (LET about 1.5 keV/μm), increases several fold as the

LET of the radiation increases to 100 to 200 keV/μm, and then decreases (BARENDSEN et al., 1963). This phenomenon presumably arises from the fact that with increasing LET there is more energy deposition during the passage of a single particle through the structure (target) whose damage results in the biological effect under study. Indeed, the shape of the dose-survival curve changes with LET such that the shoulder disappears and the curve approaches a pure exponential. As the LET increases still further, the efficiency of the process decreases because the probability of multiple traverses of a given target increases, and the RBE drops.

A second factor affecting the response of cells is temporal fractionation of the dose. It was found by ELKIND and coworkers (ELKIND and SUTTON, 1959) that the effect of a given dose is diminished if the radiation is delivered in two or more fractions separated by several hours, and that the phenomenon is intimately related to the shoulder portion of the dose-survival curve. That is, the damage, whose accumulation is responsible for the smaller response to x-rays at low doses, is in part sublethal, and the cell can recover from it. Fractionation of the dose permits that recovery to take place, so that the dose needed to obtain a given amount of cell killing is increased. Recovery is generally maximal in two hours; it is inhibited at 5° (BERRY and OLIVER, 1964), and possibly by anoxia (RÉVÉSZ and LITTBRAND, 1964). Under conditions in which a single exponential dose-survival curve obtains, as with high-LET radiations, there is no sublethal damage accumulated, and fractionation of the dose does not affect the response (BARENDSEN, 1962). This phenomenon has obvious implications for the radiotherapy of tumors, where fractionation of the dose is the usual practice.

Given the vast number of chemical changes that can be expected following radiation insult of the chemically complex cell, together with the operation of repair processes, it is not surprising that modulation of the response to a given dose of radiation can be effected by a variety of chemical agents; irradiation in their presence can either increase or decrease the response to x-rays. Oxygen has long been known to modify the effect of a given dose, typically increasing it by a factor of two to three over that obtained when the radiation is delivered under anoxic conditions. Sensitization occurs at low oxygen tension; it is maximal at a partial pressure of only 30 mm Hg (DEWEY, 1963). Presumably, the formation of free radicals is enhanced, thereby increasing the amount of primary damage to the system. Nitric oxide appears to act in a similar fashion, and the action of the stable free radical triacetoneamine *N*-oxyl (PARKER et al., 1969) might possibly be related. The oxygen effect is presumably quite important in the radiotherapy of solid tumors, the interior of which may be poorly vascularized and hence severely hypoxic (e. g. POWERS and TOLMACH, 1964). Clinical exploitation of differences in the state of oxygenation of tumor and normal tissue has been under study for some time. (See WITHERS, 1973, for a recent discussion of the basis for the clinical application of high-LET radiations, with which cells show a smaller sensitivity enhancement by oxygen than they do with x-rays.)

Certain other agents, such as actinomycin D, presumably enhance the action of x-rays by themselves contributing lesions similar to and/or in the same molecules as those produced by the radiation (ELKIND, 1971). Still other agents, such as *N*-ethyl maleimide, may inactivate protective agents that are normally present in cells. Treatment of cells with nontoxic concentrations of any of a number of metabolic inhibitors can influence survival. Often, survival can be modified by either pre- or postirradiation treatment (e. g. PHILLIPS and TOLMACH, 1966). The irradiated cell contains damage that is only potentially lethal; its expression presumably depends in part on the particular metabolic state of the cell.

A very different sort of sensitization of cells to x-rays can be brought about by growing them previously in the presence of halogenated derivatives of uracil, such as bromodeoxyuridine, which are substituted for the thymidine in the newly synthesized cellular DNA (Djordjevic and Szybalski, 1960). This sensitization constitutes one indication that the target for the lethal action of the radiation is DNA.

Protective agents (i. e. those whose presence at the time of irradiation results in a smaller cellular response to a given dose) include a number of sulfhydryl-containing compounds such as cysteamine, and certain polyalcohols. Such agents presumably react with short-lived free radicals that are produced by the ionization.

A number of biological factors affect the response to x-rays. For example, the growth status of a cell culture at the time of irradiation [i. e. whether it is actively proliferating (log phase) or in a resting state (stationary phase)] affects the survival curve parameters (Little, 1969; Hahn, 1970).

The age of the cell in the generation cycle is another significant determinant of its response to radiation (Terasima and Tolmach, 1961, 1963) and to virtually all other cytotoxic agents that have been examined (Mauro and Madoc-Jones, 1970). Study of this phenomenon is greatly facilitated by applying some sort of synchronization procedure to permit all of the cells of a culture to progress through the cycle more or less in phase. Using mitosis and DNA synthesis to mark their progress, it has been found that the survival curve parameters fluctuate in a

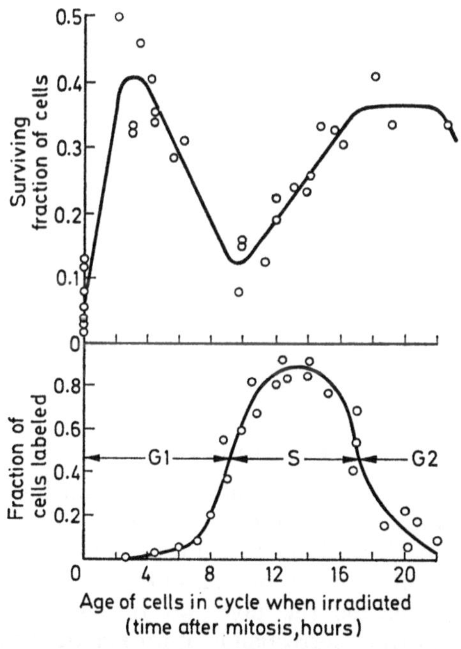


Fig. 2. Upper curve: Changes in the lethal response of HeLa S3 cells to a 500 rad dose of 220 kV x-rays as the cells progress through the generation cycle (the age-response for loss of proliferative ability). Samples of synchronous cells were irradiated at different times after mitotic collection. The fraction of cells giving rise to colonies was scored after 10 days of incubation. In this system $D_0$ shows greater age dependence than does $n$. Lower curve: The position of the cell population in the cycle at the time of irradiation was determined by measuring the fraction of cells, in parallel cultures, labeled by a 20 min exposure to $^3$H-thymidine. The median durations of the phases are shown. For both curves, data have been combined from several experiments after normalization for variations in the generation time

regular fashion as the cells traverse the cycle. Changes in either $D_0$ or $n$, or both, are found, the former varying more than 3-fold between the most and least sensitive stages. It is convenient to choose one particular dose and measure changes in survival as a function of age at that dose (the age-response, Fig. 2). Since either $n$ or $D_0$ may vary, the age-response will depend on the dose selected, changes in $n$ predominating at small doses, and in $D_0$ at large doses.

Changes in sensitivity appear to occur continuously throughout the cycle, often exhibiting complicated patterns (e. g. HeLa S3 cells show two maxima and two minima in $D_0$ during a single cycle). Nevertheless, certain generalizations may be valid (Sinclair, 1968): cells are most sensitive when they are in mitosis, and sensitivity decreases as cells progress through $S$, and increases again in $G_2$. Behavior during $G_1$ is more difficult to characterize; this phase is the most variable in duration among different cell lines, as well as among the cells of a given culture. In those lines with a long $G_1$ phase (i. e. $>6$ h), there is usually a resistant period in the early part, with sensitivity increasing to a maximum at the transition from $G_1$ to $S$. While most age-response studies have been carried out with cells in culture, analogous responses have been found *in vivo* for lymphoma cells (Mauro and Madoc-Jones, 1969; Madoc-Jones and Mauro, 1970) and bone marrow stem cells (Chaffey and Hellman, 1971). Though age-response functions must play a role in the response of tumors to radiation therapy, it has not yet been possible to exploit them clinically (Withers, 1973). They are, however, an important consideration in the chemotherapy of leukemia (Skipper, 1971).

## Postirradiation Growth and Cell Disintegration

Measurement of cell killing in terms of loss of colony forming ability provides little information about the cytological processes and molecular mechanisms by which cell death occurs. As mentioned earlier, lethally irradiated cells, except for lymphoid cells, are generally able to divide at least once before the cessation of proliferation and, ultimately, anabolic activity; in the original experiments of Puck and Marcus (1956), abortive colonies, in which the cells had permanently stopped proliferating, were observed several days after irradiation, as were giant cells. Clearly, the "death" of an irradiated cell is a prolonged and complicated process, and study of the behavior of the irradiated population during the post-irradiation period is pertinent to its elucidation. Indeed, several radiation induced perturbations in cell growth and in macromolecular synthesis are readily observed.

### A. Mitotic Delay

The most obvious perturbation in cell proliferation following irradiation is a delay in mitosis: the mitotic index temporarily falls to zero in an asynchronous population within about $^1/_2$ h after exposure (Whitmore et al., 1961; Yamada and Puck, 1961). Cells this close to mitosis enter into and complete the process without delay, but cells behind this point are reversibly inhibited from further progression. The critical time corresponds approximately to the point at which inhibition of protein synthesis prevents the cell from entering mitosis (Walters and Petersen, 1968). This point of blockade in $G_2$ is independent of dose and apparently of cell line. The duration of the delay is dose-dependent and usually seems to be approximately linear with dose, with a proportionality constant often in the range 0.3 to 1.0 min per rad. Release from the $G_2$ blockade is spontaneous; it does not occur in the absence of protein synthesis, nor at low temperature. After release, the cells proceed through mitosis in seemingly normal fashion and divide. In most instances the mitotic index then exceeds the normal level. This occurs because the duration of the mitotic delay is age-dependent; after an initial drop in the duration of delay for cells irradiated early in $G_1$ as compared with those irradiated in $M$, cells show increasing delay on being irradiated at progressively later stages in the cell cycle, at least until late S phase, as shown in Fig. 3 for HeLa cells (TERASIMA and TOLMACH, 1963). Indeed, with a large enough dose,

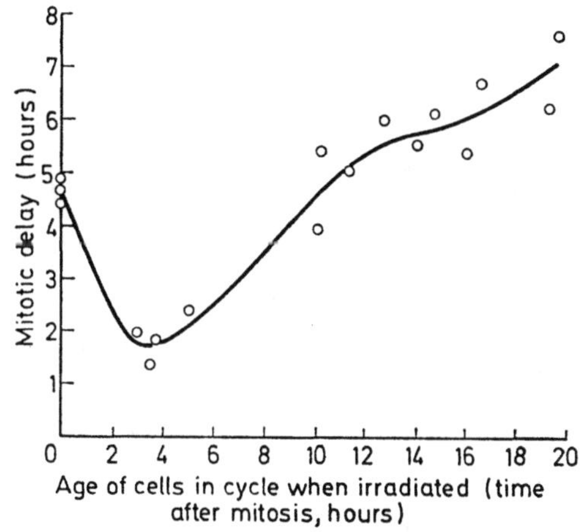


Fig. 3. Changes in mitotic delay as HeLa S3 cells are irradiated with 300 rad doses of 220 kV x-rays at different times in the generation cycle (age-response for mitotic delay). Data from a number of experiments are shown, after normalization for variations in the generation time of the controls. Cell survival (i. e. colony forming ability) after this dose is given in Fig. 2. These data were obtained by repetitive scoring of the number of cells in selected microscopic fields

cells that are in early $S$ at the time of irradiation can overtake those in $G_2$. Thus, a large fraction of the population can reach $M$ at about the same time (i. e. they are partially synchronized), with consequent overshoot of the normal mitotic index. It is noteworthy that all of the cells of an irradiated population show mitotic delay, irrespective of whether or not they will give rise to colonies; delay can be detected at doses as small as 9 rads (PUCK and STEFFEN, 1963).

Whereas all cell lines examined show a postirradiation block in $G_2$, the effect of irradiation on progression through the other phases of the cycle is not completely clear. The general finding is that cells in $M$ at the time of irradiation pass normally into $G_1$, and the duration of $G_1$ is only slightly altered, since cells pass into $S$ with minimal delay (LEEPER et al., 1973). However, a delay in $S$ is regularly observed: this is accompanied by a decreased rate of DNA synthesis (LAJTHA et al., 1958; PAINTER, 1962). The phenomenon persists for several hours after irradiation, but is not constant during this period; a plot of incorporation of radioactive precursors of DNA into acid-insoluble form decreases to a minimum, compared to controls, 1 to 3 h after irradiation, and then recovers as shown in Fig. 4 (WEISS, 1971). In fact, the curve surpasses 100% because the $S$ phase is prolonged in the irradiated cells. Thus, the cell makes DNA at a lower rate and for an extended time, thereby synthesizing a full complement. This is not true in subsequent generations; for example, the average rate and amount of synthesis in HeLa S3 cells irradiated with 500 rads during $G_1$ is about 65% of normal in the generation following irradiation (the $S$ phase is not prolonged), and analogous behavior occurs in Chinese hamster cells (Fig. 5). Deficient DNA synthesis in the postirradiation generations has been correlated with failure of the cell to complete mitosis (i. e. permanent mitotic arrest) (Hopwood and Tolmach, 1971).

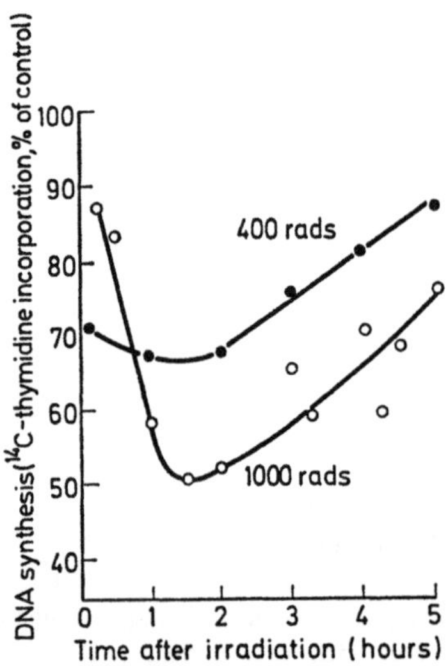


Fig. 4

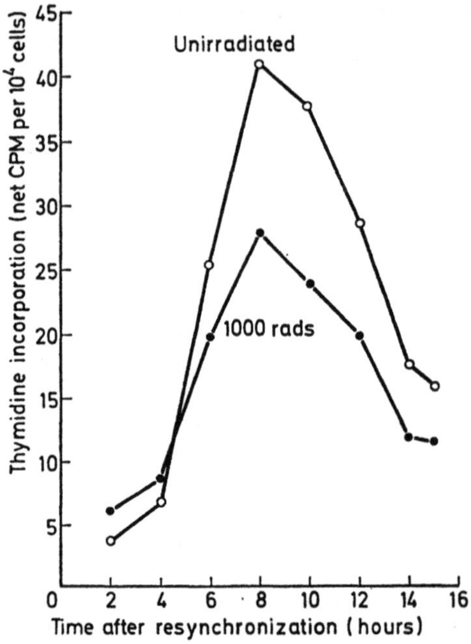


Fig. 5

Fig. 4. DNA synthesis in cultures of HeLa S3 cells shortly after irradiation with either 400 or 1000 rads of 220 kV x-rays. $^{14}$C-Thymidine was added to parallel cultures for 30 min at the times indicated, after which the cultures were washed with trichloroacetic acid and counted for radioactivity. The data presented are averages for several experiments, some employing randomly dividing cultures and others using synchronous cultures in the *S* phase. Though greater inhibition, relative to the unirradiated controls examined at the same times, occurs at the higher dose, the initial fall in the rate is faster at the lower dose, and the minima occur at the same time

Fig. 5. DNA synthesis in cultures of Chinese hamster CHO cells during the generation subsequent to the one in which they were irradiated with 1000 rads of 220 kV x-rays during $G_1$. Synchronous cultures were irradiated 2.5 h after mitotic collection; mitotic selection was repeated at the next wave of mitosis (i. e. resynchronization), and $^{14}$C-thymidine was added to parallel samples for 30 min at the times indicated. Cultures were monitored by cinemicrography to confirm that no significant loss of cells occurred up to the end of the experiment. The area under the curve for 1000 rads is 71% of that under the control curve

## B. Cell Disintegration (Physiological Death)

With the aid of time-lapse cinemicrography, it is possible to observe the permanent cessation of proliferation in lethally irradiated cells. This can usually be correlated with gross morphological alterations, or with loss of normal physiological activity (e. g. cell movement). That is, cells that fail to complete a generation and divide, usually undergo some observable degenerative process, though there have been reports of cells ceasing to divide without exhibiting any obvious disintegration during observation over several generation times (Thompson and Suit, 1969). In this section we shall refer to cell disintegration as death.

Cell death may occur when the cell is in either mitosis or interphase. Under certain conditions there is a high incidence of death in mitosis; e. g. in HeLa S3 cells that have received a dose of 500 rads, the first observable death occurs during the second postirradiation mitosis, and 75% of the cells that ultimately die (roughly 5% of the cells yield colonies at this dose) do so in mitosis (HURWITZ and TOLMACH, 1969a). At larger doses death occurs sooner after irradiation, and a larger fraction of cells undergoes interphase death. The moribund HeLa cell may remain in mitotic arrest for up to 24 h before dying, and there is no preferred time of death during this period, but recognizable disintegration always occurs. Examination of the arrested cells reveals abnormal metaphase configurations: fused chromatin, and scattered or lagging chromosomes (TOLMACH, 1961; HOPWOOD, 1971). Multipolar mitoses are frequent, but many of these are completed. Since these abnormal configurations are also evident in the mitosis preceding the fatal one, they are not necessarily immediately fatal *per se*. Death of a cell in interphase may occur at any time during the intermitotic period. Because there is no way to predict its occurrence, cells destined to die in interphase cannot be isolated, and study of the phenomenon is therefore difficult.

The ability of cells to complete division at the end of the generation in which they are irradiated is dependent on the dose to which they are exposed. At very large doses (i. e. greater than 20 krads) proliferating cells immediately lose their structural integrity, as evidenced by their failure to exclude substances such as

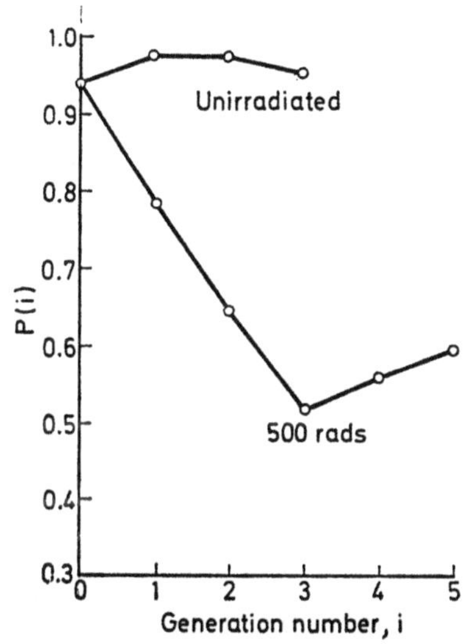


Fig. 6. Cell division in the first six generations after irradiation of HeLa S3 cultures with a 500 rad dose of 220 kV x-rays. *P(i)* is the frequency with which a cell that enters generation *i* completes the next division. These data were obtained from time-lapse cinemicrographs of six separate synchronous cultures irradiated at various times in the cell cycle

trypan blue, and by their loss of intracellular macromolecules (GOLDSTEIN and OKADA, 1969). This response may be equivalent to that of nonproliferating cells that lose functional integrity at similar doses. In the 5 to 20 krad dose range, most cells fail to divide even once, but loss of morphological integrity is delayed for several hours, after which the cells die in interphase. In the dose region below 5 krads, the cell may be able to undergo one or more rounds of division before morphological and physiological death occurs in either interphase or mitosis (Fig. 6).

Because the modes of death are so dissimilar, extrapolation of radiation effects from large doses to the small dose region, where the dose-survival response is measured, is unjustified; the mechanism(s) responsible for death at large doses may not occur at small doses.

## C. Other Kinetic Parameters

Postirradiation growth can be further characterized by the duration of the postirradiation generations, the number of divisions completed, the occurrence of cell fusion and giant cell formation. The increased duration of the irradiated generation has already been discussed. The durations of the postirradiation generations are also increased, though that of the first postirradiation generation may be close to normal, as seen in Fig. 7 (Froese, 1966; Hurwitz and Tolmach,

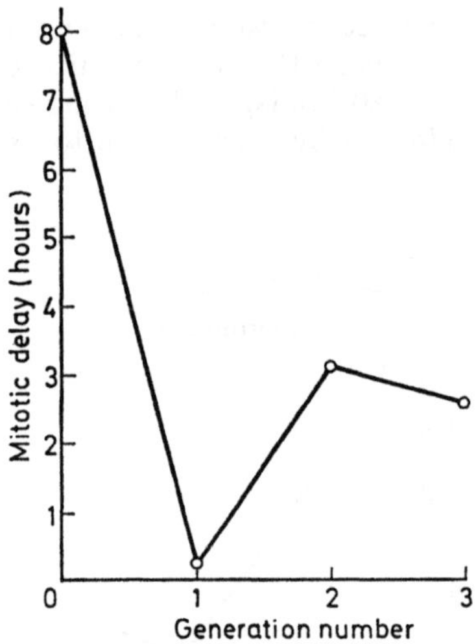


Fig. 7. Average mitotic delay in the first four generations after irradiation of HeLa S3 cells with a 500 rad dose of 220 kV x-rays. These data were obtained from the same time-lapse cinemicrographs as were examined in the experiment shown in Fig. 6

1969a). These delays appear to differ from delay in the irradiated generation in that they lack strong age or dose dependences, are of shorter duration, and are most pronounced in those cells that are destined to undergo fewest additional divisions (Hurwitz and Tolmach, 1969a; Thompson and Suit, 1969).

For HeLa S3 cells receiving doses of less than about 800 rads, virtually all cells complete one division (Hurwitz and Tolmach, 1969a); for mouse L cells the corresponding dose is 400 rads (Trott and Hug, 1970), while for Chinese hamster V-79 or CHO cells it is about 1000 rads (Hopwood, unpublished data). Some studies have shown an age dependence for the probability of cell division in the first few divisions after irradiation, but this disappears in later generations (Thompson and Suit, 1967; Trott and Hug, 1970). The ability to continue dividing decreases progressively in the generations following irradiation until the survivors constitute the majority of the cell population and begin to raise the division probability to normal (Fig. 6).

Following division of an irradiated cell, there is a high probability of fusion of the resulting sister cells (Marin and Bender, 1966; Hurwitz and Tolmach, 1969b). A cytoplasmic bridge can often be detected between them, and the presence of chromatin within the bridge can sometimes be inferred (Levis,1962). Fusion is generally followed by one or more multipolar divisions and fusions. Giant cells are thereby produced, but these may also be formed, particularly at larger doses, without division and fusion; it is not clear whether they can arise without the intervention of some kind of aberrant mitotic event.

## Conclusions

Kinetic studies of the kinds described here can suggest possible mechanisms by which radiations kill and otherwise affect cells, though they do not establish these mechanisms; detailed molecular studies are generally needed. Nevertheless, analysis of the effects of antineoplastic agents in cellular terms has been most effective in providing an understanding of the mechanisms by which these agents give rise to observed sequalae at the tissue, organ and organismic levels. For example, the acute lethal mammalian bone-marrow radiation syndrome can be traced to the loss of proliferative capacity of the stem cells from which lymphocytes, granulocytes, and magakaryocytes develop, while the gastrointestinal syndrome can be attributed to the death of crypt stem cells (Bond et al., 1956). It is clear that the depletion of cells from a given self-renewing tissue after irradiation follows a time-course directly predictable from the measured normal turn-over time of those cells (Puck, 1966).

While tumor regression after therapy cannot be analyzed in similar fashion because the tumor cells do not in general turn over, and the rate of cellular disintegration after treatment is a complex function of cell type, radiation dose, and, presumably, nutritional status, there is no doubt that destruction of reproductive capacity is the crucial cellular response in the treatment of neoplasia (see Reinhold, 1966; Powers et al., 1967). In providing quantitative description of the lethal responses of cells to toxic agents, kinetic studies like those discussed in the preceding sections permit comparisons among different cell types and assessment of the effects of different treatment conditions. The kinds of information discussed are therefore potentially of great significance to the clinical application of these agents in the treatment of neoplasia. The kinetic findings provide impetus to exploit differences among the pertinent cell types with respect to the many factors affecting the lethal response, so as to enhance the killing of cancer cells relative to the normal stem cells of the patient's cell renewal systems. While the problems are formidable because of the complexity of the systems, the heterogeneity of the cell populations in question, and the difficulty in obtaining the necessary *in vivo* data, progress is nevertheless being made along several lines: analysis of the systems in terms of the relevant parameters (e. g. Bond et al., 1970), acquisition of pertinent data (see Tubiana, 1971), and formulation and application of mathematical models that can yield numbers predictive of the outcome of any particular treatment regimen (e. g. Steward and Hahn 1971). The reorientation of the clinician's approach to the therapy of cancer that has resulted from an appreciation of the cellular aspects of the disease and its treatment, deriving largely from the developments in cellular radiation biology surveyed here, will hopefully be followed by significantly increased therapeutic success derived from those same developments (Kaplan, 1970), and from the understanding that is being gained about the molecular basis of the cell's response to irradiation.

## References

ALPER, T., FOWLER, J. F., MORGAN, R. L., VONBERG, D. D., ELLIS, F., OLIVER, R.: The characterization of the "type C" survival curve. Brit. J. Radiol. 35, 722—723 (1962).

BARENDSEN, G. W.: Dose survival curves of human cells in tissue culture irradiated with alpha-, beta-, 20kV x-, and 200 kV x-radiation. Nature (Lond.) 193, 1153—1155 (1962).

BARENDSEN, G. W., BEUSKER, L. J., VERGROESEN, A. J., BUDKE, L.: Effects of different ionizing radiations on human cells in tissue culture. II. Biological experiments. Radiat. Res. 13, 841—849 (1960).

BARENDSEN, G. W., WALTER, H. M. D., FOWLER, J. F., BEWLEY, D. K.: Effects of different ionizing radiations on human cells in tissue culture. III. Experiments with cyclotron-accelerated alpha-particles and deuterons. Radiat. Res. 18, 106—119 (1963).

BENDER, M. A., GOOCH, P. G.: The kinetics of x-ray survival of mammalian cells *in vitro*. Int. J. Radiat. Biol. 5, 133—145 (1962).

BERRY, R. J., OLIVER, R.: Effect of post-irradiation incubation conditions on recovery between fractionated doses of x-rays. Nature (Lond.) 201, 94—96 (1964).

BOND, V. P., FLIEDNER, T. M., ARCHAMBEAU, J. O.: Mammalian radiation lethality. New York and London: Academic 1965.

BOND, V. P., SUIT, H. D., MARCIAL, V. (Eds.): Time and dose relationships in radiation biology as applied to radiotherapy. Upton, N. Y.: Brookhaven National Laboratory 1970.

BRUCE, W. R., VAN DER GAAG, H.: A quantitative assay for the number of murine lymphoma cells capable of proliferation *in vivo*. Nature (Lond.) 199, 79—80 (1963).

CHAFFEY, J. T., HELLMAN, S.: Differing responses to radiation of murine bone marrow stem cells in relation to the cell cycle. Cancer Res. 31, 1613—1615 (1971).

DEWEY, D. L.: The x-ray sensitivity of *Serratia marcescens*. Radiat. Res. 19, 64—87 (1963).

DEWEY, W. C., HUMPHREY, R. M.: Restitution of radiation-induced chromosomal damage in Chinese hamster cells related to cell's life cycle. Exp. Cell Res. 35, 262—276 (1964).

DJORDJEVIC, B., SZYBALSKY, W.: Genetics of human cell lines. III. Incorporation of 5-bromo- and 5-iododeoxyuridine into the deoxyribonucleic acid of human cell lines and its effects on radiation sensitivity. J. exp. Med. 112, 509—531 (1960).

ELKIND, M. M.: Sedimentation of DNA released from Chinese hamster cells. Biophys. J. 11, 502—520 (1971).

ELKIND, M. M., SUTTON, H.: X-ray damage and recovery in mammalian cells in culture. Nature (Lond.) 184, 1293—1295 (1959).

ELKIND, M. M., WHITMORE, G. F.: The radiobiology of cultured mammalian cells. New York: Gordon and Breach 1967.

EPSTEIN, H. T.: Identification of radiosensitive volume with nucleic acid volume. Nature (Lond.) 171, 394—395 (1953).

FROESE, G.: Division delay in HeLa cells and Chinese hamster cells. A time-lapse study. Int. J. Radiat. Biol. 10, 353—367 (1966).

GOLDSTEIN, R., OKADA, S.: Interphase death of cultured mammalian cells (L5178Y). Radiat. Res. 39, 361—373 (1969).

HAHN, G. M.: Radiobiology of mammalian cells in the plateau phase of growth. In: Time and dose relationships in radiation biology as applied to radiotherapy, pp. 117—125. Upton, N. Y.: Brookhaven National Laboratory 1970.

HEWITT, H. B.: Studies on the dissemination and quantitative transplantation of a lymphocytic leukemia of CBA mice. Brit. J. Cancer 12, 378—401 (1958).

HEWITT, H. B., WILSON, C. W.: A survival curve for mammalian cells irradiated *in vivo*. Nature (Lond.) 183, 1060—1061 (1959).

HEWITT, H. B., WILSON, C. W.: Survival curves for tumor cells irradiated *in vivo*. Ann. N. Y. Acad. Sci. 95, 818—827 (1961).

HOPWOOD, L. E.: Ph. D. Thesis, Washington University, St. Louis, Mo. 1971.

HOPWOOD, L. E., TOLMACH, L. J.: Deficient DNA synthesis and mitotic death in x-irradiated HeLa cells. Radiat. Res. 46, 70—84 (1971).

HURWITZ, C., TOLMACH, L. J.: Time-lapse cinemicrographic studies of x-irradiated HeLa S3 cells. I. Cell progression and cell disintegration. Biophys. J. 9, 607—633 (1969a).

HURWITZ, C., TOLMACH, L. J.: Time-lapse cinemicrographic studies of x-irradiated HeLa S3 cells. II. Cell fusion. Biophys. J. 9, 1131—1143 (1969b).

HUTCHINSON, F.: Molecular basis for action of ionizing radiations. Science 134, 533—538 (1961).

KAPLAN, H. S.: Radiobiology's contribution to radiotherapy: Promise or mirage? Radiat. Res. 43, 460—476 (1970).

KAPLAN, H. S., MOSES, L. E.: Biological complexity and radiosensitivity. Science 145, 21—25 (1964).

LAJTHA, L. G., OLIVER, R., KUMATORI, T., ELLIS, F.: On the mechanism of radiation effect on DNA synthesis. Radiat. Res. 8, 1—16 (1958).

LEA, D. E.: Actions of radiations on living cells, 2nd ed. Cambridge: University Press 1955.
LEEPER, D. B., SCHNEIDERMAN, M. H., DEWEY, W. C.: Radiation induced cycle delay in synchronized Chinese hamster cells: Comparison between DNA synthesis and division. Radiat. Res. **53**, 326—337 (1973).
LEVIS, A. G.: Effetti dei raggi x sulla mitosi di cellule di mammiferi coltivate *in vitro*. Caryologia **15**, 59—87 (1962).
LITTLE, J. B.: Differential response of rapidly and slowly proliferating human cells to x-irradiation. Radiology **93**, 307—313 (1969).
McCULLOCH, E. A., TILL, J. E.: The radiation sensitivity of normal mouse bone marrow cells, determined by quantitative marrow transplantation into irradiated mice. Radiat. Res. **13**, 115—125 (1960).
McCULLOCH, E. A., TILL, J. E.: The sensitivity of cells from normal mouse bone marrow to gamma radiation *in vitro* and *in vivo*. Radiat. Res. **16**, 822—832 (1962).
MADOC-JONES, H., DAWSON, K. B., FIELD, E. O.: Radiosensitivity of a series of cultured primary fibrosarcomata. Radiology **90**, 541—546 (1968).
MADOC-JONES, H., MAURO, F.: Age response to x-rays, *Vinca* alkaloids, and hydroxyurea of murine lymphoma cells synchronized *in vivo*. J. nat. Cancer Inst. **45**, 1131—1143 (1970).
MARIN, G., BENDER, M. A.: A comparison of mammalian cell-killing by incorporated $^3$H-uridine. Int. J. Radiat. Biol. **7**, 235—244 (1963).
MARIN, G., BENDER, M. A.: Radiation-induced mammalian cell death: lapse-time cinemicrographic observations. Exp. Cell Res. **43**, 413—423 (1966).
MAURO, F., MADOC-JONES, H.: Age response to x-radiation of murine lymphoma cells synchronized *in vivo*. Proc. nat. Acad. Sci. (Wash.) **63**, 686—689 (1969).
MAURO, F., MADOC-JONES, H.: Age response of cultured mammalian cells to cytotoxic drugs. Cancer Res. **30**, 1397—1407 (1970).
MUNRO, T. R.: Alpha irradiation of parts of single cells in tissue culture. Exp. Cell Res. 18, 76—99 (1959).
OKADA, S.: Radiation biochemistry, Vol. 1. New York: Academic 1970.
PAINTER, R. B.: The direct effect of x-irradiation on HeLa S3 deoxyribonucleic acid synthesis. Radiat. Res. **16**, 846—859 (1962).
PARKER, L., SKARSGARD, L. D., EMMERSON, P. T.: Sensitization of anoxic mammalian cells to x-rays by triacetoneamine *N*-oxyl. Survival and toxicity studies. Radiat. Res. **38**, 493—500 (1969).
PHILLIPS, R. A., TOLMACH, L. J.: Repair of potentially lethal damage in x-irradiated HeLa cells. Radiat. Res. **29**, 413—432 (1966).
PHILPOTT, G. W., SHAEFFER, C. W., TOLMACH, L. J.: Reproductive survival of chick embryo cells irradiated *in ovo* and *in vitro*. Radiat. Res. **17**, 508—518 (1962).
POWERS, W. E., TOLMACH, L. J.: A multicomponent x-ray survival curve for mouse lymphoma cells irradiated *in vivo*. Nature (Lond.) **197**, 710—711 (1963).
POWERS, W. E., TOLMACH, L. J.: Demonstration of an anoxic component in a mouse tumor cell population by an *in vivo* assay of survival following irradiation. Radiology **83**, 328—336 (1964).
POWERS, W. E., PALMER, L. A., TOLMACH, L. J.: Cellular radiosensitivity and tumor curability. Nat. Cancer Inst. Monogr. **24**, 169—185 (1967).
PUCK, T. T.: Quantitative studies of mammalian cells *in vitro*. Rev. mod. Phys. **31**, 433—448 (1959).
PUCK, T. T.: Cellular aspects of the mammalian radiation syndrome. Radiat. Res. **27**, 272—283 (1966).
PUCK, T. T., MARCUS, P. I.: A rapid method for viable cell titration and clone production with HeLa cells in tissue culture. Proc. nat. Acad. Sci. (Wash.) **41**, 432—437 (1955).
PUCK, T. T., MARCUS, P. I.: Action of x-rays on mammalian cells. J. exp. Med. **103**, 653—666 (1956).
PUCK, T. T., MARCUS, P. I., CIECIURA, S. J.: Clonal growth of mammalian cells *in vitro*. J. exp. Med. **103**, 273—284 (1956).
PUCK, T. T., STEFFEN, J.: Life cycle analysis of mammalian cells. Biophys. J. **3**, 379—397 (1963).
RAUTH, A. M., SIMPSON, L. A.: The energy loss of electrons in solids. Radiat. Res. **22**, 643—661 (1964).
REINHOLD, H. S.: Quantitative evaluation of the radiosensitivity of cells of a transplantable rhabdomyosarcoma in the rat. Europ. J. Cancer **2**, 33—42 (1966).
RÉVÉSZ, L., LITTBRAND, B.: Variation of the relative sensitivity of closely related neoplastic cell lines irradiated in culture in the presence or absence of oxygen. Nature (Lond.) **203**, 742—744 (1964).

Silini, G., Hornsey, S.: Studies on cell-survival of irradiated Ehrlich ascites tumour. I. The effect of the host's age and the presence of nonviable cells on tumour takes. Int. J. Radiat. Biol. **4**, 127—134 (1961).

Silini, G., Hornsey, S.: Studies on cell-survival of irradiated Ehrlich ascites tumour. III. A comparison of the x-ray survival curves obtained with a diploid and a tetraploid strain. Int. J. Radiat. Biol. **5**, 147—153 (1962).

Sinclair, W. K.: Cyclic x-ray responses in mammalian cells *in vitro*. Radiat. Res. **33**, 620—643 (1968).

Skipper, H. E.: The cell cycle and chemotherapy of cancer. In: Baserga, R. (Ed.): The cell cycle and cancer, pp. 358—387. New York: Dekker 1971.

Sparrow, A. H., Underbrink, A. G., Sparrow, R. C.: Chromosomes and cellular radiosensitivity. Radiat. Res. **32**, 915—945 (1967).

Steward, P. G., Hahn, G. M.: The application of age response functions to the optimization of treatment schedules. Cell Tissue Kinet. **4**, 279—291 (1971).

Terasima, T., Tolmach, L. J., Changes in x-ray sensitivity of HeLa cells during the division cycle. Nature (Lond.) **190**, 1210—1211 (1961).

Terasima, T., Tolmach, L. J.: Variations in several responses of HeLa cells to x-irradiation during the division cycle. Biophys. J. **3**, 11—33 (1963).

Thompson, L. H., Suit, H. D.: Proliferation kinetics of x-irradiated mouse L cells studied with time-lapse photography. I. Experimental methods and data analysis. Int. J. Radiat. Biol. **13**, 391—397 (1967).

Thompson, L. H., Suit, H. D.: Proliferation kinetics of x-irradiated mouse L cells studied with time-lapse photography. II. Int. J. Radiat. Biol. **15**, 347—362 (1969).

Till, J. E.: Radiosensitivity and chromosome numbers in strain L mouse cells in tissue culture. Radiat. Res. **15**, 400—409 (1961).

Tolmach, L. J.: Growth patterns in x-irradiated HeLa cells. Ann. N. Y. Acad. Sci. **95**, 743—757 (1961).

Trott, K. R., Hug, O.: Intraclonal recovery of division probability in pedigrees of single x-irradiated mammalian cells. Int. J. Radiat. Biol. **17**, 483—486 (1970).

Tubiana, M.: The kinetics of tumor cell proliferation and radiotherapy. Brit. J. Radiol. **44**, 325—347 (1971).

Walters, R. A., Petersen, D. F.: Radiosensitivity of mammalian cells. II. Radiation effects on macromolecular synthesis. Biophys. J. 8, 1487—1504 (1968).

Weiss, B. G.: Perturbations in precursor incorporation into DNA of x-irradiated HeLa S3 cells. Radiat. Res. **48**, 128—145 (1971).

Whitmore, G. F., Stanners, C. P., Till, J. E., Gulyas, S.: Nucleic acid synthesis and the division cycle in x-irradiated L-strain mouse cells. Biochim. biophys. Acta (Amst.) **47**, 66—77 (1961).

Whitmore, G. F., Till, J. E.: Quantitation of cellular radiobiological responses. Ann. Rev. nuclear Sci. **14**, 347—374 (1964).

Withers, H. R.: The dose-survival relationship for irradiation of epithelial cells of mouse skin. Brit. J. Radiol. **40**, 187—194 (1967).

Withers, H. R.: Biological basis for high-LET radiotherapy. Radiol. **108**, 131—137 (1973).

Withers, H. R., Elkind, M. M.: Radiosensitivity and fractionation response of crypt cells of mouse jejunum. Radiat. Res. **38**, 598—613 (1969).

Yamada, M., Puck, T. T.: Action of radiation on mammalian cells. Proc. Nat. Acad. Sci. (Wash.) **47**, 1181—1191 (1961).

Chapter 25

# Clinical and Laboratory Investigation of Combination Radiation and Chemical Therapy

R. L. SCOTTE DOGGETT and MALCOLM A. BAGSHAW

With 1 Figure

## Introduction

Therapeutic radiologists have sought means of improving radiation effects on tumors relative to normal tissues for over 50 years. REGAUD (1922) demonstrated that the same biological end result could be achieved with a single large, or multiple small increments of radiation, and that the multiple smaller doses caused far less injury to normal tissues. COUTARD (1926) described favorable results of the clinical application of REGAUD'S work leading to the fractionated-dose radiotherapy techniques in use today. This discovery, along with dramatic advances in the physics and technology of radiation therapy and accumulated knowledge and experience in the application of this technology, have led to marked improvement in survival rates of patients with most forms of cancer. Although radiobiologists and radiation therapists have not made breakthroughs as significant as that of REGAUD and COUTARD, clinical investigation of methods to increase radiation response is proceeding in three major areas: (1) physiologic (i.e. increasing oxygen concentration in tumors), (2) physical (i.e. using heavy particle, high linear energy transfer radiations), and (3) chemical. The purpose of this section is to discuss the third method.

The list of chemicals used to modify radiation effects ranges from distilled water to bacterial toxins. Extensive reviews of experimental and clinical data are available (ANDREWS, 1969; BERRY, 1969; VAETH, 1969; KAPLAN, 1970). Reference to many radiation modifiers, particularly those investigated in nonmammalian systems, will be excluded, while emphasis will be placed on those agents that have had considerable clinical application, may prove to have clinical usefulness, or have been investigated by the authors in their clinics and laboratories.

It is useful to categorize agents used as radiation modifiers by the chemical mechanism resulting in cytotoxicity and the phase of the reproductive cycle in which the cells are vulnerable. There are four phases of the cell generation cycle: $M$, the process of mitosis; $G_1$, the time gap between telophase and the onset of DNA synthesis; $S$, the DNA synthetic period; and $G_2$, the interval between the end of DNA synthesis and the next mitosis. A large proportion of cells are not continuously in cycle, remaining in a prolonged $G_1$ or $G_0$ phase (MENDELSOHN, 1962). Significant variations in radiation and chemical sensitivity have been shown at different periods of the cycle (TERASIMA and TOLMACH, 1963; SKIPPER, 1964; WHITMORE et al., 1965; BRUCE et al., 1966). Perturbations resulting from radiation or chemical exposure of normal and malignant cells can alter the cell cycle in ways which can increase or decrease the therapeutic gain of combination therapy (BROWN, 1970a; DEVITA, 1971).

SKIPPER et al. (1972) classified agents into four groups relating their action to phases of the cell cycle:

(1) Cycle dependent agents which are *S*-phase specific with respect to cell killing or sensitizing (hydroxyurea; cytosine arabinoside; heavy halogenated pyrimidines).
(2) Cycle dependent agents which are *S*-phase specific, but also effect RNA and/or protein synthesis. These drugs tend to be self-limiting by slowing the progression of cells into *S* during a given exposure (methotrexate; 6-mercaptopurine; 5-fluorouracil).
(3) Cycle dependent agents without established phase specificity (vincristine; vinblastine).
(4) Agents which kill cells in nearly all portions of the generation cycle; most are cytotoxic independent of the proliferative state of the cells (actinomycin D; alkylating agents; procarbazine).

## Sensitizing and Additive Effects

Definition of mechanisms of combined action of chemical and x-rays have been vague, mostly because complex interactions are not understood well enough to justify precision. The introduction of clonal culture techniques by PUCK and MARCUS (1956) provided a method by which radiation and chemical effects could be quantified. When plotted semilogarithmically, radiosensitivity of the cells can be characterized by dose-log cell survival curves, in which the reciprocal of the slope of the straight line portion of the curve indicates the basic sensitivity and

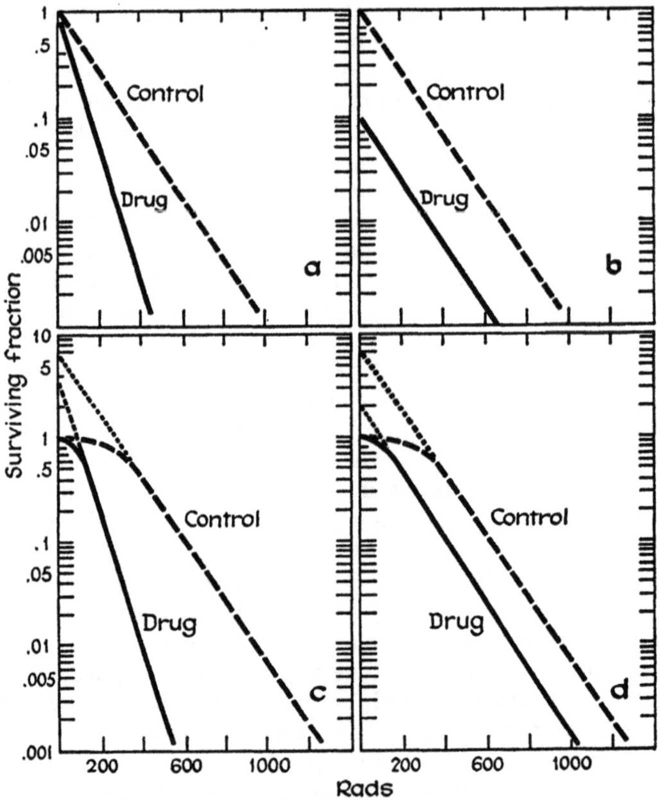


Fig. 1. Patterns of cell survival following combined treatment. See text for detailed explanation. (Reproduced from BAGSHAW and DOGGETT, 1969, by permission of S. Karger, Basel-New York)

the width of the shoulder provides an index of cellular capacity to recover from sublethal radiation effects. The use of cell survival curves to relate chemical and radiation effects on cells *in vitro* is shown in Fig. 1, in which the response to radiation alone (i.e. the control) is characterized by the dashed line. In example (b), the cell population has been depleted by a chemical effect before radiation exposure. With increasing doses of radiation, the slope of the cell survival curve is unchanged, indicating a similar cellular radiosensitivity, as when there is no chemical in the culture medium. The combined radiation-drug effect is therefore additive, as has been shown to be the case with nitrogen mustard and radiation (MARIN and LEVIS, 1964). In example (a), there is no killing of cells by the chemical alone. The dose-response curve of radiation in the presence of the chemical exhibits an altered slope, indicating a basic alteration in cell radiation sensitivity, as has been shown by KAPLAN et al. (1961) for purine and pyrimidine analogs. Example (c) more precisely characterized the increased radiation sensitivity of cells incubated with heavy halogenated pyrimidines prior to radiation. The slope is steep, and the extrapolation number (i.e. the intercept of the extrapolation of the straight line portion of the curve with the ordinate) is reduced, which, in effect, narrows the shoulder, indicating that either less sublethal radiation damage must be accumulated for cell killing, or repair of sublethal radiation is inhibited. Survival curves of the general type shown in example (d) demonstrate increased radiation sensitivity due to a reduction in the extrapolation number as in (c), without alteration of the slope of the survival curve. ELKIND and SAKAMOTO (1969) have shown that interactions of this general nature occur with actinomycin D and fractionated radiation of late $S$ in Chinese hamster cells.

Chemicals may have both sensitizing and additive effects, and more than one mechanism leading to sensitization may be in effect. Limited knowledge of these mechanisms and difficulty in quantitating them in solid tumor systems make simple distinction between sensitization and additivity sufficient for purposes of this discussion.

## Alkylating Agents

Alkylating agents that have been used in combination with radiation therapy include nitrogen mustard ($HN_2$), phenylalanine mustard, chlorambucil, cyclophosphamide (cytoxan), triethylenethiophosphoramide (thioTEPA), and triethylene melamine (TEM). Although differing in action, all have the capacity to replace hydrogen atoms by alkyl radicals. The purine base, guanine, in DNA is the preferential site, but not the only site of attack (BROOKES and LAWLEY, 1961). Such reactions result in cross links, either between different groups in the same molecule, or between different molecules.

Mammalian cells cultured in the presence of $HN_2$ exhibit an x-ray dose-response with a slope identical to that of cells radiated without $HN_2$ present (MARIN and LEVIS, 1964). A similar additive effect was shown when $HN_2$ was introduced following a single exposure of cells to radiation. ELKIND and SAKAMOTO (1969) showed that Chinese hamster cells in $G_1$ and $G_2$ were more sensitive to both $HN_2$ and radiation than were cells in $S$-phase. Radiation and $HN_2$ acted independently, both when combined as single treatments and when fractionated. When $HN_2$ was injected intravenously 24 h prior to irradiating mice with lymphocytic leukemia, CORREA and ANDREWS (1964) demonstrated an additive or independent effect of the chemical and the radiation. Combined single dose radiation treatment and regional cytoxan and $HN_2$ perfusion of rabbit hind legs bearing transplanted tumors resulted in greater normal tissue injury, without improving the tumor response seen following optimal radiation or chemical treatment alone (CLAPP et al., 1964).

A large number of clinical trials have failed to demonstrate improved results with combination alkylating agent and radiation therapy. In a series of patients with lung cancer, tumor regression rates and survival times were not increased by adding $HN_2$ to radiation therapy when the results were compared to a control group receiving radiation alone (Chalmers, 1962; Krand et al., 1963). Paterson (1958, 1960) was unable to discern any improvement in the results of treatment of localized Hodgkin's disease, when comparing patients who had received radiation alone with those who had received radiation plus $HN_2$. Combined cyclic administration of $HN_2$, vincristine, procarbazine, and prednisone (MOPP) has been reported to bring about long term control of patients with advanced Hodgkin's disease following failure of radiation therapy (DeVita and Serpick, 1967). Subsequent authors have suggested this multiple drug program is of value when given routinely following radiation therapy for patients with lymphoma; however, there is no evidence that the combination of radiation and MOPP therapy in planned sequence offers any advantage over radiation therapy given alone to be followed by MOPP therapy when recurrence of disease becomes evident (Kaplan, personal communication).

Cassady et al. (1969) reviewed 230 patients with retinoblastoma. Of 120 patients undergoing radiation therapy for early stage disease, 29 underwent regional arterial infusion of TEM, 37 received TEM intramuscularly, and 54 patients were treated with radiation alone. The local tumor control rate was essentially the same for each group (74%). Of 103 patients receiving radiation therapy for advanced disease, 69 underwent arterial infusion of TEM, 7 received intramuscular TEM, and 27 were treated with radiation only. The local tumor control rate was 20%, 0%, and 26%, respectively. This review fails to suggest that TEM is of any value for either early or late stage retinoblastoma. Furthermore, the potentially dangerous nature of the drug is indicated in that two patients died of complications directly related to TEM.

Despite initial failures in the clinic, there has been a renewed interest in agents which appear to act independently of the cell cycle such as alkylating agents, as the significance of nonproliferating tumor cells ($G_0$) has become more evident. Methylmethane sulfonate (MMS), a monofunctional alkylating agent, appears to kill cells by inducing single strand breaks in DNA. Such breaks can be repaired in exponentially growing cells more readily than in non-cycling cells grown in culture beyond the period of exponential growth (Lett et al., 1966). Using Chinese hamster cells in this stationary or plateau phase, Hahn (1969) showed a slightly greater increase in killing effect when the cells were exposed to MMS and x-ray, than was predicted from the additive effects of x-ray and MMS. Although MMS alone would not appear to be of clinical value, it is predicted that the tolerance of more rapidly proliferating normal tissue (i.e. bone marrow and intestinal epithelium) to MMS will be high, so that the agent could be given continuously in an effort to affect non-cycling cells while a cell cycle dependent agent is used with radiation to treat cells in the exponential growth phase. *In vivo* experimentation is necessary to assess this hypothesis.

## Actinomycin D

Actinomycin D interferes with RNA and protein synthesis by binding to DNA, excluding the enzyme RNA polymerase from its normal binding site (Goldberg and Rabinowitz, 1962; Reich, 1964). Radiosensitization by actinomycin D has been observed in mammalian cell culture systems (Bases, 1959; Elkind and Sakamoto, 1969). The characteristics of the survival curve for late *S* Chinese hamster cells undergoing fractionated x-irradiation in the presence of actinomycin D is shown in Fig. 1, example (c).

D'ANGIO et al. (1959) noted accelerated skin reactions in patients and mice receiving combined radiation-actinomycin D treatment and recall of previous skin changes by late administration of actinomycin D. FARBER (1966) described the initial results of combination surgical, radiation, and short-term actinomycin D treatment of 53 children with WILMS' tumor without evidence of metastasis when first seen. Thirty-five children (66%) were free of disease at two years. Ten (63%) of the 16 children developing pulmonary metastases after primary treatment were without evidence of disease two years following additional radiation-actinomycin D therapy. In a recent review of this expanded clinical material, CASSADY (1973) reports 73% (68/93) over all two year disease free survival rate; 48% (20/42) of patients developing pulmonary metastases after primary therapy appear to have been cured with combination radiation-actinomycin D therapy.

A controlled cooperative investigation to test the efficacy of single versus multiple doses of actinomycin D following surgery and radiation therapy for WILMS' tumor suggests prolonged actinomycin D administration is superior (WOLFF et al., 1968). Nineteen of 22 patients in this group (86%) were without evidence of tumor at the time of this writing, as compared to 48% of children who had received single dose therapy (11/23). This favorable differential effect has persisted well beyond the termination of the 15 month course of actinomycin D (WOLFF, personal communication). Although other authors have published results which do not indicate a need for combination radiation-actinomycin D therapy for low stage tumors (MAIER et al., 1969), it is generally accepted that actinomycin D in combination with radiation therapy does improve survival rates in patients with more advanced primary or metastatic WILMS' tumor.

## Methotrexate

Methotrexate interferes with DNA synthesis, and thereby prevents cell replication by interfering with the synthesis of the folic acid coenzyme necessary for the formation of the DNA precursor, thymidylic acid. BERRY (1970) demonstrated increased radiosensitivity of HeLa cells irradiated in a culture medium containing nontoxic doses of methotrexate under anoxic conditions. With toxic doses of methotrexate, a radiation dose-survival curve was steeper in the anoxic than in the oxic state. Subsequent experiments with HeLa cells in the stationary or plateau phase showed an increased radiation sensitivity that was also partially independent of oxygen effect. It is postulated that the mechanism for increased radiosensitivity is the same in the two experiments (i.e. methotrexate interferes with DNA synthesis, resulting in an increased proportion of late $G_1$ cells). The increased overall radiosensitivity is a result of the greater sensitivity of cells in this phase of the generation cycle.

Clinically, methotrexate is most commonly used in the treatment of acute leukemia in children and of choriocarcinoma and related trophoblastic tumors in adult females (HERTZ et al., 1961). Methotrexate is of limited value when used alone to treat patients with epidermoid carcinoma, particularly when gastrointestinal and bone marrow toxicity is assessed following conventional oral or intravenous administration (PAPAC et al., 1963). Oral administration generally results in the greatest morbidity, presumably because of slow absorption and more prolonged maintenance of toxic blood levels. A more favorable therapeutic ratio has been reported after large doses of methotrexate are infused by vein over 6 to

24 h, followed by leucovorin (citrovorum factor), the "antidote" for methotrexate (Capazzi et al., 1970; Djerassi et al., 1972).

Friedman et al. (1970) treated 168 patients with previously untreated stage III and IV head and neck cancer with oral methotrexate (5 to 10 mg daily for two weeks) resulting in a tumor volume reduction of 25% in 75% of patients. By combining curative radiation therapy with oral methotrexate, 25% (17/67) of patients were disease free two years following completion of therapy. Kramer (1969) treated a similar group of patients with advanced cancer of the head and neck using oral methotrexate (7.5 mg/day) 5 to 7 days before and during radiation therapy until systemic toxicity occurred. Although local tumor control was achieved in 63% of patients (36/57), only 32% (18/57) survived intercurrent illness or disseminated metastatic disease. A similar group of patients with advanced head and neck cancer received two courses of radiation therapy of 1800 to 2500 rads in 3 days, separated by 4 weeks (i.e. 3600 to 5000 rads in 31 elapsed days). Intravenous methotrexate (1 to 4 mg/kg) was given at intervals of two weeks for a total of four doses (Condit, 1968). Although the overall response appeared to be more favorable in the 20 patients included in the combination group, the difference was not significant when compared to a control group. Publication of results of a national prospective randomized clinical trial to evaluate methotrexate and radiation therapy in the treatment of patients with head and neck cancer should be forthcoming as the study nears completion at this writing.

In 1961, a program was started at Stanford University in which prolonged, external carotid arterial infusion of methotrexate and, later, 5-bromodeoxyuridine was combined with aggressive radiation therapy of patients with advanced, previously untreated head and neck cancer (Bagshaw et al., 1967; Doggett et al., 1967). In these patients, the intra-arterial catheter was usually introduced into the external carotid artery through the superior thyroid artery. The position of the tip of the polyethylene or polyvinyl catheter was monitored and a qualitative assessment of tumor and normal tissue infusion was made by injecting fluorescein and observing the circulatory bed of the external carotid artery by fluorescence of the infused tissues during illumination with ultraviolet light (Nelsen et al., 1963).

Twenty of 25 patients receiving methotrexate required bilateral external carotid artery catheters to infuse the entire tumor bed. Methotrexate (25 mg/catheter/day) and citrovorum factor (6 mg intramuscularly every 6 h) were given throughout the course of x-ray therapy, unless the severity of local and/or systemic reaction required interruption or discontinuation. Total doses of methotrexate ranged from 700 mg in 18 days to 2160 mg in 44 days, the average being 1263 mg in 35 days. All patients received no less than 6000 rads to the primary lesions and involved cervical node areas; bilateral neck irradiation was necessary in all but 3 patients.

Table 1 presents the long term results of three groups of patients, including a group which received 6-mercaptopurine and radiation (to be described later) and a group randomly assigned to receive x-ray therapy alone. Although 6 of 22 patients completing methotrexate-radiation therapy appeared to have successful treatment locally, one of these was considered a failure as she died of intercurrent illness, without evidence of tumor, at too short an interval after treatment (i.e. 13 months) to be considered a favorable result of combination therapy. Only one of these patients is now living. In the control group (i.e. radiation only), 6 patients (33%) had control of local disease, and 4 are alive and well for over 6 years. Although the preponderance of lesions originated in the oropharynx, including the base-of-tongue, there were insufficient numbers of patients at each tumor site to compare results between the experimental and control groups. Using a modification of the staging system of Daly and Friedman (1964) the long term control rates of patients receiving combination methotrexate-radiation therapy were 1 of 2 patients (stage II), 2 of 4 patients (stage III) and 2 of 16 patients (stage IV). There was no relationship between the total amount of methotrexate given and the results of treatment. The onset of patchy mucositis occurred at 12 and 22 days in patients receiving radiation with and without methotrexate, respectively; the mucositis occurred earlier in the successfully treated patients in both groups. Tumor regression occurred more rapidly in the patients receiving methotrexate; however, there was no difference in the extent of tumor regression between the experimental and control groups after 4 weeks.

Of concern is the late recurrence of cancer in two patients and the development of acute myelogenous leukemia in a third. In one patient, the primary tumor, an anaplastic carcinoma of the anterior floor-of-mouth (classified as $T_4-N_2$) had been well infused and apparently controlled at the time of death. A midcervical lymph node metastasis was first detected ten years after combination therapy, was outside of the infusion bed, and progressed rapidly, resulting in the patient's demise. The second patient has a recurrence of an oral tongue carcinoma (classified $T_4-N_3$) which had been infused satisfactorily and appeared controlled for 9 years; no regional node recurrence has been detected. She is undergoing a second course of combination therapy currently. Although the incidence of acute myelogenous leukemia 6 years following successful radiation-methotrexate therapy is of interest, it would be speculative to relate the leukemia and previous therapy in this single instance.

## Purine Analogs

6-Mercaptopurine (6-MP) and 6-thioguanine are the two major analogs of the normally occurring purine bases which have had clinical application. 6-MP and 6-thioguanine interfere with the *de novo* pathway of purine nucleotide synthesis and with purine interconversion; both are also incorporated into RNA and DNA. The radiosensitivity of purine-requiring *E. coli* was increased 2 to 3-fold by less than 1% replacement of guanine in DNA by its analog, 6-thioguanine (KAPLAN et al., 1964). Radiosensitization by these purine analogs is highly oxygen dependent, in contrast to the situation with certain pyrimidine analogs.

Table 1. *Results of radiation therapy of advanced head and neck cancer with and without arterial antimetabolite infusion*

| | Methotrexate and x-ray | 6-Mercaptopurine and x-ray | X-ray therapy alone |
|---|---|---|---|
| Patients Completing Therapy/ Patients Starting Therapy | 22/25 | 9/11 | 18/18 |
| Primary and Regional Node Tumor Controlled | 5 | 2 | 6 |
| Alive without Tumor | 1 (7 years) | — | 4 (6+ years) |
| Dead of Intercurrent Disease | 4[a] | 1 (21 months) | 2 (2[c], 6 years) |
| Dead of Distant Metastases | 1 (21 months) | 1 (5 years) | — |
| Primary Recurrence Controlled | 1 (9 years) | 1 (7 years) | 1 (6 years)[d] |
| Primary and/or Regional Tumor not Controlled | 15[b] | 6 | 11 |
| Primary and Regional Tumor Therapy Successful | 5/25 (20%) | 2/11 (18%) | 6/18 (33%) |

[a] Tumor free at death at 13 (score as therapy failure), 40, 63 (leukemia), and 80 months.
[b] Two patients with recurrence at 9 and 10 years.
[c] Carcinoma of the esophagus.
[d] Tumor free 6 years after radiation to lung metastases; 5 years after excision of primary recurrence.

The authors have conducted a limited clinical investigation using prolonged arterial infusion of 6-MP with radiation therapy in the treatment of patients with advanced carcinomas of the head and neck (Table 1). Doses of 6-MP ranged between 0.3 and 1 mg/kg/day with total doses ranging from 380 mg in 20 days to 1190 mg in 37 days (average dose, 760 mg in 33 days). As with methotrexate, 6-MP was given at the beginning of radiation therapy and was continued until local or systemic complications necessitated its discontinuation. Although two patients are thought to have been controlled locally, one of these patients died of intercurrent disease in less than two years, while the other died of distant metastases at 5 years. The systemic complications with 6-MP were significantly greater than with methotrexate, as no antidote is available.

## Fluorinated Pyrimidines

HEIDELBERGER et al. (1957) synthesized several pyrimidine analogs and tested them for antitumor activity. 5-Fluorouracil (5-FU) has proved to be the most useful of this series of compounds, which are most commonly used in the treatment of carcinoma of the gastrointestinal tract and breast. This agent interrupts DNA synthesis after conversion to the deoxynucleotide level by competitively inhibiting the enzyme thymidylate synthetase. 5-FU and 5-fluoro-2′-deoxyuridine (FUdR) are not incorporated into DNA, although 5-FU is incorporated into RNA. HeLa cells incubated in medium containing 5-FU before and after radiation exposure proved more sensitive than cells receiving radiation alone (BAGSHAW, 1962; BERRY, 1965). Radiation potentiating effects of 5-FU in transplanted rodent tumor systems have been suggested by a number of investigators (HEIDELBERGER et al., 1958; VERMUND et al., 1961). VIETTI et al. (1971) showed leukemic cell killing by radiation *in vivo* to be enhanced to the greatest degree when 5-FU was injected within 8 h following radiation.

MOERTEL et al. (1969) describe their experience in a randomized clinical investigation using 5-FU given by rapid intravenous injection (15 mg/kg/day) for the first three days of radiation therapy for the palliation of unresectable gastrointestinal cancer. Mean survival times were significantly increased in patients receiving combination therapy, as compared with radiation therapy alone for adenocarcinoma of the stomach (13 versus 5.9 months, respectively), pancreas (10.4 versus 6.3 months, respectively), and large bowel (22.8 versus 16.8 months, respectively). The authors speculate that survival rates (4/89 or 4.5% disease-free over 5 years) may be increased with changes in the drug schedule or total radiation dose which, in this group of patients, was 3500 to 4000 rads.

EDLAND (1970) and PROUT et al. (1970) failed to demonstrate an advantage of combination 5-FU and radiation therapy for patients with bladder malignancy. EDLAND et al. (1971) also describe failure to improve the results in the treatment of patients with incompletely excised astrocytomas, grades III and IV, when comparing survival of patients receiving radiation alone or in combination with intravenous 5-FU.

Improved three year survival incidence is reported (GOLLIN et al., 1972) for patients with advanced oral cavity and oropharyngeal squamous cell carcinomas treated with simultaneous intravenous 5-FU and curative radiation therapy (17/43 or 40%), compared with a control group of patients treated with radiation only (3/48) or 6%). A similar improvement in survival could not be shown for patients with carcinoma of the nasopharynx, hypopharynx, larynx, or lymph nodes without known primary. In a nonrandomized trial, the same group (GOLLIN and JOHNSON, 1971) could not show any advantage of external carotid artery infusion of 5-FU followed by curative radiation therapy over radiation therapy alone for patients with advanced head and neck cancer.

FLETCHER et al. (1963) found no difference in the short-term results following intravenous 5-FU with radiation or radiation alone in the treatment of patients with advanced carcinomas of the pharyngeal wall or anterior pharnyx. The same group (JESSE, 1969) compared the results of arterial methotrexate infusion preceding curative radiation therapy with arterial 5-FU infusion during radiation therapy of patients with advanced cancer of the head and neck. 5-FU appeared to be superior to methotrexate at a mean follow-up period of 42 months (i.e. 6/24 compared with 0/14 local tumor control, respectively). The authors suggest dense scarring, which results from 5-FU and radiation therapy, could entrap viable cancer cells, explaining late local recurrences in two patients (24 and 34 months).

No difference in survival could be detected in a well controlled clinical investigation in which radiation therapy was given with and without 5-FU in the treatment of patients with lung cancer (COHEN et al., 1971). In this clinical investigation, the control group (i.e. radiation alone) received 4000 rads as compared to the 5-FU-radiation treated group which received 2000 rads only. After treating patients with pulmonary metastases, which could be used as an "internal control" to evaluate combination 5-FU and radiation treatment, x-ray therapy alone was found to be more effective than 5-FU alone, and no advantage could be demonstrated in 14 patients in whom the effects of x-ray could be compared with those of 5-FU plus radiation (VON ESSEN et al., 1963).

## Hydroxyurea

Hydroxyurea (HU) is a cell-cycle-dependent, phase-specific agent that inhibits DNA synthesis, without affecting RNA or protein formation. Although it is generally accepted that HU prevents the conversion of ribonucleotides to deoxyribonucleotides by inhibiting ribonucleoside diphosphate reductase (FRENKEL and ARTHUR, 1967), multiple sites of action may be involved (YARBRO, 1968). Chinese hamster cells exposed to HU during DNA synthesis (i.e. $S$ phase) are killed; $G_1$ cells are prevented from beginning DNA synthesis. Cells exposed during $G_2$ and mitosis survive and progress until just before DNA synthesis (SINCLAIR, 1965). The effect of HU is not constant in all cell lines, since the drug has no toxic action on HeLa $S_3$ cells during either $S$ or $G_1$ phases (PHILLIPS and TOLMACH, 1966). Blocking DNA biosynthesis without affecting RNA or protein synthesis results in a significant degree of cell synchronization.

The investigation of radiation response characteristics of HU synchronized, or $G_1$ to $S$ interphase cells, may have clinical significance as a cell system at an age possibly equivalent to $G_0$ cells. HU blocked Chinese hamster cells have limited ability to repair sublethal radiation damage (ELKIND and KANO, 1971), similar to plateau-phase Chinese hamster cells (HAHN et al., 1968a), which tend to gather in $G_1$ and mimic solid tumors in a variety of parameters. Murine lymphoma cells irradiated *in vivo* after HU exposure were shown to have similar age response curves with greatest radiosensitivity when cells were at the $G_1$ to $S$ interphase block (MADOC-JONES and MAURO, 1970). Postradiation cell-killing enhancement by HU or a closely related chemical has been shown in bacterial systems (KAPP and SMITH, 1971) and in cell culture models (PHILLIPS and TOLMACH, 1966).

Clinical investigators predicted that HU would augment radiation effects by blocking cells in the $G_1$ to $S$ interphase where they are relatively radiosensitive, by killing cells in $S$ where they are generally radioresistent, and by interfering with the repair of sublethal radiation injury. The last mechanism of augmentation was suggested clinically by the observation of reactivation of postirradiation epidermitis (Sears, 1964). HU can be taken orally with limited bone marrow and gastrointestinal toxicity, particularly when administered in an intermittent high dose schedule (Lerner et al., 1969a). Lerner et al. (1969b) described the results of treating 60 patients with advanced head and neck cancer with combination HU and radiation treatment. HU (80 mg/kg every third day) was given one week before, during, and indefinitely following conventional radiation therapy. The value of combination HU and radiation in this series could not be accurately evaluated, as nearly one-half of the patients subsequently underwent surgery. However, in a second series of patients with advanced head and neck cancer undergoing combination HU-radiotherapy without subsequent surgery, 17 of 32 (53%) are without evidence of disease for periods ranging from 4 to 44 months post-treatment (Lipshutz and Lerner, 1969). HU can be recovered from the cerebrospinal fluid when given in standard doses. In a preliminary report, one of six patients is alive 22 months following combined surgical, radiation, and HU treatment of primary brain tumors (Lerner et al., 1970). Hreshchyshyn (1968) reports favorable preliminary experience with combination HU and radiation therapy of six patients with stages III-B and IV carcinomas of the cervix.

## Other Halogenated Pyrimidine Analogs

Since the demonstration by Greer and Zamenhof (1957) that bromouracil (BU) possesses the property of sensitizing *E. coli* to ultraviolet irradiation, a number of investigators have sought to elucidate this action and others to discover a clinical situation in which it might be exploited. The halogenated pyrimidine analogs 5-bromodeoxyuridine (BUdR), 5-chlorodeoxyuridine (CUdR), and 5-iododeoxyuridine (IUdR) were shown to increase the radiation sensitivity of cells cultured in media containing these analogs, the degree of radiosensitization being related directly to the extent of incorporation of the analog into DNA (Djordjevic and Szybalski, 1960; Erikson and Szybalski, 1961). The dose modifying factor of these analogs could be increased to as great as three by varying the concentration of the analog. IUdR was the most effective radiation sensitizer and the most toxic. BUdR resulted in the greatest radiosensitization with the least toxicity. Similar properties were demonstrated for 5-bromodeoxycytidine (BCdR) which is converted intracellularly into BUdR (Prusoff et al., 1961; Bagshaw, 1962). BUdR concentration influences the extrapolation number more than the slope of the cell survival curve (Mohler and Elkind, 1963). Although the extrapolation number was constant at concentrations of BUdR below $10^{-7}$ M, there was a rapid fall to one as the concentration was increased to $2 \times 10^{-6}$ M. One would predict from this finding that there would be little or no recovery between fractions, and that the extent of radiation sensitization would be more the result of limited sublethal injury repair than change in slope of the survival curve. The importance of inhibition of repair mechanisms by BUdR has been emphasized by Lett et al. (1964). By using FUdR to block *de novo* thymine deoxyribonucleotide synthesis, Erikson and Szybalski (1963a) were able to increase DNA-thymine replacement by a pyrimidine analog. This was also demonstrated by Maruyama et al. (1963) by exposing ascites lymphoma cells to BCdR injected intraperitoneally prior to radiation exposure. The dose modifying factor was 1.7 when 7% of the thymine was replaced by BUdR in the DNA in ascites lymphoma cells. Administration of FUdR in combination with BCdR resulted in an increase in DNA-thymine replacement by BUdR to 14% with a rise in the dose modifying factor to 2.4.

SZYBALSKI and LORKIEWICZ (1962) established that incorporation of the halopyrimidines into DNA was a prerequisite for radiosensitization. Although it was initially thought that bifilar labeling of DNA was necessary to induce radiosensitization, KAPLAN et al. (1962) demonstrated significant sensitization of *E. coli* after unifilar labeling. DEWEY and HUMPHREY (1965) also showed the same degree of radiation sensitization could be obtained with single as with double strand incorporation of BUdR in a mammalian cell system.

The exact mechanism by which the halogenated pyrimidine deoxyribonucleosides increase radiation sensitivity after DNA incorporation has not been discovered. Experiments by ERICKSON and SZYBALSKI (1963b) would appear to have ruled out a greater photoelectric absorption by fraudulent DNA as the explanation. RAGNI and SZYBALSKI (1962) incorporated $P^{32}$ in one strand of DNA and BU into the second strand, increasing the lethal effects of the nuclear transmutation of the $P^{32}$. This suggested that the halogenated thymine analog weakened the phosphate ester bonds, increasing the likelihood that double strand breaks might occur during irradiation (ELKIND and WHITMORE, 1967). Comparing the viscosity of normal DNA and BU-DNA after x-irradiation, LETT et al. (1964) were unable to show differences in double strand breaks in DNA and suggested that BU incorporation may inhibit postirradiation repair mechanisms rather than increase radiation induced scission of phosphate ester bonds. WHITMORE and TILL (1964) proposed the theory that the exposure of cells to both x-irradiation and halopyrimidines reduces the probability that a cell will carry out successive divisions. This condition probably prevails for larger drug concentrations, although BAGSHAW (1962) and MOHLER and ELKIND (1963) demonstrated augmented cell killing by irradiation at apparent nontoxic concentrations of the sensitizing agents.

ZIMBRICK et al. (1969a, b) have carried out a series of radiation chemistry experiments which support the contention that strand breaks in DNA are easier to produce in BU-substituted DNA than in native DNA. Irradiation of BU-DNA converted the BU to a uracil moiety. Apparently, the BU is split during a series of reactions into $Br^-$ and a uracil-5-yl radical. It is suggested that the highly reactive uracil radical forms uracil by removing the hydrogen atom from the 2′-carbon of the adjacent deoxyribose, probably leading to a single strand break. These reactions were not observed for the thymine in normal DNA.

The radiosensitization elicited by the halogenated pyrimidines has been shown to be oxygen-independent (KAPLAN et al., 1962). SUIT (1969) points out that a significant proportion of cells of a solid tumor remain hypoxic, even after administration of oxygen under pressure. He proposed that the halogenated pyrimidines might prove ineffective clinically, as those factors which limit accessibility of oxygen to cell populations would have the same adverse effect on radiation sensitizing agents. He demonstrated that 22% of tumor cells remain hypoxic in a mouse mammary carcinoma, despite breathing oxygen at 30 pounds/inch$^2$. Results of these experiments indicated that 80% of these hypoxic cells are effectively sensitized 8 h following completion of a 6 dose injection schedule carried out over 48 h. The authors suggest that an explanation for this encouraging discovery will probably relate to rapid cell movements between oxic and hypoxic compartments.

Recently, DJORDJEVIC (1970) has demonstrated a dose modifying factor for BUdR when administered after irradiation. Synchronized HeLa cells were exposed to radiation during the $S$ phase followed by BUdR administration during $G_1$. The dose-modifying effect in these experiments was less than when BUdR is incorporated into DNA prior to irradiation. In these experiments, a small amount of FUdR was used with BUdR. It is possible that inhibition of repair of sublethal radiation damage was itself inhibited by the FUdR-BUdR combination. The discovery of unscheduled DNA synthesis (RASMUSSEN and PAINTER, 1966) and repair replication of DNA after irradiation (PAINTER and CLEAVER, 1967) raised the possibility that a means could be found to induce incorporation of the halogenated pyrimidine into DNA without the limitation of cell cycle dependence. HAHN et al. (1968b) induced unscheduled DNA synthesis in Chinese hamster cells by treatment with MMS. Attempts to increase the dose modification factor by treatment of cells with radiation or MMS prior to administration of BUdR have not proved successful to this time.

Arterial infusion of both BUdR and BCdR into the tumor bed seems preferable to intravenous administration because of the efficient debromination that takes place in the liver and the conversion of BCdR to BUdR which occurs rapidly in the blood (KRISS and REVESZ, 1962; KRISS et al., 1964). Desquamation of palmar and plantar epithelium and sloughing of finger and toenails have been observed in patients undergoing intra-arterial therapy to other regions of the body in clinical trials, both in Japan and at Stanford University, suggesting that detoxication is incomplete, or that toxic by-products are produced. In these patients, there have been no signs of cytotoxic effects on bone marrow or gastrointestinal epithelium.

In an effort to develop an experimental model that would more closely parallel the use of intra-arterial radiosensitizers in man, BROWN and GOFFINET (1970b) developed a method for performing prolonged arterial infusions in the mouse. They have employed this technique to study the preferential radiosensitization of a transplanted mouse sarcoma relative to normal skin by combining long term arterial infusion of halogenated pyrimidine deoxyribonucleoside and irradiation (BROWN et al., 1971). Infusion of BCdR was carried out continuously and concomitantly with the administration of ten daily fractions of x-radiation. After initial regression of the tumor, the time required by the tumor to regrow to a standard size was determined. The dose modifying factor (DMF) for the transplanted KHT sarcoma was 1.3, whereas sensitization of skin was insignificant, indicating an overall therapeutic gain. The effect of the halogenated pyrimidine deoxyribonucleoside infusion was equivalent to delivering 23 to 31% more radiation to the transplanted tumor, without increase in damage to the normal cutaneous structures. The relative degree of substitution of DNA-thymine after BCdR infusion with and without FUdR was determined. Although FUdR increased the percent replacement of DNA-thymine from 5 to 17%, this was not accompanied by a significant increase in DMF, as was anticipated (MARUYAMA et al., 1964). The authors postulate that dose modification resulted more from a drop in the extrapolation number than an increase in the slope of the cell survival curve, as has been shown to occur *in vitro* with as little as 5% replacement of DNA-thymine (MOHLER and ELKIND, 1963). Another explanation could be that cell population radiation sensitization is influenced more by the proportion of replicating cells with thymine of DNA replaced than by the amount of analog substituted per cell as SUIT (1970) showed in mouse mammary carcinomas.

In 1964, a randomized clinical study was initiated at Stanford University for the purpose of evaluating the potentiating effect of BUdR in combination with external irradiation in patients with advanced carcinoma of the head and neck (BAGSHAW and DOGGETT, 1969). The infusion technique was identical to that described earlier for combination methotrexate- or 6-MP-irradiation of patients with advanced head and neck cancers. Several different dosage regimens were investigated. These included continuous daily infusion of up to one gram of BUdR per day for as long as thirty days, together with daily irradiation at the rate of 200 rads per day. Radiation therapy started on the fifth day of the infusion in order to permit pre-irradiation incorporation of the analog into the DNA of the neoplastic cells. In another regimen, the BUdR was infused twice daily in 30 min pulses, one in the morning and one in the afternoon for two consecutive days, followed by large fraction (i.e. 500 rads) irradiation on the third day, followed by one day of rest before repeating the cycle. It was thought that BUdR incorporation would be increased by limiting the number of radiation treatments and delaying infusion of BUdR until inhibition of DNA synthesis by irradiation had lessened. In the third technique, the patient received 3000 rads of conventional irradiation (i.e. 1000 rads per week) followed by a two week rest interval. BUdR arterial infusion was begun the sixth week and conventional radiation therapy was resumed the seventh week. By this means, it was hoped that tumor blood supply would improve after most of the neoplastic cells had been destroyed by the first half of radiation therapy, and that nonproliferating cells would return to the proliferating pool during the rest period.

No significant differences were observed between the various modes of BUdR administration and irradiation. A significant increase in radiation reaction of normal tissues undergoing both BUdR infusion and radiation therapy was demonstrated. The volume of tissue undergoing combination therapy could be precisely defined by the distribution of infused fluorescein and the radiation treatment portals. For example, radiation mucositis developed earlier and became more severe on the half of the tongue receiving combined therapy when compared to the other half which received the same dose of radiation alone. Similar differences in radiation reaction were observed in the skin. In one patient, there was sufficient tumor tissue following combination therapy for DNA extraction and analysis; 4.9% of the thymine of DNA had been replaced by BU. In spite of this favorable extent of analog incorporation, there was no greater evidence of local control of neoplasm or increase in survival than in patients receiving the same dose of radiation alone. Long term follow-up data for these patients is presented in Table 2.

Table 2. *Results of radiation therapy of advanced head and neck cancer with and without arterial 5-bromo-2′-deoxyuridine (BUdR) infusion*

| | Radiation and BUdR | X-ray therapy alone |
|---|---|---|
| Patients Completing Therapy/ Patients Starting Therapy | 19/19 | 18/18 |
| Primary and Regional Node Tumor Controlled | 4 | 6 |
| Alive without Tumor | 3 (5+ years) | 4 (6+ years) |
| Dead of Intercurrent Disease | 1 (6 years) | 2 (4 and 6 years) |
| Dead of Distant Metastases | 1 (9 months)[a] | — |
| Primary Recurrence Controlled | 1 (4 years) | 1 (6 years) |
| Primary and/or Regional Tumor Not Controlled | 13 | 11 |
| Primary and Regional Tumor Therapy Successful | 4/19 (21%) | 6/18 (33%) |

[a] Score as therapy failure as post-therapy interval short.

The local tumor and regional control rate for patients receiving combined therapy was 21% (4/19), while for those receiving radiotherapy alone it was 33% (6/18). It was concluded that, although a substantial dose modifying factor was observed, there was no therapeutic gain.

TANAKA and TAKAHASI (1970) have investigated the use of intra-arterial BUdR and external irradiation in the treatment of 36 patients with advanced carcinomas of the head and neck. BUdR (250 mg/day) and 5-FU (50 mg/day) were infused simultaneously during conventional radiation therapy. As in the Stanford University series, a marked increase in mucositis within the infused bed was observed; however, it was believed that the mucositis was less than observed in a previous group of patients treated with intra-arterial 5-FU plus irradiation. The authors suggest that a therapeutic gain has resulted on the basis of accelerated tumor regression; however, they have not published either local control rates or survival statistics.

SANO et al. (1966) and HOSHINO and SANO (1969) have recognized that the rapid turnover of normal cells adjacent to the tumor may prevent therapeutic gain when both the normal and malignant cells are in the combined treatment volume. They reasoned that there is a significant difference between the proportion of cells undergoing DNA synthesis in the central nervous system compared with that of malignant cells in more aggressive brain tumors. This reasoning is supported by the work of JOHNSON et al. (1960) who showed labeling of 0.6% of neoplastic cells of a human brain tumor after injection of $^3$H-thymidine; only occasional endothelial cell labeling was noted. HOSHINO et al. (1972) studied the degree of tritiated thymidine uptake in the brain tumors of 12 patients. In the glioblastomas, labeling varied from near 0% in the necrotic areas to approximately 20% of the cells in the more viable parts of the tumor. For less malignant astrocytomas, they found a more even distribution of thymidine uptake, but a lower labeling index of about 1%. The duration of $S$-phase was found to be 7 to 10 h in the majority of tumors.

GOFFINET et al. (1972) have carried out simultaneous carotid artery infusion of BCdR with and without FUdR and radiation treatment (300 rads/day for 7 consecutive days) of mice following intracerebral implantation of SK-26 glioma. Using time of death as the major parameter of effect, BCdR with or without FUdR proved to be a significant radiation sensitizer equivalent to an additional 45 rads per day (i.e. a 12% increase in dose effect was obtained). These authors also showed significant *in vivo* $^3$H-thymidine incorporation in transplanted tumors with only rare endothelial and glial cell labeling immediately adjacent to the tumor. This evidence suggests a long term therapeutic gain will result from differential brain tumor sensitization.

By the end of 1969, some 200 patients with brain tumors had been treated by prolonged arterial infusion of BUdR and irradiation in several different neurological clinics in Japan. In the subgroup of those patients who were treated in the Department of Neurosurgery at the University of Tokyo, 16 of 48 patients who had completed treatment by February, 1971, had been at risk for more than 18 months. Of these, 7 were living for periods up to or greater than 36 months, while 9 were dead with malignancy (HOSHINO, 1972). Considering the lethal nature of the neoplasms investigated, these preliminary observations are impressive and should stimulate others to try to verify them.

## Conclusions

The radiation oncologist is investigating four basic ways to improve the therapeutic gain factor: (1) modifying dose fractionation regimens; (2) increasing the $pO_2$ of tumor relative to adjacent normal tissue; (3) using high-linear energy transfer (LET) irradiation; and (4) combining chemical adjuvants with radiation therapy. The use of fractionated radiation dose schedules rather than single large increments has proven to be the most effective of these methods and warrants continued investigation (SUIT, 1972). The rapid re-establishment of the hypoxic/oxic cell ratio (reoxygenation) after doses of radiation comparable to those used clinically (KALLMAN, 1972) and the limited capacity for hypoxic cells to accumulate sublethal injury are the major factors in achieving the favorable results of fractionated radiation and also explain the failure of randomized clinical trials to reveal a significant advantage of hyperbaric oxygen. Clinical investigations of high-LET irradiation are under way (CATTERALL and ROGERS, 1971), but the widespread use of this modality is years in the future. Therefore, combination chemical and radiation therapy remains an important area for laboratory and clinical investigation, but with differing emphasis based on the knowledge and experience accrued over the past few years.

The choice of a chemical adjuvant can now be related to the interrelationship of cytokinetic parameters of the malignancy and the normal tissue included within the volume to be irradiated. Of the major parameters of tumor and normal tissue kinetics (i.e. growth fraction, generation time, and cell loss factor), the normal tissue growth factor seems most important clinically, as it is known in many organs from $^{3}$H-thymidine-labeling, that the latter is usually the limiting factor in the amount of radiation which can be given and is relatively constant and predictable. Human tumors of the same histologic type and size have widely varying cytokinetic parameters (FREI et al., 1970). There is evidence that irradiation of mucosa results in a compensatory expansion of the small, normal mucosa progenitoı compartment (BROWN, 1970a). Under these circumstances, BUdR would appear to be a poor adjuvant to radiation of patients with head and neck cancer. A relative increase in the sensitivity of mucosa would result, possibly lessening the therapeutic gain achieved by fractionation alone. We believe this occurred in the small series of patients so treated by BAGSHAW and DOGGETT (1967). Japanese investigators have led the way in this new approach to combination therapy by irradiating tumors with a large growth fraction within normal tissue (i.e. brain) which has a small proportion of proliferating cells, while infusing a cell cycle dependent nontoxic halogenated pyrimidine deoxyribonucleoside (BUdR).

Occult or early pulmonary metastases present another clinical situation in which the advantages of radiosensitization by pyrimidine analogs might be realized. When large volumes of lung are to be irradiated, the radiation sensitivity of pulmonary tissue imposes a serious limitation on the radiation dose which may be applied. However, the cellular composition of lung is such that there should be a significant and possibly exploitable difference in growth fractions and cell cycle times between normal endothelium and alveolar cells and tumor cells in microscopic foci. The major blood supply of small metastases is derived from pulmonary rather than bronchial arteries (MILNE et al., 1969) so that dose-modifying agents could be administered by simple intravenous injection. This means of administration is appropriate for halogenated pyrimidine deoxyribonucleosides, as they would infuse the tumor bed before undergoing debromination by the liver. Animal experiments are in progress at Stanford University to determine whether a favorable therapeutic ratio can be achieved using intravenous BUdR and total lung radiation therapy for occult metastases.

An important area of molecular radiobiological investigation involves the quantitative estimation of radiation induced single- and double-strand breaks in DNA and the identification of enzymatic DNA repair systems (KAPLAN, 1972). Chemicals which inhibit DNA repair increase the lethality of given doses of x-rays while blocking the repair of single strand breaks during the postirradiation incubation period. Among the agents identified are a hydroxyurea derivative (KAPP and

SMITH, 1971), acriflavine (KAPP and SMITH, 1970) and quinacrine (FUKS and SMITH, 1971). For these agents and possibly the pyrimidine analogs to be of therapeutic value, a means may be required to selectively affect tumor cells. Conceivably, this could be achieved by complexing the radiation sensitizing agent with certain polycations which concentrate along the altered cell membrane of tumor cells (WOODMAN, 1968).

Finally, there is steadily growing evidence for the value of radiation therapy as an adjuvant for chemotherapy. This has been most dramatically demonstrated in children with acute lymphocytic leukemia (AUR et al., 1972). Following rapid induction of complete remission with prednisone and vincristine, 2400 rads is directed to the cranio-spinal axis. The authors believe that they have increased the 5 year leukemia-free survival rate of children from 20 to 50—55% at five years utilizing radiation to kill cells which are not exposed to adequate concentrations of chemotherapeutic agents because of the "blood brain barrier." A similar program is being investigated for the treatment of children with EWING's sarcoma (JOHNSON and POMEROY, 1972). Radiation therapy is directed to the primary tumor and systemic actinomycin D, cytoxan, and vincristine therapy is carried out. Whole brain radiation therapy and intrathecal methotrexate is given to kill occult central nervous system metastases. In a limited number of patients, an actuarial analysis predicts 40% five year tumor-free survival rates.

## References


ANDREWS, J. R.: Combined cancer radiotherapy and chemotherapy: the relevance of cell population kinetics and pharmacodynamics. Cancer Chemother. Rep. 53, 313—324 (1969).

AUR, J. A., SIMONE, J. V., HUSTU, H. O., VERZOSA, M. S.: A comparative study of central nervous system irradiation and intensive chemotherapy early in remission of childhood acute lymphocytic leukemia. Cancer 29, 381—391 (1972).

BAGSHAW, M. A.: Modification of the radiosensitivity of hamster cells *in vitro*. Nature (Lond.) 193, 389—391 (1962).

BAGSHAW, M. A., DOGGETT, R. L. S.: A clinical study of chemical radiosensitization. Frontiers of Radiation Therapy and Oncology, Vol. 4. Basel, New York: Karger. San Francisco: Vaeth 1969.

BAGSHAW, M. A., DOGGETT, R. L. S., SMITH, K. C., KAPLAN, H. S., NELSEN, T. S.: Intra-arterial 5-bromodeoxyuridine and x-ray therapy. Amer. J. Roentgenol. 99, 886—894 (1967).

BASES, R.: Modification of radiation response by single-cell technics: Actinomycin D. Cancer Res. 19, 1223—1233 (1959).

BELLI, J. A.: Proliferation kinetics of normal and tumor cells. Radiology 105, 143—149 (1972).

BERRY, R. J.: Modification of radiation effects. Radiol. Clin. N. Amer. 3, 249—264 (1965).

BERRY, R. J.: Growing points in mammalian radiobiology and their implications for radiotherapy. Radiol. Clin. N. Amer. 2, 281—292 (1969).

BERRY, R. J., HALL, E. J., CAVANAGH, J.: Radiosensitivity and the oxygen effect for mammalian cells cultured *in vitro* in stationary phase. Brit. J. Radiol. 43, 81—90 (1970).

BRUCE, W. R., MEEKER, B. E., VALERIOTE, F. A.: Comparison of the sensitivity of normal hematopoietic and transplanted lymphoma colony-forming cells to chemotherapeutic agents administered *in vivo*. J. nat. Cancer Inst. 37, 233—245 (1966).

BROOKES, P., LAWLEY, P. D.: The alkylation of guanosine and guanylic acid. J. chem. Soc. 3923—3932 (1961).

BROWN, J. M.: The effect of acute X-irradiation on the cell proliferation kinetics of induced carcinomas and their normal counterpart. Radiat. Res. 43, 627—653 (1970a).

BROWN, J. M., BERRY, R. J.: Effect of X-irradiation on the cell population kinetics in a model tumor and normal tissue system: implications for the treatment of human malignancies. Brit. J. Radiol. 42, 372—377 (1969).

BROWN, J. M., GOFFINET, D. R.: A technique for intra-arterial infusion of tumor bearing mice. J. Lab. clin. Med. 76, 175—180 (1970b).

BROWN, J. M., GOFFINET, D. R., CLEAVER, J. E., KALLMAN, R. F.: Preferential radiosensitization of mouse sarcoma relative to normal skin by chronic intraarterial infusion of halogenated pyrimidine analogues. J. nat. Cancer Inst. 47, 75—89 (1971).

CAPIZZI, R. L., DECONTI, R. C., MARSH, J. C., BERTINO, J. R.: Methotrexate therapy of head and neck cancer: improvement in therapeutic index by the use of leucovorin "rescue." Cancer Res. **30**, 1782—1788 (1970).
CASSADY, J. R.: Considerations in radiation therapy of WILMS' tumor. Cancer **32**, 598—608 (1973).
CASSADY, J. R., SAGERMAN, R. H., TRETTER, P., ELLSWORTH, R. M.: Radiation therapy in retinoblastoma. Radiology **93**, 405—409 (1969).
CATTERALL, M., ROGERS, C.: An investigation into the clinical effects of fast neutrons. Brit. J. Radiol. **44**, 603—611 (1971).
CHALMERS, T. C.: Combination of radiotherapy and chemotherapy in the treatment of carcinoma of the lung. Cancer Chemother. Rep. **16**. 463—471 (1962).
CLAPP, P., TAYAO, M. S., TYREE, E. B., NICKSON, J. J., CLARKSON, B., LAWRENCE, W., JR.: An experimental study of simultaneous irradiation and regional chemotherapeutic perfusion. J. surg. Res. **4**, 371—376 (1964).
COHEN, J. L., KRANT, M. J., SHNIDER, B. I., MATIAS, P. I., HORTON, J., BAXTER, D.: Radiation plus 5-fluorouracil (NCS-19893): clinical demonstration of an additive effect in bronchogenic carcinoma. Cancer Chemother. Rep. **55**, 253—258 (1971).
CONDIT, P. T.: Treatment of carcinoma with radiation therapy and methotrexate. Missouri Med. **65**, 823—835 (1968).
CORREA, J. N., ANDREWS, J. R.: Modification of radiation effect of ascitic tumor cells by pharmacologic agents injected intravenously. Nature (Lond.) **203**, 200—208 (1964).
COUTARD, H.: Roentgen therapy of epitheliomas of the tonsillar region, hypopharynx and larynx from 1920 to 1926. Amer. J. Roentgenol. **28**, 313—331 (1932).
DALY, J. F., FRIEDMAN, M.: Combination irradiation and chemotherapy in the treatment of squamous cell carcinoma of the head and neck. Trans. Amer. Acad. Opthal. **68**, 625—643 (1964).
D'ANGIO, G. J., FARBER, S., MADDOCK, C. L.: Potentiation of x-ray effects by Actinomycin D. Radiology **73**, 175—182 (1959).
DEVITA, V. T.: Cell kinetics and the chemotherapy of cancer. Cancer Chemother. Rep. **2**, 23—33 (1971).
DEVITA, V. T., SERPICK, A.: Combination chemotherapy in the treatment of advanced Hodgkin's disease. Proc. Amer. Assoc. Cancer Res. 8, 13 (1967).
DEWEY, W. C., HUMPHREY, R. M.: Increase in radiosensitivity of ionizing radiation related to replacement of thymidine in mammalian cells with 5-bromodeoxyuridine. Radiat. Res. **26**, 538—547 (1965).
DJERASSI, I., ROMINGER, C. J., KIM, J. S., TURCHI, J., SUVANSRI, U., HUGHES, D.: Phase I study of high doses of methotrexate with citrovorum factor in patients with lung cancer. Cancer **30**, 22—30 (1972).
DJORDJEVIC, B.: Sensitization by BUdR and repair of radiation damage in synchronized cells. Livre. Des. Resumes, 4th International Congress of Radiat. Research (1970).
DOGGETT, R. L. S., BAGSHAW, M. A., KAPLAN, H. S.: Combined therapy using chemotherapeutic agents and radiotherapy. Modern trends in radiotherapy, Vol. 1. London: Butterworths 1967.
DONALDSON, S. S., CASTRO, J. R., WILBUR, J. R., JESSE, R. H., JR.: Rhabdomyosarcoma of head and neck in children: combination treatment by surgery, irradiation and chemotherapy. Cancer **31**, 26—35 (1973).
EDLAND, R. S., JAVID, M., ANSFIELD, F. J.: Glioblastoma multiforme: an analysis of the results of postoperative radiation therapy alone vs. radiotherapy and concomitant 5-fluorouracil; a prospective randomized study of 32 cases. Amer. J. Roentgenol. **111**, 337—342 (1971).
EDLAND, R. S., WEAR, J. B., JR., ANSFIELD, F. J.: Advanced cancer of the urinary bladder: an analysis of the results of radiotherapy alone vs. radiotherapy and concomitant 5-fluorouracil; a prospective randomized study of 36 cases. Amer. J. Roentgenol, **108**, 124—129 (1970).
ELKIND, M. M., SAKAMOTO, K.: Combined effects of X-irradiation and chemotherapeutic drugs (nitrogen mustard and actinomycin D). Frontiers of Radiation Therapy and Oncology, Vol. 4. Basel-New York: Karger; San Francisco: Vaeth 1969.
ELKIND, M. M., KANO, E.: Radiation-induced age-response changes in Chinese-hamster cells: evidence for a new form of damage and its repair. Int. J. Radiat. Biol. **19**, 547—560 (1971).
ELKIND, M. M., WHITMORE, G. F.: Radiobiology of cultured mammalian cells. New York: Gordon and Greech 1967.
ERIKSON, R. L., SZYBALSKI, W.: Molecular radiobiology of human cell lines. I. Comparative sensitivity to X-ray and ultraviolet light of cells containing halogen substituted DNA. Biochem. biophys. Res. Comm. **4**, 258—267 (1961).
ERIKSON, R. L., SZYBALSKI, W.: Molecular radiobiology of human cell lines. III. Radiation sensitizing properties of 5-iododeoxyuridine. Cancer Res. **23**, 122—131 (1963a).

ERIKSON, R. L., SZYBALSKI, W.: Molecular radiobiology of human cell lines. V. Comparative radiosensitizing properties of 5-halodeoxycytidines and 5-halodeoxyuridines. Radiat. Res. **20**, 252—261 (1963b).

FARBER, S., D'ANGIO, G., EVANS, A., MITUS, A.: Clinical studies of actinomycin D with special reference to Wilms' tumor in children. Ann. N. Y. Acad. Sci. **89**, 421—440 (1960).

FLETCHER, G. H., SUIT, H. D., HOWE, C. D., SAMUELS, M., JESSE, R. H., JR., VILLAREAL, R. U.: Clinical method of testing radiation-sensitizing agents in squamous cell carcinoma. Cancer **16**, 355—363 (1963).

FREI, E., SHIRAKAWA, S., LUCE, J. K., TANNOCK, I.: Cell proliferation in human melanoma. J. Clin. Invest. **49**, 1188—1199 (1970).

FRENKEL, E. P., ARTHUR, C.: Induced ribotide reductive conversion defect by hydroxyurea and its relationship to megaloblastosis. Cancer Res. **27**, 1016—1019 (1967).

FRIEDMAN, M., DENARVAES, F. N., DALY, J. F.: Treatment of squamous cell carcinoma of the head and neck with combined methotrexate and irradiation. Cancer **26**, 711—721 (1970).

FUKS, Z., SMITH, K. C.: Effects of quinacrine on x-ray sensitivity and the repair of damaged DNA in *E. coli* K-12. Radiat. Res. 48, 63—73 (1971).

GOFFINET, D. R., BROWN, J. M., BAGSHAW, M. A., KAPLAN, H. S.: Prolonged carotid arterial radiosensitizer infusion and radiation therapy of mouse gliomas. Amer. J. Roentgenol. **114**, 7—15 (1972).

GOLDBERG, I. H., RABINOWITZ, M.: Actinomycin D inhibition of deoxyribonucleic acid-dependent synthesis of ribonucleic acid. Science **136**, 315—331 (1962).

GOLLIN, F. F., ANSFIELD, F. J., BRANDENBURG, H. H., VERMUND, H.: Combined therapy in advanced head and neck cancer: a ramdozied study. Amer. J. Roentgenol. **114**, 83—88 (1972).

GOLLIN, F. F., JOHNSON, R. O.: Pre-irradiation 5-fluorouracil infusion in advanced head and neck carcinomas. Cancer **27**, 768—770 (1971).

GREER, S., ZAMENHOF, S.: Effect of 5-bromouracil in deoxyribonucleic acid of *E. coli* on sensitivity to ultraviolet radiation. Abstr. Amer. chem. Soc., 131st Meeting, p. 3c (1957).

HAHN, G. M.: Radiochemotherapy of cell cultures containing cycling and non-cycling cells. Frontiers of Radiation Therapy and Oncology, Vol. 4. Basel-New York: Karger; San Francisco: Vaeth 1969.

HAHN, G. M., STEWARD, J. R., YANG, S. J., PARKER, V.: Chinese hamster cell monolayer cultures. I. Changes in cell dynamics and modification of the cell cycle with period of growth. Exp. Cell Res. **49**, 285—292 (1968a).

HAHN, G., YANG, S. J., PARKER, V.: Repair of sublethal damage and unscheduled DNA synthesis in mammalian cells treated with monofunctional alkylating agents. Nature (Lond.) **220**, 1142—1151 (1968b).

HEIDELBERGER, C., CHAUDHURI, N. K., DANNEBERG, P., MOOREN, D., GREISBACH, L., DUSCHINSKY, R., SCHNITZER, R. J., PLEVEN, E., SCHEINER, J.: Fluorinated pyrimidines. A new class of tumor-inhibitory compounds. Nature (Lond.) **179**, 663—677 (1957).

HEIDELBERGER, C., GREISBACH, L., MONTAG, B. J., MOOREN, D., CRUZ, O.: Studies of fluorinated pyrimidines. II. Effects on transplanted tumors. Cancer Res. 18, 305—314 (1958).

HERTZ, R. J., LEWIS, J., LIPPSETT, M. B.: Five years' experience with chemotherapy of metastatic choriocarcinoma and related trophoblastic tumors in women. Amer. J. Obstet. Gynec. **82**, 631—643 (1961).

HOSHINO, T., BARKER, N. S., WILSON, C. V., BOLDERK, E. W., FEWER, D.: Cell kinetics of human gliomas. J. Neurosurg. **37**, 15—26 (1972).

HOSHINO, T., SANO, K.: Radiosensitization of malignant brain tumors with bromouridine (thymidine analogue). Acta radiol. 8, 98—113 (1969).

HRESHCHYSHYN, M. M.: Hydroxyurea (NSC-32065) with irradiation for cervical carcinoma-preliminary report. Cancer Chemother. Rep. **52**, 601—602 (1968).

JESSE, R. H.: Combined intra-arterial infusion and radiotherapy for treatment of advanced cancer of the head and neck. Frontiers of Radiation Therapy and Oncology, Vol. 4. Basel-New York: Karger; San Francisco: Vaeth 1969.

JOHNSON, H. A., HAYMAKER, W. E., RUBINI, J. R., FLIEDNER, T. M., BOND, V. P., CRONKITE, E. P., HUGHES, W. L.: A radiographic study of a human brain and glioblastoma multiforme after the *in vivo* uptake of tritiated thymidine. Cancer **13**, 636—642 (1960).

JOHNSON, R. E., POMEROY, T. C.: Integrated therapy for Ewing's sarcoma. Amer. J. Roentgenol. **114**, 532—535 (1972).

KALLMAN, R. F.: The phenomenon of reoxygenation and its implications for fractionated radiotherapy. Radiology **105**, 135—142 (1972).

KAPLAN, H. S.: Radiobiology's contribution to radiotherapy: promise or mirage? Failla Memorial Lecture. Radiat. Res. **43**, 460—476 (1970).

KAPLAN, H. S.: Enzymatic repair of radiation-induced strand breakage in cellular DNA and its chemical inhibition. Radiology **105**, 121—126 (1972).

KAPLAN, H. S., EARLE, J. D., HOWSDEN, F. L.: The role of purine and pyrimidine bases and their analogues in radiation sensitivity. J. cell. comp. Physiol. 64, 69—90 (1964).
KAPLAN, H. S., SMITH, K. C., TOMLIN, P. A.: Radiosensitization of *E. coli* by purine and pyrimidine analogues incorporated in deoxyribonucleic acid. Nature (Lond.) 190, 794—803 (1961).
KAPLAN, H. S., SMITH, K. C., TOMLIN, P. A.: Effects of halogenated pyrimidines on the radiosensitivity of *E. coli*. Radiat. Res. 16, 98—107 (1962).
KAPP, D. S., SMITH, K. C.: Lack of *in vitro* repair of x-ray induced chain breaks in DNA by the polynucleotide-joining enzymes. Int. J. Radiat. Biol. 14, 567—571 (1969).
KAPP, D. S., SMITH, K. C.: The chemical inhibition of the repair of single-strand breaks in DNA: post-irradiation sensitization to x-rays. Int. J. Radiat. Biol. 19, 255—262 (1971).
KRAMER, S.: Use of methotrexate and radiation therapy for advanced cancer of the head and neck. Frontiers of Radiation Therapy and Oncology, Vol. 4. Basel-New York: Karger; San Francisco: Vaeth 1969.
KRANT, M. J., CHALMERS, T. C., DEDERICK, M. M., HALL, T. C., LEVELE, M. B., MUENCH, H., SHNIDER, B. I., GOLD, G. L., HUNTER, C., BERSAK, S. R., OWENS, A. H., DELEON, N., DICKSON, R. J., BUNDLEY, C., BRACE, K. C., FREI, E., GEHAN, E., SAVIN, L.: Comparative trial of chemotherapy and radiotherapy in patients with non-resectable cancer of the lung. Amer. J. Med. 35, 363—370 (1963).
KRISS, J. P., REVESZ, L.: The distribution and fate of bromodeoxyuridine and bromodeoxycytidine in the mouse and rat. Cancer Res. 22, 254—263 (1962).
KRISS, J. P., SHAW, R. K., LOVINGER, R., EDMONDS, N.: Measurement of the *in vivo* degradation of carbon-14-labeled thymidine and its halogenated analogues in man by continuous monitoring of expired carbon-14-carbon dioxide. Nature (Lond.) 202, 1021—1030 (1964).
LERNER, H. J., BECKLOFF, G. L., GODWIN, M. C.: Hydroxyurea (NSC-32065) intermittent therapy in malignant diseases. Cancer Chemother. Rep. 53, 385—395 (1969a).
LERNER, H. J., BECKLOFF, G. L., GODWIN, M. C.: Concomitant hydroxyurea and radiotherapy in the management of 60 patients with head and neck cancer. Amer. Surgeon 35, 525—534 (1969b).
LERNER, H. J., BECKLOFF, R. L., GODWIN, M. C.: Treatment of astrocytoma with hydroxyurea and irradiation: report of six patients with 18-month follow-up. Amer. Surgeon 36, 401—402 (1970).
LETT, C. J., FELDSCHREIBER, P., LETT, J. T.: Repair of x-ray damage to the deoxyribonucleic acid in *Micrococcus radiodurans*. Nature (Lond.) 209, 59—62 (1966).
LETT, J. T., PARKINS, G., ALEXANDER, P., ORMEROD, M. G.: Mechanisms of sensitization to x-rays of mammalian cells by 5-bromodeoxyuridine. Nature (Lond.) 203, 593—602 (1964).
LIPSHUTZ, H., LERNER, H.: Three year observation of combined treatment for far advanced cancer of the head and neck. Amer. J. Surg. 118, 698—700 (1969).
MADOC-JONES, H., MAURO, F.: Age responses to x-rays, vinca alkaloids, and hydroxyurea of murine lymphoma cells synchronized *in vivo*. J. nat. Cancer Inst. 45, 1131—1143 (1970).
MAIER, J. G., AARESTAD, N. O.: Concepts in the treatment of WILMS' tumor. Frontiers of Radiation Therapy and Oncology, Vol. 4. Basel-New York: Karger; San Francisco: Vaeth 1969.
MARIN, G., LEVIS, A. G.: X-radiation and nitrogen mustard interaction in mammalian cells grown *in vitro*. Radiat. Res. 23, 192—201 (1964).
MARUYAMA, Y., SILINI, G., KAPLAN, H. S.: Studies of the LSA ascites lymphoma of C-57B1 mice. II. Radiosensitization *in vivo* with 5-bromodeoxycytidine and combined 5-fluorodeoxyuridine and 5-bromodeoxycytidine. Int. J. Radiat. Biol. 7, 453—462 (1963).
MENDOLSOHN, M. L.: Autoradiographic analysis of cell proliferation in spontaneous breast cancer of the C3H mouse. III. The growth fraction. J. nat. Cancer Inst. 28, 1015—1029 (1962).
MILNE, E. N., NOONAN, C. D., MARGULIS, A. R., STOUGHTON, J. A.: Vascular supply of pulmonary metastases. Experimental study in rats. Invest. Radiol. 4, 215—229 (1969).
MOERTEL, C. G., CHILDS, D. S., JR., REITEMEIER, R. J., COLBY, M. Y., JR., HOLBROOK, M. A.: Combined 5-fluorouracil and supervoltage radiation therapy of locally unresectable gastrointestinal cancer. Lancet 25, 865—867 (1969).
MOHLER, W. C., ELKIND, M. M.: Radiation response of mammalian cells grown in culture. III. Modification of x-ray survival of Chinese hamster cells by 5-bromodeoxyuridine. Exp. Cell Res. 30, 481—491 (1963).
NELSEN, T. S., EIGENBROT, E. H., BAGSHAW, M. A.: Low-flow fail-safe intra-arterial infusion. Arch. Surg. 87, 124—128 (1963).
PAINTER, R. B., CLEAVER, J. R.: Repair replication in HeLa cells after large doses of x-irradiation. Nature (Lond.) 216, 369—378 (1967).
PAPAC, R. J., JACOBS, E. M., FAYE, L. V., JR., DONAHUE, D. M.: Systemic therapy with amethopterin in squamous carcinoma of the head and neck. Cancer Chemother. Rep. 32, 47—53 (1963).

Paterson, E.: Evaluation of chemotherapeutic compounds in the reticuloses. Brit. J. Cancer **12**. 332—342 (1958).

Paterson, E.: Evaluation of chemotherapeutic compounds in the reticuloses. Acta un. int. cancr. **16**, 518—523 (1960).

Phillips, R. A., Tolmach, L. J.: Repair of potentially lethal damage in x-irradiated HeLa cells. Radiol. Res. **20**, 413—432 (1966).

Prout, G. R., Jr., Slack, N. H., Bross, I. D. J.: Irradiation and 5-fluorouracil as adjuvants in the management of invasive bladder carcinoma. A cooperative group report after 4 years. J. Urol. **104**, 116—129 (1970).

Prusoff, W. H., Cramer, J. W., Chu, M. Y., Welch, A. D.: 5-Bromo-2′-deoxycytidine (BCdR). I. Studies on metabolism *in vitro* and in mice. Biochem. Pharmacol. **8**, 324—326 (1961).

Puck, T. T., Marcus, P. I.: Action of x-rays on mammalian cells. J. exp. Med. **103**, 653—666 (1956).

Ragni, G., Szybalski, W.: Molecular radiobiology of human cell lines. II. Effects of thymidine replacement by halogenated analogues on cell inactivation by decay of incorporated radiophosphorus. J. molec. Biol. **4**, 338—346 (1962).

Rasmussen, R. E., Painter, R. B.: Radiation-stimulated DNA synthesis in cultured mammalian cells. J. cell. Biol. **29**, 11—19 (1966).

Regaud, C.: Influence de la durée d'irradiation sur les effects déterminés dans le testicule par le radium. C. R. Soc. Biol. (Paris) **86**, 787—790 (1922).

Reich, E.: Actinomycin: correlation of structure and function of its complexes with purines and DNA. Science **143**, 684—693 (1964).

Sano, K., Hoshino, T., Nagai, M.: Studies on incorporation of a radiosensitizer 5-bromo-2′-deoxyuridine into brain tumor cells and their clinical application. Neurol. Radiol. (Tokyo) **7**, 4—11 (1966).

Sears, M. E.: Erythema in areas of previous irradiation in patients treated with hydroxyurea (NSC-32065). Cancer Chemother. Rep. **40**, 31—32 (1964).

Sinclair, W. K.: Hydroxyurea: differential lethal effects on cultured mammalian cells during the cell cycle. Science **150**, 1729—1731 (1965).

Skipper, H. E.: Perspectives in cancer chemotherapy: therapeutic design. Cancer Res. **24**, 1295—1302 (1964).

Skipper, H. E., Hutchison, D. J., Schabel, F. M., Jr., Schmidt, L. H., Boldin, A., Brockman, R. W., Venditti, J. M., Wodinsky, I.: A quick reference chart on cross resistance between anticancer agents. Cancer Chemother. Rep. **56**, 493—498 (1972).

Suit, H. D.: Consideration of fractionation schedules for radiation dose. Radiology **105**, 151—156 (1972).

Suit, H. D., Hewitt, R., Urano, M., Muruyama, Y.: Effects of radiosensitizing agents in radiation therapy of mouse mammary carcinoma. Radiology **94**, 180—195 (1970).

Suit, H. D., Lindberg, R., Fletcher, G. H.: Prognostic significance of extent of tumor regression at completion of radiation therapy. Radiology **84**, 1100—1107 (1965).

Suit, H. D., Urano, M., Hewitt, R.: Effect of radiation sensitizing agents in radiation therapy of a mouse mammary carcinoma. Frontiers of radiation therapy and oncology, Vol. 4. Basel-New York: Karger; San Francisco: Vaeth 1969.

Szybalski, W., Lorkiewicz, Z.: On the nature of the principle target of lethal and mutagenic radiation effects. Abhand. Deut. Akad. Wiss., Berlin, Kl, Med. **1**, 61—71 (1962).

Tanaka, Y., Takahasi, M.: Clinical studies of intra-arterial infusion of 5-bromodeoxyuridine plus 5-fluorouracil and radiation. Radiation Protection and Sensitization. London: Taylor and Francis 1970.

Terasima, T., Tolmach, L. J.: Variations in several responses of HeLa cells to x-irradiation during the division cycle. Biophys. J. **3**, 11—33 (1963).

Vaeth, J. M.: Frontiers of Radiation Therapy and Oncology, Vol. 4. Basel-New York: Karger; San Francisco: Vaeth 1969.

Vermund, H., Hodgett, J., Ansfield, F. J.: Effects of combined roentgen irradiation and chemotherapy on transplanted tumors in mice. Amer. J. Roentgenol. **85**, 559—571 (1961).

Vietti, T., Eggerding, F., Valeriote, F.: Combined effect of X-radiation and 5-fluorouracil on survival of transplanted leukemic cells. J. nat. Cancer Inst. **47**, 865—870 (1971).

von Essen, C. F., Kligerman, M. M., Calabresi, P.: Radiation and 5-fluorouracil: a controlled clinical study. Radiology **81**, 1018—1030 (1963).

Whitmore, G. F., Gulyas, S., Botond, J.: Radiation sensitivity throughout the cell cycle in its relationship to recovery. Cellular Radiation Biology. Baltimore: Williams and Wilkins 1965.

Whitmore, G. F., Till, J. E.: Quantitation of cellular radiobiological response. Ann. Rev. nucl. Med. **14**, 347—374 (1964).

WOLFF, J. A., KRIVIT, W., NEWTON, W. A., JR., D'ANGIO, G. J.: Single versus multiple dose dactinomycin therapy of Wilms' tumor. N. Engl. J. Med. **279**, 290—322 (1968).

WOODMAN, R. J.: Localized incorporation of iododeoxyuridine from polycation-complexed iododeoxycytidylic acid into DNA of several murine and hamster tumors. Cancer Res. **28**, 2007—2016 (1968).

YARBRO, J. W.: Further studies on the mechanism of action of hydroxyurea. Cancer Res. **28**, 1082—1087 (1968).

ZIMBRICK, J. D., WARD, J. F., MYERS, L. S., JR.: Studies on the chemical basis of cellular radiosensitization in DNA. I. Pulse- and steady-state radiolysis of 5-bromouracil and thymine. Int. J. Radiat. Biol. **16**, 505—523 (1969a).

ZIMBRICK, J. D., WARD, J. F., MYERS, L. S., JR.: Studies on the chemical basis of cellular radiosensitization in DNA. II. Pulse- and steady-state radiolysis of bromouracil-substituted and unsubstituted DNA. Int. J. Radiat. Biol. **16**, 525—534 (1969b).

Chapter 26

# Tumor Immunotherapy

A. FEFER

## Introduction

Inclusion of a chapter on tumor immunotherapy in this handbook may be premature or may reflect an optimistic assessment of its future clinical potential. However, the subject is relevant to a consideration of both antineoplastic and immunosuppressive agents because (a) immunotherapy is most effective as an adjunct to other modes of therapy which may be, or indeed may *have* to be, immunosuppressive and (b) it is likely that the therapeutic results obtained with drugs, x-irradiation, and/or surgery represent the end result, not only of their antitumor activity, but also the degree to which they do or do not affect the host's immunologic response to residual tumor cells.

The increasing interest in tumor immunotherapy is reflected in a proliferation of reviews and editorials (OLD and BOYSE, 1968; ALEXANDER, 1968, 1970; JAMES, 1969; MARDINEY, 1969; EDITORIAL, 1970, 1971; HUMPHEREY, 1970; JAGARLAMOODY and MCKHANN, 1970; KEAST, 1970; SYMES, 1970; WOODRUFF, 1970; MATHÉ, 1970; MILES, 1970; MORTON, 1971; MORTON et al., 1970; SANTOS, 1970b; OETTGEN et al., 1971; BURNETT, 1971; FEFER, 1971b; HUMPHREY et al., 1971a; HUNT, 1971; JOHNSON, 1971; MITCHISON, 1971; SOPHOCLES and NADLER, 1971). The interest is attributable to an accumulation of evidence implicating immunologic factors in human as well as animal carcinogenesis (SMITH, 1968; HELLSTROM and HELLSTROM, 1969, 1971a, b; PIESSENS, 1970; FAIRLEY, 1970; GOLD, 1970). In animals, a major determinant of susceptibility or resistance to tumor induction by viruses or chemicals is the immunologic competence of the host. Thus, immunologically immature newborn animals or immunologically suppressed adults are far more susceptible to oncogenesis by a given virus than are genetically identical (syngeneic) immunologically competent adult animals (KLEIN, 1969a; LAW, 1969; ALLISON, 1970; SJOGREN and BORUM, 1971; MCCOY et al., 1972b). Therefore, the latter either develop fewer tumors and/or exhibit immunologically mediated regression of the palpable tumors induced (HAREL and CONSTANTIN, 1954; RUBIN, 1962; MCCOY et al., 1967a, 1972a; SHACHAT et al., 1968; FEFER et al., 1968; FEFER, 1969; KLEIN, 1969; LAW, 1969; ALLISON, 1971; CASAZZA et al., 1971). The importance of immunologic reactivity in oncogenesis has been explained by the demonstration that tumor cells possess tumor specific antigens (TSA) on their cell surface which are not present, either quantitatively or qualitatively, on nontumor tissue, but which can evoke a rejection response which, like a homograft reaction, is mediated largely by lymphoid cells and, to a lesser degree, by humoral antibody (FEFER et al., 1968; KLEIN, 1969b; ALLISON, 1970, 1971; MCCOY et al., 1972b).

Similar or analogous observations have recently been reported in man. Thus, patients with several congenital immunologic deficiency states (DOLL and KINLEN,

1970), as well as patients given immunosuppressive agents for organ transplantation (PENN, 1970; STARZL et al., 1970) develop an abnormally high incidence of neoplasms, especially of the lymphoreticular type. Conversely, spontaneous regression of tumors in man, after no therapy or inadequate therapy, has been reported in sufficient frequency to lend credence to the view that the regressions are immunologically mediated (EVERSON and COLE, 1966). Finally, and most significantly, many studies have strongly suggested that human tumors possess TSA detectable by *in vitro* assays which are assumed to reflect an immunologic reaction operative *in vivo* (GOLD and FREEDMAN, 1965; HELLSTROM et al., 1968; FRIDMAN and KOURILSKY, 1969; THOMSON et al., 1969; BUBENIK et al., 1970; FAIRLEY, 1970; PIESSENS, 1970; VIZA et al., 1970; HELLSTROM and HELLSTROM, 1971b; JAGARLAMOODY et al., 1971; KLEIN, 1971a, b; MORTON, 1971; OETTGEN et al., 1971; POWLES et al., 1971).

The existence of TSA is the *sine qua non* for any consideration of specific immunotherapy and provides the possibility that immunotherapy directed against TSA can preferentially or selectively kill residual tumor cells with a higher degree of antitumor specificity than can be achieved with chemotherapy. Two additional unusual features of immunotherapy, in contrast to most chemotherapy, deserve emphasis: (a) its efficacy apparently may not depend entirely upon the cell cycle of the tumor cells, and (b) it is not limited by the first order kinetics rule – it will destroy a given *number*, not a given fraction, of tumor cells. Obviously, these two features of immunotherapy, as well as its unique antitumor specificity, potentially render it especially useful as an adjunct to other modes of therapy.

I would now like to discuss the principal approaches to immunotherapy as used in animals other than humans, in which some approaches have been successful, and in humans in whom no approach has yet been convincingly effective. The emphasis will be on studies performed in etiologically and antigenically well-defined animal tumor models and on immunotherapy directed against tumors which are already clinically detectable so as to derive principles potentially relevant to immunotherapy in humans. Only the problem of eradicating cells already transformed to the malignant state will be discussed. The problem of prophylaxis or interference with the process of malignant transformation, or eradication of the oncogenic agent, a problem which may ultimately be the limiting factor in tumor immunotherapy (FIALKOW et al., 1971; ALLEN and COLE, 1972; THOMAS et al., 1972a) will not be discussed.

## Active Immunotherapy

### A. Non-Specific

The approach receiving the most attention, and recently reviewed exhaustively (FAIRLEY et al., 1970; MATHÉ, 1971a; YASHPHE, 1971; ROSENTHAL, 1972) has been active immunotherapy with Bacillus Calmette-Guerin (BCG) or other non-specific stimulants of the reticuloendothelial system which are known to enhance immunologic reactivity against a variety of antigens (HAVAS et al., 1958; BIOZZI et al., 1959; OLD et al., 1959, 1961; MALKIEL and HARGIS, 1961; HALPERN et al., 1966). BCG or other adjuvants administered before challenge with syngeneic tumor cells often retards and occasionally prevents their subsequent growth, especially if the number of tumor cells inoculated is low (HAVAS and DONNELLY, 1961; WEISS et al., 1961, 1966; WOODRUFF and BOAK, 1966; AMIEL, 1967; MATHÉ, 1968; YASHPHE, 1971). However, such stimulants have less effect if administered shortly after tumor inoculation and virtually no effect if given after tumors are already clinically detectable (Haddow and Alexander, 1964; Mathé et al., 1969b; Mathé and Pouillart, 1970; Fisher et al., 1971). Similarly, although BCG administered to animals early during the latency period after infection with oncogenic virus decreases the incidence of subsequent primary tumors, no significant effect with BCG has been reported in animals bearing detectable primary tumors (Lemonde and Clode-Hyde, 1966; Sjogren and Ankerst, 1969; Schwartz et al., 1971). The chief potential drawback of this approach, however, is that it can induce "enhancement" rather than inhibition of growth of primary or transplanted tumors (Kaliss, 1962; Weiss et al., 1966; Floersheim, 1967; Lappe, 1968; Piessens et al., 1970, 1971a).

Active immunotherapy, as an adjunct to chemotherapy or surgery, has recently been reported to be effective in mice against clinically established transplantable sarcomas (Currie and Bagshawe, 1970) or leukemias (Amiel and Berardet, 1970) and against mammary carcinomas (Martin et al., 1970; Piessens et al., 1971b). Since the determinants of success in these studies remain unknown and the same approach failed when active immunotherapy was given *before* chemotherapy (Amiel and Berardet, 1969; Currie and Bagshawe, 1970), more fundamental studies are needed to analyse the *in vivo* phenomena observed. Correlative *in vitro* studies of various components of the immune response as a function of tumor growth, chemotherapy, and immunotherapy, may ultimately reveal the prerequisites for successful "active chemoimmunotherapy." For example, although good results were reported with cyclophosphamide (Currie and Bagshawe, 1970) and procarbazine (Amiel and Berardet, 1969), nonspecific active immunotherapy may be far more effective if used in combination with drugs possessing *less* immunosuppressive activity [e.g. 1,3-*bis*(2-chloroethyl)-1-nitrosourea (BCNU) (Bonmassar et al., 1969; Fass and Fefer, 1972b)].

By analogy with the animal studies, Mathé et al. (1969a) attempted immunotherapy with BCG in patients with minimal residual disease. Patients with acute lymphoblastic leukemia in complete chemotherapy-induced remission were treated with BCG. The duration of unmaintained remission was significantly longer in the 8 patients treated with BCG than in the 10 untreated patients receiving no immunotherapy. Attempts to confirm these encouraging results with more patients are certainly warranted. To date, an English study (Leukemia Committee, 1971) on 177 patients, utilizing a different preparation of BCG administered differently, has failed to confirm Mathé's results. Similar attempts to prolong the duration of remission of acute myelogenous leukemia with BCG (Crowther, 1971), or of acute lymphoblastic leukemia with injections of *Bordetella pertussis* (Guyer and Crowther, 1969) were unsuccessful. Variable results have also been reported in patients with various cancers given BCG (Villasor, 1965). Attempts to confirm Mathé's results in man by using *his* BCG in *his* way deserve perhaps a higher priority than a search for other adjuvants (Mathé, 1971a,b), since it is quite likely that different BCG administered differently will have a different effect on immunologic reactivity.

Based on studies in a guinea pig tumor model (Zbar et al., 1971; Zbar and Tanaka, 1971), intralesional BCG has also been explored in patients with melanoma and osteogenic sarcoma (Morton et al., 1970; Morton, 1971). Local antitumor effects were observed, but with only occasional effects on distant, uninjected lesions. More such attempts will be required, with concurrent ancillary immunologic testing, before the usefulness of this approach can be evaluated. Local intratumor or systemically administered Coley's bacterial toxins have also been used in patients with terminal malignancies, with variable and generally questionable effects (Johnston, 1962; Johnston and Novales, 1962). Finally, a uniquely successful approach to local tumor immunotherapy in man has involved the treatment of multiple cutaneous carcinomas with skin-sensitizing chemicals such as 1-chloro-2,4-dinitrobenzene (DNCB), which evokes a local response more effective against local tumor than nontumor tissue (KLEIN, 1969; WILLIAMS and KLEIN, 1970).

## B. Specific

Immunization with a vaccine prepared from tumors possessing TSA induces resistance to a subsequent tumor transplant in animals (KLEIN, 1966). Since each chemically induced tumor possesses largely unique TSA (OLD et al., 1962), the vaccine must be derived from the same tumor as the one used for challenge. By contrast, since all tumors induced by a given virus possess TSA in common (KLEIN, 1969a), animals immunized with vaccine derived from any tumor induced by a given virus will become resistant to any other tumor induced by the same virus (McCOY et al., 1967a; GLYNN et al., 1968; KLEIN, 1968).

As with BCG, active immunotherapy with tumor vaccines alone or in combination with nonspecific stimulants is effective prophylactically against transplanted tumors, but is not effective once a tumor is clinically detectable (RHODES, 1962; MATSUYAMA et al., 1963; MATHÉ et al., 1969b; ELLMAN and GREEN, 1971; MATHÉ, 1971a). The use of tumor vaccines in combination with chemotherapy has received too little attention, but has shown impressive results against an established Gross leukemia (AMIEL and BERARDET, 1970). Specific active immunotherapy has more often been aimed at primary rather than transplanted tumors. The approach has often prevented development of primary tumors if initiated before or after inoculation of an oncogenic virus, but has been ineffective if instituted in animals with detectable primary tumors (FINK and RAUSCHER, 1964; GOLDNER et al., 1964; GIRARDI, 1966; SJOGREN and ANKERST, 1969; BONNEAU et al., 1970a). One exception was reported by EVANS et al. (1962a) who found that the incidence of regression of Shope papillomas was greatly increased by injecting rabbits bearing papillomas with a vaccine of their own papillomas.

Many attempts have been made to modify the tumor cell surface by coupling polysaccharides or other chemicals with foreign proteins so as to increase its immunogenicity, i.e. its ability to immunize against a tumor transplant, with relatively inconsistent results (APFFEL et al., 1966; CZAJKOWSKI et al., 1966; McENANY et al., 1968; MITCHISON, 1971). The use of tumor cells infected with unrelated viruses such as influenza (BOONE et al., 1971) or treated with *Vibrio cholerae* neuraminidase (SANFORD, 1967; BAGSHAWE and CURRIE, 1968; CURRIE and BAGSHAWE, 1969; BEKESI et al., 1971; SANFORD and CODINGTON, 1971; SIMMONS et al., 1971b) or concanavalin A (MARTIN et al., 1971) is also being explored with encouraging results. More recently, impressive regressions of established transplantable chemically-induced sarcomas were obtained by active immunotherapy using the same tumor cells treated with neuraminidase (SIMMONS et al., 1971a; RIOS and SIMMONS, 1972). Addition of BCG to the treatment regimen improved the therapeutic results (SIMMONS and RIOS, 1971). Indeed, the combination of nonspecific and specific active immunotherapy has occasionally been claimed to be preferable to either one alone (MATHÉ et al., 1969b; MATHÉ, 1971a).

Since 1902, patients with various malignancies have been actively immunized with various vaccines from their own tumor or other patients' tumors, without convincing clinical benefit attributable to the immunotherapy (LEYDEN and BLUMENTHAL, 1902; KELLOCK et al., 1922; GRAHAM and GRAHAM, 1959, 1962; CZAJKOWSKI et al., 1967; CUNNINGHAM et al., 1969; SKURKOVICH et al., 1969a; HUGHES et al., 1970; IKONOPISOV et al., 1970; BONNEAU et al., 1970b; NADLER and MOORE, 1970; CURRIE et al., 1971). NADLER and MOORE (1970), for example, treated 73 patients with advanced cancer with vaccines of irradiated or unirradiated cultured human tumor cells with no significant effect. CZAJKOWSKI et al. (1967) reported increased antitumor reactivity and some therapeutic effect in 14 patients injected with their own tumor cells coupled with rabbit gamma globulin. However, this approach had no effect on 42 patients studied by CUNNINGHAM et al. (1969). In a more controlled study, SOUTHAM (1972) treated patients after amputation for osteogenic sarcoma with irradiated extracts of their own tumors. The time to appearance of pulmonary metastases was not significantly different than that of historical untreated controls. The most encouraging results were reported by MATHÉ et al. (1969a) who treated patients with acute lymphoblastic leukemia in remission with inactivated blood from a pool of leukemic donors. Five patients thus treated remained in remission longer than did 10 untreated controls. This immunotherapeutic effect, if valid, probably does not reflect a specific immunization with hypothetical TSA, since the 5 patients did no better than did 8 patients treated with BCG or 7 patients treated with both BCG and leukemic cell vaccine. The results await confirmation.

Results from studies in animal systems raise additional problems, reservations, and recommendations concerning specific or nonspecific active immunotherapy in humans: (a) The use of nonautologous human tissue in any form as the immunogen is predicated on a viral rather than chemical etiology for human tumors, resulting in antigens shared by all tumors of a given histologic type. Although a viral etiology has not been shown, shared antigens have been detected (PIESSENS, 1970; HELLSTROM and HELLSTROM, 1971b; OETTGEN et al., 1971). (b) The immunogenicity of a tumor vaccine may be lost or destroyed in the course of its preparation due to the cellular location of the TSA or their sensitivity to various procedures, as observed in many animal tumor systems (EVANS et al., 1962a; OLD and BOYSE, 1964; NATALE et al., 1971; CHECK et al., 1971). In humans, the antigenicity of any tumor preparation to be used for active immunotherapy (whether it is cellular, subcellular, or acellular) should ideally be documented by testing the ability of the preparation to adsorb known antitumor antibodies. Furthermore, since one of the potential advantages of a tumor vaccine over BCG is the assumed specificity of the immunogen, i.e. that the tumor vaccine used contains TSA, well controlled immunotherapy studies in humans should ideally include, but to date have not, a control group of patients immunized with a comparable vaccine from comparable *nontumor* tissue. Indeed, such controls with nontumor tissue are also indicated in studies purporting to *specifically* increase humoral or cellular reactivity against autologous tumors by immunization with tumor preparations (FAIRLEY, 1970; IKONOPISOV et al., 1970; MORTON et al., 1970; MORTON, 1971; CURRIE et al., 1971; POWLES et al., 1971). (c) Finally, specific as well as nonspecific active immunotherapy can induce enhancement of tumor growth (GIRARDI, 1966; MCCOY et al., 1967b). Unfortunately, too little is known about the factors which predispose to inhibition versus enhancement in any given tumor model. It used to be assumed that active immunotherapy would act by inducing or bolstering a cellular reaction against a tumor by a host who either had no response or a woefully inadequate one. Recent studies, however, suggest that lymphocytes from tumor bearing animals are in fact reactive against tumor cells *in vitro* but that "blocking antibody" interferes with that reaction (HELLSTROM and HELLSTROM, 1969, 1971a; HELLSTROM et al., 1971a). The hypothesis must be tested that tumor inhibition or enhancement after active immunotherapy reflects an effect on blocking or nonblocking antibody rather than on cellular reactivity. Although it is not yet known whether the problem of tumor enhancement is likely to be encountered in patients, one must be aware of its potential occurrence. Additional problems and guidelines for active immunotherapy in humans have recently been outlined by GROSS (1971).

## Passive Immunotherapy (Serotherapy)

Although rejection of antigenic tumor cells is generally thought to be mediated largely by a cellular rather than a humoral response (KLEIN, 1966), sporadic but significant evidence of some effect of serotherapy has been reported and reviewed (MOTTA, 1971). Immune serum incubated with graded doses of transplanted tumor cells or administered a few days before or after challenge with a small number of tumor cells will retard or inhibit the growth of most lymphoid and some non-lymphoid tumors (ALEXANDER et al., 1966; ALEXANDER, 1968; OLD et al., 1967; VARET et al., 1968; LAW and STANTON, 1968; MCCOY et al., 1968; BUBENIK et al., 1969; MIHICH, 1969). However, serotherapy is generally not effective against a large number of tumor cells or against clinically detectable tumors (EVANS et al., 1962b; OLD et al., 1967). Until recently, the only exceptions had been reported in the primary Moloney sarcoma system (FEFER, 1969, 1970) in which young mice bearing palpable primary Moloney sarcoma virus (MSV)-induced tumors were injected with serum from adult mice hyperimmunized with MSV. Thirty-five of 102 tumors treated with immune serum completely disappeared, whereas regression was observed in only 6/71 tumors untreated or treated with non-immune serum. The possibility exists that the limiting factor in the success of serotherapy may be the amount of complement circulating in the host. This possibility has not yet been adequately tested. Other possibilities have been raised by the reported existence of serum factors which block the cytotoxic activity of immune lymphocytes, and serum factors which are themselves cytotoxic and/or capable of "unblocking" the blocking serum (HELLSTROM and HELLSTROM, 1969, 1971b; HELLSTROM et al., 1971a). The serum which was so effective against primary Moloney sarcomas had been obtained in a manner which would be expected to yield serum with cytotoxic or unblocking activity. Furthermore, serum with demonstrable "unblocking" activity *in vitro*, was recently shown to have some therapeutic effect against transplanted polyoma virus-induced tumors *in vivo* (BANSAL and SJOGREN, 1971). The possible importance of immunoglobulin type, the role of complement or properdin, and the possibility of using antibodies as carriers of drugs or radioactivity is discussed by MOTTA (1971).

Unfortunately, serotherapy can also enhance tumor growth, as shown in many tumor systems with sera directed against normal host isoantigens or, more importantly, against TSA (BOYSE et al., 1962; MOLLER, 1964; BUBENIK and KOLDOVSKY, 1965; ATTIA and WEISS, 1966; BALDWIN and BARKER, 1967; BUBENIK and TURANO, 1968; KALISS, 1968; MCCOY et al., 1968; BANSAL et al., 1972). Controlled and methodical correlative studies *in vivo* and *in vitro* concerning cytotoxic and blocking antibody will hopefully shed light on the factors which predispose to inhibition or enhancement. The enhancement in animals is sufficiently impressive to warrant caution in applying serotherapy to humans, and to encourage monitoring of such attempts with appropriate *in vitro* tests. However, the successful serotherapy against clinically established primary Moloney sarcoma virus (MSV)-induced tumors in young mice (FEFER, 1969) and in immunologically-suppressed adult mice (FEFER, 1970), as well as against polyoma tumors (BANSAL and SJOGREN, 1971) is sufficiently impressive to encourage cautious attempts in humans.

Serotherapy has been attempted in patients with various tumors with generally unimpressive and unconvincing results (MOTTA, 1971). The attempts are interesting, however, because the choice of sera used reflects the entire spectrum of assumptions derived logically from animal studies. Serum from animals has occasionally been reported to cause tumor regression in patients, but in uncontrolled studies (Murray, 1958; McCredie et al., 1959). Cytotoxic sera directed against normal isoantigens of the host (Djerassi, 1968; Laszlo, 1968; Herberman et al., 1969), or sera from volunteers immunized with host leukemic cells (Izawa et al., 1966) and therefore directed against normal host tissue as well as against hypothetical TSA have usually induced a significant but rather transient drop in the recipient's leukocyte count. Furthermore, transient remissions were reported in Burkitt's lymphoma patients infused with serum from patients in remission (Burkitt, 1967; Ngu, 1967). However, well-controlled studies showed no significant effect of parental plasma in patients with acute lymphocytic leukemia in remission (Albo et al., 1968), nor of remission plasma in patients with untreated Burkitt's lymphoma (Fass et al., 1970). Finally, serum from a patient whose melanoma had spontaneously regressed, reportedly caused regression in another melanoma patient (Sumner and Foraker, 1960), and, more recently, a patient treated surgically for a hypernephroma remained free of disease longer than expected after treatment with serum from a relative whose own hypernephroma had been eradicated (Horn and Horn, 1971). Although the regressions cannot with certainty be attributed to the serotherapy, since melanomas and hypernephromas are especially prone to regress spontaneously (Everson and Cole, 1966), the results are, nevertheless, encouraging. Additional controlled studies are indicated with remission sera or with sera from volunteers immunized with tumor or with sera from relatives whose sera can be demonstrated *in vitro* to have cytotoxic or unblocking activity (Hellstrom et al., 1968, 1971b; Morton, 1971) in patients with a minimal hematologic or non-hematologic tumor load.

## Adoptive Immunotherapy

### A. Syngeneic

The fourth approach to immunotherapy involves the adoptive transfer of lymphocytes. Immune syngeneic lymphocytes incubated with tumor cells (Old and Boyse, 1964; Klein, 1966; Rosenau and Morton, 1966; Fefer et al., 1967c; Alexander, 1968; Varet et al., 1968; Vadlamudi et al., 1971; Fass and Fefer, 1972a) or administered to animals shortly before or shortly after challenge with a small number of tumor cells (Old et al., 1962; Mitkulska et al., 1966; Mihich, 1969; Bard and Pilch, 1969; Deckers et al., 1971; Ellman and Green, 1971) will consistently and often impressively inhibit tumor growth regardless of whether the tumor is a sarcoma or a lymphoma of viral or chemical etiology, but only if the lymphocytes are immune to TSA. Unfortunately, immune cells are *not* usually effective if administered *after* the transplanted tumors are already clinically detectable, even if only 3 to 5 mm in size (Bard and Pilch, 1969; Hellstrom and Hellstrom, 1969; Ellman and Green, 1971; Fefer, 1971a; Fisher et al., 1971; Fass and Fefer, 1972a). The principal exceptions to this generalization were reported by Alexander and his associates (Alexander, 1968; Alexander and Hall, 1970), who showed that $8 \times 10^6$ immune spleen cells given intraperitoneally 2 days after intraperitoneal inoculation of $1 \times 10^3$ lymphoma cells inhibited the growth of the latter and also produced temporary regression of early transplants of a chemical sarcoma in rats following transfer of immune syngeneic thoracic duct lymphocytes.

Immune syngeneic lymphocytes are quite effective prophylactically against primary tumors if administered during the latency period to tumor formation

(Sparck and Volkert, 1965; Law et al., 1967; Chang et al., 1968; Varet et al., 1968; Wahren, 1968). This was perhaps best shown (Law et al., 1967) in C5 7Bl/6 mice thymectomized neonatally so as to render them immunologically suppressed and susceptible to oncogenesis by polyoma virus. Viable immune syngeneic spleen cells administered during the latency period often prevented the development of detectable tumors. Unimmunized lymphocytes exerted a much less significant effect, and only if administered early during the latency period.

Attempts to use syngeneic lymphoid cells immune to TSA to treat clinically detectable primary tumors have been limited to the demonstration (Delorme and Alexander, 1964) that the growth of chemically-induced sarcomas in rats can be inhibited by syngeneic immune thoracic duct lymphocytes, and that clinically established and detectable primary MSV-induced tumors in mice can be eradicated with syngeneic immune spleen cells (Fefer, 1969). Among the unique features of tumors induced by MSV is a high incidence of complete regression mediated by immunologic reaction of the primary host against TSA (Fefer et al., 1967a,b; Hellstrom et al., 1969). Therefore, MSV inoculated into immunologically competent adult mice induces tumors which ultimately regress and render the host resistant to subsequent challenge with MSV or MSV-induced tumor cells (Fefer et al., 1968), whereas MSV inoculated into young mice (Fefer et al., 1967b) or into adult mice immunologically suppressed by x-irradiation (Fefer et al., 1967b, 1968; Pollack, 1971), cyclophosphamide (Fefer, 1969), daunomycin (Casazza et al., 1971), cortisone (Shachat et al., 1968), or antilymphocyte serum (Varet et al., 1968) induces tumors, almost all of which grow progressively and kill. Accordingly, tumors were induced in young BALB/c mice and, when grossly palpable, were treated with spleen cells from adult BALB/c mice whose own primary MSV-induced tumors had regressed. The results showed that only 3 of 71 untreated mice exhibited tumor regression (68 of 71 young mice died with progressively growing tumors within 1 to 2 weeks); treatment with nonimmune cells had no effect (only 4 of 83 tumors regressed), but treatment with immune cells caused complete regression of 29 of 78 tumors.

More impressive results were obtained in similar studies with immune syngeneic cells in tumor-bearing adult mice immunosuppressed with cyclophosphamide (CY) (Fefer, 1970). Adult mice received 180 mg CY/kg and, 1 day later, MSV. Six days later, mice with palpable tumors received syngeneic spleen cells. Only 3 of 22 mice receiving no cells exhibited regression, as did 2 of 20 mice receiving nonimmune cells. By contrast, 22 of 24 mice treated with immune spleen cells exhibited complete tumor regression.

Attempts to treat tumors in patients by infusing "immune" syngeneic lymphocytes have been limited to one intriguing but negative study (Nagel et al., 1970). A patient with malignant melanoma received lymphocytes from his identical twin whose *own* melanoma had been cured and whose lymphocytes were reactive to his brother's melanoma cells by the MLC test. No therapeutic effect was noted.

### B. Allogeneic

Although lymphoid cells from allogeneic or xenogeneic donors can protect a host against a subsequent tumor challenge (Cater and Waldmann, 1967; Hill et al., 1971; Ellman et al., 1972; Katz et al., 1972), adoptive immunotherapy with such lymphoid cells sensitized against TSA has, with rare exceptions (Balme et al., 1962; Woodruff et al., 1963b; Delorme and Alexander, 1964; Woodruff and Boak, 1965; Alexander et al., 1966; Alexander, 1968), been impressively ineffective when instituted after inoculation of even a small number of tumor cells, regardless of the type of tumor or the degree of donor-host histoincompatibility (EVANS et al., 1962b; LAW et al., 1967; FEFER, 1969, 1971a, 1973b; GLYNN et al., 1969; GLYNN and KENDE, 1971). Some of the successes (WOODRUFF et al., 1963b; WOODRUFF and BOAK, 1965) involved $F_1$ hosts that could not reject the infused parental lymphocytes, while the failures may in part be attributed to the inability of totally foreign lymphoid cells to survive in an immunologically competent host – an explanation predicated on the assumption that immune cells may have to persist in the host, even if only transiently, in order to be therapeutically effective against the tumors. This view is supported by studies in which syngeneic lymphoid cells, which persist, were quite effective, whereas identically immunized allogeneic cells were not (LAW et al., 1967), and studies in which specifically sensitized allogeneic cells were therapeutically effective if they persisted, but were ineffective if they were rapidly rejected by the host (FEFER, 1970).

The principal evidence against the necessity of lymphoid cell persistence for therapeutic efficacy is provided by the studies of ALEXANDER (1968) and ALEXANDER and HALL (1970). They induced temporary regression of established primary chemically-induced sarcomas in rats by infusing thoracic duct lymphocytes from unrelated rats or sheep preimmunized with the tumor tissue. The results were somewhat surprising not only because the unrelated lymphocytes could not persist in the incompatible host, but also because it was not expected that the sheep would distinguish TSA among the large array of foreign antigens carried by the rat tumors used to immunize the sheep. However, since the same investigators (ALEXANDER et al., 1967) reported that RNA from the immunized sheep lymphocytes was also therapeutically effective, the results with lymphocytes were attributed to a transfer of information to host immunocompetent cells. Although the therapeutic efficacy of such RNA infused *in vivo* has not yet been generally established in other tumor systems by other investigators, the transfer of immunity to TSA by incubation of nonimmune lymphocytes with RNA from specifically immune lymphocytes has recently been reported (PILCH and RAMMING, 1970; PILCH et al., 1971). Presumably, if the tumor cells are killed by the lymphocytes infused, at least transient survival of the latter may be essential, whereas it may not be essential if the function of the infused cells is to transfer information to host cells which, in turn, kill the tumor. Nevertheless, the important question of lymphoid cell persistence and efficacy remains unresolved.

Lymphocytes from peripheral blood (ISRAEL et al., 1967), spleen (WOODRUFF and NOLAN, 1962), or thoracic duct (NEWTON and DONALDSON, 1969) of normal allogeneic donors have been administered to patients with various nonhematologic malignancies, and leukocytes from patients with chronic myelogenous leukemia or from multitransfused donors have been infused into patients with leukemia (SCHWARZENBERG et al., 1966; DJERASSI, 1968; MATHÉ et al., 1970), all without convincing therapeutic benefit. The relative lack of effect must be viewed in light of the several apparent prerequisites for successful immunotherapy as derived from animal studies, namely viable immune lymphocytes which persist at least transiently in a host bearing a *small* tumor load. In humans, lymphocytes from normal identical or foreign donors have been infused into patients with a large tumor load.

The most extensive clinical studies with foreign immune cells (KREMENTZ and SAMUELS, 1967; NADLER and MOORE, 1968, 1969) have involved cross immunization with killed tumor cells (never killed normal tissue) from patients with the same type of tumor, followed by cross transfusion of white blood cells. Although 20% of the patients exhibited objective responses, no controls of any kind were included, so that the responses could not be clearly attributed to the infused cells. Although the lymphocytes infused were probably immune to the hypothetical TSA, the lymphocytes were likely to be rejected quite rapidly by the host, because the host, exposed to donor tumor cells, had been immunized not only against donor tumor antigens, but also against the normal histocompatibility antigens of the donor. It is also unlikely that the lymphocytes transferred a specific sensitivity to the host since no transfer of sensitivity to any skin test was detectable (SOPHOCLES and NADLER, 1971). Although similar studies are being continued in the hope that the type of vaccine and quantity of cells used may improve the results (HUMPHREY et al., 1971 b), other approaches using cultured allogeneic lymphocytes exposed *in vitro* to killed tumor cells (MOORE and GERNER, 1970) or using lymphocytes from patients whose own tumors have been eradicated (McPEAK, 1971) are being explored.

## Adoptive Immunotherapy as an Adjunct to Whole Body x-Irradiation (Adoptive Radioimmunotherapy)

### A. Syngeneic

Since adoptive immunotherapy provides the potential of unique antitumor specificity, but is limited quantitatively by an inability to cope with a large tumor load, while whole body x-irradiation or chemotherapy can destroy a large tumor load, but are limited by a relative nonspecificity of the antitumor versus anti-normal tissue effects, the possibility of employing adoptive immunotherapy to specifically destroy residual tumor cells remaining after x-ray or chemotherapy has been investigated (FEFER, 1972b, c). Indeed, the combined approach was attempted in the early days of tumor immunology with a somewhat different rationale, namely that tumors might be eradicated by lethal doses of whole body x-irradiation and that bone marrow from normal syngeneic donors would repopulate the host and prevent x-ray-induced deaths.

BARNES et al. (1956) were the first to show that an established mouse leukemia could in fact be eradicated with lethal whole body x-irradiation plus normal syngeneic bone marrow cells. The same approach was occasionally effective against other murine lymphoid tumors, especially if instituted shortly after inoculation of a small number of tumor cells (TRENTIN, 1957) and especially if lymph node cells were also added (DEVRIES and VOS, 1958). There followed, however, several reports in which this approach was rather ineffective (MATHÉ and BEVNASE, 1959; VAN BEKKUM and DEVRIES, 1967; BORANIC, 1968; BORANIC and TONKOVIC, 1970). Unfortunately, most of the early studies involved tumors of unknown etiology and of undefined antigenic composition. Therefore, the successes and failures probably reflected the variable radiosensitivity and the relative antigenicity of the various tumors studied by different investigators at different times. Furthermore, no attempt was made to maximize the potential immunotherapeutic effect, if any, of syngeneic cells by preimmunizing the donors to TSA. More recently (FLOERSHEIM, 1969; FEFER, 1971 a), two lymphomas of known etiology and antigenicity were reported not to be susceptible to eradication by lethal whole body x-irradiation plus bone marrow and spleen cells from normal syngeneic mice, but neither lymphoma was very sensitive to the antitumor effect of x-rays per se. Additional studies are warranted in mice with different kinds of tumors of known etiology and antigenicity, with x-rays plus syngeneic cells which are nonimmune or immune to demonstrable TSA, because it is likely that whole body x-irradiation will not eradicate the tumor cells (BURCHENAL et al., 1960) and that the infused lymphoid cells will have to exert an immunotherapeutic effect against the residual tumor for cure to occur.

By analogy with the animal studies, patients with acute leukemia in relapse have been treated with supralethal whole body x-irradiation plus bone marrow from normal identical twins and have experienced disappointingly short remissions of 7 to 12 weeks (Thomas et al., 1959, 1961). The results, like the results in mice, suggest that even supralethal irradiation will not eradicate leukemia and that non-immune identical bone marrow, although quite effective in preventing death from x-rays, is immunotherapeutically ineffective against the residual tumor cells. This has stimulated efforts (Fefer et al., 1973; Rudolph et al., 1973) to add lymphocytes from normal identical twins to the regimen of x-irradiation and bone marrow transplantation and to immunize the infused donor lymphoid cells against host leukemic cells after the donor bone marrow and lymphocytes are already in the x-irradiated host. The results show that the total approach is therapeutically effective, but the contribution of the immunotherapy to the overall effect has not yet been documented (Fefer et al., 1973b).

## B. Allogeneic

Barnes et al. (1956) also postulated that *allogeneic* bone marrow infused into a tumor-bearing lethally x-irradiated mouse would colonize the host and would "destroy by the action of the immunity these residual leukemic cells, and perhaps the host." In their classic studies (Barnes et al., 1956; Barnes and Loutit, 1957), mice with a transplanted leukemia received lethal whole body x-irradiation plus bone marrow from a normal histoincompatible donor. A few mice were cured but almost all ultimately died with diarrhea and wasting, a syndrome subsequently shown to be a result of a graft-versus-host (GVH) reaction or disease (Elkins, 1971). Many similar studies with grossly histoincompatible cells have confirmed these results (DeVries and Vos, 1958; Mathé and Bernard, 1958; Mathé and Benvase, 1959; Mathé et al., 1960; Boranic and Tonkovic, 1970), and have shown that GVH disease is to be expected, that it will exert an anti-tumor effect against lymphoid and myeloid tumors, especially demonstrable by bioassy, and that it will usually kill the host. The possibility was suggested (Mathé et al., 1962) that one might use the GVH reaction against the tumor, but then treat the GVH disease and thereby save the cured host. Unfortunately, it is extremely difficult to control a GVH reaction once it is established, even in non-tumor-bearing mice (Owens and Santos, 1971; Glucksberg and Fefer, 1972), and it is likely that a GVH reaction might not exert an antitumor effect if it is controlled before it is established. Thus, the principal therapeutic possibilities have been (a) to control the GVH reaction (i.e., somehow permit it to exert its anti-tumor effect and then to stop it) or (b) to somehow confer a perferential anti-tumor specificity onto the GVH reaction. The first possibility has been explored to some extent and remains formidable (Boranic, 1968; Boranic and Tonkovic, 1970; Mathé et al., 1970; Elkins, 1971). The second possibility will hopefully receive serious attention (Fefer, 1970, 1973b).

A series of early studies (Woodruff and Symes, 1962; Woodruff et al., 1963a, b) highlighted the two problems. They showed that mice bearing long-transplanted tumors and treated with sublethal whole body x-irradiation plus lymphoid cells from histoincompatible mice or rats, died with GVH disease but often with smaller tumors. The antitumor effect was somewhat greater if the donors had been preimmunized with the tumor cells, but the mice died earlier with GVH disease. The addition of early treatment with methotrexate for the anti-cipated GVH disease was associated with an even earlier death but with much smaller tumors. Unfortunately, the contribution of the methotrexate to the overall antitumor effect observed was not clear, tumor-specific antigens were not demonstrated, and the immunity induced was both against normal host isoantigens as well as against any TSA which might have been present.

The most recent attempt to control and use the GVH reaction in tumor-bearing hosts was reported by BORANIC and TONKOVIC (1971) who treated mice bearing a myeloid or lymphoid leukemia with lethal whole body x-irradiation and spleen cells from normal histoincompatible donors. Although the GVH reaction exerted an antitumor effect demonstrable by bioassay, attempts to treat such mice prophylactically with cyclophosphamide were relatively unsuccessful and resulted in few tumor-free survivors. This relative failure was especially disappointing in view of the previously reported (BORANIC, 1968) successful eradication of the same leukemia with the same approach, but using *sublethal* instead of lethal doses of irradiation.

Attempts at allogeneic bone marrow transplantation in man have been associated with problems predictable from animal studies. Patients with acute leukemia treated with lethal whole body x-irradiation and bone marrow from normal HL-A-incompatible donors have, with rare exceptions (MATHÉ et al., 1965), done poorly because the graft either failed to "take" or induced fatal GVH disease (THOMAS et al., 1961; BORTIN, 1970; CONGDON, 1970). Attempts at bone marrow transplantation into HL-A-compatible patients with acute leukemia have, on the other hand, shown that engraftment (after lethal x-ray or cyclophosphamide) is not as significant a problem, that the GVH reaction can be modified by very early immunosuppressive therapy but remains the significant and often fatal problem, and that although a remission is the rule, leukemia occasionally recurs, which suggests an immunotherapeutic failure on the part of the normal infused allogeneic cells (GRAW et al., 1970, 1971; GRAW and SANTOS, 1970; SANTOS, 1971; FEFER et al., 1973b; THOMAS et al., 1973). It is certainly likely that this approach might be more successful if initiated in leukemic patients who are in remission and are clinically better able to tolerate the procedures (BUCKNER et al., 1973). However, special investigative attention should be provided for the detection of HL-A or non-HL-A-determined antigens not detectable by available techniques, and to cope with the problem of the extraordinary susceptibility of transplanted patients to infections which kill them in the presence or absence of leukemia recurrence (MATHÉ et al., 1965; NEIMAN et al., 1973; CLIFT et al., 1973). Above all, however, the bone marrow transplantation approach to the treatment of malignancies must be reexamined from the viewpoint of immunotherapy with its implied selective antitumor specificity, especially in view of the encouraging results obtained with transplanted HL-A-compatible bone marrow in aplastic anemia (THOMAS et al., 1972b; STORB et al., 1973), a condition which presumably requires no immunotherapeutic function on the part of the infused marrow cells.

## Adoptive Immunotherapy as an Adjunct to Chemotherapy (Adoptive Chemoimmunotherapy)

This approach has until recently received little attention. Studies with *lethal* chemoimmunotherapy are limited to a few reports (SARTORELLI and LEPAGE, 1957; FLOERSHEIM, 1969) that mice bearing transplanted tumors can often be cured with lethal dimethylmyleran or 6-thioguanine and bone marrow and spleen cells from normal syngeneic donors. The results should stimulate further studies in the same model and studies of the same approach with other drugs and other tumors.

More recent and extensive studies have involved adoptive immunotherapy as an adjunct to *sublethal* chemotherapy (Fefer, 1973a), an approach in which the only function of the infused donor cells is to destroy tumor cells immunologically, since hemopoietic repopulation by donor cells is not necessary for host survival. The results to date have been consistent in the several tumor models studied and show that clinically established tumors of known etiology and antigenicity can indeed be eradicated by sublethal adaptive chemoimmunotherapy, but only if the lymphoid cells infused are viable and derived from donors preimmunized against TSA.

Some of the most extensive studies were performed against a rapidly growing transplantable Moloney virus-induced lymphoma of BALB/c origin, designated LSTRA (Fefer, 1971a). Adult BALB/c mice were inoculated with LSTRA cells on day. Six days later, mice with palpable lymphomas and with demonstrable systemic spread received a single injection of sublethal cyclophosphamide (CY) and, 4 to 6 h later, spleen cells from adult BALB/c donors immune to cross-reacting TSA because of preimmunization with MSV. The results showed that all untreated tumor-bearing mice died by day 12, that CY doubled the median survival time, that mice treated with CY plus cells from nonimmune mice or from mice immunized with unrelated antigens did no better than those treated with CY alone, but that mice treated with CY plus cells immune to MSV survived significantly longer or were completely cured. Lethal x-irradiation of the immune cells with 5000 rads abrogated their immunotherapeutic efficacy.

The need for viable and specifically immune syngeneic cells for successful adoptive chemoimmunotherapy was more cogently demonstrated by similar studies (Fass and Fefer, 1972a, c) in which adult C57Bl/6 mice bearing a disseminated C57Bl/6 transplantable Friend virus-induced lymphoma (FBL-3) possessing potent TSA, were treated with sublethal CY plus spleen cells from adult C57Bl/6 donors preimmunized against FBL/3. Untreated mice died in 2 weeks, mice treated with CY alone or with CY plus nonimmune or nonspecifically immune control cells died in 4 weeks, while 79 of 88 mice treated with CY plus cells immune to FBL/3 survived tumor-free beyond 200 days. Freeze-thawing of the immune cells abolished their efficacy.

Thus, syngeneic adoptive chemoimmunotherapy could eradicate two different disseminated transplantable lymphomas in two strains of mice, but only if the syngeneic lymphoid cells were viable and immune to TSA. This prerequisite has also been borne out by studies of primary MSV-induced tumors (Fefer, 1969, 1970) and of other tumors. For example, L1210 leukemias were eradicated by sublethal chemotherapy plus lymphoid cells from histocompatible donors immunized with L1210 cells (Mihich, 1969; Vadlamudi et al., 1971), while an established Moloney lymphoma could not be eradicated by sublethal dimethyl myleran plus lymphoid cells from nonimmune syngeneic donors (Floersheim, 1969). It is not known, however, whether under comparable conditions immune cells would have been effective. Therefore, until well controlled studies compare the immunotherapeutic efficacy of immune and nonimmune syngeneic cells against antigenically well-defined and clinically established lymphomas and sarcomas after sublethal x-rays or drugs, one can only conclude that syngeneic lymphoid cells immune to TSA are liable to be effective when nonimmune cells are totally ineffective, and are liable to be *more* effective in the rare situation when nonimmune cells are *somewhat* effective.

The need for spleen cells specifically immune to TSA for effective chemoimmunotherapy has also been amply documented with hemisyngeneic donors. Thus, spleen cells from (BALB/c × DBA/2) $F_1$ or (BALB/c × C57Bl/6) $F_1$ donors immune to

MSV have been shown to eradicate palpable primary MSV-induced tumors in CY-treated adult BALB/c mice (FEFER, 1969), to eradicate progressively growing transplantable MSV-induced tumors (FEFER, 1969), and to eradicate a disseminated transplantable Moloney lymphoma (FEFER, 1971a).

The specificity of the immunization was further illustrated by good results obtained in the same BALB/c Moloney lymphoma model with CY plus intravenously administered spleen cells from (BALB/c × DBA/2) $F_1$ donors specifically immunized solely to the Moloney lymphoma antigens by exposure to a Moloney lymphoma of C57B1/6 origin (GLYNN et al., 1969). Such therapy caused 68 of 142 mice to survive more than 70 days and 30% of them to survive the entire observation period of up to 300 days. By contrast, nonimmune $F_1$ cells infused after CY were totally ineffective.

The possibility was considered that lymphoid cells from nonimmune but totally allogeneic donors might be effective in chemoimmunotherapy, especially if they induced a mild or subclinical GVH reaction. Experiments performed in LSTRA-bearing BALB/c mice treated with CY plus allogeneic but H-2 compatible DBA/2 spleen cells did not bear this out (FEFER, 1971a). Half the mice receiving CY plus cells from DBA donors preimmunized with MSV survived day 70 and 35% beyond day 100, whereas all mice died by day 30 if treated with CY alone, or with CY plus spleen cells from nonimmune DBA controls or even from DBA mice immune to normal BALB/c isoantigens. The results, independently confirmed by GLYNN and KENDE (1971), showed that allogeneic lymphoid cells, like syngeneic cells, had to be viable and immune to TSA in order to be immunotherapeutically effective.

The results observed with DBA/2 lymphoid cells against the transplanted BALB/c Moloney lymphoma are quite similar to those observed against primary BALB/c Moloney sarcomas which could be eradicated only by viable spleen cells from DBA mice preimmunized with MSV or with a transplanted Moloney sarcoma of BALB/c origin (FEFER, 1970). The possibility could not be ruled out that a subclinical GVH reaction did, in fact, occur and that although it was by itself immunotherapeutically ineffective when induced by nonimmune cells or cells immune to normal host isoantigens it added to the immunotherapeutic efficacy of spleen cells immune to TSA. Unfortunately, no comparable studies have been reported of adoptive chemoimmunotherapy of other well defined tumors with lymphoid cells from variably immunized H-2 compatible donors. It is interesting that lymphoid cells from nonimmune BALB/c donors had no effect on L1210 leukemia in DBA mice treated with cyclophosphamide (VADLAMUDI et al., 1971). However, immune cells were not tested. Similarly, no chemoimmunotherapeutic effect was noted in comparable studies against a spontaneous mammary adenocarcinoma of unknown antigenic composition using nonimmune allogeneic cells (SANTOS, 1970a).

In the chemoimmunotherapy models developed, CY was used to decrease the tumor load against which infused lymphocytes have to react and to depress the host's immunologic reactivity so as to delay rejection of allogeneic lymphocytes by the host. The drug may, however, have additional presently unknown but beneficial effects. It may, for example, have a selective effect on some component of the immune response such as blocking antibody formation, it may injure tumor cells and render them more susceptible to immunologic eradication, or it may destroy host lymphoid tissue and thereby provide needed space for the infused immune lymphoid cells. It is interesting that the successful chemoimmunotherapy results reported were obtained with a drug which is not only known to depress cellular and humoral reactivity against a variety of antigens, but, in the case of the Moloney sarcoma model (FEFER, 1969, 1970) and the Friend lymphoma model

(Fass and Fefer, 1972), the drug is also demonstrably able, in the dose used, to interfere with the immunological reaction of the host against the TSA of the treated tumor. Whether the immunosuppressive activity of the drug employed is necessarily bad and, therefore, the successful eradication is occurring despite the immunosuppressive activity of the drug, or whether the drug has additional functions as suggested above is not clear. It is certainly possible that adoptive chemoimmunotherapy with *syngeneic* lymphoid cells may be more effective if the chemotherapy has little or no immunosuppressive activity, whereas chemoimmunotherapy with *allogeneic* lymphoid cells may be more effective if the chemotherapy has an immunosuppressive activity so as to delay the rejection of the infused donor lymphoid cells by the host.

If the latter formulation is valid, the combined allogeneic adoptive chemoimmunotherapy approach utilized in several models should theoretically be applicable to other tumors, assuming that the tumor is antigenic and somewhat sensitive to the drug used, that the lymphoid cell donors are well-immunized to TSA, and that the drug is immunosuppressive. The principal problem to be encountered in the application of this approach to grossly histoincompatible donor-host combinations is likely to be severe or fatal GVH disease which may or may not exert an antitumor effect. However, the role or efficacy of even a severe GVH reaction as an immunotherapeutic tool depends strongly upon the kind of tumor to be treated. Thus, a severe GVH reaction induced by nonimmune allogeneic lymphoid cells exerted no detectable effect on primary Moloney sarcomas (Fefer, 1970) or on adenocarcinomas in mice (Santos, 1970a), whereas lymphoid tumors are quite susceptible to inhibition or eradication by severe and unfortunately uncontrollable GVH reactions (Barnes et al., 1956; Barnes and Loutit, 1957; DeVries and Vos, 1958; Mathé and Bernard, 1958; Mathé et al., 1960; Owens and Santos, 1965; Boranic, 1968; Boranic and Tonkovic, 1970; Glasspiegel et al., 1971).

The potential importance of tumor-specific immunity even in a setting of GVH disease has unfortunately been studied only in the primary Moloney sarcoma tumor model (Fefer, 1970). Adult BALB/c mice bearing primary MSV-induced tumors received CY plus spleen cells from H-2 incompatible C57Bl/6 mice which were nonimmunized or immunized against normal BALB/c tissue or against MSV. All mice receiving no cells died with tumor by day 50. All mice treated with C57Bl/6 spleen cells of any kind died much more rapidly with the clinical hallmarks of GVH disease. However, 15 of 16 mice treated with nonimmunized cells or with cells immune only to host isoantigens died with palpable tumors, whereas 9 of 11 mice treated with cells immune to MSV died without palpable tumors. The results suggested that a fatal GVH reaction had little effect on these non-lymphoid tumors, but that the reaction could exert a significant antitumor effect if it were induced by cells immunized to TSA. The results provided hope that a controlled GVH reaction induced by lymphoid cells specifically immunized to TSA would eradicate lymphoid tumors more effectively than would a GVH reaction induced by nonimmune cells. Preliminary results of studies in the Moloney lymphoma model support this hypothesis (Fefer, 1973b).

Adoptive chemoimmunotherapy has not yet been adequately attempted in humans. Five patients with advanced tumors have been treated with Melphalan and spleen cells from normal people or lymph node cells from pigs immunized with the tumor, and no significant effect was noted (Symes and Riddell, 1968). Another attempt involved mild chemotherapy plus infusion of thoracic duct lymphocytes, from a relative sensitized to irradiated tumor cells. No distinct therapeutic effect was noted in two patients with acute leukemia (Edwards et al., 1966), while one patient with melanoma died with a possible GVH reaction and another one exhibited no clinical change after receiving nitrogen mustard and unsensitized cells (ANDREWS et al., 1967). Further trials are indicated in more homogeneous groups of patients under more controlled conditions. However, more effort must be expended towards developing better or newer approaches to controlling or preventing the anticipated GVH reaction, and finding *in vivo* or *in vitro* ways to confer preferential antitumor specificity onto the GVH reaction, so as to either increase the reactivity of the foreign lymphoid cells to tumor cells or to decrease their reactivity to normal host cells. Steps in this direction are represented by recent studies of *in vitro* immunization (KOLDOVSKY, 1966; COHEN et al., 1971), of transfer of tumor immunity by RNA (PILCH and RAMMING, 1970; PILCH et al., 1971), of the role of soluble lymphocyte mediators of tumor destruction (BERNSTEIN et al., 1971; BRANDES et al., 1971; MACKLER, 1971), and of selective *in vitro* elimination of human lymphocytes reactive, by mixed leukocyte culture, to HL-A antigens (SALMON et al., 1971; ZOSCHKE and BACH, 1971).

Additional approaches to clinical tumor immunotherapy have been suggested, such as infusion of autologous lymphocytes incubated with tumor cells (AUST et al., 1970), with phytohemagglutinin (PHA) (FRENSTER and ROGOWAY, 1968; COSTACHEL et al., 1971), obtained in remission (SKURKOVICH et al., 1969b; FEFER, 1971c), or using such lymphocyte infusions in conjunction with high dose chemotherapy (FEFER, 1971c). These approachs involve no risk to healthly subjects and little risk to the patients, but do not yet have a solid basis in analogous animal studies.

Totally different approaches may have to be considered if and when blocking antibodies are shown in animals to be operative *in vivo* (i.e. they can interfere with the immunotherapeutic efficacy of immune cells *in vivo*) and especially when double blind studies confirm and extend the impressive association which the HELLSTROMS have reported between tumor load and blocking antibody in animals and in man (HELLSTROM et al., 1971c). The approaches may take the form of somehow removing the blocking antibody, enhancing the production of competing antibody, or conceivably using chemotherapeutic or other agents when such agents are shown in experimental systems to have an adverse effect on blocking antibody formation or activity. At this time, however, while additional animal tumor immunotherapy models are being developed and studied, some approaches to tumor immunotherapy can and should be explored in humans, but only if the studies are rigidly designed, well-controlled, and accompanied by correlative *in vitro* tests. Unfortunately, the patients who are most likely to respond to immunotherapy and are most suitable for immunotherapy are those with the smallest tumor load and are therefore patients in whom risks potentially associated with immunotherapy are more difficult to justify, whereas patients who are most readily available and most needing of experimental therapy are often those least likely to benefit from the therapy and the least likely to yield useful information.

Both ethical and scientific considerations dictate that attempts at immunotherapy of cancer in humans should not compete with other forms of therapy which have a high probability of success, but should be performed as an adjunct to and in the context of other potentially effective modes of therapy. In fact, since the patients who are most appropriate for immunotherapy are also most appropriate on theoretical grounds for adjuvant chemotherapy, the possibility of a study comparing adjuvant chemotherapy and immunotherapy in selected patient populations should be considered.

In conclusion, developments in tumor immunology in animals and humans suggest that concurrent with appropriate studies in animal models, exploratory attempts at tumor immunotherapy are warranted in humans, especially in patients whose tumor load has been reduced by other modes of therapy. Realistically, perhaps, the aim of immunotherapy attempts should not be initially to eradicate a tumor but rather to prolong a remission induced by other forms of therapy. The prerequisites for such limited success can then be determined and applied for optimal immunotherapeutic efficacy. All *in vivo* studies should, if possible, be accompanied by correlative immunologic studies *in vitro*, so as to assess the various kinds of immunologic responses elicited by the tumor or by unrelated antigens and to determine how the responses are affected by the clinical course of the disease, by conventional therapy, and by immunotherapeutic manipulations. Data thus obtained should ultimately lend rational direction to the design of scientific and therapeutic approaches to the immunotherapy of cancer in man.

This chapter is primarily based on literature published by early 1972.

## References


Albo, V., Krivit, W., Hartmann, J.: Fresh plasma as an adjuvant to the chemotherapy of acute lymphatic leukemia in children. Proc. Amer. Ass. Cancer Res. **9**, 2 (1968).

Alexander, P.: Immunotherapy of cancer. Experiments with primary tumors and syngeneic tumor grafts. Progr. exp. Tumor Res. **10**, 22—71 (1968).

Alexander, P.: Immunological aspects of cancer — II. Prospects for immunotherapy of cancer. Experience in experimental systems. Brit. med. J. **4**, 484—486 (1970).

Alexander, P., Connell, D. I., Mikulska, Z. B.: Treatment of a murine leukemia with spleen cells or sera from allogeneic mice immunized against the tumor. Cancer Res. **26**, 1508—1515 (1966).

Alexander, P., Hall, J. G.: The role of immunoblasts in host resistance and immunotherapy of primary sarcomata. Adv. Cancer Res. **13**, 1—37 (1970).

Alexander, P., Hamilton, L. D., Hall, J. G.: Effect of nucleic acids from immune lymphocytes on rat sarcomata. Nature (Lond.) **213**, 509—511 (1967).

Allen, D. W., Cole, P.: Viruses and human cancer. New Engl. J. Med. **286**, 70—82 (1972).

Allison, A. C.: Immunological aspects of cancer — part I. Potentiation of viral carcinogenesis by immunosuppression. Brit. med. J. **4**, 419—420 (1970).

Allison, A. C.: New cell antigens induced by viruses and their biological significance. Proc. Roy. Soc. (Lond.) B, **177**, 23—39 (1971).

Amiel, J. L.: Immunothérapie active non spécifique par le B.C.G. de la leucémie virale E♂G2 chez des receveurs isogénique. Rév. Fránc. Étude. clin. Biol. **12**, 912—914 (1967).

Amiel, J. L., Berardet, M.: An experimental model of active immunotherapy preceded by cytoreductive chemotherapy. Europ. J. Cancer **6**, 557—559 (1970).

Amiel, J. L., Berardet, M.: Essais de traitements de la leucémie E♂G2 associant chimiothérapie et immunothérapies actives non spécifique et spécifique. Rév. Fránc. Étud. clin. Biol. **14**, 685—688 (1969).

Andrews, G. A., Congdon, C. C., Edwards, C. L., Gengozian, N., Nelson, B., Vodopick, H.: Preliminary trials of clinical immunotherapy. Cancer Res. **27**, 2535—2541 (1967).

Apffel, C. A., Arnasson, B. G., Peters, J. H.: Induction of tumor immunity with tumor cells treated with iodoacetate. Nature (Lond.) **209**, 694—696 (1966).

Attia, M. A. M., Weiss, D. W.: Immunology of spontaneous mammary carcinomas in mice. V. Acquired tumor resistance and enhancement in strain A mice injected with mammary tumor virus. Cancer Res. **26**, 1787—1800 (1966).

Aust, J. C., Jagarlamoody, S., McKhann, C. F.: Immunization of lymphocytes *in vitro* for immunotherapy of malignant disease. Surg. Forum **21**, 118—120 (1970).

Bagshawe, K. D., Currie, G. A.: Immunogenicity of L1210 murine leukemia cells after treatment with neuraminidase. Nature (Lond.) **218**, 1254—1255 (1968).

Baldwin, R. W., Barker, C. R.: Antigenic composition of transplanted rat hepatomas originally induced by 4-dimethylaminoazobenzene. Brit. J. Cancer **21**, 338—345 (1967).

Balme, R. H., Dockerty, M. B., Grindlay, J. H., Litzow, T. J.: The use of immune lymph in the treatment of mouse cancer. Minnesota Med. **45**, 892—899 (1962).

Bansal, S. C., Hargreaves, R., Sjogren, H. O.: Facilitation of polyoma tumor growth in rats by blocking sera and tumor eluate. Int. J. Cancer **9**, 97—108 (1972).

Bansal, S. C., Sjogren, H. O.: "Unblocking" serum activity *in vitro* in the polyoma system may correlate with antitumour effects of antiserum *in vivo*. Nature (Lond.) **233**, 76—78 (1971).

Bard, D. S., Pilch, Y. H.: The role of the spleen in the immunity to a chemically induced sarcoma in C3H mice. Cancer Res. **29**, 1125—1131 (1969).

BARNES, D. W. H., LOUTIT, J. F.: Treatment of murine leukemia with x-rays and homologous bone marrow. Brit. J. Hemat. 3, 241—252 (1957).
BARNES, D. W. H., LOUTIT, J. F., NEAL, F. E.: Treatment of murine leukemia with x-rays and homologous bone marrow. Brit. med. J. 2, 626—630 (1956).
BEKESI, J. G., ARNEAULT, G. S., HOLLAND, J. F.: Increase of leukemia L1210 immunogenicity by vibrio cholerae neuraminidase treatment. Cancer Res. 31, 2130—2132 (1971).
BERNSTEIN, I. D., THOR, D. E., ZBAR, B., RAPP, H. J.: Tumor immunity. Tumor suppression *in vivo* initiated by soluble products of specifically stimulated lymphocytes. Science 172, 729—731 (1971).
BIOZZI, G., STIFFEL, C., HALPERN, B. N., MOUTON, D.: Éffect de l'inoculation du Bacille de Calmette-Guerin sur le dévelopment de la tumeur ascitique d'Ehrlich chez la souris. C. R. Soc. Biol. (Paris) 153, 987—989 (1959).
BONMASSAR, E., VADLAMUDI, S., VIEIRA, V., GOLDIN, A.: Influence of Tween 80 on the antileukemic activity of 1,3-*bis*(2-chloroethyl)-1-nitrosourea. Arch. Ital. Patol. clin. Tumori 12, 163—175 (1969).
BONNEAU, H., COCHET, G., FAVRE, R., MEYER, G.: Éssai d'un traitement immunitaire par éxtraits tumoraux irradiés aux rayons u.v. des tumeurs de hamster à virus polyome. Bull. Cancer (Paris) 57, 55—68 (1970a).
BONNEAU, H., PEYRONEL, J. C., FAVRE, R., ROBERT-VAGUE, D.: Éssais de traitement auxiliaire de cèrtains cancers humains par injections d'éxtraits tumoraux autologues irradiés aux rayons ultra-violets. Bull. Cancer (Paris) 57, 69—78 (1970b).
BOONE, C., BLACKMAN, K., BRANDCHAFT, P.: Tumour immunity induced in mice with cell-free homogenates of influenza virus-infected tumor cells. Nature (Lond.) 231, 265—266 (1971).
BORANIC, M.: Transient graft-versus-host reaction in the treatment of leukemia in mice. J. nat. Cancer Inst. 41, 421—437 (1968).
BORANIC, M., TONKOVIC, I.: Time pattern of the antileukemic effect of the graft-versus-host reaction in mice. Cancer Res. 31, 1140—1147 (1970).
BORTIN, M.: A compendium of reported human bone marrow transplants. Transplantation 9, 571—587 (1971).
BOYSE, E. A., OLD, L. J., STOCKERT, E.: Immunological enhancement of a leukemia. Nature (Lond.) 194, 1142—1144 (1962).
BRANDES, L. J., GALTON, D. A. G., WILTSHAW, E.: New approach to immunotherapy of melanoma. Lancet 2, 293—295 (1971).
BUBENIK, J., KOLDOVSKY, P.: Factors influencing the induction of enhancement and resistance to methylcholanthrene-induced tumors in a syngeneic system. Folio biol. (Praha) 11, 258—265 (1965).
BUBENIK, J., PERLMANN, P., HELMSTEIN, K., MOBERGER, G.: Cellular and humoral immune responses to human urinary bladder carcinomas. Int. J. Cancer 5, 310—319 (1970).
BUBENIK, J., TURANO, A.: Enhancing effect on tumor growth of humoral antibodies against TSTA in tumors induced by murine sarcoma virus (Harvey). Nature (Lond.) 220, 928—930 (1968).
BUBENIK, J., TURANO, A., FADDA, G.: Prevention of carcinogenesis by murine sarcoma virus (Harvey) following injection of immune sera during the latency period. Int. J. Cancer 4, 648—654 (1969).
BUCKNER, C. D., JOHNSON, F. L., THOMAS, E. D., STORB, R., CLIFT, R. A., CHARD, R. L., FUNK, D. D., NEIMAN, P., FEFER, A.: Allogeneic marrow grafting in acute lymphoblastic leukemia during marrow remission. Biomedicine 18, 295—303, 1973.
BURCHENAL, J. H., OETTGEN, H. F., HOLMBERG, E. A. D., HEMPHILL, S. C., REPPERT, J. A.: Effect of total body irradiation on the transplantability of mouse leukemia. Cancer Res. 20, 425—430 (1960).
BURKITT, D.: Clinical evidence suggesting the development of an immunological response against African lymphoma. UICC Monogr. Ser. 8, 197—203 (1967).
BURNET, F. M.: Implications of immunological surveillance for cancer therapy. Israel J. med. Sci. 7, 9—16 (1971).
CASAZZA, A. M., DIMARCO, A., DICUONZO, G.: Interference of Daunomycin and Adriamycin on the growth and regression of murine sarcoma virus (Moloney) tumors in mice. Cancer Res. 31, 1971—1976 (1971).
CATER, D. B., WALDMANN, H.: The effect on the growth of BP8 ascites tumour in C3H/C57F1 or C3H mice of "lymphocyte preparations" from C57 mice injected with BP8 cells and Freund's adjuvant. Brit. J. Cancer 21, 124—136 (1967).
CHANG, S. S., HILDEMANN, W. H., RASMUSSEN, A. F., JR.: Immunogenetic aspects of polyoma virus susceptibility in mice. J. nat. Cancer Inst. 40, 363—375 (1968).
CHECK, J. H., CHILDS, T. C., BRADY, L. W., DERASSE, A. R., FUSCALDO, K. E.: Protection against spontaneous mouse mammary adenocarcinoma by inoculation of heat-treated syngeneic mammary tumor cells. Int. J. Cancer 7, 403—408 (1971).

Clift, R. A., Buckner, C. D., Fefer, A., Lerner, K. G., Neiman, P. E., Storb, R., Murphy, M., Thomas, E. D.: Infectious complications of marrow transplantation. Transpl. Proc., 1973.
Cohen, I. R., Globerson, A., Feldman, M.: Rejection of tumor allografts by mouse spleen cells sensitized *in vitro*. J. exp. Med. **133**, 821—833 (1971).
Congdon, C. C.: Cooperative group on bone marrow transplantation in man. Transpl. Proc. **2**, 342—360 (1970).
Costachel, O., Iosub, A., Gutulescu, N., Mogos, I., Liciu, F.: Our experience in associated immunotherapy of cancer. Arch. Geschwulstforsch. **37**, 19—32 (1971).
Crowther, D.: Treatment of acute myelogenous leukemia in adults. Brit. J. Hematol. **21**, 360—361 (1971).
Cunningham, T. J., Olson, K. B., Laffin, R., Horton, J., Sullivan, J.: Treatment of advanced cancer with active immunization. Cancer **24**, 932—937 (1969).
Currie, G. A., Bagshawe, K. D.: Active immunotherapy with Corynebacterium parvum and chemotherapy in murine fibrosarcomas. Brit. med. J. **1**, 541—544 (1970).
Currie, G. A., Bagshawe, K. D.: Tumor-specific immunogenicity of methylcholanthrene-induced sarcoma cells after incubation in neuraminidase. Brit. J. Cancer **23**, 141—149 (1969).
Currie, G. A., Lejeune, F., Fairley, G. H.: Immunization with irradiated tumour cells and specific lymphocyte cytotoxicity in malignant melanoma. Brit. med. J. **2**, 305—310 (1971).
Czajkowski, N. P., Rosenblatt, M., Cushing, F. R., Vazquez, J., Wolf, P. L.: Production of active immunity to malignant neoplastic tissue. Cancer **19**, 739—749 (1966).
Czajkowski, N. P., Rosenblatt, M., Wolf, P. L., Vazquez, J.: A method of active immunization to autologous human tumor tissue. Lancet **2**, 905—909 (1967).
Deckers, P. J., Edgerton, B. W., Thomas, B. S., Pilch, Y. H.: The adoptive transfer of concomitant immunity to murine tumor isografts with spleen cells from tumor-bearing animals. Cancer Res. **31**, 734—742 (1971).
Delorme, E. J., Alexander, P.: Treatment of primary fibrosarcoma in the rat with immune lymphocytes. Lancet **2**, 117—120 (1964).
DeVries, M. J., Vos, P.: Treatment of mouse lymphosarcoma by total body x-irradiation and by injection of bone marrow and lymph node cells. J. nat. Cancer Inst. **21**, 1117—1129 (1958).
Djerassi, I.: Transfusion of lymphocyte antibody and lymphocytes from multitransfused donors. Clin. Pediat. **7**, 272—273 (1968).
Doll, R., Kinlen, L.: Immunological aspects of cancer — Part I. Immunosurveillance and cancer. Epidemiological evidence. Brit. med. J. **4**, 420—422 (1970).
*Editorial:* Immunologic aspects of neoplasia. Cancer Bull. **22**, 91—96 (1970).
*Editorial:* Immunotherapy of cancer. Med. J. Austral. **2**, 289—291 (1971).
Edwards, C. L., Congdon, C. C., Gengozian, N., Vodopick, H., Andrews, G. A.: Treatment of acute leukemia: An experimental immunologic approach. Exp. Hematol. **9**, 23—24 (1966).
Elkins, W. L.: Cellular immunology and the pathogenesis of the graft-versus-host reactions. Progr. Allergy **15**, 78—187 (1971).
Ellman, L., Green, I.: L2C guinea pig leukemia: Immunoprotection and immunotherapy. Cancer **28**, 647—654 (1971).
Ellman, L., Katz, D. H., Green, I., Paul, W. E., Benacerraf, B.: Mechanisms involved in the antileukemic effect of immunocompetent allogeneic lymphoid cell transfer. Cancer Res. **32**, 141—148 (1972).
Evans, C. A., Gorman, L. R., Ito, Y., Weiser, R. S.: Antitumor immunity in the Shope papilloma-carcinoma complex of rabbits. I. Papilloma regression induced by homologous and autologous tissue vaccines. J. nat. Cancer Inst. **29**, 277—285 (1962a).
Evans, C. A., Weiser, R. S., Ito, Y.: Antiviral and antitumor immunologic mechanisms operative in the Shope papilloma-carcinoma system. Cold Spr. Harb. Symp. quant. Biol. **27**, 453—462 (1962b).
Everson, T. C., Cole, W. H.: Spontaneous Regression of Cancer. Philadelphia: W. B. Saunders 1966.
Fairley, G. H.: Immunological aspects of cancer — II. Evidence for antigenicity in human tumours with reference to both melanoma and acute leukaemia. Brit. med. J. **4**, 483—484 (1970).
Fairley, G. H., Crowther, D., Guyer, J. G., Hardisty, R. M., Kay, H. E. M., Knapton, P. J., McElwain, T. J., Parr, I. B.: Active immunotherapy in the treatment of leukemia and other malignant diseases in animals and man. Rec. Results Cancer Res. **30**, 138—141 (1970).
Fass, L., Fefer, A.: Studies of adoptive chemoimmunotherapy of a Friend virus induced lymphoma. Cancer Res. **32**, 997—1001 (1972a).

FASS, L., FEFER, A.: Application of an *in vitro* cytotoxicity test to studies of the effects of drugs on the cellular immune response in mice. I. Primary response. J. Immunol. **109**, 749—753 (1972b).

FASS, L., FEFER, A.: Factors related to therapeutic efficacy in adoptive chemoimmunotherapy of a Friend virus-induced lymphoma. Cancer Res., **32**, 2427—2431 (1973).

FASS, L., HERBERMAN, R. B., ZIEGLER, J., MORROW, R. H.: Evaluation of the effect of remission plasma on untreated patients with Burkitt lymphoma. J. nat. Cancer Inst. **44**, 145—149 (1970).

FEFER, A.: Immunotherapy and chemotherapy of Moloney sarcoma virus-induced tumors in mice. Cancer Res. **29**, 2177—2183 (1969).

FEFER, A.: Immunotherapy of primary Moloney sarcoma virus-induced tumors. Int. J. Cancer **5**, 327—337 (1970).

FEFER, A.: Adoptive chemoimmunotherapy of a Moloney lymphoma. Int. J. Cancer 8, 364—373 (1971a).

FEFER, A.: Experimental approaches to immunotherapy of cancer. In: Current concepts in the management of leukemia and lymphoma. Rec. Results Cancer Res. **36**, 182—192 (1971b).

FEFER, A.: Guest Editorial: Immunotherapy of cancer. J. nat. Cancer Inst. **47**, VII—XII (1971c).

FEFER, A.: Adoptive tumor immunotherapy in mice as an adjunct to whole body x-irradiation or chemotherapy — A review. Israel J. med. Sci. **9**, 350—365 (1973a).

FEFER, A.: Immunotherapy of cancer in mice. In: Frontiers Radiation Therapy Oncology, Vol. 7. pp. 35—49. Basel: S. Karger 1972.

FEFER, A.: Treatment of a Moloney lymphoma with cyclophosphamide and H-2-incompatible spleen cells. Cancer Res. **33**, 641—644 (1973b).

FEFER, A., BUCKNER, C. D., CLIFT, R. A., FASS, L., LERNER, K. G., MICKELSON, E. M., NEIMAN, P., RUDOLPH, R., STORB, R., THOMAS, E. D.: Marrow grafting in identical twins with hematologic malignancies. Transpl. Proc. **5**, 927—931 (1973a).

FEFER, A., MCCOY, J. L., GLYNN, J. P.: Antigenicity of a virus-induced murine sarcoma (Moloney). Cancer Res. **27**, 962—967 (1967a).

FEFER, A., MCCOY, J. L., GLYNN, J. P.: Induction and regression of primary Moloney sarcoma virus-induced tumors in mice. Cancer Res. **27**, 1626—1631 (1967b).

FEFER, A., MCCOY, J. L., GLYNN, J. P.: Studies on the growth and regression of a transplantable Moloney sarcoma. Cancer Res. **27**, 2207—2211 (1967c).

FEFER, A., MCCOY, J. L., PERK, K., GLYNN, J. P.: Immunologic, virologic and pathologic studies of regression of autochthonous Moloney sarcoma virus (MSV)-induced tumors in mice. Cancer Res. **28**, 1577—1585 (1968).

FEFER, A., THOMAS, E. D., BUCKNER, C. D., STORB, R., NEIMAN, P., GLUCKSBERG, H., CLIFT, R. A., LERNER, K. G.: Marrow Transplants in Aplastic Anemia and Leukemia. Seminars in Hematology, (1973b).

FIALKOW, P. J., THOMAS, E. D., BRYANT, J. I., NEIMAN, P. E.: Leukaemic transformation of engrafted human marrow cells *in vivo*. Lancet **1**, 251—255 (1971).

FINK, M. A., RAUSCHER, F. J.: Immune reactions to a murine leukemia virus. I. Induction of immunity to infection with virus in the natural host. J. nat. Cancer Inst. **32**, 1075—1082 (1964).

FISHER, B., SAFFER, E. A., FISHER, E. R.: Experiences with lymphocyte immunotherapy in experimental tumor systems. Cancer **27**, 771—781 (1971).

FLOERSHEIM, G. L.: Facilitation of tumor growth by Bacillus pertussis. Nature (Lond.) **216**, 1235—1237 (1967).

FLOERSHEIM, G. L.: Treatment of Moloney lymphoma with lethal doses of dimethyl myleran combined with injection of hemopoietic cells. Lancet **1**, 228—233 (1969).

FRENSTER, J. H., ROGOWAY, W. M.: *In vitro* activation and reinfusion of autologous human lymphocytes. Lancet **2**, 979—980 (1968).

FRIDMAN, W. H., KOURILSKY, E. M.: Stimulation of lymphocytes by autologous leukaemia cells in acute leukaemia. Nature (Lond.) **224**, 277—279 (1969).

GIRARDI, A. J.: Tumor resistance and tumor enhancement with $SV_{40}$ virus-induced tumors. Germinal Centers in Immune Responses. Proc. of a Symposium held at the University of Bern, Switzerland, June 22—24, 1966, pp. 422—427. Heidelberg: Springer-Verlag 1966.

GLASSPIEGEL, J. S., SALTZSTEIN, E. C., RIMM, A. A., GILLER, R. H., BORTIN, M. M.: Graft-versus-leukemia: Adoptive immunotherapy for the eradication of murine leukemia. Exp. Hematol. **21**, 23—24 (1971).

GLUCKSBERG, H., FEFER, A.: Chemotherapy of established graft-versus-host (GVH) disease in mice. Transplantation **13**, 300—305 (1972).

GLYNN, J. P., HALPERN, B. L., FEFER, A.: An immunochemotherapeutic model for the treatment of a transplanted Moloney virus-induced lymphoma in mice. Cancer Res. **29**, 515—520 (1969).

Glynn, J.P., Kende, M.: Treatment of Moloney virus-induced leukemia with cyclophosphamide and specifically sensitized allogeneic cells. Cancer Res. 31, 1383—1388 (1971).
Glynn, J.P., McCoy, J.L., Fefer, A.: Cross-resistance to the transplantation of syngeneic Friend, Moloney and Rauscher virus-induced tumors. Cancer Res. 28, 434—439 (1968).
Gold, P.: The role of immunology in human cancer research. Canad. med. Ass. J. 103, 1043—1051 (1970).
Gold, P., Freedman, S.: Demonstration of tumor-specific antigens of the human colonic carcinomata by immunological tolerance and absorption techniques. J. exp. Med., 121, 439—462 (1965).
Goldner, H., Girardi, A.J., Larsen, D.M., Hilleman, M.R.: Interruption of $SV_{40}$ virus tumorigenesis using irradiated homologous tumor antigens. Proc. Soc. exp. Biol. 117, 851—857 (1964).
Graham, J.B., Graham, R.M.: The effect of vaccine on cancer patients. Surg. Gynec. Obstet. 109, 131—138 (1959).
Graham, J.B., Graham, R.M.: Autogenous vaccine in cancer patients. Surg. Gynec. Obstet. 114, 1—4 (1962).
Graw, R.G., Jr., Herzig, G.P., Rogentine, G.N., Jr., Yankee, R.A., Leventhal, B., Whang-Peng, J., Halterman, R.H., Kruger, G., Berard, C., Henderson, E.S.: Graft-versus-host reaction complicating HL-A matched bone marrow transplantation. Lancet 2, 1053—1055 (1970).
Graw, R.G., Jr., Leventhal, B.G., Yankee, R.A., Rogentine, G.N., Wang-Peng, J., Ginnif, M.H., Herzig, G.P., Halterman, R.H., Henderson, E.S.: HL-A and mixed leukocyte culture matched allogeneic bone marrow transplantation in patients with acute leukemia. Transplant. Proc. 3, 405—408 (1971).
Graw, R.G., Jr., Santos, G.W.: Bone marrow transplantation in patients with leukemia. Incidence and severity of graft-versus-host disease in successful HL-A-matched transplants. Transplantation 11, 197—199 (1971).
Gross, L.: Tentative guidelines referring to inoculation of homologous cancer extracts in man. Int. J. Cancer 7, 182—185 (1971).
Guyer, R.J., Crowther, D.: Active immunotherapy in treatment of acute leukemia. Brit. med. J. 2, 406—407 (1969).
Haddow, A., Alexander, P.: An immunological method of increasing the sensitivity of primary sarcomas to local irradiation with x-ray. Lancet 1, 452—457 (1964).
Halpern, B.N., Biozzi, G., Stiffel, C., Mouton, D.: Inhibition of tumor growth by administration of killed Corynebacterium parvum. Nature (Lond.) 212, 853—854 (1966).
Harel, J., Constantin, T.: Sur la malignité des tumeurs provoquées par le virus fibromateaux de Shope, chez le lapin nouveau-né et le lapin adulte traité par des doses massives de cortisone. Bull. Ass. Franc. Cancer 41, 483—489 (1954).
Havas, H.F., Donnelly, A.J.: Mixed bacterial toxins in the treatment of tumors. IV. Response of methylcholanthrene-induced, spontaneous, and transplanted tumors in mice. Cancer Res. 21, 17—25 (1961).
Havas, H.F., Groesbeck, M.E., Donnelly, A.J.: Mixed bacterial toxins in the treatment of tumors. I. Methods of preparation and effects on normal and sarcoma 37-bearing mice. Cancer Res. 18, 141—148 (1958).
Hellstrom, I., Hellstrom, K.E., Pierce, G.E., Bill, A.H.: Demonstration of cell-bound and humoral immunity against neuroblastoma cells. Proc. nat. Acad. Sci. (Wash.) 60, 1231—1238 (1968).
Hellstrom, I., Hellstrom, K.E., Pierce, G.E., Fefer, A.: Studies on immunity to autochthonous mouse tumors. Transplant. Proc. 1, 90—94 (1969).
Hellstrom, I., Hellstrom, K.E., Sjogren, H.O.: Some recent information on "blocking antibodies" as studied *in vitro*. Transplant. Proc. 3, 1221—1227 (1971a).
Hellstrom, I., Hellstrom, K.E., Sjogren, H.O., Warner, G.A.: Serum factors in tumor-free patients cancelling the blocking of cell-mediated tumor immunity. Int. J. Cancer 8, 185—191 (1971b).
Hellstrom, I., Sjogren, H.O., Warner, G., Hellstrom, K.E.: Blocking of cell-mediated tumor immunity by sera from patients with growing neoplasms. Int. J. Cancer 7, 226—237 (1971c).
Hellstrom, K.E., Hellstrom, I.: Cellular immunity against tumor antigens. Adv. Cancer Res. 122, 167—223 (1969).
Hellstrom, K.E., Hellstrom, I.: Some aspects of the immune defense against cancer. I. *In vitro* studies on animal tumors. Cancer 28, 1266—1268 (1971a).
Hellstrom, K.E., Hellstrom, I.: Some aspects of the immune defense against cancer. II. *In vitro* studies on human tumors. Cancer 28, 1269—1271 (1971b).
Herberman, R., Rogentine, G.N., Oren, M.E.: Bioassay of antitumor effects of human alloantisera. Clin. Res. 17, 328 (1969).

HILL, G., LITTLEJOHN, K., KELLY, G., ATKINS, R., GREER, J., EISEMAN, B.: Effects of pig leukocytes on mouse lymphatic leukemia. J. Surg. Oncol. 3, 569—579 (1971).
HORN, L., HORN, H. L.: An immunological approach to the therapy of cancer. Lancet 2, 465—469 (1971).
HUGHES, L. E., KEARNEY, R., TULLY, M.: A study in clinical cancer immunotherapy. Cancer 26, 269—278 (1970).
HUMPHREY, L. J.: Tumor immunity. J. surg. Res. 10, 493—512 (1970).
HUMPHERY, L. J., JEWELL, W. R., MURRAY, D. R., GRIFFEN, W. O., JR.: Immunotherapy for the patient with cancer. Ann. Surg. 173, 47—54 (1971a).
HUMPHREY, L. J., MURRAY, D. R., BOEHM, O. R.: Effect of tumor vaccines in immunizing patients with cancer. Surg. Gyn. Obstet. 132, 437—442 (1971b).
HUNT, P. S.: Immunity in cancer. Aust. New Zeal. J. Surg. 40, 369—373 (1971).
IKONOPISOV, R. L., LEWIS, M. G., HUNTER-CRAIG, I. D., BODENHAM, D. C., PHILLIPS, T. M., COOLING, C. I., PROCTOER, J., FAIRLEY, G. H., ALEXANDER, P.: Autoimmunization with irradiated tumour cells in human malignant melanoma. Brit. med. J. 2, 752—754 (1970).
ISRAEL, L., MANNONI, P., MAWAS, C., GINESTE, J., GROSS, B., SORS, C.: 70 perfusions de lymphocytes homologues dans 25 cas de cancers avancés. Path. Biol. (Paris) 15, 603—606 (1967).
IZAWA, T., SAKURAI, M., ATSUTA, Y., YOSHIZUMI, P.: Antigenicity of leukemia and antiserum therapy. Ann. Paediat. Jap. 12, 346—362 (1966).
JAGARLAMOODY, S. M., AUST, S. C., TEW, R. H., MCKHANN, C. F.: *In vitro* detection of cytotoxic cellular immunity against tumor specific antigens by a radioisotope technique. Proc. nat. Acad. Sci. (Wash.) 68, 1346—1350 (1971).
JAGARLAMOODY, S. M., MCKHANN, C. F.: Immunotherapy of cancer-current status. Geriatrics 25, 155—160 (1970).
JAMES, K. W.: Tumor immunology and response to radiation therapy. Radiol. Clin. N. Amer. 7, 353—364 (1969).
JOHNSON, F. L.: Immunological aspects of malignant disease. Med. J. Aust. 2, 317—325 (1971).
JOHNSTON, B. J.: Clinical effect of Coley's toxin — I. A controlled study. Cancer Chemother. Rep. 21, 19—41 (1962).
JOHNSTON, B. J., NOVALES, E. T.: Clinical effect of Coley's toxin — II. A seven year study. Cancer Chemother. Rep. 21, 43—68 (1962).
KALISS, N.: Immunological enhancement in tumor homografts in mice. A review. Cancer Res. 18, 992—1003 (1958).
KALISS, N.: The elements of immunologic enhancement. A consideration of mechanisms. Ann. N. Y. Acad. Sci. 101, 64—79 (1962).
KATZ, D. H., ELLMAN, L., PAUL, W. E., GREEN, I., BENACERRAF, B.: Resistance of guinea pigs to leukemia following transfer of immunocompetent allogeneic lymphoid cells. Cancer Res. 32, 133—140 (1972).
KEAST, D.: Immunosurveillance and cancer. Lancet 2, 710—712 (1970).
KELLOCK, T. H., CHAMBERS, H., RUSS, S.: An attempt to procure immunity to malignant disease in man. Lancet 1, 217—219 (1922).
KLEIN, G.: Tumor antigens. Ann. Rev. Microbiol. 20, 223—252 (1966).
KLEIN, G.: Tumor-specific transplantation antigens. Cancer Res. 28, 625—635 (1968).
KLEIN, G.: Experimental studies in tumor immunology. Fed. Proc. 28, 1739—1753 (1969a).
KLEIN, G.: Hypersensitivity reactions at tumor sites. Cancer Res. 29, 2351—2362 (1969b).
KLEIN, G.: Immunological studies on a human tumor. Dilemmas of the experimentalist. Israel J. med. Sci. 7, 111—131 (1971a).
KLEIN, G.: Immunological studies on Burkitt's lymphoma. Leukemia research fund lecture. Postgrad. med. J. 47, 141—155 (1971b).
KOLDOVSKY, P.: An attempt at *in vitro* sensitization of immunologically competent cells against tumour specific antigens. Folia biol. (Praha) 12, 238—247 (1966).
KREMENTZ, E. T., SAMUELS, M. T.: Tumor cross-transplantation and cross-transfusion in the treatment of advanced malignant disease. Bull. Tulane med. Fac. 26, 263—270 (1967).
LAPPE, M. A.: Evidence for the antigenicity of papillomas induced by 3-methylcholanthrene. J. nat. Cancer Inst. 40, 823—846 (1968).
LASZLO, J., BUCKLEY, C. E., III, AMOS, B. D.: Infusion of isologous immune plasma in chronic lymphocytic leukemia. Blood 31, 104—110 (1968).
LAW, L. W.: Studies of the significance of tumor antigens in induction and regression of neoplastic diseases. Cancer Res. 29, 1—21 (1969).
LAW, L. W., TING, R. C., LECKBAND, E.: Prevention of virus-induced neoplasms in mice through passive transfer of immunity by sensitized syngeneic lymphoid cells. Proc. nat. Acad. Sci. (Wash.) 57, 1068—1075 (1967).
LAW, L. W., TING, R. C., STANTON, M. S.: Some biologic, immunogenic and morphologic effects in mice after infection with murine sarcoma virus. I. Biologic and immunogenic studies. J. nat. Cancer Inst. 40, 1101—1112 (1968).

Lemonde, P., Clode-Hyde, M.: Influence of Bacillus Calmette-Guerin infection on polyoma in hamsters and mice. Cancer Res. 26, 585—589 (1966).
*Leukemia Committee:* Treatment of acute lymphoblastic leukemia: Comparison of immunotherapy (BCG) — intermittent methotrexate on therapy after a 5-month intermittent cytotoxic regimen. (Concord Trial.) Brit. med. J. 4, 189—194 (1971).
Leyden, E. von, Blumenthal, F.: Attempts to immunize humans by inoculation of their own cancer. Deutsch. Med. Wschr. 28, 637—638 (1902).
Mackler, B. F.: Role of soluble lymphocyte mediators in malignant-tumour destruction. Lancet 2, 297—301 (1971).
Malkiel, S., Hargis, B. J.: Influence of B pertussis on host survival following S-180 implantation. Cancer Res. 21, 1461—1464 (1961).
Mardiney, M. R., Jr., Block, J. B., Serpick, A. A.: Immunotherapy for leukemia: Quantitative aspects and adjuvant relationship to chemotherapy. Cancer Chemother. Rep. 53, 3—12 (1969).
Martin, D. S., Hayworth, P. E., Fugman, R. A.: Enhanced cures of spontaneous murine mammary tumors with surgery, combination chemotherapy and immunotherapy. Cancer Res. 30, 709—716 (1970).
Martin, W. J., Wunderlich, J. R., Fletcher, F., Inman, J. K.: Enhanced immunogenicity of chemically-coated syngeneic tumor cells. Proc. nat. Acad. Sci. (Wash.) 68, 469—472 (1971).
Mathé, G.: Immunotherapie active de la leucémie L1210 appliquées après la greffe tumorale. Rév. Fránc. Étud. clin. Biol. 13, 881—883 (1968).
Mathé, G.: Immunological aspects of cancer — II. Immunological treatment of leukaemias. Brit. med. J. 4, 487—488 (1970).
Mathé, G.: Active immunotherapy. Adv. Cancer Res. 14, 1—36 (1971a).
Mathé, G.: Immunotherapy in the treatment of acute lymphoid leukemia. Hosp. Pract. 6, 43—51 (1971b).
Mathé, G., Amiel, J. L., Bernard, J.: Traitement de souris AKR à l'age de six mois par irradiation totale suivie de transfusion de cellules hématopoiétiques allogéniques incidences respectives de la leucémie et du syndrome secondaire. Bull. Cancer 47, 331—340 (1960).
Mathé, G., Amiel, J. L., Niemetz, J.: Greffe de moelle osseuse après irradiation totale chez des souris leucémiques suivie de l'administration d'un antimitotique pour réduire la fréquence du syndrome secondaire et ajouter à l'effet antileucémique. C. R. Acad. Sci. (Paris) 254, 3603—3605 (1962).
Mathé, G., Amiel, J. L., Schwarzenberg, L., Cattan, A., Schneider, M., DeVries, M. J., Tubiana, M., Lalanne, C., Binet, J. L., Papeirnik, M., Seman, G., Matsukura, M., Schwarzmann, V., Flaisler, A.: Successful allogeneic bone marrow transplantation in man: Chimerism, induced specific tolerance and possible antileukemic effects. Blood 25, 179—196 (1965).
Mathé, G., Amiel, J. L., Schwarzenberg, L., Schneider, M., Cattan, A., Schlumburger, A. R., Hayat, M., DeVassal, F.: Active immunotherapy for acute lymphoblastic leukemia. Lancet 1, 697—699 (1969a).
Mathé, G., Bernard, J.: Essai de traitement, par l'irradiation X suivie de l'administration de cellules myeloides homologues, de souris AK atteintes de leucémie spontanée très avancée. Bull. Cancer 45, 289—300 (1958).
Mathé, G., Bevnase, J.: Essai de traitement de la leucémie greffe L1210 par l'irradiation X suivie de transfusions de cellules hématopoiétique normales. Rév. Fránc. Étud. clin. Biol. 4, 442—446 (1959).
Mathé, G., Pouillart, P.: Active immunotherapy of L1210 leukemia applied after the graft of tumor cells. Rec. Results Cancer Res. 30, 64—75 (1970).
Mathé, G., Pouillart, P., Lapeyraque, F.: Active immunotherapy of L1210 leukemia applied after the graft of tumor cells. Brit. J. Cancer 23, 814—824 (1969b).
Mathé, G., Schwarzenberg, L., Amiel, J. L., Pouillart, P., Schneider, M., Cattan, A.: Experimental basis and clinical results of leukemia adoptive immunotherapy. Rec. Results Cancer Res. 30, 76—84 (1970).
Matsuyama, M., Maekawa, A., Horikawa, H., Suzumori, K., Sogal, K., Iwai, K.: Ineffectiveness of autotransplantation on growth of the methylcholanthrene sarcoma in rats and mice. Nature (Lond.) 197, 805—807 (1963).
McCoy, J. L., Fefer, A., Glynn, J. P.: Comparative studies on the induction of transplantation resistance in BALB/c and C57 B1/6 mice in three murine leukemia systems. Cancer Res. 27, 1743—1748 (1967a).
McCoy, J. L., Fefer, A., Glynn, J. P.: Influence of infectious virus on the induction of transplantation resistance in the Friend tumor system. Cancer Res. 27, 2267—2271 (1967b).
McCoy, J. L., Fefer, A., Glynn, J. P.: Inhibition and enhancement of syngeneic Friend virus-induced lymphoma cells by passively transferred anti-Friend serum. Exp. Hematol. 16, 24—26 (1968).

McCoy, J. L., Fefer, A., McCoy, N. T., Kirsten, W. H.: Immunobiologic studies of tumors induced by murine sarcoma virus (Kirsten). Cancer Res. **32**, 343—349 (1972a).
McCoy, J. L., Fefer, A., Ting, R. C., Glynn, J. P.: The development of specific cellular and humoral immunity in mice infected with Rauscher leukemia virus as neonates or adults. Cancer Res. 1671—1678 (1972b).
McCredie, J. A., Brown, E. R., Cole, W. H.: Immunologic treatment of tumors. Proc. Soc. exp. Biol. (N. Y.) **100**, 31—33 (1959).
McEnany, M. T., Kelly, M. G., Fahey, J. L.: Effects of immunization with tumor-cell-foreign-protein conjugates on growth of syngeneic tumor grafts. Proc. Amer. Ass. Cancer Res. **9**, 46 (1968).
McPeak, C. J.: Intralymphatic therapy with immune lymphocytes. Cancer **28**, 1126—1128 (1971).
Mihich, E.: Combined effects of chemotherapy and immunity against leukemia L1210 in DBA/2 mice. Cancer Res. **29**, 848—854 (1969).
Mikulska, Z. B., Smith, C., Alexander, P.: Evidence for an immunological reaction of the host directed against its own actively growing primary tumor. J. nat. Cancer Inst. **36**, 29—35 (1966).
Miles, A. E.: The immunological treatment of malignant disease. S. Afr. med. J. **44**, 1116—1119 (1970).
Mitchison, N. A.: Immunologic approach to cancer. Transplant. Proc. **2**, 92—103 (1971).
Moller, G.: The effects on tumor growth in syngeneic recipients of antibodies against tumor-specific antigens in methylcholanthrene-induced mouse sarcomas. Nature (Lond.) **204**, 846—847 (1964).
Moore, G. E., Gerner, R. E.: Cancer immunity-hypothesis and clinical trial of lymphocytotherapy for malignant disease. Ann. Surg. **172**, 733—739 (1970).
Morton, D. L.: Immunological aspects of neoplasia: A rational basis for immunotherapy. Ann. int. Med. **74**, 587—604 (1971).
Morton, D. L., Eilber, F. R., Joseph, W. L., Wood, W. C., Trahan, E., Ketcham, S.: Immunological factors in human sarcomas and melanomas. A rational basis for immunotherapy. Ann. Surg. **172**, 740—749 (1970).
Motta, R.: Passive immunotherapy of leukemia and other cancer. Adv. Cancer Res. **14**, 161—179 (1971).
Murray, G.: Experiments in immunity in cancer. Canad. med. Assoc. J. **79**, 249—259 (1958).
Nadler, S. H., Moore, G. E.: Immunotherapy of malignant melanoma. Geriatrics. **23**, 150—153 (1968).
Nadler, S. H., Moore, G. E.: Immunotherapy of malignant disease. Arch. Surg. **99**, 376—381 (1969).
Nadler, S. H., Moore, G. E.: Response to injection of cultured human tumor cells. Arch. Surg. **100**, 244—248 (1970).
Nagel, G. A., Arneault, G. S., Holland, J. F., Kirkpatrick, D., Kirkpatrick, R.: Cell-mediated immunity against malignant melanoma in monozygous twins. Cancer Res. **30**, 1828—1832 (1970).
Natale, N., Reiner, J., Southam, C. M.: Immunogenic efficacy of various syngeneic tumor cell preparations. Cancer **28**, 1118—1125 (1971).
Neiman, P., Wasserman, P. B., Wentworth, B. B., Kao, G. F., Lerner, K. G., Storb, R., Buckner, C. D., Clift, R. A., Fefer, A., Fass, L., Glucksberg, H., Thomas, E. D.: Interstitial pneumonia and cytomegalovirus infection as complications of human marrow transplantation. Transplantation **15**, 478—485 (1973).
Newton, W. T., Donaldson, R. C.: Lymph transfusion in patients with cancer. Amer. J. Surg. **118**, 988—991 (1969).
Ngu, V.: Host defences to Burkitt tumours. Brit. med. J. **1**, 345—347 (1967).
Oettgen, H. F., Old, J. L., Boyse, E. A.: Human tumor immunology. Med. Clin. N. Amer. **55**, 761—785 (1971).
Old, L. J., Benacerraf, B., Clarke, D. A., Carswell, E. A., Stockert, E.: The role of the reticuloendothelial system in the host reaction to neoplasia. Cancer Res. **121**, 1281—1300 (1961).
Old, L. J., Boyse, E. A.: Immunology of experimental tumors. Ann. Rev. Med. **15**, 167—186 (1964).
Old, L. J., Boyse, E. A.: Prospects for immunotherapy of human cancer. Ann. int. Med. **69**, 393—396 (1968).
Old, L. J., Boyse, E. A., Clarke, D. A., Carswell, E. A.: Antigenic properties of chemically induced tumors. Ann. N. Y. Acad. Sci. **101**, 80—106 (1962).
Old, L. J., Clarke, D. A., Benacerraf, B.: Effect of Bacillus Calmette-Guerin (BCG) infection on transplanted tumors in the mouse. Nature (Lond.) **184**, 291—292 (1959).

Old, L. J., Stockert, E., Boyse, E. A., Geering, G.: A study of passive immunization agains a transplanted G+ leukemia with specific antigens. Proc. Soc. exp. Biol. (N. Y.) **124**, 63—68 (1967).
Owens, A. H., Jr., Santos, G. W.: The effect of cyclophosphamide and allogeneic and parental spleen cells on the course of L1210 leukemia. Exp. Hemat. 8, 15—17 (1965).
Owens, A. H., Jr., Santos, G. W.: The effect of cytotoxic drugs on graft-versus-host disease in mice. Transplantation 11, 378—382 (1971).
Penn, I.: Malignant tumors in organ transplant recipients. Rec. Results Cancer Res. **35**, 1—51 (1970).
Piessens, W. F.: Evidence for human cancer immunity. A review. Cancer **26**, 1212—1220 (1970).
Piessens, W. F., Heimann, R., Legros, N., Heuson, J.: Effect of Bacillus Calmette-Guerin on mammary tumor formation and cellular immunity in dimethylbenz(a)anthracene-treated rats. Cancer Res. **31**, 1061—1065 (1971a).
Piessens, W. F., Heimann, R., Legros, N., Heuson, J.: Effects of Bacillus Calmette-Guerin (BCG) infection on residual disease of the rat mammary tumor after ovariectomy. Europ. J. Cancer **7**, 377—380 (1971b).
Piessens, W. F., Lachapelle, F. L., Legros, N., Heuson, J.: Facilitation of rat mammary tumour growth by BCG. Nature (Lond.) **228**, 1210—1211 (1970).
Pilch, Y. H., Ramming, K. P.: Transfer of tumor immunity with ribonucleic acid. Cancer **26**, 630—637 (1970).
Pilch, Y. H., Ramming, K. P., Deckers, P. J.: Transfer of tumor immunity with RNA. Israel J. med. Sci. **7**, 246—258 (1971).
Pollack, S. B.: Effect of host sex and splenectomy on Moloney virus-induced sarcomas. Int. J. Cancer **8**, 264—271 (1971).
Powles, R. L., Balchin, L. A., Fairley, G. H., Alexander, P.: Recognition of leukaemia cells as foreign before and after autoimmunization. Brit. med. J. **1**, 486—489 (1971).
Rhodes, E. L.: An attempt to obtain autoimmunity to tumors with Freund's adjuvant and tetanus toxoid. Nature (Lond.) **193**, 1091 (1962).
Rios, A., Simmons, R. L.: Comparative effect of mycobacterium bovis- and neuraminidase-treated tumor cells on the growth of established methylcholanthrene fibrosarcomas in syngeneic mice. Cancer Res. **32**, 16—21 (1972).
Rosenau, W., Morton, D. L.: Tumor-specific inhibition of growth of methylcholanthrene-induced sarcomas *in vivo* and *in vitro* by sensitized isologous lymphoid cells. J. nat. Cancer Inst. **36**, 825—836 (1966).
Rosenthal, S. R.: BCG in cancer and leukemia. Bull. Inst. Pasteur **70**, 29—50 (1972).
Rubin, J.: The immunological basis for non-infective Rous sarcomas. Cold Spr. Harb. Symp. quant. Biol. **27**, 441—452 (1962).
Rudolph, R. H., Fefer, A., Thomas, E. D., Buckner, C. D., Clift, R. A., Storb, R.: Isogeneic marrow grafts for hematologic malignancy in man. Arch. int. Med. **132**, 279—285 (1973).
Salmon, S. E., Drakauer, R. S., Whitmore, W. F.: Lymphocyte stimulation. Selective destruction of cells during blastogenic response to transplantation antigens. Science **172**, 490—492 (1971).
Sanford, B. H.: An alteration in tumor histocompatibility induced by neuraminidase. Transplantation **4**, 1273—1279 (1967).
Sanford, B. H., Codington, J. F.: Further studies on the effect of neuraminidase on tumor cell transplantability. Tissue Antigens **1**, 153—161 (1971).
Santos, G. W.: Effect of graft-versus-host disease on a spontaneous adenocarcinoma. Exp. Hematol. **20**, 46—48 (1970a).
Santos, G. W.: Immunologic concepts and their potential role in cancer therapy. Postgrad. Med. **48**, 194—198 (1970b).
Santos, G. W.: Application of marrow grafts in human disease. Amer. J. Path. **65**, 653—668 (1971).
Sartorelli, A. C., LePage, G. A.: Modification of thioguanine toxicity in tumor-bearing mice with bone marrow transplants. Proc. Amer. Ass. Cancer Res. **26**, 246 (1957).
Schwartz, D. B., Zbar, B., Gibson, W. T., Chirigos, M. A.: Inhibition of murine sarcoma virus oncogenesis with living BCG. Int. J. Cancer **8**, 320—325 (1971).
Schwarzenberg, L., Mathé, G., Schneider, M., Amiel, J. L., Cattan, A., Schlumburger, J. R.: Attempted adoptive immunotherapy of acute leukemia by leukocyte transfusions. Lancet **2**, 365—368 (1966).
Shachat, D. A., Fefer, A., Moloney, J. B.: Effect of cortisone on oncogenesis by murine sarcoma virus (Moloney). Cancer Res. **28**, 517—520 (1968).
Simmons, R. L., Rios, A.: Immunotherapy of cancer: Immunospecific rejection of tumors in recipients of neuraminidase-treated tumor cells plus BCG. Science **174**, 591—593 (1971).

SIMMONS, R. L., RIOS, A., LUNGREN, G., RAY, P. K., MCKHANN, C. F., HAYWOOD, G. R.: Immunospecific regression of methylcholanthrene fibrosarcoma with the use of neuraminidase. Surgery **70**, 38—46 (1971a).

SIMMONS, R. L., RIOS, A., RAY, P. K., LUNDGREN, G.: Effect of neuraminidase on the growth of methylcholanthrene fibrosarcoma in normal and immunosuppressed syngeneic mice. J. nat. Cancer Inst. **47**, 1087—1094 (1971b).

SJOGREN, H. O., ANKERST, J.: Effect of BCG and allogeneic tumor cells on adenovirus Type 12 tumorigenesis in mice. Nature (Lond.) **221**, 863—864 (1969).

SJOGREN, H. O., BORUM, K.: Tumor-specific immunity in the course of primary polyoma and Rous tumor development in intact and immunosuppressed rats. Cancer Res. **31**, 890—988 (1971).

SKURKOVICH, S. V., KISLJAK, N. S., MACHONOVA, L. A., BEGUNENKO, S. A.: Active immunization of children suffering from acute leukemia in acute phase with live allogeneic leukemic cells. Nature (Lond.) **223**, 509—511 (1969a).

SKURKOVICH, S. V., MACHONOVA, L. A., REZNICHENKO, F. M., CHERVONSKY, G. I.: Treatment of children with acute leukemia by passive cyclic immunization with autoplasma and autoleukocytes operated during the remission period. Blood **33**, 186—197 (1969b).

SMITH, R. T.: Tumor-specific immune mechanisms. New Engl. J. Med. **278**, 1207—1214, 1268—1275 and 1326—1331 (1968).

SOPHOCLES, A. M., NADLER, S. H.: Immunologic aspects of cancer. Surg. Gyn. Obst. **133**, 321—331 (1971).

SOUTHAM, C. M.: Immunotherapy of sarcoma patients. Frontiers of Radiation Therapy and Oncology, Vol. 7. Basel: Karger 1972.

SPARCK, J. V., VOLKERT, M.: Effect of adoptive immunity on experimentally-induced leukemia in mice. Nature (Lond.) **206**, 578—579 (1965).

STARZL, T. E., PENN, I., HALGRIMSON, C. G.: Immunosuppression and malignant neoplasms. New Engl. J. Med. **283**, 934—935 (1970).

STORB, R., THOMAS, E. D., BUCKNER, C. D., CLIFT, R. A., JOHNSON, F. L., FEFER, A., GLUCKSBERG, H., GIBLETT, E. R., LERNER, K. G., NEIMAN, P.: Allogeneic Marrow Grafting for Treatment of Aplastic Anemia. Blood, **43**, 157—180 1973.

SUMNER, W. C., FORAKER, G.: Spontaneous regression of human melanoma, clincal and experimental studies. Cancer **13**, 79—81 (1960).

SYMES, M. O.: Immunological problems in the treatment of malignant disease. Proc. roy. Soc. Med. **63**, 135—136 (1970).

SYMES, M. O., RIDDELL, A. G.: Immunologically competent cells in the treatment of malignant disease. Lancet **1**, 1054—1056 (1968).

THOMAS, E. D., BRYANT, J. I., BUCKNER, C. D., CLIFT, R. A., FEFER, A., JOHNSON, F. L., NEIMAN, P., RAMBERG, R. E., STORB, R.: Leukaemic transformation of engrafted human marrow cells in-vivo. II. Lancet I: 1310—1313 (1972a).

THOMAS, E. D., BUCKNER, C. D., RUDOLPH, R. H., FEFER, A., STORB, R., NEIMAN, P. E., BRYANT, J. I., CHARD, R. L., CLIFT, R. A., EPSTEIN, R. B., FIALKOW, P. J., FUNK, D. D., GIBLETT, E. R., LERNER, K. G., REYNOLDS, R. A., SLICHTER, S.: Allogeneic marrow grafting for hematologic malignancy using HL-A matched donor-recipient sibling pairs. Blood **38**, 267—287 (1971).

THOMAS, E. D., BUCKNER, C. D., CLIFT, R. A., FASS, L., FEFER, A., LERNER, K. G., NEIMAN, P., ROWLEY, N., STORB, R.: Marrow grafting in patients with acute leukemia. Transpl. Proc. **5**, 917—922 (1973).

THOMAS, E. D., BUCKNER, C. D., STORB, R., NEIMAN, P. E., FEFER, A., CLIFT, R. A., SLICHTER, S. J., FUNK, D. D., BRYANT, J. I., LERNER, K. E.: Aplastic anemia treated by marrow transplantation. Lancet **I**, 284—289 (1972b).

THOMAS, E. D., HERMAN, E. C., JR., GREENOUGH, W. B., III., HAGER, E. B., CANNON, J. H., SAHLER, O. D., FERREBEE, J. W.: Irradiation and marrow infusion in leukemia. Arch. int. Med. **107**, 829—845 (1961).

THOMAS, E. D., LOCHTE, H. L., CANNON, J. H., SAHLER, O. D., FERREBEE, J. W.: Supralethal whole-body irradiation and isologous marrow transplantation in man. J. clin. Invest. **38**, 1709 (1959).

THOMSON, D. M. P., KRUPEY, J., FREEDMAN, S. O., GOLD, P.: The radioimmunoassay of circulating carcinoembryonic antigen of the human digestive system. Proc. nat. Acad. Sci. (Wash.) **64**, 161—167 (1969).

TRENTIN, J. J.: Whole body x-ray and bone marrow therapy of leukemia in mice. Proc. Amer. Assoc. Cancer Res. **2**, 54 (1957).

VADLAMUDI, S., PADARATHSINGH, M., BONMASSAR, E., GOLDIN, A.: Effect of combination treatment with cyclophosphamide and isogeneic or allogeneic spleen and bone marrow cells in leukemic (L1210) mice. Int. J. Cancer **7**, 160—166 (1971).

VAN BEKKUM, D. W., DEVRIES, M. J.: Radiation chimeras. London: Logos Press (1967).

Varet, B., Levy, J. P., Leclerc, J. C., Senik, A.: Rôle de l'immunité dans le rejet des tumeurs induites par le virus MSV. Effect des serums antithymocytes. Int. J. Cancer 3, 727—733 (1968).
Villasor, R.: The clinical use of BCG vaccine in stimulating host resistance to cancer. Philipp. med. Assoc. 41, 619—632 (1965).
Viza, D., Davies, D. A. L., Tood, R., Bernard-Degani, P., Bernard, C., Harris, R.: Mise en évidence, isolement et purification partielle d'antigénes leucémiques chez l'homme. Presse Med. 78, 2259—2264 (1970).
Wagner, H., Rollinghoff, M.: In Vitro Induction of Tumor-Specific Immunity. J. exp. Med., 138, 1—15 (1973).
Wahren, B.: Immunotherapy in Friend virus leukemia. II. Prevention of Friend leukemia by passive administration of immune serum and cells to young mice. J. nat. Cancer Inst. 41, 931—938 (1968).
Weiss, D. W., Bonhag, R. S., Deome, K. R.: Protective activity of fractions of tubercule bacilli against isologous tumors in mice. Nature (Lond.) 190, 889—891 (1961).
Weiss, D. W., Bonhag, R. S., Leslie, P.: Studies on the heterologous immunogenicity of a methanol-insoluble fraction of attentuated tubercle bacilli (BCG). II. Protection against tumor isografts. J. exp. Med. 124, 1039—1065 (1966).
Williams, A. C., Klein, E.: Experiences with local chemotherapy and immunotherapy in pre-malignant and malignant skin lesions. Cancer 25, 450—462 (1970).
Woodruff, M.: Immunological aspects of cancer. II. Immunotherapy of cancer. Brit. med. J. 4, 486—487 (1970).
Woodruff, M. F. A., Boak, J. L.: Inhibitory effect on pre-immunized CBA spleen cells on transplants of A-strain mouse mammary carcinoma in (CBA × A) $F_1$ hybrid recipients. Brit. J. Cancer 19, 411—417 (1965).
Woodruff, M. F. A., Boak, J. L.: Inhibitory effect of injections of Corynebacterium parvum on the growth of tumor transplants in isogeneic hosts. Brit. J. Cancer 20, 345—352 (1966).
Woodruff, M. F. A., Nolan, B.: Preliminary observations on treatment of advanced cancer by injection of allogeneic spleen cells. Lancet 2, 426—429 (1963).
Woodruff, M. F. A., Symes, M. O.: The use of immunologically competent cells in the treatment of cancer. Experiments with a transplantable mouse tumor. Brit. J. Cancer 16, 707—715 (1962).
Woodruff, M. F. A., Symes, M. O., Anderson, N. F.: The effect of intraperitoneal injection of thoracic duct lymphocytes from normal and immunized rats in mice inoculated with the Landschutz ascites tumour. Brit. J. Cancer 17, 482—487 (1963a).
Woodruff, M. F. A., Symes, M. O., Stuart, A. E.: The effect of rat spleen cells on two transplanted mouse tumours. Brit. J. Cancer 17, 320—327 (1963b).
Yashphe, D. J.: Immunological factors in nonspecific stimulation of host resistance to syngeneic tumors. A review. Israel J. med. Sci. 7, 90—107 (1971).
Zbar, B., Bernstein, I. D., Rapp, H. J.: Suppression of tumor growth at the site of infection with living Bacillus Calmette-Guerin. J. nat. Cancer Inst. 46, 831—839 (1971).
Zbar, B., Tanaka, T.: Immunotherapy of cancer. Regression of tumors after intralesional injection of living Mycobacterium bovis. Science 172, 271—273 (1971).
Zoschke, D. C., Bach, F. H.: Specificity of allogeneic cell recognition by human lymphocytes *in vitro*. Science 172, 1350—1352 (1971).

Chapter 27

# Evaluation of Immunosuppressive Agents

MALCOLM S. MITCHELL

With 2 Figures

## Introduction

Immunosuppressive agents are not by and large a unique class of compounds, but are rather a variety of chemical and biological substances that share the common property of inhibiting the immune response. A knowledge of the biochemical locus of action of a new agent enables a reasonable prediction of its effectiveness as an immunosuppressant, particularly if it is known to inhibit DNA, RNA, or protein synthesis. Yet in light of the need for highly selective agents, capable of affecting only immunity to a defined antigen without general cytocidal effects, or capable of inhibiting only one element of the immune response, empiricism and the testing of a variety of different agents have a distinct place in addition to careful deductive reasoning. Biological agents, such as antibodies or antisera, that work against the types of cells involved in immunity, also require testing in a variety of immunological systems and should not be assumed to work in only one of them. Thus, antilymphocyte serum has been ascertained to inhibit cellular immunity while leaving antibody production relatively unaffected, a feature that was not readily predictable *a priori*.

As with all pharmacological agents, toxicity must be measured together with the therapeutic response, in order to gain insight into the potential usefulness of the agent. Potency achieved at the expense of prohibitive toxicity is obviously of no benefit, either in an investigation of the immune response itself, or in an evaluation of the clinical effects of the compound on a disorder of altered immunity. It should be obvious, too, that a failure to achieve immunosuppression with nearly "homeopathic" doses of a drug proves nothing either, as emphasized by HITCHINGS and ELION (1963) in their early review on this subject. One should have some knowledge of the magnitude of the dosage of an agent that causes death, such as the $LD_{50}$, and especially the $LD_{10}$, in order to determine the limits and general range of dosage allowable in animal experimentation. Measurements of peripheral white blood cell counts, weights, and observations on the general physical condition of test subjects concomitant with immunological measurements are essential information in animal experiments and are as easily obtainable in rodents as in larger animals. Comparisons among several agents based upon the use of a fixed percentage of the $LD_{50}$ or of the $LD_{10}$ allow a valid estimation of relative potency impossible with more arbitrary doses.

A variety of dosages and dosage schedules should always be used in testing a new potential immunosuppressive agent. Effects of single and multiple doses, given before, together with, or after the antigen, should always be investigated, because past experience has shown radically different effects upon immunity depending upon such variations in scheduling. For example, effects ranging from immunological tolerance, through immunosuppression, to augmentation of antibody synthesis have been observed with 6-mercaptopurine (6-MP) (Schwartz et al., 1959; Schwartz and Dameshek, 1963; Sahiar and Schwartz, 1965; Chanmougan and Schwartz, 1966), cytarabine (cytosine arabinoside) (Harris and Hersh, 1968; Gordon et al., 1969; Mitchell et al., 1969b, c), and actinomycin D, (Claman and Bronsky, 1965; Ambrose, 1969; Uyeki and Llacer, 1969, 1970). Some agents are effective as immunosuppressants only before the antigen, notably busulfan (Berenbaum, 1967), some such as cytoxan are suppressive before or after the antigen (Aisenberg, 1967) and those dependent upon the inhibition of DNA synthesis (the antimetabolites) are suppressive when given after the antigen (Schwartz et al., 1959; Buskirk et al., 1965; Santos and Owens, 1966; Berenbaum, 1967; Harris and Hersh, 1968; Mitchell et al., 1969b), with unusual effects, such as augmentation, sometimes seen with courses given before the antigen. Different qualitative effects upon the immune response depend at least as much upon the magnitude and scheduling of the dosage as upon the type of drug itself.

Similarly, more than one immunological system should be examined before accepting or rejecting a compound as an immunosuppressive agent, preferably including delayed hypersensitivity as well as antibody synthesis. *In vivo* administration of the agent should always be included in any screening, since a substance proved to affect immunity in a certain way *in vitro* may have paradoxical *in vivo* effects. An example is the *in vivo* immunosuppressive properties of phytohemagglutinin (Gamble, 1966; Elves, 1967; Jennings and Oates, 1967), a stimulator of nonspecific lymphocytic transformation into lymphoblasts *in vitro* (Nowell, 1960).

Since the immunological response to an antigen may be divided conveniently into two categories, we will consider separately methods that could be used to determine whether a new agent can inhibit (1) humoral antibody synthesis or (2) cellular immunity (delayed hypersensitivity). "Standard" methods that have been used successfully by a number of investigators will be outlined, but improvements and newer procedures that offer better quantification or greater simplicity will also be indicated. Finally, ways of deciding whether the agent represents a potentially useful addition to the clinical armamentarium will be examined.

## Synthesis of Antibody

The synthesis of humoral antibody by plasma cells derived from "bursa-dependent" small lymphocytes (see recent review by Craddock et al., 1971) consists of the production of 19S IgM antibody followed by 7S IgG antibody. This sequence is characteristic of a primary response to an antigen, while a secondary (anamnestic) response usually consists of the production of 7S IgG antibody only (Uhr and Finkelstein, 1963). A "feedback" inhibition of IgM by IgG has been described (Uhr and Finkelstein, 1963), such that the production of IgG during an immune response ordinarily shuts off the synthesis of IgM, probably by more than one mechanism. Immunosuppressive agents have been shown to exert differential effects upon the synthesis of IgM and IgG (Sahiar and Schwartz, 1965; Santos and Owens, 1966; Mitchell et al., 1969b) with a greater suppressive effect upon IgG than upon IgM. Inhibition of IgG synthesis has led secondarily to a breakdown in the feedback suppression of IgM, with a consequent persistence of IgM in the serum for at least several weeks. Occasionally, effects primarily upon IgM synthesis, both suppressive and augmentative, have been demonstrated (Mitchell et al., 1969b). As already noted, augmentation of the total humoral immune response has also been described with several agents.

## A. Testing in Animals

The preliminary screening of agents for possible immunosuppressive effects upon antibody synthesis may involve histological examination of lymphoid tissues after administration of the agents. Depletion of lymphocytes from germinal centers, or the medullary region (red pulp in the spleen) may give some indication of the agent's potential effects, but agents which act on DNA synthesis of antibody-producing cells often do not elicit such gross effects and would be missed entirely. In addition, long-lived lymphocytes and plasma cells are resistant to the effects of several potent agents (MILLER and COLE, 1967).

Table 1. *Points to be considered in testing effects of an agent upon antibody synthesis*

1. Antibody-producing cells:
   a) Plaque-forming cells (PFC)
   b) Rosette-forming cells (RFC)
2. Titration of serum antibodies:
   a) Hemolysins
   b) Hemagglutinins
   c) "Passive" hemagglutinins
   d) Isohemagglutinins (esp. mouse and rat)
   e) Cytotoxic antibodies
   f) Cytophilic antibodies
3. Effects of synthesis of IgM and IgG:
   a) "Developed" PFC or mercaptoethanol-degradable RFC
   b) Mercaptoethanol-degradable and -resistant serum antibodies
   c) Sucrose gradient ultracentrifugation of serum antibodies
   d) Sephadex G-200 column chromatography of serum antibodies
4. Effects on the secondary (anamnestic) response:
   a) Antigenic challenge of previously suppressed animals
   b) Treatment of previously sensitized ("primed") animals with drug after secondary challenge with antigen
5. Induction of immunological tolerance:
   a) Serial challenges in the absence of the immunosuppressive agent, of animals previously given a high dosage of the agent and of the antigen
   b) Challenge with a second antigen to determine specificity

For these reasons, the effects of an agent upon antibody synthesis is best judged by administering a specific antigen and measuring specific antibody produced in response. Xenogeneic red blood cells, usually sheep or goat, have been a favorite antigen for titration of serum antibody because of the simplicity of microtechnics (SEVER, 1962; MITCHELL et al., 1969a), and because of the development of two sorts of assay for the quantitation of antibody-producing cells in this system. Lymphoid cells forming "plaques" of hemolysis when plated upon agar (JERNE et al., 1963), or carboxymethyl cellulose (INGRAHAM and BUSSARD, 1964) impregnated with red blood cells, have been termed "plaque-forming cells" (PFC), and are those synthesizing and releasing complement-dependent hemolysins. Lymphoid cells forming "rosettes" by attaching red blood cells to their surface after *in vitro* incubation represent antigen-binding cells with the potential to make antibody as well as active antibody-producing cells themselves during the course of the response (ZAALBERG, 1964; BIOZZI et al., 1967; GERY et al., 1970; MOAV and HARRIS, 1970). These cells have been termed "rosette-forming cells" (RFC). PFC reach their peak during the primary response on the fourth day after antigen (JERNE et al., 1963; MOAV and HARRIS, 1970), while RFC usually increase to a maximum a day or two later (BIOZZI et al., 1967; GERY et al., 1970). As might be anticipated, the peaks during a secondary response are usually reached 1 to 2 days earlier in both sorts of assay (Figs. 1 and 2).

Although originally the only PFC identifiable were those producing 19S (IgM) antibodies, modification of the original technics by using antibody to IgG has allowed the "development" of plaques formed by 7S (IgG) antibodies too (DRESSER and WORTIS, 1965; STERZL and RIHA, 1965). RFC appear to involve both 7S and 19S antibodies, so that degradation of 19S by mercaptoethanol (DEUTSCH and MORTON, 1957; SAHIAR and SCHWARTZ, 1965) permits identification of RFC containing 7S antibodies (MOAV and HARRIS, 1970).

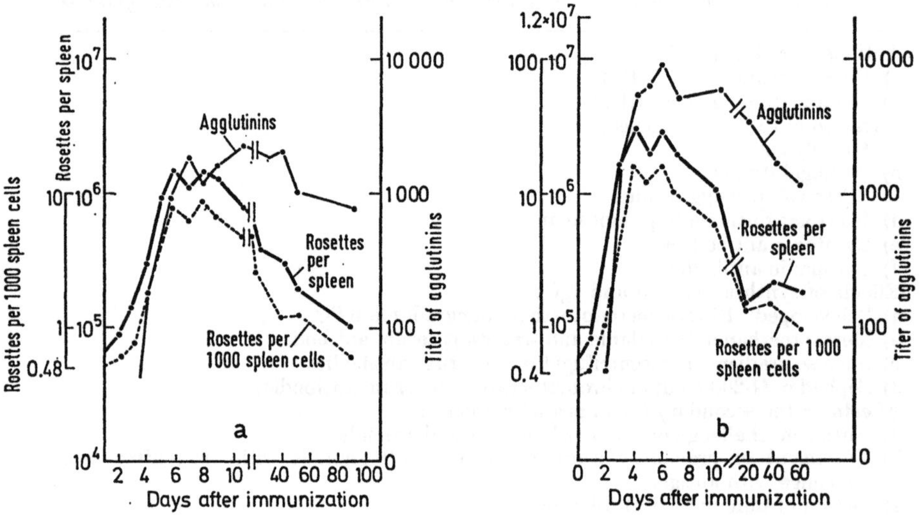


Fig. 1. Kinetics of production of rosette-forming cells (RFC) and of serum hemagglutinins in the mouse spleen after injection of $10^8$ sheep RBC. a) Primary response. b) Secondary response of a mouse primed with $10^5$ RBC 25 days earlier. Adapted, with permission, from BIOZZI et al. (1967)

Changes in RFC and PFC after immunization or after immunosuppressive therapy have been closely paralleled by changes in titers of the homologous antibodies (i.e. agglutinins or hemolysins, respectively) (Figs. 1 and 2), but not necessarily by other kinds of antibody. More explicitly, changes in the number of PFC's (hemolysin-producing cells) resulting from immunosuppression have not always been concordant with changes in serum hemagglutinins (HARRIS and HERSH, 1968). RFC's and hemolysins have shown some concordance, however, during early immunization. During the decline phase in antibody synthesis, both agglutinin and hemolysin titers fail to show a correlation with RFC's (BIOZZI et al., 1967).

Adaptations of the basic PFC and RFC technics have expanded their usefulness in immunological investigations, both in terms of simplicity of performance and of the range of antigenic systems that can now be studied. It is now possible to perform the test on microscope slides using thin-layer agarose as a support medium (GOLUB et al., 1968) or without any supporting medium (CUNNINGHAM and SZENBERG, 1968), the latter test requiring only 30 min to perform. NOSSAL et al. (1970) have modified the procedure to allow manipulation of the cells in open microcultures, while KLESIUS (1970) has introduced optical density reading of the hemoglobin released into the supernatant fluid, to allow more rapid screening of a number of agents. Of these, only the procedure of GOLUB et al. (1968) allows a permanent record and is the one closest to the original JERNE-NORDIN technic, but it requires a longer time to perform than the CUNNINGHAM-SZENBERG or the KLESIUS modification (4 h). Perhaps even more significant adaptations now permit the use

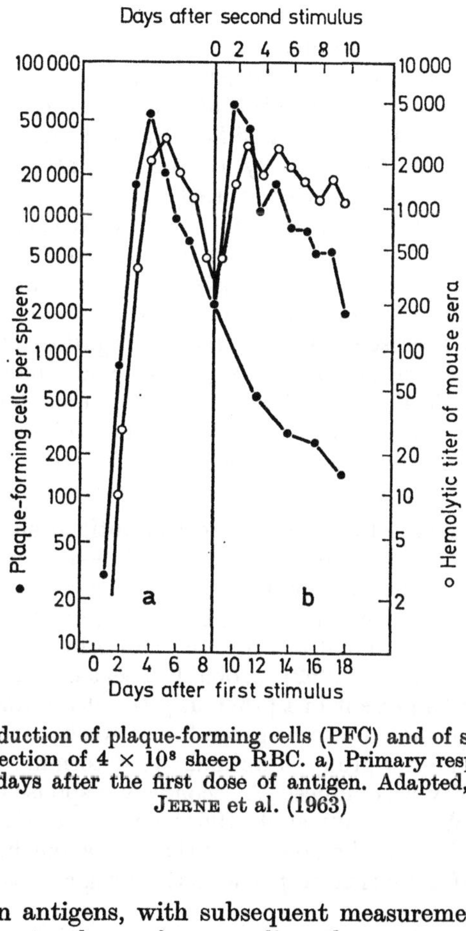


Fig. 2. Kinetics of production of plaque-forming cells (PFC) and of serum hemolysins in the mouse spleen after injection of $4 \times 10^8$ sheep RBC. a) Primary response. b) Secondary response: reinjection 8 days after the first dose of antigen. Adapted, with permission, from JERNE et al. (1963)

of protein or hapten antigens, with subsequent measurement of lymphoid cells producing antibodies to them after coupling the antigen to the erythrocytes (MERCHANT and HRABA, 1966; BIOZZI et al., 1967; GOLUB et al., 1968). The basic PFC and RFC procedures may now be useful in elucidating the effects of many immunosuppressive agents in a variety of antigenic systems with only minimal changes in laboratory screening procedures.

Titration of serum antibodies should be performed wherever feasible in disposable round-bottomed plastic microtrays, now available from a number of suppliers (e.g. Cooke "Microtiter" plates, Cooke Engineering Co., Arlington, Va., USA and Linbro "Dispotray", Linbro Chemical Co., New Haven, Conn., USA). These trays require only 25 μl quantities of each reagent and allow rapid simultaneous titration of 8 antisera per tray, with results available within 2 h. After serial dilution of the test antiserum, xenogeneic red blood cells, either uncoated (when used as the antigen) or coupled with proteins after tannic acid treatment

(Herbert, 1967), with haptens (Bullock and Kantor, 1965), or with polysaccharides (Landy and Lamb, 1953) are added as the test reagent. It should be emphasized that the use of formalinized red blood cells (Difco Laboratories, Detroit, Michigan, USA), preferably goat red blood cells, which have been maximally sensitive in our hands, has allowed the maintenance of antigen coupled to erythrocytes in a stable preparation for up to 6 months in many instances. Formalinized cells can also be used in direct hemagglutination reactions, but they are not susceptible to hemolysis.

After titration of hemagglutinins or hemolysins, one should then estimate the proportion of 19S (IgM) and 7S (IgG) present in the antibody reacting to the specific antigen. The simplest method is that of degradation by 2-mercaptoethanol (Deutsch and Morton, 1957), as modified by Sahiar and Schwartz (1965), which destroys polymeric 19S antibody leaving IgG intact. Incubation of serum for one hour at 37°, preferably diluted at least 1 : 2 to avoid precipitation, with an equal volume of 0.2 *M* 2-mercaptoethanol in buffered saline, is sufficient to inactivate IgM. Very often minimal decreases in total antibody synthesis mask profound selective effects of an agent upon IgG synthesis, which are detectable after mercaptoethanol degradation of the serum. More precise discrimination between IgM and IgG requires sucrose gradient ultracentrifugation (Stanworth, 1967), or Sephadex G-200 column chromatography (Fahey and Terry, 1967), principally because IgA antibody is also partially sensitive to mercaptoethanol. The various fractions from either the gradient or column should each be subjected to mercaptoethanol individually for the greatest precision in identification of the classes of antibody containing residual activity after immunosuppression.

The secondary (anamnestic) response to the antigen should also be studied. Animals previously primed with antigen 3 to 4 weeks earlier should be treated with the putative immunosuppressive agent after a challenge dose of antigen, to determine what levels of the agent are required to suppress the response. Secondary responses have been more difficult to suppress than primary responses (Schwartz et al., 1959; La Plante et al., 1962), probably because of the greater number of antibody-producing cells present in a previously sensitized animal after challenge. An antigenic challenge should also be given 3 to 4 weeks after suppression of the primary response in another group of animals, to determine whether a persistent suppression of immunity was induced. A secondary response usually occurs under these circumstances (Weisburger et al., 1964; Sterzl, 1967; Finger et al., 1949; Mitchell et al., 1969b), but the possibility that the agent has induced tolerance should be considered if there is no response to the antigen in the absence of further drug treatment.

Drug-induced immunological tolerance is defined as a state of specific unresponsiveness to an antigen, as measured by the inability of the animal to respond with detectable immunity to the specific antigen in the absence of the inducing agent. These considerations require that several challenges be made with the original antigen, after the period of immunosuppression, and that a second antigen be tested to rule out a prolonged state of general hyporesponsiveness. The absence or profound reduction of antibody titers and of antibody-producing cells after challenge with the "tolerogenic" material, together with a primary response to the new antigen, establish the presence of tolerance. To test specifically for the ability of a new agent to induce immunological tolerance, a high dose of the antigen and of the agent should be used (Schwartz and Dameshek, 1962; Aisenberg, 1967; Gordon et al., 1969), for it has been under these circumstances that such drug-induced tolerance has most easily been achieved in the past.

## B. Antibodies to Allogeneic Tumor Cells

Transplantable murine tumors are cellular immunogens that can be used to test the effects of a new agent upon both humoral and cellular immunity. They are particularly valuable for that reason, as well as for their importance in studying the problem of immunosuppression of the host during tumoricidal chemotherapy. Methods of carrying the tumors and of transplanting them to allogeneic hosts have been described by FISCHER and SARTORELLI (1964). Isohemagglutinins against the H-2 (histocompatibility) antigens carried by the tumors are titratable in the serum (STIMPFLING, 1964; MITCHELL et al., 1969a) 10 days after transplantation and reach their peak at 2 to 3 weeks. Titration of cytotoxic antibodies (BOYSE et al., 1964), which are capable of lysing tumor cells in the presence of complement, is less sensitive than titration of isohemagglutinins, but identifies a group of antibodies that appear to be important in the rejection of ascites tumors *in vivo*. Measurement of $^{51}$Cr release and the use of microtitration (WIGZELL, 1965; KALISS, 1969) have substantially simplified the titration procedure, which may also be performed as originally described by enumeration of the percentage of dead cells stained by trypan blue (BOYSE et al., 1964). Cytophilic antibodies capable of arming macrophages to attach and sometimes to ingest tumor cells *in vitro* may also be titrated in the serum of the same mice (HOY and NELSON, 1969). Such antibodies are also proving to be of great importance in the rejection of ascites tumors. Like isohemagglutinins, cytophilic antibodies rise to a peak at 2 weeks after injection of antigenic tumor cells.

The transplantable tumors suitable and easily obtainable for study of the antibodies mentioned include leukemia L1210 (DBA/2), mastocytoma P815Y (DBA/2), leukemia L5178Y (DBA/2), leukemia EL-4 (C57Bl/6), sarcoma BP-8 (C3H), and sarcoma-I (A). (The strain of mouse in which the tumor originated and in which it should be passed is in parentheses). Solid tumors, such as those induced by carcinogens or viruses, are also appropriate for study, particularly of the effects on antibodies causing "enhancement" (HUTCHIN, 1968; SNELL, 1970), since enhancement with ascites tumors has been difficult to obtain (HUTCHIN et al., 1967). Cellular immunity to these murine tumors may be measured by one of the methods referred to on pp. 8—10. Procedures for the quantification of antibody-producing cells have not yet been described with allogeneic tumors as the antigen. The usual sequence of IgM to IgG antibody probably occurs with all of the antibodies described above. Our own unpublished data indicates that this is true at least for the response to leukemia L1210 in allogeneic mice given one or several injections of the tumor.

## C. *In Vitro* Culture Methods

It is possible to cultivate dissociated lymphoid cells from rabbits (MICHAELIDES and COONS, 1963), or mice (MISHELL and DUTTON, 1966; MARBROOK, 1967) *in vitro*, allowing the investigation of immunosuppressive agents directly upon the cells that are synthesizing antibody. The procedure has been most helpful in "dissections" of the immune response using immunosuppressive agents with known effects, but is equally useful in evaluation of the locus of action of new agents. Only substances that do not require conversion to an active form in the plasma or in nonlymphoid tissues such as the liver are suitable for this sort of investigation. Lymphoid cells from normal or "primed" animals are incubated with sheep red blood cells, and are treated with drug at various times during the incubation period, after which the cells are removed, washed and tested for antibody production by rosette or plaque formation. This system allows giving "pulses" of an agent, usu-

ally after preliminary determination of its inhibitory capacity *in vivo*, permitting
usually after preliminary determination of its inhibitory capacity *in vivo*, permiting more precise definition of the agent's mode of action, although always with the proviso that *in vitro* culture systems never completely reflect the situation *in vivo* where free exchange of cells from distant lymphoid areas can occur. Nevertheless, useful information about a number of agents has been garnered by this or similar methods (O'Brien and Coons, 1963; Ambrose and Coons, 1963; Uyeki and Llacer, 1969, 1970). Attempts to assay the effects of antimetabolites by addition directly to plaque-forming cells during the assay procedure on agar have not been entirely successful (Gavin et al., 1969).

Within the past two years, technics for studying the percentage of "thymus-dependent" (T) and "bursa-dependent" (B) lymphocytes in human peripheral blood have been adapted from studies in animals. These involve spontaneous rosette formation with sheep erythrocytes, for thymus dependent cells (Jondal et al., 1972; Wybran et al., 1972) and labeling of immunoglobulin receptors on "bursa-dependent" cells by fluorescent antibody to human immunoglobulins (Gray et al., 1971). These methods permit enumeration of the two types of cells during and after immunosuppressive therapy, a use whose potential has not yet been fully realized.

## D. Investigations in Man

There are a number of different antigens suitable for immunizing human beings. *Escherichia coli* Vi antigen, from a rare strain (5396/38) of the organism has been used by several investigators (Levin et al., 1964; Santos et al., 1964; Mitchell et al., 1969c) to test the primary immune response, since the antigen is one to which most people have never been exposed. This polysaccharide antigen is fairly weak, with 70 to 100 μg giving rise to peak titers, detectable by passive hemagglutination (Landy and Lamb, 1953), of 1 : 8 to 1 : 128 depending upon the serological technic and the endpoint chosen, but has the advantage of sensitivity in detecting immunosuppressive activity. Vi antigen is obtainable from Dr. Marion Webster, National Institutes of Health, Bethesda, Maryland, USA, and must be sterilized by heating the solution in saline (100 μg/ml) to 80° C for 5 min on 3 successive days. A newer antigen, which gives somewhat higher titers than Vi antigen [1 : 256 in cancer patients in "good condition," 1 : 32 to 1 : 64 in those in "poor condition" (Curtis et al., 1970)] is keyhole limpet hemocyanin (Pacific Biomarine Co., Venice, California, USA). An additional advantage of this antigen is its ability to sensitize the individual for delayed hypersensitivity, allowing the investigation of two sorts of "primary" response at once (Curtis et al., 1970). Details on its preparation are given elsewhere (Campbell et al., 1964), as is a complete description of its use (Swanson and Schwartz, 1967; Curtis et al., 1970).

Many individuals have not been exposed to *Salmonella typhi* O and H antigens. Exposure to the latter leads to easily detectable 7S agglutinins as well as 19S agglutinins. We have obtained results parallel with those found with Vi antigen using Salmonella, but the considerable local reaction at the site of injection, as well as a moderate systemic reaction, has limited its usefulness. Xenogeneic (alligator) red blood cells have been used without untoward effects in man to test the primary response (Harris et al., 1970). Hapten-protein conjugates have also been used for this purpose, and like hemocyanin lead to skin reactivity (Kantor and Bullock, 1969).

Toxoids have been useful in the investigation of the secondary immune response. Fluid tetanus or diphtheria toxoid in individuals previously immunized with the antigen leads within 7 to 10 days to a pronounced IgG "booster" response titratable by passive hemagglutination that is delayed or prevented by immunosuppressive therapy (MITCHELL et al., 1969c). Those individuals who have never been immunized show a primary response similar to those with the other antigens mentioned. It is sometimes possible and is highly desirable to immunize subjects with toxoid 3 weeks prior to their entry into a study of immunosuppression, in order to insure that one may study the secondary response. This also allows for study of the primary response in the same subject in the absence of therapy.

It is important to have a matched set of control subjects in any investigation of immunosuppression in man, which means not simply age-matched individuals, but also individuals with a similar pathologic condition wherever possible. Usually that implies a group of patients, with cancer or autoimmune disease, not undergoing systemic therapy, since these groups are the ones most often investigated. It should be noted that while cellular immunity is most usually decreased in patients with widespread carcinoma (HUTCHIN, 1968; AL-SARRAF et al., 1970), patients with severe debilitating carcinoma may also have decreased humoral immunity (LYTTON et al., 1964). Patients in good general condition have nearly normal humoral antibody responses, even patients with lymphoma or leukemia (LARSON and TOMLINSON, 1953), excluding chronic lymphocytic leukemia.

This study of human subjects, like that of simpler animals, should encompass not only the immediate period around the immunosuppressive treatment, but should continue for at least 4 weeks after cessation of therapy, to discern whether delayed rises in titer occur. Rechallenge with the antigen given initially, and then a new antigen, should be performed in any situation where tolerance is suspected. Most studies in man heretofore have not applied the rigid criteria for tolerance as in other animal models, and possible demonstrations of tolerance have been only presumptive.

## Cellular Immunity (Delayed Hypersensitivity)

Cellular immunity is mediated by thymus-dependent small lymphocytes (see review by CRADDOCK et al., 1971), secondarily involving macrophages attracted by mediators released from the lymphocytes (DAVID, 1971; WAKSMAN, 1971). Among the types of reaction involved here are skin sensitivity to microbial allergens, including tuberculin, rejection of allografts and xenografts (although antibodies may also be involved), rejection of neoplasms, and engulfment of microbial cells such as *Listeria*. Spontaneously occurring autoimmune disorders have been suspected

Table 2. *Techniques used in testing effects of an agent upon cellular immunity*

1. Induction of cellular immunity (delayed hypersensitivity):
   a) Skin testing
   b) Measurement of paw or ear swelling
   c) Analysis of histological changes in site of reaction and in regional nodes
2. Skin grafting:
   a) Rejection time
   b) Histology of graft
3. Graft versus host reaction:
   a) Injection of parental lymphoid cells into $F_1$ recipients
   b) Injection of lymphoid cells into irradiated allogeneic or xenogeneic recipients
4. Quantitative measurement of cellular immunity *in vitro:*
   a) Lymphoid cell-mediated cytotoxicity of murine mastocytoma P-815Y cells
5. Nonspecific inflammatory response:
   a) Induction of chronic inflammation by injection of FREUND's adjuvant, cotton pellets, or turpentine

but not yet proved to be the result of altered cellular immunological reactivity of the host against his own tissues, in those disorders in which immune complexes have not been shown to be involved. In the production of a lesion of delayed hypersensitivity there is a large inflammatory component involving migration of sensitized lymphocytes and later of macrophages, so that statements on the effectiveness of an "immunosuppressive" regimen must often be qualified by the possibility that the suppression was on inflammation and not on an immunological event. This question will be considered later.

## A. Testing in Animals

The simplest and most common method of evaluating delayed hypersensitivity has been gross or histological examination of skin lesions produced after intradermal injection of an antigen. The guinea pig has for some time been used in this sort of experiment (Brent, 1959; Kaplan and Dienes, 1959), reacting with erythema and induration that are measurable with a micrometer caliper. The lesions show distinct histological changes between 24 and 36 h after intradermal challenge. In other rodents, particularly mice, swelling of the paw (Uyeki et al., 1969), or of the ear (Asherson and Zembala, 1970), have been used for a comparable purpose. The usual procedure is to sensitize the animal, by painting the skin with a known amount of antigen, or by injecting it intradermally if the material does not produce extensive necrosis, and 3 to 4 weeks later to challenge the animal in a similar fashion to test his responsiveness. If the putative immunosuppressive agent is administered at the time of initial sensitization, a failure to react upon challenge is evidence for a suppression of *de novo* sensitization of small lymphocytes. Histological examination of lesions from these animals may reveal a diminished or absent inflammatory response (Kaplan and Dienes, 1959), and the regional lymph nodes may show an absence of the progression of change from (competent) small lymphocytes through large pyroninophilic lymphoblasts to (committed) small lymphocytes that are characteristically seen (André et al., 1962; Turk and Stone, 1963).

There are now quantitative methods for measuring directly the extent to which small lymphocytes are sensitized to react against the antigen. These involve direct cytotoxicity, in the absence of complement, of lymphocytes directed against cellular antigens, usually tumor cells. Several variations have been described (Brunner et al., 1966, 1970; Hellstrom et al., 1968; Takasugi and Klein, 1970; Heppner and Kopp, 1971), which all basically allow the reaction of lymphocytes with target cells and then measure either cytolysis or cloning ability (viability) of the target cells. Brunner et al. (1966, 1970) have published a simple test system in which lymphocytes from sensitized mice are reacted against the DBA/2 mastocytoma P815Y in fluid medium for 48 h *in vitro*, after which mastocytoma cells are counted in a hemocytometer. A "percentage of lysis" may be calculated by comparing remaining cells in experimental tubes with those remaining in tubes containing normal (unsensitized) lymphocytes, permitting quantification of the effects of several dosage regimens of immunosuppressive agent administered to the mice *in vivo*. The mastocytoma P815Y can be used to determine immunity to H-$2^d$ antigens (from DBA/2 mice) developed against a variety of other DBA/2 tumors, including Leukemia L1210 (Mitchell, 1971). By the use of radioactive chromium release as an indicator (Brunner et al., 1966, 1970), the length of the procedure can be shortened to 4 to 6 h, and many other tumors can be used as targets, including those whose size is not very different from small lymphocytes and which could not therefore be counted easily in a hemocytometer. We have found the release of radioactive chromium less sensitive in discriminating among treatment groups, however, and BRUNNER himself has recently reported similar findings (at the First International Congress of Immunology). It is important in experiments with tumor cells as antigen *in vivo* to use tumor cells killed by exposure to ultraviolet light or x-irradiation, in order to establish that direct effects upon immunity occurred rather than simply inhibition of multiplication of the tumor cells by the cytotoxic agent tested. CALABRESI (1967) was among the first to study the immunosuppressive effects of several cytotoxic agents using this system. HENNEY (1970) has recently described an adaptation of the technic that can be used to identify the cellular immune response to soluble antigens, such as haptens, when these are coupled to the target mast cells.

An ingenious method of enumerating cells concerned with delayed hypersensitivity reactions has been devised by BLOOM et al. (1970). Their assay is analogous to the PFC procedure mentioned earlier for antibody-producing cells, and takes advantage of the property of antigen-stimulated lymphocytes to support the growth of RNA viruses, which in turn form the plaques. The procedure has much to recommend it as a quantitative procedure for cellular immunity and seems relatively easy to perform.

Skin grafting has been used extensively in the past to test new immunosuppressive agents but is a very stringent test of a drug's effectiveness. Considerable immunosuppression is required to allow the graft to live only a day or two more since the growth rate of skin cells is relatively slow. Revascularization of the graft and other factors also influence its survival. Its major value is less as an initial screening test than as a final "preclinical" test, since a major use of immunosuppressive agents is in prolongation of the survival of allografts. Standard technics of skin grafting have been described in detail (BILLINGHAM, 1961). The diameter of the transferred grafts should be the same in experimental and control groups to equalize the dose of antigen. Grafts of tumor cells (subcutaneous or intraperitoneal) that are resistant to the tested agent provide a more sensitive assay system *in vivo*, for when the host's immunity is suppressed, the tumor cells grow rapidly and may kill the animal (HUMPHREY et al., 1961). It is not always possible to obtain such a resistant tumor cell line, but if available, the results may amplify subtle effects on cellular immunity and prevent their being overlooked.

The graft-versus-host reaction (see review by MCBRIDE, 1966), is a phenomenon of rejection of a recipient's tissues by injected immunocompetent lymphoid cells that the recipient is unable to recognize as foreign. Parental strain lymphocytes transferred into $F_1$ hybrids (GOWANS, 1962; MATHÉ et al., 1963; GRAY et al., 1968), or allogeneic or xenogeneic lymphocytes injected into irradiated recipients (SALEH et al., 1969) predictably lead to such a reaction in a number of strain combinations. The immunosuppressive agent may be given in various dosage schedules and the intensity of the graft versus host reaction may be measured by spleen weight assay (SIMONSEN, 1962; GRAY et al., 1968), histological examination of various organs such as spleen, intestine and skin (VAN BEKKUM and DEVRIES, 1967), or by comparison of the degree of runting and time of death of groups of drug-treated with untreated recipients (SIMONSEN, 1962; MCBRIDE, 1966).

The induction of immunological tolerance in cellular immunity, to transplantation antigens for example, has been extremely difficult to obtain except with strong alkylating agents such as cytoxan or procarbazine, or with antilymphocyte serum. The use of soluble transplantation or tumor antigens may soon be possible, and it is probable that many of the same principles applying to the induction of tolerance in antibody synthesis will then apply. Many states of "tolerance" in cellular immunity currently described may in fact be examples of immunological "enhancement," i.e., the inhibition by serum antibodies of cellular immune rejection of foreign tissue (see recent reviews by HUTCHIN, 1968; and SNELL, 1970). The factors influencing these "blocking" or "enhancing" antibodies, which are for the most part IgG globulins, are probably similar to those influencing other IgG antibodies. There is some hope for selective inhibition of enhancing antibodies in the future by immunosuppressive agents in order to aid rejection of tumors. At present, however, there is a good deal of basic work required in the field of enhancement, such that assay of enhancing antibodies cannot yet be recommended for routine use in evaluating a new agent.

Induction of a complex autoimmune disease in animals, such as experimental allergic encephalomyelitis (EAE) (WAKSMAN, 1959), aspermatogenesis (POKORNA, 1970) or thyroiditis (SPIEGELBERG and MIESCHER, 1963) by injection of appropriate antigenic material in Freund's adjuvant, or induction of adjuvant arthritis due to Freund's adjuvant itself (PEARSON, 1959), provide test systems in which the potency of an agent in diseases analogous to those in man can be assessed, even though its mode of action may not easily be evaluable. Delay in the onset of disease, or prevention of gross or microscopic histological changes may be measured. Several investigators have reported such studies (HOYER et al., 1962; SPIEGELBERG and MIESCHER, 1963; GIBBONS, 1969; LEVINE et al., 1970).

New Zealand (NZB) mice or $F_1$ derivatives (NZB × NZW), develop autoimmune diseases "spontaneously" throughout their lifetime, including hemolytic anemia and a lupus erythematosus-like syndrome (EAST, 1969) which can be studied as natural models of disease. Thus far their use as experimental subjects for the investigation of immunosuppressive drugs is largely unexploited except for work with cyclophosphamide (RUSSELL et al., 1966; STAPLES and TALAL, 1970).

It is highly desirable to include a test upon one of these autoimmune diseases in the final preclinical evaluation of a new immunosuppressive agent, since such a test allows a more direct extrapolation to conditions in man than does a simple *in vitro* test of lymphocyte cytotoxicity upon target cells.

## B. *In Vitro* Methods

Inhibition of the migration of macrophages by sensitized lymphocytes in the presence of specific antigen (DAVID et al., 1964; GEORGE and VAUGHAN, 1964) provides a test of cellular immunity in which a number of drugs may be tested *in vitro*. A migration inhibitory factor (BLOOM and BENNETT, 1968) released by the lymphocytes is synthesized after stimulation by antigen and can itself be inhibited by immunosuppressive agents that block protein synthesis. Results in this system with antimitotic agents thus far have been in connection with the elucidation of mechanisms of production and release of migration inhibitory factor (DAVID et al., 1968), but at least one study was specifically concerned with testing the immunosuppressive agents themselves (KAPLAN and CALABRESI, 1965). This test has the same limitations as the *in vitro* culture methods for antibody synthesis, viz. that only drugs which do not require previous *in vivo* activation in nonlymphoid tissues are testable. In addition, it is not strictly comparable to *in vitro* cultures of antibody-producing cells since lymphocytes from normal donors cannot be sensitized *in vitro*.

## C. Investigations in Man

Testing of induction *de novo* of delayed hypersensitivity in man has usually been accomplished with 1-chloro-2,4-dinitrobenzene (DNCB) (KLIGMAN and EPSTEIN, 1959; LEVIN et al., 1964; WALDORF et al., 1968; MITCHELL et al., 1969c; AL-SARRAF et al., 1970), but *p*-nitrosodimethylaniline (MAIBACH and EPSTEIN,

1965; KANTOR and BULLOCK, 1969) and conjugated haptens have also been used. DNCB should be applied in acetone solution, usually as 2000 μg in 0.1 ml, directly to the skin of the arm or forearm (WALDORF et al., 1968), or on an Elastopatch® bandage (Duke Laboratories, South Norwalk, Conn. USA). Two weeks later, the challenge dose, usually 50 or 100 μg, should be administered to the opposite arm or forearm and the reaction is read at 48 and 72 h. The presence of induration indicates a "positive" reaction. Erythema alone constitutes a "1+" reaction, which is below the threshold for positivity, and is often the reaction seen with immunosuppressive agents. A direct vesicant action of the 2000 μg sensitizing dose is usually seen, even in subjects who do not exhibit delayed hypersensitivity on challenge. It is important, therefore, to apply the sensitizing dose to an area of skin that is not cosmetically important to the patient. The sensitizing dose of immunogen should be given during the period of administration of the agent to be tested, either on the day of an infusion or on the first or second day of a several-day course. The challenge dose should be given during a drug-free interval, to distinguish effects upon induction of immunity from those on the peripheral expression of the inflammatory response. Nearly 100% of a normal population responds to DNCB, although responsiveness decreases with age (WALDORF et al., 1968), but patients with late stage HODGKIN'S disease (AISENBERG, 1966) and metastatic carcinoma (AL-SARRAF et al., 1970) often lack reactivity. It is important to have carefully matched control subjects with a similar disease, particularly since the test should not be repeated in a single subject, to be certain one is measuring the induction of delayed hypersensitivity by the original stimulus.

Table 3. *Antigens and tests applicable to the study of human subjects*

1. Antibody synthesis:
   a) Primary response
      1) Escherichia coli 5396/38 Vi antigen
      2) Keyhole limpet hemocyanin (KLH)
      3) Salmonella typhi H antigen
      4) Conjugated haptens
      5) Tetanus toxoid (if not previously immunized)
      6) Xenogeneic erythrocytes
   b) Secondary response
      1) Tetanus toxoid or diphtheria toxoid
      2) Salmonella typhi H antigen
2. Cellular immunity:
   a) Induction of delayed hypersensitivity
      1) Dinitrochlorobenzene (DNCB)
      2) Keyhole limpet hemocyanin (KLH)
      3) Protein-conjugated haptens
      4) Paranitrosodimethylaniline (NDMA)
   b) Established delayed hypersensitivity
      1) Candida
      2) Mumps
      3) Trichophyton
      4) Purified protein derivative of tuberculin (PPD)
      5) Streptokinase-streptodornase (Varidase)
   c) Nonimmunological inflammatory response
      1) Rebuck-Crowley "skin window" (acute and chronic inflammation)

Administration of keyhole limpet hemocyanin leads both to the production of humoral antibodies and the development of delayed hypersensitivity. CURTIS et al. (1970) were able to sensitize 94% of their experimental subjects with neoplasia, using skin reactivity as a criterion. Thirty-one (89%) of 35 patients showed *in vitro* transformation of lymphocytes in the presence of the antigen, using another criterion of responsiveness. KANTOR and BULLOCK (1969) achieved 100% skin sensitization in 26 patients using an injection of protein-conjugated haptens (picryl-HSA). Mercaptoethanol-sensitive antibodies were elicited in 24 of 26, but mercaptoethanol-resistant antibodies were not usually detectable.

Established delayed hypersensitivity reactions usually have been resistant to immunosuppressive agents (LEVIN et al., 1964; SANTOS et al., 1964; MITCHELL et al., 1969c), but there have been reported exceptions (AL-SARRAF et al.,1970; MITCHELL and DECONTI, 1970). Occasionally, the percentage of patients reacting has increased after successful therapy (of leukemia) with "immunosuppressive" agents (DUPUY et al., 1971). The most commonly used skin tests that have been used to determine established reactivity have been candida, mumps, trichophyton, purified protein derivative of tuberculin (PPD), and streptokinase-streptodornase (Varidase). The choice of antigen is based upon the likelihood that the person will have had exposure previously and be reactive initially, to enable a comparison of skin tests before, during, and after therapy. The proportion of a population of individuals reacting has ranged from approximately 80% in normal subjects (DUPUY et al., 1971), to only about 10% in some cancer patients (AL-SARRAF et al., 1970), with a third study showing intermediate results (MITCHELL et al., 1969c). In dealing with patients, and particularly with those who have a neoplasm, it is wise to use a panel of 4 or 5 antigens to increase the probability that an individual patient will be reactive to at least one of them. Five mm of induration after 48 to 72 h is usually accepted as a "positive" reaction in these tests, in response to 0.1 ml of the intradermally injected antigen.

When peripheral blood lymphocytes, or lymphocytes obtained from lymphoid tissue, are incubated with certain antigens to which the individual has been sensitized previously, such as tuberculin, hemocyanin, or streptolysin-O, they undergo enlargement to pyroninophilic "blasts" and synthesize DNA and RNA. A variety of plant mitogens, notably phytohemagglutinin (PHA), produce the same "blastic transformation" (NOWELL, 1960). Blastic transformation of lymphocytes is a measurement of one property of thymus-dependent cells involved in cellular immunity and has the distinct advantage of not requiring manipulation of the patient beyond the drawing of his blood. Cancer chemotherapeutic agents given *in vivo* have suppressed transformation of lymphocytes incubated *in vitro* with PHA (HERSH and OPPENHEIM, 1967; HEINE et al., 1969), or with streptolysin-O (HEINE et al., 1969), in patients with neoplasia or nonmalignant disease. Cytotoxic agents (LOPES-CARDOZO, 1970) and antilymphocyte serum (TURSI et al., 1969) have been similarly effective in mice. Complete methods of tissue culture and quantification of results by incorporation of radiolabeled nucleotides are described in papers by HERSH and his collaborators (HERSH and OPPENHEIM, 1967; CURTIS et al., 1970). It should be cautioned, however, that there is not always a good correlation between the strength of skin test reactivity and the degree of blastogenesis *in vitro* (CURTIS et al., 1970), even though the correlation has sometimes been found (HERSH and OPPENHEIM, 1965). It appears that the basic ability of lymphocytes from many patients with neoplasia to respond to PHA is probably unaltered (SUTHERLAND et al., 1971).

Skin grafting between two test subjects may be used to test suppression of delayed hypersensitivity by a new agent, but carries the risk of transmission of serum hepatitis. To obviate this we have transferred grafts of neonatal foreskin brought sterilely from the delivery room in tissue culture medium containing penicillin and streptomycin. A test graft, 2 cm in diameter, may be applied to one forearm, while the skin removed for placement of the graft may be applied to the opposite forearm as a control for technic. The day on which the graft is completely rejected with formation of an eschar is the endpoint. This occurs in approximately 2 weeks if the agent is ineffective. Histological examination after a punch biopsy of sites showing long term survival of a test graft is highly desirable.

## D. Effects upon "Nonspecific" Aspects of Inflammation

Even well-established immunosuppressive agents such as azathioprine and methotrexate have not been demonstrated conclusively to act upon clinical conditions by virtue of their known immunosuppressive properties (Swanson and Schwartz, 1967). It has been suggested (Page et al., 1962) that such agents may be effecting a beneficial result by suppressing inflammatory components of the cellular immune response. In defense of a more specific mechanism of action upon immunity, however, it should be recalled that established delayed hypersensitivity reactions are usually retained during chemotherapy, indicating that chronic inflammatory responses can occur. Furthermore, Stevens and Willoughby (1969) have clearly established in direct experimentation with several immunosuppressive agents that chronic inflammatory reactions are very little affected, whereas acute inflammation is completely inhibited. The chronic inflammatory granulomatous reactions studied were similar histologically to those seen with immunological stimuli. Since the altered immunological reactions responsible for most autoimmune diseases have not been elucidated, it is impossible to ascribe beneficial therapeutic effects specifically to immunosuppression. Yet it is equally impossible to state with confidence that beneficial effects are due completely to a suppression of inflammation.

There are, nevertheless, a few known effects of immunosuppressive agents upon macrophages, the recruited "nonspecific" elements in the lesion of cellular immunity (Waksman, 1971). Hurd and Ziff (1968) have demonstrated that 6-mercaptopurine inhibits the multiplication of bone marrow monocytes. Since the peritoneal macrophages are derived from this population of cells (Volkman and Gowans, 1965), this cytotoxic effect of 6-mercaptopurine could inhibit participation of macrophages in delayed hypersensitivity. Hurd and Ziff (1968) in fact found a correlation between late infiltration of macrophages and cytotoxic effects on bone marrow cells. *In vitro* experiments (Kaplan and Calabresi, 1965; David, 1968) suggest that the synthesis of mediators (migration inhibitory factor) in sensitized lymphocytes may be impaired by immunosuppressive agents, including not only inhibitors of protein synthesis, but inhibitors of the formation of DNA and RNA as well. Synthesis of antibodies cytophilic for macrophages may also be impaired by immunosuppressive agents, although there are presently no published data on this point. Such antibodies may also play a significant role in certain kinds of cellular immune response involving macrophages (Nelson, 1969).

In testing the effects of an immunosuppressive agent upon delayed hypersensitivity, to help separate the immunological from the inflammatory aspects, it is helpful to have as a control a "nonimmunological" chronic inflammatory response, such as that to cotton implanted pellets, Freund's adjuvant, or turpentine (Stevens and Willoughby, 1969). In man, croton oil painted on the skin has been used (Johnson et al., 1971), but this leads to acute inflammation and the test substance is itself immunosuppressive (Bluestein and Green, 1970). A better method for studying both acute and chronic exudates is the "skin window" technique described by Rebuck and Crowley (1955). This technique has been used to successfully study the effects of 6-mercaptopurine on late (mononuclear) infiltration into an inflammatory site (Page et al., 1964). An abrasion with a scalpel is made on the forearm and sterile coverslips are applied, to allow serial observation of the resulting inflammatory exudate which is removed and stained at intervals (Rebuck and Crowley, 1955). It is probable that with the rapid elucidation of mediators liberated from lymphocytes during delayed hypersensitivity currently taking place (Waksman, 1971; David, 1971), very specific methods of identifying immunosuppression of cellular immunity that will circumvent the difficulties discussed above will soon be available in man and lower animals.

## Clinical Trials of Immunosuppressive Agents in Autoimmune Diseases

Once an agent is established as effective in preclinical trials, and its toxicity is found to be acceptable within a certain dosage range in man, trials of the agent in autoimmune disorders may be attempted. As with any new compound, however, established agents of known effectiveness should be used first in the disorders, with the new agent reserved for resistant cases. The autoimmune disease should be treated for at least 3 months to allow perceptible improvement to occur. Polyvasculitides that frequently show a distinct improvement under therapy, such as polyarteritis nodosa and Wegener's granulomatosis, often require several months before beginning to regress, but may continue to improve thereafter. The dosage chosen should be in the middle to upper portion of the presumptive therapeutic range, with the usual precautions taken of following complete blood counts, liver and renal function tests, and tests of other organs particularly affected by the agent in question. Biological agents (sera or enzymes) that might elicit an immune response to themselves should be monitored by serial titrations of specific antibodies (Peterson et al., 1971).

Trials of established agents, such as azathioprine, methotrexate, and cytoxan, known by individual case reports or uncontrolled series to be effective in a disorder ascribed to altered immunity, must ultimately be performed by a "double-blind" technique. In this sort of investigation, "other" therapy of the disorder (usually including corticosteroids) is manipulated according to the clinical condition of the patient by one investigator, while the immunosuppressive agent under trial or a placebo is administered at a constant dosage to all patients. A disinterested investigator should follow laboratory tests, making adjustments if necessary in the dosage of the active agent if toxicity (such as leukopenia) supervenes, without regard to clinical results. Subjects should be allocated randomly to the group receiving placebo or active drug, with a cross-over to the other group after 3 or 4 months. By this means all patients will at some time receive the active compound. It also allows those patients who have had their dosage of active compound adjusted, because of toxicity while initially taking the drug, to have a similar "adjustment" of the placebo to continue to conceal the identity of the substances. The proviso that investigators concerned with the clinical care of the patients provide all therapy that would usually be given if the patient were not in a study, insures that there will be no breach of ethics.

A battery of antigens should be administered during at least one half of the study to test primary and secondary humoral antibody responses, as well as *de novo* and established cellular reactivity. The results of these tests should be known only to the "disinterested" investigator following laboratory data. Even though one may not be able to prove that effectiveness was due to immunosuppression, and even though the response to exogenous antigens may not completely reflect changes in response to the etiological immunogen, it is helpful to know the dose of drug chosen was immunosuppressive in a particular patient. That is especially true if the regimen is not effective, to provide evidence that the dosage was adequate.

It should be emphasized that most of the agents known to be immunosuppressive in animals and many of those proved of value in man, including even azathioprine at the time of this writing, have not yet been released for use in autoimmune disorders. Any of the trials mentioned here must necessarily be performed according to protocols approved by the appropriate committees within or outside the hospital.

## References


AISENBERG, A. C.: Manifestations of immunologic unresponsiveness in Hodgkin's disease. Cancer Res. **26**, 1152—1160 (1966).

AISENBERG, A. C.: Studies on cyclophosphamide-induced tolerance to sheep erythrocytes. J. exp. Med. **125**, 833—845 (1967).

AL-SARRAF, M., WONG, P., SARDESAI, S., VAITKEVICIUS, V. K.: Clinical immunologic responsiveness in malignant disease. I. Delayed hypersensitivity reaction and the effect of cytotoxic drugs. Cancer **26**, 262—268 (1970).

AMBROSE, C. T.: Regulation of the secondary antibody response *in vitro*. Enhancement by actinomycin D and inhibition by a macromolecular product of stimulated lymph node cultures. J. exp. Med. **130**, 1003—1029 (1969).

AMBROSE, C. T., COONS, A. H.: Studies on antibody production. VIII. The inhibitory effect of chloramphenicol on the synthesis of antibody in tissue culture. J. exp. Med. **117**, 1075—1087 (1963).

ANDRÉ, J. A., SCHWARTZ, R. S., MITUS, W. J., DAMESHEK, W.: The morphologic responses of the lymphoid system to homografts. II. The effects of antimetabolites. Blood **19**, 334—348 (1962).

ASHERSON, G. L., ZEMBALA, M.: Contact sensitivity in the mouse. IV. The role of the lymphocytes and macrophages in passive transfer and the mechanism of the interaction. J. exp. Med. **132**, 1—15 (1970).

BERENBAUM, M. C.: Immunosuppressive agents and the cellular kinetics of the immune response: In: MIHICH, E. (Ed.): Immunity, cancer and chemotherapy, pp. 217—237. New York: Academic Press 1967.

BILLINGHAM, R. E.: Free skin grafting in mammals. In: BILLINGHAM, R. E., SILVERS, W. R. (Eds.): Transplantation of tissues and cells, pp. 1—26. Philadelphia: Wistar Institute 1961.

BIOZZI, G., STIFFEL, C., MOUTON, D.: A study of antibody-containing cells in the course of immunization. In: MIHICH, E. (Ed.): Immunity, cancer and chemotherapy, pp. 103—131. New York: Academic Press 1967.

BLOOM, B. R., BENNETT, B.: Migration inhibitory factor associated with delayed-type hypersensitivity. Fed. Proc. **27**, 13—20 (1968).

BLOOM, B. R., JIMENEZ, L., MARCUS, P. I.: A plaque assay for enumerating antigen-sensitive cells in delayed-type hypersensitivity. J. exp. Med. **132**, 16—30 (1970).

BLUESTEIN, H. G., GREEN, I.: Croton oil induced suppression of the immune response of guinea pigs. Nature (Lond.) **228**, 871—872 (1970).

BOYSE, E. A., OLD, L. J., CHOUROULINKOV, I.: Cytotoxic test for demonstration of mouse antibody. In: Methods in medical research, Vol. 10, pp. 39—47. Chicago: Yearbook Medical Publishers 1964.

BRENT, L.: Transplantation immunity and hypersensitivity. In: Mechanisms of hypersensitivity, pp. 555—568. Boston: Little, Brown and Co. 1959.

BRUNNER, R. T., MAUEL, J., RUDOLF, H., CHAPUIS, B.: Studies of allograft immunity in mice. I. Induction, development and *in vitro* assay of cellular immunity. Immunology **18**, 501—515 (1970).

BRUNNER, R. T., MAUEL, J., SCHINDLER, R.: *In vitro* studies of cell-bound immunity; cloning assay of the cytotoxic action of sensitized lymphoid cells on allogeneic target cells. Immunology **11**, 499—506 (1966).

BULLOCK, W. E., KANTOR, F. S.: Hemagglutination reactions of human erythyocytes conjugated covalently with dinitrophenyl groups. J. Immunol. **94**, 317—322 (1965).

BUSKIRK, H. H., CRIM, J. A., PETERING, H. G., MERRITT, K., JOHNSON, A. G.: Effect of uracil mustard and several antitumor drugs on the primary antibody response in rats and mice. J. nat. Cancer Inst. **34**, 747—758 (1965).

CALABRESI, P.: New techniques for measuring the effects of chemotherapeutic agents upon neoplastic and normal host cells. Proc. int. Congr. Chemother. (Vienna) **5**, 409—421 (1967).

CAMPBELL, D. H., GARVEY, J. S., CREMER, N. E., SUSSADORF, D. H.: Methods in immunology. New York: Benjamin pp. 69—70 (1964).
CHANMOUGAN, D., SCHWARTZ, R. S.: Enhancement of antibody synthesis by 6-mercaptopurine. J. exp. Med. **124**, 363—378 (1966).
CLAMAN, H. N., BRONSKY, E. A.: Inhibition of antibody production and acquired immunologic tolerance by actinomycin. J. Immunol. **95**, 718—721 (1965).
CRADDOCK, C. G., LONGMIRE, R., MCMILLAN, R.: Lymphocytes and the immune response. New Engl. J. Med. **285**, 324—331, 378—384 (1971).
CUNNINGHAM, A. J., SZENBERG, A.: Further improvements in the plaque technique for detecting single antibody-forming cells. Immunology **14**, 599—600 (1968).
CURTIS, J. E., HERSH, E. M., HARRIS, J. E., MCBRIDE, C., FREIREICH, E. J.: The human primary immune response to keyhole limpet hemocyanin: interrelationships of delayed hypersensitivity, antibody response and *in vitro* blast transformation. Clin. exp. Immunol. **6**, 473—490 (1970).
DAVID, J. R.: Macrophage migration. Fed. Proc. **27**, 6—12 (1968).
DAVID, J. R.: Lymphocytic factors in cellular hypersensitivity. In: Immunobiology. Stanford: Sinauer, 146—156 (1971).
DAVID, J. R., AL-ASKARI, S., LAWRENCE, H. S., THOMAS, L. J.: Delayed hypersensitivity *in vitro*. I. The specificity of inhibition of cell migration by antigens. J. Immunol. **93**, 264—273 (1964).
DEODHAR, S. D., CRILE, G., JR.: Enhancement of metastases by antilymphocyte serum in allogeneic murine tumor system. Cancer Res. **29**, 776—779 (1969).
DEUTSCH, H. F., MORTON, J. I.: Dissociation of human serum macroglobulins. Science **125**, 600—601 (1957).
DIETRICH, F. M., DUKOR, P.: The immune response to heterologous red cells in mice. III. Cyclophosphamide-induced tolerance to multispecies red cells. Pathol. Microbiol. **30**, 909—917 (1967).
DRESSER, D. W., WORTIS, H. H.: Use of an antiglobulin serum to detect cells producing antibody with low haemolytic efficiency. Nature (Lond.) **208**, 859—861 (1965).
DUPUY, J. M., KOURILSKY, F. M., FRADELIZZI, D., FEINGOLD, N., JACQUILLAT, C., BERNARD, J., DAUSSET, J.: Depression of immunologic reactivity of patients with acute leukemia. Cancer **27**, 323—331 (1971).
EAST, J.: Viruses and autoimmunity. Vox Sang. (Basel) **16**, 318—324 (1969).
ELVES, M. W.: Suppression of antibody production by phytohaemagglutinin. Nature (Lond.) **213**, 495—496 (1967).
FAHEY, J. L., TERRY, E. W.: Ion exchange chromatography and gel filtration. In: Handbook of Experimental Immunology, pp. 19—43. Philadelphia: F. A. Davis 1967.
FINGER, H., EMMERLING, P., BRUSS, E.: The influence of cyclophosphamide on the process of priming for the secondary response. Experientia (Basel) **25**, 1183—1184 (1969).
FISCHER, G. A., SARTORELLI, A. C.: Development, maintenance and assay of drug resistance. In: Methods in medical research, Vol. 10, pp. 247—262. Chicago: Yearbook Medical Publishers 1964.
FRISCH, A. V., DAVIES, G. H.: Inhibition of hemagglutinin synthesis by cytoxan: specificity and drug-induced "tolerance." J. Lab. clin. Med. **68**, 103—112 (1966).
GAMBLE, C. N.: The effect of phytohemagglutinin on the primary antibody response of mice to rat erythrocytes and human gamma globulin. Int. Arch. Allergy Appl. Immunol. **29**, 470—477 (1966).
GAVIN, J., WATERBURY, W., FRIEDMAN, H.: Antibody plaque reduction *in vitro* and *in vivo*: a rapid assay for immunosuppressive agents. Transplant. Proc. **1**, 413—415 (1969).
GEORGE, M., VAUGHAN, J. H.: *In vitro* cell migration as a model for delayed hypersensitivity. Proc. Soc. exp. Biol. (N. Y.) **111**, 514—521 (1962).
GERY, I., EYAL, O., BENEZRA, D.: The relationship between lymphocyte transformation and immune response. III. Kinetics of production of antibody forming cells. Immunology **19**, 97—104 (1970).
GOLUB, E. S., MISHELL, R. I., WEIGLE, W. O., DUTTON, R. W.: A modification of the hemolytic plaque assay for use with protein antigens. J. Immunol. **100**, 133—137 (1968).
GORDON, R. O., WADE, M. E., MITCHELL, M. S.: The production of tolerance to human erythrocytes in the rat with cytosine arabinoside or cyclophosphamide. J. Immunol. **103**, 233—243 (1969).
GOWANS, J. L.: The fate of parental strain small lymphocytes in $F_1$ hybrid rats. Ann. N. Y. Acad. Sci. **99**, 432—455 (1962).
GRAY, G. D., CRIM, J. A., MICKELSON, M. M.: The immunosuppressive effects of ara-cytidine. II. Effects on the graft versus host reaction. Transplantation **6**, 818—825 (1968).
GRAY, H. M., RABELLINO, E., PIROFSKY, B.: Immunoglobulins on the surface of lymphocytes. J. clin. Invest. **50**, 2368—2375 (1971).

Greig, M. E., Gibbons, A. J.: Effects of cytarabine and adamantoyl cytarabine on experimental allergic encephalomyelitis in rats. Arch. int. Pharmacodyn. **182**, 364—369 (1969).
Harris, J. E., Hersh, E. M.: The effect of 1-Beta-D-arabinosylfuranosyl-cytosine on the immune response of mice to sheep red blood cells. Cancer Res. **28**, 2432—2436 (1968).
Harris, J. E., Hersh, E. M., Huggins, S.: Human immune response to a xenogeneic nucleated cell. Transplantation **9**, 440—446 (1970).
Heine, K. M., Stobbe, H., Klatt, R., Apostoloff, E., Dutz, W.: Lymphocyte transformation tests in patients under therapy with immunosuppressive drugs. Helv. med. Acta **35**, 140—145 (1969).
Hellstrom, I., Hellstrom, K. E., Pierce, G. E., Bill, A. H.: Demonstration of cell-bound and humoral immunity against neuroblastoma cells. Proc. nat. Acad. Sci. (Wash.) **60**, 1231—1238 (1968).
Henney, C. S.: *In vitro* cytotoxic test for detecting cell mediated immunity to soluble antigen. Nature (Lond.) **226**, 1167—1169 (1970).
Heppner, G. H., Kopp, J. S.: A dilute agar colony-inhibition (CI) test for studying cell-mediated immune responses against tumor cells. Int. J. Cancer **7**, 26—33 (1971).
Herbert, W. J.: Passive haemagglutination. In: Handbook of experimental immunology, pp. 720—744. Philadelphia: F. A. David 1967.
Hersh, E. M., Oppenheim, J. J.: Impaired *in vitro* lymphocyte transformation in Hodgkin's disease. New Engl. J. Med. **273**, 1006—1012 (1965).
Hersh, E. M., Oppenheim, J. J.: Inhibition of *in vitro* lymphocyte transformation during chemotherapy in man. Cancer Res. **27**, 98—105 (1967).
Hitchings, G. H., Elion, G. B.: Chemical suppression of the immune response. Pharmacol. Rev. **15**, 365—405 (1963).
Hoy, W. E., Nelson, D. S.: Studies on cytophilic antibodies. V. Alloantibodies cytophilic for mouse macrophages. Aust. J. exp. Biol. med. Sci. **47**, 525—537 (1969).
Hoyer, L. W., Good, R. A., Condie, R. M.: Experimental allergic encephalomyelitis: the effect of 6-mercaptopurine. J. exp. Med. **116**, 311—327 (1962).
Humphreys, S. R., Chirigos, M. A., Milstead, K. L., Mantel, N., Goldin, A.: Studies on the suppression of the homograft response with folic acid antagonists. J. nat. Cancer Inst. **27**, 259—276 (1961).
Hurd, E. R., Ziff, M.: Studies of the anti-inflammatory action of 6-mercaptopurine. J. exp. Med. **128**, 785—800 (1968).
Hutchin, P.: Mechanisms and functions of immunologic enhancement. Surg. Gynec. Obstet. **126**, 1331—1356 (1968).
Hutchin, P. D., Amos, B., Prioleau, W. H., Jr.: Interactions of humoral antibodies and immune lymphocytes. Transplantation **5**, 68—75 (1967).
Ingraham, J., Bussard, A.: Application of a localized hemolysin reaction for specific detection of individual antibody-forming cells. J. exp. Med. **119**, 667—684 (1964).
Jennings, J. F., Oates, C. M.: The effect of phytohemagglutinin on the immune response *in vivo*. Clin. exp. Immunol. **2**, 445—453 (1967).
Jerne, N. K., Nordin, A. A., Henry, C.: The agar plaque technique for recognizing antibody-producing cells. In: Amos, B., Koprowski, H. (Eds.): Cell-bound antibodies, pp. 109—125. Philadelphia: Wistar Institute Press 1963.
Johnson, M. W., Maibach, H. I., Salmon, S. E.: Skin reactivity in patients with cancer; impaired delayed hypersensitivity or faulty inflammatory response? New Engl. J. Med. **284**, 1255—1257 (1971).
Jondal, M., Holm, G., Wigzell, H.: Surface markers on human T and B lymphocytes. I. A large population of lymphocytes forming nonimmune rosettes with sheep red blood cells. J. exp. Med. **136**, 207—215 (1972).
Kaliss, N.: Micromethod for assaying immune cytolysis by the release of $^{51}$Cr. Transplantation **8**, 526—530 (1969).
Kantor, F. S., Bullock, W. E.: Hapten-protein conjugates as antigens for evaluation of immunological competence in man. J. Allergy **43**, 349—357 (1969).
Kaplan, M. H., Dienes, L.: The cellular response in forms of delayed- or immediate-type skin reactions in the guinea pig. In: Mechanisms of hypersensitivity, pp. 435—450. Boston: Little, Brown and Co. 1959.
Kaplan, S. R., Calabresi, P.: Suppression of delayed hypersensitivity *in vivo* and *in vitro* by cytosine arabinoside. Clin. Res. **13**, 543 (1965).
Klesius, P. H.: A rapid method for *in vitro* screening of immunosuppressants using mouse spleen cells. Proc. Soc. exp. Biol. (N. Y.) **135**, 155—159 (1970).
Kligman, A. M., Epstein, W. L.: Some factors affecting contact sensitization in man. In: Shaffer, J. H., LoGrippo, G. A., Chase, M. W. (Eds.): Mechanisms of hypersensitivity, pp. 713—722. Boston: Little, Brown and Co. 1959.

LANDY, M., LAMB, E.: Estimation of Vi antibody employing erythrocytes treated with purified Vi antigen. Proc. Soc. exp. Biol. (N. Y.) **82**, 593—598 (1953).

LAPLANTE, E. S., CONDIE, R. M., GOOD, R. A.: Prevention of secondary immune response with 6-mercaptopurine. J. Lab. clin. Med. **59**, 542—549 (1962).

LARSON, D. L., TOMLINSON, L. J.: Quantitative antibody studies in man. III. Antibody response in leukemia and other malignant lymphomata. J. clin. Invest. **32**, 317—321 (1953).

LEVIN, R. H., LANDY, M., FREI, E.: The effect of 6-mercaptopurine on immune response in man. New Engl. J. Med. **271**, 16—22 (1964).

LEVINE, S., HOENIG, E. M., KIES, M. W.: Allergic encephalomyelitis: immunologically specific inhibition of cellular passive transfer by encephalotogenic basic proteins. Clin. exp. Immunol. **6**, 503—517 (1970).

LOPES-CARDOZO, E.: The effect of cytostatic therapy with cyclophosphamide alone or in combination with methotrexate on the phytohemagglutinin lymphocyte culture and on the immunoglobulins. Oncology **24**, 261—272 (1970).

LYTTON, B., HUGHES, L. E., FULTHORPE, E. J.: Circulating antibody response in malignant disease. Lancet **1**, 69—71 (1964).

MCBRIDE, R. A.: Graft versus host reaction in lymphoid proliferation. Cancer Res. **26**, 1135—1151 (1966).

MAIBACH, H. I., EPSTEIN, W. L.: Immunologic responses of healthy volunteers receiving azathiopurine (Imuran). Int. Arch. Allergy appl. Immunol. **27**, 102—109 (1965).

MARBROOK, J.: Primary immune response in cultures of spleen cells. Lancet **2**, 1279—1281 (1967).

MATHÉ, G., AMIEL, J. L., SCHWARZENBERG, L., MERY, A. M.: A method of reducing the incidence of the secondary syndrome in allogenic marrow. Blood **22**, 44—52 (1963).

MERCHANT, M. S., HRABA, T.: Lymphoid cells producing antibody against simple haptens: detection and enumeration. Science **152**, 1378—1379 (1966).

MICHAELIDES, M. A., COONS, A. H.: Studies on antibody production. V. The secondary response *in vitro*. J. exp. Med. **117**, 1035—1051 (1963).

MILLER, J. J., III., COLE, L. J.: Resistance of long-lived lymphocytes and plasma cells in rat lymph nodes to treatment with prednisone, cyclophosphamide, 6-mercaptopurine and actinomycin D. J. exp. Med. **126**, 109—125 (1967).

MISHELL, R. I., DUTTON, R. W.: Immunization of dissociated spleen cell cultures from normal mice. J. exp. Med. **126**, 423—442 (1967).

MITCHELL, M. S.: Central inhibition of cellular immunity to leukemia L1210 by isoantibody. Cancer Res. **32**, 825—831 (1972).

MITCHELL, M. S., BOVE, J. R., CALABRESI, P.: Simplified estimation of mouse isohemagglutinins by microassay. Transplantation **1**, 294—296 (1969a).

MITCHELL, M. S., KAPLAN, R., CALABRESI, P.: Alteration of antibody synthesis in the rat by cytosine arabinoside. Cancer Res. **29**, 896—904 (1969b).

MITCHELL, M. S., WADE, M. E., DECONTI, R. C., BERTINO, J. R., CALABRESI, P.: Immunosuppressive effects of cytosine arabinoside and methotrexate in man. Ann. intern. Med. **70**, 535—547 (1969c).

MOAV, N., HARRIS, T. N.: Rosette formation in relation to active synthesis of antibody. J. Immunol. **105**, 1501—1511 (1970).

NELSON, D. S.: Macrophages and immunity. Amsterdam: North Holland Press 1969.

NOSSAL, G. J. V., BUSSARD, A. E., LEWIS, H., MAZIE, J. C.: *In vitro* stimulation of antibody formation by peritoneal cells. I. Plaque technique of high sensitivity enabling access to the cells. J. exp. Med. **131**, 894—916 (1970).

NOWELL, P. C.: Phytohemagglutinin: an initiator of mitosis in cultures of normal human leukocytes. Cancer Res. **20**, 462—466 (1960).

O'BRIEN, T. F., COONS, A. H.: Studies on antibody production. VII. The effect of 5-bromodeoxyuridine on the *in vitro* anamnestic antibody response. J. exp. Med. **117**, 1063—1074 (1963).

PAGE, A. R., CONDIE, R. M., GOOD, R. A.: Effect of 6-mercaptopurine on inflammation. Amer. J. Path. **40**, 519—530 (1962).

PAGE, A. R., CONDIE, R. M., GOOD, R. A.: Suppression of plasma cell hepatitis with 6-mercaptopurine. Amer. J. Med. **36**, 200—213 (1964).

PEARSON, C. M.: Development of arthritis in the rat following injection with adjuvant. In: Mechanisms of hypersensitivity, pp. 647—671. Boston: Little, Brown and Co. 1959.

POKORNA, Z.: Induction of experimental autoimmune aspermatogenesis by immune serum fractions. Folia Biol. (Kraków) **16**, 320—329 (1970).

REBUCK, J. W., CROWLEY, J. H.: A method of studying leukocytic functions *in vivo*. Ann. N. Y. Acad. Sci. **59**, 757—805 (1955).

RUSSELL, P. J., HICKS, J. D., BURNET, F. M.: Cyclophosphamide treatment of kidney disease in (NZB × NZW) $F_1$ mice. Lancet 1, 1279—1284 (1966).

SAHIAR, K., SCHWARTZ, R. S.: The immunoglobulin sequence. I. Arrest by 6-mercaptopurine and restitution by antibody, antigen or splenectomy. J. Immunol. **95**, 345—354 (1965).

SALEH, W. S., MACLEAN, D., GORDON, J., LAMOUREUX, G.: A test to measure the immunosuppressive potency of antilymphocyte sera. Transplantation 8, 524—526 (1969).

SANTOS, G. W., OWENS, A. H., JR., SENSENBRENNER, L. L.: Effects of selected cytotoxic agents on antibody production in man; a preliminary report. Ann. N. Y. Acad. Sci. **114**, 404—423 (1964).

SANTOS, G. W., OWENS, A. H., JR.: 19S and 7S antibody production in the cyclophosphamide- or methotrexate-treated rat. Nature (Lond.) **209**, 622—624 (1966).

SCHWARTZ, R. S., EISNER, A., DAMESHEK, W.: The effect of 6-MP on primary and secondary immune responses. J. clin. Invest. **38**, 1394—1403 (1959).

SCHWARTZ, R. S., DAMESHEK, W.: The role of antigen dosage in drug-induced immunological tolerance. J. Immunol. **90**, 703—710 (1963).

SEVER, J. L.: Application of a micro technique to viral serological investigations. J. Immunol. **88**, 320—329 (1962).

SIMONSEN, M.: Graft versus host reactions. Their natural history and applicability as tools of research. In: Progress in allergy, Vol. 6, pp. 349—467. Basel: Karger 1962.

SNELL, G.: Immunologic enhancement. Surg. Gynec. Obstet. **130**, 1109—1119 (1970).

SPIEGELBERG, H. L., MIESCHER, P. A.: The effect of 6-mercaptopurine and aminopterin on experimental immune thyroiditis in guinea pigs. J. exp. Med. **118**, 869—890 (1963).

STANWORTH, D. R.: Ultracentrifugation of immunoglobulins. In: Handbook of experimental immunology, pp. 44—111. Philadelphia: F. A. David 1967.

STAPLES, P. J., TALAL, N.: Impaired recovery of plaque-forming cells in New Zealand mice given cyclophosphamide. J. Immunol. **104**, 1101—1107 (1970).

STERZL, J.: The effect of immunosuppressive drugs at various stages of differentiation of immunologically competent cells. In: Immunity, cancer and chemotherapy, pp. 71—99. New York-London: Academic Press 1967.

STERZL, J., RIHA, I.: Detection of cells producing 7S antibodies by the plaque technique. Nature (Lond.) **208**, 858—859 (1965).

STEVENS, J. E., WILLOUGHBY, D. A.: The anti-inflammatory effect of some immunosuppressive agents. J. Path. **97**, 367—373 (1969).

STIMPFLING, J. H.: Methods for detection of hemagglutinins in mouse isoantisera. In: Methods in medical research, Vol. 10, pp. 22—26. Chicago: Year Book Medical Publishers 1964.

SUTHERLAND, R. M., INCH, W. R., MCCREDIE, J. A.: Phytohemagglutinin (PHA) induced transformation of lymphocytes from patients with cancer. Cancer **27**, 574—578 (1971).

SWANSON, M. A., SCHWARTZ, R. S.: Immunosuppressive therapy. The relation between clinical response and immunologic competence. New Engl. J. Med. **277**, 163—170 (1967).

TAKASUGI, M., KLEIN, E.: A microassay for cell-mediated immunity. Transplantation **9**, 219—227 (1970).

TURK, J. L., STONE, S. H.: Implication of the cellular changes in lymph nodes during the development and inhibition of delayed type hypersensitivity. In: Cell-bound antibody, pp. 51—60. Philadelphia: Wistar Institute Press 1963.

TURSI, A., GREAVES, M. F., TORRIGIANI, G.: Response to phytohemagglutinin of lymphocytes from mice treated with anti-lymphocyte globulin. Immunology **17**, 801—811 (1969).

UHR, J. W., FINKELSTEIN, M. S.: Antibody formation. IV. Formation of rapidly and slowly sedimenting antibodies and immunological memory to bacteriophage øX-174. J. exp. Med. **117**, 457—477 (1963).

UYEKI, E. M., KLASSEN, R. S., LLACER, V.: Analysis of dextran- and methylated albumin-induced hypersensitivity by mouse paw swelling. Proc. Soc. exp. Biol. (N. Y.) **132**, 1140—1146 (1969).

UYEKI, E. M., LLACER, V.: Effect of antibiotics on antibody-forming cells *in vitro*. Biochem. Pharmacol. **18**, 948—951 (1969).

UYEKI, E. M., LLACER, V.: Antitumour agents on antibody-producing cells *in vitro*. Biochem. Pharmacol. **19**, 2419—2424 (1970).

VAN BEKKUM, D. W., DEVRIES, M. J.: Secondary disease following bone marrow transplantation: In: Radiation chimeras, pp. 79—126. London: Logos-Academic Press 1967.

VOLKMAN, A., GOWANS, J. L.: The origin of macrophages from bone marrow in the rat. Brit. J. exp. Path. **46**, 62—70 (1965).

WAKSMAN, B. H.: Experimental allergic encephalomyelitis as prototype of the class of auto-allergic diseases. In: Mechanisms of hypersensitivity, pp. 679—691. Boston: Little, Brown and Co. 1959.

WAKSMAN, B. H.: Delayed hypersensitivity: immunologic and clinical aspects. In: Immunobiology, pp. 28—34. Stanford: Sinauer 1971.
WALDORF, D. S., WILLKENS, R. S., DECKER, J. L.: Impaired delayed hypersensitivity in an aging population. J. Amer. med. Assoc. **203**, 831—834 (1968).
WEISBURGER, A. S., DANIEL, T. M., HOFFMAN, A.: Suppression of antibody synthesis. J. exp. Med. **120**, 183—196 (1964).
WIGZELL, H.: Quantitative titrations of mouse H-2 antibodies using $Cr^{51}$-labeled target cells. Transplantation **3**, 423—431 (1965).
WYBRAN, J., CARR, M. C., FUDENBERG, H. H.: The human rosette-forming cell as a marker of a population of thymus derived cells. J. clin. Invest. **51**, 2537—2543 (1972).

Chapter 28

# Immunosuppressive Agents

EVAN M. HERSH

## Introduction

The field of chemical immunosuppression, now approximately 14 years old, has become an important component of several major basic and clinical scientific disciplines. In experimental systems, the use of chemical immunosuppressive agents has permitted a kinetic and biochemical analysis and characterization of the immune response and host defense mechanisms which would not have been possible without them. While chemical immunosuppression lacks a complete degree of immunological specificity (because of hematological, gastrointestinal, cutaneous, hepatic, renal, and neurological toxicity), appropriate regimens of drug administration have still proven very useful in the study of immunity.

The utility of chemical immunosuppression in fundamental immunological experiments is based on the fact that the various chemotherapeutic agents with immunosuppressive properties have specific and, more important, different mechanisms of action. Furthermore, different tissues have different degrees of susceptibility to some of these agents. Thus, there are specific inhibitors of various components of DNA synthesis, DNA-dependent RNA synthesis, and protein synthesis. Within these major classes of inhibitors, there are agents which appear to effect only one defined step within a synthetic process. For example cytosine arabinoside is activated by deoxycytidine kinase, inhibits cellular proliferation by inhibiting DNA polymerase, and is degraded by a specific deaminase (COHEN, 1966). Since it has a very short half-life in the circulation and tissues before degradation, and since lymphoid tissue is particularly susceptible to its action (having a high kinase-deaminase ratio), it can be used as a chemical scalpel to dissect the immune response. Since the immune response, from the time of antigen injection to the time of the production of antibody, consists of a series of cellular events involving different cell populations, appropriately timed doses of an agent like cytosine arabinoside can be used to explore the nature of each step sequentially. Recently, the development of methods with which the immune response can be explored *in vitro* (DUMONDE et al., 1969) has permitted the use of the chemical immunosuppressants *in vitro* to further dissect the response. The mechanisms of action of the various agents are described in other sections of this book and will not be detailed here.

The characterization of the immunosuppressive properties of a variety of specific anticancer and related agents has led to their clinical use in two areas of therapeutics, in the maintenance of organ and tissue allografts and in the treatment of autoimmune or inflammatory diseases. Clinically, chemical immunosuppression is of interest, not only as immunosuppressive therapy, but also from the point of view that chemical immunosuppression is an undesirable side effect of cancer chemotherapy. Thus, the cancer chemotherapist and the clinical immunologist have disparate interests in chemical immunosuppression, based on the objectives of their therapy. The clinical transplantation immunologist tries to identify drugs, doses, and schedules which will suppress cell-mediated immunity and the cellular component of the inflammatory reaction, since these are the basis of the mechanism of the rejection of organ and tissue allografts (DAMMIN, 1968). The clinical immunologist, dealing with autoimmune, allergic, or inflammatory diseases, may wish to suppress both cell-mediated and humoral immunity. In contrast, because tumor immunity is based mainly on cell-mediated host defense mechanisms (KLEIN, 1969) and indeed, antibody may be of the disadvantageous blocking type (KALISS, 1958), the cancer chemotherapist attempts to identify drugs, doses, and schedules which tend to preserve cell-mediated immunity. Of course, all clinical regimens are designed to minimize the undesirable side effects, particularly the myelosuppressive phenomena of granulocytopenia and thrombocytopenia.

The major immunological concern of the cancer chemotherapist is the immunological surveillance mechanism which must be spared by his various regimens of cancer chemotherapy. The surveillance mechanism (BURNET, 1970), based on the ability of circulating lymphocytes to recognize and react against foreign cell surface antigens, is presumed to be involved in the elimination of early primary tumors and in the elimination of many metastatic deposits (when they are only a few cells in number). If a regimen interferes with the circulation and/or function of these effector lymphocytes, surveillance will be impaired and metastatic disease will be promoted. This has been demonstrated in a number of animal systems, in which immunosuppressive therapy increases the rate and number of both primary tumors and metastatic deposits (ALLISON and LAW, 1968). Also, there is an increased incidence of malignancy in patients on chronic immunosuppressive therapy (STARZL et al., 1970). Thus, regimens that do not impair surveillance are desired.

In the current chapter an attempt will be made to evaluate the present state of the field of chemical immunosuppression. This evaluation and review will be oriented mainly towards immunosuppression in humans, but pertinent animal experiments will also be reviewed. The major areas to be covered will include the nature of the normal human immune response, the relationship of drug action to the mechanism of the immune response, various approaches to classification of immunosuppressive drugs, and the characteristics of the specific immunosuppressive phenomena. Finally, the interrelationship of chemotherapy, chemical immunosuppression, tumor response, and prognosis will be discussed. No attempt will be made to provide a complete review of the literature on chemical immunosuppression; rather, selected papers with typical results, or covering the important major areas, will be reviewed. For more detailed reviews on basic immunology, mechanism of drug action, biochemical pharmacology, and various aspects of immunosuppression, several pertinent reviews are available in the literature (HITCHINGS and ELION, 1963; BERENBAUM, 1964a; AISENBERG, 1965; MAKINODAN et al., 1965; SCHWARTZ, 1965; GABRIELSON and GOOD, 1967; MIHICH, 1967; HERSH and FREIREICH, 1968; SCHWARTZ, 1968; SORKIN and DEWECK, 1969).

## Relationship of Chemical Immunosuppression to the Normal Immune Response

During the last two decades, many of the fundamental cellular features of the mammalian immune response have been identified (GOWANS and MCGREGOR, 1965). Also, the mediation of the host defense mechanisms by the products of the immune response and by associated nonspecific mechanisms have been fairly well characterized. The immune response and the resultant or associated specific and nonspecific immune mechanisms can be described as a series of cellular events taking place in lymph nodes, followed by a series of cellular and humoral events in the periphery, resulting in defense of the body against the invasion of foreign matter. Since these phenomena take place sequentially, the effects of chemical immunosuppressive agents on the various steps can, in many instances, be studied separately.

The major steps in the adult mammalian immune response are as follows. When antigen is injected, inhaled, ingested, absorbed through the skin, or released into the tissues, it reaches the draining lymph nodes through their afferent lymphatics. Subsequently, antigen localizes in both the cortical and the medullary macrophages. In the latter, it is rapidly degraded to a nonantigen state and digested. In contrast, the antigen may localize for long periods in the cortical dendritic macrophages (FISHMAN and ADLER, 1967). The antigen trapping mechanism in the latter is apparently very important in the immune response, and drug regimens which interfere with this trapping mechanism can suppress the immune response. The events which occur subsequent to this antigen trapping are not entirely clear. The antigen is partially degraded (processed) and apparently coupled to a preformed RNA. This immunogenic RNA remains at the surface of the cortical dendritic macrophages and is brought into contact with the precursors of the antibody forming cells. These cells, which have the morphology of small lymphocytes, subsequently undergo a lymphoblastoid transformation. The next step is a wave of proliferation among these lymphoblastoid cells resulting first in a population of immunologically committed large lymphoblasts and subsequently, a population of effector cells, either small lymphocytes or plasma cells. The duration of this wave of proliferation varies greatly according to the species and according to the nature, dose, and route of antigen injection. However, some generalizations about it can be made. It usually starts approximately 24 to 48 h after the introduction of antigen and lasts from between 4 and 14 days (SISKIND and BENACERRAF, 1969).

Detailed comments are necessary about the cells produced by this wave of lymphoblastoid transformation. First, it can produce up to $10^{10}$ or more cells per responding lymph node during a single response. The cells produced include the committed large lymphoblastoid cells, differentiated effector small lymphocytes, small lymphocytes carrying immunological memory, and plasma cells.

Large numbers of the committed large lymphoblasts are relased from the node during the first 4 to 10 days after immunization (HALL, 1969). They pass out through the efferent lymphatics, then into the thoracic duct and from there they pass into the blood. These are short lived cells, and they localize in the gut, the lung, and also at sites of specific antigen localization. These cells do not recirculate, but leave the circulation at the level of the post capillary venule by crawling between the endothelial cells. HALL, who has done the most work on this phase of the response, has hypothesized that this population of cells provides the first line of host defense of extravascular immunity against foreign antigens. This is achieved through the mechanism of local antibody production by these cells.

The effector small lymphocytes and memory cells are also released from the node through the efferent lymphatics into the thoracic duct. In contrast to the large lymphoblastoid cells, they constantly recirculate through the blood, the tissues, and back through the lymph nodes (GOWANS, 1969). These are the cells that provide immunological surveillance for the body, through their capacity to recognize foreign histocompatibility antigens and react against them. It has been hypothesized that these cells recognize and destroy not only foreign tissue grafts but also spontaneous antigenic tumors as they arise. The mechanism by which these effector small lymphocytes carry out the reactions of cell-mediated immunity include the following: localization at the antigen site, antigen recognition, lymphoblastoid transformation at the local site, and release of soluble mediators (including macrophage chemotactic factor, migration inhibitory factor, blastogenic factor, and lymphocyte cytotoxin) (LAWRENCE and LANDY, 1969). These factors attract and localize macrophages at the site of antigen localization. These mediators also activate the macrophages which destroy the antigen by phagocytosis, intracellular killing, and digestion.

The plasma cells, produced subsequent to the wave of lymphoblastoid transformation, remain in the lymph node. These cells produce the bulk of the antibody which is released into the circulation, but antibody production actually begins at the point when committed lymphoblastoid cells first appear. Two major classes of circulating antibodies are produced. IgM or 19S antibody is produced first and is followed by the production of IgG or 7S antibody (BAUER et al., 1963). This sequence of events can be referred to as the productive phase of the immune response. IgM production is transient, peaking at one to two weeks and usually subsiding by 28 days, while IgG production may continue for months or even years. The IgG antibody, as it is produced, exerts feed-back control over the IgM production. Therefore, it is actually the cause of the early decline in IgM synthesis and release (BYSTRYN, 1970). IgG antibody leaves the circulation and reacts with antigen. Antigen-antibody reactions destroy antigen by a number of mechanisms including complement fixation and lysis (in the case of cellular antigen), opsinization for phagocytosis or by the mechanism of vascular damage, mediator release and subsequent acute inflammation (HERSH and BODEY, 1970).

Another important aspect of the immune system is the role of the thymus and bursa derived lymphocytes. Embryologically, competent lymphoid cells arise from or come under the differentiating influence of the central gut-associated lymphoid tissue, the analog of which, in the bird, is the Bursa of Fabricius (COOPER et al., 1965), and the thymus (COOPER et al., 1967). Both thymus-derived and gut-associated cells are involved in the antibody response. The antibody is actually synthesized by the gut-associated lymphocytes. These antibody forming cells, in the adult, are derived from the bone marrow and can be referred to as B cells (ROITT et al., 1969). Reactions of cell-mediated immunity, such as delayed hypersensitivity and homograft rejection are mediated by the thymus derived lymphocytes. These are also the cells which constantly recirculate from blood, through nodes, to thoracic duct lymph, and back to blood. These recirculating thymus derived cells can be referred to as T cells (RAFF and WORTIS, 1970). Recently, several methods have been developed to differentiate T and B cells in the peripheral circulation (ROITT et al., 1969; RAFF and WORTIS, 1970). Thus, it is now possible to reevaluate chemical immunosuppression, not only for its overall effect on the lymphocyte population, but as to whether it differentially effects the T and B cell subpopulations.

In summary, the immune response and the reactions of its immunological products include several interrelated components. Each would be subject, in a unique fashion, to the action of different chemotherapeutic agents. The major cellular components of the immune response in this regard are as follows: first, precursor immunocompetent but uncommitted lymphoid cells in their resting state (stem cells), recent evidence indicates that these are very slowly turning over in the nodes (AISENBERG and WILKES, 1967); second, the cortical dendritic macrophages which take up, process and store antigen; third, lymphoid cells in the process of lymphoblastoid transformation and proliferation; fourth, the plasma cells during the phase of active antibody production; fifth, the circulating and fixed committed large lymphoblasts, committed small effector lymphocytes and memory cells. The main divisions of the immune response relevant to chemical immunosuppression include the stage of uncommitted non-stimulated immunocompetence, the stage of antigen uptake and processing, the induction phase during which immunological committment is conferred on the responding cells, the phase of lymphoblastoid transformation and proliferation, the phase of lymphoblast release, the phase of antibody synthesis and release, the phase of circulation of antibody and specifically committed effector lymphocytes, and finally, the phase of effector reactions of both cell-mediated and humoral immunity in the periphery.

From the above outline of the immune response, it is apparent that chemotherapeutic agents with different mechanisms of action, administered at various times relative to the time of antigen administration, will have varying but specific effects on immunity. Each phase of the immune response will be particularly subject to the action of specific agents of one or another class. Some drugs will have a unique action against one phase, while others may have action against several phases.

A classification of immunosuppressive drugs according to the phase or phases of the immune response which they effect is given in Table 1. The phase of antigen uptake and processing was originally thought to be resistant to modification by chemotherapeutic drugs. However, recent studies in animal systems indicate that the phagocytic activity of the cortical dendritic macrophages, or the antigen processing capacity, may be sensitive to certain drugs. Thus, the activity of the reticuloendothelial system for the uptake of both particulate and soluble antigen is impaired by corticosteroids, cyclophosphamide, methotrexate, and chloroambucil (NETTESHEIM and HAMMONS, 1970).

Precursor cell populations (uncommitted but immunologically competent stem cells) are inhibited or destroyed by alkylating agents such as nitrogen mustard. This conclusion results from the observation that nitrogen mustard is immunosuppressive only when administered prior to, or at the latest, simultaneous with antigen (GREEN, 1958). Presumably, resting precursor lymphocytes are killed. It is also possible that through the cross-linking of their DNA, a lethal event occurs during subsequent antigen-induced proliferation. Precursor lymphoid cell populations can also be inhibited and/or destroyed by radiation (TALIAFERRO et al., 1964), corticosteroids (ROSE, 1959), or antilymphocyte serum or globulin (ALS or ALG) (TAUB, 1970).

The proliferative phase of the immune response is inhibited by some of the lympholytic agents mentioned above, but most important by the cell cycle phase specific drugs. In other words, it is inhibited by

Table 1. *Sites of action of immunosuppressive agents on the steps of the immune response*

| Antigen uptake and/or processes | Antigen recognition and precursor cells | Blastogenesis | Proliferation | Antibody production | Effector reactions |
|---|---|---|---|---|---|
| Actinomycin D<br>Corticosteroids<br>Cyclophosphamide<br>X-irradiation | Alkylating agents<br>Antilymphocyte serum (ALS)<br>Corticosteroids<br>X-irradiation | L-Asparaginase<br>Actinomycin D<br>Cyclophosphamide<br>5-Fluorouracil<br>6-Mercaptopurine | Actinomycin D<br>Arabinosylcytosine<br>MTX<br>Periwinkle alkaloids | Cyclophosphamide | Steroids<br>ALS |

drugs which inhibit cellular proliferation. Most of the antimetabolites including the purine, pyrimidine, pyrimidine nucleoside, and folic acid analogs fall into this class. These drugs are immunosuppressive only when administered during the proliferative phase, and if given before antigen administration, or more than one week after antigen administration, they are not immunosuppressive. Because they inhibit or kill only proliferating cells, profound immunosuppression can often be achieved without severe destruction of the majority of the lymphoid cells. The responding lymphoid cells are blocked from entering or proceeding through the proliferative phase. Thus, when the drug is stopped, the immune response often resumes without further antigen stimulation (SCHWARTZ, 1965). However, permanent suppression or even tolerance can be induced by cell cycle phase specific agents, particularly when the dose and duration of treatment are extended (SCHWARTZ, 1965).

The nonspecific inflammatory reaction, which is a component of both humoral and cell-mediated immunological reactions, as well as a component of the response to trauma or infection, is also susceptible to the action of chemotherapeutic agents. The nonspecific inflammatory response consists of two main phases (REBUCK and CROWLEY, 1955); i.e., an initial phase of granulocyte exudation followed by a phase of mononuclear cell exudation (monocytes and macrophages). During this phase of mononuclear cell exudation, the granulocytes disappear. Ordinarily, the granulocytic phase of the inflammatory response is diminished only under circumstances when the granulocyte count falls below 1000 (BODEY et al., 1966). However, the mononuclear cell phase is inhibited by cancer chemotherapeutic agents, even when the total leukocyte count is not reduced (HERSH et al., 1966). This suppression is apparently due to a reduction in the numbers of circulating monocytes (HURD and ZIFF, 1968) which is due to a selective reduction of their proliferation in and release from the bone marrow. Agents that can suppress the mononuclear cell phase of the inflammatory response include the cell cycle specific antimetabolites, corticosteroids, and inhibitors of protein synthesis, such as actinomycin D (HERSH and FREIREICH, 1968).

## Interrelationship of Chemotherapy, Immunosuppression, and Prognosis During the Treatment of Human Disease

No discussion of chemical immunosuppression for the treatment of human disease is complete without a consideration of the interaction of the immunocompetence of the patient, the host defense mechanisms that may be suppressed, and the effects of the chemotherapy on the course of the patient's disease. This relationship is complex and difficult to evaluate, particularly because patients with either cancer, autoimmune disease, or renal failure treated by transplantation have disease-associated immunological deficiencies of various degrees (HERSH et al., 1971b). Depending upon the disease state, these spontaneous deficiencies may be of cell-mediated or humoral immunity, or both. During the progression of malignant disease in patients with leukemia, lymphoma, or solid tumors, immunological deficiency involving both cell-mediated and humoral immunity develops (HERSH et al., 1970). Cell-mediated and humoral immunity are affected to different degrees, and the patterns of deficiency are unique and specific, depending upon the underlying tumor (HERSH et al., 1970). Patients with early disease are relatively normal immunologically, whereas patients with advanced disease (even untreated) have severe immunological deficiency.

The effects of chemotherapy are then superimposed on these immunological defects. Several investigators have shown that chemotherapy administered to patients who already have an underlying immunological defect is more immunosuppressive than the same doses of drugs administered to patients who have no pre-existing immunological defect. For example, azathioprine therapy suppresses the immune response of normal volunteers much less than the same dose administered to patients with sarcoidosis (EPSTEIN and MAIBACH, 1965).

The degree of chemical immunosuppression also depends upon whether the therapy is intermittent or continuous. Continuous immunosuppressive therapy (i.e. daily drug doses) is usually administered to patients who have received organ transplants. Typically, they receive daily oral azathioprine and prednisone, and daily parenteral antilymphocytic globulin (ALG) (SCHWARTZ, 1968). In contrast, intermittent chemotherapy is often administered to patients with malignancy and is the schedule of choice for many tumors. For example, patients may receive 5 day courses of 6-mercaptopurine, methotrexate, vincristine, and prednisone in combination, separated by 9 to 14 day rest periods (FREIREICH et al., 1968). Studies of the response to primary immunization given during these two types of therapy indicate that continuous therapy is more suppressive of the development of new delayed hypersensitivity and less suppressive of the antibody response, while intermittent therapy has little effect on the development of new delayed hypersensitivity but is markedly suppressive of the development of the antibody response (HERSH et al.,1966). Thus, these types of therapy are appropriately suited to the maintenance of organ homografts or the protection of the antitumor surveillance mechanism. Indeed, the suppression of the latter mechanism by continuous chemotherapy may explain why there is an increased incidence of malignancy among renal homograft recipients who are on chronic continuous immunosuppressive treatment (STARZL et al., 1970).

Intensive intermittent chemotherapy commonly administered to cancer patients has such a limited effect on cell-mediated host defense mechanisms that not only is the development of new cell-mediated immunity not inhibited, but the transient suppression of established cell-mediated immunity during the actual time of drug administration, usually recovers rapidly and may overshoot. This overshoot involves cell-mediated immunity and can be demonstrated *in vivo* and *in vitro* (CHEEMA and HERSH, 1971). Indeed, patients who exhibit this overshoot of immunological reactivity may have a better prognosis than those who do not (CHEEMA and HERSH, 1971). Patients may be immunologically incompetent prior to therapy and may regain their competence subsequent to therapy. These patients also have a better prognosis than those who do not recover or who lose their competence (HERSH et al., 1971a). Thus, at least for cancer chemotherapy, there seems to be a relationship between the maintenance, recovery, or overshoot of immunocompetence and a positive effect of the chemotherapy.

These observations do not indicate a causal relationship. Immunocompetence or response to chemotherapy may be under the influence of the same factors. Regardless, evaluation of the degree of effect of chemotherapy on the specific immune response and on the general immunocompetence of the patient, before and after therapy, may determine his prognosis.

## Comparative Studies of Immunosuppression by Different Agents

Of the numerous studies of chemical immunosuppression, very few compare the effects of different agents within a class, or different classes of agents with each other, particularly using one antigen in one animal species. This is surprising since this approach is clearly important in the search for more effective, less cytotoxic cancer chemotherapeutic agents. Comparative studies seem mandatory in selection

Table 2. *Effect of drug on host defense*

| Species | Host defense parameter | Normal value | Cyclo or HN2 | 6 MP, 6 TG or azathioprine | MTX | Ara-C or 5FU | Vinca alkaloid | Miscell-aneous | Reference |
|---|---|---|---|---|---|---|---|---|---|
| Mouse[1] | Skin graft survival | 11.7 | 15.3 (C) | 16.1 (M) | — | — | — | — | AMIEL et al. (1964) |
| Mouse[2] | Mean antibody titer | 5.5 | 0.0 (C) | 3.0 (M) | 2.5 | 5.0 (F) | 5.5 | — | BERENBAUM and BROWN (1964) |
| Guinea pig[3] | Anaphylaxis (survivors) | 3/30 | 20/21 (C) | 3/18 (M) | — | — | 3/18 | 0/14 | MAIBACH and MAGUIRE (1962) |
| Guinea pig[4] | Antibody titer | 5120 | 10 (C) | 5120 (A) | — | 5120 (F) | — | — | MAIBACH and MAGUIRE (1966) |
| Rat[5] | Mean peak | 7.2 | 2.4 (C) | 5.7 (M) | 0.0 | 7.4 (F) | — | 6.0 | SANTOS and OWENS (1964) |
| Rat[6] | Mean peak antibody titer | 7.2 | 3.4 (C) | 8.2 (M) | 4.7 | 7.2 (F) | 8.7 | — | SANTOS and OWENS (1964) |
| Man[7] | Mean peak antibody titer | 7.7 | 0.0 (C)<br>9.6 (N) | 0.0 (M) | 0.0 | 6.0 (F) | — | — | SANTOS and OWENS (1964) |
| Mouse[8] | Skin graft survival | 9.2 | 15.7 (C) | 11.4 (A) | — | — | — | 12.6[9] | DIETRICH and DUKOR (1968) |
| Mouse[10] | HPFC/$10^6$<br>spleen cells | 462[11]<br>462[12] | 11 (C)<br>4 (C) | 115 (M)<br>605 (M) | 117<br>601 | —<br>— | 119<br>505 | —<br>— | UYEKI (1967) |
| Guinea pig[13] | Delayed hypersensitivity | 9/9[14] | 0/9 | — | 0/5 | — | — | — | BOREK (1968) |
| Mouse[15] | HPFC/spleen $\log_{10}$ fraction of control | 0 | —3.0 (C)<br>—4.0[16]<br>—4.0[17] | —2.3 (T) | —2.6 | —2.8 (F) | — | — | BERENBAUM and BROWN (1964) |
| Rat[18] | Burn<br>Pleurisy<br>CFA | 100<br>100<br>100 | 24 (C)<br>100 (C)<br>90 (C) | 28 (M)<br>100 (M)<br>47 (M) | 0<br>100<br>45 | —<br>—<br>— | —<br>—<br>— | 40[19]<br>100[19]<br>100[19] | STEVENS and WILLOUGHBY (1969) |
| Mouse[20] | Antigen retention in spleen | $2.4 \times 10^3$ | $1.9 \times 10^3$ (C) | — | — | — | — | $0.7 \times 10^3$ [9]<br>$1.5 \times 10^3$ [21]<br>$1.5 \times 10^3$ [22] | NETTESHEIM and HAMMONS (1970) |
| Mouse[23] | Relative immunosuppression | 0<br>+0.16[17] | +1.61 (C) | +0.11 (M) | +0.44 | +0.36 (A) | —1.01 | —0.05[9]<br>—0.05[21] | FLOERSHEIM (1970) |
| Rat[24] | Eosinophilia | 650 | 100 | — | 100 | — | — | 150 | BOYER et al. (1970) |
| Mouse[25] | GVH | 100 | 0 (C) | 93 (M) | 80 | — | — | 85[9] | OWENS and SANTOS (1971) |

[1] Drugs given at 1/6 $LD_{50}$ per day, daily on day 1—6, then on alternate days to day 14.

[2] Drugs given at various doses over wide range, data in Table is effect of 1/10 of $LD_{20}$. Drug given 2 days after antigen, titer determined 9 days after antigen.

[3] Animals given ovalbumin on day 1 and challenged 3 weeks later, drugs given day 1—10.

[4] Drug given day 1—5, antigen given day 4 and 5, titer measured on day 19.

[5] Drugs given daily × 5 starting 48 h after antigen (sheep RBC IP).

[6] Drugs given daily × 5 starting 4 h before antigen (sheep RBC IP).

[7] Drugs given daily × 7 starting 4 h after antigen (100 μg Vi SC) except HN2 given × 1.

[8] Survival in days of SKI grafts on C3H recipients, drugs given daily × 5 starting day of graft.

[9] Cortisone acetate.

[10] Drug given × 1 before or after antigen (sheep RBC) response measured 5 days after antigen.

[11] Drug 3 days after antigen.

[12] Drug 2 days before antigen.

[13] Drug given day 2—10 after antigen (synthetic amino acid co-polymer), skin test day 10.

[14] No positive/no tested.

[15] Drug given 2 days after antigen (sheep RBC) plaques measured 5 days after antigen.

[16] Analine mustard.

[17] Phenylalanine mustard.

[18] Drug given in 3 day course starting day of thermal burn, turpentine induced pleurisy or skin response to complete Freund's adjuvant (CFA) and measured as percent of control.

[19] Antilymphocyte serum.

[20] Drug given 3 days before $I^{125}$ HGG given IV and retention measured at CPM per spleen at 7 days after antigen.

[21] Actinomycin D.

[22] Irradiation.

[23] Relative effect on HPFC response and erythropoiesis when drug given daily × 4 starting day of antigen and functions measured day 5. Positive value indicates predominant immunosuppressive effect and negative value the opposite.

[24] Effect of single dose of drug on eosinophil count 7 days after challenge with trichinella larvae.

[25] Percent mortality from GVH in animals given drug on days 5, 8, 11, and 14 after cell transfer.

of the agent best suited for a particular immunosuppressive objective and also for the evaluation of potential new immunosuppressive agents.

Several investigators have outlined the principles which should be applied to such comparative studies in order to make them interpretable. AMIEL et al. (1964) suggested that comparative studies could only be done when a standard fraction of the $LD_{50}$, in standard courses, and resulting in a standard degree of toxicity, was used. SANTOS and OWENS (1964) and SANTOS et al. (1964) suggested that the effects of maximally tolerable doses of each drug should be compared using a standard antigen in a standard species. They also emphasize the fact that the relative timing of drug and antigen administration must be comparable. Thus, there is no point in comparing the effects of two drugs, both given after antigen, if one is immunosuppressive only when given before antigen. BERENBAUM and BROWN (1964) proposed that dose response curves for each drug in terms of both myelosuppressive and immunosuppressive properties and survival of treated animals must be determined before the immunosuppressive effects of one drug can be compared with those of another. MAKINODAN et al. (1965) pointed out that not only must these pharmacological considerations be taken into account, but also an optimal antigen dose and the most sensitive test to detect the immune response must be used before immunosuppressive effects or their absence can be confidently evaluated. However, one could argue from the opposite point of view, that a weak antigen and/or a system characterized by a weak immune response should be used. With such a system, minor or weak degrees of immunosuppression could be detected.

A sample of some of the more important comparative studies of chemical immunosuppression are outlined in Table 2. A criterion for the selection of these specific studies for inclusion in this review was that the doses and schedules of the several drugs used in a given study were comparable in terms of $LD_{10}$, myelosuppression, reduction in spleen size or splenic cell number, weight loss of the animal, or other important side effects. Most studies have been done in the mouse and rat, but SANTOS and OWENS (1964) have also studied the comparative pharmacology of immunosuppression in humans. In general, the most immunosuppressive agents available appear to be cyclophosphamide, methotrexate, and 6-mercaptopurine.

A particularly important and relevant approach to the comparative evaluation of different chemical immunosuppressants was recently presented by FLOERSHEIM (1970). The antibody response of mice was determined by measurement of the numbers of hemolytic plaque forming cells in the spleen, and the bone marrow proliferative activity was measured by the appearance of $Fe^{59}$ incorporating cells in the peripheral blood. These were studied simultaneously. An index which related the relative degrees of immunosuppression and myelosuppression to each other was established. In this system, in the mouse, cyclophosphamide was superior as a specific immunosuppressant (at doses which were not myelosuppressive) to radiation, methotrexate, cytosine arabinoside, 6-mercaptopurine, procarbazine, prednisolone, actinomycin D, and the vinca alkaloids. The vinca alkaloids, mitomycin C, actinomycin D, prednisolone, and chlorambucil had relatively more myelosuppressive than immunosuppressive effects. Cyclophosphamide, 6-mercaptopurine, methotrexate, cytosine arabinoside, and procarbazine had more immunosuppressive than myelosuppressive effects. These studies have also revealed that, depending upon its mechanism of action, a given agent is immunosuppressive either when given after antigen or before antigen, but not both. The one exception was cyclophosphamide which was an effective immunosuppressant when given either before or after the antigen.

This observation, that cyclophosphamide is the most potent chemical immunosuppressant, was first made in 1964 and has been repeatedly confirmed since that time. Cyclophosphamide has shown itself to be superior to the other agents in suppression of the antibody response of mice to TAB vaccine (BERENBAUM and BROWN, 1964), in suppression of the antibody response of mice to human serum albumin or polio virus (AMIEL et al., 1964), in suppression of the rejection of skin grafts (AMIEL et al., 1964; FLOERSHEIM, 1969), in suppression of the graft-versus-host disease in mice (OWENS and SANTOS, 1971), in reduction of the response of rats to sheep red blood cells (SANTOS and OWENS, 1964) and in suppression of the response of guinea pigs to foreign albumin (MAIBACH and MAGUIRE, 1966). It was as effective as any other agent in suppressing the response of man to the Vi antigen (SANTOS and OWENS, 1964).

These and other experimental results have recently led STARZL and his group to investigate the use of cyclophosphamide in the maintenance of renal homografts (STARZL et al., 1971). Using historical controls, this group has determined (in preliminary studies) that patients treated with cyclophosphamide have fewer and more easily controlled rejection episodes than subjects treated with azathioprine.

In summary, new immunosuppressive agents or regimens cannot be evaluated without relating the results to some standard. Antigens, test systems, and drug schedules should be used which take into account the mechanism of drug action and which can be compared to concurrent or previous results with the same system.

## A. Alkylating Agents

The alkylating agents are the most interesting and potentially the most important class of chemical immunosuppressive agents. Their effects on the immune response are varied, both quantitatively and qualitatively, depending upon the specific agent, its dose, and schedule. In general, the more potent alkylating agents are effective against both primary and secondary and both cell-mediated and humoral immune responses in a number of animal species, including mice, rats, rabbits, guinea pigs, and humans. Comparative studies (mentioned above) have indicated that one of the alkylating agents, cyclophosphamide, is the most potent immunosuppressive agent of any class currently available.

The alkylating agents were among the first classes of chemical substances evaluated for their immunosuppressive properties. Nitrogen mustard was one of the first specific agents studied and was found to be a relatively weak inhibitor of the immune response. It had to be used in doses near the toxic level or actually in the toxic range to be effective. Thus, HEKTOEN and CORPER (1921), in one of the initial demonstrations of the immunosuppressive effects of chemicals, showed that mustard gas, administered before or simultaneous with antigen, inhibited the formation of agglutinins and hemolysins to sheep red blood cells in rabbits. Interestingly, treatment after antigen exposure was not effective. This has been confirmed by several investigators. For instance, GREEN (1958) showed that nitrogen mustard inhibited the immune response of rabbits to *Salmonella typhi* H antigen, but only when given 24 to 48 h before antigen. PHILLIPS et al. (1947) and SPURR (1947) found that the effect of nitrogen mustard was to delay and lower the peak titer and that treatment with this drug at any dose could not completely abolish the immune response to antigen.

The alkylating agents, because of their action in cross-linking the DNA of both dividing and resting cells, particularly the latter, have been referred to as radiomimetic (ALEXANDER et al., 1957; WHEELER and ALEXANDER, 1964a, b). Their lympholytic properties are also similar to those of radiation (SCHREK, 1961;

STEFANI and SCHREK, 1964). Finally, nitrogen mustard is similar to radiation in that both types of treatment are capable of suppressing the immune response only when given prior to the administration of antigen. The immune response, once initiated, is relatively or completely resistant to the action of both radiation and mustard (GREEN, 1958). This suggests that both kill or damage nondividing (or slowly dividing) precursor or stem cells selectively.

This timing effect is variable, depending upon which alkylating agent is under study. Two of these agents, cyclophosphamide and phenylalanine mustard (Melphalan), are highly potent. They completely suppress several types of cell-mediated or humoral immune responses, when administered either before, simultaneously with, or after antigen injection (BROWN and BERENBAUM, 1964; FRISCH and DAVIES, 1965). On the other hand, agents such as uracil mustard, nitrogen mustard, mustard gas, and triethylene melamine are weak immunosuppressants and do not completely abolish the immune response. Uracil mustard is effective only when given after antigen, while nitrogen mustard, mustard gas, and triethylene melamine are mainly effective when given before antigen (BUSKIRK et al., 1965; HERSH and FREIREICH, 1968).

Because cyclophosphamide is the most potent immunosuppressive alkylating agent, and because it has been one of the most extensively studied of the immunosuppressive agents, the remainder of this discussion of alkylating agents will focus on its effects. Cyclophosphamide has been shown to be capable of completely suppressing the primary antibody response (BERENBAUM and BROWN, 1970), the secondary antibody response (FRISCH and DAVIES, 1965; FINGER et al., 1969), the development of new delayed hypersensitivity (TURK and STONE, 1963), the homograft response (AMIEL et al., 1964), the production of interferon (ROBINSON and HEATH, 1968), the antigen trapping mechanism in the lymph node (NETTESHEIM and HAMMONS, 1970), and the local inflammatory response (STEVENS and WILLOUGHBY, 1969). Thus, under the appropriate experimental circumstances of dose and schedule it has broad suppressive effects against host defense mechanisms. Of particular interest is the fact that cyclophosphamide can suppress an ongoing immunological reaction (FRISCH and DAVIES, 1965) and that it can induce tolerance which is both immunologically specific and permanent (AISENBERG and WILKES, 1967). Also, with the appropriate timing of drug and antigen, these specific effects can be achieved while the general host defenses are partially spared. These features will be discussed in detail below.

The schedule of administration of cyclophosphamide is of great interest in terms of its immunosuppressive properties. In several species, as mentioned above, it has been shown to be immunosuppressive whether administered before, simultaneous with, or after antigen administration (FRISCH and DAVIES, 1965). The most sensitive period runs from 72 h before to 48 h after antigen. Also, FRISCH and DAVIES (1965) showed that the primary immune response could be suppressed by drug administration starting up to 15 days after antigen administration. Subsequent to this time the antibody response became refractory. Since BRUCE et al. (1966) showed that the effects of cyclophosphamide in the mouse are mainly on proliferating cells, the following hypothesis has been proposed by several workers in the field (AISENBERG and WILKES, 1967; AISENBERG, 1967; AISENBERG and DAVIS, 1968). The immunosuppressive properties of cyclophosphamide administered before antigen probably result from the killing of slowly proliferating antigen-reactive precursor cells. Immunosuppression induced by cyclophosphamide given after antigen administration must be the result of effects on the rapidly proliferating specifically stimulated responding cells. After 15 days (at least in the mouse) proliferation again falls off and there develops a nondividing, resistant population of antibody producing plasma cells. At this point cyclophosphamide ceases to be effective.

The effects of cyclophosphamide on the proliferating lymphoid cells can be so marked that the entire responding clone of cells is killed. This has led to the development of a special approach to immunosuppression and tolerance induction based on the work of several investigators (SANTOS and OWENS, 1966; AISENBERG and WILKES, 1967; SANTOS and OWENS, 1968). The essentials of this approach are to immunize the animal or subject and to follow that immunization in approximately 24 h with a large, relatively short, one to 5 day course of drug. Tolerance often results. Twenty-four hours after the end of this course, another dose of the same antigen may be given. If this dose is large, it should reinforce the effect. Presumably, the cyclophosphamide given after antigen administration kills the rapidly proliferating, specifically responsive clone of cells. This approach has been used clinically by SANTOS and others to establish bone marrow allografts in man using courses of 40 mg/kg/day for 4 days (SANTOS et al., 1971).

Through several studies, a number of important features of cyclophosphamide-induced immunological tolerance have been established. First, tolerance can be induced by drug administered either before or after antigen. In one study, drug administration 72 h before antigen was most effective (SANTOS and OWENS, 1966); in another study, drug given 24 to 72 h after antigen was most effective (AISENBERG and WILKES, 1967), while in still another investigation the effective period was from 60 h before to 48 h after antigen (AISENBERG, 1967). These studies were in the same species, but with different antigens. Second, the larger the antigen dose the better (AISENBERG, 1967), particularly when the antigen is very foreign to the responding individual (e.g., sheep red blood cells to the mouse). It was hypothesized that a large dose of antigen permits some fraction of it to reach sequestered sites of antigen reactive cells, without the mediation of macrophages. This type of antigen (unprocessed) has been hypothesized to inactivate the antigen reactive precursor lymphoid cells (SANTOS and OWENS, 1968). Third, drug used as a tolerance-inducing agent and given prior to antigen has been observed to eliminate background hemolytic plaque-forming cells in the spleens of nonimmunized animals (AISENBERG and WILKES, 1967). This suggests that its major action in tolerance induction (in the schedule in which drug is given before antigen) is to eliminate the slowly proliferating antigen reactive precursor cells. Fourth, tolerance induction also depends upon antigen strength. Thus, a weak antigen (e.g., red cells of a closely related species) is tolerogenic in cyclophosphamide-treated animals, even at a relatively low dose (DIETRICH and DUKOR, 1968). It was hypothesized that the close relatedness of antigen to recipient allowed for delayed clearance and prolonged circulation of antigen and therefore permitted antigen to get to the sequestered sites (mentioned above) without being processed. Finally, the thymus seems necessary for the recovery from drug induced immunological tolerance, at least for certain antigens. Thus, in the mouse, tolerance induced to sheep red blood cells by cyclophosphamide reverses to a state of active immunity only in the presence of the thymus, and is permanent in thymectomized animals (AISENBERG and DAVIS, 1968).

Evidence that the immunosuppressive effects of cyclophosphamide are primarily the result of damage to proliferating cells is as follows. In nonthymectomized mice, tolerance is induced by cyclophosphamide but not by radiotherapy. In contrast, in previously thymectomized animals, tolerance cannot be induced by cyclophosphamide (AISENBERG and MURRAY, 1971). It is known that previous thymectomy also reduces the background proliferation of antigen reactive cells to zero in nonimmunized animals. It is also known that both x-ray therapy and cyclophosphamide therapy have nonspecific immunosuppressive properties. However, cyclophosphamide fails, while x-ray therapy succeeds, in bringing out the immunological defect in previously thymectomized animals when these therapies are given before antigen. This further supports the hypothesis. Finally, bone marrow cells administered after treatment, protect animals from radiotherapy but not from cyclophosphamide in terms of survival, and BRUCE et al. (1966) have shown that nondividing marrow stem cells are sensitive to x-ray therapy but insensitive to cyclophosphamide.

Several studies in a number of species have shown that cyclophosphamide is a potent inhibitor of the rejection of various types of grafts (AMIEL et al., 1964; SANTOS, 1966; FLOERSHEIM, 1969). Thus, it is surprising that more attention has not been paid to cyclophosphamide as a primary drug in the maintenance of renal allografts. In part, this has been due to the fact that one of the complications of cyclophosphamide treatment is hemorrhagic cystitis. Recently, STARZL et al. (1971), have studied a small group of kidney transplant patients in whom daily oral cyclophosphamide, prednisone, and ALG therapy were combined. Eleven had renal allografts and one had a hepatic allograft, and most of them were poor histocompatibility antigen (HLA) matches. Cyclophosphamide treatment impressed STARZL and his colleagues as being highly potent compared to their previous regimen of azathioprine, prednisone, and ALG. The majority of these patients had no postgraft rejection episodes (at least in the first 3 posttransplant months) and this was achieved at relatively nontoxic doses of drug. In addition, renal biopsies suggested that histological evidence of rejection was less severe in the cyclophosphamide-treated patients compared to their previously studied patients. A basis for this finding has been suggested by LEMMEL et al. (1971) who compared the hematological effects of the thiopurine, 6-mercaptopurine, with cyclophosphamide in NZB mice. Animals received equally toxic doses, daily for 5 to 8 weeks. 6-Mercaptopurine decreased the levels of circulating polymorphonuclear leukocytes, monocytes, and large lymphocytes. Counts of small and medium sized lymphocytes remained unchanged. In contrast, cyclophosphamide decreased the numbers of small and medium lymphocytes, leaving the other cell types unchanged. 6-Mercaptopurine produced a marked fall in hematocrit while cyclophosphamide did not. Finally, cyclophosphamide had some beneficial effects on the autoimmune disease process to which these mice are subject, while 6-mercaptopurine was inactive. These results suggested to the authors that 6-mercaptopurine exerted an antiproliferative action on the bone marrow as shown by a decrease of short lived cells, while cyclophosphamide had its main effects on circulating cells, resulting in depletion of long lived small lymphocytes. This led to an inhibition of autoantibody formation and immune complex deposition in the kidney. Cyclophosphamide would therefore appear to be preferable when suppression of ongoing cellular or humoral immune reactions is desired.

At this point, it would be useful to summarize the data concerning the effects of cyclophosphamide on various autoimmune states at the experimental and clinical level. Cyclophosphamide is highly potent in the suppression of the development of such experimental autoimmune diseases as thyroiditis (NAKAMURA and WEIGLE, 1970) and allergic encelphalomyelitis (PATERSON et al., 1967; PATERSON and HANSON, 1969). Even a single large dose of drug, given 24 to 48 h after the sensitizing antigen, can suppress the appearance of the autoimmune state for over 100 days. Of greater interest is the fact that several of these states can be reversed by drug after they are already firmly established. Thus, allergic encephalomyelitis in some strains of rats, can be reversed when drug treatment is started after the disease is established and after profound paralysis of the animal exists (PATERSON, 1971).

This is achieved by daily treatment with drug for approximately 10 days. Disease activity may remain suppressed for over 100 days. In animals with established thyroiditis, if repeated courses of thyroid antigen followed by doses of cyclophosphamide are given, circulating levels of thyroid antibody become markedly suppressed (NAKAMURA and WEIGLE, 1970). This suggests that the antigen doses induce immunological stimulation of the memory cells, which results in their entering the proliferative phase, at which time they are killed by the drug. In NZB mice, which have circulating levels of antibodies to DNA and RNA, if repeated courses of Poly-I, Poly-C followed by cyclophosphamide are given, the levels of circulating DNA antibodies fall markedly (STEINBERG and TALAL, 1970).

Of great interest is the observation that prophylactic therapy can stop the development of spontaneous autoimmune disease in NZB/NZW mice (RUSSELL and HICKS, 1968). Thus, 1.8 mg/kg/week of cyclophosphamide started at 150 days of life and continued for one year, reduces the incidence of autoimmune renal disease in these animals from 100% to approximately 7%.

These observations have been extended to man. Autoimmune, or autoimmune related diseases which can be ameliorated by cyclophosphamide therapy include the nephrotic syndrome (DRUMMOND et al., 1968), lipoid nephrosis (ETTELDORF et al., 1967), rheumatoid arthritis (MAINLAND and SUTCLIFFE, 1970), WEGENER'S granulomatosis (NOVACK and PEARSON, 1971) and peripheral uveitis (BUCKLEY and GILLS, 1969). The majority of patients shown to be responsive to cyclophosphamide, had previously been shown to be refractory to high doses of corticosteroids.

SANTOS' work with cyclophosphamide has brought to a culmination many of the earlier studies with this drug (SANTOS and OWENS, 1964; SANTOS et al., 1964). These authors initially showed that cyclophosphamide was immunosuppressive with respect to the primary immune response in animals and man. They subsequently showed that graft-versus-host disease could be induced by lymphocyte injection into cyclophosphamide-treated animals (OWENS and SANTOS, 1968). Of great importance was the fact that as the cyclophosphamide dose or transferred cell dose were increased independently, the resultant graft-versus-host disease was worsened. Finally, important studies were carried out in man in which it was shown that antigen given 24 h after a dose or course of cyclophosphamide failed to induce an immune response, whereas antigen one week after cyclophosphamide did induce such a response (SANTOS et al., 1970). Effective doses were 7 mg/kg/day for 7 days, 17 mg/kg for 3 days, or 25 mg/kg for 2 days.

These results have led to the design of the bone marrow transplant scheme used by SANTOS and others (GRAW et al., 1970; SANTOS et al., 1971). Patients are primed with a unit of whole blood from the potential donor and 24 h later a 4 day course of cyclophosphamide at 40 mg/kg is started. Twenty-four hours after the last dose, bone marrow is given, and in the majority of subjects, tolerance is induced and the graft takes. These studies depend upon the fact that (a) antigen rapidly localizes in the lymph nodes and induces proliferation of specific antigen reactive clones of cells and (b) the effects of a given dose of cyclophosphamide and circulating levels of active cyclophosphamide (or its active metabolite) are gone within 6 h after injection of the drug. The takes, even in HLA incompatible subjects are remarkable; however, graft-versus-host disease, even in HLA compatible donor-recipient pairs has been a severe problem. The utility of this approach is also limited by the myelosuppressive and cardiotoxic effects of these large doses of drug.

In summary, the potency and specificity of properly timed courses of cyclophosphamide make it likely that this agent will become more widely used not only as a tool to study the immune response but also as the agent of choice for clinical chemical immunosuppression of autoimmune disease and for the control of allograft rejection.

## B. Purinethiols and Purinethiol Nucleosides

Both historically and in terms of current clinical usage, the thiopurines are the most important class of immunosuppressive agents. The modern era of experimental and clinical chemical immunosuppression began in 1958 when Schwartz studied the immunosuppressive effects of 6-mercaptopurine on the antibody response of rabbits (Schwartz et al., 1958). Azathioprine, a member of the thiopurine class, is currently the most widely used chemical immunosuppressive drug, although it may eventually be replaced by cyclophosphamide. This is both for the treatment of autoimmune disease (Michael et al., 1967) and for the maintenance of organ homografts (Schwartz, 1968). In fact, for the latter, and in spite of the development and use of antilymphocyte serum, azathioprine remains the drug of choice. As will be outlined below, the characteristics of the cell-cycle-specific immunosuppressive agents (including the thiopurines, folic acid antagonists, vinca alkaloids, nucleoside analogs and certain alkylating agents) were worked out to a significant extent by Schwartz and others, through a study of the effects of 6-mercaptopurine on the immune response. The thiopurines which have received most attention include 6-mercaptopurine, azathioprine and thioguanine.

6-Mercaptopurine was shown to completely inhibit development of the primary antibody response after antigenic stimulation (Schwartz et al., 1958, 1959; Sterzl, 1960). 6-Mercaptopurine has been shown to be effective in rabbits (Schwartz et al., 1958, 1959), guinea pigs (Hoyer et al., 1962), and mice (Amiel et al., 1964; Berenbaum and Brown, 1964). The timing of the administration of 6-mercaptopurine is critical, and this feature was recognized during the initial studies. Maximum inhibition of the antibody response occurs when the drug is given during the early proliferative phase of the immune response, that is, during the first 48 h after the injection of the antigen. Schwartz et al. (1958, 1959) found that neither pretreatment with 6-mercaptopurine nor treatment after antibody had appeared, had a suppressive effect on the response. A typical potent immunosuppressive regimen was administration of maximally tolerated doses of drugs from immediately after antigen injection to approximately 7 days after antigen injection. Similar effects were shown for thioguanine in mice (Frisch and Davies, 1962; Frisch et al., 1962).

Proof that 6-mercaptopurine exerted its effects through an antiproliferative activity was given by André et al. (1962a, b). They studied the effects of 6-mercaptopurine on the histologic features of the lymph nodes draining sites of skin graft placement in rabbits. 6-Mercaptopurine not only prolonged skin graft survival, but completely prevented the development and proliferation of large pyroninophilic lymphoblastoid cells in the draining lymph nodes. If, after 7 to 14 days, histologic studies showed that the appearance and proliferation of these large lymphoblastoid cells had escaped the immunosuppressive effects, evidence of graft rejection subsequently appeared. Similar histologic and gross changes occurred if the drug was stopped.

Not only timing, but dose of drug also had an important influence on the degree of effectiveness of immunosuppression. Low doses of drug were ineffective. Doses just below the toxic range were effective and doses in the markedly toxic range were highly effective. For instance, Berenbaum and Brown (1964) found in mice that a single dose of 200 mg/kg was necessary to completely suppress the response to TAB vaccine and that this was approximately the $LD_{10}$ dose. Twice this dose, or 400 mg/kg, was the $LD_{80}$ dose. This illustrates an important principle which applies to most chemical immunosuppressive agents, namely that the dose response curve is steep.

These dose-response considerations also bear on the efficacy of 6-mercaptopurine in suppression of the secondary antibody response and its effectiveness in tolerance induction. BUTLER and COONS (1964) found that 6-mercaptopurine, although capable of suppressing the primary antibody response of mice, and of inhibiting the priming response for the secondary antibody response, was completely incapable of suppressing the secondary response itself, if given only during the induction phase of the latter. In contrast, several investigators found that in rabbits, the secondary antibody response to a number of protein antigens could be completely inhibited by a course of drug in the toxic dose range (SCHWARTZ et al., 1959). As in suppression of the primary response, the drug must be administered during the proliferative phase. Larger doses of 6-mercaptopurine, given in courses of one to two weeks, starting on the day of antigen administration, have also been shown to induce specific immunological tolerance (SCHWARTZ and DAMESHEK, 1959, 1963). Tolerance induction is augmented by increasing antigen dose. Thus, SCHWARTZ and DAMESHEK (1963) demonstrated that, in rabbits given protein antigens immediately before a course of 6-mercaptopurine, the antibody response was suppressed to any antigen dose, but only the highest antigen doses combined with chemotherapy resulted in tolerance. This observation has been confirmed, particularly in experiments where living and proliferating antigen is administered subsequent to the tolerance induction. It forms the basis for successful marrow transplantation in a number of species. The mechanism of tolerance induction is presumably the killing of the proliferating antigen reactive clone of cells by the administration of the drug during the proliferative phase. Another possibility is that the drug reduces the population of lymphoid cells, producing a state of relative immunological paralysis (SCHWARTZ and DAMESHEK, 1963).

The thiopurines have also been shown to be immunosuppressive in man. LEVIN et al. (1964) showed that a one month course of 6-mercaptopurine, administered to patients with solid tumors, at doses which produced only mild myelosuppression, could completely suppress the primary antibody response and the development of delayed hypersensitivity. Not only were the primary cell-mediated and humoral immune responses suppressed in these patients, but tolerance was apparently produced in some, since they did not respond to second doses of antigen. The antigens used were tularemia vaccine and the Vi antigen of *E. coli*. EPSTEIN and MAIBACH (1965) have also demonstrated in man, with plague vaccine as the antigen, that the primary and secondary antibody response can be suppressed by modest doses of azathioprine (100 mg/subject/day).

Although azathioprine is widely used in the maintenance of organ allografts and in the treatment of autoimmune disease, and although the immune responses of patients so treated are often suppressed during treatment, it is usually impossible to specifically evaluate the effects of chemical immunosuppression with thiopurines in those patients for a number of reasons. First, the patients may be uremic (MOYNIHAN and JACKSON, 1966). Second, their disease state may be associated with naturally occurring immunological deficiency (LEVENTHAL et al., 1967). Third, these patients often receive combined therapy with other immunosuppressive agents such as corticosteroids and/or antilymphocyte serum. Therefore, the effects of one agent cannot be identified precisely.

6-Mercaptopurine and the other thiopurines also have major effects on cell mediated as well as humoral immunity. Some studies in man (LEVIN et al., 1964) and in rabbits (ANDRÉ et al., 1962a, b) have already been described. The effects of 6-mercaptopurine on delayed hypersensitivity in guinea pigs have been studied (HOYER et al., 1962). Fifty mg/kg/day starting on the day of Bacillus Calmette-Guerin (BCG) administration completely suppressed development of delayed hypersensitivity in approximately 50 to 75% of animals. Half that dose suppresses delayed hypersensitivity in only 20% of animals, approximately the same percentage as normally do not develop delayed hypersensitivity after a single BCG inoculation. After cessation of therapy, most animals eventually did develop delayed hypersensitivity.

Recent studies have indicated some surprising features of this suppression of delayed hypersensitivity. The results suggest that the apparent specific immunological effect may be due to the effects of 6-mercaptopurine on the nonspecific inflammatory response. Thus, ZWEIMAN and PHILLIPS (1970), have investigated the effects of treatment with maximally tolerated doses of 6-mercaptopurine on the development of immunity to tuberculin in guinea pigs. In their initial study, these authors found that the effect of the drug after BCG inoculation was to completely suppress the development of delayed hypersensitivity tested *in vivo*. However, *in vitro*, the lymphocytes of the treated animal were able to undergo a normal blastogenic response to tuberculin. Furthermore, these lymphocytes could transfer tuberculin sensitivity to other animals. This suggested that a nonlymphoid feature of delayed hypersensitivity was being affected. Macrophage exudation was a good candidate. They subsequently showed that the nonspecific inflammatory response was inhibited in these animals by 6-mercaptopurine treatment (PHILLIPS and ZWEIMAN, 1970).

These recent findings are not entirely surprising, since the potent anti-inflammatory effects of 6-mercaptopurine have been documented by others. The administration of 6-mercaptopurine to rabbits (PAGE et al., 1962) and to man (HERSH et al., 1966) inhibits the mononuclear phase of the inflammatory response.

Other agents, including methotrexate, cyclophosphamide, chlorambucil, and actinomycin D, also suppress the mononuclear phase of the inflammatory response (HERSH and FREIREICH, 1968). Once the drug is stopped, the inflammatory response returns to normal within a few days (HERSH et al., 1966). This inhibition of the nonspecific inflammatory response has been shown to be due to a change in the circulating leukocyte population. 6-Mercaptopurine treatment markedly reduces the production and release of mononuclear phagocytic cells from the marrow (HURD and ZIFF, 1968). This rapidly turning over population releases monocytes into the peripheral blood, which enter inflammatory sites and become macrophages (VOLKMAN and GOWANS, 1965a, b; VOLKMAN, 1966). This population is selectively suppressed by 6-mercaptopurine therapy. It is the depletion of this population from the blood which results in the loss of the inflammatory response during 6-mercaptopurine treatment. Since monocyte and macrophage exudation are an important component of specific delayed hypersensitivity, it is not surprising that this nonspecific effect can manifest itself in depression of this specific immunological phenomenon. It has also been hypothesized that suppression of the inflammatory response is also responsible for the prolongation of graft survival by 6-mercaptopurine (PAGE et al., 1962).

The thiopurines have also been shown to suppress organ and tissue graft survival in a number of animal systems. This includes graft survival in the rabbit (ANDRÉ et al., 1962a, b), rat (TINBERGER, 1968; VAN BEKKUM, 1969), and mouse (MEEKER et al., 1960; POWELL et al., 1962) to mention just a few. Certain aspects of treatment to prolong allograft survival are important. Large doses of drugs are certainly more effective than small doses. In addition, weak antigenic differences are more easily suppressed than strong antigen differences (McQuarrie et al., 1965; Harrison and Bartlett, 1970). Thus, in partially inbred animals, skin graft survival in mice was prolonged an average of 60 to 70 days across a weak histocompatability barrier compared to only 30 to 40 days across a strong barrier. In some of the treated animals, grafted across a weak barrier, graft survival over 120 days was occasionally observed. In addition, across the weak barrier, the effective dose was as low as 2 mg/kg compared to 12 mg/kg in outbred animals.

A number of other thiopurines are even more effective than 6-mercaptopurine or azathioprine in skin graft protection, in mice. Kimball et al. (1965) compared the effects of 6-mercaptopurine, $\alpha$-thioguanine deoxyribonucleoside and arabinosyl-6-mercaptopurine on skin graft survival. 6-Mercaptopurine prolonged graft survival only 4 days over the control, while the latter two drugs prolonged skin graft survival 10 and 11 days, respectively, at completely nontoxic doses.

Treatment with 6-mercaptopurine can also modulate the immune response in several ways. Thus, if small doses of 6-mercaptopurine are given from day 0 to day 7 after antigen administration, the IgG antibody response may be selectively prevented from developing (Borel et al., 1965; Sahir and Schwartz, 1966). In contrast, the IgM, or first antibody response, may be only slightly delayed, may then appear, may reach even supranormal levels, and may be prolonged compared to the duration of the IgM response in untreated animals. This modulation is presumably due to the fact that the switchover from IgM to IgG production is prevented, and since IgG never appears, the normal feed-back suppression of IgM by IgG is blocked.

Therapy with 6-mercaptopurine can actually augment the immune response. Thus, if a dose of antigen is given approximately one week following the end of a one week course of 6-mercaptopurine, the subsequent antibody response may be two or three times that of the untreated animal (Chanmougan and Schwartz, 1966). It was originally hypothesized by these authors, who discovered this phenomenon, that the release of nucleic acid breakdown products, from cells damaged by the thiopurine treatment, served as an adjuvant to the subsequent immune response. More recent data concerning the proliferation and competence of lymphoid cells following chemotherapy, suggests that this phenomenon might have been due to rebound and overshoot in the numbers of precursor cells capable of responding to antigen (Cheema and Hersh, 1971). Further research on this phenomenon is needed to accurately determine its etiology.

No discussion of immunosuppression with thiopurines is complete without some mention of the effects of thiopurines on autoimmune disease. Schwartz and Dameshek (1962) were the first to use thiopurine therapy in the treatment of an autoimmune phenomenon. They observed that 6-mercaptopurine therapy was effective in the control of autoimmune hemolytic anemia. Subsequently, most investigators have used azathioprine, given on a daily oral schedule, in doses of 100 to 200 mg/day. Patients with Crohn's disease (Brooke et al., 1969, 1970), patients with autoimmune erythroid aplasia (Safdar et al., 1970), and patients with pemphigus vulgaris (Burton et al., 1970) have all shown dramatic responses to azathioprine therapy. Immunological renal disease including lupus nephritis (Maher and Schreiner, 1970) and the nephrotic syndrome of childhood (Abramowicz et al., 1970) have shown variable positive responses to azathioprine therapy. Subacute and chronic glomerular nephritis have also responded to azathioprine treatment (Bardana et al., 1970). Some workers report significant clinical benefit, while others report treatment failure. The efficacy of treatment relates, at least in part, to the dose and duration with which the drug is used, with aggressive therapy being most effective. Other disease states that have shown some response to azathioprine treatment include Wegener's granulomatosis (CHOY et al., 1969), steroid refractory idiopathic thrombocytopenic purpura (SUSSMAN, 1967), and several others, including allergic vasculitis, Goodpasture's syndrome, systemic lupus erythematosus, and lupoid hepatitis (CORLEY et al., 1966).

Therapy of autoimmune diseases with azathioprine or any other immunosuppressive agent must be done with caution and only in disease states known to be refractory to conventional therapy. This is because these agents are myelosuppressive and increase the susceptibility of the patients to infection. Most important, however, is the recent disturbing finding that patients on chronic immunosuppressive therapy with azathioprine and prednisone have a markedly increased incidence of malignant disease (STARZL et al., 1970). These patients tend to get malignant lymphomata and cutaneous or mucocutaneous malignancies; many other types of malignancy have also been described. The incidence of malignancy may be as high as 5% in patients who have been treated from between one to 5 years with chemical immunosuppressive agents. Therefore, the use of these agents in nonlife threatening autoimmune states must be limited to patients with disease severe enough to justify this risk.

In summary, the thiopurines are a group of highly active chemical immunosuppressive agents which have been widely studied and which have been used to characterize the various components of chemical immunosuppression. They are the most widely used chemical immunosuppressive agents today and are effective in the treatment of autoimmune disease and in the maintenance of organ homografts. Until more specific immunosuppressive therapy is available, which will not require the use of general antiproliferative agents, the thiopurines will probably remain a mainstay of this type of treatment.

## C. Folic Acid Antagonists

Folic acid antagonists including aminopterin and amethopterin (methotrexate) have been extensively investigated for their immunosuppressive properties (HITCHINGS and ELION, 1963; GABRIELSON and GOOD, 1967; HERSH and FREIREICH, 1968). Most studies have been done with methotrexate, and the findings for both antagonists are essentially the same.

As might be expected from its known antiproliferative effects, methotrexate has potent immunosuppressive properties. In general, methotrexate therapy can suppress the primary antibody response (UYEKI, 1967), the secondary antibody response (BRANDRISS et al., 1965), the development of delayed hypersensitivity (BOREK, 1968), the homograft reaction (BERENBAUM, 1963), the graft-versus-host response (UPHOFF, 1961; SCHWARTZ and BELDOTTI, 1965), experimental autoimmune disease (BRANDRISS, 1963), experimental inflammation (HERSH et al., 1966), and the activity of the reticuloendothelial system (MEGIRIAN and LEONARDI, 1966) in a variety of animal species.

In terms of its ability to suppress the primary antibody response, methotrexate is approximately as potent as some of the other immunosuppressants such as cyclophosphamide and 6-mercaptopurine (AMIEL et al., 1964; SANTOS and OWENS, 1964; BERENBAUM and BROWN, 1964; FLOERSHEIM, 1970). In comparison with the other immunosuppressive chemotherapeutic agents, the activity of methotrexate is somewhat variable, depending upon the species and test system. Thus, it is one of the most potent suppressors of the development of new delayed hypersensitivity (BOREK, 1968) and a potent suppressor of the antibody response (UYEKI, 1967). However, it is less effective as a suppressoı of the homograft reaction (GLYNN et al., 1963) except in the case of graft-versus-host disease (BRANDRISS, 1965; BOREK,

1968). In man, a one week course of methotrexate, at maximally tolerable doses, completely inhibits the primary antibody response (as does an equally toxic course of 6-mercaptopurine or cyclophosphamide (SANTOS et al., 1964).

In comparative studies, relative efficacy has also been shown to depend upon the timing of administration. Thus, when administered to rats to suppress the primary antibody response to sheep red blood cells, a course of methotrexate was more potent than cyclophosphamide if the drugs were started 48 h after antigen, but cyclophosphamide was more potent than methotrexate when the drugs were started 4 h after antigen (SANTOS and OWENS, 1964). This is presumably due to the fact that methotrexate is almost entirely a cell-cycle specific agent and as such would have its major effect at the height of the proliferative phase of the immune response.

A unique feature of methotrexate activity is its special ability to suppress the development of delayed hypersensitivity. At least in the guinea pig, and probably in several other species, methotrexate and cyclophosphamide are the most potent drugs in this regard (BOREK, 1968). A completely nontoxic course of methotrexate will completely suppress the development of this response. This may be due in part to the agent's anti-inflammatory, as well as its immunosuppressive effects (HERSH et al., 1966). Methotrexate therapy and adoptive transfer have been used to study the mechanism of this suppression of delayed hypersensitivity (FRIEDMAN and BUCKLER, 1963; FRIEDMAN, 1964). Methotrexate blocked proliferation of a population of sensitive cells which could express delayed hypersensitivity in the periphery, but did not prevent the development of sensitivity. Thus, methotrexate treated recipients of sensitized cells showed suppression of delayed hypersensitivity, but, methotrexate treatment of the donor so that he could not express delayed hypersensitivity did not prevent his cells from transferring this immunological reactivity to an untreated animal. The mechanism of action was also studied by TURK and STONE (1963) using histological methods. They showed that methotrexate, in doses which suppressed the development of detectable delayed hypersensitivity, did not block the development of large pyroninophilic cells in the lymph nodes after primary immunization. Therefore, the mechanism of action of methotrexate was to block the proliferation and production of antigen reactive small lymphocytes from these pyroninophilic cells. In contrast, cyclophosphamide induced inhibition of delayed hypersensitivity occurred at the step prior to the development of these large pyroninophilic cells and none appeared in the lymph nodes of the suppressed animals.

For effective immunosuppression with an antiproliferative drug like methotrexate, the timing of its administration is critical. If a dose or course of methotrexate precedes antigen administration, and no drug is given after antigen, the immune response is either unaffected or is actually augmented (UYEKI, 1967). In contrast, if a course of methotrexate is started at the time of, or a day or two after, antigen administration and continued through the time of the major proliferation in the responding lymphoid tissue, the immune response is at least partially and often completely suppressed. However, tolerance induction is rare, probably because toxicity supervenes before an adequate dose of drug is given.

A particularly interesting feature of the use of methotrexate as an immunosuppressant, is the reversibility of the drug effect with its specific antagonist folinic acid (citrovorum factor). If immunosuppressive doses of methotrexate are followed within 24 h by appropriate doses of this antagonist, the toxic side effects of methotrexate are inhibited, while the immunosuppressive properties proceed in an almost unaltered fashion (BERENBAUM, 1964b; BERENBAUM and BROWN, 1965).

If the specific antagonist is administered too soon after the antimetabolite, both immunosuppressive and myelosuppressive effects are abrogated.

In contrast to the major effects of methotrexate on delayed hypersensitivity, homograft reaction is only weakly inhibited by this agent. This may be due to its relatively narrow therapeutic ratio, and the intervention of toxic effects prior to an adequate course. For example, only modest prolongation of skin homograft survival is achieved in the mouse, even in the toxic range (Glynn et al., 1963). Gabrielson and Good (1967), in their review of chemical immunosuppression, point out that the mouse may not be the ideal species in which to study the effects of methotrexate. However, even in other species, suppression of homograft reactivity to skin, lung, bone marrow, and heart homografts is mainly achieved in the toxic range (Gabrielson and Good, 1967). With antigen overloading at the time of grafting, the immunosuppressive potency of methotrexate can be augmented (Medawar, 1963).

In contrast to the above, methotrexate has potent suppressive effects on the graft-versus-host reaction. In mice, the graft-versus-host reaction produced by injection of parental lymphoid cells into neonatal $F_1$ hybrids is vigorously suppressed by methotrexate treatment (Uphoff, 1958). In adult mice (Lochte et al., 1962) and dogs (Thomas et al., 1962), methotrexate also suppresses this reactivity. In animals which are successfully suppressed, surviving members of the treated group are chimeras (Thomas et al., 1962).

Methotrexate is also a potent inhibitor of experimental autoimmune disease. Both allergic encephalomyelitis (Brandriss, 1963) and thyroiditis (Spiegelberg and Miescher, 1963) are inhibited by treatment with the drug. Suppression is achieved even after the disease activity has become established, and even gross symptomatic disease activity can be reversed by daily treatment.

Related observations have been made in man. Methotrexate is particularly useful in the treatment of advanced refractory polymyositis (Malaviya et al., 1968; Sokoloff et al., 1971) and advanced refractory peripheral uveitis (Wong and Hersh, 1965). Patients who were either paralyzed or blind have had relatively normal function restored by weekly or bi-weekly administration of the drug in minimally myelosuppressive doses (20 mg/M$^2$ twice weekly). While comparative studies have not been done, this effect is certainly more complete and more rapid in onset than that observed during the treatment of other autoimmune diseases with such drugs as cyclophosphamide or azathioprine. Treatment may be limited by gastrointestinal and hematological toxicity and by the fact that use of the drug in the face of poor renal function is contraindicated.

The mechanism responsible for these effects is unknown. Their rapid onset (9 to 14 days) and their lack of effect on established delayed hypersensitivity and antibody levels suggests anti-inflammatory rather than immunosuppressive effects. Indeed, Wong and Hersh (1965) have found that therapeutic benefit was associated with suppression of the mononuclear phase of the inflammatory response.

A final role for methotrexate has been in the investigation of experimental infection. The data suggest that, with reservations, its use be considered in human infections where the pathogenesis is related to an immunological reaction. An early observation was the conversion of attenuated to virulent disease. Thus, methotrexate treatment in the dog converts distemper vaccination into a fatal infection (Thomas et al., 1963). If methotrexate treatment is given to the guinea pig, concurrent with inoculation of tubercle bacilli, local control is abrogated and disseminated virulent disease results (Pritchard and Hayes, 1961). In contrast, if methotrexate treatment is given to guinea pigs who are immune, but who are undergoing necrotizing cutaneous lesions after local inoculation of tubercle bacilli, the violent local reaction (delayed hypersensitivity) is abolished and the lesions heal (PRITCHARD and HAYES, 1961). Similarly, lymphocytic chorio-meningitis (a progressive fatal viral disease in the mouse, the pathogenesis of which has been demonstrated to be due to the lymphocytic immune response to the viral infection) can be controlled by methotrexate therapy (LEVY and HAAS, 1958). Methotrexate facilitates the viremia, but abolishes the lymphocytic response and, therefore, completely does away with the neurological signs and symptoms. Of course, all of the above may be due to anti-inflammatory rather than specific immunosuppressive effects. Regardless, the use of methotrexate in immunological inflammatory reactions in man, even those associated with infectious agents, should be considered seriously.

## D. Cytosine Arabinoside and Related Nucleoside Analogs

The nucleoside analog and specific inhibitor of DNA synthesis, cytosine arabinoside, has potent immunosuppressive properties in several species including the mouse (GRAY et al., 1968), rat (GRAY and MICKELSON, 1970a), hamster (FISCHER and GERSHON, 1966), rabbit (KAPLAN et al., 1966), and human (MITCHELL et al., 1969). In a variety of rodent species, the primary antibody response to sheep red blood cells, measured by the formation of hemolysins or hemagglutinins or the development of hemolytic plaque-forming cells in the spleen, was suppressed by relatively nontoxic doses of drug. The hemolytic plaque-forming cell response 4 days after antigen injection was completely abolished, but the antibody response between 6 and 12 days after antigen injection was only partially suppressed (HARRIS and HERSH, 1968). This differential was related to the fact that cytosine arabinoside is an inhibitor of DNA synthesis and the major effect of cytosine arabinoside was to delay the proliferation of the antibody forming cells. The proliferation of both IgM and IgG forming cells was inhibited. Once the drug effect ceases, the inhibited proliferative activity resumes and antibody is produced. The secondary antibody response could also be suppressed by appropriately timed doses of drug (GRAY et al., 1968a).

Under special circumstances, more profound and long lasting suppression of the immune response has been achieved. In the mouse, if drug was administered daily, from days 1 to 11 after antigen administration, the primary response was completely abolished and did not reappear after therapy was stopped (GRAY et al., 1968a). Tolerance was not induced. In the rat, when higher doses of drug and repeated doses of antigen were given, specific immunological tolerance to sheep red blood cells could be induced (GORDON et al., 1969).

Cytosine arabinoside does not prolong skin allograft survival in mice and rats, nor does it suppress renal allograft survival in the dog (ALEXANDER et al., 1969; GRAY et al., 1969a). In contrast, it does suppress the development of graft-versus-host (GVH) disease in the mouse (GRAY et al., 1968b). These effects are all moderate, and permanent graft survival or permanent suppression of GVH is not achieved. Comparative studies generally indicate that cytosine arabinoside is a weak immunosuppressant.

In humans, schedules of cytosine arabinoside, similar to those which are optimal for the treatment for malignancy, partially suppressed the primary and secondary antibody response and the development of delayed hypersensitivity (MITCHELL et al., 1969). The continuous 5 day infusion of approximately 100 mg/$M^2$/day is one of the most effective regimens (VALLEJOS et al., in preparation).

The immunosuppressive properties of cytosine arabinoside could be inhibited by the concurrent administration of deoxycytidine (FISCHER et al., 1966). Thus, the daily administration of 40 mg/kg of cytosine arabinoside given alone for 7 days reduced the index of response from the control value of 1.0 to 0.10, while the concurrent administration of 89 mg/kg of deoxycytidine restored this response to an index of 0.68. These data suggest that, in a fashion similar to methotrexate followed by folinic acid, the sequential administration of daily doses of cytosine arabinoside and deoxycytidine might protect the subject from the myelosuppressive effects of the drug while maintaining its immunosuppressive activity. This point has not yet been explored.

Because cytosine arabinoside is an inhibitor of DNA synthesis, and since the proliferative phase of the immune response to primary immunization is precisely timed, the timing of cytosine arabinoside administration determines whether a given dose and schedule of administration will be immunosuppressive. This has been studied in detail in the mouse. Single doses or one day courses of drug (given every 8 h) inhibited the antibody response and graft-versus-host disease when given 48 to 72 h after antigen (Gray et al., 1968b; Harris and Hersh, 1968). This has been confirmed by an *in vitro* study of the primary response to sheep red blood cells by mouse spleen fragments (Holtermann and Nordin, 1969). Drug, when present in the incubation mixture from 0 to 12 h after antigen exposure, had no effect on the *in vitro* antibody response. If drug exposure was continued from 9 to 18 h, there was a 40% reduction in the number of antibody forming cells. If continued for 24 h after antigen exposure, there was a 70% reduction in the number of antibody forming cells, and if continued for 48 h, there was complete suppression of the *in vitro* antibody response. Thus, the drug is ineffective if given before the proliferative phase begins.

The immunosuppressive effects of various other pyrimidine nucleoside analogues were compared by Fischer et al. (1966). Cytosine arabinoside was found to be more potent in suppressing the immune response of mice to sheep erythrocytes than 5-fluorodeoxyuridine or 5-bromodeoxyuridine. 5-Iododeoxyuridine was essentially inactive. 6-Azauridine was also a relatively weak immunosuppressant.

The immunosuppressive properties of cytosine arabinoside are generally limited by the short half-life of the drug. Recently, certain esterified derivatives, which are slowly hydrolyzed to release cytosine arabinoside, have been shown to possess significantly greater immunosuppressive activity than the native compound. This has been studied extensively by Gray et al. (1972). The stearate, palmitate, 4-methoxybenzoate, and adamantoyl derivatives are the most active. Single daily doses of these drugs can maintain therapeutic blood levels for at least 24 h after each dose, due to the slow release of the active compound. Moderate nontoxic doses of these derivatives can completely suppress the hemagglutinin response of mice and hamsters to sheep red blood cells, at doses at which cytosine arabinoside itself produces only a 10% reduction of the response. The immunosuppressive properties of these derivatives, relative to cytosine arabinoside, are identical to their anti-leukemic properties against L1210 leukemia relative to cytosine arabinoside. Equimolar courses of the derivatives prolong skin allograft survival in rats remarkably well. Skin graft survival among the controls was 14 days; among animals treated with cytosine arabinoside, 16 days; among animals treated with the adamantoyl derivative, 23 days; while among animals treated with the palmitate derivative it was 34 days. These data suggest that the palmitate derivative should be explored in all of the currently available experimental transplant systems, and subsequently its use in man should be carefully considered.

The adamantoyl derivative also has several unique properties (Gray et al., 1969; Greig and Gibbons, 1969; Gray and Mickelson, 1970b). While it suppresses skin graft survival in rats and mice, and the development of allergic encephalomyelitis in mice, it has a more variable effect on the antibody response. In the rat, it suppresses the antibody response to bovine serum albumin (BSA) but does not suppress the response to sheep red blood cells or flagellen. These effects are similar to those seen in neonatally thymectomized animals. Thymic atrophy with spleen sparing has been noted in histologic studies of rats treated with this drug. The investigators hypothesize that since deoxycytidine kinase, the enzyme which activates cytosine arabinoside, is present in greatest activity in the thymus and marrow, this particular drug has a selective action on the thymus-dependent, bone marrow-derived lymphocytes (GRAY, 1972).

In summary, while the parent compound cytosine arabinoside has limited immunosuppressive effects, mainly because of its short half-life, the newer esters of the drug offer promise as potent immunosuppressants.

## E. Vinca Alkaloids

The Vinca alkaloids have potent antitumor activity in a variety of human and animal neoplasms, including the ability to induce complete remission when used alone. Surprisingly they are weak immunosuppressants. This is in spite of the fact that their major tissue specificity, in terms of antitumor activity, is against lymphoid neoplasms. For example, in man, vincristine can rapidly induce complete remission in acute lymphocytic leukemia, but has not been demonstrated to have any immunosuppressive activity (SANTOS et al., 1964). In part, this may be related to the schedule of administration (single injections once or twice weekly). These would be associated with only transient blood levels of the drug. In contrast, in animal systems in which immunosuppressive properties have been demonstrated, effective schedules usually involve daily administration of the drug during the proliferative phase of the immune response (AISENBERG and WILKES, 1964).

There is also a major species difference in the immunosuppressive properties of the Vinca alkaloids. Potent immunosuppressive effects have been observed in the rat (SANTOS and OWENS, 1964), while only weak immunosuppressive effects have been reported in the mouse (AMIEL et al., 1964). No clinical utility of the Vinca alkaloids as immunosuppressive drugs for use in man has been observed.

The weak immunosuppressive activity of the Vinca alkaloids has been observed in several studies. BERENBAUM and BROWN (1964) observed that complete or near complete suppression of the antibody response of mice to TAB vaccine was achieved only at approximately the $LD_{90}$ dose, when drug was given as a single dose during the proliferative phase. MAIBACH and MAGUIRE (1963) observed that the development of anaphylactic antibodies in the guinea pig after ovalbumin injection was blocked by cyclophosphamide but not vinblastine. (FLOERSHEIM (1970) observed that on a relative basis, the immunosuppressive activity of the Vinca alkaloids in the mouse was less than their myelosuppressive activity. They had only 1/10 to 1/100 of the immunosuppressive activity of a potent drug such as cyclophosphamide. However, very large doses of drug in the mouse (3 mg/kg/day for 3 days, administered during the proliferative phase) were able to reduce the hemolytic plaque forming cell response to sheep red blood cells by about 75%. There was no effect on the circulating antibody titer.

Potent activity has been observed in the mouse, in one system, which may or may not be related directly to immunosuppression. NORTH (1970) studied the effect of a single dose of 100 μg of vinblastine on the resistance of mice to *Listeria monocytogenes* infection. When this pulse was given during the first 24 h after experimental infection, the development of resistance was blocked. Specifically, the migration of macrophages into infected foci was inhibited. He did not determine whether this was due to a hematopoietic effect or whether it was due to an inhibition of the immune response and of the subsequent specific immunological inflammatory reaction.

The most extensive studies of the immunosuppressive properties of the Vinca alkaloids have been done in the rat by AISENBERG and WILKES (1964). They observed progressively more potent immunosuppression as the dose of the Vinca alkaloids was raised to 0.2 mg/kg/day (the $LD_{10}$ dose). The primary antibody response and the development of delayed hypersensitivity to BSA were both completely inhibited by this dose of either vincristine or vinblastine. The homograft response was also markedly suppressed by this dose and skin graft survival of up to 30 days was observed in approximately 10% of the animals, compared to 6 days in the control. Of great interest was the fact that both early ongoing antibody production and early but established delayed hypersensitivity could be turned off by treatment started as late as 3 to 5 days after antigen administration. These observations were partially confirmed by SANTOS and OWENS (1964) who found that the rat's immune response to sheep red blood cells was partially blocked by vinblastine. The induction time of the antibody response was prolonged from approximately 6 days in the control to approximately 18 days in the treated animals. This was a modest effect since it was prolonged 32 days with cyclophosphamide and 42 days with methotrexate. There was no effect of this therapy on the mean peak titer.

The timing of administration of the drug was also critical (SANTOS and OWENS, 1964). The effects of vinblastine therapy were seen only when a single dose of drug was administered 48 h after antigen. There was no effect if the drug was administered before antigen or if it was administered only 4 h after the antigen.

In summary, the Vinca alkaloids are moderately immunosuppressive in the rat, provided that they are given in toxic doses during the proliferative phase. They do not appear to be very immunosuppressive in the mouse or guinea pig, and have not been demonstrated to be immunosuppressive in man. In the latter situation, the schedule of administration for therapy in man is such that weak immunosuppressive properties may not have been revealed.

## F. Actinomycin D and other Antibiotics

While many antibiotics have been tested for their immunosuppressive properties, only a few have been shown to have significant immunosuppressive effects. Antibiotics of particular interest include puromycin, mitomycin C, the actinomycins, chloramphenicol, and azaserine. While all of these have been shown to have immunosuppressive properties, either *in vivo* or *in vitro*, only the actinomycins warrant extensive comment. The others are either so weak or so toxic in their immunosuppressive range *in vivo* that they are of little interest.

*In vivo*, the actinomycins are weak immunosuppressive agents. Thus, NATHAN et al. (1950), STERZL (1961), BUTLER and COONS (1964), and WITTE et al. (1966) found that there was only slight or no suppression of the antibody responses of mice or rabbits with toxic doses of these drugs. In most of these systems, the serum antibody responses to bacterial or erythrocyte antigens were studied. In contrast, JERNE et al. (1963) observed that single doses of actinomycin, given one day after sheep red blood cells, suppressed the hemolytic plaque-forming cell response in the mouse spleen. It is likely, however, that if they had studied the peripheral antibody response, it would have shown only slight suppression. Some authors have reported striking suppressive effects of actinomycin D treatment *in vivo*. Thus SPEIRS (1965) found that if toxic doses of actinomycin D were given weekly with tetanus toxoid to mice, complete inhibition of the antibody response for at least 3 weeks was observed. Tolerance was not induced. The most critical study of the use of actinomycin for *in vivo* immunosuppression was that of FLOERSHEIM (1970), who compared its immunosuppressive and myelosuppressive properties. It fell into the class of drugs that he characterized as having potent myelosuppressive and relatively weak immunosuppressive effects.

In addition to suppression of the antibody response, KOLIN and LANDI (1970) found that actinomycin D could reduce the intensity of cell-mediated immune reactions. Thus, if administered to guinea pigs just prior to delayed hypersensitivity skin testing, the intensity of the delayed reaction could be reduced approximately 75%. This could have been a nonspecific effect. Thus, using *in vitro* methods, DAVID (1965) showed that actinomycin D could inhibit the synthesis and release of migration inhibitory factor, a mediator of delayed hypersensitivity known to be important *in vivo*. In contrast, PAGE (1964), studying the nonspecific local inflammatory response in rabbits, found that the administration of actinomycin D immediately following the inflammatory injury completely inhibited the mononuclear cell phase of the response. This suggests that the inhibition of the delayed hypersensitivity may be in part due to the effect on mononuclear infiltration and in part to the effects on the immunologically specific components of the response.

One or both of these effects may be the basis for the supposed effectiveness of the actinomycins on organ allograft rejection. Although it has now ceased to be used to any extent, actinomycin C was once commonly used to reverse acute rejection crises (MURRAY et al., 1963). However, its effectiveness was never documented in a controlled experiment.

In spite of the fact that actinomycin is not really useful for *in vivo* immunosuppression, it has been used extensively for the study of the immune response *in vitro*. This is a consequence of the fact that the biochemical mechanism of action of actinomycin D has been precisely described and it is known to inhibit specifically DNA-dependent RNA synthesis and, therefore, the early phases of protein synthesis. For this reason, *in vitro*, where myelosuppressive toxicity is not a consideration, it can be used to explore the cellular events of the immune response. A relatively large series of studies has been done which can be summarized as follows. The drug can suppress both the primary and the secondary antibody response to a variety of antigens (UHR, 1963; SVEHAG, 1964). Concentrations in the range of 1 mg/ml are effective. When cells in the midst of an ongoing antibody response are exposed to drugs in culture, it is ineffective for the first 24 h. Subsequently, its effect increases progressively. This has suggested that the life span of the messenger RNA for antibody synthesis is approximately 24 h (LAZDA and STARR, 1965). In contrast, when actinomycin D is added to cells after primary or secondary antigenic stimulation, it has profound effects when given during the first 5 h and has progressively diminishing effects when administered after that time period (HERSCOWITZ et al., 1971). This suggested that early developmental cell types were most sensitive to the antiproliferative activity of the antibiotic and that as the cells matured into functional types, they became less sensitive to the antibiotic.

In summary, actinomycin D is not particularly useful for immunosuppression *in vivo* since it does not have potent immunosuppressive properties. However, because its specific mechanism of biochemical action is known, it can be useful *in vitro* in the exploration of specific stages of the immune response.

## G. Immunosuppressive Enzymes

A completely new area has developed in the field of chemical immunosuppression during the last 4 years. This is a result of the discovery that the enzyme

L-asparaginase has immunosuppressive properties. This is important, first because of the potential for combining therapy with this nonmyelosuppressive agent and full doses of myelosuppressive drugs such as azathioprine and, second, it indicates the necessity for reinvestigation of the amino acid requirements of the immune response and for an investigation of the effects of specific amino acid depletion on immunity.

Kidd (1953) observed that guinea pig serum caused regression of lymphomas in animal systems. After the observation that this activity was due to L-asparaginase (Broome, 1968), this enzyme was prepared, and used successfully in the treatment of animal and human lymphoid malignancies (Adamson and Fabro, 1968; Whitecar et al., 1970). At approximately this time, investigations *in vitro* showed that L-asparaginase blocked the blastogenic response of peripheral blood lymphocytes to both nonspecific mitogens and specific mitogenic antigens (Ohno and Hersh, 1970a). Subsequently, *in vivo* immunosuppressive properties were demonstrated.

L-Asparaginase is indeed a potent suppressor of lymphocyte blastogenic response *in vitro*. Doses as low as 1 I.U./ml completely suppressed the response to phytohemagglutinin, Streptolysin-O and also the allogeneic mixed leukocyte culture (Ohno and Hersh, 1970a). This activity was shown to be specific since it was reversed by L-asparagine. In addition, the enzyme was completely noncytotoxic and the blastogenic response recovered if the enzyme was washed from the cultures.

L-Asparaginase also suppresses the primary antibody response *in vivo*. In the mouse, a single dose of 1000 I.U., or a 5 day course of 10 to 100 I.U. per day suppressed the formation of hemolytic plaque-forming cells after immunization with sheep red blood cells (Ohno et al., 1970). This effect could also be reversed by L-asparagine (Chakrabarty and Friedman, 1970), the major effect of the drug being to delay the antibody response. Although peripheral blood titers were completely suppressed 4 to 7 days after antigen administration, they recovered between 7 and 20 days whether or not drug administration was continued. This effect can be explained through an understanding of the mechanism of action of the enzyme. By degrading peripheral blood L-asparagine, a deficiency of this amino acid is produced and those tissues lacking asparagine synthetase undergo complete suppression of proliferation (Miller et al., 1970). In contrast, those tissues with adequate asparagine synthetase levels are unaffected. In the normal mouse, lymphoid tissue (spleen) is completely lacking in the latter enzyme (Prager and Bachynsky, 1968). However, asparagine deficiency rapidly induces asparagine synthetase in the spleen and once it has been induced, recovery of immune responses occurs (Horowitz et al., 1968).

L-Asparaginase treatment also suppresses the human immune response. Twenty-five to 100000 I.U./M²/day inhibited the primary antibody response to high molecular weight protein and synthetic amino acid copolymer antigens (Ohno and Hersh, 1970b). The immunosuppression was dose-dependent and was most profound in those patients who received a longer course. Both antibody production and the development of delayed hypersensitivity were inhibited. Lymphocytes from the peripheral blood of treated patients failed to respond to mitogens *in vitro*, unless first washed and cultured in the absence of patients' serum.

Of great interest to the transplantation immunologist is the fact that L-asparaginase also suppresses cell-mediated immunity. The development of delayed hypersensitivity to protein antigens in the rabbit (Kahn and Hill, 1970), allergic encephalomyelitis in the rat (Kahn et al., 1970), graft-versus-host disease in the mouse (HOBIK, 1969), tumor allograft survival in the mouse (BRAMBILLA et al., 1970) and skin graft survival in several rodent species (BERTELLI et al., 1968; ETHEREDGE et al., 1971), were either suppressed or prolonged by L-asparaginase treatment. This suppression or prolongation was achieved without major toxicity, except for weight loss. Recent reports of prolonged organ allograft survival induced by L-asparaginase treatment also have appeared. RAPAPORT et al. (1971) used L-asparaginase alone at 150 to 200 I.U./kg/day for 9 to 21 days and prolonged renal allograft survival in mongrel dogs. There was a 30% increase in graft survival time. In another study, LEVIN and MERRILL (1971) transplanted kidneys from Lewis-Brown Norway $F_1$ rats into bilaterally nephrectomized Lewis rats. The treated animals received 1000 I.U./kg/day of L-asparaginase for 7, 14, or 21 days. The 7 day course of treatment prolonged graft survival, but all animals eventually experienced rejection. In contrast, half or more of the animals treated for 14 to 21 days had indefinite survival of functional grafts. Again, the major toxicity was weight loss. These findings, along with the lack of myelosuppressive activity of the enzyme, suggests that it should be seriously considered as adjunctive therapy for the maintenance of renal homografts in man or for attempts at graft tolerance induction during the immediate post-transplant period.

An interesting aspect of the toxicity of L-asparaginase is the development of immunity and clinical allergy to the enzyme. This has been studied fairly extensively in man. Prior to treatment, no individuals are allergic or have antibody or positive skin tests. However, after one course of treatment, positive skin reactivity is observed. In one study, wheal and flare reactivity and delayed hypersensitivity were noted in 40% of the patients (OETTGEN et al., 1970). Circulating precipitating antibody was also detected in the blood. Clinical evidence of allergy has included urticaria, abdominal cramps, dyspnea, facial edema, anaphylactic shock, and serum sickness.

The development of immunity to an agent which itself is immunosuppressive is of great interest. Since the material is a bacterial protein, it of course would be immunogenic in man. Since none of these patients were studied with respect to the kinetics of the development of immunity relative to their blood levels of the enzyme, it is possible that immunity developed only after immunosuppressive levels of the enzyme disappeared.

Another enzyme with the potential for potent immunosuppressive activity is L-glutaminase. This material has only been studied *in vitro*. It has been found to have potent effects on the *in vitro* lymphocyte blastogenic response to mitogen such as phytohemagglutinin, Streptolysin-O and the mixed leukocyte culture (HERSH, 1971). The inhibition is complete at doses as low as 0.5 I.U./ml, but is completely reversible if the enzyme is washed from the cultures up to 72 h. The *in vitro* immunosuppressive activity of L-glutaminase is entirely specific. Thus, doses of 0.5 I.U./ml are completely reversed by 20 μmol L-glutamine. When high specific activity neutral L-glutaminase becomes available, it is hoped that this material will also be shown to be immunosuppressive *in vivo*.

The findings reviewed in this section are important for several reasons. They indicate that the specific requirements of a tissue for so-called nonessential nutrients can be exploited to advantage in both antitumor and immunosuppressive therapy. They also indicate the need to intensively investigate the nutritional requirements of individual normal and neoplastic tissues from the point of view of their content of synthetic enzymes (e.g. asparagine synthetase). Finally, these studies of L-asparaginase and L-glutaminase indicate the need for further work on synthetic amino acid analogs as antitumor and immunosuppressive agents.

### H. Miscellaneous Agents

In addition to the immunosuppressive agents described in the above section, there are many other drugs which fall into the previously described classes which are immunosuppressive, and which are either accepted cancer chemotherapeutic agents or are antineoplastic agents under development. There are many other purine, pyrimidine, folic acid, and nucleoside antagonists, as well as other alkylating agents which have immunosuppressive properties. However, since the behaviors of these drugs follows the principles described in the preceding sections, they will not be discussed in detail in this section. Rather, drugs which have interesting immunosuppressive properties, but which cannot be classified under any of the categories mentioned above, will be described.

One of the most potent immunosuppressive agents in this category is the antitumor agent procarbazine. This drug is a likely candidate for an immunosuppressant in man, since its main antitumor activity is against the lymphoid malignancy, Hodgkin's disease. Several reports have appeared recently concerning its effectiveness against organ or skin xenograft survival from hamsters to mice resulting in an increase of from 4.5 days in untreated animals to 12.5 days in procarbazine-treated animals (Cerilli et al., 1970). Floersheim (1966, 1967) reported that procarbazine can prolong the survival of skin allograft across a strong histocompatibility barrier in mice and even induce tolerance in adult mice if allogeneic lymphocyte cells are injected as well. Stewart and Cohen (1969) have recently reported that as an immunosuppressant, procarbazine was as potent as antiserum to lymphocytes in mice. Both agents significantly prolonged survival of skin allografts by 4 to 6 weeks. Procarbazine can also suppress the development and expression of inflammatory or autoimmune states such as allergic encephalomyelitis (Georgi et al., 1963), and Floersheim (1964) showed that it can suppress the expression of established delayed hypersensitivity in guinea pigs. This drug was one of the few which could suppress both the erythema and the induration associated with this response.

In addition, procarbazine can produce potent suppression of the antibody response. It appears to be active in suppressing the antibody response either when given before (day 21 to day 2) or after (day 1 to day 7) the antigen (Stewart and Cohen, 1969). Therefore, its effects are somewhat related to those of cyclophosphamide, to other alkylating agents, and even to radiation.

Only one report of the use of this drug in human inflammatory conditions has been reported. Witte et al. (1966) found that it had activity in man against autoimmune hemolytic anemia and lupus erythematosus.

These findings suggest that procarbazine is a potent agent which may have its major effects against circulating thymus-derived lymphocytes. As such, its use in autoimmune states, inflammatory states, and in transplantation immunology should be considered. However, the agent is a potent carcinogen in animal systems, and this finding may limit its use in patients who do not have malignant disease (Kelley et al., 1964). Another potential limitation is species variation, since the drug does not prolong skin graft survival in the dog (MacDonald et al., 1971).

Another new immunosuppressive agent of great interest is the antiserotonin agent Cinanserin. This apparently has no bone marrow toxicity and has been evaluated both *in vitro* against lymphocyte function and *in vivo* by the same group against the homograft reaction in mice. *In vitro*, Cinanserin at a concentration of $7 \times 10^{-5}$ M inhibits phytohemagglutinin-stimulated protein and DNA synthesis by greater than 60% (Schwartz et al., 1969). A concentration of $1 \times 10^{-4}$ M is more than 90% inhibitory. At equal molar concentrations, this material was more active than azathioprine. It was only effective when added initially and was not active when added late. These findings prompted an investigation of the effects of Cinanserin alone or in combination with azathioprine *in vivo* in the mouse (AMBINDER et al., 1969). Cinanserin suppressed antibody formation to sheep red blood cells and has the significant effect of prolonging mouse skin homografts across the strong histocompatibility barrier. First set skin graft rejection time was increased from 9 to 11.3 days compared to 11.1 days by azathioprine alone and to 12.0 days by the combination of azathioprine and Cinanserin. Since this material is nonmyelosuppressive, its use in the prolongation of organ allograft survival should be considered.

Another agent of interest is amantadine hydrochloride. This material, an antiviral agent marketed for the prevention of infection by influenza virus, was found to inhibit human lymphocytes stimulated with phytohemagglutinin (RAWLS et al., 1967). The concentration which effectively inhibited the response to phytohemagglutinin was similar to that which maximally inhibited virus replication. The drug inhibited the mitogenic response without affecting the ability of phytohemagglutinin to agglutinate leukocytes. The authors concluded that phytohemagglutinin, amantadine and certain lipid containing RNA viruses take part in cell membrane interactions of a common nature. This finding may be related to the observation of MATHÉ et al. (1971) that amantadine blocks the immunotherapeutic effects of BCG inoculation in patients undergoing active immunotherapy for acute leukemia.

A number of tranquilizing agents are immunosuppressive, both *in vivo* and *in vitro*. The mechanism of their action is not known. However, it is thought that they exert their action, at least in part, by membrane effects. Some examples of these immunosuppressive effects are as follows. In rabbits, pretreatment with propiomazine reduced the antibody response of rabbits approximately 50% when given for 5 to 8 weeks before immunization (HENSON and BRUNSON, 1969). Chlorpromazine and other phenothiazines are also known to inhibit *in vitro* lymphocyte transformation (KAMADA et al., 1971) and to inhibit the development of antibody producing cells *in vitro*. Thus, these agents should be used with caution in patients undergoing chemical immunosuppressive treatment or receiving immunosuppressive cancer chemotherapy because of the danger of additive immunosuppressive effects. The thalidomide drugs have also been described to be immunosuppressive (HELLMAN, 1966). This has been most clearly documented for the graft-versus-host disease in the chicken embryo (FIELD et al., 1966) but also for the splenomegaly induced in the hybrid rats following the injection of parenteral strain spleen cells (FIELD et al., 1966).

Thus, many miscellaneous chemical agents used for a variety of medical purposes have immunosuppressive properties which are both unexpected and surprising. Therefore, in patients undergoing chemical immunosuppression or immunosuppressive anticancer treatment, any other agent should be used with extreme caution. An effort should be made to evaluate the immunosuppressive properties of drugs of many classes not usually thought to be immunosuppressive.

## Conclusions

The subject of chemical immunosuppression is important today because of (a) the widespread use of chemotherapeutic agents in the treatment of cancer and (b) the use of immunosuppressive cancer chemotherapeutic agents in the maintenance of organ homografts and the treatment of autoimmune and inflammatory diseases in man. An understanding of chemical immunosuppression must be based on an understanding of the nature of the normal human immune response, particularly its cellular basis, and on an understanding of the patterns of circulation of small lymphocytes on which the mechanism of immunological surveillance is based.

Multiple cell types and multiple stages of metabolic activity are involved and therefore drugs with specific mechanisms of action will have different effects on the quality and quantity of the immune response. In general, drugs can be classified according to whether they affect the stage of antigen uptake and processing, interaction of macrophages with antigen-reactive cells, lymphoblastoid transformation and proliferation, antibody production, or the stages of immune reactant-antigen interaction in the periphery.

Immunosuppressive chemotherapeutic agents can also be classified according to the drug type; each class, including alkylating agents, purine antagonists, pyrimidine antagonists, folic acid antagonists, plant alkaloids and enzymes, has its unique action on immunological mechanisms.

The properly timed administration of the appropriate immunosuppressive antitumor agent can (a) inhibit the primary and secondary immune responses of both humoral and cell-mediated types, (b) suppress established immunological reactivity, (c) induce immunological tolerance, or (d) modulate the immune response so that one component is inhibited while another component is augmented. If antigen administration follows certain types of chemotherapy, the immune response to that antigen may actually be moderately enhanced.

There are classes of immunosuppressive agents other than the well known cancer chemotherapeutic agents, and these may play a role in both the clinical transplantation and the cancer field in the future. They include heterologous antilymphocyte serum, specific immunosuppressive antibody, specific and nonspecific mitotic inhibitors, and specific antigen.

Because immunocompetence is impaired in patients with certain types of neoplastic disease and becomes progressively more impaired in all patients with advanced metastatic disease, there is an extremely important interaction between the immunosuppressive properties of chemotherapeutic agents, the disease associated immunosuppression, and the effects of the chemotherapy on the size of the tumor. The specific nature of this interaction determines whether a patient will have immunosuppression and/or a tumor response as a result of a specific course or series of courses of chemotherapy. Since cell-mediated immunity is responsible for effective tumor immunity, regimens of chemotherapy which preserve this type of responsiveness are to be sought by the cancer chemotherapist. The intensive intermittent chemotherapy used today partially fulfills this objective.

## References

Abramowicz, M., Barnett, H. L., Edelmann, C. M., Jr., Greifer, I., Kobayashi, O., Arneil, G. C., Barron, B. A., Gordillo, P. G., Hallman, N., Tiddens, H. A.: Controlled trial of azathioprine in children with nephrotic syndrome. Lancet I, 959—961 (1970).

Adamson, R. H., Fabro, S.: Antitumor activity and other biologic properties of L-asparaginase. A Review. Cancer Chemother. Rep. 52, 617—626 (1968).

Aisenberg, A. C.: Drugs employed for the suppression of immunologic responsiveness. New Engl. J. Med. 272, 1114—1117 (1965).

Aisenberg, A. C.: Studies on cyclophosphamide-induced tolerance to sheep erythrocytes. J. exp. Med. 125, 833—845 (1967).

Aisenberg, A. C., Davis, C.: The thymus and recovery from cyclophosphamide-induced tolerance to sheep erythrocytes. J. exp. Med. 128, 35—46 (1968).

Aisenberg, A. C., Murray, C.: The contrasting effects of cyclophosphamide and radiation on the immune responses of the mouse. J. exp. Med. 133, 877—884 (1971).

Aisenberg, A. C., Wilkes, B.: Studies on the suppression of immune responses by the periwinkle alkaloids. J. clin. Invest. 43, 2394—2403 (1964).

AISENBERG, A. C., WILKES, B.: Immunological tolerance induced by cyclophosphamide assayed by plaque spleen cell method. Nature (Lond.) **213**, 498—499 (1967).

ALEXANDER, P., COUSENS, S. F., STACEY, K. A.: The reactions of the mutagenic alkylating agents with proteins and nucleic acids. In: WOLSTENHOLME, G. E. W., O'CONNOR, C. (Eds.): Drug resistance in microorganisms, pp. 294—322. Boston: Little, Brown and Co. 1957.

ALEXANDER, J. L., HALL, T. C., DIETHELM, A. G., MURRAY, J. E.: The effects of cytosine arabinoside on canine renal allografts. Transplantation **7**, 210—215 (1969).

ALLISON, A. C., LAW, L. W.: Effects of antilymphocyte serum on virus oncogenesis. Proc. Soc. exp. Biol. (N. Y.) **127**, 207—212 (1968).

AMBINDER, E. P., SCHWARTZ, G. H., RUBIN, A. L., STENZEL, K. H.: Prolongation of survival of skin homografts in mice with Cinanserin alone and in combination with azathioprine. Transplantation **7**, 127—129 (1969).

AMIEL, J. L., MATHÉ, G., MATSUKURA, M., MERY, A. M., DAGUET, G., TENENBAUM, R., GARATTINI, S., BREZIN, C., PALMA, V.: Tests for the determination of the effect of antimitotic products on immune reactions. Immunology **7**, 511—526 (1964).

ANDRE, J. A., SCHWARTZ, R. S., MITUS, W. J., DAMESHEK, W.: The morphologic responses of the lymphoid system to homografts. I. First and second set responses in normal rabbits. Blood **19**, 313—333 (1962a).

ANDRE, J. A., SCHWARTZ, R. S., MITUS, W. J., DAMESHEK, W.: The morphologic responses of the lymphoid system to homografts. II. The effects of antimetabolites. Blood **19**, 334—348 (1962b).

BARDANA, E. J., JR., PORTER, G. A., PIROFSKY, B., GOURLEY, R. T., BAYRAKCI, C.: Azathioprine in steroid-insensitive nephropathy. Amer. J. Med. **49**, 789—800 (1970).

BAUER, D. C., MATHIES, M. J., STAVITSKY, A. B.: Sequence of synthesis of gamma$_1$-macroglobulin and gamma$_2$-globulin antibodies during primary and secondary responses to proteins, salmonella antigens and phage. J. exp. Med. **117**, 889—907 (1963).

BERENBAUM, M. C.: Prolongation of homograft survival in guinea pigs treated with amethopterin. Nature (Lond.) **198**, 606—607 (1963).

BERENBAUM, M. C.: Effects of carcinogens on immune processes. Brit. med. Bull. **20**, 159—164 (1964a).

BERENBAUM, M. C.: Prolongation of homograft survival by methotrexate with protection against toxicity by folinic acid. Lancet II, 1363—1365 (1964b).

BERENBAUM, M. C., BROWN, I. N.: Dose-response relationships for agents inhibiting the immune response. Immunology **7**, 65—71 (1964).

BERENBAUM, M. C., BROWN, I. N.: The effect of delayed administration of folinic acid on immunological inhibition by methotrexate. Immunology **8**, 251—259 (1965).

BERTELLI, A., DONATI, L., TRABUCCHI, E., JR.: Prolonged survival of allo- and xeno-grafts of skin by means of an antitumoral compound. The L-asparaginase. Arch. Ital. Patol. clin. Tumori. **11**, 457—469 (1968).

BODEY, G. P., BUCKLEY, M., SATHE, Y. S., FREIREICH, E. J.: Quantitative relationships between circulating leukocytes and infection in patients with acute leukemia. Ann. intern. Med. **64**, 328—340 (1966).

BOREK, F.: Specific suppression of immune response to a synthetic antigen capable of evoking exclusively delayed-type sensitivity in guinea pigs. Int. Arch. Allergy. **34**, 479—487 (1968).

BOREL, Y., FAUCONNET, M., MIESCHER, P. A.: Effect of 6-mercaptopurine (6-MP) on different classes of antibody. J. exp. Med. **122**, 263—275 (1965).

BOYER, M. H., BASTEN, A., BEESON, P. B.: Mechanisms of eosinophilia. Part III. Suppression of eosinophilia by agents known to modify immune responses. Blood **36**, 458—469 (1970).

BRAMBILLA, G., PARODI, S., CAVANNA, M., CARACENI, C. E., BALDINI, L.: The immunodepressive activity of *Escherichia coli* L-asparaginase in some transplantation systems. Cancer Res. **30**, 2665—2670 (1970).

BRANDRISS, M. W.: Methotrexate: suppression of experimental allergic encephalomyelitis. Science **140**, 186—187 (1963).

BRANDRISS, M. W., SMITH, J. W., WELSH, P.: Suppression of immune response by methotrexate; *in vivo* and *in vitro* studies. Fed. Proc. **24**, 377 (1965).

BROOKE, B. N., HOFFMANN, D. C., SWARBRICK, E. T.: Azathioprine for CROHN's disease. Lancet **II**, 612—614 (1969).

BROOKE, B. N., JAVETT, S. L., DAVISON, O. W.: Further experience with azathioprine for CROHN's disease. Lancet **II**, 1050—1053 (1970).

BROOME, J. D.: L-Asparaginase: the evolution of a new tumor inhibitory agent. Trans. N. Y. Acad. Sci. **30**, 690—704 (1968).

BROWN, I. N., BERENBAUM, M. C.: Inhibition of immune processes by Melphalan. Nature (Lond.) **201**, 1340 (1964).

Bruce, W. R., Meeker, B. E., Valeriote, F. A.: Comparison of the sensitivity of normal hematopoietic and transplanted lymphoma colony-forming cells to chemotherapeutic agents administered *in vivo*. J. nat. Cancer Inst. **37**, 233—245 (1966).
Buckley, C. E., III., Gills, J. P., Jr.: Cyclophosphamide therapy of peripheral uveitis. Arch. intern. Med. **124**, 29—34 (1969).
Burnet, F. M.: The concept of immunological surveillance. In: Schwartz, R. S. (Ed.): Progress in experimental tumor research, Vol. B, pp. 1—27. Basel: S. Karger 1970.
Burton, J. L., Greaves, M. W., Marks, J., Dawber, R. P. R.: Azathioprine in pemphigus vulgaris. Brit. med. J. **3**, 84—86 (1970).
Buskirk, H. H., Crim, J. A., Petering, H. G., Merritt, K., Johnson, A. G.: Effect of uracil mustard and several antitumor drugs on the primary antibody response in rats and mice. J. nat. Cancer Inst. **34**, 747—758 (1965).
Butler, W. T., Coons, A. H.: Studies on antibody production. XII. Inhibition of priming by drugs. J. exp. Med. **120**, 1051—1060 (1964).
Bystryn, J. C., Graf, M. W., Uhr, J. W.: Regulation of antibody formation by serum antibody. II. Removal of specific antibody by means of exchange transfusion. J. exp. Med. **132**, 1279—1287 (1970).
Cerilli, J., Gideon, L., Hattan, D.: Effect of immunosuppression and cellular antigen on xenograft survival. Transpl. Proc. **2**, 516—521 (1970).
Chakrabarty, A. K., Friedman, H.: L-Asparaginase-induced immunosuppression: effects on antibody-forming cells and serum titers. Science **167**, 869—870 (1970).
Chanmougan, D., Schwartz, R. S.: Enhancement of antibody synthesis by 6-mercaptopurine. J. exp. Med. **124**, 363—378 (1966).
Cheema, A. R., Hersh, E. M.: Patient survival after chemotherapy and its relationship to *in vitro* lymphocyte blastogenesis. Cancer **28**, 851—855 (1971).
Choy, D. S. J., Gould, W. J., Gearhart, R. P., Sauer, J.: Remission in Wegener's granulomatosis treated with steroids and azathioprine. N. Y. State J. Med. **69**, 1205—1209 (1969).
Cohen, S. S.: Introduction to the biochemistry of D-arabinosyl nucleosides. Molec. Biol. **5**, 1—88 (1966).
Cooper, M. D., Gabrielsen, A. E., Good, R. A.: The development of the immune system in the chicken. In: Smith, R. T., Miescher, P., Good, R. A., (Eds.): Phylogeny of immunity, pp. 243—252. Gainesville, Fl.: University of Florida Press 1967.
Cooper, M. D., Peterson, R. D. A., Good, R. A.: Delineation of the thymic and bursal lymphoid system in the chicken. Nature (Lond.) **205**, 143—146 (1965).
Corley, C. C., Jr., Lessner, H. E., Larsen, W. E.: Azathioprine therapy of "autoimmune" diseases. Amer. J. Med. **41**, 404—412 (1966).
Dammin, G. J.: The pathology of human renal transplantation. In: Rapaport, F. T., Dausset, J. (Eds.): Human transplantation, pp. 170—200. New York: Grune and Stratton 1968.
David, J. R.: Suppression of delayed hypersensitivity *in vitro* by inhibitors of protein synthesis. J. exp. Med. **122**, 1125—1134 (1965).
Dietrich, F. M., Dukor, P.: The immune response to heterologous red cells in mice. IV. Induction of unresponsiveness to weakly immunogenic red cells by cyclophosphamide and cortisone acetate. Clin. exp. Immunol. **3**, 783—793 (1968).
Drummond, K. N., Hillman, D. A., Marchessault, J. H. V., Feldman, W.: Cyclophosphamide in the nephrotic syndrome of childhood: its use in two groups of patients defined by clinical, light microscopic and immunopathologic findings. Canad. med. Ass. J. **98**, 524—531 (1968).
Dumonde, D. C., Wolstencroft, R. A., Panayi, G. S., Matthew, M., Morley, J., Howson, W. T.: "Lymphokines": non-antibody mediators of cellular immunity generated by lymphocyte activation. Nature (Lond.) **224**, 38—42 (1969).
Epstein, W. L., Maibach, H. I.: Immunologic competence of patients with psoriasis receiving cytotoxic drug therapy. Arch. Derm. **91**, 599—606 (1965).
Etheredge, E. E., Shons, A., Harris, N., Najarian, J. S.: Prolongation of skin xenograft survival by L-asparaginase. Transplantation **11**, 353—354 (1971).
Etteldorf, J. N., Roy, S., III., Summit, R. L., Sweeney, M. J., Wall, H. P., Berton, W. M.: cyclophosphamide in the treatment of idiopathic lipoid nephrosis. J. Pediat. **70**, 758—766 (1967).
Field, E. O., Gibbs, J. E., Tucker, D. F., Hellmann, K.: Effect of thalidomide on the graft versus host reaction. Nature (Lond.) **211**, 1308—1310 (1966).
Finger, H., Emmerling, P., Bruss, E.: The influence of cyclophosphamide on the process of priming for the secondary response. Experientia (Basel) **25**, 1183—1184 (1969).
Fischer, D. S., Gershon, R. K.: Immune response and immunosuppression in the hamster. Clin. Res. **14**, 331 (1966).
Fischer, D. S., Cassidy, E. P., Welch, A. D.: Immunosuppression by pyrimidine nucleoside analogs. Biochem. Pharmacol. **15**, 1013—1022 (1966).

FISHMAN, M., ADLER, F. L.: The role of macrophage RNA in the immune response. Cold Spr. Harb. Symp. Quant. Biol. 32, 343 (1967).
FLOERSHEIM, G. L.: Screening auf antirheumatica am modele der tuberkulin reaktion. Helv. physiol. pharmacol. Acta 22, 92—109 (1964).
FLOERSHEIM, G. L.: Effect of methylhydrazine derivatives on the survival of second-set skin homografts. Nature (Lond.) 211, 638—639 (1966).
FLOERSHEIM, G. L.: Drug-induced tolerance for skin homografts across the H-2 barrier in adult mice. Science 156, 951—954 (1967).
FLOERSHEIM, G. L.: A study of combined treatment with chemical immunosuppressants and antilymphocytic serum to prolong skin allograft survival. Transplantation 8, 392—402 (1969).
FLOERSHEIM, G. L.: A comparative study of the effects of antitumour and immunosuppressive drugs on antibody-forming and erythropoietic cells. Clin. exp. Immunol. 6, 861—870 (1970).
FREIREICH, E.J., HENDERSON, E.S., KARON, M.R., FREI, E., III.: The treatment of acute leukemia considered with respect to cell population kinetics. In: The Proliferation and Spread of Neoplastic Cells, pp. 441—452. (A Collection of Papers Presented at the Twenty-First Annual Symposium on Fundamental Cancer Research, 1967, at the University of Texas M. D. Anderson Hospital and Tumor Institute at Houston, Houston, Texas.) Baltimore: Williams and Wilkins Co. 1968.
FRIEDMAN, R.M., BUCKLER, C.E.: Methotrexate inhibition of tuberculin hypersensitivity in inbred guinea pigs. J. Immunol. 91, 846—850 (1963).
FRIEDMAN, R.M.: Role of interferon in viral interference. Nature (Lond.) 201, 848—849 (1964).
FRISCH, A.W., DAVIES, G.H.: The inhibition of hemagglutinin formation in mice by purine and pyrimidine analogues. J. Immunol. 88, 269—273 (1962).
FRISCH, A.W., DAVIES, G.H.: Inhibition of hemagglutinin synthesis by cytoxan. Cancer Res. 25, 745—751 (1965).
FRISCH, A.W., DAVIES, G.H., MILSTEIN, V.: The inhibition of hemagglutinin formation in mice by thioguanine. J. Immunol. 89, 300—305 (1962).
GABRIELSON, A.E., GOOD, R.A.: Chemical suppression of adaptive immunity. In: DIXON, F.J., HUMPHREY, J.H. (Eds.): Advances in immunology, Vol. 6, pp. 92—230. New York: Academic Press 1967.
GEORGI, F., HONEGGER, C.G., REIDER, H.P., WUTHRICH, R.: Beeinflussung der experimentellen allergischen Encephalomyelitis durch ein Cytostaticum der Methylhydrazinreike. Helv. physiol. pharmacol. Acta 21, 381—393 (1963).
GLYNN, J.P., BIANCO, A.R., GOLDIN, A.: Effect of "Methotrexate" and "Melphalan" on the survival of tumour and skin homografts. Nature (Lond.) 198, 1003—1004 (1963).
GORDON, R.O., WADE, M.E., MITCHELL, M.S.: The production of tolerance to human erythrocytes in the rat with cytosine arabinoside or cyclophosphamide. J. Immunol. 103, 233—243 (1969).
GOWANS, J.L., MCGREGOR, D.D.: The immunological activities of lymphocytes. In: Progress in allergy, Vol. 9, pp. 1—78. Basel: S. Karger 1965.
GOWANS, J.L.: The recirculation of lymphocytes from blood to lymph in the rat. J. Physiol. 164, 54—69 (1969).
GRAW, R.G., JR., ROGENTINE, G.N., JR., LEVENTHAL, B.G., HALTERMAN, R.H., BERARD, C., HERZIG, G.P., YANKEE, R.A., WHANG-PENG, J., KRUGER, G., HENDERSON, E.S.: Graft-versus-host reaction complicating HL-A matched bone-marrow transplantation. Lancet II, 1053—1055 (1970).
GRAY, G.D.: Lymphocyte phosphorylation of cytarabine: an organ and species survey. Biochem. Pharmacol. 21, 2227—2236 (1972).
GRAY, G.D., CRIM, J.A., MICKELSON, M.M.: The immunosuppressive activity of ara-cytidine. II. Effects on the graft-versus-host reaction. Transplantation 6, 818—825 (1968b).
GRAY, G.D., MICKELSON, M.M.: The immunosuppressive effects of adamantoyl cytarabine. II. Effects on skin allograft rejection by rats and mice. Transplantation 9, 177—179 (1970a).
GRAY, G.D., MICKELSON, M.M.: The immunosuppressive activity of adamantoyl cytarabine. III. Immunosuppressive specificity in rats. Immunology 19, 417—428 (1970b).
GRAY, G.D., MICKELSON, M.M., CRIM, J.A.: The immunosuppressive activity of ara-cytidine. Transplantation 6. 805—817 (1968a).
GRAY, G.D., MICKELSON, M.M., CRIM, J.A.: Immunosuppressive effects of adamantoyl cytarabine. I. Inhibition of hemagglutinin formation and graft-versus-host reactions in mice. Biochem. Pharmacol. 18, 2163—2169 (1969b).
GRAY, G.D., PERPER, R.J., MICKELSON, M.M., CRIM, J.A., ZUKOWSKI, C.F.: The immunosuppressive activity of ara-cytidine (cytarabine). III. Effects of canine renal allograft rejection and hemagglutinin formation. Transplantation 7, 183—187 (1969a).

Gray, G.D., Nichol, F.R., Mickelson, M.M., Camiener, G.W., Gish, D.T., Kelly, R.C., Wechter, W.J., Moxley, T.E., Neil, G.L.: The immunosuppressive, antiviral and antitumor activities of cytarabine derivatives. Biochem. Pharmacol. **21**, 465—475 (1672).

Green, D.M.: The effects of nitrogen mustard (methyl bis (β-chloro ethyl)amine HCl) on the immunological response of the rabbit. I. The effects of nitrogen mustard on the primary response to a bacterial antigen. Brit. J. exp. Pathol. **39**, 192—198 (1958).

Greig, M.E., Gibbons, A.J.: Effects of cytarabine and adamantoyl cytarabine on experimental allergic encephalomyelitis in rats. Arch. int. Pharmacodyn. **182**, 364—369 (1969).

Hall, J.G.: Effector mechanisms in immunity. Lancet I, 25—28 (1969).

Harris, J.E., Hersh, E.M.: The effect of 1-β-D-arabinofuranosylcytosine on the immune response of mice to sheep red blood cells. Cancer Res. **28**, 2432—2436 (1968).

Harrison, H.W., Bartlett, J.A.: Immunosuppression across weak histocompatibility barriers. Transplantation **10**, 358—360 (1970).

Hektoen, L., Corper, H.J.: Effect of mustard gas (dichlorethylsulphid) on antibody formation. J. infect. Diseases **28**, 279 (1921).

Hellman, K.: Immunosuppression by thalidomide. Implications for teratology. Lancet I, 1136—1137 (1966).

Henson, E.C., Brunson, J.G.: Inhibition of circulating antibody formation induced by propiomazine and epinephrine combination. Nature (Lond.) **222**, 593—594 (1969).

Herscowitz, H.B., Stavitsky, A.B., Tew, J.G.: Effects of actinomycin D, mitomycin C, and 5-bromodeoxyuridine on the *in vitro* anamnestic response to keyhole limpet hemocyanin. In: Cellular immunology, Vol. 2, pp. 259—268. New York: Academic Press 1971.

Hersh, E.M.: L-Glutaminase: suppression of lymphocyte blastogenic responses *in vitro*. Science **172**, 736—738 (1971).

Hersh, E.M., Freireich, E.J.: Host defense mechanisms and their modification by cancer chemotherapy. In: Busch, H. (Ed.): Methods in cancer research, Vol. IV., pp. 355—451. New York: Academic Press 1968.

Hersh, E.M., Wong, V.G., Freireich, E.J.: Inhibition of the local inflammatory response in man by antimetabolites. Blood **27**, 38—47 (1966).

Hersh, E.M., Bodey, G.P.: Leukocytic mechanism of inflammation. Ann. Rev. Med. **21**, 105—132 (1970).

Hersh, E.M., Curtis, J.E., Cheema, A.R.: Host defense failure in the etiology and pathogenesis of malignant disease. Proc. 24th Ann. Symp. Fund. Cancer Res. — Environment and Cancer, pp. 407—427. Baltimore: Williams and Wilkins 1972.

Hersh, E.M., Curtis, J.E., Harris, J.E., McBride, C.M., Alexanian, R., Rossen, R.: Host defense mechanisms in lymphoma and leukemia. In: Leukemia-Lymphoma, pp. 149—167. (A Collection of Papers Presented at the Fourteenth Annual Clinical Conference on Cancer, 1969, at the University of Texas M. D. Anderson Hospital and Tumor Institute at Houston, Houston, Texas.) Chicago: Yearbook Medical Publishers 1970.

Hersh, E.M., Whitecar, J.P., Jr., McCredie, K.B., Bodey, G.P., Sr., Freireich, E.J.: Chemotherapy, immunocompetence, immunosuppression and prognosis in acute leukemia. New Engl. J. Med. **285**, 1211—1216 (1971a).

Hitchings, G.H., Elion, G.B.: Chemical suppression of the immune response. Pharmacol. Rev. **15**, 365—405 (1963).

Hobik, H.P.: Immunosuppressive Wirkung von L-Asparaginase in der Graft-Versus-Host-Reaktion. Naturwiss. **56**, 217 (1969).

Holtermann, O.A., Nordin, A.A.: The effect of cytosine arabinoside upon the primary immune response *in vitro*. Proc. Soc. exp. Biol. (N. Y.) **132**, 1003—1005 (1969).

Horowitz, B., Madras, B.K., Meister, A., Old, L.J., Boyse, E.A., Stockert, E.: Asparagine synthetase activity of mouse leukemias. Science **160**, 533—535 (1968).

Hoyer, J.R., Hoyer, L.W., Good, R.A., Condie, R.M.: The effect of 6-mercaptopurine on delayed hypersensitivity in guinea pigs. J. exp. Med. **116**, 679—685 (1962).

Hurd, E.R., Ziff, M.: Studies on the anti-inflammatory action of 6-mercaptopurine. J. exp. Med. **128**, 785—800 (1968).

Jerne, N.K., Nordin, A.A., Henry, C.: The agar plaque technique for recognizing antibody-producing cells. In: Amos, B., Koprowski, H. (Eds.): Cell bound antibodies, pp. 109—122. Philadelphia: Wistar Inst. Press 1963.

Kaliss, N.: A review. Immunological enhancement of tumor homografts in mice. Cancer Res. **18**, 992—1003 (1958).

Kamada, N., Brecher, G., Tjio, J.H.: *In vitro* effects of chlorpromazine and meprobamate on blast transformation and chromosomes. Proc. Soc. exp. Biol. (N. Y.) **136**, 210—214 (1971).

Kaplan, S., Northrup, J., DeConti, R.C., Calabresi, P.: Suppression of immunological responses by cytosine arabinoside. Clin. Res. **14**, 483 (1966).

KELLEY, M. G., O'GARA, R. W., GUDEKAR, K., YANCEY, S. T., OLIVERIO, V. T.: Carcinogenic activity of a new anti-tumor agent, *N*-isopropyl-alpha (2-methylhydrazino)-*p*-toluamide HCl. Cancer Chemother. Rep. **39**, 77—80 (1964).

KHAN, A., HILL, J. M.: Suppression of skin hypersensitivity and antibody formation by L-asparaginase. J. Immunol. **104**, 679—684 (1970).

KHAN, A., HILL, J. M., ADACHI, M.: L-Asparaginase in experimental auto-immune disease: Inhibition of allergic encephalomyelitis. J. Immunol. **105**, 256—258 (1970).

KIDD, J. G.: Regression of transplanted lymphomas induced *in vivo* by means of normal guinea pig serum. I. Course of transplanted cancers of various kinds in mice and rats given guinea pig serum, horse serum or rabbit serum. J. exp. Med. **98**, 565—582 (1953).

KIMBALL, A. P., LEPAGE, G. A., BOWMAN, B., HERRIOT, S. J.: Suppression of the homograft response by purinethiol nucleosides. Proc. Soc. exp. Biol. (N. Y.) **119**, 248—252 (1965).

KLEIN, G.: Experimental studies in tumor immunology. Fed. Proc. **28**, 1739—1753 (1969).

KOLIN, A., LANDI, S.: Effect of actinomycin D on the tuberculin skin reaction in guinea pigs. Int. Arch. Allergy **38**, 607—617 (1970).

LAWRENCE, H. S., LANDY, M.: Mediators of cellular immunity. New York: Academic Press **1969**.

LAZDA, V., STARR, J. L.: The stability of messenger ribonucleic acid in antibody synthesis. J. Immunol. **95**, 254—261 (1965).

LEMMEL, E., HURD, E. R., ZIFF, M.: Differential effects of 6-mercaptopurine and cyclophosphamide on autoimmune phenomena in NZB mice. Clin. exp. Immunol. **8**, 355—362 (1971).

LEVENTHAL, B. G., WALDORF, D. S., TALAL, N.: Impaired lymphocyte transformation and delayed hypersensitivity in Sjogren's syndrome. J. clin. Invest. **46**, 1338—1345 (1967).

LEVIN, B., MERRILL, J. P.: Immunosuppressive activity of L-asparaginase. Transplantation **12**, 141—144 (1971).

LEVIN, R. H., LANDY, M., FREI, E., III: The effect of 6-mercaptopurine on immune response in man. New Engl. J. Med. **271**, 16—22 (1964).

LEVY, H. B., HASS, V. H.: Alteration of the course of lymphocytic choriomeningitis in mice by certain antimetabolites. Virology **5**, 401—407 (1958).

LOCHTE, H. L., JR., LEVY, A. S., GUENTHER, D. M., THOMAS, E. D., FERREBEE, J. W.: Prevention of delayed foreign marrow reaction in lethally irradiated mice by early administration of methotrexate. Nature (Lond.) **196**, 1110—1111 (1962).

MACDONALD, A. S., CHAN, C. C., FALVEY, C. F.: Use of procarbazine hydrochloride (Natulan) and procarbazine hydrochloride and azathioprine in canine renal allografts. Transplantation **11**, 103—104 (1971).

MAHER, J. F., SCHREINER, G. E.: Treatment of lupus nephritis with azathioprine. Arch. intern. Med. **125**, 293—298 (1970).

MAIBACH, H. I., MAGUIRE, H. C.: Role of species specificity in failure of inhibition of guinea pig anaphylactic sensitization with cancer chemotherapy drugs. Nature (Lond.) **197**, 82—83 (1962).

MAIBACH, H. I., MAGUIRE, H. C., JR.: Studies on the inhibition of antibody formation in the guinea-pig with cyclophosphamide, azathioprine, 5-fluorouracil and urethane. Int. Arch. Allergy **29**, 209—212 (1966).

MAINLAND, D., SUTCLIFFE, M. I.: Report of cooperating clinics committee of The American Rheumatism Association. A controlled trial of cyclophosphamide in rheumatoid arthritis. New Engl. J. Med. **283**, 883—889 (1970).

MAKINODAN, T., ALBRIGHT, J. F., PERKINS, E. H., NETTESHEIM, P.: Suppression of immunologic responses. Med. Clin. N. Amer. **49**, 1569—1596 (1965).

MALAVIYA, A. N., MANY, A., SCHWARTZ, R. S.: Treatment of dermatomyositis with methotrexate. Lancet II, 485—488 (1968).

MATHÉ, G., AMIEL, J. L., SCHWARZENBERG, L., SCHNEIDER, M., HAYAT, M., DEVASSAL, F., JASMIN, C., ROSENFELD, C., POUILLART, P.: Preliminary result of a new protocol for the active immunotherapy of acute lymphoblastic leukaemia: inhibition of the immunotherapeutic effect by vincristine or amantadine. Rev. Europ. Etudes clin. Biol. **16**, 216—224 (1971).

MCQUARRIE, D. G., SARGEANT, J. R., VARCO, R. L.: The effect of homograft antigen strength on the emergence of 6-mercaptopurine-resistant, immune competent cells. J. Surg. Res. **5**, 79—89 (1965).

MEDAWAR, P. B.: The use of antigenic tissue extracts to weaken the immunological reaction against skin homographs in mice. Transplantation **1**, 21—38 (1963).

MEEKER, W. R., JR., CONDIE, R. M., GOOD, R. A., VARCO, R. L.: Alteration of the homograft response by antimetabolites. Ann. N. Y. Acad. Sci. **87**, 203—213 (1960).

MEGIRIAN, R., LEONARDI, D.: Effect of methotrexate on the blood clearances of carbon after india ink. J. Reticuloendothelial Soc. **3**, 295—304 (1966).

Michael, A. F., Vernier, R. L., Drummond, K. N., Levitt, J. I., Herdman, R. C., Fish, A. J., Good, R. A.: Immunosuppressive therapy of chronic renal disease. New Engl. J. Med. **276**, 817—828 (1967).

Mihich, E.: Immunity, cancer and chemotherapy. New York: Academic Press 1967.

Miller, H. K., Krakoff, I. H., Salser, J. S., Balis, M. E.: Sensitivity to L-asparaginase and amino acid metabolism. J. nat. Cancer Inst. **44**, 1120—1139 (1970).

Mitchell, M. S., Wade, M. E., DeConti, R. C., Bertino, J. R., Calabresi, P.: Immunosuppressive effects of cytosine arabinoside and methotrexate in man. Ann. intern. Med. **70**, 535—547 (1969).

Moynihan, P. C., Jackson, J. F.: Lymphocyte transformation in acute uraemia. Nature (Lond.) **212**, 206 (1966).

Murray, J. E., Merrill, J. P., Harrison, J. H., Wilson, R. E., Dammin, Q. J.: Prolonged survival of human-kidney homografts by immunosuppressive drug therapy. New Engl. J. Med. **268**, 1315—1323 (1963).

Nakamura, R. M., Weigle, W. O.: Suppression of thyroid lesions in rabbits by treatment with cyclophosphamide after the induction of thyroiditis. Clin. exp. Immunol. **7**, 541—550 (1970).

Nathan, H. C., Bieber, S., Elion, G. B., Hitchings, G. H.: Detection of agents which interfere with the immune response. Proc. Soc. exp. Biol. (N. Y.) **197**, 796—799 (1961).

Nettesheim, P., Hammons, A. S.: Effect of immunosuppressive agents on retention of antigen in the mouse spleen. Proc. Soc. exp. Biol. (N. Y.) **133**, 696—701 (1970).

North, R. J.: Suppression of cell-mediated immunity to infection by an antimitotic drug. Further evidence that migrant macrophages express immunity. J. exp. Med. **132**, 535—545 (1970).

Novack, S. N., Pearson, C. M.: Cyclophosphamide therapy in Wegener's granulomatosis. New Engl. J. Med. **284**, 938—940 (1971).

Oettgen, H. F., Stephenson, P. A., Schwartz, M. K., Leeper, R. D., Tallal, L., Tan, C. C., Clarkson, B. D., Golbey, R. B., Krakoff, I. H., Karnofsky, D. A., Murphy, M. L., Burchenal, J. H.: Toxicity of *E. coli* L-asparaginase in man. Cancer **25**, 253—278 (1970).

Ohno, R., Harris, J. E., Hersh, E. M.: L-Asparaginase: suppression of the immune response of mice to sheep red blood cells. Clin. exp. Immunol. **7**, 221—227 (1970).

Ohno, R., Hersh, E. M.: The inhibition of lymphocyte blastogenesis by L-asparaginase. Blood **35**, 250—262 (1970a).

Ohno, R., Hersh, E. M.: Immunosuppressive effect of L-asparaginase in man. Cancer Res. **30**, 1605—1611 (1970b).

Owens, A. H., Jr., Santos, G. W.: The induction of graft versus host disease in mice treated with cyclophosphamide. J. exp. Med. **128**, 277—291 (1968).

Owens, A. H., Jr., Santos, G. W.: The effect of cytotoxic drugs on graft-versus-host disease in mice. Transplantation **11**, 378—382 (1971).

Page, A. R.: Inhibition of the lymphocyte response to inflammation with anti-metabolites. Amer. J. Pathol. **45**, 1029—1044 (1964).

Page, A. R., Condi, R. M., Good, R. A.: Effect of 6-mercaptopurine on inflammation. Amer. J. Pathol. **40**, 519—530 (1962).

Paterson, P. Y.: Cyclophosphamide treatment of experimental allergic encephalomyelitis in Lewis rats. J. Immunol. **196**, 1473—1479 (1971).

Paterson, P. Y., Hanson, M. A.: Studies of cyclophosphamide suppression of experimental allergic encephalomyelitis in Wistar rats. J. Immunol. **103**, 795—803 (1969).

Paterson, P. Y., Hanson, M. A., Gerner, E. W.: Cyclophosphamide inhibition of experimental allergic encephalomyelitis in Wistar rats. Proc. Soc. exp. Biol. (N. Y.) **124**, 928—932 (1967).

Phillips, F. S., Hopkins, F. H., Freeman, M. L. A.: Effect of tris (beta-chloroethyl)amine on antibody production in goats. J. Immunol. **55**, 289—296 (1947).

Phillips, S. M., Zweiman, B.: Cellular mechanisms in the depression of delayed hypersensitivity by 6-mercaptopurine. Fed. Proc. **29**, 701 (1970).

Powell, A., Hubay, C. A., Holden, W. D.: A rational screening program for studies in homotransplantation. Surg. Gynec. Obstet. **114**, 167—172 (1962).

Prager, M. D., Bachynsky, N.: Asparagine synthetase in asparaginase resistant and susceptible mouse lymphomas. Biochem. biophys. Res. Commun. **31**, 43—47 (1968).

Prichard, R. W., Hayes, D. M.: The effects of aminopterin on guinea pig tuberculoses. Amer. J. Pathol. **38**, 325—333 (1961).

Raff, M. C., Wortis, H. H.: Thymus dependence of $\Theta$ bearing cells in the peripheral lymphoid tissues of mice. Immunology **18**, 931—942 (1970).

Rapaport, F. T., Shimada, T., Watanabe, K.: Prolongation of canine renal allograft survival by L-asparaginase. Transplantation **12**, 217—222 (1971).

RAWLS, W. E., MELNICK, J. L., OLSON, G. B., DEN, P. B., GOOD, R. A.: Effect of amantadine hydrochloride on the response of human lymphocytes to phytohemagglutinin. Science **158**, 506—507 (1967).
REBUCK, J. W., CROWLEY, J. H.: A method of studying leukocytic functions *in vivo*. II. Techniques in the study of leukocytic function. Ann. N. Y. Acad. Sci. **59**, 757—805 (1955).
ROBINSON, T. W. E., HEATH, R. B.: Effect of cyclophosphamide on the production of interferon. Nature (Lond.) **217**, 178—179 (1968).
ROITT, I. M., GREAVES, M. F., TORRIGIANI, G., BROSTOFF, J., PLAYFAIR, J. H. L.: The cellular basis of immunological responses. A synthesis of some current views. Lancet II, 367—371 (1969).
ROSE, B.: Hormones and allergic responses. In: SHAFFER, J. H., LOGRIPPO, G. A., CHASE, M. W. (Eds.): Mechanisms of hypersensitivity, pp. 599—612. Boston: Little Brown and Co. 1959.
RUSSELL, P. J., HICKS, J. D.: Cyclophosphamide treatment of renal disease in (NZB × NZW) $F_1$ hybrid mice. Lancet I, 440—446 (1968).
SAFDAR, S. H., KRANTZ, S. B., BROWN, E. B.: Successful immunosuppressive treatment of erythroid aplasia appearing after thymectomy. Brit. J. Haematol. **19**, 435—443 (1970).
SAHIR, K., SCHWARTZ, R. S.: The immunoglobulin sequence. I. Arrest by 6-mercaptopurine and restitution by antibody, antigen or splenectomy. J. Immunol. **95**, 345—354 (1966).
SANTOS, G. W.: Adoptive transfer of immunologically competent cells. III. Comparative ability of allogeneic and syngeneic spleen cells to produce a primary antibody response in the cyclophosphamide pretreated mouse. J. Immunol. **97**, 587—593 (1966).
SANTOS, G. W., BURKE, P. J., SENSENBRENNER, L. L., OWENS, A. H., JR.: Rationale for the use of cyclophosphamide as an immunosuppressant for marrow transplants in man. In: BERTELLI, A., MONACO, A. P. (Eds.): Pharmacological treatment in organ and tissue transplantation, pp. 24—31. Amsterdam: Excerpta Medica Foundation 1970.
SANTOS, G. W., OWENS, A. H., JR.: A comparison of the effect of selected cytotoxic agents on the primary agglutinin response in rats injected with sheep erythrocytes. Bull. Johns Hopkins Hosp. **114**, 384—401 (1964).
SANTOS, G. W., OWENS, A. H., JR.: Adoptive transfer of immunologically competent cells. I. Quantitative studies of antibody formation by syngeneic spleen cells in the cyclophosphamide pre-treated mouse. Bull. Johns Hopkins Hosp. **118**, 109—126 (1966).
SANTOS, G. W., OWENS, A. H., JR.: Syngeneic and allogeneic marrow transplants in the cyclophosphamide pre-treated rat. In: DAUSSET, J., HAMBERGER, J., MATHÉ, G. (Eds.): Advances in transplantation, pp. 431. Proceedings of the First International Congress of the Transplantation Society, Paris, 27—30 June 1967. Copenhagen: Munksgaard 1968.
SANTOS, G. W., OWENS, A. H., JR., SENSENBRENNER, L. L.: Effects of selected cytotoxic agents on antibody production in man. A preliminary report. Ann. N. Y. Acad. Sci. **114**, 404—423 (1964).
SANTOS, G. W., SENSENBRENNER, L. L., BURKE, P. J., COLVIN, M., OWENS, A. H., JR., BIAS, W. B., SLAVIN, R. E.: Marrow transplantation in man following cyclophosphamide. Transplant. Proc. **3**, 400—404 (1971).
SCHREK, R.: Qualitative and quantitative reactions of lymphocytes to x-rays. Ann. N. Y. Acad. Sci. **95**, 839—848 (1961).
SCHWARTZ, R. S.: Immunosuppressive drugs. In: Progress in allergy, Vol. 9, pp. 246—303. Basel: S. Karger 1965.
SCHWARTZ, R. S.: Immunosuppressive drug therapy. In: RAPAPORT, F. T., DAUSSET, J. (Eds.): Human transplantation, pp. 440—471. New York: Grune and Stratton 1968.
SCHWARTZ, R. S., ANDRE, J.: Pharmacological studies. The chemical suppression of immunity. In: GRABER, P., MIESCHER, P. (Eds.): Mechanisms of cell and tissue damage produced by immune reactions, pp. 385—409. Basel: Benno Schwabe 1962.
SCHWARTZ, R. S., BELDOTTI, L.: The treatment of chronic murine homologous disease. A comparative study of four "immunosuppressive" agents. Transplantation **3**, 79—97 (1965).
SCHWARTZ, R. S., DAMESHEK, W.: Drug-induced immunological tolerance. Nature (Lond.) **183**, 1682—1683 (1959).
SCHWARTZ, R. S., DAMESHEK, W.: The treatment of autoimmune hemolytic anemia with 6-mercaptopurine and thioguanine. Blood **19**, 483—500 (1962).
SCHWARTZ, R. S., DAMESHEK, W.: The role of antigen dosage in drug-induced immunologic tolerance. J. Immunol. **90**, 703—710 (1963).
SCHWARTZ, R., EISNER, A., DAMESHEK, W.: The effect of 6-mercaptopurine on primary and secondary immune responses. J. clin. Invest. **38**, 1394—1403 (1959).
SCHWARTZ, R., STACK, J., DAMESHEK, W.: Effect of 6-mercaptopurine on antibody production. Proc. Soc. exp. Biol. (N. Y.) **99**, 164—167 (1958).
SCHWARTZ, G. H., STENZEL, K. H., RUBIN, A. L.: Depression of lymphocyte transformation by drugs *in vitro*. Transplantation 8, 704—711 (1969).

Siskind, G. W., Benacerraf, B.: Cell selection by antigen in the immune response. In: Dixon, F. J., Humphrey, J. H. (Eds.).: Advances in immunology, Vol. 10, pp. 1—50. New York: Academic Press 1969.
Sokoloff, M. C., Goldberg, L. S., Pearson, C. M.: Treatment of corticosteroid-resistant polymyositis with methotrexate. Lancet I, 14—16 (1971).
Sorkin, E., DeWeck, A.: The immune response and its suppression. Basel: S. Karger 1969.
Speirs, R. S.: Effect of actinomycin D upon the immune responses to tetanus toxoid. Life Sci. **4**, 343—349 (1965).
Spiegelberg, H. L., Miescher, P. A.: The effect of 6-mercaptopurine and aminopterin on experimental immune thyroiditis in guinea pigs. J. exp. Med. **118**, 864—890 (1963).
Spurr, C. L.: Influence of nitrogen mustards on the antibody response. Proc. Soc. exp. Biol. (N. Y.) **64**, 259—261 (1947).
Starzl, T. E., Penn, I., Schroter, G., Putnam, C. W., Halgrimson, C. G., Martineau, G., Amemiya, H., Groth, C. G.: Cyclophosphamide and human organ transplantation. Lancet II, 70—74 (1971).
Starzl, T. E., Porter, K. A., Andres, G., Halgrimson, C. G., Hurwitz, R., Giles, G., Terasaki, P. I., Penn, I., Schroter, G. T., Lilly, J., Starkie, S. J., Putnam, C. W.: Long-term survival after renal transplantation in human: with special reference to histocompatibility matching, thymectomy, homograft glomerulonephritis, heterologous ALG, and recipient malignancy. Ann. Surg. **172**, 437—472 (1970).
Stefani, S., Schrek, R.: *In vitro* effect of phytohemagglutinin on the sensitivity of human lymphocytes to nitrogen mustard ($HN_2$). J. Lab. clin. Med. **63**, 1027—1032 (1964).
Steinberg, A. D., Talal, N.: Suppression of antibodies to nucleic acids with polyinosinic polycytidylic acid and cyclophosphamide in murine lupus. Clin. exp. Immunol. **7**, 687—691 (1970).
Sterzl, J.: Inhibition of the inductive phase of antibody formation by 6-mercaptopurine examined by the transfer of isolated cells. Nature (Lond.) **185**, 256—257 (1960).
Sterzl, J.: Effect of some metabolic inhibitors in antibody formation. Nature (Lond.) **189**, 1022—1023 (1961).
Stevens, J. E., Willoughby, D. A.: The anti-inflammatory effect of some immunosuppressive agents. J. Pathol. **97**, 367—373 (1969).
Stewart, P. B., Cohen, V.: Antiserum to lymphocytes and procarbazine compared as immunosuppressants in mice. Science **164**, 1082—1083 (1969).
Sussman, L. N.: Azathioprine in refractory idiopathic thrombocytopenic purpura. J. Amer. med. Assoc. **202**, 259—263 (1967).
Svehag, S. E.: Antibody formation *in vitro* by separated spleen cells: inhibition by actinomycin or choramphenicol. Science **146**, 659—661 (1964).
Taliaferro, W. H., Taliaferro, L. G., Jaroslow, B. N.: Radiation and immune mechanisms. New York: Academic Press 1964.
Taub, R. N.: Biological effects of heterologous antilymphocyte serum. In: Progress in allergy, Vol. 14, pp. 208—258. Basel: S. Karger 1970.
Thomas, E. D., Baker, J. A., Ferrebee, J. W.: The effect of methotrexate on the production of antibodies against attenuated distemper virus in the dog. J. Immunol. **90**, 324—328 (1963).
Thomas, E. D., Collins, J. A., Herman, E. C., Jr., Ferrebee, J. W.: Marrow transplants in lethally irradiated dogs given methotrexate. Blood **19**, 217—228 (1962).
Tinberger, W. J.: The effects of some immunosuppressive agents on kidney graft survival in rats. Transplantation **6**, 203—207 (1968).
Turk, J. L., Stone, S. H.: Implications of the cellular changes in lymph nodes during the development and inhibition of delayed type hypersensitivity. In: Amos, B., Koprowski, H. (Eds.): Cell bound antibodies, pp. 51—60. Philadelphia: Wistar Institute Press 1963.
Uhr, J. W.: Actinomycin D. Its effect on antibody formation *in vitro*. Science **142**, 1476—1477 (1963).
Uphoff, D. E.: Alteration of homograft reaction by A-methopterin in lethally irradiated mice treated with homologous marrow. Proc. Soc. exp. Biol. (N. Y.) **99**, 651—653 (1958).
Uphoff, D. E.: Drug induced immunological "tolerance" for homotransplantation. Transplant. Bull. **28**, 12—16 (1961).
Uyeki, E. W.: Effects of several antitumour agents on spleen hemolysin plaque-forming cells. Biochem. Pharmacol. **16**, 53—58 (1967).
Vallejos, C., Cheema, A. R., Hersh, E. M.: Immunosuppressive effects of continuous 5-day arabinosyl cytosine infusion in man (unpublished).
Van Bekkum, D. W., Heystek, G. A., Marquet, R. L.: Effects of immunosuppressive treatment on rejection of heart allografts in rats. Transplantation 8, 678—688 (1969).
Volkman, A.: The origin and turnover of mononuclear cells in peritoneal exudates in rats. J. exp. Med. **124**, 241—254 (1966).

Volkman, A., Gowans, J. L.: The origin of macrophages from bone marrow in the rat. Brit. J. exp. Pathol. **46**, 62—70 (1965a).
Volkman, A., Gowans, J. L.: The production of macrophages in the rat. Brit. J. exp. Pathol. **46**, 50—61 (1965b).
Wheeler, G. P., Alexander, J. A.: Studies with mustards. V. *In vivo* fixation of $C^{14}$ labeled alkylating agents by bilaterally grown sensitive and resistant tumors. Cancer Res. **24**, 1331—1337 (1964a).
Wheeler, G. P., Alexander, J. A.: Studies with mustards. VI. Effects of alkylating agents upon nucleic acid synthesis in bilaterally grown sensitive and resistant tumors. Cancer Res. **24**, 1338—1346 (1964b).
Whitecar, J. P., Jr., Bodey, G. P., Harris, J. E., Freireich, E. J.: L-Asparaginase. New Engl. J. Med. **282**, 732—734 (1970).
Witte, S., Martin, H., Schubert, J. C. F.: Über die cytostatische Therapie mit einem Methylhydrazinderivat. Schweiz. med. Wschr. **96**, 93—99 (1966).
Wong, V. G., Hersh, E. M.: Methotrexate in the therapy of cyclitis. Trans. Amer. Acad. Ophthal. Otolaryng. **69**, 279—293 (1965).
Zweiman, B., Phillips, S. M.: *In vitro* lymphocyte reactivity during depression of tuberculin hypersensitivity by 6-mercaptopurine. Science **169**, 284—285 (1970).

Chapter 29

# Clinical Utility of Immunosuppressive Agents

JULES E. HARRIS and RAMESH C. BAGAI

## Introduction

Immunosuppressive drugs have two principal applications in clinical medicine. They are used in organ transplantation and autoimmune disease. The chemical suppression of the immune response has played an important part in human organ transplantation. Except where identical twins are involved, it is allogeneic grafts that are transplanted. Even with good tissue matching, there is some degree of histocompatibility difference between donor and recipient. In general, the less the histocompatibility difference the longer will be the survival of the grafted organ (VAN ROOD, 1969; FESTENSTEIN et al., 1971; SACHS et al., 1971). Survival is further improved by the use of immunosuppressive drugs to abolish or impair the allograft rejection reaction of the recipient (MURRAY et al., 1963). The rationale for the use of drugs in a transplant situation is clear, and based on sound immunological considerations. In the case of autoimmune disease, however, the argument for the use of immunosuppressive drugs is less cogent. Many diseases are believed to be autoimmune in nature, that is, they are presumed to represent instances of humoral and cell-mediated immune reactivity within the body against antigenic determinants carried by normal tissue. Such an aberrant immune response against self is considered to be both initially responsible for the pathogenesis of the disease and for persisting tissue destruction during the later course of it. The situation is rarely this clearcut and certain diseases termed autoimmune might more properly be described as diseases of unknown etiology with associated immunological phenomena. Immunosuppressive drugs may be effective in these diseases, but it is by no means definitively established that their successful action is due solely or even in part to suppression of the immune function. Prior to the introduction of cytotoxic drugs with immunosuppressive activity, steroids constituted the therapeutic mainstay in autoimmune disease. Steroids have a lympholytic effect and will suppress lymphocytopoiesis (DOUGHERTY et al., 1960). They have, though, numerous other effects, any of which might affect disease processes with associated immunological features. They suppress local inflammatory reactions. In pharmacological doses steroids impair the development of epitheloid and giant cells from mononuclear cells and prevent fibrosis. They also interfere with the diapedesis of neutrophils (GERMUTH, 1956). Steroids are known to prevent disruption of lysosomes and the release of proteolytic enzymes (WEISSMAN, 1965). The stabilizing effect of steroids on lysosomal membranes may be inhibitory to the afferent limb of the immune response by interfering with the uptake and processing of antigen (DE DUVE, 1964). Steroids will impair the transit of immune complexes across glomerular capillaries, as well as the adherence of polymorphonuclear leucocytes to vascular endothelium (GERMUTH et al., 1968). Steroids may have anticomplement activity (GEWURZ et al., 1965). These nonspecific effects may play as important a part in suppressing the clinical and laboratory manifestations of autoimmune disease as any direct effect on the immune apparatus. Moreover, although there are numerous studies reporting immunosuppressive activity of steroids in experimental animals there are no such studies in man. Cytotoxic drugs were introduced for the therapy of autoimmune disease partly because steroids provided usually temporary and incomplete relief and partly because of the serious side-effects of "iatrogenic hypercorticism" (BRAVO et al., 1967; EREMIN et al., 1969). Whereas suppression of the normal immune response has been noted with the use of cytotoxic immunosuppressive drugs in autoimmune disease there is no correlation between their ability to impair normal immune function and their effect on the disease for which they have been used (SWANSON and SCHWARTZ, 1967; PIROFSKY et al., 1969; WONG, 1969; DENMAN et al., 1970; ALEPA et al., 1970). In autoimmune disease, secondary immune responses may be more important in perpetuating pathology than are primary reactions. In animal studies, agents such as 6-mercaptopurine, actinomycin D, and cyclophosphamide have little effect on long-lived lymphocytes and plasma cells perhaps responsible for secondary immune reactions (MILLER and COLE, 1967). Immunosuppressive drugs under certain circumstances may actually stimulate rather than suppress immune reactivity (CHANMOUGAN and SCHWARTZ, 1966; LABORDE and BACH, 1971). These drugs, then, may not be affecting the course of immunological disease solely by an effect on humoral and cell-mediated immunity. Their anti-inflammatory activity may play an important part in mediating their clinical effects (MOENS and BROCTEUR, 1965; HERSH et al., 1966; PATTERSON et al., 1971). [Anti-inflammatory activity may be involved in cytotoxic drug suppression of allograft rejection. Indeed, indomethacin, an anti-inflammatory agent, will prolong skin graft survival in guinea pigs (COPPOLA et al., 1970).] There may, too, be some poorly defined action on pharmacologic substances such as histamine, bradykinin, and serotonin which are involved in immediate hypersensitivity (SWANSON and SCHWARTZ, 1967). The problem remains unsettled, and therapy, although frequently beneficial, continues to be empiric. Dosage schedules are also empiric. The drugs are not given to obtain so many units of immunosuppression – there is, in fact, no way at present of obtaining such a measurement – but rather they are given in arbitrary dosage schedules which time and experience in their use have established. The attainment of peripheral lymphocytopenia is no effective guide to therapy (DENMAN et al., 1970; STEINBERG et al., 1971).

## Complications of Immunosuppressive Therapy

### A. Infection

The use of cytotoxic drugs for immunosuppression in chronic disease is not without risk. Infectious complications, as the direct result of impaired host defense due to these drugs, are major problems in transplantation patients. Sepsis in the post-transplantation period is the principal cause of death in renal allograft recipients (KELLY et al., 1967; RIFKIND et al., 1967; NAKAMOTO, 1967; MOORE and HUME, 1969a; MCDONALD, 1971). It is the cause of death in 50% or more of post-transplantation fatalities (HILL et al., 1964). In the first three months after transplantation, death due to infection is largely caused by bacterial organisms; in later months nonbacterial (i.e. viral, fungal, protozoan) infection is important (STARZL et al., 1970). Bacterial pneumonia and septicemia are the most common types of infection which develop. Infection of the genitourinary tract occurs with high frequency (KELLY et al., 1967; PROUT et al., 1967; MCDONALD, 1971). Most infections are caused by gram-negative bacteria. *Pseudomonas aeruginosa* is the commonest pathogen (PLETKA et al., 1969); infection with *Proteus morganii*, *Klebsiella aerogenes*, and *Escherichia coli* is also common. Multiple organism infection is not unusual. Fungal infection may develop and is difficult to diagnose antemortem in the immunosuppressed patient. Pulmonary involvement by *Candida*, *Aspergillus*, and *Nocardia* may be found (HILL et al., 1967). *Pneumocystis carinii* may complicate the clinical course (PLETKA et al., 1969; COHEN et al., 1971).

Viral disease may develop but is less frequent than bacterial infection. Varicella has been reported (FINE et al., 1969). It may have a hemorrhagic pattern in the immunosuppressed patient. Cytomegalovirus infection has been diagnosed both antemortem (BALAKRISHNAN et al., 1969) and at autopsy (RIFKIND, 1965) in renal transplantation patients but the clinical significance of this infection in transplant patients is not clearly defined. Herpes zoster has an increased incidence following transplantation and appears to be particularly common after local irradiation of the allograft for rejection crises (RIFKIND, 1967). The incidence of warts *(Verrucae vulgaris)* seems also to be increased in renal transplant patients receiving immunosuppressive drugs (SPENCER, 1969). Severe and sometimes fatal herpes simplex may occur (MONTGOMERIE et al., 1969) and herpes labialis is common. Progressive multifocal leukoencephalopathy has been reported following renal transplantation (MANZ et al., 1971).

Infection encountered following hepatic and cardiac allotransplantation is similar to that seen with kidney transplants (STINSON et al., 1969; FULGINITI et al., 1969). Following heart transplantation gram-negative bacterial pneumonia with sepsis is common. *Pseudomonas aeruginosa* is most frequently implicated as the causative organism. Septicemia caused by *Enterococcus* has been reported. *Serratia marcescens* septicemia may occur. *Pneumocystis carinii* may cause extensive pulmonary involvement. Multiple organism infection, especially of the lungs, is common and may be recognized only at autopsy (STINSON et al., 1971). The most valuable procedure in establishing the cause of pulmonary infections has been percutaneous transtracheal aspiration because of the high frequency with which mixed flora may be cultured from sputum specimens. The use of antilymphocyte globulin in cardiac transplant patients may predispose to widespread herpes simplex infection. In liver allograft recipients the liver may become infected with organisms from the *Aerobacter-Klebsiella* group, *Escherichia coli* and *Bacteroides*. Extrahepatic sepsis has been caused by gram-negative bacilli such as *Escherichia coli*, *Aerobacter-Klebsiella* species, *Proteus* species, and *Pseudomonas aeruginosa*. Prophylactic antibiotic sterilization of the bowel reduces neither the incidence nor the severity of infectious complications and may encourage the emergence of resistant strains of bacteria (FULGINITI et al., 1969). Disseminated *Candida albicans* infection has been seen. Widespread cytomegalovirus disease and *Pneumocystis carinii* infection have been documented.

Infectious complications result in the death of many recipients of bone marrow grafts (BORTIN, 1970; SOLBERG et al., 1971). Infection with multiple organisms is not uncommon. Most septicemia is caused by enteric gram-negative bacilli. *Staphylococcus aureus*, *Klebsiella* species, *Bacteroides* species, *Candida albicans*, and *Pneumocystis carinii* may be causative organisms. A problem peculiar to bone marrow transplantation has been the complication of graft-versus-host disease in the recipient (GRAW et al., 1970a, b; GONGDON, 1971; GRAW and SANTOS, 1971). Leukemic transformation of engrafted bone marrow cells in a case where the recipient had leukemia has been reported (FIALKOW et al., 1971).

## B. Cytogenetic Changes

Cytotoxic drugs used in autoimmune disease may produce chromosome damage in patients to whom they are given. This potentially dangerous side-effect must be weighed carefully against any possible benefit of therapy. Chromosome changes may be found in bone marrow cells after azathioprine administration (JENSEN and SØBORG, 1966; JENSEN, 1970). Azathioprine may be mutagenic to the fetus when given to a mother during pregnancy (LEB et al., 1970). Chromosome abnormalities have been found in the lymphocytes of both the mother and the child following birth. Methotrexate will produce chromosomal damage *in vitro* (VOORHEES et al., 1969). Cytogenetic abnormalities have been found in patients with psoriasis treated with methotrexate (RYAN et al., 1965; LOCHER and FRÄNZ, 1967; JENSEN, 1967). Cytotoxic drugs used for immunosuppression may have teratogenic effects in pregnant women (SOKAL and LESSMANN, 1960). Such effects have been recorded for 6-mercaptopurine and busulfan when given in alternating courses (SOKAL and LESSMANN, 1960), chlorambucil (SHOTTON and MONIE, 1963), methotrexate (SOKAL and LESSMANN, 1960; SUTHERLAND and LIGHT, 1965; CURLESS, 1971), and cyclophosphamide (COATES, 1970; TOLEDO et al., 1971). Renal transplant patients who receive immunosuppressive medication throughout pregnancy have experienced normal pregnancies without fetal malformations (MUSSET et al., 1971). Of interest is the observation that immunosuppressive agents such as cyclophosphamide, methotrexate and 6-mercaptopurine do not prevent a normal rate of linear growth (SUNDERMAN and PEARSON, 1969). Azathioprine and steroid in combination do not inhibit wound healing (ARUMUGAM et al., 1971).

## C. Malignancy in the Immunosuppressed Patient

BURNET (1970) has advanced the following theory of "immunological surveillance" – "... when aberrant cells with proliferative potential arise in the body, they will carry new antigenic determinants on their surface. When a significant amount of new antigen has developed, a thymus-dependent immunological response will be initiated which eventually eliminates the aberrant cells in essentially the same way as a homograft is destroyed." Should such an immune mechanism in fact exist in man it might be expected that drugs which interfere with the normal expression of the immune response would, if given over a prolonged interval, lead to an increased incidence of cancer. This appears to be the case, at least in human allograft recipients. Neoplastic disease, in patients undergoing prolonged immunosuppression following a graft procedure, occurs with an incidence of about 100 times greater than in the general population (GUPTA et al., 1969; McKHANN, 1969; KAY et al., 1970; STARZL et al., 1970; FAHEY, 1971; PENN et al., 1971; SCHNECK and PENN, 1971; WALKER et al., 1971). The risk of primary cancer in transplant recipients is 5 per 1000 under the age of 40, greatly exceeding the risk in the general population of 8.2 per 100000. The most common tumor reported is reticulum cell sarcoma with an unusual intracerebral origin. Most of the others which occur are epithelial in origin and include squamous carcinoma of the lip, squamous or basal cell carcinoma of the skin, carcinoma of the colon, testis, ovary, and stomach. Lymphosarcoma, gastrointestinal leiomyosarcoma, and Kaposi's sarcoma also occur. This increased risk of neoplasia does not appear related to the use of any one agent. Patients developing malignancy received azathioprine, prednisone, and antilymphocyte globulin in varied combinations and with a variety of dosage schedules. The question as to whether immunosuppressive medication should be reduced in the hope that the patient will reject the *de novo* tumor is unsettled (STARZL et al., 1970; SIMMONS et al., 1970). Such a move may lead to the rejection of the graft itself. In a few instances, cancers from the kidney donor have been unknowingly transplanted to the allograft recipient (GATTI and GOOD, 1971). These tumors have regressed with discontinuation of immunosuppressive medication.

An increased risk of malignancy may be associated with long-term administration of methotrexate (HARRIS, 1971; CRAIG and ROSENBERG, 1971). Prolonged administration of cyclophosphamide may lead to transitional cell carcinoma of the bladder (WORTH, 1971).

### D. Other Complications Associated with Immunosuppressive Drugs

Treatment with methotrexate for periods ranging from 1 to 5 years may be associated with postnecrotic fibrosis and cirrhosis (O'ROURKE and ECKERT, 1964; EPSTEIN and CROFT, 1969; MULLER et al., 1969). Signs of cirrhosis may develop insidiously. Portal hypertension and esophageal varices have been reported to occur (SHARP et al., 1967; COE and BULL, 1968). The amount of hepatic damage incurred appears to be a function of the duration of therapy and the total amount of drug given (HERSH et al., 1966). Liver function tests may return to normal with cessation of therapy, but hepatic fibrosis may nonetheless persist.

Myocarditis with interstitial fibrosis has been reported to occur in a number of patients who had been on immunosuppressive therapy for kidney transplantation (CHATTY and DEODHAR, 1969). Opportunistic viral infection in a host with compromised host defense is suspect in these cases.

## Immunosuppressive Drugs in Human Transplantation

### A. Kidney

Azathioprine is the drug most widely used in human transplantation for suppression of the allograft rejection reaction. Azathioprine is an *S*-substituted derivative of 6-mercaptopurine. It was synthesized with the intention of protecting 6-mercaptopurine from rapid methylation and oxidation and to provide a carrier compound from which active drug could be slowly released *in vivo* (ELION, 1967). The *S*-linkage is split by thioglucosidases *in vivo* and the cytotoxic and immunosuppressive activity of azathioprine is believed to be due to the release of 6-mercaptopurine in tissue. In immunosuppression studies using the hemagglutinin response of mice to sheep red blood cells, azathioprine is active at a lower fraction of the $LD_{50}$ than is 6-mercaptopurine (ELION, 1967). Azathioprine is more effective than 6-mercaptopurine in inhibiting the formation of spontaneous mouse spleen rosette-forming cells with sheep red blood cells (BACH et al., 1969). Studies of immunosuppression in canine renal allografting have shown azathioprine to be superior to 6-mercaptopurine (CALNE, 1961; CALNE et al., 1962). The above considerations have led to the widespread use of azathioprine in human transplantation. There is, however, no study available comparing the immunosuppressive properties of 6-mercaptopurine and azathioprine in man. When administered to healthy male adult volunteers, azathioprine in a dosage of 100 mg daily failed to suppress a primary humoral immune response to plague vaccine but did block the formation of a secondary immune response to the vaccine (MAIBACH and EPSTEIN, 1965). In the same study azathioprine failed to inhibit established and newly induced contact dermatitis.

In early programs of immunosuppression for renal transplantation, azathioprine was used in combination with prednisone (WOODRUFF et al., 1969; PLETKA et al., 1969). Animal experiments have shown azathioprine and prednisone in combination to be more effective than either drug used alone in suppressing allograft rejection (ADELSBERGER et al., 1970) and in suppressing humoral antibody responses (FRIEDMAN et al., 1971). Dosage schedules were arbitrary and variable. In general, high doses of both drugs (i.e. azathioprine 5 mg/kg/day; prednisone 4 mg/kg/day) were given in the immediate postoperative period. Drug doses were then scaled downward and adjusted on the basis of clinical considerations and leucocyte and platelet counts. Maintenance immunosuppressive therapy usually consisted of prednisone 10 to 20 mg/day and azathioprine 1 to 2 mg/kg/day. Recently, cyclophosphamide has been used with good results as the primary immunosuppressant in kidney allograft recipients (STARZL et al., 1971). Cyclophosphamide has also been used to replace azathioprine in circumstances where azathioprine toxicity was suspected. The drug is used in combination with prednisone and antilymphocyte globulin. Following loading doses of about 2 to 6 mg/kg/day, maintenance doses of about 1 mg/kg/day are established.

Two major problems in organ transplantation have been the detection and the reversal of rejection crises. Most of these occur within the first few postoperative months (PLETKA et al., 1969). Late rejection may also occur (FLANIGAN et al., 1971). Most tests used to detect renal allograft rejection have involved a measurement of deteriorating renal function (KINCAID-SMITH, 1967; RIGGIO et al., 1968; CHISHOLM et al., 1969; MACLEAN et al., 1969; MOOKERJEE et al., 1969; SAMPSON, 1969; CLARKSON et al., 1970; SALAMAN, 1970; SHEHADEH, 1970; ZUHLKE and HERMAN, 1970; MURPHY et al., 1971). These have been useful, but do not serve to evaluate changes in host immune response which give rise to the rejection reaction. These changes may have begun sometime before impaired renal function is detected. Moreover, tests of function alone do not provide an immunologic rationale for "titration" with immunosuppressive drugs. One approach to the immunological detection of renal allograft rejection in man has involved serial monitoring of the peripheral blood of allograft recipients for the detection of lymphoid cells with increased DNA synthesis. These cells appear in association with renal allograft rejection (TENNENBAUM et al., 1968; HERSH et al., 1970; PARKER et al., 1970; PARKER and MOWBRAY, 1971; PAGE et al., 1971). They may appear prior to clinical or biochemical manifestations of rejection and allow for not only the recognition of these but also for prediction of them. The detection of these cells may allow, too, for judging the adequacy of immunosuppressive therapy used to treat rejection reactions (PAGE et al., 1971). Monitoring of lymphocyte responsiveness to phytohemagglutinin appears to be of no value in evaluating the efficacy of immunosuppression in renal transplantation (POSEN et al., 1971). The migration inhibition test with purified glomerular basement membrane antigen and guinea pig peritoneal exudate cells as indicator has been used to assay allograft immunity in human renal transplant patients (MELNICK and FRIEDMAN, 1970). The leucocyte migration technique using donor white blood cells or extracts of donor tissue may be used to identify rejection crises and to monitor their reversal with immunosuppressive drugs (SMITH et al., 1969; MAGIL et al., 1971). The migration inhibition test has been used to follow the immunosuppressive effect of antilymphocyte globulin in human liver transplantation (EDDLESTON et al., 1969). The rosette inhibition test has been used in renal allotransplantation to detect allograft rejection and to regulate the dosage of immunosuppressive medication (MUNRO et al., 1971).

Rejection crises in renal transplantation have been managed by the use of actinomycin C (CALNE et al., 1968; WOODRUFF, 1969; OWEN, 1969; PLETKA et al., 1969), increasing the dose of oral steroids (CALNE et al., 1968; OWEN, 1969; DOAK et al., 1969; WOODRUFF, 1969), giving local graft irradiation (GLEASON and MURRAY, 1967; OWEN, 1969; WOODRUFF, 1969) or by administration of antilymphocyte globulin (WOODRUFF, 1967, 1969; CALNE et al., 1968). It is unsettled whether antilymphocyte globulin is truly effective in rejection crises (MEE and EVANS, 1970). These measures have been used singly or in combination. A single large dose (1 g) of intravenous prednisolone has been suggested as a means of reversing rejection crises (BELL et al., 1971). A success rate of 86% has been obtained with no toxic side-effects. Up to 3 doses may be given over a period of 4 days. Failure to respond following such a course is believed to represent an instance of "irreversible" rejection and is an indication for removal of the graft without further compromising patient survival. Cyclophosphamide has been used to reverse rejection reactions which had failed to respond to treatment with prednisone, azathioprine, local irradiation, actinomycin C, and anticoagulants (ULDALL et al., 1971).

A special word is in order about the use of antilymphocyte globulin (ALG) in transplantation. ALG has been employed for immunosuppression in clinical organ transplantation since 1966 (STARZL et al., 1967).

The preparation and properties of antilymphocyte sera have been reviewed by JOOSTE (1970) and the application of ALG in clinical transplantation has been recently reviewed by NAJARIAN and SIMMONS (1971).The activity of ALG is believed due to its ability to selectively deplete lymphocytes primarily concerned with cell-mediated immune responses (LANCE, 1970). Such lymphocytes, once covered with ALG, are probably either phagocytosed by the reticuloendothelial system of the liver or lysed (HARRIS et al., 1971). ALG is more effective in suppressing cell-mediated immunity than in blocking humoral immune responses. Immune memory and second-set allograft rejection reactions may also be inhibited. ALG will suppress established delayed hypersensitivity reactions in patients to whom it is given (BRUNSTETTER and CLAMAN, 1968). In kidney transplant patients ALG will prevent the development of sensitivity to dinitrochlorobenzene and keyhole limpet hemocyanin (MANNICK et al., 1971).

Difficulties are posed in accurately assessing the potency of any particular batch of ALG (MEDAWAR, 1968). Some batches of ALG may not be as biologically active as others. Workers use a variety of cell preparations (thymocytes, peripheral blood lymphocytes, thoracic duct lymphocytes, spleen cells, lymphoblastoid cell lines) and a number of different animal species (horse, rabbit, goat) in which to prepare ALG. Immunization procedures differ and the actual method of processing the ALG obtained has not been standardized. There is no definitive guidance as to the correct dose of ALG to use in man, particularly when it is given as adjunct therapy to other immunosuppressive drugs. To be most effective ALG must be given at, or perhaps before, transplantation. Treatment for longer than 3 to 4 months may not be necessary (STARZL et al., 1970; SHEIL et al., 1971). Primary doses given for only 2 to 3 weeks with cessation of ALG thereafter may be all that is required to obtain whatever improved immunosuppression ALG is capable of producing (NAJARIAN and SIMMONS, 1971). Longterm treatment with ALG may actually interfere with the activity of other immunosuppressive drugs.

Numerous groups have been impressed with the effectiveness of ALG in prolonging graft survival when used in combination with conventional immunosuppressive agents (STARZL et al., 1967; SHORTER et al., 1968; NAJARIAN et al., 1969; DOAK et al., 1969; COSIMI et al., 1970). The average one year survival of cadaver renal allografts using conventional immunosuppression is 42%. Claims of survival ranging from 76 to 90% have been made where ALG was also used (MOORE and HUME, 1969b; STARZL et al., 1970; MANNICK et al., 1971). The final place of ALG in transplantation immunosuppression remains, however, unsettled (VAN ROOD, 1969; SELL, 1969). Much of the early success attributed to the use of ALG might have been due to improved tissue matching techniques or to the benefit of greater experience in the use of immunosuppressive agents. However, one controlled clinical trial (SHEIL et al., 1971), using both ALG of horse and goat origin as adjunct immunosuppressive therapy, has resulted in a decreased rate of graft rejection, a greater percentage of grafts which survived with good function, and a reduced mortality from infectious complications in ALG-treated patients compared to a group of allograft recipients who received no ALG.

ALG may be given intravenously or intramuscularly, although when given intramuscularly it may cause severe pain, erythema, and tenderness at the point of injection. Certain preparations of ALG may cause anemia and thrombocytopenia. The one consistent hematological effect of ALG is to cause profound lymphocytopenia. This will occur within 6 h of first injection. Slight temperature elevations may be observed. Features of serum sickness with arthralgia, urticarial eruptions, and periorbital edema have been described. Anaphylactic reactions have been reported (MEDAWAR, 1968; NAJARIAN et al., 1969; COSIMI et al., 1970). Allergic reactions may occur in about 40% of patients treated for longer than 2 weeks (NAJARIAN and SIMMONS, 1971). Goat ALG appears to be less toxic than equine ALG (SHEIL et al., 1971). There is, though, some cross-reactivity between horse and goat protein. Some 25% of persons allergic to horse globulin will also be allergic to goat globulin. Patients receiving ALG make antibodies to it and immune elimination could in time make ALG inactive (BUTLER et al., 1969). Some workers report the production of immune tolerance to ALG following the intravenous administration of normal aggregate-free horse gamma globulin (TAUB et al., 1969; BRENDEL et al., 1969; WEKSLER et al., 1970). Others have been unsuccessful with this approach (MOBERG et al., 1970). The tolerance produced may not be complete enough to prevent the development of antibody which leads to anaphylactic reactions (WEKSLER et al., 1969).

## B. Liver

Programs of immunosuppression for liver transplantation are similar to those used in kidney transplantation: combinations of azathioprine, steroid, and xenogeneic ALG (STARZL et al., 1968; CALNE et al., 1968). The dose of azathioprine must be kept low because of the potential hepatotoxicity of the drug. The serum immunosuppressive activity of azathioprine may fall with the mixed cholestatic and hepatocellular type of jaundice associated with liver transplant rejection (MITCHELL et al., 1970). The use of early intensive courses of ALG may allow for a lower dose of azathioprine and steroid in the immediate postoperative period when patients seem most susceptible to infectious complications. Actinomycin C and local irradiation of the graft have been used to combat rejection crises. High dose steroid administration can be rapidly effective when rejection occurs.

## C. Heart and Lung

Immunosuppression in heart transplant programs resembles that used with renal and hepatic allografting with the exception that the regular use of ALG is more routine with heart transplants (BARNARD. 1969; BOTHA, 1969; COOLEY et al., 1969; NORA et al., 1969; STINSON et al., 1969a). Acute rejection episodes have generally been managed with actinomycin D and increased doses of steroid (STINSON et al., 1969b).

Clinical experience with lung transplantations is limited and the results obtained have been uniformly disappointing. The effectiveness of immunosuppression cannot be assessed. Immunosuppression regimens have used combinations of azathioprine, steroid, actinomycin C, and ALG (WHITE et al., 1966; COOLEY et al., 1967).

### D. Bone Marrow

Bone marrow grafting in man depends heavily on the presence of histocompatibility between donor and recipient (Meuwissen et al., 1969; De Koning et al., 1969). Improved "takes" have been reported following "conditioning" of recipients with antilymphocyte serum (Mathé et al., 1970). Patients may be prepared by pregraft "priming" with cyclophosphamide (Bach et al., 1968). Immunosuppression to prevent graft rejection and to combat graft-versus-host disease has involved combinations of antilymphocyte serum, prednisone, azathioprine and steroid (Solberg et al., 1971).

## Immunosuppressive Drugs in Autoimmune Disease

### A. Autoimmune Blood Disease

#### I. Autoimmune Hemolytic Anemia

Autoimmune hemolytic anemia in infancy has been successfully treated with azathioprine (Hitzig and Massimo, 1966). Treatment allowed for either a reduction in dose of steroid or complete remission requiring no additional therapy. The therapeutic approach used is one which may be applicable to other autoimmune conditions which have failed to respond to steroids. Steroids should be reduced slowly only after azathioprine has been given for 1 to 2 months. If there is no exacerbation of disease with cessation of steroid, azathioprine is continued for an additional 3 to 4 months in full dosage and only then is gradually reduced. Careful adjustment in the dosages of both steroid and azathioprine may be necessary. Occasionally, optimum results will only be obtained when both drugs are used together, although in amounts lower than their usual dose if used alone.

#### II. Idiopathic Thrombocytopenic Purpura

The documentation of platelet antibodies in this condition has suggested an autoimmune etiology (Karpatkin and Suskind, 1969). The disease, in instances where it has not responded to either or both steroid and splenectomy, has been controlled with cytotoxic immunosuppressive drugs (Dameshek, 1962; Corley et al., 1966; Sussman, 1967; Laros and Penner, 1968; Kuzemko and Keidan, 1968; Bouroncle and Doan, 1969). Good responses have been obtained with azathioprine in doses ranging from 1 to 6 mg/kg/day. In some patients, continued treatment with small doses of steroid appeared to improve the azathioprine response. Cyclophosphamide in a dose of 50 to 200 mg/day has induced permanent remissions which allow for discontinuation of therapy (Laros and Penner, 1971). Vinblastine may have value in cases which fail to respond to azathioprine or where steroids and splenectomy are contraindicated (Marmont et al., 1971).

#### III. Hyperglobulinemic Purpura

Successful management of this unusual condition has been reported with the use of thioguanine (Weiss et al., 1963). Good clinical responses may be obtained, but with little alteration in laboratory abnormalities. Cryoglobulinemia not responsive to prednisone has shown clinical improvement following treatment with cyclophosphamide (Mathison et al., 1971).

## B. Autoimmune Renal Disease

### I. Systemic Lupus Erythematosus (SLE)

Immunologic mechanisms may play a role in the glomerulonephritis of SLE (KOFFLER et al., 1967). Cytotoxic drugs have had a role in the management of SLE since nitrogen mustard was first used for this condition in 1954 (DUBOIS, 1954). The drug was found to be effective in the nephrotic syndrome of SLE. The combination of azathioprine and steroids may give both clinical and histologic improvement in lupus nephritis (DRINKARD et al., 1970). Significant symptomatic and objective relief of the systemic manifestations of SLE has been reported with the use of azathioprine alone (LEE et al., 1961; CORLEY et al., 1966). In the study of LEE et al. (1961) a normal humoral immune response to Brucella vaccine was noted despite azathioprine-induced fall in anti-A and anti-B titers, total serum gamma globulin, and antinuclear antibodies. Cyclophosphamide has been used to control the renal manifestations of SLE (CAMERON et al., 1970; STEINBERG et al., 1971). It is effective alone or given in conjunction with low dose steroids. The cyclophosphamide effect may be dose-dependent and the simultaneous administration of steroid may permit larger doses of cyclophosphamide to be given. The best responses in lupus nephritis were seen in those patients with the highest creatinine clearances and the least severe nephritis by biopsy evaluation. The response, in lupus nephritis with impaired renal function, to the combination of azathioprine and steroid is also poor (MAHER and SCHREINER, 1970). Progressive lupus nephropathy has been treated successfully with goat antihuman antilymphocyte and antithymocyte serum (PIROFSKY et al., 1969). A therapeutic response in lupus hemolytic anemia has been obtained with the same preparations (PIROFSKY et al., 1971).

### II. Glomerulonephritis

Immune mechanisms may be involved in the pathogenesis of many forms of glomerulonephritis (DIXON, 1968; CHRISTIAN, 1969). Immunoglobulin and complement components may be found in the glomerular basement membrane in proliferative glomerulonephritis. "Idiopathic" nephrotic syndrome may be an immunological disease as well (NGU et al., 1970). Proliferative, membranous and mixed forms of glomerulonephritis may respond to the combination of steroid and azathioprine in situations where steroid alone was ineffective (ADAMS et al., 1967; MICHAEL et al., 1967; BARDANA et al., 1970). Steroid-resistant proliferative glomerulonephritis has responded well to cytotoxic therapy with cyclophosphamide (WHITE, 1967). The cyclophosphamide was withdrawn without causing relapse. Forms of glomerulonephritis resistant to steroids alone may stabilize when treated with the combination of prednisone and azathioprine (WHITE, 1967; LEVITT, 1970). On the other hand, BOOTH and ABER (1970) have reported no improvement in either renal function or renal histology in adult patients with proliferative glomerulonephritis treated for up to 12 months with cyclophosphamide or azathioprine. ABRAMOWICZ et al. (1970) have found the combination of azathioprine and steroid to be of no value in children with the nephrotic syndrome. However, patients with steroid-sensitive relapsing nephrotic syndrome treated with cyclophosphamide relapse less frequently than those treated with steroids (BARRATT and SOOTHILL, 1970). The authors of this last report offer it as the first example of a positive controlled trial of cytotoxic therapy in human nephritis. Goat antihuman thymocyte antisera has given a therapeutic response in glomerulonephritis (PIROFSKY et al., 1971).

### III. Goodpasture's Syndrome

A considerable body of evidence has been presented to show that Goodpasture's syndrome is an autoimmune disease (HILL and CRUICKSHANK, 1953; DE GOWIN et al., 1963; SCHEER and GROSSMAN, 1964; DUNCAN et al., 1965). Steroids provide inadequate control for this condition. They fail to prevent the progression of renal insufficiency (LERNER et al., 1967). Azathioprine has been used to control the disease (CORLEY et al., 1966). The combination of azathioprine and prednisone has arrested renal deterioration and reversed pulmonary changes (HAYSLETT et al., 1971). Prednisone and 6-mercaptopurine have resulted in improved renal function which persisted following cessation of therapy (EVERETT et al., 1970). Renal function may be improved with antilymphocyte antiserum when previous treatment with prednisone and azathioprine have been unsuccessful (PIROFSKY et al., 1969).

## C. Gastrointestinal Disease

### I. Ulcerative Colitis

Azathioprine has been of benefit in supplementing standard therapy for ulcerative colitis. The drug may be useful in patients who are unable to tolerate or who fail to respond to treatment with steroids, surgery, or sulfasalazine (PATTERSON et al., 1971). Systemic manifestations such as pyoderma gangrenosum and arthritis have been ameliorated and steroid requirements reduced (BOWEN et al., 1966). Occasionally, complete remissions have been obtained allowing for medication free intervals or treatment with sulfasalazine alone (JONES, 1969). Remissions induced by azathioprine in steroid-resistant disease may be followed by early relapse if steroids are too quickly withdrawn (THEODOR et al., 1968). The response of ulcerative colitis to azathioprine is unpredictable. Disease may recur at variable times after therapy is discontinued. MACKAY and WALL (1968) suggest that treatment with steroid and azathioprine is better than with azathioprine alone.

### II. Regional Enteritis

Azathioprine has been used successfully to treate cases of regional enteritis resistant to conventional management, including surgery (BROOKE et al., 1969, 1970; DRUCKER and JEEJEEBHOY, 1970). Treatment has led to healing of fistulae and ulcers together with marked symptomatic improvement. Good responses have been obtained at all stages of the disease. Some workers, however, have reported poor responses for azathioprine in regional enteritis (RHODES et al., 1970). A major consideration in azathioprine treatment for this bowel lesion is the appreciation that no experimental or clinical evidence has been adduced to show that regional enteritis is an immunological disease. Azathioprine could exert its effect through an anti-inflammatory action. Also, COOKE (1970) cautions against azathioprine in a disease which in most patients eventually "burns itself out."

### III. Liver Disease

Chronic active hepatitis has been effectively managed with azathioprine (POWELL, 1969; GROS and ZWIRNER, 1969). Too abrupt withdrawal of drug may lead to severe recurrence of disease. In some cases subsidence of acute inflammatory hepatic changes was followed by the development of hepatic cirrhosis. Low dose steroid administered concurrently may prevent this transition. Prednisolone and azathioprine have been found equally effective in maintaining disease quiescence in cases of active chronic autoimmune hepatitis (MACKAY, 1968). Steroid and azathioprine given together may give substantial clinical and biochemical improvement (FORSTER et al., 1971).

Immune mechanisms have been implicated in the pathogenesis of primary biliary cirrhosis (PARONETTO et al., 1964; WALKER et al., 1965), and responses have been obtained in this condition with azathioprine (FISCHER and SCHMID, 1967). The administration of azathioprine may give prompt relief of pruritus before any possible immunosuppressive effect of the drug could be exerted (ALARCON-SEGOVIA et al., 1970).

The radiological features of primary sclerosing cholangitis have been restored to normal with azathioprine treatment (JAVETT, 1971).

## D. Wegener's Granulomatosis

This disease process may represent a hypersensitivity state (FAHEY et al., 1954; TUHY et al., 1958; BEIDLEMAN, 1963). Antigen-antibody complexes have been found in the glomeruli of affected patients (LERMAN and CASTLEMAN, 1969). Cytotoxic drugs given early in the course of the disease may arrest its progress and in some cases reverse its effects (RAITT, 1971). An occasional patient may enter a remission with no relapse after withdrawal of immunosuppressive drugs. Responses have been obtained with nitrogen mustard (AUNGST and LESSMANN, 1962), chlorambucil (McILVANIE, 1966), azathioprine alone (BOURONCLE et al., 1967; ALDO et al., 1970) or in combination with steroid (NORTON et al., 1968) or duazomycin A (KAPLAN et al., 1968). Intermittent methotrexate therapy may act more rapidly than steroids, alkylating agents, or azathioprine and may then be the treatment of choice in acutely ill patients (CAPIZZI and BERTINO, 1971).

## E. Collagen Diseases

### I. Rheumatoid Arthritis

Autoimmune mechanisms have been postulated to be implicated in the pathogenesis of rheumatoid arthritis (HOLLANDER et al., 1965; OSGOOD, 1966; STANFIELD et al., 1966; FOSDICK, 1968). Although alkylating agents were first used for rheumatoid arthritis in 1951 (DIAZ et al., 1957), it has only been over the past decade that cytotoxic drugs have been widely employed for control of severe forms of this disease (KAHN et al., 1967). The hazards and advantages of immunosuppressive therapy for rheumatoid arthritis have been reviewed by BAUM and VAUGHAN (1969). Azathioprine has been useful in the management of cases of rheumatoid arthritis resistant to other forms of therapy (DODSON and BENNETT, 1969). In patients receiving steroids, azathioprine may have a "steroid-sparing" effect allowing for a decrease in daily steroid requirements (MASON et al., 1969). Chlorambucil has given clinical responses in rheumatoid arthritis refractory to conventional treatment (RENIER et al., 1967; DE SEZE et al., 1967). Treatment of rheumatoid arthritis with either azathioprine or chlorambucil has little effect on either cellular or humoral immunity despite inducing peripheral lymphocytopenia (DENMAN et al., 1970). Cyclophosphamide is effective in controlling both adult and childhood forms of rheumatoid arthritis (FOSDICK et al., 1968; SKOGLUND et al., 1971; RAU, 1971; JARLOR and SORENSEN, 1971). No direct correlation has been found between the degree of clinical response with cyclophosphamide and the extent of depression of immune function (ALEPA et al., 1970). Although cyclophosphamide offers substantial benefits, its use is only advocated when more standard forms of therapy have failed (Cooperating Clinics, 1970). Cyclophosphamide in conjunction with prednisone has been used to clear ocular lesions occurring in severe rheumatoid arthritis (HURD et al., 1970). Responses in rheumatoid arthritis have been obtained with the use of antilymphocyte globulin (PIROFSKY et al., 1971).

Capillary migration inhibition using peripheral blood leucocytes has been demonstrated with synovial extracts in patients with rheumatoid arthritis (ROTHENBERGER and THIELE, 1970). The test may have potential value in monitoring the effects of cytotoxic drugs.

### II. Dermatomyositis-Scleroderma

A dramatic response in patients with dermatomyositis has been obtained through the intermittent intravenous administration of methotrexate (MALAVIYA et al., 1968). Responses were obtained in patients resistant to steroids and persisted following cessation of drug. SOKOLOFF et al. (1971) have reported responses to intermittent intravenous methotrexate in steroid-resistant polymyositis. Muscle strength improved and skin lesions resolved. This was associated with recovery of serum enzyme levels to normal.

Chlorambucil given in association with steroids and vasodilating agents has proven effective in controlling many of the manifestations of scleroderma (MACKENZIE, 1970). Thioguanine has also been used effectively in scleroderma (DEMIS et al., 1964).

## F. Ocular Disease

Ocular inflammatory diseases of an "autoallergic" nature such as peripheral uveitis and chorioretinitis have been treated with methotrexate or cyclophosphamide (WONG, 1969; BUCKLEY and GILLS, 1969a). The use of cyclophosphamide and steroids in combination was found to be more effective than the use of either drug alone.

An autoimmune pathogenesis has been suggested for Behcet's disease (OSHIMA et al., 1963). The condition has responded to azathioprine (ROSSELET et al., 1968) and to the combination of steroid and cyclophosphamide (CHAOUAT et al., 1968; BUCKLEY and GILLS, 1969b).

## G. Skin Disease

### I. Pemphigus

An immunological basis for pemphigus has been advanced (JORDON et al., 1967; BEUTNER et al., 1968; HURST, 1970; WHITTINGHAM and MACKAY, 1971; MULLER et al., 1971). Azathioprine has been used successfully to treat this disease (KRAKOWSKI et al., 1969; WOLFF and SCHREINER, 1969; BURTON et al., 1970; GREAVES et al., 1971). Azathioprine appears to act slowly in this illness and steroids should be used concurrently or not withdrawn too rapidly during initial phases of therapy. Steroids may be in time completely withdrawn or their total dose reduced to a tolerable level. In some cases remissions may persist with withdrawal of all therapy. Methotrexate may be used to maintain steroid-induced remissions (LEVNER and GOLDBERG, 1969). Cyclophosphamide may be effective in instances where neither steroids nor azathioprine produce control of active disease (EBRINGER and MACKAY, 1969).

## H. Neuromuscular Disease

Cases of polyneuropathy resistant to steroid therapy have been carried into remission with azathioprine (YUILL et al., 1970). Remissions were maintained following withdrawal of the drug.

Various combinations of azathioprine, 6-mercaptopurine, methotrexate, and actinomycin C used in conjunction with cholinesterase inhibitors have been reported to give significant remissions in myasthenia gravis (MERTENS et al., 1969). Remissions have been claimed with the use of antilymphocyte globulin in myasthenia gravis (PIROFSKY et al., 1971).

### I. Asthma

Thioguanosine and 6-mercaptopurine have given symptomatic improvement in patients with intermittent asthma of recent onset (ASMUNDSSON et al., 1971). Patients with chronic asthma failed to benefit.

## Conclusions

The use of cytotoxic drugs with immunosuppressive activity in man has been reviewed. These agents confer great clinical benefit in human transplantation. In this area sound immunological considerations govern their application. In autoimmune disease their use is less clearly based on any sound immunological rationale. Their effect in this group of diseases is not well understood. The correct duration of treatment in autoimmune disease is not known. Their advantages here must be balanced against their potential and actual toxic side effects. Their use in chronic disease is only warranted where other more conventional forms of therapy have been ineffective.

### References


ABRAMOWICZ, M., BARNETT, H. L., EDELMANN, C. M., JR., GREIFER, I., KOBAYASHI, O., ARNEIL, G. C., BARRON, B. A., GORDILLO, P. G., HALLMAN, N., TIDDENS, H. A.: Controlled trial with azathioprine in children with nephrotic syndrome. A report for the International Study of Kidney Disease in Children. Lancet I, 959—961 (1970).

ADAMS, D. A., GORDON, A., MAXWELL, M. H.: Azathioprine treatment of immunological renal disease. J. Amer. med. Assoc. **199**, 459—463 (1967).

ADELSBERGER, B., SINIOS, A., DEICHER, H.: Suppression der Transplantationsreaktion durch gleichzeitige Gabe von Azathioprin und Prednisolon. Zeitschrift für Immunitätsforschung. Allergie klin. Immunol. **139**, 277—289 (1970).

ALARCON-SEGOVIA, D., MAYORGA-CORTES, A., WOLPERT, E.: Primary biliary cirrhosis. Prompt relief of pruritus with azathioprine treatment. J. Amer. med. Assoc. **214**, 367—368 (1970).

ALDO, M. A., BENSON, M. D., COMERFORD, F. R., COHEN, A. S.: Treatment of Wegener's granulomatosis with immunosuppressive agents. Arch. intern. Med. **126**, 298—305 (1970).

ALEPA, F. P., ZVAIFLER, N. J., SLIWINSKI, A. J.: Immunologic effects of cyclophosphamide treatment in rheumatoid arthritis. Arthritis Rheum. **13**, 754—760 (1970).

ARUMUGAM, S., NIMMANNIT, S., ENQUIST, I. F.: The effect of immunosuppression on wound healing. Surg. Gynec. Obst. **133**, 72—74 (1971).

ASMUNDSSON, T., KILBURN, K. H., LASZLO, J., KROCK, C. J.: Immunosuppressive therapy of asthma. J. Allergy **47**, 136—147 (1971).

AUNGST, C. W., LESSMANN, E. M.: WEGENER's granulomatosis treated with nitrogen mustard. N. Y. J. Med. **62**, 3302—3310 (1962).

BACH, F. H., ALBERTINI, R. J., ANDERSON, J. L., JOO, P., BORTIN, M. M.: Bone-marrow transplantation in a patient with the Wiskott-Aldrich syndrome. Lancet II, 1364—1366 (1968).

BACH, J. F., DARDENNE, M., FOURNIER, C.: In vitro evaluation of immunosuppressive drugs. Nature (Lond.) **222**, 998—999 (1969).

BALAKRISHNAN, S. L., ARMSTRONG, D., RUBIN, A. L., STENZEL, K. H.: Cytomegalovirus infection after renal transplantation. J. Amer. med. Assoc. **207**, 1712—1714 (1969).

BARDANA, E. J., PORTER, G. A., PIROFSKY, B., GOURLEY, R. T., BAYRAKCI, C.: Azathioprine in steroid-insensitive nephropathy. Amer. J. Med. **49**, 789—800 (1970).

BARNARD, C. N.: Human heart transplantation. Canad. med. Ass. J. **100**, 91—104 (1969).

BARRATT, T. M., SOOTHILL, J. F.: Controlled trial of cyclophosphamide in steroid-sensitive relapsing nephrotic syndrome of childhood. Lancet II, 479—482 (1970).

BAUM, J., VAUGHAN, J.: Immunosuppressive drugs in rheumatoid arthritis. Ann. intern. Med. **71**, 202—204 (1969).

BEIDLEMAN, B.: Wegener's granulomatosis. J. Amer. med. Assoc. 186, 827—830 (1963).
BELL, P. R. F., BRIGGS, J. D., CALMAN, K. C., PATON, A. M., WOOD, R. F. M., MACPHERSON, S. G., KYLE, K.: Reversal of acute clinical and experimental organ rejection using large doses of intravenous prednisolone. Lancet I, 876—880 (1971).
BEUTNER, E. H., JORDON, R. E., CHORZELSKI, T. P.: Autoantibodies in pemphigus vulgaris: response to an intercellular substance of epidermis. J. Amer. med. Assoc. 192, 682—688 (1965).
BOOTH, L. J., ABER, G. M.: Immunosuppressive therapy in adults with proliferative glomerulonephritis. Lancet II, 1010—1013 (1970).
BORTIN, M. M.: A compendium of reported human bone marrow transplants. Transplantation 9, 571—587 (1970).
BOTHA, M. C.: Leucocyte-antigen matching in donor selection for heart transplantation. Lancet II, 508—512 (1969).
BOURONCLE, B. A., DOAN, C. A.: Treatment of refractory idiopathic thrombocytopenic purpura. J. Amer. med. Assoc. 207, 2049—2052 (1969).
BOURONCLE, B. A., SMITH, E. J., CUPPAGE, F. E.: Treatment of Wegener's granulomatosis with Imuran. Amer. J. Med. 42, 314—318 (1967).
BOWEN, G. E., IRONS, G. V., JR., RHODES, J. B., KIRSNER, J. B.: Early experience with azathioprine in ulcerative colitis. J. Amer. med. Assoc. 195, 460—464 (1966).
BRAVO, J. F., HERMAN, J. H., SMYTH, C. J.: Musculoskeletal disorders after renal homotransplantation. Ann. intern. Med. 66, 87—104 (1967).
BRENDEL, W., LAND, W., HOPF, U., SEIFERT, J.: Induction of tolerance in man to horse-IgG. Lancet II, 1141—1142 (1969).
BROOKE, B. N., HOFFMANN, D. C., SWARBRICK, E. T.: Azathioprine for CROHN's disease. Lancet II, 612—615 (1969).
BROOKE, B. N., JAVETT, S. L., DAVISON, O. W.: Further experience with azathioprine for CROHN's disease. Lancet II, 1050—1053 (1970).
BRUNSTETTER, F. H., CLAMAN, H. N.: Impairment of delayed hypersensitivity in uremic patients by antilymphocyte serum. Transplantation 6, 485—487 (1968).
BUCKLEY, C. E., III., GILLS, J. P., JR.: Cyclophosphamide therapy of peripheral uveitis. Arch. intern. Med. 124, 29—35 (1969a).
BUCKLEY, C. E., III., GILLS, J. P., JR.: Cyclophosphamide therapy of BEHCET's disease. J. Allergy 43, 273—283 (1969b).
BURNET, F. M.: The concept of immunological surveillance. Progr. exp. Tumor. Res. 13, 1—27 (1970).
BURTON, J. L., GREAVES, M. W., MARKS, J., DAWBER, R. P. R.: Azathioprine in pemphigus vulgaris. Brit. med. J. 3, 84—86 (1970).
BUTLER, W. T., ROSSEN, R. D., KNIGHT, V., BROOKS, E. B., NORA, J. J., LEACHMAN, R. D., MORGEN, R. O., JUDD, K., TRENTIN, J. J., COOLEY, B. A., DEBAKEY, M. E.: Antilymphocyte globulin turnover rates in heart transplant patients. Clin. Res. 17, 72 (1969).
CALNE, R. Y.: Inhibition of the rejection of renal homografts in dogs by purine analogues. Transplant. Bull. 28, 65—81 (1961).
CALNE, R. Y., ALEXANDRE, G. P. J., MURRAY, J. E.: A study of the effects of drugs in prolonging survival of homologous renal transplants in dogs. Ann. N. Y. Acad. Sci. 99, 743—761 (1962).
CALNE, R. Y., EVANS, D. B., HERBERTSON, B. M., JOYSEY, V., MCMILLAN, R., MAGINN, R. R., MILLARD, P. R., PENA, J. R., SALAMAN, J. R., WHITE, H. J. O., WITHYCOMBE, J. F. R., YOFFA, D. E.: Survival after renal transplantation in man: an interim report on 54 consecutive transplants. Brit. med. J. 2, 404—406 (1968).
CALNE, R. Y., WILLIAMS, R., DAWSON, J. L., ANSELL, I. D., EVANS, D. B., FLUTE, P. T., HERBERTSON, P. M., JOYSEY, V., KEATES, G. H. W., KNILL-JONES, R. P., MASON, S. A., MILLARD, P. R., PENA, J. R., PENTLOW, B. D., SALAMAN, J. R., SELLS, R. A., CULLUM, P. A.: Liver transplantation in man. II. A report of two orthotopic liver transplants in adult recipients. Brit. med. J. 4, 541—546 (1968).
CAMERON, J. S., ROBINSON, R., BOULTON-JONES, M., OGG, C.: Treatment of lupus nephritis with cyclophosphamide. Lancet II, 846—849 (1970).
CAPIZZI, R. L., BERTINO, J. R.: Methotrexate therapy of Wegener's granulomatosis. Ann. intern. Med. 74, 74—79 (1971).
CHANMOUGAN, D., SCHWARTZ, R. S.: Enhancement of antibody synthesis by 6-mercaptopurine. J. exp. Med. 124, 363—379 (1966).
CHAOUAT, Y., PAQUET, J., PELISSON, J., KANOVITCH, B., RASCORSCKI, S.: Le cyclophosphamide au long cours à petites doses dans le traitement des rheumatismes inflammatoires graves. Rev. Rhum. 35, 649—656 (1968).
CHATTY, M. E., DEODHAR, S. D.: Myocardial changes and kidney transplantation. Lesions in patients receiving immunosuppressive therapy. Arch. Path. 88, 602—608 (1969).

CHISHOLM, G.D., PAPADIMITRIOU, M., KULATILAKE, A.E., SHACKMAN, R.: The diagnosis of renal allotransplants in man. Lancet I, 904—906 (1969).
CHRISTIAN, C.L.: Immune-complex disease. New Engl. J. Med. **280**, 878—884 (1969).
CLARKSON, A.R., MORTON, J.B., CASH, J.D.: Urinary fibrin/fibrinogen degradation products after renal homotransplantation. Lancet II, 1220—1223 (1970).
COATES, A.: Cyclophosphamide in pregnancy. Aust. N. Z. Obstet. Gynaec. **10**, 33—34 (1970).
COE, R.O., BULL, F.E.: Cirrhosis associated with methotrexate treatment of psoriasis. J. Amer. med. Assoc. **206**, 1515—1520 (1968).
COHEN, M.L., WEISS, E.B., MONACO, A.P.: Successful treatment of *Pneumocystis carinii* and *Nocardia asteroides* in a renal transplant patient. Amer. J. Med. **50**, 269—276 (1971).
CONGDON, C.C.: Bone marrow transplantation. Science **171**, 1116—1124 (1971).
COOKE, W.T.: Azathioprine in CROHN's disease. Lancet II, 1195—1196 (1970).
Cooperating Clinics Committee of the American Rheumatism Committee: A controlled trial of cyclophosphamide in rheumatoid arthritis. New Engl. J. Med. **17**, 883—889 (1970).
COOLEY, D.A., BLOODWELL, R.D., HALLMAN, G.L., LEACHMAN, R.D., NORA, J.J., MILAM, J.D.: Cardiac transplantation: general considerations and results. Ann. Surg. **169**, 892—903 (1969).
COOLEY, D.A., BLOODWELL, R.D., HALLMAN, G.L., NORA, J.J., HARRISON, G.M., LEACHMAN, R.D.: Organ transplantation for advanced cardiopulmonary disease. Ann. Thorac. Surg. **8**, 30—46 (1969).
COPPOLA, E.D., HEMSTREET, G.P., VILLEGAS, G.R.: Pharmacological treatment. In: BERTELLI, A., MONACO, A.P. (Eds.): Organ and tissue transplantation, p. 79. Amsterdam: Excerpta Medica Foundation 1970.
CORLEY, C.C., JR., LESSNER, H.E., LARSEN, W.E.: Azathioprine therapy of "autoimmune" diseases. Amer. J. Med. **41**, 404—412 (1966).
CRAIG, S.R., ROSENBERG, E.W.: Methotrexate-induced carcinoma? Arch. Derm. **103**, 505—506 (1971).
CURLESS, R.G.: Methotrexate in young women with psoriasis. New Engl. J. Med. **285**, 296—297 (1971).
DAMESHEK, W.: Treatment of autoimmune disease with antipurine drugs. Blood **20**, 119 (1962).
DE DUVE, C.: In: THOMAS, L., UHR, J.W., GRANT, L. (Eds.): Injury, inflammation and immunity. Baltimore: Williams and Wilkins **1964**.
DE GOWIN, R.L., ODA, Y., EVANS, R.H.: Nephritis and lung hemorrhage, Goodpasture's syndrome. Arch. intern. Med. **111**, 62—68 (1963).
DE KONING, J., VAN BEKKUM, D.W., DICKE, K.A., DOOREN, L.J., VAN ROOD, J.J., RADL, J.: Transplantation of bone-marrow cells and fetal thymus in an infant with lymphopenic immunological deficiency. Lancet I, 1223—1227 (1969).
DEMIS, D.J., BROWN, C.S., CROSBY, W.H.: Thioguanine in the treatment of certain autoimmune immunologic and related diseases. Amer. J. Med. **37**, 195—205 (1964).
DENMAN, E.J., DENMAN, A.M., GREENWOOD, B.M., GALL, D., HEATH, R.B.: Failure of cytotoxic drugs to suppress immune responses of patients with rheumatoid arthritis. Ann. rheum. Dis. **29**, 220—231 (1970).
DE SEZE, S., BEDOISEAU, M., DEBEYRE, N., KAHN, M.F.: Résultats de la thérapeutique a visée immunodépressive chez 40 malades atteints de polyarthrite rheumatoide grave. Sem. Hop. Paris **43**, 3084—3091 (1967).
DIAZ, C.J., GARCIA, E.L., MERCHANTE, A., PERIANES, J.: Treatment of rheumatoid arthritis with nitrogen mustard: preliminary report. J. Amer. med. Assoc. **147**, 1418—1419 (1951).
DIXON, F.J.: The pathogenesis of glomerulonephritis. Amer. J. Med. **44**, 493—498 (1968).
DOAK, P.B., DALTON, N.T., MEREDITH, J., MONTGOMERIE, J.Z., NORTH, J.D.K.: Use of antilymphocyte globulin after cadaveric renal transplantation. Brit. med. J. **4**, 522—525 (1969).
DODSON, W.H., BENNETT, J.C.: Possible usefulness of azathioprine (Imuran) in severe rheumatoid arthritis. J. clin. Pharmacol. **9**, 251—258 (1969).
DOUGHERTY, T.F., BERLINER, M.L., BERLINER, D.L.: Hormonal influence on lymphocyte differentiation from RES cells. Ann. N. Y. Acad. Sci. **88**, 78—82 (1960).
DRINKARD, J.P., STANLEY, T.M., DORNFELD, L., AUSTIN, R.C., BARNETT, E.V., PEARSON, C.M., VERNIER, R.L., ADAMS, D.A., LATTA, H., GONICK, H.C.: Azathioprine and prednisone in treatment of adults with lupus nephritis. Medicine **49**, 411—432 (1970).
DRUCKER, W.R., JEEJEEBHOY, K.N.: Azathioprine: adjunct to surgical therapy of granulomatous enteritis. Ann. Surg. **172**, 618—626 (1970).
DUBOIS, E.L.: Nitrogen mustard in treatment of systemic lupus erythematosus. Arch. intern. Med. **93**, 667—672 (1954).
DUNCAN, D.A., DRUMMOND, K.N., MICHAEL, A.F.: Pulmonary hemorrhage and glomerulonephritis: report of six cases and study of renal lesion by fluorescent antibody technique and electron microscopy. Ann. intern. Med. **62**, 920—938 (1965).

Ebringer, A., MacKay, I. R.: Pemphigus vulgaris successfully treated with cyclophosphamide. Ann. intern. Med. 71, 125—127 (1969).

Elion, G. B.: Biochemistry and pharmacology of purine analogues. Fed. Proc. 26, 898—904 (1967).

Epstein, E. H., Croft, J. D.: Cirrhosis following methotrexate administration for psoriasis. Arch. Derm. 100, 531—534 (1969).

Eremin, J., Swaney, W. E., Marshall, V. C.: Avascular necrosis in cadaveric renal allografts. Aust. N. Z. J. Surg. 39, 41—46 (1969).

Everett, D., Newcomer, K. L., Anderson, J., Bergin, J., Overholt, E. L.: Goodpasture's syndrome. Response to mercaptopurine and prednisone. J. Amer. med. Assoc. 213, 1849—1852 (1970).

Fahey, J. L.: Cancer in the immunosuppressed patient. Ann. intern. Med. 75, 310—312 (1971).

Fahey, J. L., Leonard, E., Churg, J., Godman, G. C.: Wegener's granulomatosis. Amer. J. Med. 17, 168—179 (1954).

Festenstein, H., Oliver, R. T. D., Sachs, J. A., Burke, J. M., Adams, E., Divver, W., Hyams, A., Pegrum, G. D., Balfour, I. C., Moorhead, J. F.: Multicenter collaboration in 162 tissue-typed renal transplants. The London and regional transplant group, March, 1969 to December, 1970. Lancet II, 225—228 (1971).

Fialkow, P. J., Bryant, J. I., Thomas, E. D., Neiman, P. E.: Leukaemic transformation of engrafted human marrow cells in vivo. Lancet I, 251—255 (1971).

Fine, R. N., Wright, H. T., Jr., Lieberman, E., Gordon, A.: Azathioprine and varicella. J. Amer. med. Assoc. 207, 147—148 (1969).

Fischer, J. A., Schmid, M.: Treatment of primary biliary cirrhosis with azathioprine. Lancet I, 421—424 (1967).

Flanigan, W. J., Caldwell, F. T., Williams, G. D., Brewer, T. E., Glenn, W. E., Headstream, J. W., Campbell, G. S.: Clinical patterns of renal allograft rejection. Ann. Surg. 173, 733—747 (1971).

Forster, E., Maas, D., Beck, K., Oehlert, W., Birnbaum, F.: Das histologische Bild der chronisch-aggressiven Hepatitis bei immunsuppressiver Therapie. Dtsch. med. Wschr. 96, 1—5 (1971).

Fosdick, W. M.: Cytotoxic therapy in rheumatoid arthritis. Med. Clin. N. Amer. 52, 747—757 (1968).

Fosdick, W. M., Parsons, J. L., Hill, D. F.: Long-term cyclophosphamide therapy in rheumatoid arthritis. Arth. Rheum. 11, 151—161 (1968).

Friedman, E. A., Gelfand, M., Bernheimer, H. P.: Synergism in immunosuppression. I. Effect of methylprednisolone, azathioprine, chlorambucil and radiation on tetanus antitoxin production. Transplantation 11, 479—486 (1971).

Fulginiti, V. A., Scribner, R., Groth, C. G., Putman, C. W., Brettschneider, L., Gilbert, S. Porter, K. A., Starzl, T. E.: Infection in recipients of liver homografts. New Engl. J. Med. 279, 619—626 (1969).

Gatti, R. A., Good, R. A.: Occurrence of malignancy in immunodeficiency diseases. A literature review. Cancer 28, 89—98 (1971).

Germuth, F. G., Jr.: Role of adrenocortical steroids in infection, immunity and hypersensitivity. Pharmacol. Rev. 8, 1—24 (1956).

Germuth, F. G., Jr., Valdes, A. J., Senterfit, L. B., Pollack, A. D.: A unique influence of cortisone in the transit of specific macromolecules across vascular walls in immune complex disease. Johns Hopkins med. J. 122, 137—153 (1968).

Gewurz, H., Wernick, P. R., Quie, P. G., Good, R. A.: Effects of hydrocortisone succinate on the complement system. Nature (Lond.) 208, 755—757 (1965).

Gleason, R. E., Murray, J. E.: Report from Kidney Transplant Registry: analysis of variables in the function of human kidney transplants. Transplantation 5, 360—373 (1967).

Graw, R. G., Jr., Rogentine, G. N., Jr., Halterman, R. H., Berard, C., Herzig, G. P., Yankee, R. A., Whang-Peng, J., Kruger, G., Henderson, E. S.: Graft-versus-host reaction complicating HL-A matched bone-marrow transplantation. Lancet II, 1053—1055 (1970a).

Graw, R. G., Jr., Santos, G. W.: Bone-marrow transplantation in patients with leukemia. Transplantation 11, 197—199 (1971).

Graw, R. G. Jr., Whang-Peng, J., Kruger, G., Buckner, C. D., Leventhal, B. G., Berard, C., Henderson, E. S.: Complication of bone-marrow transplantation. Graft-versus-host disease resulting from chronic-myelogenous-leukaemia leucocyte transfusions. Lancet II, 338—340 (1970).

Greaves, M. W., Burton, J. L., Marks, J., Dawber, R. P. R.: Azathioprine in treatment of bullous pemphigoid. Brit. med. J. 1, 144—145 (1971).

GROSS, H., ZWIRNER, K.: Immuodepressorische Therapie der chronischaggressiven Hepatitis. Münch. Med. Wschr. III, 2481—2485 (1969).
GUPTA, P.K., PINN, V.M., TAFT, P.D.: Cervical dysplasia associated with azathioprine (Imuran) therapy. Acta cytol. 13, 373—376 (1969).
HARRIS, C.C.: Malignancy during methotrexate and steroid therapy for psoriasis. Arch. Derm. 103, 501—504 (1971).
HARRIS, N.S., MERINO, G., NAJARIAN, J.S.: Mode of action of antilymphocyte sera (ALS). Transplant. Proc. 3, 797—799 (1971).
HAYSLETT, J.P., BERTE, J.B., KASHGARIAN, M.: Successful treatment of renal failure in GOODPASTURE's syndrome. Arch. intern. Med. 127, 953—957 (1971).
HERSH, E.M., BUTLER, W.T., ROSSEN, R.D., MORGEN, R.O.: Activated lymphocytes (AL): a rapid test to detect allograft rejection. Clin. Res. 18, 425 (1970).
HERSH, E.M., WONG, V.G., FREIREICH, E.J.: Inhibition of the local inflammatory response in man by antimetabolites. Blood 27, 38—48 (1966).
HERSH, E.M., WONG, V.G., HENDERSON, E.S., FREIREICH, E.J.: Hepatotoxic effect of methotrexate. Cancer 19, 600—606 (1966).
HILL, A.G.S., CRUICKSHANK, B.: A study of antigenic components of kidney tissue. Brit. J. exp. Path. 34, 27—34 (1953).
HILL, R.B., JR., DAHRLING, B.E., STARZL, T.E., RIFKIND, D.: Death after transplantation. Amer. J. Med. 42, 327—334 (1967).
HILL, R.B., JR., ROWLANDS, D.T., JR., RIFKIND, D.: Infectious pulmonary disease in patients receiving immunosuppressive therapy for organ transplantation. New Engl. J. Med. 271, 1921—1927 (1965).
HITZIG, W.H., MASSIMO, L.: Treatment of autoimmune hemolytic anemia in children with azathioprine (Imuran). Blood 28, 840—850 (1966).
HOLLANDER, J.L., MCCARTY, D.J., JR., ASTORGA, G., CASTRO-MURILLO, E.: Studies on the pathogenesis of rheumatoid joint inflammation: I. The "R.A. Cell" and a working hypothesis. Ann. intern. Med. 62, 271—280 (1965).
HURD, E.R., SNYDER, W.B., ZIFF, M.: Choroidal nodules and retinal detachments in rheumatoid arthritis: improvement with fall in immunoglobulin levels following prednisolone and cyclophosphamide therapy. Amer. J. Med. 48, 273—278 (1970).
HURST, H.G.: Pemphigus and pemphigoid: some current concepts. Canad. med. Ass. J. 103, 1279—1282 (1970).
JARLOV, N.V., SORENSEN, K.: Behandling af reumatoid arthritis med cyklofosfamid (Endoxin). Ugeskr. Laeg. 133, 587—589 (1971).
JAVETT, S.L.: Azathioprine in primary sclerosing cholangitis. Lancet I, 810 (1971).
JENSEN, M.K.: Chromosome studies in patients treated with azathioprine and amethopterin. Acta med. scand. 182, 445—455 (1967).
JENSEN, M.K.: Effect of azathioprine on the chromosome complement of human bone marrow cells. Int. J. Cancer 5, 147—151 (1970).
JENSEN, M.K., SØBORG, M.: Chromosome aberrations in human cells following treatment with Imuran. Acta med. scand. 179, 249—250 (1966).
JONES, R.A.: Immunosuppressive therapy in ulcerative colitis. Proc. roy. Soc. Med. 62, 499—501 (1969).
JOOSTE, S.V.: Review. Immunological effects of heterologous antilymphocytic sera. Lymphology 3, 79—103 (1970).
KAHN, M.F., BEDOISEAU, M., DE SEZE, S.: Immunosuppressive drugs in the management of malignant and severe rheumatoid arthritis. Proc. roy. Soc. Med. 60, 130—133 (1967).
KAPLAN, S.R., HAYSLETT, J.P., CALABRESI, P.: Treatment of advanced WEGENER's granulomatosis with azathioprine and duazomycin A. New Engl. J. Med. 278, 239—244 (1968).
KARPATKIN, S., SUSKIND, G.W.: In vitro detection of platelet antibody in patients with idiopathic thrombocytopenic purpura and systemic lupus erythematosis. Blood 33, 795—812 (1969).
KASHIWAGI, N., BRANTIGAN, C.O., BRETTSCHNEIDER, L., GROTH, C.G., STARZL, T.E.: Clinical reactions and serologic changes after the administration of heterologous antilymphocyte globulin to human recipients of renal homografts. Ann. intern. Med. 68, 275—286 (1968).
KAY, S., FRABLE, W.J., HUME, D.M.: Cervical dysplasia and cancer developing in women on immunosuppression therapy for renal homotransplantation. Cancer 26, 1048—1052 (1970).
KELLY, W.D., LILLEHEI, R.C., AUST, J.B., VARIO, R.L., LEONARD, A.S., GRIFFEN, W.O., MARKLAND, L., HERDMAN, R.C., VERMER, R.L., MICHAEL, A.F., LEVITT, J.: Kidney transplantation: experience at the University of Minnesota Hospitals. Surgery 62, 704—720 (1967).

Kincaid-Smith, P.: Histological diagnosis of rejection of renal homografts in man. Lancet II, 849—852 (1967).
Koffler, D., Schur, P. H., Kunkel, H. G.: Immunological studies concerning the nephritis of systemic lupus erythematosus. J. exp. Med. **126**, 607—624 (1967).
Krakowski, A., Covo, J., Rozanski, Z.: Pemphigus vulgaris. Arch. Derm. **100**, 117 (1969).
Kuzemko, J. A., Keidan, M. B.: Treatment of chronic idiopathic thrombocytopenic purpura with azathioprine and prednisone: a clinical trial with three children. Clin. Pediat. **7**, 216—219 (1968).
Laborde, M. A., Bach, J. F.: Inhibition et stimulation par l'azathioprine de l'incorporation de thymidine par les lymphocytes en culture mixte. C. R. Acad. Sci. (Paris) **272**, 509—512 (1971).
Lance, E. M.: Mode of action of antilymphocyte serum. Fed. Proc. **29**, 209—211 (1970).
Laros, R. K., Penner, J. A.: "Refractory" thrombocytopenic purpura treated successfully with cyclophosphamide. J. Lab. clin. Med. **72**, 987—988 (1968).
Laros, R. K., Penner, J. A.: "Refractory" thrombocytopenic purpura treated successfully with cyclophosphamide. J. Amer. med. Assoc. **215**, 445—449 (1971).
Leb, D. E., Kanovitz, B. S., Weisskopf, B.: Azathioprine called mutagenic. J. Amer. med. Assoc. **212**, 969—970 (1970).
Lee, S. L., Meiselas, L. E., Zingale, S. B., Richman, S. M.: Effect of 6-mercaptopurine administration on antibody production and clinical course in systemic lupus erythematosus; report of a case. Arthritis Rheum. **4**, 56—63 (1961).
Lerman, J., Castleman, B.: Draining ears and renal failure in a thirty-six-year-old man. New Engl. J. Med. **280**, 828—834 (1969).
Lerner, R. A., Glassock, R. J., Dixon, F. J.: The role of antiglomerular basement membrane antibody in the pathogenesis of human glomerulonephritis. J. exp. Med. **126**, 989—1004 (1967).
Lever, W. F., Goldberg, H. S.: Treatment of pemphigus vulgaris with methotrexate. Arch. Derm. **100**, 70—78 (1969).
Levitt, J. I.: Deterioration of renal function after discontinuation of long-term prednisone-azathioprine therapy in primary renal disease. New Engl. J. Med. **282**, 1125—1127 (1970).
Locher, H., Franz, J.: Chromosomenveränderungen bei Methotrexatebehandlungen. Med. Welt. **34**, 1965—1966 (1967).
MacKay, I. R.: Chronic hepatitis: Effect of prolonged suppressive treatment and comparison of azathioprine with prednisolone. Quart. J. Med. **147**, 379—392 (1968).
MacKay, I. R., Wall, A. J.: Azathioprine therapy of ulcerative colitis. Amer. J. dig. Dis. **13**, 850—851 (1968).
MacKenzie, A. H.: Scleroderma responds to chlorambucil therapy. J. Amer. med. Assoc. **213**, 1117—1118 (1970).
MacLean, L. D., MacKinnon, K. G., Inglis, F. G., Dossetor, J. B.: When should renal allografts be removed? Arch. Surg. **99**, 269—274 (1969).
Magil, A., Hancock, D. J., Zabriskie, J. B., Guttmann, R. P., Falk, R. E.: A rapid method of assessment of cellular immunity with human blood leukocytes. Proc. Canad. Fed. Biol. Soc. **14**, 152 (1971).
Maher, J. F., Schreiner, G. E.: Treatment of lupus nephritis with azathioprine. Arch. intern. Med. **125**, 293—298 (1970).
Maibach, H. I., Epstein, W. L.: Immunologic responses of healthy volunteers receiving azathioprine (Imuran). Int. Arch. Allergy **27**, 102—109 (1965).
Malaviya, A. N., Many, A., Schwartz, R. S.: Treatment of dermatomyositis with methotrexate. Lancet II, 485—488 (1968).
Mannick, J. A., Davis, R. C., Cooperband, S. R., Glasgow, A. H., Williams, L. F., Harrington, J. T., Cavallo, T., Schmitt, G. W., Idelson, B. A., Olsson, C. A., Nabseth, D. C.: Clinical use of rabbit antihuman lymphocyte globulin in cadaver-kidney transplantation. New Engl. J. Med. **284**, 1109—1115 (1971).
Manz, H. J., Dinsdale, H. B., Morrin, P. A. F.: Progressive multifocal leukoencephalopathy after renal transplantation. Ann. intern. Med. **75**, 77—81 (1971).
Marmont, A. M., Damasio, E. E., Gori, E.: Vinblastine sulphate in idiopathic thrombocytopenic purpura. Lancet II, **94** (1971).
Mason, M., Curry, H. F. L., Barnes, C. G., Dunne, J. F., Hezleman, B. L., Strickland, I. D.: Azathioprine in rheumatoid arthritis. Brit. med. J. **1**, 420—422 (1969).
Mathé, G., Amiel, J. L., Schwarzenberg, L., Choay, J., Trolard, P., Schneider, M., Hayat, M., Schlumberger, J. R., Jasmin, C.: Bone marrow graft in man after conditioning by antilymphocytic serum. Brit. med. J. **2**, 131—136 (1970).

MATHISON, D. A., CONDEMI, J. J., LEDDY, J. P., CALLERAME, M. L., PANNER, B. J., VAUGHAN, J. H.: Purpura, arthralgia, and IgM-IgG cryoglobulinemia with rheumatoid factor activity. Response to cyclophosphamide and splenectomy. Ann. intern. Med. **74**, 383—390 (1971).

McDONALD, J. C., RITCHEY, R. J., FUSELIER, P. F., LINDSEY, E. S., McCRACKEN, B. H.: Sepsis in human renal transplantation. Surgery **69**, 189—193 (1971).

McILVANIE, S. K.: Wegener's granulomatosis: successful treatment with chlorambucil. J. Am. med. Assoc. **197**, 90—92 (1966).

McKHANN, C. F.: Primary malignancy in patients undergoing immunosuppression for renal transplantation. Transplantation **8**, 209—212 (1969).

MEDAWAR, P. B.: In: RAPAPORT, F. T., DAUSSET, J. (Eds.): Biological effects of heterologous antilymphocyte sera. Human transplantation, pp. 501—509. New York: Grune and Stratton 1968.

MEE, A. D., EVANS, D. B.: Antilymphocyte-serum preparations in treatment of renal-allograft rejection. Lancet II, 16—19 (1970).

MELNICK, H., FRIEDMAN, H.: Inhibition of macrophage-migration as an in vitro correlate of hypersensitivity to a kidney antigen during allograft immunity. Fed. Proc. **29**, 785 (1970).

MERTENS, H. G., BALZEREIT, F., LEIPERT, M.: The treatment of severe myasthenia gravis with immunosuppressive agents. Europ. Neurol. **2**, 321—339 (1969).

MEUWISSEN, H. J., GATTI, R. A., TERASAKI, P. I., HONG, R., GOOD, R. A.: Treatment of lymphopenic hypogammaglobulinemia and bone-marrow aplasia by transplantation of allogeneic marrow. New Engl. J. Med. **281**, 691—697 (1969).

MICHAEL, A. F., VERNIER, R. L., DRUMMOND, K. N., LEVITT, J. I., HERDMAN, R. C., FISH, A. J., GOOD, R. A.: Immunosuppressive therapy of chronic renal disease. New Engl. J. Med. **276**, 817—828 (1967).

MILLER, J. J., III., COLE, L. J.: Resistance of long-lived lymphocytes and plasma cells in rat lymph nodes to treatment with prednisone, cyclophosphamide, 6-mercaptopurine and actinomycin D. J. exp. Med. **126**, 109—125 (1967).

MITCHELL, C. G., SMITH, M. G. M., EDDLESTON, A. L. W. F., WILLIAMS, R.: Serum immunosuppressive activity due to azathioprine and its relation to hepatic function after liver transplantation. Lancet I, 1196—1199 (1970).

MOBERG, A. W., GEWURZ, H., SIMMONS, R. L., NAJARIAN, J. S.: Desensitization to horse-globulin before immunosuppressive treatment. Lancet II, 214 (1970).

MOENS, C., BROCTEUR, J.: Treatment of rheumatoid arthritis with immunosuppressive drugs. I. Clinical study. Acta rheum. scand. **11**, 212—220 (1965).

MONTGOMERIE, J. Z., BECROFT, D. M. O., CROXSON, M. C., DOAK, P. B., NORTH, J. D. K.: Herpes-simplex-virus infection after renal transplantation. Lancet II, 867—871 (1969).

MOOKERJEE, B., GAULT, M. H., DOSSETOR, J. B.: Hyperchloremic acidosis in early diagnosis of renal allograft rejection. Ann. intern. Med. **71**, 47—58 (1969).

MOORE, T. C., HUME, D. M.: The period and nature of hazard in clinical renal transplantation. I. The hazard to patient survival. Ann. Surg. **170**, 1—11 (1969a).

MOORE, T. C., HUME, D. M.: The period and nature of hazard in clinical renal transplantation. III. The hazard to transplant kidney survival. Ann. Surg. **170**, 25—29 (1969b).

MULLER, H. K., SUTHERLAND, R. C., JAMIESON, W. J., DE BOER, W. G. R. M.: Autoantibodies in bullous pemphigoid. Med. J. Aust. **1**, 429—431 (1971).

MULLER, S. A., FARROW, G. M., MARTALOCK, D. L.: Cirrhosis caused by methotrexate in the treatment of psoriasis. Arch. Derm. **100**, 523—530 (1971).

MUNRO, A., BEWICK, M., MANUEL, L., CAMERON, J. S., ELLIS, F. G., BOULTON-JONES, M., OGG, C. S.: Clinical evaluation of a rosette inhibition test in renal allotransplantation. Brit. med. J. **3**, 271—275 (1971).

MURPHY, G. P., HESSE, V. E., REYNOSO, G. D., MOORE, R. H., COHEN, E., KENNY, G. M.: Human renal allotransplants. Value of physical examination, biochemical, hematologic, and immunochemical testing. N. Y. State J. Med. **71**, 956—960 (1971).

MURRAY, J. E., MERRILL, J. P., HARRISON, J. H., WILSON, R. E., DAMMIN, G. J.: Prolonged survival of human kidney homograft by immunosuppressive drug therapy. New Engl. J. Med. **268**, 1315—1323 (1963).

MUSSET, R., PITOUT, P., LAMBERT-NETTER, A.: Transplantation rénale et grossesse. Presse Med. **79**, 1273—1276 (1971).

NAJARIAN, J. S., SIMMONS, R. L.: The clinical use of antilymphocyte globulin. New Engl. J. Med. **285**, 158—166 (1971).

NAJARIAN, J. S., SIMMONS, R. L., GEWURZ, H., MOBERG, A., MERKEL, F., MOORE, G. E.: Antiserum to cultured human lymphoblasts: preparation, purification and immunosuppressive properties in man. Ann. Surg. **170**, 617—632 (1969).

Nakamoto, S., Straffon, R. A., Kolff, W. J.: Three years' clinical experience with cadaver kidney transplantation. Transplantation 5, 854—858 (1967).

Ngu, J. L., Barratt, T. M., Soothill, J. F.: Immunoconglutinin and complement changes in steroid sensitive relapsing nephrotic syndrome of children. Clin. exp. Immun. 6, 109—116 (1970).

Nora, J. J., Cooley, D. A., Fernbach, D. J., Rochelle, G. D., Milam, J. D., Montgomery, J. R., Leachman, R. D., Butler, W. T., Rossen, R. D., Bloodwell, R. B., Hallman, G. L., Trentin, J. J.: Rejection of the transplanted human heart; indexes of recognition and problems in prevention. New Engl. J. Med. 280, 1079—1086 (1969).

Norton, W. L., Suki, W., Strunk, S.: Combined corticosteroid and azathioprine therapy in two patients with Wegener's granulomatosis. Arch. intern. Med. 121, 554—560 (1968).

O'Rourke, R. A., Eckert, G. E.: Methotrexate-induced hepatic injury in an adult. Arch. intern. Med. 113, 191—194 (1964).

Osgood, E. E.: Cross-immunity, not antoimmunity, as the mechanism of rheumatoid arthritis and related diseases. In: Stephens, C. A. L., Jr., Stanfield, A. B. (Eds.): Cellular concepts in rheumatoid arthritis, pp. 137—154. Springfield: Charles C. Thomas 1966.

Oshima, Y., Shimuzu, T., Yokohari, R., Matsumoto, T., Kano, K., Kagami, T., Nagaya, H.: Clinical studies in Behcet's syndrome. Ann. rheum. Dis. 22, 36—45 (1963).

Owen, K.: Renal transplantation. Brit. J. Hosp. Med. 2, 1216—1219 (1969).

Page, D., Posen, G., Stewart, T., Harris, J.: Immunologic detection of renal allograft rejection in man: increased DNA synthesis by peripheral lymphoid cells. Transplantation 12, 341—347 (1971).

Parker, J. R., Ellis, F. G., Cameron, J. S., Ogg, C. S.: Detection of rejection of human renal allografts by increased RNA synthesis in peripheral lymphocytes. Proc. Europ. Dialysis Transplant Ass. 7, 331—335 (1970).

Parker, J. R., Mowbray, J. F.: Peripheral blood leucocyte changes during human renal allograft rejection. Transplantation 11, 201—209 (1971).

Paronetto, F., Schaffner, F., Popper, H.: Immunocytochemical and serologic observations in primary biliary cirrhosis. New Engl. J. Med. 271, 1123—1128 (1964).

Patterson, J. F., Norton, R. A., Schwartz, R. S.: Azathioprine treatment of ulcerative colitis, granulomatous colitis and regional enteritis. Amer. J. dig. Dis. 16, 327—332 (1971).

Penn, I., Halgrimson, C. G., Starzl, T. E.: De novo malignant tumors in organ transplant recipients. Transplantation Proc. 3, 773—778 (1971).

Pirofsky, B., Bardana, E. J., Jr., Bayracki, C.: Antilymphocyte antisera in immunologically mediated renal disease. J. Amer. med. Assoc. 210, 1059—1064 (1969).

Pirofsky, B., Reid, R. H., Bardana, E. J., Jr., Bayracki, C.: Antithymocyte antisera therapy in nonsurgical immunologic disease. Transplant. Proc. 3, 769—772 (1971).

Pletka, P., Cohen, S. L., Hulme, B., Kenyon, J. R., Owen, K., Thompson, A. E., Snell, M., Mowbray, J. F., Porter, K. A., Leigh, D. A., Peart, W. S.: Cadaveric renal transplantation: an analysis of 65 cases. Lancet I, 1—5 (1969).

Posen, G., Harris, J., Page, D., Stewart, T.: Reaction lymphocyte blastogenesis (RLB) in the immunologic assessment of human renal allograft recipients. Proc. E.D.T.A. pp. 270—278, 1971.

Prout, G. R., Jr., Hume, D. M., Lee, H. M., Williams, G. M.: Some urological aspects of 93 consecutive renal homotransplants in modified recipients. J. Urol. 97, 409—425 (1967).

Raitt, J. W.: Wegener's granulomatosis: treatment with cytotoxic agents and adrenocorticoids. Ann. intern. Med. 74, 344—356 (1971).

Rau, R.: Cyclophosphamid-Behandlung der progredient-chronischen Polyarthritis, unter besonderer Berücksichtigung des sauren α-Glycoproteins und der Immunoglobuline. Dtsch. med. Wschr. 96, 992—1001 (1971).

Renier, J. C., Deshayes, P., Besson, J., Barazer, C. I., Delahaya, D., Bregeon, C.: Traitement de la polyarthrite rheumatoide par le chlorambucil: à propos de 48 observations. Presse Med. 75, 2527—2530 (1967).

Rhodes, J., Dainton, D., Beck, P.: Azathioprine in Crohn's disease. Lancet II, 1142 (1970).

Rifkind, D.: Cytomegalovirus infection after renal transplantation. Arch. intern. Med. 116, 554—558 (1965).

Rifkind, D.: The activation of varicella-zoster virus infection by immunosuppressive therapy. J. Lab. clin. Med. 68, 463—474 (1966).

Rifkind, D., Marchioro, T. L., Schneck, S. A., Hill, R. B., Jr: Systemic fungal infections complicating renal transplantation and immunosuppressive therapy. Amer. J. Med. 43, 28—38 (1967).

Rifkind, D., Marchioro, T. L., Waddell, W. R., Starzl, T. E.: Infectious diseases associated with renal homotransplantation. I. Incidence, types, and predisposing factors. II. Differential diagnosis and management. J. Amer. med. Assoc. 189, 397—407 (1964).

RIGGIO, R. R., SCHWARTZ, G. H., STENZEL, K. H., RUBIN, A. L.: Alpha-2-hyperglobulinaemia as a humoral indicator of the homograft reaction. Lancet I, 1218—1221 (1968).

ROSSELET, E., SAUDAN, Y., ZENKLUSEN, G.: Les effects de l'azathioprine (Imuran) dans la maladie de Behcet. Premiers résultats thérapeutiques. Ophthalmologica (Basel) **156**, 218—226 (1968).

ROTHENBERGER, W., THIELE, H. G.: In vitro-Studie zur Pathogenese der primär-chronischen Polyarthritis mittels des Migrations-Inhibitionstests. Klin. Wschr. **48**, 1308—1311 (1970).

RYAN, T. J., BODDINGTON, M. M., SPRIGGS, A. I.: Chromosomal abnormalities produced by folic acid antagonists. Brit. J. Derm. **77**, 541—555 (1965).

SACHS, J. A., OLIVER, R. T. D., FESTENSTEIN, H., BLANDY, J. P., SALAMAN, J. R., BALFOUR, I. C., PEGRUM, G. D., WILLIAMS, G. B., HOPEWELL, J. P., MOORHEAD, J. F., BARNES, A. D., BEWICK, M.: International collaboration in renal transplantation. Lancet II, 228—230 (1971).

SALAMAN, J. R.: Use of radioactive fibrinogen for detecting rejection of human renal transplants. Brit. med. J. **2**, 517—521 (1970).

SAMPSON, D.: Ultrasonic method for detecting rejection of human renal allotransplants. Lancet II, 976—978 (1969).

SCHEER, R. L., GROSSMAN, M. A.: Immune aspects of the glomerulonephritis associated with pulmonary hemorrhage. Ann. intern. Med. **60**, 1009—1021 (1964).

SCHNECK, S. A., PENN, I.: De-novo brain tumours in renal-transplant recipients. Lancet I, 983—986 (1971).

SELL, S.: Antilymphocyte antibody effects in experimental animals and problems in human use. Ann. intern. Med. **71**, 177—196 (1969).

SHARP, H., WHITE, J., KRIVIT, W.: Methotrexate induced liver injury. Proc. Amer. Ass. Cancer Res. **8**, 60 (1967).

SHEHADEH, I. H., CARPENTER, C. B., MONTERIO, C. H., MERRILL, J. P.: Renal allograft rejection. An analysis of lysozymuria serum complement, lymphocyturia and heterophil antibodies. Arch. intern. Med. **125**, 850—857 (1970).

SHEIL, A. G. R., KELLY, G. E., STOREY, B. G., MAY, J., KALOWSKI, S., MEARS, D., ROGERS, J. H., JOHNSON, J. R., CHARLESWORTH, J., STEWART, J. H.: Controlled clinical trial of antilymphocyte globulin in patients with renal allografts from cadaver donors. Lancet I, 359—363 (1971).

SHORTER, R. G., HALLENBECK, G. A., NAVA, C., O'KANE, H. O., DEWEERD, J. H., JOHNSON, W. J.: Antilymphoid sera in renal allotransplantation. Arch. Surg. **97**, 323—329 (1968).

SHOTTON, D., MONIE, I. W.: Possible teratogenic effect of chlorambucil on a human fetus. J. Amer. med. Assoc. **186**, 74—75 (1963).

SIMMONS, R. L., KELLY, W. D., TALLENT, M. B., NAJARIAN, J. S.: Care of dysgerminoma with widespread metastases appearing after renal transplantation. New Engl. J. Med. **283**, 190—191 (1970).

SKOGLUND, R. R., SCHANBERGER, J. E., KAPLAN, J. M.: Cyclophosphamide therapy for severe juvenile rheumatoid arthritis. Amer. J. Dis. Child. **121**, 531—533 (1971).

SMITH, M. G. M., EDDLESTON, A. L. W. F., DOMINGUEZ, J. A., EVANS, D. B., BEWICK, M., WILLIAMS, R.: Changes in leucocyte migration after renal transplantation. Brit. med. J. **3**, 275—278 (1969).

SOKAL, J. E., LESSMANN, E. M.: Effects of cancer chemotherapeutic agents on the human fetus. J. Amer. med. Assoc. **172**, 1765—1771 (1960).

SOKOLOFF, M. C., GOLDBERG, L. S., PEARSON, C. M.: Treatment of corticosteroid-resistant polymyositis with methotrexate. Lancet I, 14—16 (1971).

SOLBERG, C. O., MEUWISSEN, H. J., NEEDHAM, R. N., GOOD, R. A., MATSEN, J. M.: Infectious complications in bone-marrow transplant patients. Brit. med. J. **1**, 18—23 (1971).

SPENCER, E. S.: Immunosuppression and cancer. Lancet I, 777—778 (1969).

STANFIELD, A. B., STEPHENS, C. A. L., JR., HILL, D. F.: Tissue culture investigations in rheumatoid arthritis. In: STEPHENS, C. A. L., JR., STANFIELD, A. B. (Eds.): Cellular concepts in rheumatoid arthritis, pp. 155—177. Springfield: Charles C. Thomas 1966.

STARZL, T. E., GROTH, C. G., BRETTSCHNEIDER, L., PENN, I., FULGINITI, V. A., MOON, J. B., BLANCHARD, H., MARTIN, A. J., PORTER, K. A.: Orthotopic homotransplantation of the human liver. Ann. Surg. **168**, 392—415 (1968).

STARZL, T. E., GROTH, C., BRETTSCHNEIDER, L., SMITH, O. G. V., PENN, I., KASHIWAGI, N.: Perspectives in organ transplantation (Proceedings of the Swiss Society of Immunology). Antibiot. Chemother. **15**, 349—383 (1969).

STARZL, T. E., MARCHIORO, T. L., HUTCHINSON, O. E., PORTER, K. A., CERILLI, G. J., BRETTSCHNEIDER, L.: The clinical use of antilymphocyte globulin in renal transplantation. Transplantation **5**, 1100—1105 (1967).

STARZL, T. E., PENN, I., HALGRIMSON, C. G.: Immunosuppression and malignant neoplasms. New Engl. J. Med. **283**, 934—935 (1970).

Starzl, T. E., Penn, I., Schroter, G., Putman, C. W., Halgrimson, C. G., Martineau, G., Amemiya, H., Groth, C. G.: Cyclophosphamide and human organ transplantation. Lancet II, 70—74 (1971).

Starzl, T. E., Porter, K. A., Andres, G., Halgrimson, C. G., Hurwitz, R., Giles, G., Terasaki, P. I., Penn, I., Schroter, G. T., Lilly, J., Starkie, S. J., Putnam, C. W.: Long-term survival after renal transplantation in humans (with special reference to histocompatibility matching, thymectomy, homograft glomerulonephritis, heterologous ALG, and recipient malignancy). Ann. Surg. 172, 437—472 (1970).

Steinberg, A. D., Kaltreider, H. B., Staples, P. J., Goetzl, E. J., Talal, N., Decker, J. L.: Cyclophosphamide in lupus nephritis: a controlled trial. Ann. intern. Med. 75, 165—171 (1971).

Stinson, E. B., Bieber, C. P., Griepp, R. B., Clark, D. A., Shumway, N. E., Remington, J. S.: Infectious complications after cardiac transplantation in man. Ann. intern. Med. 74, 22—36 (1971).

Stinson, E. B., Dong, E., Jr., Bieber, C. P., Popp, R. L., Shumway, N. E.: Cardiac transplantation in man. II. Immunosuppressive therapy. J. thorac. cardiovasc. Surg. 58, 326—337 (1969a).

Stinson, E. B., Dong, E., Jr., Bieber, C. P., Schroeder, J. S., Shumway, N. E.: Cardiac transplantation in man. I. Early rejection. J. Amer. med. Assoc. 207, 2233—2242 (1969b).

Sunderman, C. R., Pearson, H. A.: Growth effects of long-term antileukemic therapy. J. Pediat. 75, 1058—1062 (1969).

Sussman, L. N.: Azathioprine in refractory idiopathic thrombocytopenic purpura. J. Amer. med. Assoc. 202, 259—263 (1967).

Sutherland, J. M., Light, I. J.: The effect of drugs upon the developing fetus. Pediat. Clin. N. Amer. 12, 781—806 (1965).

Swanson, M. A., Schwartz, R. S.: Immunosuppressive therapy — the relation between clinical response and immunologic competence. New Engl. J. Med. 277, 163—170 (1967).

Taub, R. N., Kochwa, S., Brown, S. M., Rubin, A. D., Dameshek, W.: Antigen-induced immunological tolerance in man to equine anti-human-thymocyte gamma-globulin. Lancet II, 521—523 (1969).

Tennenbaum, J. I., St. Pierre, R. L., Cerilli, G. J.: Evaluation of immunosuppressive therapy and clinical course in renal transplants by in vitro lymphocyte transformation. Transplantation 6, 986—990 (1968).

Theodor, E., Gilon, E., Waks, U.: Treatment of ulcerative colitis with azathioprine. Brit. med. J. 4, 741—743 (1968).

Toledo, T. M., Harper, R. C., Moser, R. H.: Fetal effects during cyclophosphamide and irradiation therapy. Ann. intern. Med. 74, 87—91 (1971).

Trepel, F., Pichlmayr, R., Kimura, J., Brendel, W., Begemann, H.: Therapieversuche mit Antilymphocytenserum bei Autoaggressions-Krankheiten des Menschen. Klin. Wschr. 46, 856—864 (1968).

Tuhy, J. E., Maurice, G. L., Niles, N. R.: Wegener's granulomatosis. Amer. J. Med. 25, 638—646 (1958).

Uldall, R., Taylor, R., Swinney, J.: Cyclophosphamide in human organ transplantation. Lancet II, 258—259 (1971).

Van Rood, J. J.: Tissue typing and organ transplantation. Lancet I, 1142—1146 (1969).

Voorhees, J. J., Janzen, M. K., Harrell, E. R., Chakrabarti, S. G.: Cytogenetic evaluation of methotrexate-treated psoriatic patients. Arch. derm. 100, 269—274 (1969).

Walker, D., Gill, T. J., III., Corson, J. M.: Leiomyosarcoma in a renal allograft recipient treated with immunosuppressive drugs. J. Amer. med. Assoc. 215, 2084—2086 (1971).

Walker, J. G., Doniach, D., Roitt, I. M., Sherlock, S.: Serological tests in diagnosis of primary biliary cirrhosis. Lancet I, 827—831 (1965).

Weiss, H. J., Demis, D. J., Elgart, M. L., Brown, E. S., Crosby, W. H.: Treatment of two cases of hyperglobulinemic purpura with thioguanine. New Engl. J. Med. 268, 753—756 (1963).

Weissmann, G.: Lysosomes. New Engl. J. Med. 273, 1143—1149 (1965).

Weksler, M. E., Bull, G., Schwartz, G. H., Stenzel, K. H., Rubin, A. L.: Immunologic responses of graft recipients to antilymphocyte globulin: effect of prior treatment with aggregate-free gamma globulin. J. clin. Invest. 49, 1589—1595 (1970).

Weksler, M. E., Schwartz, G., Stenzel, K., Rubin, A.: Anaphylactic reaction to A.L.G. after induction of tolerance. Lancet II, 1361 (1969).

White, J. J., Tanser, P. H., Anthonisen, N. R., Wynands, J. E., Pare, J. A. P., Becklake, M. R., Munro, D. D., MacLean, L. D.: Human lung homotransplantation. Canad. med. Ass. J. 94, 1199—1209 (1966).

WHITE, R. H. R.: Cytotoxic drug therapy in steroid-resistant glomerulonephritis. Proc. roy Soc. Med. **60**, 1164—1168 (1967).
WHITTINGHAM, S., MACKAY, I. R.: The "pemphigus" antibody and immunopathies affecting the thymus. Brit. J. Derm. **84**, 1—6 (1971).
WOLFF, K., SCHREINER, E.: Immunosuppressive Therapie bei Pemphigus vulgaris. Vorläufige Erfahrungen mit Azathioprin (Imurel). Arch. klin. exp. Derm. **235**, 63—77 (1969).
WONG, V. G.: Immunosuppressive therapy of ocular inflammatory disease. Arch. Ophthal. **81**, 628—637 (1969).
WOODRUFF, M. F. A.: Antilymphocyte serum: summary and further observations. Transplantation **5**, 1127—1133 (1967).
WOODRUFF, M. F. A., NOLAN, B., ROBSON, J. S., MACDONALD, M. K.: Renal transplantation in man; experience in 35 cases. Lancet I, 6—12 (1969).
WORTH, P. H. L.: Cyclophosphamide and the bladder. Brit. med. J. **3**, 182 (1971).
YUILL, G. M., SWINBURN, W. R., LIVERSEDGE, L. A.: Treatment of polyneuropathy with azathioprine. Lancet II, 854—856 (1970).
ZUHLKE, V., HERMAN, G.: Diagnose der Abstoßungsreaktion transplantierter Nieren durch immunologische Untersuchungen der Harneuveisse. Münch. med. Wschr. **112**, 61—64 (1970).

# Author Index

Page numbers in *italics* refer to the bibliography

# Subject Index

## Recent Results in Cancer Research

Sponsored by the Swiss League against Cancer
Editor-in-chief: P. Rentchnick

**Vol. 1** R. Schindler
Die tierische Zelle in Zellkultur

**Vol. 2** Neuroblastomas – Biochemical Studies
Edited by C. Bohuon

**Vol. 3** W. C. Hueper
Occupational and Environmental Cancers of the Respiratory System

**Vol. 4** L. Goldman
Laser Cancer Research

**Vol. 5** D. Metcalf
The Thymus

**Vol. 6** Malignant Transformation by Viruses
Edited by W. H. Kirsten

**Vol. 7** Ch. G. Moertel
Multiple Primary Malignant Neoplasms

**Vol. 8** New Trends in the Treatment of Cancer
Edited by L. Manuila, S. Moles, and P. Rentchnick

**Vol. 9** J. Lindenmann and P. A. Klein
Immunological Aspects of Viral Oncolysis

**Vol. 10** R. S. Nelson
Radioactive Phosphorus in the Diagnosis of Gastrointestinal Cancer

**Vol. 11** R. G. Freeman and J. M. Knox
Treatment of Skin Cancer

**Vol. 12** H. T. Lynch
Hereditary Factors in Carcinoma

**Vol. 13** Tumours in Children
Edited by H. B. Marsden and J. K. Steward

**Vol. 14** N. Odartchenko
Production Cellulaire Erythropoiétique

**Vol. 15** B. Sokoloff
Carcinoid and Serotonin

**Vol. 16** M. L. Jacobs
Malignant Lymphomas and their Management

**Vol. 17** Normal and Malignant Cell Growth
Edited by R. J. Fry, M. L. Griem, and W. H. Kirsten

**Vol. 18** E. Anglesio
The Treatment of Hodgkin's Disease

**Vol. 19** P. Bannasch
The Cytoplasm of Hepatocytes during Carcinogenesis

**Vol. 20** Rubidomycin
Edited by J. Bernard, R. Paul, M. Boiron, C. Jacquillat, and R. Maral

**Vol. 21** Scientific Basis of Cancer Chemotherapy
Edited by G. Mathé

**Vol. 22** P. Koldovsky
Tumor Specific Transplantation Antigen

**Vol. 23** W. A. Fuchs, J. W. Davidson, and H. W. Fischer
Lymphography in Cancer

**Vol. 24** J. Hayward
Hormones and Human Breast Cancer

**Vol. 25** P. Roy-Burman
Analogues of Nucleic Acid Components

**Vol. 26** Tumors of the Liver
Edited by G. T. Pack and A. H. Islami

**Vol. 27** J. Szymendera
Bone Mineral Metabolism in Cancer

**Vol. 28** E. S. Meek
Antitumour and Antiviral Substances of Natural Origin

**Vol. 29** Aseptic Environments and Cancer Treatment
Edited by G. Mathé

**Vol. 30** Advances in the Treatment of Acute (Blastic) Leukemias
Edited by G. Mathé

**Vol. 31** P. Denoix
Treatment of Malignant Breast Tumors

**Vol. 32** R. S. Nelson
Endoscopy in Gastric Cancer

**Vol. 33** Experimental and Clinical Effects of L-Asparaginase
Edited by E. Grundmann and H. F. Oettgen

**Vol. 34** Chemistry and Biological Actions of 4-Nitroquinoline 1-Oxide
Edited by H. Endo, T. Ono, and T. Sugimura

**Vol. 35** I. Penn
Malignant Tumors in Organ Transplant Recipients

**Vol. 36** Current Concepts in the Management of Leukemia and Lymphoma
Edited by J. E. Ultmann, M. L. Griem, W. H. Kirsten, and R. W. Wissler

**Vol. 37** S. Chiappa, R. Musumeci, and C. Uslenghi
Endolymphatic Radiotherapy in Malignant Lymphomas

**Vol. 38** P. C. Koller
The Role of Chromosomes in Cancer Biology

**Vol. 39** Current Problems in the Epidemiology of Cancer and Lymphomas
Edited by E. Grundmann and H. Tulinius

**Vol. 40** F. A. Langley and A. C. Crompton
Epithelial Abnormalities of the Cervix Uteri

**Vol. 41** Tumours in a Tropical Country
Edited by A. C. Templeton

**Vol. 42** Breast Cancer: A Challenging Problem
Edited by M. L. Griem, E. V. Jensen, J. E. Ultmann, and R. W. Wissler

**Vol. 43** Nomenclature, Methodology and Results of Clinical Trials in Acute Leukemias
Edited by G. Mathé, P. Pouillart, and L. Schwarzenberg.

**Vol. 44** Special Topics in Carcinogenesis
Edited by E. Grundmann

**Vol. 45** P. Koldovsky
Carcinoembryonic Antigens

**Vol. 46** Diagnosis and Therapy of Malignant Lymphoma
Edited by K. Musshoff

**Special Supplement**
Biology of Amphibian Tumors
Edited by M. Mizell

**Springer-Verlag**
**Berlin**
**Heidelberg**
**New York**

München Johannesburg
London Madrid New Delhi
Paris Rio de Janeiro Sydney
Tokyo Utrecht Wien

MIX
Papier aus verantwortungsvollen Quellen
Paper from responsible sources
FSC® C105338

If you have any concerns about our products,
you can contact us on
**ProductSafety@springernature.com**

In case Publisher is established outside the EU,
the EU authorized representative is:
**Springer Nature Customer Service Center GmbH**
**Europaplatz 3, 69115 Heidelberg, Germany**

Printed by Libri Plureos GmbH
in Hamburg, Germany